Motor Control

Translating Research into Clinical Practice

Fourth Edition

Anne Shumway-Cook
PT, PhD, FAPTA
Professor
Division of Physical Therapy
Department of Rehabilitation Medicine
University of Washington
Seattle, Washington

Marjorie Woollacott
PhD
Professor
Department of Human Physiology
Institute of Neuroscience
University of Oregon
Eugene, Oregon

Wolters Kluwer Health | Lippincott Williams & Wilkins
Philadelphia • Baltimore • New York • London
Buenos Aires • Hong Kong • Sydney • Tokyo

Acquisitions Editor: Emily Lupash
Product Manager: Meredith L. Brittain, with Laura Horowitz of Hearthside Publishing Services
Marketing Manager: Allison M. Noplock
Designer: Doug Smock
Production Services: SPi Technologies

Fourth Edition

351 West Camden Street
Baltimore, MD 21201

Two Commerce Square
2001 Market Street
Philadelphia, PA 19103

Printed in China

Library of Congress Cataloging-in-Publication Data
Shumway-Cook, Anne, 1947-
Motor control : translating research into clinical practice / Anne Shumway Cook and Marjorie H. Woollacott. — 4th ed.
p. ; cm.
Includes bibliographical references and index.
ISBN 9781451117103
1. Motor ability. 2. Motor learning. 3. Medical rehabilitation. 4. Brain damage—Patients—Rehabilitation. I. Woollacott, Marjorie H., 1946- II. Title.
[DNLM: 1. Motor Skills—physiology. 2. Movement—physiology. 3. Movement Disorders—therapy. 4. Physical Therapy Modalities. 5. Posture—physiology. WE 103]

QP301.S535 2010
612′.04—dc22

2010029395

To purchase additional copies of this book, call our customer service department at **(800) 638-3030** or fax orders to **(301) 223-2320**. International customers should call **(301) 223-2300**.

Visit Lippincott Williams & Wilkins on the Internet: http://www.lww.com. Lippincott Williams & Wilkins customer service representatives are available from 8:30 am to 6:00 pm, EST.

9 8 7 6 5 4 3 2

RRS1205

It is with great love and gratitude that we dedicate this book to the many people, including professional colleagues and patients, who have contributed to the development of the ideas presented here. We also gratefully acknowledge the divine source of our enthusiasm, wisdom, and joy. The sweet mix of inspiration and effort involved in the creation of this book was truly a delight.

CONTENTS

PART IV

PREFACE

In recent years there has been great interest among clinicians regarding the tremendous expansion of research in the field of motor control and the implications of this research to clinical practice. This explosion of new research in the field of neuroscience and motor control has created a gap between research and clinical practice. *Motor Control: Translating Research into Clinical Practice,* Fourth Edition is dedicated to reducing this gap by reviewing current research in the area of motor control and exploring the translation of this research into best clinical practices.

AN OVERVIEW OF THE FOURTH EDITION

This book is divided into four parts. Part I, Theoretical Framework, reviews current theories of motor control, motor learning, and recovery of function after neurological insult. The clinical implications of various theories of motor control are discussed, as are the physiological basis of motor control and motor learning. This part also includes a suggested conceptual framework for clinical practice and a framework for understanding and examining impairments in the patient with neurological deficits. The first part is the foundation for the major thrust of the book, which addresses motor control issues as they relate to the control of posture and balance (Part II), mobility (Part III), and upper-extremity function (Part IV).

The chapters in each of these parts follow a standard format. The first chapter in each part discusses issues related to normal control processes. The second chapter (and in some cases the third) describes age-related issues. The third chapter presents research on abnormal function, and the final chapters discuss the clinical applications of current research, including methods for examining and treating patients with motor dyscontrol in each of the three functional areas.

This book will be of use in several ways. First, we envision it as a textbook used in both undergraduate and graduate courses on normal motor control, motor development across the lifespan, and rehabilitation in the area of physical and occupational therapy, as well as kinesiology and exercise science. We also envision that the book will assist clinicians in staying connected to some of the research that serves as the foundation for evidence-based clinical practice. A strength of *Motor Control: Translating Research into Clinical Practice,* Fourth Edition is its summary of a broad range of research papers and the translation of this research into clinical practice. However, reading summaries cannot replace the insights that are gained by delving into the original research papers. A book by its very nature summarizes only research available before its publication; therefore it is critical that clinicians and students alike continue to read emerging research.

CHANGES TO THE FOURTH EDITION

This fourth edition of *Motor Control* includes updated research in each of the three key areas: postural control, mobility, and upper extremity function. Laboratory activities have been expanded and, as in the third edition, answer keys are at the end of each chapter. Five case studies with associated videos have been added to assist the reader in understanding underlying impairments associated with specifc neurological diagnoses, and the use of selected clinical measures to assess aspects of postural control, mobility, and upper extremity function. Each of the clinical chapters includes an extensive review of the research on the efficacy of assessment and treatment procedures presented.

Additional Resources

Motor Control, Fourth Edition includes additional resources for both students and instructors that are available on the book's companion website at http://thepoint.lww.com/Shumway-Cook4e. The student resources are also available via the Student Resource DVD-ROM packaged with this text.

Students

Students who have purchased *Motor Control,* Fourth Edition have access to the following additional resources on a back-of-book DVD and at http://thepoint.lww.com/Shumway-Cook4e:

- Videos that examine motor control deficits, including deficits in postural control, mobility, and upper extremity function in different types of neurologic pathology (chronic stroke, cerebellar pathology, cerebral palsy, and Parkinson's disease) as well as in balance-impaired elders. These videos can be viewed in their entirety or in the following segments: impairments, postural control, mobility, and upper extremity control.
- The searchable Full Text On-line.

Instructors

Approved adopting instructors will be given access to the following additional resources:

- Videos as described above
- A test generator with 380 questions
- An image bank of all the images and tables in the book
- Full Text On-line as described above

A FINAL NOTE

Motor Control: Translating Research into Clinical Practice, Fourth Edition, seeks to provide a framework that will enable the clinician to incorporate current theory and research on motor control into clinical practice. More importantly, it is our hope that the book will serve as a springboard for developing new, more effective approaches to examining and treating patients with motor dyscontrol.

Anne Shumway-Cook
Marjorie H. Woollacott

PART I

THEORETICAL FRAMEWORK

Movement is essential to our ability to walk, run, and play; to seek out and eat the food that nourishes us; to communicate with friends and family; to earn our living—in essence to survive.

TERRI NASH, M.S., C.P.M.

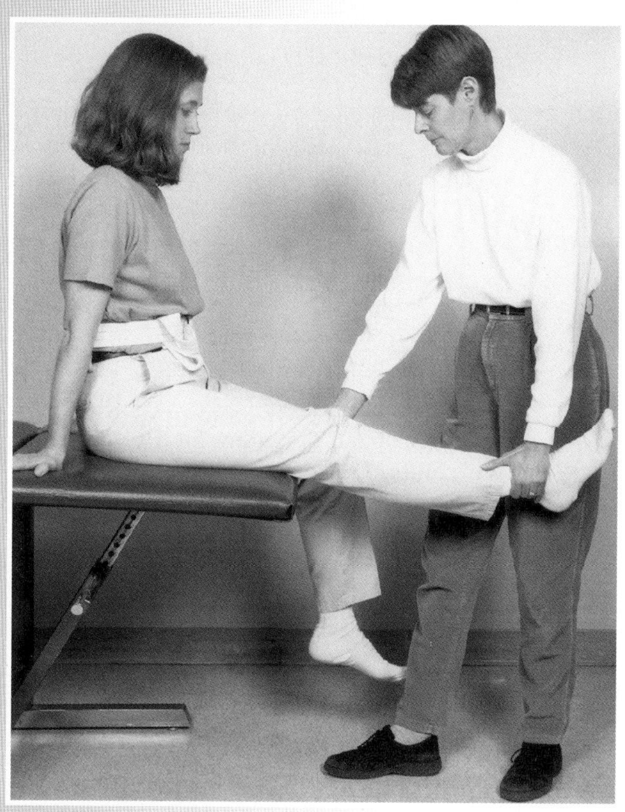

CHAPTER 1

MOTOR CONTROL: ISSUES AND THEORIES

LEARNING OBJECTIVES

Following completion of this chapter, the reader will be able to:

1. Define motor control, and discuss its relevance to the clinical treatment of patients with movement pathology.
2. Discuss how factors related to the individual, the task, and the environment affect the organization and control of movement.
3. Define what is meant by a theory of motor control, and describe the value of theory to clinical practice.
4. Compare and contrast the following theories of motor control: reflex, hierarchical, motor programming, systems, dynamic systems, and ecological, including the individuals associated with each theory, critical elements used to explain the control of normal movement, limitations, and clinical applications.
5. Discuss the relationship between theories of motor control and the parallel development of clinical methods related to neurologic rehabilitation.
6. Compare and contrast the neurofacilitation approaches to the task-oriented approach with respect to assumptions underlying normal and abnormal movement control, recovery of function, and clinical practices related to assessment and treatment.

INTRODUCTION

What is Motor Control?

Movement is a critical aspect of life. It is essential to our ability to walk, run, and play; to seek out and eat the food that nourishes us; to communicate with friends and family; to earn our living—in essence to survive. The field of motor control is directed at studying the nature of movement, and how movement is controlled. **Motor control** is defined as the ability to regulate or direct the mechanisms essential to movement. It addresses questions such as how does the central nervous system (CNS) organize the many individual muscles and joints into coordinated functional movements? How is sensory information from the environment and the body used to select and control movement? How do our perceptions of ourselves, the tasks we perform, and the environment in which we are moving influence our movement behavior? What is the best way to study movement, and how can movement problems be quantified in patients with motor control problems?

Why Should Therapists Study Motor Control?

Physical and occupational therapists have been referred to as "applied motor control physiologists" (Brooks, 1986). This is because therapists spend a considerable amount of time retraining patients who have motor control problems producing functional movement disorders. Therapeutic intervention is often directed at changing movement or increasing the capacity to move. Therapeutic strategies are designed to improve the quality and quantity of postures and movements essential to function. Thus, understanding motor control and, specifically, the nature and control of movement is critical to clinical practice.

We will begin our study of motor control by discussing important issues related to the nature and control of movement. Next, we will explore different theories of motor control, examining their underlying assumptions and clinical implications. Finally, we will review how theories of motor control relate to past and present clinical practices.

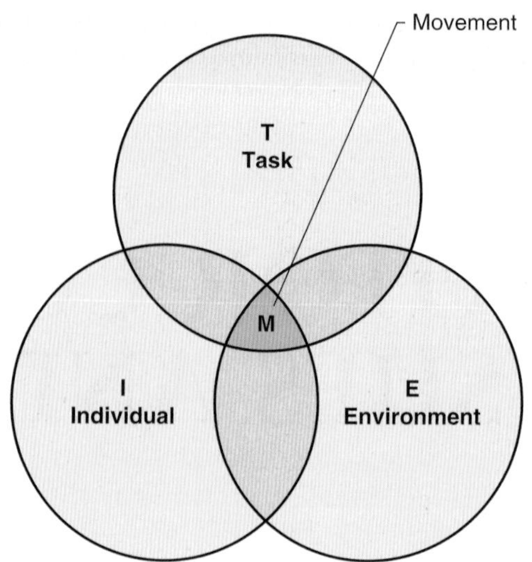

FIGURE 1.1 Movement emerges from interactions between the individual, the task, and the environment.

UNDERSTANDING THE NATURE OF MOVEMENT

Movement emerges from the interaction of three factors: the individual, the task, and the environment. Movement is organized around both task and environmental demands. The individual generates movement to meet the demands of the task being performed within a specific environment. In this way, we say that the organization of movement is constrained by factors within the individual, the task, and the environment. The individual's capacity to meet interacting task and environmental demands determines that person's functional capability. Motor control research that focuses only on processes within the individual without taking into account the environment in which that individual moves or the task that he or she is performing will produce an incomplete picture. Thus, in this book our discussion of motor control will focus on the interactions of the individual, the task, and the environment. Figure 1.1 illustrates this concept.

Factors within the Individual That Constrain Movement

Within the individual, movement emerges through the cooperative effort of many brain structures and processes. The term *"motor" control* in itself is somewhat misleading, since movement arises from the interaction of multiple processes, including those that are related to *perception, cognition,* and *action.*

Movement and Action

Movement is often described within the context of accomplishing a particular action. As a result, motor control is usually studied in relation to specific actions or activities. For example, motor control physiologists might ask: how do people walk, run, talk, smile, reach, or stand still? Researchers typically study movement control within the context of a specific activity, like walking, with the understanding that control processes related to this activity will provide insight into principles for how all of movement is controlled.

Understanding the control of action implies understanding the motor output from the nervous system to the body's effector systems, or muscles. The body is characterized by a high number of muscles and joints, all of which must be controlled during the execution of coordinated, functional movement. There are also multiple ways a movement can be carried out (multiple equivalent solutions). This problem of choosing among equivalent solutions and then coordinating the many muscles and joints involved in a movement has been referred to as the "degrees of freedom problem" (Bernstein, 1967). It is considered a major issue being studied by motor control researchers and will be discussed in later chapters. So the study of motor control includes the study of the systems that control *action.*

Movement and Perception

Perception is essential to action, just as action is essential to perception. **Perception** is the integration of sensory impressions into psychologically meaningful information. Perception includes both peripheral sensory mechanisms and higher-level processing that adds interpretation and meaning to incoming afferent information. Sensory/perceptual systems provide information about the state of the body (e.g., the position of different body parts in space) and features within the environment critical to the regulation of movement. Sensory/perceptual information is clearly integral to the ability to act effectively within an environment (Rosenbaum, 1991). Thus, understanding movement requires the study of systems controlling *perception* and the role of perception in determining our actions.

Movement and Cognition

Since movement is not usually performed in the absence of intent, cognitive processes are essential to motor control. In this book, we define cognitive processes broadly to include attention, planning, problem solving, motivation, and emotional aspects of motor control that underlie the establishment of intent or goals. Motor control includes perception and action systems that are organized to achieve specific goals or intents. Thus, the study of motor control must include the study of *cognitive* processes as they relate to perception and action.

So within the individual, many systems interact in the production of functional movement. While each of these components of motor control—perception, action, and cognition—can be studied in isolation, we believe a true picture of the nature of motor control cannot be achieved without a synthesis of information from all three. This concept is shown in Figure 1.2.

Task Constraints on Movement

In addition to constraints related to the individual, tasks can also impose constraints on the neural organization of movement. In everyday life, we perform a tremendous variety of functional tasks requiring movement. The nature of the task being performed in part determines the type of movement needed. Thus, understanding motor control requires an awareness of how tasks regulate neural mechanisms controlling movement.

Recovery of function following CNS damage requires that a patient develop movement patterns that meet the demands of functional tasks in the face of sensory/perceptual, motor, and cognitive impairments. Thus, therapeutic strategies that help the patient (re)learn to perform functional tasks, taking into consideration underlying impairments, are essential to maximizing the recovery of functional independence. But what tasks should be taught, in what order, and at what time? An understanding of task attributes can provide a framework for structuring tasks. Tasks can be sequenced from least to most difficult based on their relationship to a shared attribute.

The concept of grouping tasks is not new to clinicians. Within the clinical environment, tasks are routinely grouped into functional categories. Examples of

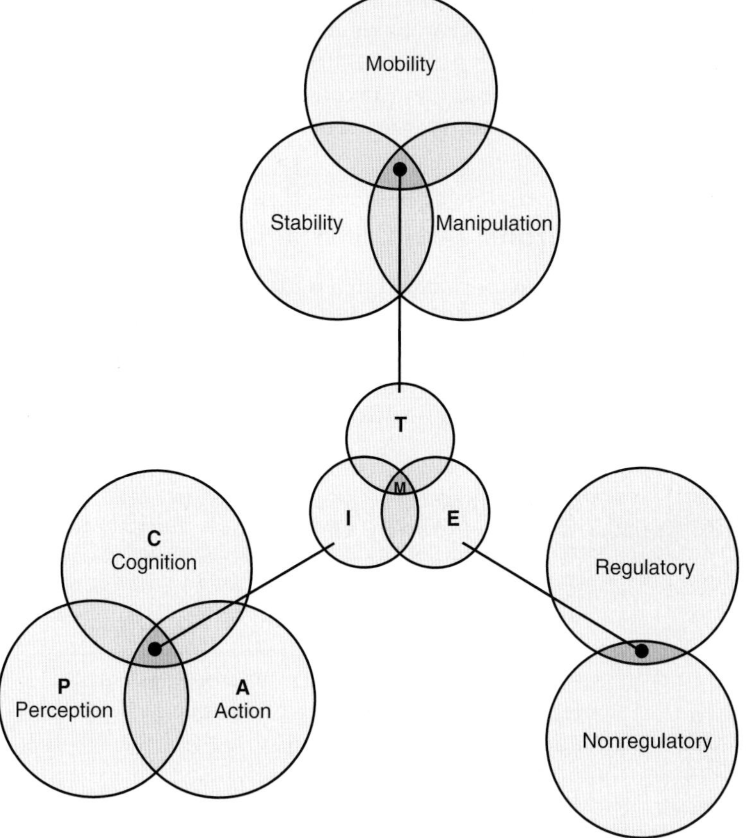

FIGURE 1.2 Factors within the individual, the task, and the environment affect the organization of movement. Factors within the individual include the interaction of *perception, cognition,* and *action (motor) systems.* Environmental constraints on movement are divided into regulatory and nonregulatory factors. Finally, attributes of the task contribute to the organization of functional movement.

functional task groupings include bed mobility tasks (e.g., moving from a supine to a sitting position, moving to the edge of the bed and back, as well as changing positions within the bed); transfer tasks (e.g., moving from sitting to standing and back, moving from chair to bed and back, moving onto and off of a toilet), and activities of daily living (ADLs) (e.g., dressing, toileting, grooming, and feeding).

An alternative to classifying tasks functionally is to categorize them according to the critical attributes that regulate neural control mechanisms. For example, movement tasks can be classified as discrete or continuous. Discrete movement tasks, such as kicking a ball or moving from sitting to standing or lying down, have a recognizable beginning and end. In continuous movements such as walking or running, the end point of the task is not an inherent characteristic of the task but is decided arbitrarily by the performer (Schmidt, 1988b).

Movement tasks have also been classified according to whether the base of support is still or in motion (Gentile, 1987). "Stability" tasks such as sitting or standing are performed with a nonmoving base of support, while "mobility" tasks such as walking and running have a moving base of support. In the clinic, tasks involving a nonmoving base of support (e.g., sitting and standing) are often practiced prior to mobility tasks such as walking, on the premise that stability requirements are less demanding in the tasks that have a nonmoving base of support. Support for this type of hierarchical ordering of postural tasks comes from research demonstrating that attentional resources increase as stability demands increase. For example, tasks that have the lowest attentional demand are those with a nonmoving base of support (often called "static postural control tasks") such as sitting and standing; attentional demands increase in mobility tasks such as walking and obstacle clearance (Chen et al., 1996; LaJoie et al., 1993).

The presence of a manipulation component has also been used to classify tasks (Gentile, 1987). The addition of a manipulation task increases the demand for stability beyond that demanded for the same task lacking the manipulation component. Thus, tasks might be sequenced in accordance with the hierarchy of stability demands (e.g., standing, standing and lifting a light load, standing and lifting a heavy load).

Finally, tasks have been classified according to movement variability (Gentile, 1987; Schmidt, 1988b). Open movement tasks such as playing soccer or tennis require performers to adapt their behavior within a constantly changing and often unpredictable environment. In contrast, closed movement tasks are relatively stereotyped, showing little variation, and they are performed in relatively fixed or predictable environments. The training for closed movement tasks is often performed prior to that for open movement tasks, which require adapting movements to changing environmental features. Figure 1.2 shows three of the task components we are concerned with in this book.

Understanding important attributes of tasks allows a therapist to develop a taxonomy of tasks that can provide a useful framework for functional examination; it allows a therapist to identify the specific kinds of tasks that are difficult for the patient to accomplish. In addition, the set of tasks can serve as a progression for retraining functional movement in the patient with a neurologic disorder. An example of a taxonomy of tasks using two attributes, stability–mobility and environmental predictability is shown in Table 1.1. However, as discussed above, a taxonomy of tasks can be developed using other attributes as well. Lab Activity 1-1 offers you an opportunity to develop your own taxonomy of tasks. The answers to this activity may be found at the end of this chapter.

Environmental Constraints on Movement

Tasks are performed in a wide range of environments. Thus, in addition to attributes of the task, movement is also constrained by features within the environment. In order to be functional, the CNS must take into consideration attributes of the environment when

TABLE 1.1 A Taxonomy of Tasks Combining the Stability–Mobility and Closed–Open Task Continua

	Stability	Quasimobile	Mobility
Closed predictable environment	Sit/stand/ nonmoving surface	Sit to stand/kitchen chair w/arms	Walk/nonmoving surface
Open unpredictable environment	Stand/rocker board	Sit to stand/Rocking chair	Walk on uneven or moving surface

LAB ACTIVITY 1-1

Objective: To develop your own taxonomy of movement tasks.

Procedure: Make a graph like the one illustrated in Table 1.1. Identify two continua you would like to combine. You can begin by using one or more of the continua described above, or alternatively you can create your own continuum based on attributes of movement tasks we have not discussed. In our example, we combined the stability—mobility continuum with the open—closed continuum.

Assignment

1. Fill in the boxes with examples of tasks that reflect the demands of each of the continua.
2. Think about ways you could "progress" a patient through your taxonomy. What assumptions do you have about which tasks are easiest and which the hardest? Is there a "right" way to move through your taxonomy? How will you decide what tasks to use and in what order?

planning task-specific movements. As shown in Figure 1.2, attributes of the environment that affect movement have been divided into regulatory and nonregulatory features (Gordon, 1987). Regulatory features specify aspects of the environment that shape the movement itself. Task-specific movements must conform to regulatory features of the environment in order to achieve the goal of the task. Examples of regulatory features of the environment include the size, shape, and weight of a cup to be picked up and the type of surface on which we walk (Gordon, 1997). Nonregulatory features of the environment may affect performance, but movement does not have to conform to these features. Examples of nonregulatory features of the environment include background noise and the presence of distractions.

Features of the environment can in some instances enable or support performance, or alternatively, they may disable or hinder performance. For example, walking in a well-lit environment is much easier than walking in low light conditions or in the dark because the ability to detect edges, sizes of small obstacles, and other surface properties is compromised when the light level is low (Patla & Shumway-Cook, 1999).

Thus, understanding features within the environment that both regulate and affect the performance of movement tasks is essential to planning effective intervention. Preparing patients to perform in a wide variety of environments requires that we understand the features of the environment that will affect movement performance and that we adequately prepare our patients to meet the demands in different types of environments.

We have explored how the nature of movement is determined by the interaction of three factors, the individual, the task, and the environment. Thus, the movement we observe in patients is shaped not just by factors within the individual, such as sensory, motor, and cognitive impairments, but also by attributes of the task being performed and the environment in which the individual is moving. We now turn our attention to examining the control of movement from a number of different theoretical views.

THE CONTROL OF MOVEMENT: THEORIES OF MOTOR CONTROL

Theories of motor control describe viewpoints regarding how movement is controlled. A **theory of motor control** is a group of abstract ideas about the control of movement. A **theory** is a set of interconnected statements that describe unobservable structures or processes and relate them to each other and to observable events. Jules Henri Poincare (1908) said, "Science is built up of facts, as a house is built of stone; but an accumulation of facts is no more a science than a heap of stones is a house." A theory gives meaning to facts, just as a blueprint provides the structure that transforms stones into a house (Miller, 2002).

However, just as the same stones can be used to make different houses, the same facts are given different meaning and interpretation by different theories of motor control. Different theories of motor control reflect philosophically varied views about how the brain controls movement. These theories often reflect differences in opinion about the relative importance of various neural components of movement. For example, some theories stress peripheral influences, others may stress central influences, while still others may stress the role of information from the environment in controlling behavior. Thus, motor control theories are more than just an approach to explaining action. Often they stress different aspects of the organization of the underlying neurophysiology and neuroanatomy of that action. Some theories of motor control look at the brain as a *black box* and simply study the rules by which this black box interacts with changing environments as a variety of tasks are performed. As you will see, there is no one theory of motor control that everyone accepts.

Value of Theory to Practice

Do theories really influence what therapists do with their patients? Yes! Rehabilitation practices reflect the theories, or basic ideas, we have about the cause and nature of function and dysfunction (Shepard, 1991). In general, then, the actions of therapists are based on assumptions that are derived from theories. The specific practices related to examination and intervention used with the patient who has motor dyscontrol are determined by underlying assumptions about the nature and cause of movement. Thus, motor control theory is part of the theoretical basis for clinical practice. This will be discussed in more detail in the last section of this chapter.

What are the advantages and disadvantages of using theories in clinical practice? Theories provide:

- a framework for interpreting behavior;
- a guide for clinical action;
- new ideas; and
- working hypotheses for examination and intervention.

Framework for Interpreting Behavior

Theory can help therapists to interpret the behavior or actions of patients with whom they work. Theory allows the therapist to go beyond the behavior of one patient and broaden the application to a much larger number of cases (Shepard, 1991).

Theories can be more or less helpful depending on their ability to predict or explain the behavior of an individual patient. When a theory and its associated assumptions does not provide an accurate interpretation of a patient's behavior, it loses its usefulness to the therapist. Thus, theories can potentially limit a therapist's ability to observe and interpret movement problems in patients.

Guide for Clinical Action

Theories provide therapists with a possible guide for action (Miller, 2002; Shepard, 1991). Clinical interventions designed to improve motor control in the patient with neurologic dysfunction are based on an understanding of the nature and cause of normal movement, as well as an understanding of the basis for abnormal movement. Therapeutic strategies aimed at retraining motor control reflect this basic understanding.

New Ideas: Dynamic and Evolving

Theories are dynamic, changing to reflect greater knowledge relating to the theory. How does this affect clinical practices related to retraining the patient with motor dyscontrol? Changing and expanding theories of motor control need not be a source of frustration to clinicians. Expanding theories can broaden and enrich the possibilities for clinical practice. New ideas related to examination and intervention will evolve to reflect new ideas about the nature and cause of movement.

Working Hypotheses for Examination and Intervention

A theory is not directly testable, since it is abstract. Rather, theories generate hypotheses, which are testable. Information gained through hypothesis testing is used to validate or invalidate a theory. This same approach is useful in clinical practice. So-called hypothesis-driven clinical practice transforms the therapist into an active problem solver (Rothstein & Echternach, 1986; Rothstein et al., 2003). Using this approach to retrain the patient with motor dyscontrol calls for the therapist to generate multiple hypotheses (explanations) for why patients move (or do not move) in ways to achieve functional independence. During the course of therapy therapists will test various hypotheses, discard some, and generate new explanations that are more consistent with their results.

Each of the many theories that will be discussed in this chapter has made specific contributions to the field of motor control, and each has implications for clinicians retraining patients with motor dyscontrol. It is important to understand that all models are unified by the desire to understand the nature and control of movement. The difference is in the approach.

Reflex Theory

Sir Charles Sherrington, a neurophysiologist in the late 1800s and early 1900s, wrote the book *The Integrative Action of the Nervous System* in 1906. His research formed the experimental foundation for a classic reflex theory of motor control. The basic structure of a reflex is shown in Figure 1.3. For Sherrington, reflexes were the building blocks of complex behavior. He believed that complex behavior could be explained through the combined action of individual reflexes that were chained together (Sherrington, 1947). Sherrington's view of a reflexive basis for movement persisted

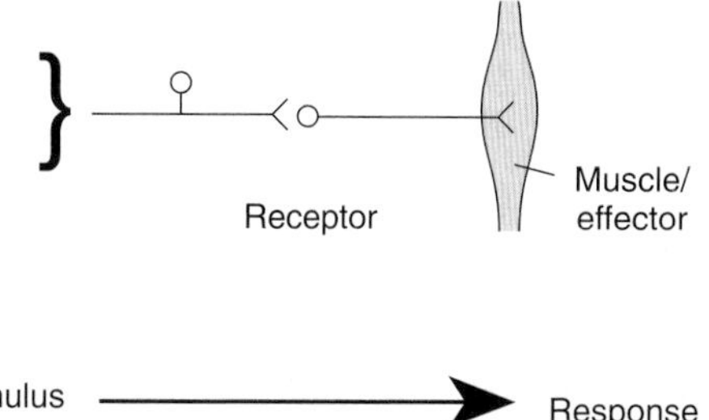

FIGURE 1.3 The basic structure of a reflex consists of a receptor, a conductor, and an effector.

unchallenged by many clinicians for 50 years, and it continues to influence thinking about motor control today.

Limitations

There are a number of limitations of a reflex theory of motor control (Rosenbaum, 1991). First, the reflex cannot be considered the basic unit of behavior if both spontaneous and voluntary movements are recognized as acceptable classes of behavior, because the reflex must be activated by an outside agent.

Second, the reflex theory of motor control does not adequately explain and predict movement that occurs in the absence of a sensory stimulus. More recently, it has been shown that animals can move in a relatively coordinated fashion in the absence of sensory input (Taub & Berman, 1968).

Third, the theory does not explain fast movements, that is, sequences of movements that occur too rapidly to allow for sensory feedback from the preceding movement to trigger the next. For example, an experienced and proficient typist moves from one key to the next so rapidly that there is no time for sensory information from one keystroke to activate the next.

Fourth, the concept that a chain of reflexes can create complex behaviors fails to explain the fact that a single stimulus can result in varying responses depending on context and descending commands. For example, there are times when we need to override reflexes to achieve a goal. Thus, normally touching something hot results in the reflexive withdrawal of the hand. However, if our child is in a fire, we may override the reflexive withdrawal in order to pull the child from the fire.

Finally, reflex chaining does not explain the ability to produce novel movements. Novel movements put together unique combinations of stimuli and responses according to rules previously learned. A violinist who has learned a piece on the violin and also knows the technique of playing the cello can play that piece on the cello without necessarily having practiced it on the cello. The violinist has learned the rules for playing the piece and has applied them to a novel situation.

Clinical Implications

How might a reflex theory of motor control be used to interpret a patient's behavior and serve as a guide for the therapist's actions? If chained or compounded reflexes are the basis for functional movement, clinical strategies designed to test reflexes should allow therapists to predict function. In addition, a patient's movement behaviors would be interpreted in terms of the presence or absence of controlling reflexes. Finally, retraining motor control for functional skills would focus on enhancing or reducing the effect of various reflexes during motor tasks.

Hierarchical Theory

Many researchers have contributed to the view that the nervous system is organized as a hierarchy. Among them, Hughlings Jackson, an English physician, argued that the brain has higher, middle, and lower levels of control, equated with higher association areas, the motor cortex, and spinal levels of motor function (Foerster, 1977).

Hierarchical control in general has been defined as organizational control that is top down. That is, each successively higher level exerts control over the level below it, as shown in Figure 1.4. In a strict vertical hierarchy, lines of control do not cross and there is never bottom-up control.

In the 1920s, Rudolf Magnus began to explore the function of different reflexes within different parts of the nervous system. He found that reflexes controlled by lower levels of the neural hierarchy are present only when cortical centers are damaged. These results were later interpreted to imply that reflexes are part of a hierarchy of motor control, in which higher centers normally inhibit these lower reflex centers (Magnus, 1925; 1926)

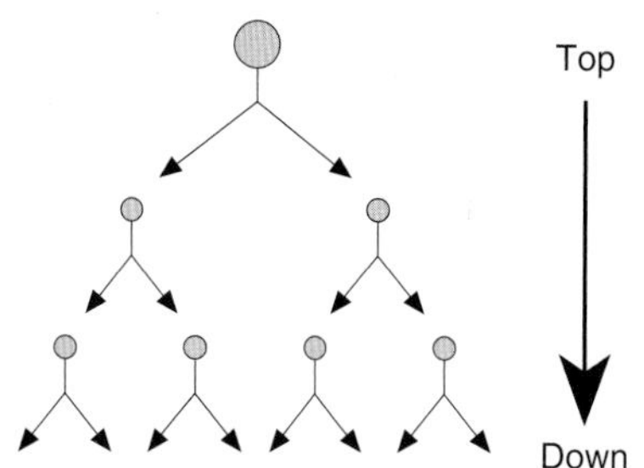

FIGURE 1.4 The hierarchical control model is characterized by a top-down structure, in which higher centers are always in charge of lower centers.

Later, Georg Schaltenbrand (1928) used Magnus's concepts to explain the development of mobility in children and adults. He described the development of human mobility in terms of the appearance and disappearance of a progression of hierarchically organized reflexes. He went on to say that pathology of the brain may result in the persistence of primitive lower level reflexes. He suggested that a complete understanding of all the reflexes would allow the determination of the neural age of a child or of a patient with motor control dysfunction.

In the late 1930s, Stephan Weisz (1938) reported on hierarchically organized reflex reactions that he thought were the basis for equilibrium in humans. He described the ontogeny of equilibrium reflexes in the normally developing child and proposed a relationship between the maturation of these reflexes and the child's capacity to sit, stand, and walk.

The results of these experiments and observations were drawn together and are often referred to in the clinical literature as a reflex/hierarchical theory of motor control. This theory suggests that motor control emerges from reflexes that are nested within hierarchically organized levels of the CNS.

In the 1940s, Arnold Gesell (Gesell, 1954; Gesell & Armatruda, 1947) and Myrtle McGraw (McGraw, 1945), two well-known developmental researchers, offered detailed descriptions of the maturation of infants. These researchers applied the current scientific thinking about reflex hierarchies of motor control to explain the behaviors they saw in infants. Normal motor development was attributed to increasing corticalization of the CNS, resulting in the emergence of higher levels of control over lower level reflexes. This has been referred to as a neuromaturational theory of development. An example of this model is illustrated in Figure 1.5. This theory assumes that CNS maturation is the primary agent for change in development. It minimizes the importance of other factors, such as musculoskeletal changes, during development.

Current Concepts Related to Hierarchical Control

Since Hughlings Jackson's original work, a new concept of hierarchical control has evolved. Modern neuroscientists have confirmed the importance of elements of hierarchical organization in motor control. The concept of a strict hierarchy, in which higher centers are always in control, has been modified. Current concepts describing hierarchical control within the nervous system recognize the fact that each level of the nervous system can act on other levels (higher and lower), depending on the task. In addition, the role of reflexes in movement has been modified. Reflexes are not considered the sole determinant of motor control, but only as one of many processes important to the generation and control of movement.

Limitations

One of the limitations of a reflex/hierarchical theory of motor control is that it cannot explain the dominance of reflex behavior in certain situations in normal adults. For example, stepping on a pin results in an immediate withdrawal of the leg. This is an example of a reflex within the lowest level of the hierarchy dominating motor function. It is an example of bottom-up control. Thus, one must be cautious about assumptions that all low-level behaviors are primitive, immature, and nonadaptive, while all higher level (cortical) behaviors are mature, adaptive, and appropriate.

Clinical Implications

Abnormalities of reflex organization have been used by many clinicians to explain disordered motor

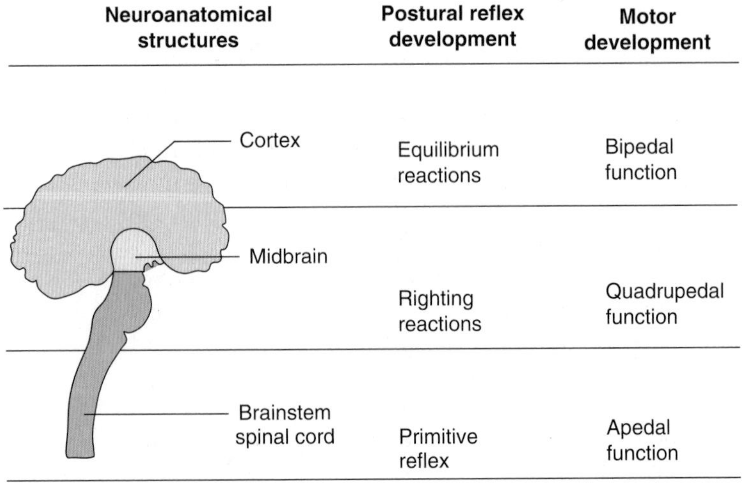

FIGURE 1.5 The neuromaturational theory of motor control attributes motor development to the maturation of neural processes, including the progressive appearance and disappearance of reflexes.

control in the patient with a neurologic disorder. Signe Brunnstrom, a physical therapist who pioneered early stroke rehabilitation, used a reflex hierarchical theory to describe disordered movement following a motor cortex lesion. She stated, "When the influence of higher centers is temporarily or permanently interfered with, normal reflexes become exaggerated and so called pathological reflexes appear" (Brunnstrom, 1970, p. 3).

Berta Bobath, an English physical therapist, in her discussions of abnormal postural reflex activity in children with cerebral palsy, stated that "the release of motor responses integrated at lower levels from restraining influences of higher centers, especially that of the cortex, leads to abnormal postural reflex activity" (Bobath, 1965; Mayston, 1992). The clinical applications of the reflex/hierarchical theory will be discussed in more detail in the last section of this chapter.

Motor Programming Theories

More recent theories of motor control have expanded our understanding of the CNS. They have moved away from views of the CNS as a mostly reactive system and have begun to explore the physiology of actions rather than the physiology of reactions. Reflex theories have been useful in explaining certain stereotyped patterns of movement. However, an interesting way of viewing reflexes is to consider that one can remove the stimulus, or the afferent input, and still have a patterned motor response (VanSant, 1987). If we remove the motor response from its stimulus, we are left with the concept of a central motor pattern. This concept of a central motor pattern, or motor program, is more flexible than the concept of a reflex because it can either be activated by sensory stimuli or by central processes. Scientists who contributed to the development of this theory include individuals from clinical, psychological, and biological backgrounds (Bernstein, 1967; Keele, 1968; Wilson, 1961).

A motor program theory of motor control has considerable experimental support. For example, experiments in the early 1960s studied motor control in the grasshopper or locust and showed that the timing of the animal's wing beat in flight depended on a rhythmic pattern generator. Even when the sensory nerves were cut, the nervous system by itself could generate the output with no sensory input; however, the wing beat was slowed (Wilson, 1961). This suggested that movement is possible in the absence of reflexive action. Sensory input, while not essential in driving movement, has an important function in modulating action.

These conclusions were further supported by work examining locomotion in cats (Grillner, 1981). The results of these experiments showed that in the cat, spinal neural networks could produce a locomotor rhythm with neither sensory inputs nor descending patterns from the brain. By changing the intensity of stimulation to the spinal cord, the animal could be made to walk, trot, or gallop. Thus, it was again shown that reflexes do not drive action, but that central pattern generators (spinally mediated motor programs) by themselves can generate such complex movements as the walk, trot, and gallop. Further experiments showed the important modulatory effects of incoming sensory inputs on the central pattern generator (Forssberg, 1975).

These experiments led to the motor program theory of motor control. This term has been used in a number of ways by different researchers, so care should be taken in determining how the term is being used. The term *motor program* may be used to identify a central pattern generator (CPG), that is, a specific neural circuit like that for generating walking in the cat. In this case, the term represents neural connections that are stereotyped and hardwired.

But the term *motor program* is also used to describe the higher level motor programs that represent actions in more abstract terms. A significant amount of research in the field of psychology has supported the existence of hierarchically organized motor programs that store the rules for generating movements so that we can perform the tasks with a variety of effector systems (Keele, 1968). You can see this for yourself in Lab Activity 1-2.

As shown in Figure 1.6, it has been hypothesized that the rules for writing a given word are stored as an abstract motor program at higher levels within the CNS. As a result, neural commands from these higher centers used to write your name could be sent to various parts of the body. Yet, elements of the written signature remain constant regardless of the part of the body used to carry out the task (Bernstein, 1967).

Limitations

The concept of central pattern generators expanded our understanding of the role of the nervous system in the control of movement. However, we must be careful to realize that the central pattern generator concept was never intended to replace the concept of the importance of sensory input in controlling movement. It simply expanded our understanding of the flexibility of the nervous system in creating movements to include its ability to create movements in isolation from feedback.

An important limitation of the motor program concept is that a central motor program cannot be considered to be the sole determinant of action

LAB ACTIVITY 1-2

Objective: To apply to concept of motor program to functional movement.

Procedure: Write your signature as you normally would on a small piece of paper. Now write it larger, on a blackboard. Now try it with your other hand.

Assignment

1. Examine the three signatures carefully, looking for common elements found in all of them.
2. Write down the common elements you found. What do you think are the causes for both the common elements and the differences? How do your results support or contradict the theory of motor programs?

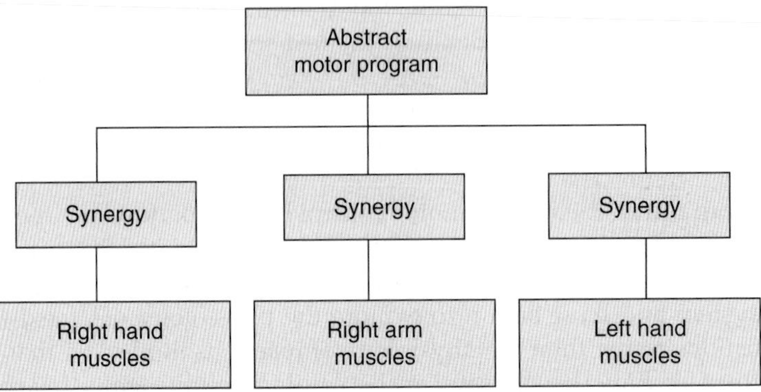

FIGURE 1.6 Levels of control for motor programs and their output systems. Rules for action are represented at the highest level, in abstract motor programs. Lower levels of the hierarchy contain specific information, including muscle response synergies, essential for effecting action.

(Bernstein, 1967). Two identical commands to the elbow flexors, for example, will produce different movements depending on whether your arm is resting at your side or you are holding your arm out in front of you. The forces of gravity will act differently on the limb in the two conditions, and thus modify the movement. In addition, if your muscles are fatigued, similar nervous system commands will yield different results. Thus, the motor program concept does not take into account that the nervous system must deal with both musculoskeletal and environmental variables in achieving movement control.

Clinical Implications

Motor program theories of motor control have allowed clinicians to move beyond a reflex explanation for disordered motor control. Explanations for abnormal movement have been expanded to include problems resulting from abnormalities in central pattern generators or in higher level motor programs. In patients whose higher levels of motor programming are affected, motor program theory suggests the importance of helping patients relearn the correct rules for action. In addition, intervention should focus on retraining movements important to a functional task, not just on reeducating specific muscles in isolation.

Systems Theory

In the early and mid-1900s Nicolai Bernstein (1896–1966), a Russian scientist, was looking at the nervous system and body in a whole new way. Previously, neurophysiologists had focused primarily on neural control aspects of movement. Bernstein, who also participated in the development of motor program theories, recognized that you cannot understand the neural control of movement without an understanding of the characteristics of the system you are moving and the external and internal forces acting on the body (Bernstein, 1967).

In describing the characteristics of the system being moved, Bernstein looked at the whole body as a mechanical system, with mass, and subject to both external forces such as gravity and internal forces such as both inertial and movement-dependent forces. He thus showed that the same central command could result in quite different movements because of the interplay between external forces and variations in the initial conditions. For the same reasons, different commands could result in the same movement. Bernstein also suggested that control of integrated movement was probably distributed throughout many interacting systems working cooperatively to achieve movement. This gave rise to the concept of a distributed model of motor control (Bernstein, 1967).

How does Bernstein's approach to motor control differ from the approaches presented previously? Bernstein asked questions about the organism in a continuously changing situation. He found answers about the nature and control of movement that were different from those of previous researchers because he asked different questions, such as: How does the body as a mechanical system influence the control process? and How do the initial conditions affect the properties of the movement?

In describing the body as a mechanical system, Bernstein noted that we have many degrees of freedom that need to be controlled. For example, we have many joints, all of which flex or extend and many of which can be rotated as well. This complicates movement control incredibly. He said, "Coordination of movement is the process of mastering the redundant degrees of freedom of the moving organism" (Bernstein, 1967). In other words, it involves converting the body into a controllable system.

As a solution to the degrees of freedom problem, Bernstein hypothesized that hierarchical control exists to simplify the control of the body's multiple degrees of freedom. In this way, the higher levels of the nervous system activate lower levels. The lower levels activate synergies, or groups of muscles that are constrained to act together as a unit. Thus, for example, when the demands of a task increase, the control signal to the synergy increases, leading to parallel increases in the activation in all muscles in the synergy. We can think of our movement repertoire to be like sentences made up of many words. The letters within the words are the muscles, the words themselves are the synergies, and the sentences are the actions themselves. Thus, Bernstein believed that synergies play an important role in solving the degrees of freedom problem. This is achieved by constraining certain muscles to work together as a unit. He hypothesized that although there are few synergies, they make possible almost the whole variety of movements we know. For example, he considered some simple synergies to be the locomotor, postural, and respiratory synergies.

Since Bernstein first proposed the concept of synergies, research has continued to examine this concept, and as a result, our understanding of the nature of synergies continues to evolve and change. For example, Latash and others (Latash et al., 2007; Latash & Anson, 2006) have proposed a new definition of the term *synergy*. In this definition, synergies are not used by the nervous system to eliminate redundant degrees of freedom, but instead to ensure flexible and stable performance of motor tasks. They call this the "principle of abundance." They define synergy as a neural organization of a multielement system (e.g., muscles) that: (a) organizes sharing of a task among a set of elemental variables (e.g., muscles); and (b) ensures covariation among elemental variables with the purpose of stabilizing performance variables (e.g., center of mass in posture control or the end point in a reaching task). Thus, synergies show both stability against perturbations and flexibility to solve concurrent tasks (Latash et al., 2007; Newell et al., 1984). Ting and colleagues (Torres-Oviedo & Ting, 2007) are examining the organization and structure of muscle synergies used for balance control. In traditional views of synergies, a muscle belongs to only one synergy, and muscles within a synergy are activated equally as a unit. Newer views of synergies suggest that a muscle can belong to multiple synergies; in addition, an individual muscle has a unique contribution to each synergy. Finally, the total activation of a muscle is dependent on both the simultaneous activation of multiple synergies containing that muscle and the relative contribution of that muscle within each of these synergies. The research examining the role of synergies in postural control is described in more detail in Chapter 7.

Since Bernstein first put forth the principles of systems theory, a number of researchers have expanded and built upon this approach, and have referred to it as the "dynamic systems theory" (Kamm et al., 1991; Kelso & Tuller, 1984; Kugler & Turvey, 1987; Perry, 1998; Thelen et al., 1987). In principle, the theories are very similar at their foundation; thus, either term may be used when people discuss this framework. The dynamic systems theory comes from the broader study of dynamics or synergetics within the physical world, and asks the questions: How do the patterns and organization we see in the world come into being from their orderless constituent parts? and How do these systems change over time? For example, we have thousands of muscle cells in the heart that work together to make the heart beat. How is this system of thousands of degrees of freedom (each cell we add contributes a new degree of freedom to the system) reduced to a system of few degrees of freedom, so that all the cells function as a unit?

These phenomena, which we see not only in the heart muscle but also in the patterns of cloud formations and the patterns of movement of water as it goes from ice to liquid to boiling to a gaseous state, are examples of the principle of "self-organization," which is a fundamental principle of dynamic systems. This principle states that when a system of individual parts comes together, its elements behave collectively in an ordered way. There is no need for a "higher" center issuing instructions or commands in order to achieve coordinated action. This principle applied to motor control predicts that movement could emerge as a result of interacting elements, without the need for specific commands or motor programs within the nervous system.

The dynamic systems perspective also tries to find mathematical descriptions of these self-organizing systems. Critical features that are examined are called "the nonlinear properties" of the system (Harbourne & Stergiou, 2009; Kugler & Turvey, 1987). What is nonlinear behavior? A nonlinear system is one whose output is not proportional to its input (Harbourne & Stergiou, 2009). A nonlinear behavior is one that transforms into a new configuration when a single parameter of that behavior is gradually altered and reaches a critical value. For example, as an animal walks faster and faster, there is a point at which, suddenly, it shifts into a trot. As the animal continues to move faster, there is a second point at which it shifts into a gallop. This is shown in Figure 1.7.

What causes this change from one behavioral pattern (e.g., a walk) to a new behavioral pattern (e.g., a trot)? Dynamic theory suggests that the new movement emerges because of a critical change in one of the systems, called a "control parameter." A **control parameter** is a variable that regulates change in the behavior of the entire system. In our example, the control parameter is velocity. When the animal's walking velocity, a control parameter, reaches a critical point there is a shift in the animal's behavior, from a walk to a trot. Thus, the dynamic action perspective has de-emphasized the notion of commands from the central nervous system in controlling movement and has sought physical explanations that may contribute to movement characteristics as well (Perry, 1998).

An important concept in describing movement from a dynamic systems theory perspective is the role of variability in the control of movement. In the dynamic systems theory, human movement, like behavior in other complex nonlinear systems, has inherent variability that is critical to optimal function (Harbourne & Stergiou, 2009). Movement variability includes variations that occur normally in motor performance across multiple repetitions of a task (Stergiou et al., 2006). However, the role of variability in motor control in dynamic systems theory is viewed differently from other theories of motor control. For example, in motor program theory, variability is considered to be the consequence of errors in motor performance, with the assumption that as performance improves during skill acquisition, error—and consequently variability—decrease. In contrast, in dynamic systems theory, variability is not considered to be the result of error, but rather as a necessary condition of optimal function. Optimal variability provides for flexible, adaptive strategies, allowing adjustment to environmental change, and as such is a central feature of normal movement. Too little variability can lead to injury (as in repetitive-strain problems), while too much variability leads to impaired movement performance, such as occurs in persons with ataxia.

In dynamic systems theory, a small amount of variability indicates a highly stable behavior. Highly stable behaviors are often viewed as an attractor state. Attractor states may be considered highly stable, preferred patterns of movement; many are used to accomplish common activities of daily life. Animals all habitually walk at a preferred pace that represents an attractor state for walking speed specific to the individual. Walking at other speeds is possible, but barring outside influences, individuals tend to walk at a preferred pace, which is energetically most efficient. The degree to which the flexibility exists to change a preferred pattern of movement is characterized as an attractor well. This concept is shown in Figure 1.8. The deeper the well, the harder it is to change the

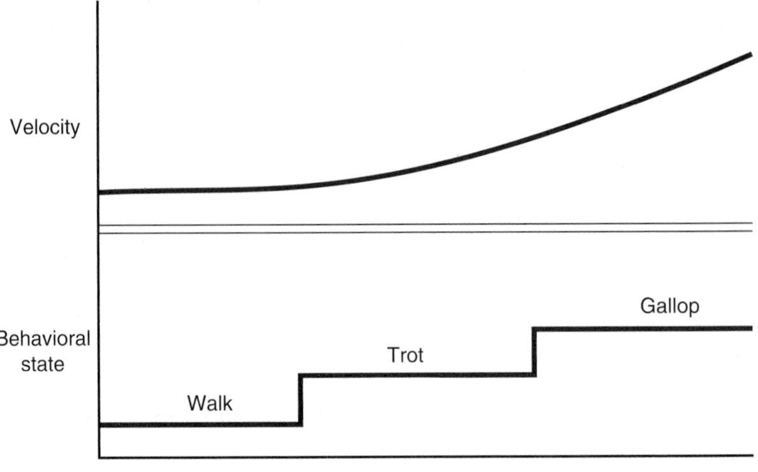

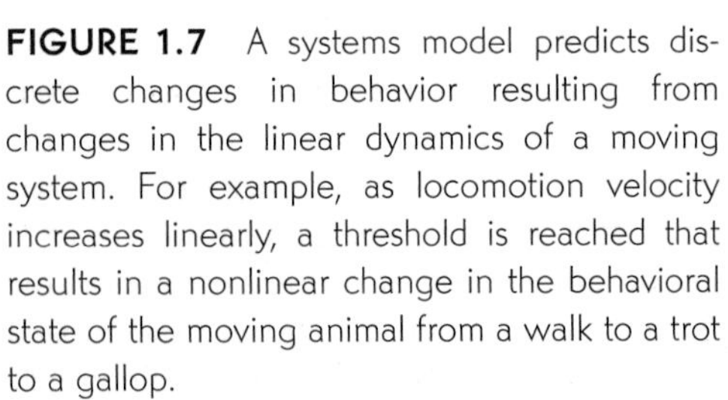
FIGURE 1.7 A systems model predicts discrete changes in behavior resulting from changes in the linear dynamics of a moving system. For example, as locomotion velocity increases linearly, a threshold is reached that results in a nonlinear change in the behavioral state of the moving animal from a walk to a trot to a gallop.

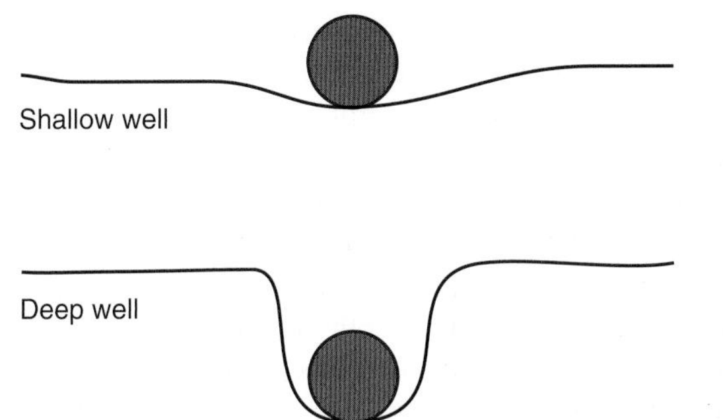

FIGURE 1.8 Attractor wells describe the variability in a preferred pattern of movement.

preferred pattern, suggesting a stable movement pattern. A shallow well suggests an unstable pattern.

Attractor wells may be viewed as riverbeds. When a riverbed is quite deep, the likelihood that the river will flow outside the established riverbed is slight. The river flows in the preferred direction established by the riverbed, which is a deep attractor well. Alternatively, if the riverbed is quite shallow, the river will be more likely to flow in areas not established by the riverbed. In this case, the shallow riverbed is a shallow attractor well. So too, movement patterns in patients could be characterized as stable or unstable based on the difficulty associated with changing them. It will be much easier to change an unstable movement pattern that has a shallow attractor well than to change a stable movement pattern that has a deep attractor well.

Kelso and Tuller (1984) have shown that stable movement patterns become more variable, or unstable, just prior to a transition to a new movement pattern. For example, if persons are asked to move their two index fingers of the right and left hand out of phase, (that is, one finger is flexing while the other is extending) while making the movements faster and faster, an abrupt phase transition occurs between the two fingers. The asymmetrical out-of-phase mode shifts suddenly to a symmetrical in-phase mode (both fingers flexing) involving a shift to activation of homologous muscle groups. Researchers have documented an increase in variability prior to the emergence of new, more stable patterns of behavior during the acquisition of new movement skills in both children and adults (Gordon, 1987; Harbourne & Stergiou, 2009; Harbourne et al., 2007; Woollacott & Shumway-Cook, 1990). Thus, it may be possible for therapists to view variability in movement behavior as an antecedent to change in some patients.

Limitations

What are some of the limitations of Bernstein's systems (including the dynamic systems) approach? Thus far, we have discussed the broadest of the approaches. Because dynamic systems theory takes into account not only the contributions of the nervous system to action, but also the contributions of the muscle and skeletal systems, as well as the forces of gravity and inertia, it predicts actual behavior much better than did previous theories. This theory reminds us that the nervous system in isolation will not allow the prediction of movement. However, a limitation of some variations of this model can be the presumption that the nervous system has a less important role in determining the animal's behavior, giving mathematical formulas and principles of body mechanics a more dominant role in describing motor control. Understanding the application and relevance of this type of analysis to clinical practice can be very difficult.

Clinical Implications

The systems theory has a number of implications for therapists. First, it stresses the importance of understanding the body as a mechanical system. Movement is not determined solely by the output of the nervous system, but is the output of the nervous system as filtered through a mechanical system, the body. When working with the patient who has a CNS deficit, the therapist must be careful to examine the contribution of impairments in the musculoskeletal system, as well as the neural system, to overall loss of motor control. The systems theory suggests that examination and intervention must focus not only on the impairments within individual systems contributing to motor control, but also on the effect of interacting impairments among multiple systems. With the use of the uncontrolled manifold (UCM) analysis it also may provide ways to test whether the patient is using particular muscle or joint movement patterns in a synergistic way, to actually enhance performance output (e.g., accurately reaching or balancing).

In addition, one of the major implications of the systems theory is the view that movement is an emergent property—that is, it emerges from the interaction of multiple elements that self-organize based on certain dynamic properties of the elements themselves. This means that shifts or alterations in movement behavior can often be explained in terms of physical principles rather than necessarily in terms of neural structures. What are the implications of this for treating motor dyscontrol in patients? If as clinicians we understood more about the physical or dynamic properties of the human body, we could make use of these properties in helping patients to regain motor control. For example, velocity can be an important contributor to the dynamics of movement. Often, patients are asked to move slowly in an effort to move safely. Yet, this approach to retraining fails to take into account the interaction between speed and physical properties of the body, which produce momentum, and therefore can help a weak patient move with greater ease.

Variability as a characteristic feature of normal movement has important clinical implications for therapists involved in retraining movement in patients with neural pathology. When variability is viewed as a consequence of error, therapists will use therapeutic strategies designed to reduce error, guiding patients toward an optimal and stable movement pattern. In contrast, when variability is viewed as a critical element of normal function, therapists will encourage patients to explore variable and flexible movement patterns that will lead to success in achieving performance goals (Harbourne & Stergiou, 2009).

Ecological Theory

In the 1960s, independent of the research in physiology, a psychologist named James Gibson was beginning to explore the way in which our motor systems allow us to interact most effectively with the environment in order to perform goal-oriented behavior (Gibson, 1966). His research focused on how we detect information in our environment that is relevant to our actions and how we use this information to control our movements. The ability to use perceptions to guide action emerges early in life. For example, by 15 weeks of age infants do not automatically reach for every object that passes by, but instead they are able to use perceptions related to velocity to determine in advance whether or not they can catch a ball (von Hofsten & Lindhagen, 1979).

This view was expanded by students of Gibson (Lee & Young, 1986; Reed, 1982) and became known as the ecological approach to motor control. It suggests that motor control evolved so that animals could cope with the environment around them, moving in it effectively in order to find food, run away from predators, build shelter, and even play (Reed, 1982). What was new about this approach? It was really the first time that researchers began focusing on how actions are geared to the environment. Actions require perceptual information that is specific to a desired goal-directed action performed within a specific environment. The organization of action is specific to the task and the environment in which the task is being performed.

Whereas many previous researchers had seen the organism as a sensory/motor system, Gibson stressed that it was not sensation per se that was important to the animal, but perception. Specifically, what is needed is the perception of environmental factors important to the task. He stated that perception focuses on detecting information in the environment that will support the actions necessary to achieve the goal. From an ecological perspective, it is important to determine how an organism detects information in the environment that is relevant to action, what form this information takes, and how this information is used to modify and control movement (Lee & Young, 1986).

In summary, the ecological perspective has broadened our understanding of nervous system function from that of a sensory/motor system, reacting to environmental variables, to that of a perception/action system that actively explores the environment to satisfy its own goals.

Limitations

Although the ecological approach has expanded our knowledge significantly with regard to the interaction of the organism and the environment, it has tended to give less emphasis to the organization and function of the nervous system that led to this interaction. Thus, the research emphasis has shifted from the nervous system to the organism/environment interface.

Clinical Implications

A major contribution of this view is in describing the individual as an active explorer of the environment. The active exploration of the task and the environment in which the task is performed allows the individual to develop multiple ways to accomplish a task. Adaptability is important not only in the way we organize movements to accomplish a task, but also in the way we use perception.

An important part of intervention is helping the patient explore the possibilities for achieving a functional task in multiple ways. The ability to develop multiple adaptive solutions to accomplishing a task requires that the patient explore a range of possible ways to accomplish a task and discover the best solution, given his or her set of limitations.

Which Theory of Motor Control is Best?

So which motor control theory best suits the current theoretical and practical needs of therapists? Which is the most complete theory of motor control, the one that really predicts the nature and cause of movement and is consistent with our current knowledge of brain anatomy and physiology?

As you no doubt can already see, there is no one theory that has it all. We believe the best theory of motor control is one that combines elements from all of the theories presented. A comprehensive or integrated theory recognizes the elements of motor control we do know about and leaves room for the things we do not. Any current theory of motor control is in a sense unfinished, since there must always be room to revise and incorporate new information.

Many people have been working to develop an integrated theory of motor control (Gordon, 1987; Horak & Shumway-Cook, 1990; Woollacott & Shumway-Cook, 1990). In some cases, as theories are modified, new names are applied. As a result, it becomes difficult to distinguish among evolving theories. For example, systems, dynamic, dynamic action, and dynamic systems theory are all terms that are often used interchangeably.

Previously we (Woollacott & Shumway-Cook 1990; 1997) have called the theory of motor control on which we base our research and clinical practice a systems approach. We have continued to use this name, although our concept of systems theory differs from Bernstein's systems theory and has evolved to incorporate many of the concepts proposed by other theories of motor control. In this book we will continue to refer to our theory of motor control as a systems approach. This approach argues that it is critical to recognize that movement emerges from an interaction between the individual, the task, and the environment in which the task is being carried out. Thus, movement is not solely the result of muscle-specific motor programs or stereotyped reflexes, but results from a dynamic interplay between perception, cognition, and action systems. This theoretical framework will be used throughout this textbook, and it is the basis for clinical methods related to examination and intervention in the patient with neurologic problems. We have found the theory useful in helping us to generate research questions and hypotheses about the nature and cause of movement.

PARALLEL DEVELOPMENT OF CLINICAL PRACTICE AND SCIENTIFIC THEORY

Much has been written about the influence of changing scientific theories on the treatment of patients with movement disorders. Several excellent articles discuss in detail the parallel developments between scientific theory and clinical practice (Gordon, 1987; Horak, 1992).

Although neuroscience researchers identify the scientific basis for movement and movement disorders, it is up to the clinician to develop the applications of this research. Thus, scientific theory provides a framework that allows the integration of practical ideas into a coherent philosophy for intervention. A theory is not right or wrong in an absolute sense, but it is judged to be more or less useful in solving the problems presented by patients with movement dysfunction (Gordon, 1987; Horak, 1992).

Just as scientific assumptions about the important elements that control movement are changing, so too, is clinical practice related to treatment of the patient with a neurologic deficit changing. New assumptions regarding the nature and cause of movement are replacing old assumptions. Clinical practice evolves in parallel with scientific theory, as clinicians assimilate changes in scientific theory and apply them to practice. This concept is shown in Figure 1.9. Let us explore in more detail the evolution of clinical practice in light of changing theories of motor control.

Neurologic Rehabilitation: Reflex-Based Neurofacilitation Approaches

In the late 1950s and early 1960s, the so-called neurofacilitation approaches were developed, resulting in a dramatic change in clinical interventions directed at the patient with neurologic impairments (Gordon, 1987; Horak, 1992). For the most part, these approaches still dominate the way clinicians treat the patient with a neurologic deficit.

Neurofacilitation approaches include the Bobath approach, developed by Karl and Berta Bobath (1975), the Rood approach, developed by Margaret Rood (Stockmeyer, 1967), Brunnstrom's approach, developed by Signe Brunnstrom (1966), proprioceptive neuromuscular facilitation (PNF), developed by Kabat and Knott (1954) and expanded by Voss et al. (1985), and sensory integration therapy, developed by Jean Ayres (1972). These approaches were based largely on assumptions drawn from both the reflex and hierarchical theories of motor control.

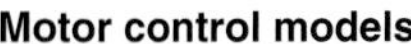

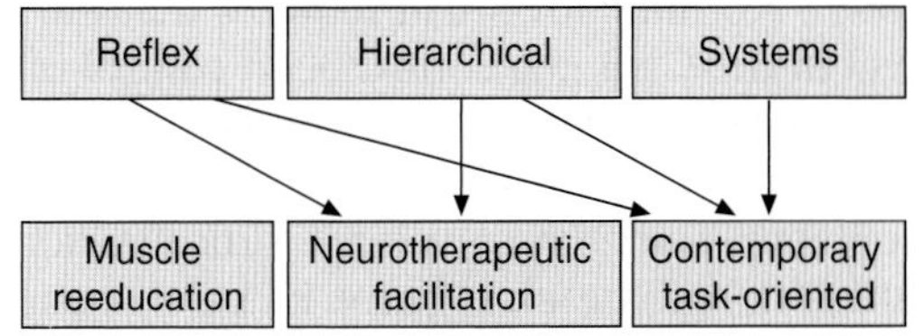

FIGURE 1.9 The parallel development of theories of motor control and clinical practices designed to examine and treat patients with motor dyscontrol. (Adapted with permission from Horak F. Assumptions underlying motor control for neurologic rehabilitation. In: Contemporary management of motor control problems. Proceedings of the II Step Conference. Alexandria, VA: American Physical Therapy Association, 1992:11.)

Prior to the development of the neurofacilitation approaches, therapy for the patient with neurologic dysfunction was directed largely at changing function at the level of the muscle itself. This has been referred to as a muscle reeducation approach to intervention (Gordon, 1987; Horak, 1992). Although the muscle reeducation approach was effective in managing movement disorders resulting from polio, it had less impact on altering movement patterns in patients with upper motor neuron lesions. Thus, the neurofacilitation techniques were developed in response to clinicians' dissatisfaction with previous modes of intervention and a desire to develop approaches that were more effective in solving the movement problems of patients with neurologic dysfunction (Gordon, 1987).

Clinicians working with patients with upper motor neuron (motor cortex and pyramidal tract) lesions began to direct clinical efforts toward modifying the CNS itself. Neurofacilitation approaches focused on retraining motor control through techniques designed to facilitate and/or inhibit different movement patterns. *Facilitation* refers to intervention techniques that increase the patient's ability to move in ways judged to be appropriate by the clinician. Inhibitory techniques decrease the patient's use of movement patterns considered to be abnormal (Gordon, 1987).

Underlying Assumptions

Neurofacilitation approaches are largely associated with both the reflex and hierarchical theories of motor control. Thus, clinical practices have been developed based on assumptions regarding the nature and cause of normal motor control, abnormal motor control, and the recovery of function.

This approach suggests that normal movement results from a chain of reflexes organized hierarchically within the CNS. Thus, control of movement is top down. Normal movement requires that the highest level of the CNS, the cortex, be in control of both intermediate (brainstem) and lower (spinal cord) levels of the CNS. This means that the process of normal development, sometimes called "corticalization," is characterized by the emergence of behaviors organized at sequentially higher and higher levels in the CNS. A great emphasis is placed on the understanding that incoming sensory information stimulates, and thus drives, a normal movement pattern.

Explanations regarding the physiological basis for abnormal motor control from a reflex and hierarchical perspective largely suggest that a disruption of normal reflex mechanisms underlies abnormal movement control. It is assumed that lesions at the highest cortical levels of the CNS cause release of abnormal reflexes organized at lower levels within the CNS. The release of these lower-level reflexes constrains the patient's ability to move normally.

Another prevalent assumption is that abnormal or atypical patterns of movement seen in patients with motor cortex lesions are the direct result of the lesion itself, as opposed to considering some behaviors as developing either secondary to the lesion or in response to the lesion (i.e., compensatory to the lesion). Thus, it is predicted that in the child with motor cortex lesions, the process of increasing corticalization is disrupted, and as a result motor control is dominated by primitive patterns of movement organized at lower levels of the CNS. In addition, in the adult with acquired motor cortex lesions, damage to higher levels of the CNS probably results in a release of lower centers from higher-center control. Likewise, primitive and pathologic behaviors organized at these levels reemerge to dominate, preventing normal patterns of movement from occurring.

A central assumption concerning the *recovery of function* in the patient with a motor cortex lesion is that recovery of normal motor control cannot occur unless higher centers of the CNS regain control over lower centers. According to this approach, recovery of function, in a sense, recapitulates development, with higher centers gradually regaining their dominance over lower centers of the CNS.

Two key assumptions are that: (a) functional skills will automatically return once abnormal movement patterns are inhibited and normal movement patterns facilitated, and (b) repetition of these normal movement patterns will automatically transfer to functional tasks.

Clinical Applications

What are some of the clinical applications of these assumptions? First, examination of motor control should focus on identifying the presence or absence of normal and abnormal reflexes controlling movement. Also, intervention should be directed at modifying the reflexes that control movement. The importance of sensory input for stimulating normal motor output suggests an intervention focus of modifying the CNS through sensory stimulation (Gordon, 1987; Horak, 1992).

A hierarchical theory suggests that one goal of therapy is to regain independent control of movement by higher centers of the CNS. Thus, intervention is geared toward helping the patient regain normal patterns of movement as a way of facilitating functional recovery.

The neurofacilitation approaches still dominate the way clinicians examine and intervene with patients who have CNS pathology. However, just as scientific theory about the nature and cause of movement has changed in the past 30 years, so too, have many of the neurofacilitation approaches changed their approach to practice. Currently within the neurofacilitation approaches, there is a greater emphasis on explicitly training function and less emphasis on inhibiting reflexes and retraining normal patterns of movement. In addition, there is more consideration of motor learning principles when developing intervention plans. The boundaries between approaches are less distinct, as each approach integrates new concepts related to motor control into its theoretical base.

Task-Oriented Approach

One of the newer approaches to retraining is the task-oriented approach to clinical intervention, based on newer theories of motor control. In previous publications we have referred to this approach as a systems approach (Woollacott & Shumway-Cook, 1990). Others have referred to these new clinical methods as a motor control or motor learning approach (Carr & Shepard, 1987). Whatever the label, these newer methods of clinical practice are based on concepts emerging from research in the fields of motor control, motor learning, and rehabilitation science. Clinical practice is dynamic, changing in response to emerging evidence. We will continue to refer to the clinical approach presented in this book as a "task-oriented" approach, although specific examination and treatment strategies will by necessity change as new research in the field emerges.

Underlying Assumptions

Assumptions underlying a task-oriented approach are quite different from those underlying the neurofacilitation techniques. In the task-oriented approach it is assumed that normal movement emerges as an interaction among many different systems, each contributing different aspects of control. In addition, movement is organized around a behavioral goal and is constrained by the environment. Thus, the role of sensation in normal movement is not limited to a stimulus/response reflex mode but is essential to predictive and adaptive control of movement as well.

Assumptions regarding abnormal motor control suggest that movement problems result from impairments within one or more of the systems controlling movement. Movements observed in the patient with a motor cortex lesion represent behavior that emerges from the best mix of the systems remaining to participate. This means that what is observed is not just the result of the lesion itself, but also of the efforts of the remaining systems to compensate for the loss and still be functional. However, the compensatory strategies developed by patients are not always optimal. Thus, a goal in intervention may be to improve the efficiency of compensatory strategies used to perform functional tasks.

Clinical Applications

These assumptions suggest that when retraining movement control, it is essential to work on identifiable functional tasks rather than on movement patterns for movement's sake alone. A task-oriented approach to intervention assumes that patients learn by actively attempting to solve the problems inherent in a functional task rather than by repetitively practicing normal patterns of movement. Adaptation to changes in the environmental context is a critical part of recovery of function. In this context, patients are helped to learn a variety of ways to solve the task goal rather than a single muscle activation pattern.

SUMMARY

1. Motor control is the ability to regulate the mechanisms essential to movement. Thus, the field of motor control is directed at studying the nature of movement and how that movement is controlled.
2. The specific practices used to examine and treat the patient with motor dyscontrol are determined by underlying assumptions about how movement is controlled, which come from specific theories of motor control.
3. A theory of motor control is a group of abstract ideas about the control of movement. Theories provide: (a) a framework for interpreting behavior, (b) a guide for clinical action, (c) new ideas, and (d) working hypotheses for examination and intervention.
4. Rehabilitation practices reflect the theories or basic ideas we have about the nature of function and dysfunction.
5. This chapter reviews many motor control theories that influence our perspective regarding examination and intervention, including the reflex theory, hierarchical theory, motor programming theories, systems theory, and ecological theory.
6. In this textbook we use a systems theory as the foundation for many clinical applications. According to systems theory, movement arises from the interaction of multiple processes, including: (a) perceptual, cognitive and motor

processes within the individual, and (b) interactions between the individual, the task, and the environment.

7. Clinical practices evolve in parallel with scientific theory, as clinicians assimilate changes in scientific theory and apply them to practice. Neurofacilitation approaches to intervention were developed in parallel with the reflex and hierarchical theories of motor control. New approaches to intervention, such as the task-oriented approach, are being developed in response to changing theories of motor control.

ANSWERS TO LAB ACTIVITY ASSIGNMENTS

Lab Activity 1-1

1. As you do this lab you will find there are many ways to organize a taxonomy of tasks, since there are many attributes you could use to order tasks. You may also find that as therapists we often order tasks according to the stability demands associated with tasks.
2. You will find that it is easy to distinguish the easiest tasks (e.g., sitting with support) from the hardest tasks (e.g., walking on uneven surfaces while holding a cup of water), but it is not always easy to order intermediate tasks. This suggests that there is no "one" way to move through a progression of tasks, particularly the tasks that reflect an intermediate level of difficulty.

Lab Activity 1-2

1. You should see that regardless of the size or hand used to write your signature, there are common elements in each of the signatures.
2. These common elements may include the relationship of one letter to another, how certain letters are formed, and the tendency to stop and start certain letters in relatively the same place. These commonalities support the theory of motor programs.

CHAPTER 2

MOTOR LEARNING AND RECOVERY OF FUNCTION

LEARNING OBJECTIVES

Following completion of this chapter, the reader will be able to:

1. Define motor learning; discuss the similarities and differences between learning, performance, and recovery of function.
2. Compare and contrast implicit and explicit forms of learning and give examples of each.
3. Discuss the basic concepts, clinical implications, and limitations of each of the following motor learning theories: Adams's closed-loop, Schmidt's schema theory, and Newell's ecological theory.
4. Compare and contrast the following theories related to stages of motor learning: Fitts and Posner's three-stage theory, systems three-stage theory, and Gentile's two-stage theory.
5. Define intrinsic versus extrinsic feedback, give examples of each, and discuss their importance in teaching motor skills.
6. Discuss factors that have an impact on the structure of practice and describe their effect on performance versus learning.
7. Define recovery of function; describe the differences between recovery and compensation.
8. Discuss the effect of preinjury and postinjury factors on recovery of function following central nervous system injury.

INTRODUCTION TO MOTOR LEARNING

Following her stroke, Mrs. Jean J received therapy for 5 weeks. She gradually regained the ability to stand, walk, and feed herself. What is the cause of her recovery of motor function? How much is due to "spontaneous recovery"? How much of her recovery may be attributed to therapeutic interventions? How many of her reacquired motor skills will she be able to retain and use when she leaves the rehabilitation facility and returns home? These questions and issues reflect the importance of motor learning to clinicians involved in retraining the patient with motor control problems.

What is Motor Learning?

In Chapter 1, we defined the field of motor control as the study of the nature and control of movement. We define the field of **motor learning** as the study of the acquisition and/or modification of movement. While *motor control* focuses on understanding the control of movement already acquired, *motor learning* focuses on understanding the acquisition and/or modification of movement.

The field of motor learning has traditionally referred to the study of the acquisition or modification of movement in normal subjects. In contrast, **recovery of function** has referred to the reacquisition of movement skills lost through injury.

While there is nothing inherent in the term *motor learning* to distinguish it from processes involved in the recovery of movement function, the two are often thought of as separate. This separation between recovery of function and motor learning may be misleading. Issues facing clinicians concerned with helping patients reacquire skills lost as the result of injury are similar to those faced by people in the field of motor learning. Questions common to both include: How can I best structure practice (therapy) to ensure learning? How can I ensure that skills learned in one context transfer to others? and Will simplifying a task (i.e., making it easier to perform) result in more efficient learning? What is the best way to promote neural plasticity and adaptation underlying the (re) acquisition of movement skills critical to the recovery of function?

In this chapter we use the term *motor learning* to encompass both the acquisition and the reacquisition of movement. We will begin our study of motor learning by discussing important issues related to the nature of motor learning. Following this, we will explore different theories of motor learning, examining their underlying assumptions and clinical implications. We will discuss the practical applications of motor learning research. Finally, we will discuss issues related to recovery of function, including the many factors that affect a patient's ability to recover from brain injury.

NATURE OF MOTOR LEARNING

Early Definitions of Motor Learning

Learning has been described as the process of acquiring knowledge about the world; *motor learning* has been described as a set of processes associated with practice or experience leading to relatively permanent changes in the capability for producing skilled action. This definition of motor learning reflects four concepts: (a) learning is a process of acquiring the capability for skilled action; (b) learning results from experience or practice; (c) learning cannot be measured directly—instead, it is inferred from behavior; and (d) learning produces relatively permanent changes in behavior; thus, short-term alterations are not thought of as learning (Schmidt & Lee, 2005).

Broadening the Definition of Motor Learning

In this chapter, the definition of motor learning has been expanded to encompass many aspects not traditionally considered part of motor learning. Motor learning involves more than motor processes; it involves learning new strategies for sensing as well as moving. Thus, motor learning, like motor control, emerges from a complex of perception/cognition/action processes.

Previous views of motor learning have focused primarily on changes in the individual. But the process of motor learning can be described as the search for a task solution that emerges from an interaction of the individual with the task and the environment. Task solutions are new strategies for perceiving and acting (Newell, 1991).

Similarly, the recovery of function involves the search for new solutions in relationship to specific tasks and environments given the new constraints imposed on the individual by neural pathology. Thus, one cannot study motor learning or recovery of function outside the context of how individuals are solving functional tasks in specific environments.

Relating Performance and Learning

Traditionally, the study of motor learning has focused solely on motor outcomes. Earlier views of motor learning did not always distinguish it from performance (Schmidt & Lee, 2005). Changes in performance that resulted from practice were usually thought to reflect changes in learning. However, this view failed to consider that certain practice effects improved performance initially but were not necessarily retained, which is a condition of learning. This led to the notion that learning could not be evaluated during practice, but rather during specific retention or transfer tests. Thus, **learning**, defined as a relatively permanent change, has been distinguished from **performance**, defined as a temporary change in motor behavior seen during practice sessions.

For example, Mrs. Jean J shows an improved ability to stand symmetrically (with weight evenly distributed to both legs) at the end of her daily therapy session, but when she returns to therapy the following day, she again stands with all her weight on her noninvolved leg. This suggests that while performance had improved in response to therapy, learning had not yet occurred. When on subsequent days Mrs. J demonstrates a more symmetric weight-bearing stance even as she arrives for therapy, we may suggest that learning (a permanent change in behavior) is occurring.

Forms of Learning

The recovery of function following injury involves the reacquisition of complex tasks. However, it is difficult to understand the processes involved in learning using the study of complex tasks. Therefore, many researchers have begun by exploring simple to more complex forms of learning, with the understanding that these more simple forms of learning are the basis for the acquisition of skilled behavior.

We begin by reviewing different forms of learning and discussing some of their clinical applications. We then consider theories of motor learning that have been developed to describe the acquisition of skilled behavior and suggest how each might be used to explain the acquisition of a skill such as reaching for a glass of water. At the outset, we provide an overview of the categories of memory and learning.

Basic Forms of Long-Term Memory: Nondeclarative (Implicit) and Declarative (Explicit)

Studies of patients with memory deficits due to bilateral medial temporal lobe lesions have shown that these patients show a profound loss of the ability to remember factual knowledge. This type of memory, usually called "declarative memory" or "explicit memory," involves the association of information related to people or things one has encountered, places one has been, and the meaning of these bits of information. On the other hand, the patients still possess other forms of long-term memory related to motor skills, and simple learning tasks such as habituation, sensitization, and classical conditioning. Figure 2.1 shows a diagram of the two major categories of long-term memory that we will discuss next, nondeclarative (or implicit) and declarative (or explicit), and the different types of learning embedded within them. We will see that much of motor learning is nondeclarative or implicit.

Nondeclarative (Implicit) Forms of Learning

As you see in Figure 2.1, nondeclarative learning can be divided into a number of subtypes, each controlled by different parts of the brain. We will begin our discussion of nondeclarative learning with nonassociative forms of learning, which are the simplest forms of learning, involving reflex pathways.

Nonassociative Forms of Learning

Nonassociative learning occurs when animals are given a single stimulus repeatedly. As a result, the nervous system learns about the characteristics of that stimulus. Habituation and sensitization are two very simple forms of nonassociative learning. **Habituation** is a decrease in responsiveness that occurs as a result of repeated exposure to a nonpainful stimulus (Kandel et al., 2000).

Habituation is used in many different ways in the clinical setting. For example, habituation exercises are used to treat dizziness in patients with certain types of vestibular dysfunction. Patients are asked to repeatedly move in ways that provoke their dizziness. This repetition results in habituation of the dizziness response. Habituation also forms the basis of therapy for children whose behavior is termed "tactile defensive," that is, children who show excessive

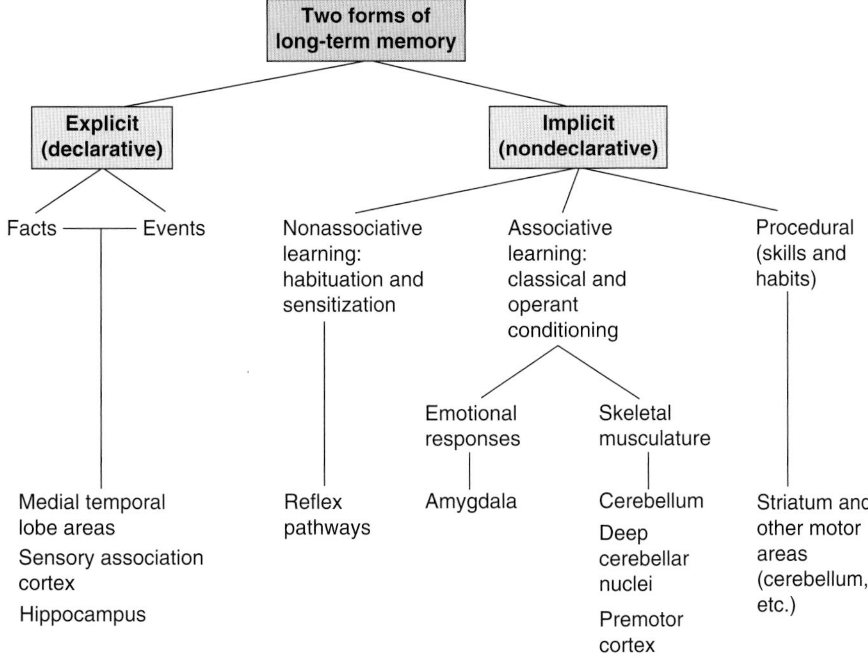

FIGURE 2.1 Different forms of memory. (Adapted from Kandel ER, Kupfermann I, Iversen S. Learning and memory. In: Kandel ER, Schwartz JH, Jessell TM, eds. Principles of neural science, 4th ed. New York: McGraw-Hill, 2000:1231.)

responsiveness to cutaneous stimulation. Children are repeatedly exposed to gradually increasing levels of cutaneous inputs in an effort to decrease their sensitivity to this stimulus.

Sensitization is an increased responsiveness following a threatening or noxious stimulus (Kandel et al., 2000). For example, if I receive a painful stimulus on the skin, and then a light touch, I will react more strongly than I normally would to the light touch. After a person has habituated to one stimulus, a painful stimulus can dishabituate the response to the first. That is, sensitization counteracts the effects of habituation.

There are times when increasing a patient's sensitivity to a threatening stimulus is important. For example, increasing a patient's awareness of stimuli indicating likelihood for impending falls might be an important aspect of balance retraining.

Associative Forms of Learning

A second type of nondeclarative or implicit learning is associative learning. What is *associative learning*? It is through associative learning that a person learns to predict relationships, either relationships of one stimulus to another (classical conditioning) or the relationship of one's behavior to a consequence (operant conditioning). For example, when a patient recovering from a stroke, through repeated practice, begins to learn to redefine their stability limits so that they do not put so much weight on their involved limb that they fall, they are undergoing associative learning, and specifically, operant conditioning. That is, they are learning that stability is associated with a new strategy of weight support.

It has been suggested that associative learning has evolved to help animals learn to detect causal relationships in the environment. Establishing lawful and therefore predictive relationships among events is part of the process of making sense and order of our world. Recognizing key relationships between events is an essential part of the ability to adapt behavior to novel situations (Kandel et al., 2000).

Patients who have suffered an injury that has drastically altered their ability to sense and move in their world have the task of reexploring their body in relationship to their world in order to determine what new relationships exist between the two. Pavlov studied how humans and animals learn the association of two stimuli through the simple form of learning that is now called "classical conditioning."

Classical Conditioning. Classical conditioning consists of learning to pair two stimuli. During classical conditioning an initially weak stimulus (the conditioned stimulus) becomes highly effective in producing a response when it becomes associated with another, stronger, stimulus (the unconditioned stimulus). The conditioned stimulus (CS) is usually something that initially produces no response (like a bell). In contrast, the unconditioned stimulus (UCS), which could be food, always produces a response. After repeated pairing of the conditioned and the unconditioned stimulus, one begins to see a conditioned response (CR) to the conditioned stimulus. Remember, it originally produced no response (Kandel et al., 2000). This relationship is shown in Figure 2.2.

What the subject is doing in this type of learning is to predict relationships between two stimuli or events that have occurred and to respond accordingly. For example, in a therapy setting, if we repeatedly give patients a verbal cue in conjunction with physical assistance when making a movement, they may eventually begin to make the movement with only the verbal cue.

Thus, as patients gain skills we see them move along the continuum of assistance, from hands-on assistance from the therapist, to performing the task with verbal cues, and eventually to performing the action unassisted.

It has been shown that we generally learn relationships that are relevant to our survival; it is more difficult to associate biologically meaningless events. These findings underscore an important learning principle: the brain is most likely to perceive and integrate aspects of the environment that are most pertinent. With regard to therapy, patients are most likely to learn tasks and in environments that are relevant and meaningful to them.

Operant Conditioning. Operant, or instrumental, conditioning is a second type of associative learning (Kandel et al., 2000). It is basically trial-and-error learning. During **operant conditioning** we learn to associate a certain response, from among many

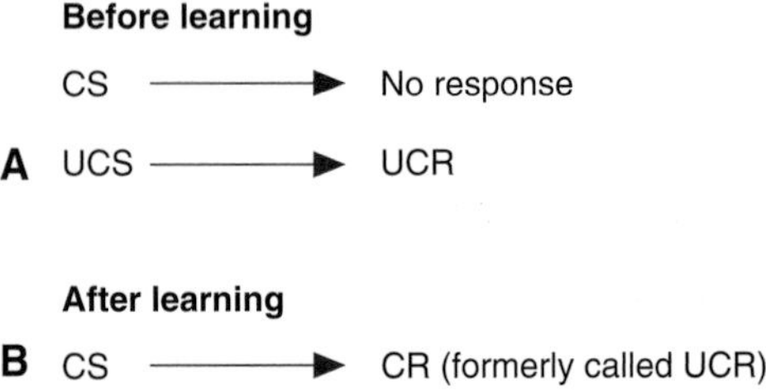

FIGURE 2.2 The process of classical conditioning is diagrammed, showing the relationship between the conditioned stimulus (CS), unconditioned stimulus (UCS), conditioned response (CR), and unconditioned response (UCR) before learning (A) and during the course of learning (B).

that we have made, with a consequence. The classic experiments in this area were done with animals that were given food rewards whenever they randomly pressed a lever inside their cages. They soon learned to associate the lever press with the presentation of food, and the frequency of lever pressing became very high.

The principle of operant conditioning could be stated as follows: Behaviors that are rewarded tend to be repeated at the cost of other behaviors. And likewise, behaviors followed by aversive stimuli are not usually repeated. This has been called the "law of effect" (Kandel et al., 2000).

Operant conditioning plays a major role in determining the behaviors shown by patients referred for therapy. For example, the frail elderly person who leaves her home to go shopping and experiences a fall is less likely to repeat that activity. A decrease in activity results in declining physical function, which in turn increases the likelihood that she will fall. This increased likelihood for falls will reinforce her desire to be inactive, and on it goes, showing the law of effect in action. Therapists may make use of a variety of interventions to assist this patient in regaining her activity level and in reducing her likelihood of falling. One intervention may be the use of desensitization to decrease her anxiety and fear of falling—for example, practicing walking in outdoor situations that have engendered fear in the past.

Operant conditioning can be an effective tool during clinical intervention. Verbal praise by a therapist for a job well done serves as a reinforcer for some (though not all) patients. Setting up a therapy session so that a particular movement is rewarded by the successful accomplishment of a task desired by the patient is a powerful example of operant conditioning.

Regions of the brain that have been shown to contribute to these types of implicit memory include the cerebellum and the deep cerebellar nuclei for movement conditioning (e.g., for certain types of classical conditioning and to gain control of reflexes, such as the vestibulo-ocular reflex), the amygdala for adaptation involving the emotions (e.g., for conditioned fear, such as the fear of falling in an older adult, after an injurious fall) and the lateral dorsal premotor areas of the cortex (for associating a particular sensory event with a specific movement) (see Fig. 2.1) (Kandel et al., 2000; Krakauer & Ghez, 2000).

Procedural Learning

Another type of nondeclarative or implicit learning is **procedural learning,** which refers to learning tasks that can be performed automatically without attention or conscious thought, like a habit. Procedural learning develops slowly through repetition of an act over many trials, and it is expressed through improved performance of the task that was practiced. Like other forms of implicit learning, procedural learning does not require awareness, attention, or other higher cognitive processes. During motor skill acquisition, repeating a movement continuously under varying circumstances would typically lead to procedural learning. That is, one automatically learns the movement itself, or the rules for moving, called a "movement schema."

For example, when teaching a patient to transfer from chair to bed, we often have the patient practice the task repeatedly in order to learn a movement strategy that is effective in performing a transfer task. To better prepare patients to transfer effectively in a wide variety of situations and contexts, patients practice under different conditions in order to learn to move from chairs of differing heights and at different positions relative to the bed. They thus begin to form the rules associated with the task of transfer. The development of rules for transferring will allow them to safely transfer in unfamiliar circumstances. Constant practice and repetition under varying contexts results in efficient procedural learning underlying the reacquisition of effective and safe transfers. As shown in Figure 2.1 the striatum of the basal ganglia is critical to procedural learning (Kandel et al., 2000).

Declarative or Explicit Learning

While nondeclarative or implicit learning is more reflexive, automatic, or habitual in character, and requires frequent repetition for its formation, **declarative learning** results in knowledge that can be consciously recalled and thus requires processes such as awareness, attention, and reflection (Kandel et al., 2000). As noted above, it involves the ability to remember factual knowledge (often related to objects, places, or events). Declarative learning can be expressed in declarative sentences, like: "First I button the top button, then the next one." Therapists often use declarative learning when helping patients reacquire functional skills. They may teach a specific sequence to a patient who is having difficulty moving from sitting to standing: first move to the edge of the chair, lean forward "nose over toes," then stand up. Constant repetition can transform declarative into nondeclarative or procedural knowledge. In our example, when patients are first learning to stand, they may verbally describe the steps as they do them. However, with repetition, the movement of standing up becomes an automatic motor activity—that is, one that does not require conscious attention and monitoring.

The advantage of declarative learning is that it can be practiced in ways other than the one in which it was learned. For example, expert ski racers, when preparing to race down a slalom hill at 120 miles an hour, rehearse in their minds the race and how they will run it. Also, prior to getting on the ice, figure skaters preparing to perform will often mentally practice the sequences they will skate.

In therapy, when helping patients reacquire skills lost through injury, should the emphasis be on procedural (implicit) learning or declarative (explicit) learning? This is a complex issue and depends in part on the location and type of central nervous system (CNS) pathology. As discussed in more detail in Chapter 5, some types of neural pathology impair implicit learning, while others affect explicit learning. Since declarative learning requires the ability to verbally express the process to be performed, it cannot easily be used with patients who have cognitive and/or language deficits that impair their ability to recall and express knowledge. Teaching movement skills declaratively would, however, allow patients to rehearse their movements mentally, increasing the amount of practice available to them when physical conditions such as fatigue would normally limit it.

Neural circuitry underlying declarative learning includes inputs from the sensory association cortices that synthesize somatosensory, visual, and auditory sensations; medial temporal lobe areas (including parahippocampal and perirhinal cortices, the entorhinal cortex, and the dentate gyrus); the hippocampus; and the subiculum. The right hippocampus is especially important for spatial representation—that is, memory for space and context—and the left hippocampus is more important for memories of words and objects. A lesion to any one of these components would have a major impact on declarative learning and memory. However, long-term memory is stored in the association cortices, so damage to these areas does not affect early memories (Kandel et al., 2000).

Declarative or explicit learning also involves four different types of processing, including encoding, consolidation, storage, and retrieval. Encoding involves the circuitry just described and requires attention. The extent of the encoding is determined by the level of motivation, the extent of attention to the information, and the ability to associate it meaningfully with information that is already in memory. Consolidation includes the process of making the information stable for long-term memory storage, and involves structural changes in neurons. Storage involves the long-term retention of memories and has a vast capacity compared to the limited capacity of short-term or working memory. Retrieval involves the recall of information from different long-term storage sites. It is subject to distortion, since an individual reconstructs the memories from a combination of different sites. Interestingly, it is most accurate when retrieved in the same context in which it was created (Kandel et al., 2000).

One last type of memory that is critical for the encoding and recall of long-term memory is working, or short-term, memory. This memory system consists of an attentional control system, also known as the central executive (located in the prefrontal cortex), and two rehearsal systems, the articulatory loop for rehearsing language and the visuospatial sketch pad for vision and action (located in different parts of the posterior parietal or visual association cortex).

This information suggests that teaching movement skills can be optimized when the patient is highly motivated, attending fully to the task, and able to relate or integrate the new information to information they already know about the task. When retraining gait, it would thus be important to find a goal that is important to the patient, such as being able to walk to the mailbox for the newspaper, work with them in an environment in which they can attend fully to the task instructions and their own performance outcome, and relate instructions for improved gait characteristics to previous knowledge so that they can remember them after the therapy session is over.

THEORIES OF MOTOR LEARNING

Just as there are theories of motor control, there are theories of motor learning, that is, a group of abstract ideas about the nature and control of the acquisition or modification of movement. Theories of motor learning, like theories of motor control, must be based on current knowledge regarding the structure and function of the nervous system. The following sections review theories of motor learning; also included is a brief discussion of several theories related to recovery of function, the reacquisition of skills lost through injury. Motor learning theories and the accompanying research that tests associated hypotheses related to learning are part of the foundation for evidence-based practice. Evidence-based practice (discussed in more detail in Chapter 6) is an approach to clinical practice that integrates the best available research with individual clinical expertise and client characteristics (Sackett et al., 1996; Jette et al., 2003). Arguments were made at a National Center for Medical Rehabilitation Research workshop that although learning is central to medical rehabilitation, many therapists use learning principles that are intuitive or the result of their personal clinical experience, rather than principles derived from research evidence. This may be partly the result of classical motor learning research having used simple laboratory tasks that are not related to more complex activities of daily living (ADLs) (McNevin et al., 2000; Fuhrer & Keith, 1998).

Schmidt's Schema Theory

In the early 1970s the main theory of motor learning was based on the concept of closed-loop processes in motor control. In a **closed-loop** process, sensory feedback is used for the ongoing production of skilled movement. This theory hypothesized that, in motor learning, sensory feedback from the ongoing movement is compared within the nervous system with the stored memory of the intended movement (Adams, 1971; Ivry, 1997). The closed-loop theory of motor learning also hypothesized that two distinct types of memory were important in this process. The first, called the **memory trace** was used in the selection and initiation of the movement. The second, which Adams (1971) called a **perceptual trace**, was then built up over a period of practice and became the internal reference of correctness. He proposed that, after movement is initiated by the memory trace, the perceptual trace takes over to carry out the movement and detect error.

The closed-loop theory of motor learning had been criticized for several reasons, including the fact that it could not explain either the accurate performance of novel movements or of open-loop movements, made in the absence of sensory feedback.

In the 1970s, in response to many of the limitations of the closed-loop theory of motor learning, Richard Schmidt, another researcher from the field of physical education, proposed a new motor learning theory, which he called the "schema theory." It emphasized open-loop control processes and the generalized motor program concept (Schmidt, 1975). Although the concept of motor programs was considered essential to understanding motor control, no one had yet addressed the question of how motor programs can be learned. As had other researchers before him, Schmidt proposed that motor programs do not contain the specifics of movements, but instead contain generalized rules for a specific class of movements. He predicted that when learning a new motor program, the individual learns a generalized set of rules that can be applied to a variety of contexts.

At the heart of this motor learning theory is the concept of schema, which has been important in psychology for many years. The term **schema** originally referred to an abstract representation stored in memory following multiple presentations of a class of objects. For example, after seeing many different types of dogs, it is proposed that we begin to store an abstract set of rules for general *dog* qualities in our brain, so that whenever we see a new dog, no matter what size, color, or shape, we can identify it as a dog. The schema theory of motor learning is equivalent to the motor programming theory of motor control. At the heart of both theories is the generalized motor program. The **generalized motor program** is considered to contain the rules for creating the spatial and temporal patterns of muscle activity needed to carry out a given movement (Schmidt & Lee, 2005).

Schmidt proposed that, after an individual makes a movement, four things are available for brief storage in short-term memory: (a) the initial movement conditions, such as the position of the body and the weight of the object manipulated; (b) the parameters used in the generalized motor program; (c) the outcome of the movement, in terms of **knowledge of results** (KR); and (d) the sensory consequences of the movement—that is, how it felt, looked, and sounded. This information is stored in short-term memory only long enough to be abstracted into two schemas, the recall schema (motor) and a recognition schema (sensory).

The **recall schema** is used to select a specific response. Schmidt and Lee (2005) suggest that it may be created in the following way. Each time a person makes a movement with a particular goal in mind, he or she uses a particular movement parameter, such as a given force, and then receives input about the movement's accuracy. After making repeated movements using different parameters causing different outcomes, the nervous system creates a relationship between the size of the parameter and the movement outcome. Each new movement adds a new data point to the internal system to refine the rule. After each movement, the sources of information are not retained in the recall schema, but only the rule that was created.

When making a given movement, the initial conditions and desired goal of the movement are inputs to the recall schema. The initial conditions (e.g., lifting a heavy vs. a light object) may alter, for example, the slope of the line, representing the rule.

The **recognition schema** is used to evaluate the response. In this case the sensory consequences and outcomes of previous similar movements are coupled with the current initial conditions to create a representation of the expected sensory consequences. This is then compared to the sensory information from the ongoing movement in order to evaluate the efficiency of the response. When a person makes a movement, he or she selects the outcome wanted and chooses the initial conditions. With the recognition schema rule, the person can determine the expected sensory consequences, which help with movement evaluation. These sensory consequences are similar to Adams's perceptual trace (Schmidt & Lee, 2005). When the movement is over, any error information is fed back into the schema and the schema is modified as a result of the sensory feedback and KR. Thus, according to this theory, learning consists of the ongoing process of updating the recognition and recall schemas with each movement that is made.

One of the predictions of schema theory is that variability of practice should improve motor learning. Schmidt hypothesized that learning was affected not only by the extent of practice but by the variability of practice. Thus, with increased variability of practice, the generalized motor program rules were made stronger. A second prediction is that a particular movement may be produced accurately, even if it has never been made before, if it is based on a rule that has previously been created as part of an earlier movement practice.

Clinical Implications

What are some of the clinical implications of schema theory? According to schema theory, when our patient Mrs. Jean J is learning a new movement task such as reaching for a glass of milk with her affected limb, optimal learning will occur if this task is practiced under many different conditions. This will allow her to develop a set of rules for reaching (recall schema), which then could be applied when reaching for a variety of glasses and cups. As she practices reaching and lifting, sensory information about the initial conditions and consequences of her reaches will be used to form a recognition schema, which will be used to evaluate the accuracy of future reaches. As rules for reaching improve, Mrs. J. will become more capable of generating appropriate reaching strategies for picking up an unfamiliar glass, with less likelihood of dropping the glass or spilling the drink. Practicing reaching under many different conditions is essential then to forming accurate recall and recognition schemas.

Limitations

Is schema theory supported by research? Yes and no. As mentioned above, one of the predictions of schema theory is that when practicing a skill, variable forms of practice will produce the most effective schema or motor program. Research to test this prediction has used the following paradigms. Two groups of subjects are trained in a new task, one given constant practice conditions and the other given variable practice conditions. Both groups are then tested on a new but similar movement. According to schema theory, the second group should show higher-level performance than the first, because they have developed a broad set of rules about the task, which should allow them to apply the rules to a new situation. On the other hand, the first group should have developed a very narrow schema with limited rules that would not be easily applicable to new situations.

In studies on normal adults, the support is mixed. Many studies show large effects of variable practice, while some studies show very small effects or no effect at all. However, with regard to studies in children, there has been strong support. For example, 7- and 9-year-old children were trained to toss beanbags over variable distances or a fixed distance. When asked to throw at a new distance, the variable practice group produced significantly better scores than the fixed practice group (Kerr & Booth, 1977). Why might there be differences between children and adults in these experiments? It has been suggested that it may be difficult to find experimental tasks for which adults do not already have significant variable practice during normal activities, while children, with much less experience, are more naive subjects (Shapiro & Schmidt, 1982). Therefore, the experiments may be more valid in children.

Another limitation of the theory is that it lacks specificity. It does not predict how the generalized motor program or the other schemata are created—i.e., how a person makes his or her first movement before any schema exists. In addition, because of its generalized nature, there are few recognizable mechanisms that can be tested. Thus, it is not clear how schema processing itself interacts with other systems during motor learning and how it aids in the control of that movement.

Another challenge to the schema theory has been its inability to account for the immediate acquisition of new types of coordination. For example, researchers have shown that if all of a centipede's limbs except for two pairs are removed, the centipede will immediately produce a quadrupedal gait (Kugler et al., 1980). It has been argued that findings such as these cannot be accounted for by schema theory (Newell, 1991).

Ecological Theory

Karl Newell drew heavily from both systems and ecological motor control theories to create a theory of motor learning based on the concept of search strategies (Newell, 1991). In the previous learning theories proposed by Adams (1971) and Schmidt (1975), practice produced a cumulative continuous change in behavior due to a gradual buildup of the strength of motor programs. It was proposed that, with practice, a more appropriate representation of action is developed.

In contrast, Newell suggests that motor learning is a process that increases the coordination between perception and action in a way that is consistent with the task and environmental constraints. What does he mean by this? He proposes that, during practice, there is a search for optimal strategies to solve the task, given the task constraints. Part of the search for optimal strategies involves not merely finding the appropriate motor response for the task, but finding the most appropriate perceptual cues as well. Thus, both perception and action systems are incorporated or mapped into an optimal task solution.

Critical to the search for optimal strategies is the exploration of the *perceptual/motor workspace*. Exploring the perceptual workspace involves exploring all the possible perceptual cues in order to identify those that are most relevant to the performance of a specific task. Perceptual cues that are critical to the way in which a task is executed are also called "regulatory cues" (Gentile, 1972). Likewise, exploring the motor workspace involves exploring the range of movements possible in order to select the optimal or most efficient movements for the task. Optimal solutions then incorporate the relevant perceptual cues and optimal movement strategies for a specific task. Newell believes that one useful outcome of his theory will be the impetus to identify critical perceptual variables essential to optimal task-relevant solutions. These critical variables will be useful in designing search strategies that produce efficient mapping of perceptual information and movement parameters.

According to the ecological theory, perceptual information has a number of roles in motor learning. In a prescriptive role, perceptual information relates to understanding the goal of the task and the movements to be learned. This information has typically been given to learners through demonstrations.

Another role of perceptual information is as feedback, both during the movement (concurrent feedback, sometimes called "knowledge of performance") and on completion of the movement (**knowledge of results**). Finally, it is proposed that perceptual information can be used to structure the search for a perceptual/motor solution that is appropriate for the demands of the task. Thus, in this approach, motor learning is characterized by optimal task-relevant mapping of perception and action, not by a rule-based representation of action.

Newell discusses ways to augment skill learning. The first is to help the learner understand the nature of the perceptual/motor workspace. The second is to understand the natural search strategies used by performers in exploring space. The third is that of providing augmented information to facilitate the search. One central prediction of this theory is that the transfer of motor skills will be dependent on the similarity between the two tasks of the optimal perceptual/motor strategies and relatively independent of the muscles used or the objects manipulated in the task.

In summary, this new approach to motor learning emphasizes dynamic exploratory activity of the perceptual/motor workspace in order to create optimal strategies for performing a task.

Clinical Implications

What are the clinical implications of the ecological theory of motor learning? As in the schema theory, when our patient Mrs. Jean J is relearning a movement with her affected arm, such as reaching for a glass, repeated practice with reaching for a variety of glasses that contain a variety of substances within them results in learning to match the appropriate movement dynamics for the task of reaching. But in addition, the ecological theory suggests that the patient learns to distinguish the relevant perceptual cues important to organizing action. Relevant perceptual cues for reaching for and lifting a glass of milk include the size of the glass, how slippery the surface is, and how full it is. Thus, in order to relearn to reach, Mrs. J. must not only develop effective motor strategies, she must also learn to recognize relevant perceptual cues and match them to optimal motor strategies. If a perceptual cue suggests a heavy glass, she will need to grasp with more force. If the glass is full, the speed and trajectory of the movement must be modified to accommodate the situation. If Mrs. J. is unable to recognize these essential sensory cues, a motor strategy that is less than optimal will be generated. That is, she may spill the fluid within the glass or the glass may slip.

Perceptual cues such as the color of the glass, are nonregulatory cues, which are not essential to the development of optimal movement strategies for grasping. Thus, during recovery of motor skills, an important part of "motor learning" is learning to discriminate relevant from irrelevant perceptual cues. Knowledge about the critical perceptual cues associated with a task is essential in dealing with a new variation of the task. When faced with a novel variation of the task, the patient must actively explore the perceptual cues to find the information necessary to solve the task problem optimally.

Limitations

Though this theory takes into account more of the variables that need to be considered in motor learning (dealing with interactions between the individual, the task, and the environment), it is still a very new theory. One of its major limitations is that it has yet to be applied to specific examples of motor skill acquisition in any systematic way.

Theories Related to Stages of Learning Motor Skills

Another set of theories focuses on motor learning from a temporal perspective and attempts to more carefully characterize the learning process. These theories begin by describing initial stages of skill acquisition and describe how learning occurs over time.

Fitts and Posner Three-Stage Model

Fitts and Posner (1967), two researchers from the field of psychology, described a theory of motor learning related to the stages involved in learning a new skill. They suggest that there are three main phases involved in skill learning. In the first stage, the learner is concerned with understanding the nature of the task, developing strategies that could be used to carry out the task, and determining how the task should be evaluated. These efforts require a high degree of cognitive activity such as attention. Accordingly, this stage is referred to as the "cognitive stage of learning."

In this stage, the person experiments with a variety of strategies, abandoning those that do not work while keeping those that do. Performance tends to be quite variable, perhaps because many strategies for performing the task are being sampled. However, improvements in performance are also quite large in this first stage, perhaps as a result of selecting the most effective strategy for the task.

Fitts and Posner call the second stage in skill acquisition "the associative stage." By this time, the person has selected the best strategy for the task and now begins to refine the skill. Thus, there is less variability in performance during this stage, and improvement also occurs more slowly. It is proposed that verbal/cognitive aspects of learning are not as important at this stage because the person focuses more on refining a particular pattern rather than on selecting among alternative strategies (Schmidt & Lee, 2005). This stage may last from days to weeks or months, depending on the performer and the intensity of practice.

The third stage of skill acquisition has been called the "autonomous stage." Fitts and Posner define this stage by the automaticity of the skill and the low degree of attention required for its performance, as shown in Figure 2.3. Thus, the person can begin to devote his or her attention to other aspects of the skill in general, like scanning the environment for obstacles that might impede performance, or he or she may choose to focus on a secondary task (like talking to a friend while performing the task) or to save his or her energy, so as not to become fatigued.

Several research studies have supported the hypothesis that during later stages of motor learning, as a motor skill becomes more automated, it requires less attentional resources, and in fact, paying too much attention to the elements of the task may reduce performance (Beilock et al., 2002; Wulf & Weigelt, 1997). For example, Perkins-Ceccato et al. (2003) have shown that when asked to focus attention on the motor elements of a task, such as focusing on the form of the golf swing and adjusting the force for the distance they were from the target (internal focus), novices who were just learning the skill became better, as compared with using an external focus (hitting the ball as close to the target as possible). In contrast, experts in the skill actually showed the opposite effect, with performance decrements when using internal focus on the elements of the swing. In a study by Beilock et al. (2002), experienced golfers were more accurate at putting under dual-task conditions than when focusing attention on step-by-step putting performance. In addition, expert soccer players performed better at dribbling under dual-task conditions with their dominant right foot, but performed better in the skill-focused condition when using their less-skilled left foot. Novices also performed better when skill-focused, regardless of the foot they used. This suggests that execution of a high-level–skill task can actually be helped by distraction by a secondary task. Why would this happen? It is possible that focusing cognitive resources on a well-learned task that has become automated actually interferes with the automatic motor control processes.

Clinical Implications. How can the three-stage model help us to understand the acquisition of motor skills in patients? This theory suggests that Mrs. J. would learn to reach for a glass in the following way. When first learning to reach for the

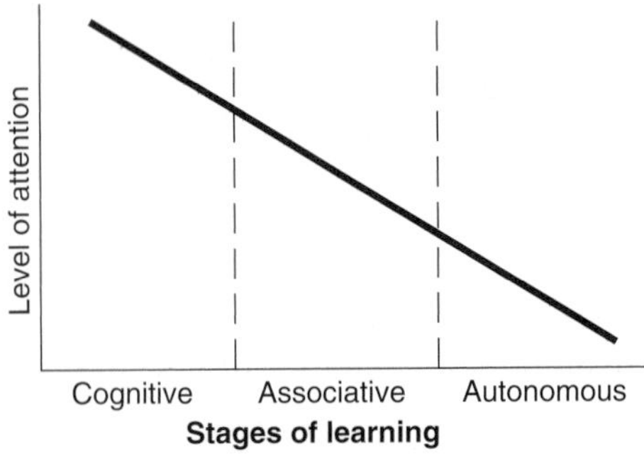

FIGURE 2.3 The changing attentional demands associated with the three stages of motor skill acquisition outlined by Fitts and Posner (1976).

glass, the task would require a great deal of attention and conscious thought. Mrs. J would initially make a lot of errors and spill a lot of water, while she experimented with different movement strategies to accomplish the task. When moving into the second stage, however, her movements toward the glass would become refined as she developed an optimal strategy. At this point, the task would not require her full attention. In the third autonomous stage, Mrs. J would be able to reach for the glass while carrying on a conversation or being engaged in other tasks.

Systems Three-Stage Model

Another theory related to stages of motor learning comes originally from work by Bernstein (1967) and was subsequently extended by researchers in the area of dynamical systems theory and motor development (Fentress, 1973; Newell & van Emmerik, 1989; Southard & Higgins, 1987). We have called this theory the "systems three-stage theory" because, like Bernstein's systems theory of motor control, the emphasis is on controlling degrees of freedom of the body segments involved in the movement as a central component of learning a new movement skill. In the first stage, there is a reduction of the number of degrees of freedom of the joints to be controlled to a minimum. This theory suggests that when a novice or an infant is first learning a new skill, the degrees of freedom of the body are constrained as they perform the task, in order to make the task easier to perform. For example, a person first learning to use a hammer may cocontract agonist and antagonist muscles at the wrist joint to stiffen this joint and primarily control hammer movement at the elbow. The learner can perform the task reasonably accurately at this stage, but the movement is not energetically efficient, and the performer is not able to deal flexibly with environmental changes. As the task is gradually mastered, the learner begins to release the degrees of freedom at the wrist and learns to coordinate the movements at the two joints, which allows for more movement efficiency, freedom, and thus, skill.

This tendency to freeze degrees of freedom during the early stages of learning a task can be seen during the development of balance control. A newly standing infant may freeze the degrees of freedom of the legs and trunk, and sway only about the ankle joints in response to threats to balance. Gradually, with experience and practice, infants may increase the degrees of freedom used, as they learn to control sway at the hip as well (Woollacott et al., 1998).

Vereijken, Newell, and colleagues (1992) have taken this approach and used it to develop a model of the stages of motor learning. They suggest that the first stage of motor learning is the **novice stage,** in which the learner simplifies the movement in order to reduce the degrees of freedom. They suggest that this is accomplished by constraining or coupling multiple joints, so they move in unison, and by fixing the angles of many of the joints involved in the movement. These constraints are made at the cost of efficiency and flexibility in response to changing task or environmental demands.

In the second stage, called the **advanced stage,** the performer begins to release additional degrees of freedom, by allowing movements at more joints involved in the task. Now the joints can be controlled independently as necessary for the task requirements. Simultaneous contraction of agonist and antagonist muscles at a joint would be reduced, and muscle synergies across a number of joints would be used to create a well-coordinated movement that is more adaptable to task and environmental demands. For example, in postural development it might be hypothesized that this would allow the infant to begin to balance using hip, knee, and ankle joints equally, as more complex balance tasks are mastered (Bernstein, 1967; Newell & Vaillancourt, 2001).

In the third stage, called the **expert stage,** the individual now has released all the degrees of freedom necessary to perform the task in the most efficient and coordinated way. Bernstein predicts that there is also an exploitation of reactive phenomena of forces of one segment that influence another segment. That is, the person uses passive forces increasingly in movement control, allowing less expenditure of active forces and more efficient use of energy, thus reducing fatigue. Thus, the individual has learned to take advantage of the mechanics of the musculoskeletal system and of the environment and to optimize the efficiency of the movement. They can exploit the mechanical and inertial properties of the limbs to increase movement characteristics such as speed and to reduce energy costs (Rose, 1997; Schmidt & Lee, 2005; Vereijken, et al., 1992).

These general hypotheses regarding stages of motor skills have been supported by a number of studies. For example, in adult skill learning, Arutyunyan et al. (1969) have shown that pistol shooters first use control at the shoulder joint in their aiming movements, but with increasing practice, the degrees of freedom of the arm to include the distal joints. In addition, Southard and Higgins (1987) found that there was a progressive release of the distal arm segments in the learning of a racquetball forehand shot. Broderick and Newell (1999) also found that the progression of skill in basketball bouncing started with movements of the shoulder and wrist and progressed to release of the previously constrained elbow joint with further training. This has also been supported in the development of leg kicking and early walking in infants, with progression from mainly proximal (hip) control with few adjustments to distal (knee and ankle) control, accompanied by increased adjustments and modulation (Jensen et al., 1995; Hallemans et al., 2007; Newell & Vaillancourt, 2001).

Interestingly, the final stage of Bernstein's motor learning model has also received supporting evidence from the motor control literature. Schneider & Zernicke (1989) found that after practicing an arm-motion task pattern, subjects were able to use active muscle forces as complementary forces to the passive interactive components of the moving limb, thus exploiting reactive forces and reducing their own need to generate tension. This was especially notable at the point of movement reversals.

The analysis of the degrees of freedom of the body segments can be applied to the level of individual joints involved in a movement (what might be called the "component level of joint space"); it can also be applied at the dynamical level of movement or the active degrees of freedom (dimension) of the attractor dynamic (Newell & Vaillancourt, 2001) that supports the control of the individual components of joint space. A dimensional analysis aims to give an index of the number of independent degrees of freedom, in terms of equations of motion, that are needed to predict the time-dependent properties of the output of the system.

Principle-component analysis has been used to estimate the number of independent dimensions required to define the spatial and temporal organization of joint-space variables (Haken 1996; Verrel et al., 2008). These dimensions might represent what has been referred to as "controlled variables" in dynamical systems theory (Latash, 1996). It has been shown that early in the learning of a motor task (a torso-and-limb coordination locomotion task called "pedalo") there were a number of principle components (i.e., independent dimensions accounting for data variance). After learning the task, the dimensionality was reduced to one.

Clinical Implications. The systems three-stage theory has a number of clinical implications. First, it suggests a possible explanation for the presence of coactivation of muscles during the early stages of acquiring a motor skill and as an ongoing strategy in patients who are unable to learn to control a limb dynamically. One explanation is that coactivation serves to stiffen a joint and therefore constrain the degrees of freedom. This strategy may in fact be a reasonable solution to the underlying problem, inability to control the degrees of freedom of a limb segment.

This theory offers a new rationale for using developmental stages in rehabilitation. Traditionally, recapitulating developmental stages in the adult patient was based on a neuromaturational rationale. Alternatively, motor development could be viewed from a biomechanical perspective as gradual release of degrees of freedom. For example, the progression from supporting oneself on all fours to upright kneeling to an independent stance can be viewed as a gradual increase in the number of degrees of freedom that must be controlled. Thus, having a patient practice maintaining an upright kneeling position before learning to control stance could be justified using this theory from a mechanical rather than a neural perspective.

Finally, this theory suggests the importance of providing external support during the early phases of learning a motor skill in patients with coordination problems. Providing external support would constrain the degrees of freedom that the patient initially has to learn to control. As coordinative abilities improve, support can be systematically withdrawn as the patient learns to control more and more degrees of freedom.

Limitations. It has been noted that little research has been focused on the autonomous or expert stage of learning, partly because it would take months or years to bring many subjects to this skill level on a laboratory task. Thus, the principles that govern motor learning processes to lead to this last stage of mastery are largely unknown (Schmidt, 1988a).

Gentile's Two-Stage Model

In contrast to the three-stage theories discussed previously, Gentile (1972, 1987) proposed a two-stage theory of motor skill acquisition that describes the goal of the learner in each stage. In the first stage, the goal of the learner is to develop an understanding of the task dynamics. At this stage, they are just getting the idea of the requirements of the movement (Gentile, 1972). This includes understanding the goal of the task, developing movement strategies appropriate to achieving the goal, and understanding the environmental features critical to the organization of the movement. An important feature of this stage of motor learning is learning to distinguish relevant, or regulatory, features of the environment from those that are nonregulatory.

In the second stage, called the "fixation/diversification stage," the goal of the learner is to refine the movement. Refining movement includes both developing the capability of *adapting* the movement to changing task and environmental demands and performing

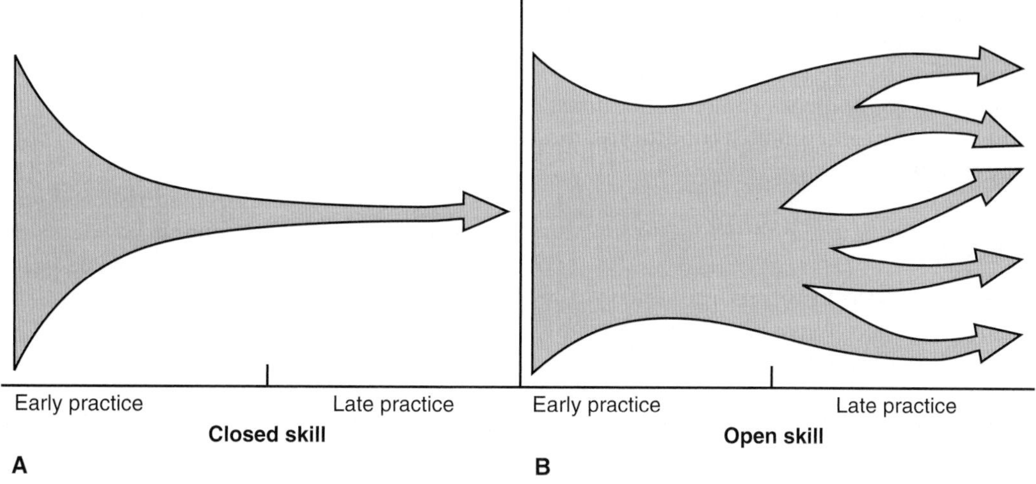

FIGURE 2.4 Schematic representation of movement patterns associated with open versus closed motor skills. Closed skills require refinement of a single or limited number of movement patterns (movement consistency); in contrast, open skills require a diversity of movement patterns (movement diversity). (Adapted from Higgens JR, Spaeth RA. Relationship between consistency of movement and environmental conditions. Quest 1979; 17:65.)

the task *consistently* and *efficiently*. The terms *fixation* and *diversification* refer to the distinct requirements of open versus closed skills. As discussed in Chapter 1, closed skills have minimal environmental variation, and thus require a consistent movement pattern with minimal variation. The concept is illustrated in Figure 2.4A, which is a representation of the movement consistency that occurs with repeated practice under unchanging conditions. Movement variability decreases with practice. In contrast, open skills are characterized by changing environmental conditions and therefore require movement diversification. This concept of movement diversification is illustrated in Figure 2.4B (Higgins & Spaeth, 1979).

Stages of Motor Program Formation

Finally, researchers have hypothesized that hierarchical changes may occur in movement control as motor programs are assembled during the learning of a new task (MacKay, 1982; Schmidt & Lee, 2005). Motor programs for controlling a complex behavior might be created by combining programs that control smaller units of the behavior, until the whole behavior is controlled as a unit. The example given by MacKay illustrates the process of learning to shift gears in a car with manual transmission. In this example, in early stages of practice each of the seven components of the skill (accelerator up, clutch down, shift lever forward, shift lever to right, shift lever forward, clutch up, accelerator down) is controlled by a separate motor program. As the learner improves his or her ability to shift, components of the behavior are grouped and controlled together, such as when we combine control of the clutch and accelerator. This is the middle practice stage. Finally, in late practice, all seven components of the gear-shifting process are controlled by a single motor program.

In our example of Mrs. J learning to move from sitting to standing, initially during early practice she may develop a motor program for each component of the movement—for example, sliding forward on the seat, shifting her feet back, leaning her trunk forward, putting her hands on the chair arms, and standing up. During middle practice she may begin to combine units of the behavior—for example, sliding forward on the seat and repositioning her feet. Finally, in late practice, all parts of the movement are combined into one program for the movement of sitting to standing.

PRACTICAL APPLICATIONS OF MOTOR LEARNING RESEARCH

Very often therapists ask themselves questions such as: What is the best way to structure my therapy sessions in order to optimize learning? How often should my patient practice a particular task? Is the type of feedback that I am giving to my patients concerning the quality of their movements really effective? Could I give a different form of feedback that might be better? Should I give feedback with every trial that the patient makes, or would it be better to withhold feedback occasionally and make the patients try to discern for themselves whether their movement is accurate or efficient? What is the best timing for feedback? In this section, we discuss research in motor learning that has attempted to answer these questions. We review the research in relation to the different motor learning factors that are important to consider when retraining patients with motor control problems, including practice frequency, feedback, practice conditions, and variability of practice.

Practice Levels

The most important factor in retraining motor skills is the amount of practice. According to research by Fitts (1964), Newell & Rosenbloom (1981), and others, practice on many different tasks, using widely different performance measures showed the same result: a logarithmic law of practice, described by Schmidt and Lee (2005) as the power law of practice. The logarithmic relationship shows that the rate of improvement during any part of practice is linearly related (on a log scale) to the amount left to improve. This means that early in practice of a new task, performance improves rapidly, while after much practice, it improves more slowly. It also shows that performance may improve for many years, although increments may be small. One application of this law has been as an explanation of the efficacy of constraint-induced therapy. It is possible that one reason for the substantial improvement in motor skills for patients undergoing this intensive training (about 6 hours a day for 2 weeks) is simply the massive numbers of practice trials they have performed (Schmidt & Lee, 2005).

Feedback

We have already discussed the importance of feedback in relation to motor learning. Clearly, some form of feedback is essential for learning to take place. In this section, we describe the types of feedback that are available to the performer and the contributions of these different types of feedback to motor learning.

The broadest definition of feedback includes all the sensory information that is available as the result of a movement that a person has produced. This is typically called **response-produced feedback** (also called "movement-produced feedback"). This feedback is usually further divided into two subclasses, intrinsic (or inherent) feedback and extrinsic (or augmented) feedback (Schmidt & Lee, 2005; Shea et al., 1993).

Intrinsic Feedback

Intrinsic (or **inherent**) **feedback** is feedback that comes to the individual simply through the various sensory systems as a result of the normal production of the movement. This includes such things as visual information concerning whether a movement was accurate, as well as somatosensory information concerning the position of the limbs as one was moving (Schmidt & Lee, 2005).

Extrinsic Feedback

Extrinsic (or **augmented**) **feedback** is information that supplements intrinsic feedback. For example, when you tell a patient that he or she needs to lift his or her foot higher to clear an object while walking, you are offering extrinsic feedback.

Extrinsic feedback can be given *concurrently* with the task and in addition, at the end of the task, in which case it is called **terminal feedback.** An example of concurrent feedback would be verbal or manual guidance to the hand of a patient learning to reach for objects. An example of terminal feedback would be telling a patient after a first unsuccessful attempt to rise from a chair, to push harder the next time, using the arms to create more force to stand up.

Knowledge of Results

Knowledge of results (KR) is one important form of extrinsic feedback. It has been defined as terminal feedback about the outcome of the movement, in terms of the movement's goal (Schmidt & Lee, 2005; Shea et al., 1993). This is in contrast to **knowledge of performance** (KP), which is feedback relating to the movement pattern used to achieve the goal.

Research has been performed to determine the types of feedback that are the best to give a subject. Almost all of the research that has been performed involves examining the efficacy of different types of knowledge of results. Typically, research has shown that knowledge of results is an important learning variable; that is, it is important for learning motor tasks (Bilodeau et al., 1959). However, there are certain types of tasks for which intrinsic feedback (e.g., visual or kinesthetic) is sufficient to provide most error information, and KR has only minimal effects. For example, in learning tracking tasks, KR only minimally improves the performance and learning of a subject.

It has also been shown that KR is a performance variable; that is, it has temporary effects on the ability of the subject to perform a task. This may be due to motivational or alerting effects on the performer, as well as guidance effects (i.e., it tells the subject how to perform the task better in the next trial).

When should KR be given for optimal results? Should it be given right after a movement? What delay is best before the next movement is made, to ensure maximum learning efficiency? Should KR be given after every movement? These are important questions for the therapist who wants to optimize the learning or relearning of motor skills in patients with motor disorders.

Experiments attempting to determine the optimal KR delay interval have found very little effect of KR delay on motor learning efficacy. The same is true of the post-KR delay interval. There may be a slight reduction in learning if the KR delay is very short, but any effects are very small. However, it has been shown that it is good not to fill the KR delay interval with other movements, since these appear to interfere with the learning of the target movements. Research on the effects of filling the post-KR delay interval with extraneous activities is less clear. Apparently, this interval is not as important as the KR delay interval for the integration of KR information. It has also been recommended that the *intertrial interval* should not be excessively short, but the literature in this area shows conflicting results (Salmoni et al., 1984) concerning the effects of different lengths of intertrial intervals on learning.

What happens to learning efficacy if KR is not given for every trial? For example, if you ask a patient to practice a reaching movement and give the patient feedback only on the accuracy of the movement every 5 or 10 trials, what do you think might happen? One might assume that decreasing the amount of KR given would have a detrimental effect on learning. However, experiments in this area have shown surprising results.

In one study Winstein and Schmidt (1990) manipulated KR to produce what they called a "fading schedule," giving more KR early in practice (50% frequency) and gradually reducing it later in practice. They compared the performance of this group to one given a 100% frequency feedback condition (feedback on every trial). No difference in performance was found during acquisition, but the 50% fading frequency condition gave better scores on a delayed-retention test. Why would this be the case? They propose that on no-KR trials, the subject needs to use other cognitive processes, such as those related to error detection. In addition, when KR is given in 100% of trials, this produces dependency on the KR (Shea et al., 1993; Winstein & Schmidt, 1990).

In another set of studies, Lavery (1962) compared the performance of: (a) subjects who had KR feedback on every trial; (b) subjects who had **summary KR,** that is, KR for each of the trials only at the end of an entire block of 20 trials; and (c) subjects who had both types of feedback. It was found that at the end of the acquisition trials, performance was best if KR was given after every trial (groups 1 and 3 had far better performance than group 2). However, when performance was then compared for the groups on transfer tests, for which no KR was given at any time, the group that was originally the least accurate, the summary-KR-only group (group 2), was now the most accurate (Lavery, 1962).

These results suggest that summary KR is the best feedback; but if this were so, group 3 should have been as good as group 2, and this was not the case. It has thus been concluded that immediate KR is detrimental to learning, because it provides too much information and allows the subject to rely on the information too strongly (Schmidt & Lee, 2005).

What is the best number of trials to complete before giving KR? This appears to vary depending on the task. For very simple movement timing tasks, in which KR was given after 1 trial, 5 trials, 10 trials, or 15 trials, the performance on acquisition trials was best for the most frequent feedback, but when a transfer test was given, the performance was best for the 15-trial summary group. In a more complex task, for which a pattern of moving lights had to be intercepted by an arm movement (like intercepting a ball with a bat), the most effective summary length for learning was 5 trials, and anything more or less was less efficient (Schmidt et al., 1989; Schmidt & Lee, 2005).

How precise must KR be in order to be most effective? The answer varies for adults versus children. For adults, quantitative KR appears to be best, with the more precise KR giving more accurate performance, up to a point, beyond which there is no further improvement. For adults, units of measure (e.g., inches, centimeters, feet, and miles) do not seem to be important, with even nonsense units being effective. However, in children, unfamiliar units or very precise KR can be confusing and reduce learning (Newell & Kennedy, 1978; Schmidt & Lee, 2005).

Practice Conditions

We have already discussed the importance of KR to learning. A second variable that is also very important is practice. Typically, the more practice you can give a patient, the more the patient learns, with other things being equal. Thus, in creating a therapy session, the number of practice attempts should be maximized. But what about fatigue? How should the therapist schedule practice periods versus rest periods? Research to answer these questions is summarized in the following sections.

Massed versus Distributed Practice

To answer the questions above, researchers have performed experiments comparing two types of practice sessions: massed and distributed. **Massed practice** is defined as a session in which the amount of practice time in a trial is greater than the amount of rest between trials. This may lead to fatigue in some tasks. **Distributed practice** is defined as a session in which the amount of rest between trials is equal to or greater than the amount of time for a trial. For continuous tasks, massed practice has been proven to decrease performance markedly while it is present, but it affects learning only slightly when learning is measured on a transfer task in distributed conditions. In this case fatigue may mask the original learning effects during massed practice, but they become apparent on the transfer tasks. For discrete tasks, the research results are not as clear, and they appear to depend considerably on the task (Schmidt & Lee, 2005).

Keep in mind that in the therapy setting a risk of injury due to fatigue will increase during massed practice for tasks that may be somewhat dangerous for the patient, such as tasks in which a fall could result. In this case, it is best not to overly fatigue the patient and risk injury.

Constant versus Variable Practice

The ability to generalize learning to novel situations is considered a very important variable in motor learning. In general, research has shown that variable practice increases this ability to adapt and generalize learning. For example, in one experiment one group of subjects practiced a timing task (they had to press a button when a moving pattern of lights arrived at a particular point) at variable speeds of 5, 7, 9, and 11 miles per hour, while a second group (constant practice) practiced at only one of those speeds. Then, all subjects performed a transfer test, in which they performed at a speed outside their previous range of experience. The absolute errors were smaller for the variable than for the constant practice group (Catalano & Kleiner, 1984; Schmidt & Lee, 2005). Thus, in this example, variable practice allowed a person to perform significantly better on novel variations of the task. Using variable practice may be most essential when learning tasks that are likely to be performed in variable conditions. Tasks that require minimal variation and will be performed in constant conditions may best be practiced in constant conditions (Rose, 1997).

Random versus Blocked Practice: Contextual Interference

Surprisingly, it has also been found that factors that make performing a task more difficult initially very often make learning more effective in the long run. These types of factors have been called "context effects." For example, if you were to ask a person to practice five different tasks in random order, versus blocking the trials (i.e., practicing one task for a block of trials then moving on to the next task), you might presume that it would be easier to learn each task in a blocked design. However, this is not the case. Although performance is better during the acquisition phase when trials are in a blocked design, when tested on a transfer task, performance is actually better in the randomly ordered conditions. Thus, contextual interference occurs when multiple skills are practiced within a single session.

Is it always the case that random practice is better than blocked practice? It appears that a number of factors related to both the task and the learner must be considered when deciding whether to use random versus blocked practice (Magill & Hall, 1990). Random practice appears to be most effective when used with skills that use different patterns of coordination, and thus different underlying motor programs (Magill & Hall, 1990). In addition, characteristics of the individual, such as level of experience and intellectual abilities, may also influence the effectiveness of random practice (Rose, 1997). Researchers have found that random practice may be inappropriate until learners understand the dynamics of the task being learned (Del Rey et al., 1983; Goode, 1986). In addition, research by Edwards et al. (1986) on motor learning in adolescents with Down syndrome suggest that random practice was not superior to blocked practice in this group of learners. To understand the clinical applications of contextual interference complete Lab Activity 2-1.

You can repeat this lab activity exploring how the structure of a therapy session would vary if you were using constant versus variable practice, guided versus discovery learning, or knowledge of results versus knowledge of performance.

Whole versus Part Training

One approach to retraining function is to break the task down into interim steps, helping the patient to master each step prior to learning the entire task. This has been called "task analysis," and it is defined as the process of identifying the components of a skill or movement and then ordering them into a sequence. How are the components of a task defined? They are defined in relation to the goals of the task. So, for example, a task analysis approach to retraining mobility would be to break down the locomotor pattern into naturally occurring components such as step initiation, stability during stance, and push-off to achieve progression. During mobility retraining, the patient

LAB ACTIVITY 2-1

Objective: To understand the clinical applications of contextual interference.

Procedure: Your patient is John C., a 33-year-old with degenerative spinocerebellar ataxia. He requires minimal assistance in most of his activities of daily living (ADL) because of dysmetria and dyscoordination. Today's therapy session is focusing on training transfers (bed to wheelchair and wheelchair to toilet) and bed mobility skills (supine to prone [rolling], and supine to sitting on edge of bed, and sitting to standing).

Assignment

Your job is to plan a therapy session showing how your therapy strategies would vary if you were considering context effects on recovery of function.

1. Outline a therapy session to teach these skills based on a random practice schedule.
2. How would your therapy session differ if you were focusing on training using a blocked practice schedule?
3. What will the effects of each approach to practice have on the initial acquisition of skills, and what effect will each approach have on long-term retention and transfer to novel conditions?

would practice each of these components in isolation, before combining them into the whole gait pattern. But each of these components must be practiced within the overall context of gait. For example, having a patient practice hip extension while prone will not necessarily increase the patient's ability to achieve the goal of stance stability, even though both require hip extension. Thus, part-task training can be an effective way to retrain some tasks, if the task itself can be naturally divided into units that reflect the inherent goals of the task (Schmidt, 1991; Winstein, 1991).

Transfer

A critical issue in rehabilitation is how training transfers, either to a new task or to a new environment. For example, will learning a task in a clinical environment transfer to a home environment? Or does practice in standing balance transfer to a dynamic balance task such as walking around the house? What determines how well a task learned in one condition will transfer to another? Researchers have determined that the amount of transfer depends on the similarity between the two tasks or the two environments (Lee, 1988; Schmidt et al., 1989). A critical aspect in both appears to be whether the neural processing demands in the two situations are similar. For example, training a patient to maintain standing balance in a well-controlled environment, such as on a firm, flat surface in a well-lit clinic, will not necessarily enable the patient to balance in a home environment that contains thick carpets, uneven surfaces, and visual distractions. The more closely the processing demands in the practice environment resemble those in the actual environment, the better the transfer will be (Schmidt & Lee, 2005; Winstein, 1991).

Mental Practice

It has been shown that mentally practicing a skill (the act of performing the skill in one's imagination, with no action involved) can produce large positive effects on the performance of the task. For example, Hird et al. (1991) taught subjects in different groups a pegboard task, putting pegs of different colors and shapes into holes in the pegboard, or a pursuit rotor task, in which the subject was asked to follow a target moving in a circular pattern. Groups were given seven sessions of training using different combinations of physical and mental practice, with a control group getting practice on a totally separate task (a stabilometer task). Results showed that the group given 100% mental practice was more effective at the task than the control group, but not nearly as effective as the group given the same amount of physical practice (100%). The groups given different combinations of mental and physical practice showed learning that was proportional to the time spent in physical practice. These results suggest that physical practice is definitely the best type of practice, but mental practice is an effective way to enhance learning during times when physical practice is not possible.

Why is this the case? One hypothesis is that the neural circuits underlying the motor programs for the movements are actually triggered during mental practice, and the subject either does not activate the final muscle response at all or activates responses at very low levels that do not produce movement. In Chapter 3, we discuss experiments showing that one part of the brain, the supplementary motor cortex, is activated during mental practice.

Guidance versus Discovery Learning

One technique often used in therapy is guidance; that is, the learner is physically guided through the task to be learned. Research has again explored the efficiency of this form of learning versus other forms of learning that involve trial-and-error discovery procedures. In one set of experiments (Schmidt & Lee, 2005), various forms of physical guidance were used in teaching a complex elbow-movement task. When performance was measured on a no-guidance transfer test, physical guidance was no more effective than simply practicing the task under unguided conditions. In other experiments (Singer, 1980), practice under unguided conditions was found to be less effective for acquisition of the skill, but was more effective for later retention and transfer. This is similar to the results just cited, which showed that the conditions that made the performance acquisition more difficult enhanced performance in transfer tests.

This does not mean that we should never use guidance in teaching skills, but it does imply that if guidance is used, it should be used only at the outset of teaching a task, to acquaint the performer with the characteristics of the task to be learned.

The Challenge Point Framework: A Framework for Optimizing Motor Learning

As you can see, there are many factors that need to be considered when planning a therapy program, including characteristics of the learner (patient), the task being taught, and the learning environment, including conditions of practice. The challenge point framework (CPF) is a theoretical framework for organizing the learning environment by taking into consideration characteristics of the learner, the task being learned, and the conditions of practice (Guadagnoli & Lee, 2004). According to CPF, learning is intimately related to the amount of information available to the person when learning a task. Information is viewed as a challenge to the performer. Optimal information leads to optimal learning; however, too little or too much information can slow the learning process. The optimal challenge point for learning is determined by characteristics of the learner (e.g., skill level), the difficulty of the task, and the environment (defined by the conditions of practice and feedback) (Guadagnoli & Lee, 2004).

In CPF, task difficulty is conceptualized as both nominal (i.e., constant) and functional. Nominal task difficulty reflects factors such as some of the perceptual and motor processing requirements of the task that are constant. In contrast, functional task difficulty is variable, depending on the skill level of the performer and the conditions under which a task is being performed. Thus, while every task contains a specific nominal level of difficulty, the conditions under which the task is practiced and the skill level of the performer will change the functional level of difficulty (Guadagnoli & Lee, 2004). For example, in the task of walking, *nominal* difficulty is determined by the perceptual and motor requirements of walking and is an invariant and inherent characteristic of the task. In contrast, *functional* difficulty will vary according to the skill level of the performer and the conditions of practice. In our example, functional difficulty associated with walking on a level, unobstructed surface is low for a healthy young adult but high for a person in the acute stages of recovering from a stroke. As recovery progresses and the skill level of the patient increases, the functional level of difficulty associated with walking on level ground declines. The therapist can increase the functional difficulty of the learning environment by changing the conditions of practice, taking into consideration the skill level of the learner and the difficulty of the task being learned.

In our example, in the acute recovery stage, when the skill level of the patient is low, walking may be best learned under blocked conditions (repetitive practice of walking on level ground, followed by repetitive practice of walking over obstacles, followed by repetitive practice of walking with a load) with high frequency KR (feedback after every repetition). As the patient's skill level increases, learning may be best when walking is practiced under random conditions (walking on level ground, obstacles, loads, and dual-task conditions) with low frequency KR. Using CPF, the therapist can optimize the potential for learning in each therapy session by manipulating the conditions of practice, taking into consideration the skill level of the patient, and the difficulty of the task.

Onla-or and Winstein (2008) tested the predictions of the CPF for motor learning in Parkinson's disease (PD) through the systematic manipulation of three factors: the learner's skill level (control vs. PD), conditions of practice (random vs. blocked practice order, and frequency of KR), and nominal task difficulty (low vs. high). Twenty adults with PD and 20 nondisabled controls practiced a goal-directed arm movement under low (1500 msec movement time) versus high (900 msec movement time) levels of nominal task difficulty, and under low-demand (blocked practice order with 100% KR) and high-demand (random practice order with 60% KR) practice conditions. The difference between goal and participant-generated movement (root mean square error) was used to quantify learning 1 day after practice. The results from this study partially supported the predictions made by the CPF. Under low-demand practice conditions, individuals with moderately severe PD demonstrated learning comparable to that of controls when nominal task difficulty was low, but demonstrated learning deficits when nominal task difficulty was high. Under high-nominal-demand practice conditions, individuals with PD demonstrated learning comparable to that of controls only when the context of the recall test was the same as that during practice (e.g., random retention test in the random practice conditions; or blocked practice retention test in the blocked practice conditions). In other words, they could not generalize or transfer learning to a new context, unlike the controls, suggesting that further refinements are needed to this model.

While the CPF provides a potentially useful framework to help therapists make decisions regarding how to organize the practice environment, taking into consideration both the skill level of the patient (learner) and the difficulty of the tasks being learned, further research is needed to validate this approach in patients with neurologic pathology.

RECOVERY OF FUNCTION

Motor learning is the study of the acquisition or modification of movement in normal subjects. In contrast, **recovery of function** has referred to the reacquisition of movement skills lost through injury. Understanding the effect of brain injury on motor control requires a good understanding of issues related to recovery of function.

Concepts Related to Recovery of Function

To understand concepts related to recovery of function it is necessary first to define terms such as *function* and *recovery*.

Function

Function is defined here as the complex activity of the whole organism that is directed at performing a behavioral task (Craik, 1992). Optimal function is characterized by behaviors that are efficient in accomplishing a task goal in a relevant environment.

Recovery

The term *recovery* has a number of different meanings pertaining to regaining function that has been lost after an injury. A stringent definition of recovery requires achieving the functional goal in the same way it was performed before injury; that is, using the same processes used prior to the injury (Almli & Finger, 1988). Less-stringent definitions define recovery as the ability to achieve task goals using effective and efficient means, but not necessarily those used before the injury (Slavin et al., 1988).

Recovery versus Compensation

Is recovery the same as or different from compensation? **Compensation** is defined as behavioral substitution; that is, alternative behavioral strategies are adopted to complete a task. Recovery is achieving function through original processes, while compensation is achieving function through alternative processes. Thus, function returns, but not in a form identical to that before injury.

A question of concern to many therapists is: Should therapy be directed at recovery of function or compensation? The response to this question has changed over the years as our knowledge about the plasticity and malleability of the adult CNS has changed (Gordon, 1987). For many years, the adult mammalian CNS was characterized as both rigid and unalterable. On maturation, function was believed to be localized to various parts of the CNS. Research at the time suggested that regeneration and reorganization were not possible within the adult CNS. This view of the CNS naturally led to therapy directed at compensation, since recovery, in the strict sense of the word, was not possible. More recent research in the field of neuroscience has begun to show that the adult CNS has great plasticity and retains an incredible capacity for reorganization. Studies on neural mechanisms underlying recovery of function are covered in Chapter 4.

Sparing of Function

When a function is not lost, despite a brain injury, it is referred to as a **spared function** (Craik, 1992). For example, when language develops normally in children who have suffered brain damage early in life, retained language function is said to be spared.

Stages of Recovery

Several authors have described stages of recovery from neural injury. Stages of recovery are based on the assumption that the process of recovery can be broken down into discrete stages. Classically, recovery is divided into spontaneous recovery and forced recovery. *Forced recovery* is recovery obtained through specific interventions designed to have an impact on neural mechanisms (Bach-y-Rita & Balliet, 1987).

The presumption is that different neural mechanisms underlie these relatively discrete stages of recovery. Chapter 4 describes how research on neural mechanisms might contribute new methods to improving and speeding the various stages of recovery.

Factors Affecting Recovery of Function

A number of factors can affect the outcome of damage to the nervous system as well as the extent of subsequent recovery, including both endogenous (within the individual) and exogenous (external to the individual) factors (Chapman & McKinnon, 2000). In addition, both preinjury and postinjury factors influence the extent of injury and the recovery of function. Figure 2.5 illustrates some of the factors that have an impact on recovery of function after brain injury. The following sections review the research examining some, but not all, of the effects of these factors on recovery of function.

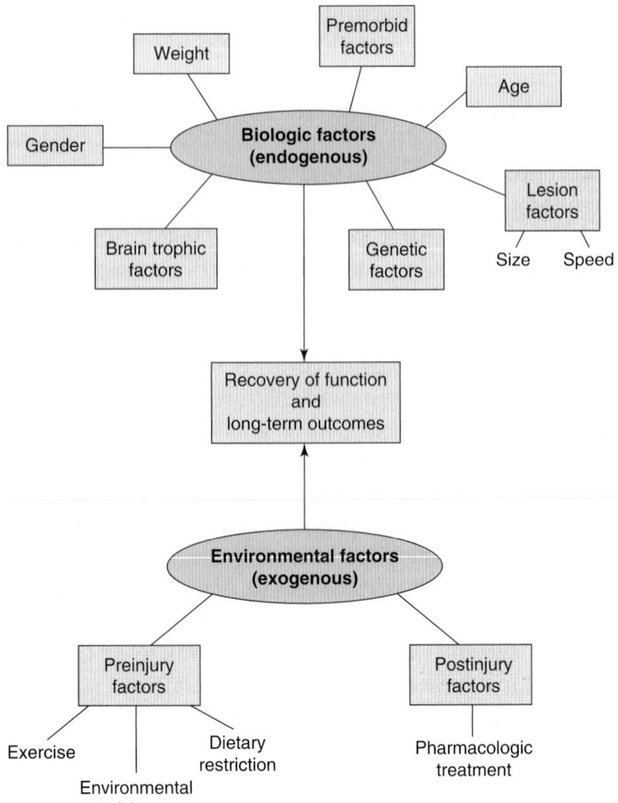

FIGURE 2.5 Factors that influence recovery of function and outcomes after CNS pathology are complex and include both endogenous (within the individual) and exogenous (external to the individual) factors occurring prior to and following injury. (Adapted from Chapman SB, McKinnon L. Discussion of developmental plasticity: factors affecting cognitive outcome after pediatric traumatic brain injury. J Commun Disord 2000;33:335.)

Effect of Age

How does age affect recovery? Does outcome vary if brain damage occurs early versus later in life? Early views on age-related effects on recovery of brain function proposed that injury during infancy caused fewer deficits than damage in the adult years. For example, in the 1940s, Kennard (1940, 1942) performed experiments in which she removed the motor cortex of infant versus adult monkeys and found that infants were able to learn to feed, climb, walk, and grasp objects, while adults were not able to recover these functions. In humans, this effect has been noted in language function, in which damage to the dominant hemisphere shows little or no effect on speech in infants but causes different degrees of aphasia in adults. However, there is research to suggest that early injury can result in reduced brain plasticity and may interfere with later emerging functions. For example, young children with injuries to the frontal areas of the cortex may appear to function normally until they reach an age at which frontal skills are more apparent (Anderson et al., 1999). Thus, the age of the individual at the time of the lesion affects recovery of function, but in a complex manner, depending on the location of the lesion and the function it subserves (Chapman & McKinnon, 2000; Held, 1987; Stein et al., 1995). If an area is mature, injury will typically cause similar damage in infants and adults. But, if another area that is functionally related is not yet mature, it may assume the function of the injured area. In addition, if an immature area is damaged and no other area assumes its function, no problems may be seen in infancy, but in later years, deficits may become apparent. In summary, what the data on age-related effects on brain injury suggest is that "the brain reacts differently to injury at different stages of development" (Stein et al., 1995, p. 77).

Characteristics of the Lesion

In addition to age, characteristics of the lesion also affect the extent of recovery from injury (Held, 1987). In general, researchers have shown a fairly strong relationship between injury severity and long-term functional outcomes; however, there is considerable variability in recovery even among individuals with severe brain injury. This suggests that the injury severity may be an indicator rather than a predictor of recovery (Chapman & McKinnon, 2000). Researchers have also found that patients with a small lesion have a greater chance of recovery, as long as a functional area has not been entirely removed. In addition, slowly developing lesions appear to cause less functional loss than lesions that happen quickly. For example, case studies have shown that a person who functioned well until near death were found on autopsy to have a large lesion in the brain tissue related to a particular function.

This phenomenon has been explored experimentally by making serial lesions in animals, with the animal being allowed to recover between lesions (Craik, 1992). If a single large lesion is made in the motor cortex (Brodmann's areas 4 and 6), animals become immobilized; in contrast, function is spared if a similar lesion is produced serially over a period of time. If serial lesions are made, the animal recovers the ability to walk, feed, and right itself with no difficulty (Travis & Woolsey, 1956). Other factors, such as the age of the animal, also influence the effect of serial lesions. In younger animals, function is spared even when serial lesions are performed close together. In contrast, older animals may not show any sparing of function, regardless of how much time has elapsed between lesions (Stein et al., 1995).

Preinjury Neuroprotective Factors

A number of preinjury factors have been shown to moderate the effect of pathology (degenerative and traumatic) on CNS function. Preinjury exercise, environmental enrichment, and dietary restriction are all examples of neuroprotective factors. Researchers have shown that preinjury exercise can protect against some of the damaging effects of aging, neurodegeneration, and brain injury. In animal studies, prestroke exercise was found to reduce infarct size, although the mechanisms underlying this finding are not clear. Neuroprotective aspects of exercise may be due to an increase in exercise-induced neuroplasticity and/or angiogenesis to support collateral blood flow. In addition, preinjury exercise may serve to decrease processes such as apoptosis, edema, and the inhibition of neurite growth-inhibiting molecules (Kleim et al., 2003).

Experiments have shown that preinjury environmental enrichment protects animals against certain deficits after brain lesions. For example, two sets of rats received lesions of the cortex, one group with preoperative enrichment and a control group. After surgery, the enriched animals made fewer mistakes during maze learning and in fact performed better than control animals without brain damage (Held, 1998).

In a second study by Held et al. (1985), the effect of preoperative and postoperative enrichment was compared for a locomotor task following removal of sensorimotor cortex. They found that preoperatively enriched rats were no different from enriched controls with sham lesions on both behavioral and fine-grained movement analyses. The group that was only postoperatively enriched was mildly impaired in locomotor skills, but recovered more quickly than the controls with lesions, although they never regained full locomotor function. Thus, postoperative enrichment is effective, but it does not allow the same extent of recovery as preoperative enrichment.

Held suggests that enriched subjects may have functional neural circuitry that is more varied than that of restricted subjects, and this could provide them with a greater ability to reorganize the nervous system after a lesion or simply to use alternative pathways to perform a task.

It appears that if environmental stimulation is to have an effect on recovery of function, it must incorporate active participation of the patient in order for full recovery to occur (Stein et al., 1995). When rats with unilateral lesions of the visual cortex were exposed to visual shapes, only the rats that were allowed to move freely in the environment and to interact with the visual cues showed good recovery of visual function. The rats that were exposed to the visual cues within their environment but were restrained from moving were very impaired (Stein et al., 1995).

Postinjury Factors

Effect of Pharmacology. Another factor that can affect recovery of function after brain injury is the use of pharmacological treatments that reduce the nervous system's reaction to injury and promote recovery of function. There are several excellent articles that review basic scientific and clinical studies on pharmacological strategies for behavioral restoration following brain damage (Feeney and Sutton, 1987; Goldstein, 1993, 2003). These studies suggest that certain drugs can have profound effects on the recovery process; however, while some drugs are beneficial to the recovery of function, others may be detrimental.

Scientists are studying the effects of a number of different types of drugs on recovery of function following brain injury, including:

1. Drugs that affect trophic factors, promoting regeneration and cell survival;
2. Drugs that replace neurotransmitters lost because of cell death;

3. Drugs that prevent the effects of toxic substances produced or released by dead or dying cells;
4. Drugs that restore blood circulation; and
5. Antioxidants, such as vitamin E, which block the effects of free radicals that destroy cell membranes (Stein et al., 1995).

Amphetamine is a well-studied drug that appears to facilitate recovery following brain injury. Amphetamine works by enhancing the effects of neurotransmitters such as adrenaline, noradrenaline, serotonin, and dopamine (Braun et al., 1986; Feeney et al., 1981, 1982; Goldstein, 2003; Hovda & Feeney, 1985; Stein et al., 1995). Several studies have shown that following stroke, treatment with amphetamines in conjunction with physical therapy produced a better outcome in motor performance on the Fugl–Meyer test than either intervention in isolation (Crisostomo et al., 1988; Walker-Batson et al., 1992).

The inhibitory neurotransmitter gamma-aminobutyric acid (GABA) also affects recovery of function—drugs that were GABA agonists impeded recovery from brain damage in the rat, while GABA antagonists were beneficial (Goldstein, 1993). Administration of cholinergic agents appears to facilitate recovery (van Woerkom et al., 1982). However, the administration of various drugs that block specific types of glutamate receptors have had mixed results (Goldstein, 1993, 2003).

There is considerable debate about the use of antioxidants such as vitamin E in both traumatic and neurodegenerative diseases such as Parkinson's disease. Considerable destruction of cell tissue that leads to the production of free radicals occurs during early stages of trauma. Free radicals are molecules of hydrogen, oxygen, and iron that have extra electrons, making them highly destructive to other living cells. Free radicals destroy the lipid membrane of a cell, allowing toxic substances to enter the cell and essential substances inside the cell to leave. Drugs such as vitamin E that block the effects of free radicals are called "antioxidants" (Stein et al., 1995). Stein and colleagues (1995) demonstrated that rats who were given vitamin E directly after frontal lobe damage were able to perform a spatial learning task as well as noninjured rats. A study by Fahn (1991) looked at the effect of vitamin E in patients in the early stages of Parkinson's disease and found that it appeared to slow the progression of the disease. Unfortunately, other studies have not been as successful in showing the beneficial effects of vitamin E on slowing the progression of Parkinson's disease.

Finally, drugs that are used to treat commonly occurring comorbidities in older patients can have a deleterious effect on recovery of function following stroke. For example, antihypertensive and sedative agents have been shown to slow recovery of motor and language functions following stroke (Goldstein, 1993, 2003; Goldstein & Davis, 1988).

In addition to drug-related factors, many factors within the individual influence the effect of drugs on brain recovery, including age, sex, health status at the time of injury, and type and extent of injury (stroke, trauma, or ischemia). For example, several researchers have shown that hormonal levels have a profound effect on both extent of damage following brain trauma and response to medication. Because of hormonal differences, the effect of a drug varies between male and female patients. Metabolic status can influence drug reactions as well. This is particularly important in light of the fact that systemic metabolism can change quickly following brain injury (Stein et al., 1995). For example, hypermetabolism can cause the breakdown of a drug too quickly, reducing its effectiveness.

Overall, results from drug studies following brain injury are very promising and suggest that pharmacologic treatment can enhance recovery of function following brain injury (Feeney & Sutton, 1987; Goldstein, 2003; Stein et al., 1995).

Neurotrophic Factors. Research on the role of neurotrophic factors and their role in brain plasticity has grown in recent years; it is a complex subject, and a complete discussion is beyond the scope of this book. Neurotrophic factors such as insulin-like growth factors may contribute to plasticity because they modulate synaptic efficacy by regulating synapse formation, neurotransmitter release, and neuronal excitability (Torres-Aleman, 1999). Other neurotrophic factors, such as brain-derived neurotrophic factor (BDNF) have been shown to have an impact on neural plasticity in animal models (Pham et al., 2002; Sherrard & Bower, 2001).

Effect of Exercise and Training. Training is a different form of exposure to enriched environments in that the activities used are specific rather than generalized (Held, 1998). Ogden and Franz (1917) performed an interesting study in which they produced hemiplegia in monkeys by making lesions in the motor cortex. They then gave four types of postoperative training: (a) no treatment, (b) general massage of the involved arm, (c) restraint of the noninvolved limb, and (d) restraint of the noninvolved limb coupled with stimulation of the involved limb to move, along with forced active movement of the animal. The last condition was the only one to show recovery, and in this condition it occurred within 3 weeks.

A study by Black et al. (1975) examined recovery from a motor cortex forelimb area lesion. They initiated training immediately after surgery or 4 months after surgery, with training lasting 6 months. They found that training of the involved hand alone, or training of the involved and normal hand together, was more effective than training the normal hand alone. When training was delayed, recovery was worse than when it was initiated immediately following the lesion.

The effect of postinjury rehabilitation training on neural plasticity and recovery of function is complex and is affected by many factors, including the location and type of injury and the timing and intensity of intervention. It is not always the case that early and intense intervention is best. In animal models of recovery of function, researchers have found that early and intense motor enrichment may promote neural plasticity in the contralesional hemisphere, but it exaggerated the effects of injury in the perilesional area. Forced motor enrichment (simulating forced-use paradigms) in the first week after injury exaggerated the extent of the cortical injury (Humm et al., 1999; Risedal et al., 1999). In contrast, a more gradual and modest increase in motor therapy facilitated neural plasticity and recovery of function in perilesional areas (Schallert et al., 2003).

Clinical Implications

By now it should be clear that the field of rehabilitation has much in common with the field of motor learning, defined as the study of the acquisition of movement. More accurately, therapists involved in treatment of the adult patient with a neurologic injury are concerned with issues related to motor relearning, or the reacquisition of movement. The pediatric patient who is born with a CNS deficit or who experiences injury early in life faces the task of acquisition of movement in the face of unknown musculoskeletal and neural constraints. In either case, the therapist is concerned with structuring therapy in ways to maximize acquisition and/or recovery of function.

Remember Mrs. Jean J from the beginning of this chapter? Mrs. J received therapy for 5 weeks following her stroke and had recovered much of her ability to function. We wanted to know more about why this happened. What is the cause of Mrs. J's recovery of motor function? How much of her recovery may be attributed to therapeutic interventions? How many of her reacquired motor skills will she be able to retain and use when she leaves the rehabilitation facility and returns home?

Mrs. J's reacquisition of function cannot be attributed to any one factor. Some of her functional return will be due to recovery, that is, regaining control of original mechanisms; some will be due to compensatory processes. In addition, age, premorbid function, site and size of the lesion, and the effect of interventions all interact to determine the degree of function regained.

Mrs. J has had excellent therapy as well. She has been involved in carefully organized therapy sessions that have contributed to her reacquisition of task-relevant behaviors. Both associative and nonassociative forms of learning may have played a role in her recovery. Habituation was used to decrease reports of dizziness associated with inner-ear problems. Trial-and-error learning (operant conditioning) was used to help her discover optimal solutions to many functional tasks. Her therapist carefully structured her environment so that optimal strategies were reinforced. For example, biofeedback was used to help her develop better foot control during locomotion.

Functionally relevant tasks were practiced under wide-ranging conditions. Under optimal conditions, this would lead to procedural learning, ensuring that Mrs. J would be able to transfer many of her newly gained skills to her home environment. Practicing tasks under varied conditions was aimed at the development of rule-governed actions or schemata. Recognizing the importance of developing optimal perceptual and motor strategies, her therapist structured the therapy sessions so that Mrs. J explored the perceptual environment. This was designed to facilitate the optimal mapping of perceptual and motor strategies for achieving functional goals. Finally, therapy was directed at helping Mrs. J repeatedly solve the sensorimotor problems inherent in various functional tasks, rather than teaching her to repeat a single solution.

SUMMARY

1. Motor learning, like motor control, emerges from a complex set of processes, including perception, cognition, and action.
2. Motor learning results from an interaction of the individual with the task and environment.
3. Forms of learning include nondeclarative or implicit learning and declarative or explicit learning. Nondeclarative learning can be divided into nonassociative learning, associative learning, and procedural learning.
4. Nonassociative learning occurs when an organism is given a single stimulus repeatedly. As a result, the nervous system learns about the characteristics of that stimulus.
5. Habituation and sensitization are two very simple forms of nonassociative learning. Habituation is a decrease in responsiveness

that occurs as a result of repeated exposure to a nonpainful stimulus. Sensitization is an increased responsiveness following a threatening or noxious stimulus.

6. In associative learning, a person learns to predict relationships, either relationships of one stimulus to another (classical conditioning) or the relationship of one's behavior to a consequence (operant conditioning).
7. Classical conditioning consists of learning to pair two stimuli. During operant conditioning we learn to associate a certain response, from among many that we have made, with a consequence.
8. *Procedural learning* refers to other nondeclarative learning tasks that can also be performed automatically without attention or conscious thought, like a habit.
9. Declarative or explicit learning results in knowledge that can be consciously recalled, and thus requires processes such as awareness, attention, and reflection.
10. Different theories of motor control include Adams's closed-loop theory of motor control, Schmidt's schema theory, the ecological theory of learning as exploration, and a number of theories on the stages of motor learning.
11. Classical recovery is divided into spontaneous recovery and forced recovery, that is, recovery obtained through specific interventions designed to have an impact on neural mechanisms.
12. Experiments show that several preinjury factors, including exercise, environmental enrichment, and nutrition, are neuroprotective; that is, they minimize the effects of neurodegenerative and traumatic brain injury.
13. Postinjury factors such as exercise and training can have a positive effect on recovery of function, but the optimal timing, frequency, and intensity of training depends on the location of injury.

ANSWERS TO LAB ACTIVITY ASSIGNMENTS

Lab Activity 2-1

1. In a random practice schedule John would practice each skill only once or twice before moving to the next skill. A random practice approach requires preplanning and a good physical setup.
2. In contrast, if you were organizing your therapy session on a blocked schedule of practice, you would practice each of the specific skills one at a time. That is, you would first have John practice wheelchair-to-bed transfers for a concentrated period of time, then switch to a different skill, wheelchair-to-toilet transfers, and practice that repeatedly before switching to the next task.
3. In the random practice schedule, if all the tasks to be practiced are not physically close to one another, too much time is wasted moving to site-specific areas for practice, which is not realistic in the amount of time available for therapy. Traditional methods for retraining motor skills by having a patient practice one skill repeatedly may initially result in the speedy acquisition of a skill, but long-term learning and the ability to transfer skills to novel conditions is limited. In contrast, encouraging the patient to practice a number of tasks in random order may slow down the initial acquisition of skills, but will be better for long-term retention (Schmidt & Lee, 2005).

CHAPTER 3

PHYSIOLOGY OF MOTOR CONTROL

LEARNING OBJECTIVES

Following completion of this chapter, the reader will be able to:

1. Discuss the differences between parallel and hierarchical processing in motor control and give examples of each.
2. Describe the anatomical connections and functional contributions to movement control for each of the major components of the brain (spinal cord, brainstem, cerebellum, basal ganglia, and each cortical area).
3. Describe the electrical properties of an action potential and a resting potential and the process of synaptic transmission.
4. Describe the components of the somatosensory system, including sensory receptors, ascending pathways, and higher-level centers that process information from this system relative to other sensory inputs.
5. Discuss elements in the dorsal versus ventral stream pathways in the visual system and explain the role of each system in visual processing.
6. Discuss the role of motor cortex, basal ganglia, and cerebellum during internally generated versus externally triggered movements.

INTRODUCTION AND OVERVIEW

Motor Control Theories and Physiology

As we mentioned in Chapter 1, theories of motor control are not simply a collection of concepts regarding the nature and cause of movement. They must take into consideration current research findings about the structure and function of the nervous system. Movement arises from the interaction of perception and action systems, with cognition affecting both systems at many different levels. Within each of these systems are many levels of processing, which are illustrated in Figure 3.1. For example, perception can be thought of as progressing through various processing stages. Each stage reflects specific brain structures that process sensory information at different levels, from initial stages of sensory processing to increasingly abstract levels of interpretation and integration in higher levels of the brain.

Some neuroscience research suggests that movement control is achieved through the cooperative effort of many brain structures that are organized both hierarchically and in parallel. This means that a signal may be processed in two ways. A signal may be processed **hierarchically**, within ascending levels of the central nervous system (CNS). In addition, the same signal may be processed simultaneously among many different brain structures, showing **parallel distributed processing.** Hierarchical processing, in conjunction with parallel distributed processing, occurs in the perception, action, and cognitive systems of movement control.

When we talk about "hierarchical" processing in this chapter, we are describing a system in which higher levels of the brain are concerned with issues of abstraction of information. For example, within the perceptual system, hierarchical processing means

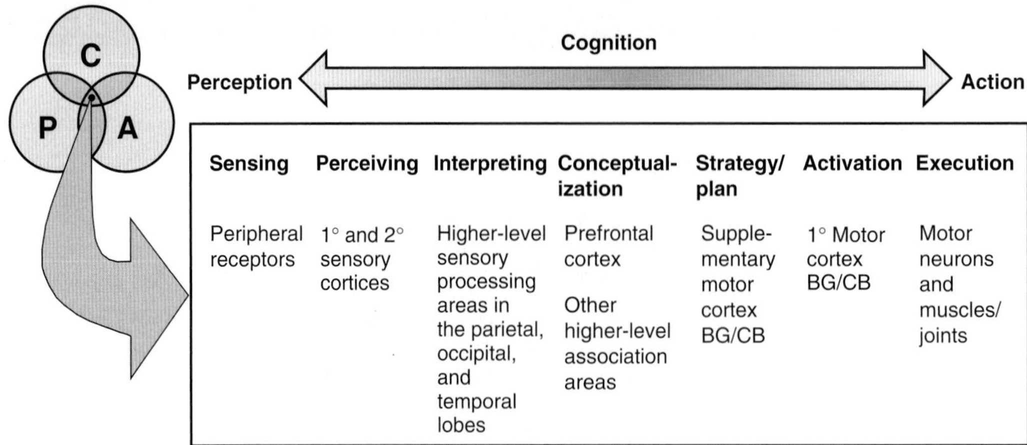

FIGURE 3.1 Model of the interaction between perceptual, action and cognitive processes involved in motor control. BG = basal ganglia; CB = cerebellum.

that higher brain centers integrate inputs from many senses and interpret incoming sensory information. On the action side of movement control, higher levels of brain function form motor plans and strategies for action. Thus, higher levels might select the specific response to accomplish a particular task. Lower levels of processing would then carry out the detailed monitoring and regulation of the response execution, making it appropriate for the context in which it is carried out. Cognitive systems overlap with perception and action systems, and involve high-level processing for both perception and action. In addition, many structures of the brain (e.g., the spinal cord, brainstem, cerebellum, and association cortex) have both perception and action components.

In parallel distributed processing, the same signal is processed simultaneously among many different brain structures, although for different purposes. For example, the cerebellum and the basal ganglia process higher-level motor information simultaneously before sending it back to the motor cortex for action.

This chapter reviews the processes underlying the production of human movement. The first section of this chapter presents an overview of the major components of the CNS and the structure and function of a neuron, the basic unit of the CNS. The remaining sections of this chapter discuss in more detail the neural anatomy (the basic circuits) and the physiology (the function) of the systems involved in the production and control of movement. The chapter follows the neural anatomy and physiology of movement control from perception into cognition and action, recognizing that it is often difficult to distinguish where one ends and others begin.

Overview of Brain Function

Brain function underlying motor control is typically divided into multiple processing levels, including the spinal cord, the brainstem (the midbrain and the hindbrain, including the medulla and pons), the cerebellum (sometimes included with the brainstem), and the forebrain, including the cerebral cortex, thalamus hypothalamus, the basal ganglia, amygdala, and hippocampus (Amaral, 2000; Patton et al., 1989).

Spinal Cord

At the lowest level of the perception/action hierarchy is the spinal cord. The circuitry of the spinal cord is involved in the initial reception and processing of somatosensory information (from the muscles, joints, and skin) and the reflex and voluntary control of posture and movement through the motor neurons. At the level of spinal cord processing, we can expect to see a fairly simple relationship between the sensory input and the motor output. At the spinal cord level, we see the organization of reflexes, the most stereotyped responses to sensory stimuli, and the basic flexion and extension patterns of the muscles involved in leg movements, such as kicking and locomotion (Amaral, 2000; Kandel, 2000b).

Sherrington (1906) called the motor neurons of the spinal cord the "final common pathway," since they are the last processing level before muscle activation occurs. Figure 3.2A shows the anatomist's view of the nervous system with the spinal cord positioned caudally. Figure 3.2B shows an abstract model of the nervous system with the spinal cord (segmental spinal networks) positioned at the bottom

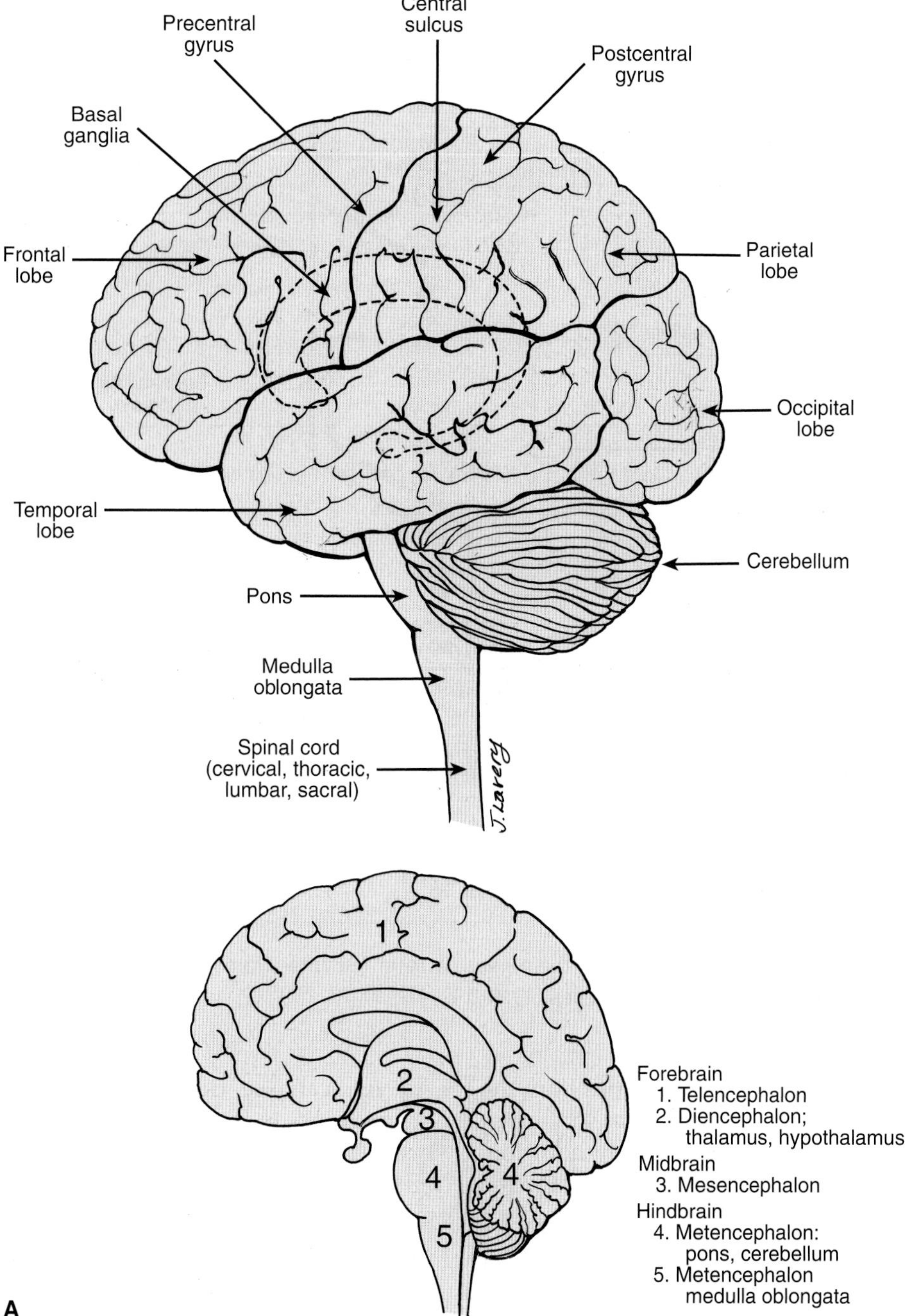

FIGURE 3.2 A, The nervous system from an anatomist's point of view. (*continued*)

of the hierarchy, with its many parallel pathways. In this view, the sensory receptors are represented by the box labeled "afferent input" and send information (represented by thin arrows) to the spinal cord (segmental spinal networks) and higher parts of the brain. After processing at many levels, including the segmental spinal networks, the output (represented by thick arrows) modulates the activity of the skeletal muscles.

Brainstem

The spinal cord extends rostrally to join the next neural processing level, the brainstem. The brainstem contains important nuclei involved in postural control and locomotion, including the vestibular nuclei, the red nucleus, and the reticular nuclei. It also contains ascending and descending pathways transmitting sensory and motor information to other parts of the CNS.

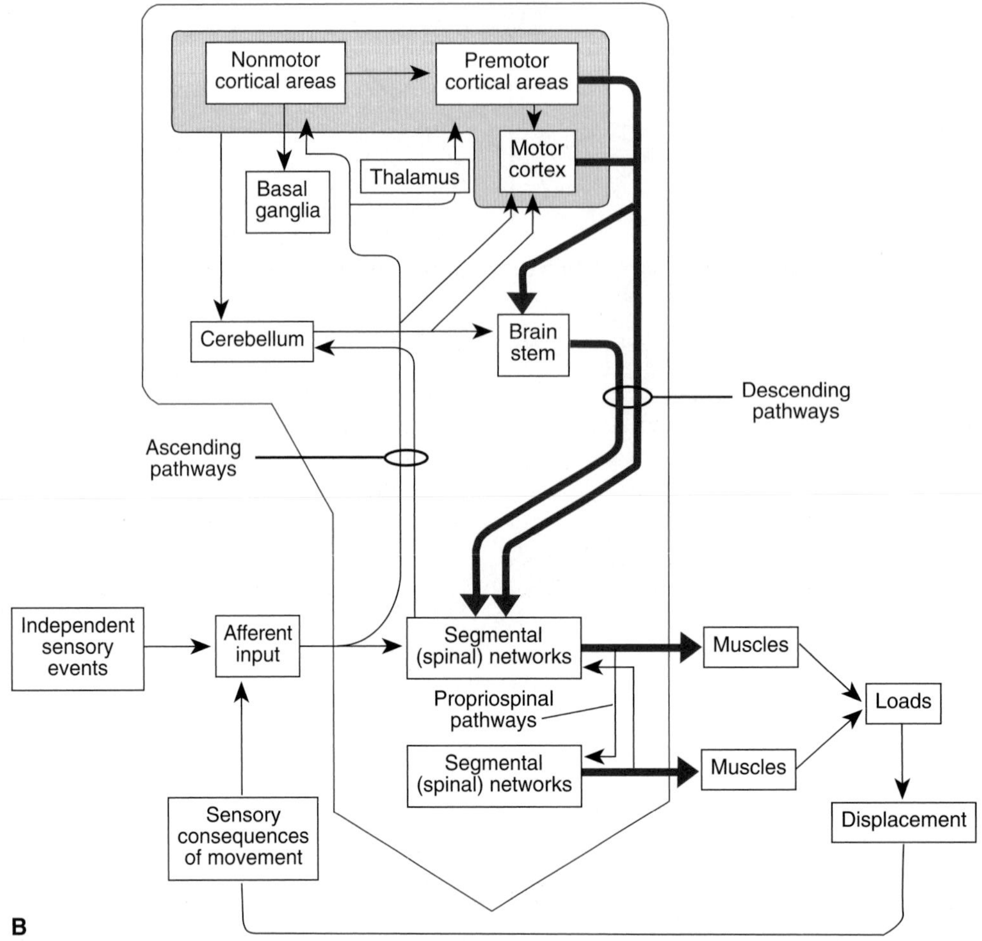

FIGURE 3.2 (*Continued*) B, An abstract model of the nervous system. (Adapted from Kandel ER, Schwartz JH, Jessell TM, eds. Principles of neuroscience, 3rd ed. New York: Elsevier, 1991:8.)

The brainstem receives somatosensory input from the skin and muscles of the head, as well as sensory input from the vestibular and visual systems. In addition, nuclei in the brainstem control the motor output to the neck, face, and eyes and are critical to the functions of hearing and taste. In fact, all the descending motor pathways except the corticospinal tract originate in the brainstem. Finally, the reticular formation, which regulates our arousal and awareness, is also found within the brainstem (Amaral, 2000).

The anatomist's view of the brainstem (Fig. 3.2A) shows divisions from caudal to rostral into the medulla, pons, and midbrain, while the abstract model (Fig. 3.2B) shows its input connections from the spinal cord and higher centers (the cerebellum and motor cortex) and its motor pathways back to the spinal cord.

Cerebellum

The cerebellum lies behind the brainstem (Fig. 3.2A) and is connected to it by tracts called "peduncles." As you can see from Figure 3.2B, the cerebellum receives inputs from the spinal cord (giving it feedback about movements) and from the cerebral cortex (giving it information on the planning of movements), and it has outputs to the brainstem. The cerebellum has many important functions in motor control. One is to adjust our motor responses by comparing the intended output with sensory signals, and then to update the movement commands if they deviate from the intended trajectory. The cerebellum also modulates the force and range of our movements and is involved in motor learning (from simple adaptation through more complex learning).

Diencephalon

As we move rostrally in the brain, we next find the diencephalon (Fig. 3.2A), which contains the thalamus and the hypothalamus. The thalamus processes most of the information coming to the cortex from the many parallel input pathways (from the spinal cord, cerebellum, and brainstem). These pathways stay segregated during the thalamic processing and during the subsequent output to the different parts of the cortex (Kandel, 2000b).

Cerebral Hemispheres (Cerebral Cortex and Basal Ganglia)

As we move higher, we find the cerebral hemispheres, which include the cerebral cortex and basal ganglia. Lying at the base of the cerebral cortex, the basal ganglia (Fig. 3.2A) receive input from most areas of the cerebral cortex and send their output back to the motor cortex via the thalamus. Some of the functions of the basal ganglia involve higher-order cognitive aspects of motor control, such as the planning of motor strategies (Kandel & Schwartz, 1991).

The cerebral cortex (Fig. 3.2A) is often considered the highest level of the motor control hierarchy. The parietal and premotor areas, along with other parts of the nervous system, are involved in identifying targets in space, choosing a course of action, and programming movements. The premotor areas send outputs mainly to the motor cortex (Fig 3.2B), which sends its commands on to the brainstem and spinal cord via the corticospinal tract and the corticobulbar system.

In light of these various subsystems involved in motor control, clearly, the nervous system is organized both hierarchically and "in parallel." Thus, the highest levels of control affect not only the next levels down, but they also can act independently on the spinal motor neurons. This combination of parallel and hierarchical control allows a certain overlap of functions, so that one system is able to take over from another when environmental or task conditions require it. This also allows a certain amount of recovery from neural injury, by the use of alternative pathways.

To better understand the function of the different levels of the nervous system, let us examine a specific action and walk through the pathways of the nervous system that contribute to its planning and execution. For example, perhaps you are thirsty and want to pour some milk from the carton in front of you into a glass. Sensory inputs come in from the periphery to tell you what is happening around you, where you are in space, and where your joints are relative to each other: they give you a map of your body in space. In addition, sensory information gives you critical information about the task you are to perform: how big the glass is and what size and how heavy the milk carton is. Higher centers in the cortex make a plan to act on this information in relation to the goal: reaching for the carton of milk.

From your sensory map, you make a movement plan (using, possibly, the parietal lobes and supplementary and premotor cortices). You are going to reach over the box of corn flakes in front of you. This plan is sent to the motor cortex, and muscle groups are specified. The plan is also sent to the cerebellum and basal ganglia, and they modify it to refine the movement. The cerebellum sends an update of the movement output plan to the motor cortex and brainstem. Descending pathways from the motor cortex and brainstem then activate spinal cord networks, spinal motor neurons activate the muscles, and you reach for the milk. If the milk carton is full, when you thought it was almost empty, spinal reflex pathways will compensate for the extra weight that you did not expect and activate more motor neurons. Then, the sensory consequences of your reach will be evaluated, and the cerebellum will update the movement—in this case, to accommodate a heavier milk carton.

Neuron—The Basic Unit of the CNS

The lowest level in the hierarchy is the single neuron in the spinal cord. How does it function? What is its structure? To explore more fully the ways that neurons communicate between the levels of the hierarchy of the nervous system, we need to review some of the simple properties of the neuron, including the resting potential, the action potential, and synaptic transmission.

Remember that the neuron, when it is at rest, always has a negative electrical charge or potential on the inside of the cell, with respect to the outside. Thus, when physiologists record from a neuron intracellularly with an electrode, they discover that the inside of the cell has a **resting potential** of about –70 mV with respect to the outside (Fig. 3.3). This electrical potential is caused by an unequal concentration of chemical ions on the inside versus the outside of the cell. Thus, K^+ ions are high on the inside of the cell and Na^+ ions are high on the outside of the cell, and an electrical pump within the cell membrane keeps the ions in their appropriate concentrations. When the neuron is at rest, K^+ channels are open and keep the neuron at this negative potential (Kandel, 1976; Koester & Siegelbaum, 2000; Patton et al., 1989).

When a neuron is excited, one sees a series of dramatic jumps in voltage across the cell membrane. These are the **action potentials**, nerve impulses, or spikes. They do not go to zero voltage, but to +30 mV (as shown in Fig. 3.3). That is, the inside of the neuron becomes positive. Action potentials are also about 1 msec in duration, and the membrane is quickly repolarized. The height of the action potential is always about the same: –70 to +30 mV = ~100 mV.

How does the neuron communicate this information to the next cell in line? It does this through the

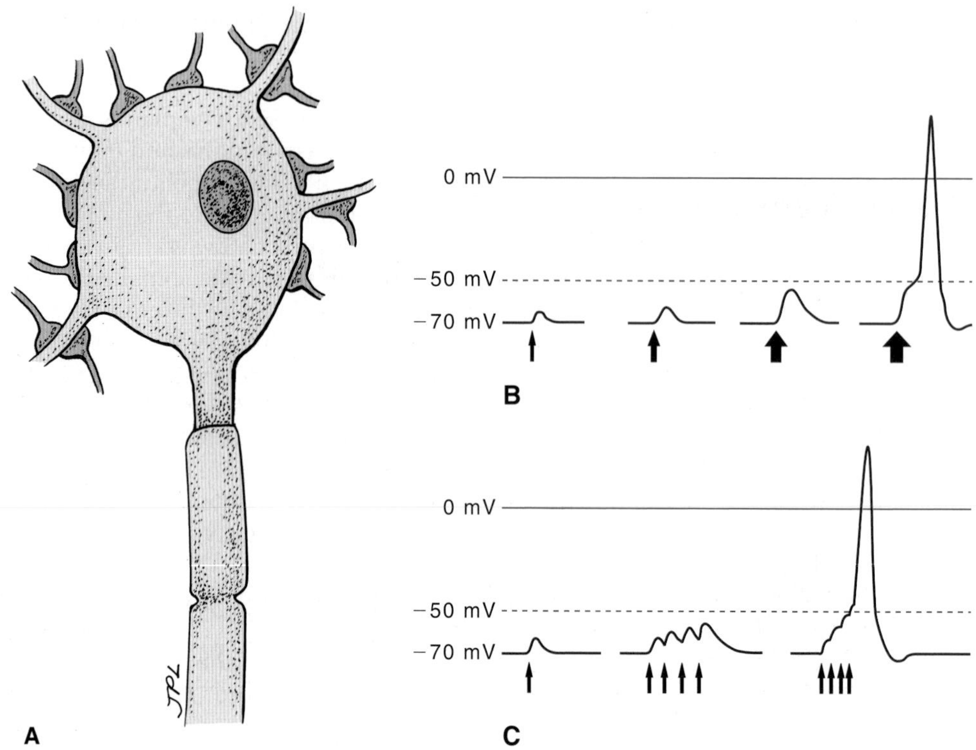

FIGURE 3.3 A, A neuron with many synaptic connections on the cell body and dendrites. B, Example of spatial summation, in which progressively larger numbers of presynaptic neurons are activated simultaneously (represented by progressively larger arrows) until sufficient transmitter is released to activate an action potential in the postsynaptic cell. C, Example of temporal summation, in which a single presynaptic neuron is activated once, four times at a low frequency, or four times at a high frequency (arrows indicate timing of presynaptic potentials). Note that with a high-frequency stimulus the postsynaptic potential does not decay back to resting levels, but each successive potential sums toward threshold, to activate an action potential.

process of **synaptic transmission.** A cleft 200 Å wide separates neurons. Each action potential in a neuron releases a small amount of transmitter substance. It diffuses across the cleft and attaches to receptors on the next cell, which open up channels in the membrane and depolarize the cell. One action potential makes only a small depolarization, called an **excitatory postsynaptic potential** (EPSP). The EPSP normally dies away after 3 to 4 msec, and as a result, the next cell is not activated (Patton et al., 1989).

But if the first cell fires enough action potentials, there is a series of EPSPs, and they continue to build up depolarization to the threshold voltage for the action potential in the next neuron. This is called **summation.** There are two kinds of summation, temporal and spatial, and these are illustrated in Figure 3.3, B and C. **Temporal summation** results in depolarization because of synaptic potentials that occur close together in time (Fig. 3.3C). **Spatial summation** produces depolarization because of the action of multiple cells synapsing on the postsynaptic neuron (Fig. 3.3B). Spatial summation is really an example of parallel distributed processing, since multiple pathways are affecting the same neuron (Kandel & Siegelbaum, 2000).

The effectiveness of a given synapse changes with experience. For example, if a given neuron is activated over a short period of time, it may show **synaptic facilitation,** in which it releases more transmitter and therefore more easily depolarizes the next cell. Alternatively, a cell may also show **defacilitation** (or **habituation**). In this case, the cell is depleted of transmitter, and thus is less effective in influencing the next cell. Many mechanisms can cause synaptic facilitation or habituation in different parts of the nervous system. Increased use of a given pathway can result in synaptic facilitation. However, in a different pathway, increased use could result in defacilitation or habituation. Variations in the coding within the neuron's internal chemistry and the stimuli activating the neuron will determine whether it will respond to these signals in one mode or another. For more information, see Chapter 4, which describes the physiology of simple and complex forms of learning (Kandel, 2000b).

With this overview of the essential elements of the nervous system, we can now turn our attention to the heart of this chapter, an in-depth discussion of the sensory/motor processes underlying motor control.

SENSORY/PERCEPTUAL SYSTEMS

What is the role of sensation in the production and control of movement? In Chapter 2, on motor control theories, there were divergent views about the importance of sensory input in motor control. Current neuroscience research suggests that sensory information plays many different roles in the control of movement.

Sensory inputs serve as the stimuli for reflexive movement organized at the spinal cord level of the nervous system. In addition, sensory information has a vital role in modulating the output of movement that results from the activity of pattern generators in the spinal cord (e.g., locomotor pattern generators). Likewise, at the spinal cord level, sensory information can modulate movement that results from commands originating in higher centers of the nervous system. The reason that sensation can modulate all these types of movement is that sensory receptors converge on the motor neurons, considered the final common pathway. But another role of sensory information in movement control is accomplished via ascending pathways, which contribute to the control of movement in much more complex ways.

Somatosensory System

The somatosensory system, from the lowest to the highest level of the CNS hierarchy, going from the reception of signals in the periphery to the integration and interpretation of those signals relative to other sensory systems in association cortex, is described in this section. Notice how both hierarchical and parallel distributed processing contribute to the analysis of somatosensory signals.

Peripheral Receptors

Muscle Spindle. Most muscle spindles are encapsulated spindle-shaped sensory receptors located in the muscle belly of skeletal muscles. They consist of: (a) specialized very small muscle fibers, called **intrafusal fibers** (**extrafusal fibers** are the regular muscle fibers); (b) sensory neuron endings (group Ia and group II afferents) that wrap around the central regions of these small intrafusal muscle fibers; and (c) gamma motor neuron endings that activate the polar contractile regions of the intrafusal muscle fibers. Figure 3.4 shows a muscle spindle with its intrafusal muscle fibers (nuclear chain and nuclear bag), the sensory neuron endings (Ia and II), and the motor neuron endings (gamma).

Muscle spindles detect both absolute muscle length and changes in muscle length, and along with the monosynaptic reflex, help to finely regulate muscle length during movement. In humans, the muscles with the highest spindle density (spindles per muscle) are the extraocular, hand, and neck muscles. It should not be surprising that neck muscles have such a high spindle density, because we use these muscles in eye/head coordination as we reach for objects and move about in the environment (Gordon & Ghez, 1991)

The different types of muscle fibers and sensory and motor neurons innervating the muscle spindle are designed to support two muscle spindle functions, the signaling of: (a) static length of the whole muscle, and (b) dynamic changes in muscle length. In the following paragraphs we will explain the way each part of the spindle supports this role.

Intrafusal Muscle Fibers. The two types of intrafusal muscle fibers are called "nuclear bag" (divided into both static and dynamic types) and "nuclear chain" (static type) fibers. The nuclear bag fiber has many spherical nuclei in its central noncontractile region (looking like an elastic bag of nuclei), which stretches quickly when lengthened because of its elasticity, while the nuclear chain fiber has a single row of nuclei, and, being less elastic, stretches slowly (Fig. 3.4A).

Groups Ia and II Afferent Neurons. These afferent neuron endings, whose cell bodies are in the dorsal-root ganglia of the spinal cord, wrap around the intrafusal muscle fibers in the following way. The Ia fiber sensory endings wrap around the equatorial region (which is most elastic) of both bag and chain intrafusal muscle fibers and thus respond quickly to stretching, sensing the rate of change of the muscle length. The group II endings wrap around the region next to the equator, which is less elastic and thus less responsive to stretching. The Ia afferents go to both bag and chain fibers, while the group II afferents go mainly to the chain fibers (Fig. 3.4A). Thus, the group Ia afferent neurons are most sensitive to the rate of change or dynamic muscle length and the group II afferent neurons are most responsive to steady-state or static muscle length. The group Ia afferents (but not the group II afferents) respond well to slight tendon taps, sinusoidal stretches, and even vibration of the muscle tendon, since these stimuli cause fast changes in muscle length (Pearson & Gordon, 2000).

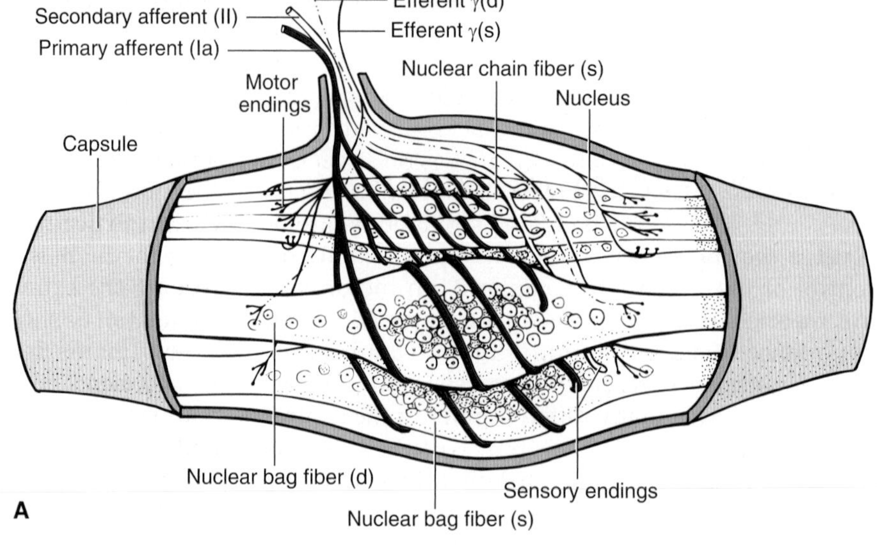

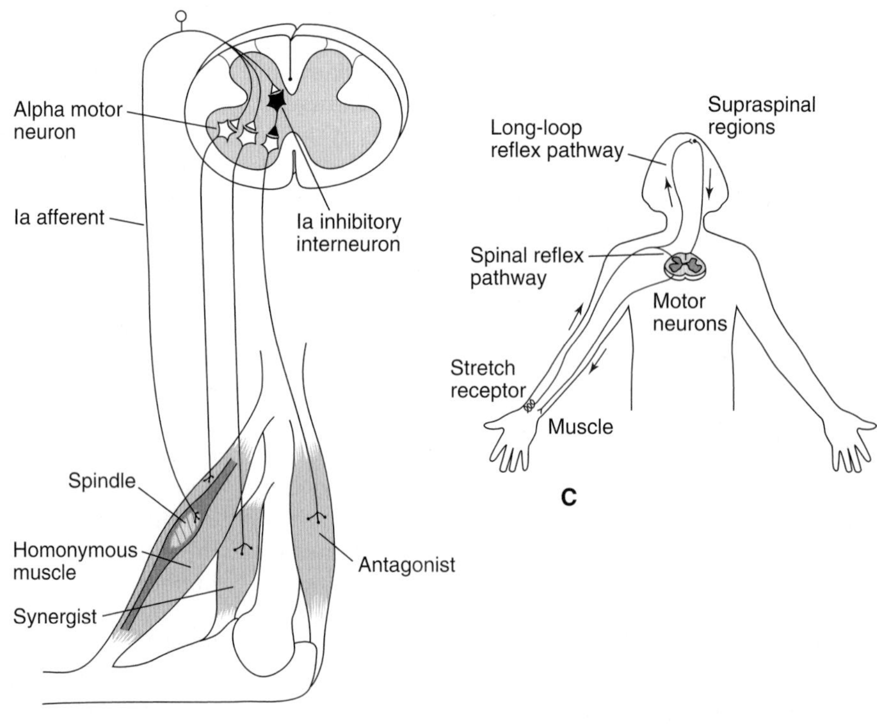

FIGURE 3.4 Anatomy of the muscle spindle. A, Drawing of a muscle spindle showing: (1) dynamic and static nuclear bag fibers and static nuclear chain muscle fibers; (2) the group Ia and II afferent neurons that wrap around their central regions, sensing muscle length and change in length; and (3) the gamma efferent motor neurons that cause their polar regions to contract in order to keep the central regions from going slack during contractions of the whole muscle in which the muscle spindle is embedded. B, Neural circuitry of the monosynaptic stretch reflex, showing the muscle spindle in the biceps muscle, the Ia afferent pathway to the spinal cord, with monosynaptic connections to the alpha motor neuron of the biceps and its synergist, and its connection to the Ia inhibitory interneuron that inhibits the motor neuron to the antagonist triceps muscle. C, Muscle spindle information contributes to both a spinal reflex pathway and a long loop reflex pathway. s = static; d = dynamic. (Parts B & C, aqdapted with permission from Kandel ER, Schwartz JH, Jessell TM, eds. Principles of neuroscience, 4th ed. New York: Elsevier, 2000.)

Gamma Motor Neurons. Both the bag and chain muscle fibers are activated by axons of the **gamma motor neurons.** The cell bodies of the gamma motor neurons are inside the ventral horn of the spinal cord, intermingled with the **alpha motor neurons,** innervating the extrafusal (regular skeletal muscle) fibers. The gamma motor neuron axons terminate at the polar, striated region of the bag and the chain muscle fibers, as shown in Figure 3.4A. There are two types of gamma motor neurons: (a) the gamma dynamic, activating only dynamic bag muscle fibers, and (b) the gamma static, innervating both static bag and chain muscle fibers. Activation of the gamma dynamic motor neurons enhances the dynamic responses of the Ia afferent neurons, while activation of the gamma static motor neurons enhances the responses of the group II afferent neurons, signaling the steady-state length of the muscles.

How is information from the muscle spindle used during motor control? Muscle spindle information is used at many levels of the CNS hierarchy. At the lowest level, it is involved in reflex activation of muscles. However, as the information ascends the CNS hierarchy, it is used in increasingly complex and abstract ways. For example, it may contribute to our perception of our sense of effort. In addition, it is carried over different pathways to different parts of the brain, in this way contributing to the parallel distributed nature of brain processing.

Stretch Reflex Loop. When a muscle is stretched, it stretches the muscle spindle, exciting the Ia afferents. Two types of reflex responses can be triggered by this Ia afferent excitation, a monosynaptic spinal reflex and a long-loop or transcortical reflex, as shown in Figure 3.4C. The spinal stretch reflex is activated by excitatory monosynaptic connections from the Ia afferent neurons to the alpha motor neurons, which activate their own muscle and synergistic muscles (Fig. 3.4B). The Ia afferents also excite Ia inhibitory interneurons, which then inhibit alpha motor neurons to the antagonist muscles (Fig. 3.4B). For example, if the gastrocnemius muscle is stretched, the muscle spindle Ia afferents in the muscle are excited, and they, in turn, excite the alpha motor neurons of the gastrocnemius, which cause it to contract. The Ia afferent also excites the Ia inhibitory interneuron, which inhibits motor neurons to the antagonist muscle, the tibialis anterior, so that if this muscle was contracting, it now relaxes. The group II afferents also excite their own muscle, but disynaptically (Patton et al., 1989; Pearson & Gordon, 2000). The long-loop or transcortical reflex (see Fig. 3.4C) is a more modifiable reflex, and therefore is often called a "functional stretch reflex." The gain of this reflex can be easily modified according to the environmental conditions or preparatory set of the subject.

What is the purpose of gamma motor neuron activity, and when are these motor neurons to the muscle spindle active? Whenever there is a voluntary contraction, there is coactivation of both alpha (activating the main muscle, i.e., the extrafusal muscle fiber) and gamma (activating the spindle muscle, i.e., the intrafusal fiber) motor neurons. Without this coactivation, spindle sensory neurons would be silent during voluntary muscle contraction. With it, in addition to the regular extrafusal fibers of the muscle, the polar regions of the nuclear bag and chain fibers contract, and thus the central region of the muscle spindle (with the group Ia and II afferent endings) cannot go slack. Because of this coactivation, if there is unexpected stretch during the contraction, the group Ia and II afferents will be able to sense it, and compensate.

Golgi Tendon Organs. Golgi tendon organs (GTOs) are spindle-shaped (1 mm long by 0.1 mm diameter) and are located at the muscle–tendon junction (Fig. 3.5A). They connect to 15 to 20 muscle fibers. Afferent information from the GTO is carried to the nervous system via the Ib afferent fibers. Unlike the muscle spindles, they have no efferent connections, and thus are not subject to CNS modulation.

The GTO is sensitive to tension changes that result from either stretch or contraction of the muscle. The GTO responds to as little as 2 to 25 *g* of force. The GTO reflex is an inhibitory disynaptic reflex, inhibiting its own muscle and exciting its antagonist (Fig. 3.5B). Note in the figure that joint receptors and cutaneous receptors may also contribute to this reflex.

Researchers used to think that the GTO was active only in response to large amounts of tension, so they hypothesized that the role of the GTO was to protect the muscle from injury. Current research has shown that these receptors constantly monitor muscle tension and are very sensitive to even small amounts of tension changes caused by muscle contraction. A newly hypothesized function of the GTO is that it modulates muscle output in response to fatigue. Thus, when muscle tension is reduced because of fatigue, the GTO output is reduced, lowering its inhibitory effect on its own muscle (Patton et al., 1989; Pearson & Gordon, 2000).

It has also been shown that the GTOs of the extensor muscles of the leg are active during the stance phase of locomotion and act to excite the extensor muscles and inhibit the flexor muscles until the GTO is unloaded (Pearson et al., 1992). This is exactly the opposite of what would be expected from the reflex when it is activated with the animal in a passive state. Thus, the reflex appears to have different properties under different task conditions.

Joint Receptors. How do joint receptors work, and what is their function? There are a number of different types of receptors within the joint itself, including Ruffini-type endings or spray endings, paciniform endings, ligament receptors, and free nerve endings. They are located in different portions of the joint capsule. Morphologically, they share the same characteristics as many of the other receptors found in the nervous system. For example, the ligament receptors are almost identical to GTOs, while the paciniform endings are identical to pacinian corpuscles in the skin.

There are a number of intriguing aspects of joint function. The joint receptor information is used at several levels of the hierarchy of sensory processing. Some researchers have found that joint receptors

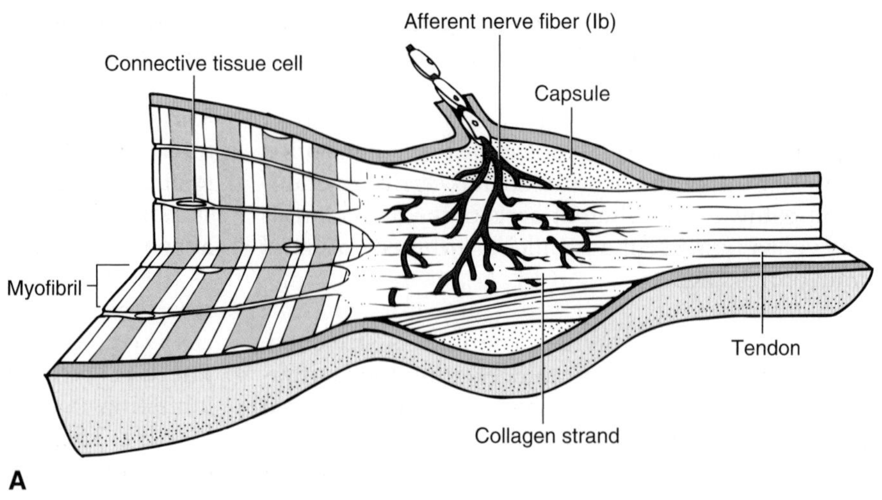

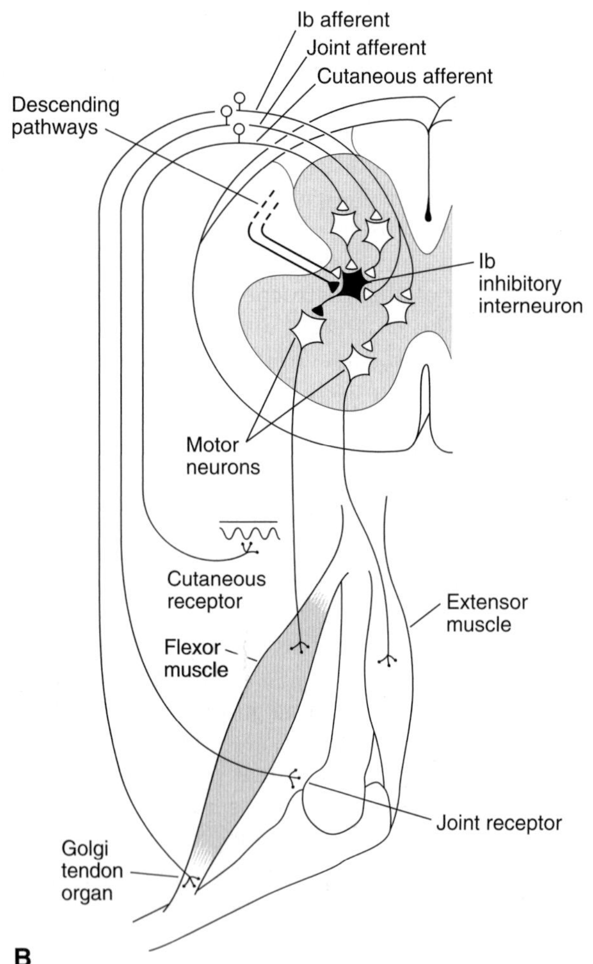

FIGURE 3.5 A, Golgi tendon organ and its Ib afferent innervation. It is located at the muscle-tendon junction and is connected to 15 to 20 muscle fibers. B, Neural circuitry of the Golgi tendon organ (GTO) reflex pathways, showing the GTO in the biceps muscle. Ib afferent information from the GTO synapses onto Ib inhibitory interneurons, which inhibit motor neurons to the agonist muscle and also disynaptically excite motor neurons in the antagonist triceps muscle. (Part B adapted with permission from Kandel ER, Schwartz JH, Jessel TM, eds. Principles of neuroscience, 3rd ed. New York: Elsevier, 1991.)

appear to be sensitive only to extreme joint angles (Burgess & Clark, 1969). Because of this, the joint receptors may provide a danger signal about extreme joint motion.

Other researchers have reported that many individual joint receptors respond to a limited range of joint motion. This phenomenon has been called "range fractionation," with multiple receptors being activated in overlapping ranges. Afferent information from joint receptors ascends to the cerebral cortex and contributes to our perception of our position in space. The CNS determines joint position by monitoring which receptors are activated at the same time, and this allows the determination of exact joint position.

Cutaneous Receptors. There are also several types of cutaneous receptors: (a) mechanoreceptors, including pacinian corpuscles, Merkel's disks, Meissner's corpuscles, Ruffini endings, and lanceolate endings around hair follicles, detecting mechanical stimuli; (b) thermoreceptors, detecting temperature changes; and (c) nociceptors, detecting potential damage to the skin. Figure 3.6 shows the location of these receptors in the skin. The number of receptors within the sensitive areas of the skin, such as the tips of the fingers, is very high, on the order of 2500 per square centimeter (Gardner et al., 2000).

Information from the cutaneous system is also used in hierarchical processing in several different ways. At lower levels of the CNS hierarchy, cutaneous information gives rise to reflex movements. Information from the cutaneous system also ascends and provides information concerning body position essential for orientation within the immediate environment.

The nervous system uses cutaneous information for reflex responses in various ways, depending on the extent and type of cutaneous input. A light, diffuse stimulus to the bottom of the foot tends to produce extension in the limb, as for example, when you touch the pad of a cat's foot lightly, it will extend it. This is called the "placing reaction," and it is found in human infants as well. In contrast, a sharp focal stimulus tends to produce withdrawal, or flexion, even when it is applied to exactly the same area of the foot. This is called the "flexor withdrawal reflex," and it is used to protect us from injury. The typical pattern of response in the cutaneous reflex is ipsilateral flexion and contralateral extension, which allows you to support your weight on the opposite limb (mediated by group III and IV afferents).

It is important to remember that even though we consider reflexes to be stereotyped, they are modulated by higher centers, depending on the task and the context. Remember our example of the flexor reflex, which typically causes withdrawal of a limb from a noxious stimulus. However, if there is more at stake than not hurting yourself, such as saving the life of your child, the CNS inhibits the activation of this

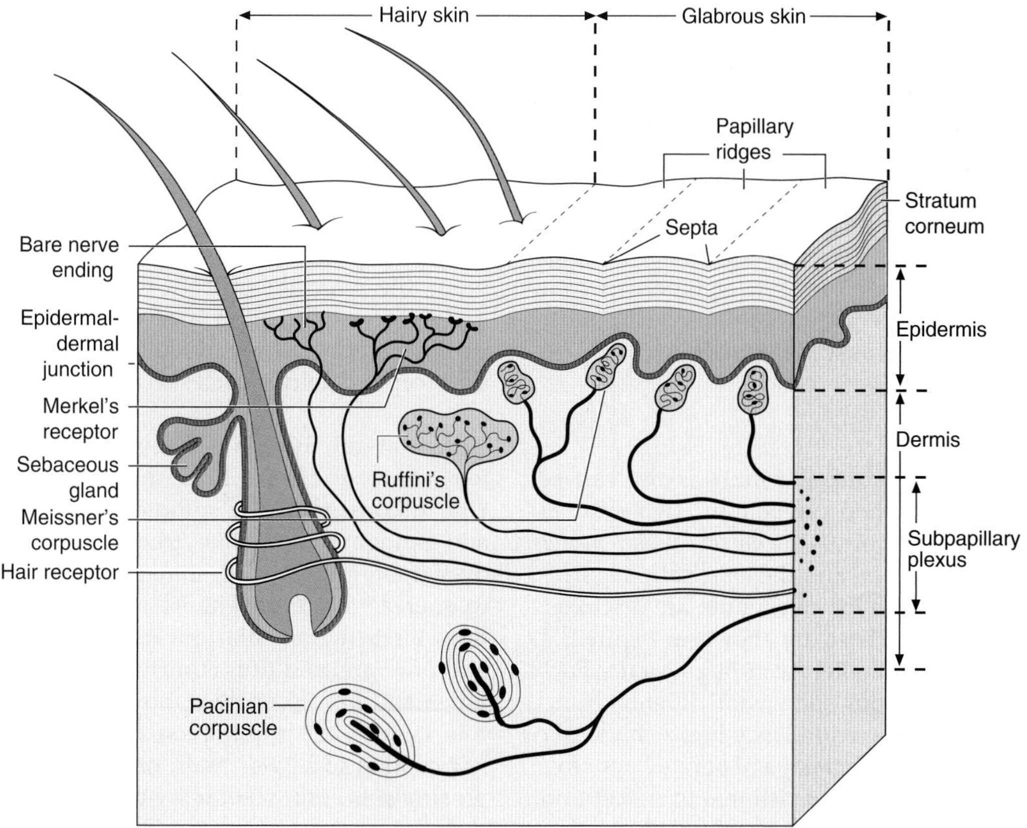

FIGURE 3.6 Location of cutaneous receptors in the skin. (Adapted with permission from Kandel ER, Schwartz JH, Jessell TM, eds. Principles of neuroscience, 3rd ed. New York: Elsevier, 1991.)

reflex movement in favor of actions more appropriate to the situation.

Role of Somatosensation at the Spinal Cord Level

Information from cutaneous, muscle, and joint receptors modifies the output of circuits at the spinal cord level that control basic activities such as locomotion. In the late 1960s, Grillner and colleagues (Grillner, 1973, 1981) performed experiments in which they cut the dorsal roots to the spinal cord of cats to eliminate sensory feedback from the periphery and made lesions to eliminate inputs from higher brain centers. They stimulated the spinal cord and were able to activate the neural pattern generator for locomotor patterns. They found that low rates of repetitive stimulation gave rise to a walk and higher rates to a trot and then a gallop. This suggests that complex movements, such as locomotion, can be generated at the spinal cord level without supraspinal influences or inputs from the periphery.

If we do not need sensory information to generate complex movement, does that mean there is no role for sensory information in its execution? No. Hans Forssberg and his colleagues (1977) have shown that sensory information modulates locomotor output in a very elegant way. When he brushed the paw of a spinalized (the spinal cord was transected at level T12) cat with a glass rod during the swing phase of walking, it caused the paw to flex more strongly and get out of the way of the rod. But during stance, the very same stimulation caused stronger extension, in order to push off more quickly and avoid the rod in this way. Thus, he found that the same cutaneous input could modulate the step cycle in different functional ways, depending on the context in which it was used. Similar findings related to the modulation of the locomotor step cycle in response to phase-specific somatosensory input has been shown in humans as well (Stein, 1991).

Ascending Pathways

Information from the trunk and limbs is also carried to the sensory cortex and cerebellum. Two systems ascend to the cerebral cortex: the *dorsal column–medial lemniscal* (DC-ML) *system* and the *anterolateral system*. (Systems that ascend to the cerebellum are discussed later in this chapter.) These are shown in Figure 3.7. They are examples of parallel ascending systems. Each relays information about somewhat different functions, but there is some redundancy between the two pathways. What is the advantage of parallel systems? They give extra subtlety and richness to perception, by using multiple modes of processing information. They also give a measure of insurance of continued function in case of injury (Gardner et al., 2000; Patton et al., 1989).

Dorsal Column–Medial Lemniscal System. The *dorsal columns* (Fig. 3.7) are formed mainly by dorsal-root ganglion neurons, and thus they are first-order neurons. The majority of the fibers branch on entering the spinal cord, synapsing on interneurons and motor neurons to modulate spinal activity, and send branches to ascend in the dorsal column pathway toward the brain. What are the functions of the dorsal column (D-C) neurons? They send information on cutaneous, muscle, tendon, and joint sensibility up to the somatosensory cortex and other higher brain centers. There is an interesting exception, however. Leg proprioceptors have their own private pathway to the brainstem, the lateral column. They join the dorsal column pathway in the brainstem. The D-C pathway also contains information from touch and pressure receptors, and codes especially for discriminative fine touch (Gardner et al., 2000).

Where does this information go, and how is it processed? The pathways synapse at multiple levels in the nervous system, including the medulla, where second-order neurons become the *medial lemniscal* pathway and cross over to the thalamus, synapsing with third-order neurons, which proceed to the somatosensory cortex. Every level of the hierarchy has the ability to modulate the information coming into it from below. Through synaptic excitation and inhibition, higher centers have the ability to shut off or enhance ascending information. This allows higher centers to selectively tune (up or down) the information coming from lower centers.

As the neurons ascend through each level to the brain, the information from the receptors is increasingly processed to allow meaningful interpretation of the information. This is done by selectively enlarging the receptive field of each successive neuron.

Anterolateral System. The second ascending system, shown in Figure 3.7, is the *anterolateral* (AL) system. It consists of the spinothalamic, spinoreticular, and spinomesencephalic tracts. These fibers cross over upon entering the spinal cord and then ascend to brainstem centers. The AL system has a dual function. First, it transmits information on crude touch and pressure, and thus contributes in a minor way to touch and limb proprioception. It also plays a major role in relaying information related to thermal and nociception to higher brain centers. All levels of the sensory processing hierarchy act on the AL system in the same manner as for the DC-ML system (Gardner et al., 2000).

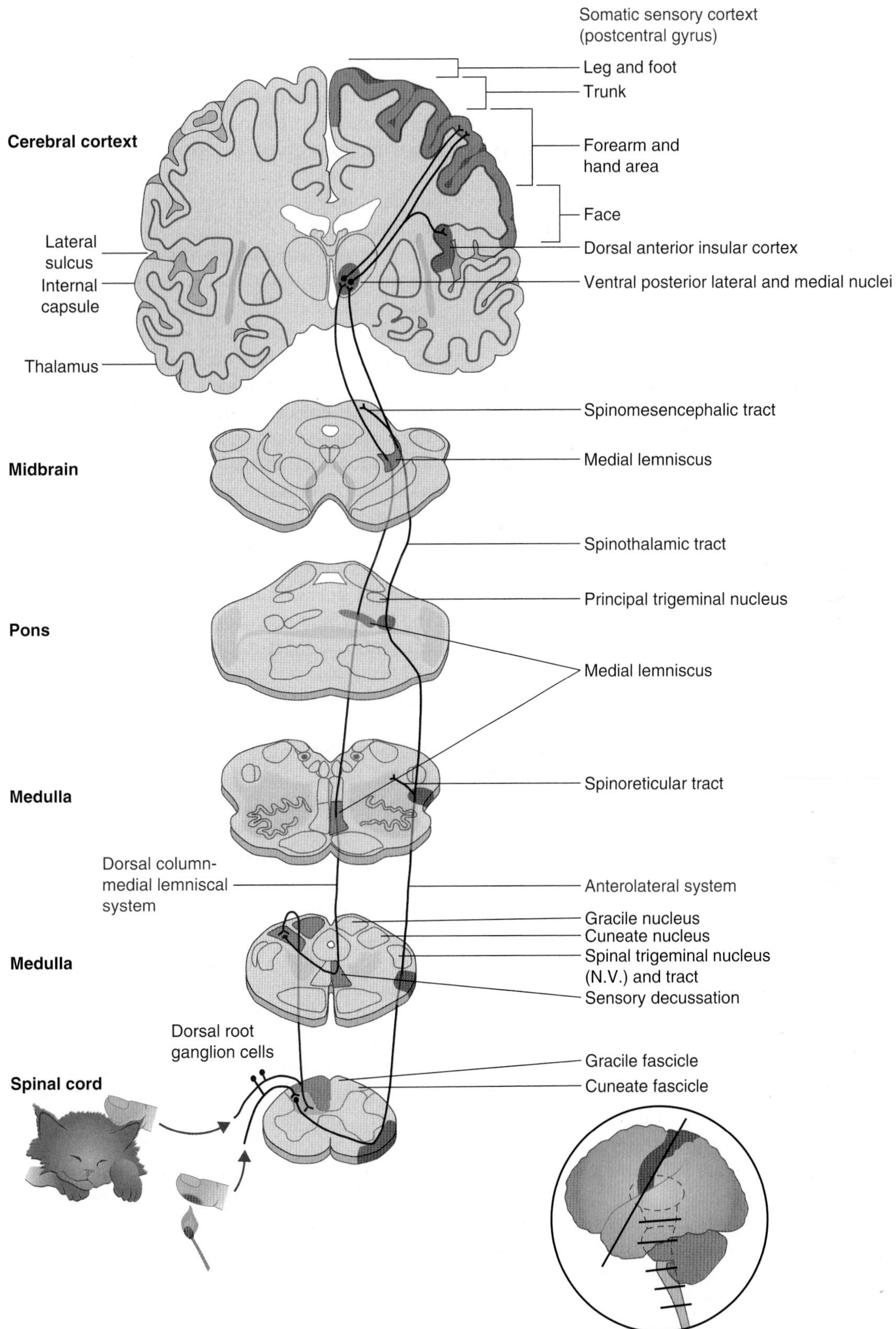

FIGURE 3.7 Ascending sensory systems, including the dorsal column–medial lemniscal pathway, which contains information from touch and pressure receptors, and the anterolateral system, which contains information on pain, temperature, crude touch, and pressure.

There is a redundancy of information in both tracts. A lesion in one tract does not cause complete loss of discrimination in any of these senses. However, a lesion in both tracts causes severe loss. Hemisection of the spinal cord (e.g., caused by a serious accident) would cause tactile sensation and proprioception in the arms to be lost on the ipsilateral side (fibers have not crossed yet), while pain and temperature sensation would be lost on the contralateral side (fibers have already crossed upon entering the spinal cord) (Gardner et al., 2000).

Thalamus

Information from both the ascending somatosensory tracts, like information from virtually all sensory systems, goes through the *thalamus*. In addition, the thalamus receives information from a number of other areas of the brain, including the basal ganglia and the cerebellum. Thus, the thalamus is a major processing center of the brain. In general, a lesion in this area will cause severe sensory (and motor) problems. The thalamus has become a target for treatments aimed at decreasing tremor in patients with Parkinson's disease.

Somatosensory Cortex

The *somatosensory cortex* is a major processing area for all the somatosensory modalities, and marks the beginning of conscious awareness of somatosensation. The somatosensory cortex is divided into two major areas: *primary somatosensory cortex* (SI) (also called Brodmann's areas 1, 2, 3a, and 3b); and *secondary somatosensory cortex* (SII) Figure 3.8A shows the location of areas SI and SII on the surface of the brain, while Figure 3.8B shows a coronal cross section of the brain indicating the location of Brodmann's areas 1, 2, 3a, and 3b within SI. Finally Figure 3.8C shows the input connections to SI, the internal connections between the various areas of SI, and the output to SII. In SI, kinesthetic and touch information from the contralateral side of the body is organized in a somatotopic manner and spans four cytoarchitectural areas, Brodmann's areas 1, 2, 3a, and 3b.

It is in this area that we begin to see cross-modality processing. This means that information from joint receptors, muscle spindles, and cutaneous receptors is now integrated to give us information about movement in a given body area. This information is laid on top of a map of the entire body, which is distorted to reflect the relative weight given sensory information from certain areas, as shown in Figure 3.8B. For example, the throat, mouth, and hands are heavily represented because we need more detailed information to support the movements that are executed by these structures. This is the beginning of the spatial processing that is essential to the coordination of movements in space. Coordinated movement requires information about the position of the body relative to the environment and the position of one body segment relative to another (Gardner & Kandel, 2000).

Contrast sensitivity is very important to movement control, since it allows the detection of the shape and edges of objects. The somatosensory cortex processes incoming information to increase contrast sensitivity so that we can more easily identify and discriminate between different objects through touch. How does it do this? It has been shown that the receptive fields of the somatosensory neurons have an excitatory center and inhibitory surround. This inhibitory surround aids in two-point discrimination through *lateral inhibition*.

How does lateral inhibition work? The cell that is excited inhibits the cells next to it, thus enhancing contrast between excited and nonexcited regions of the body. The receptors themselves do not have lateral inhibition; it happens at the level of the dorsal columns and at each subsequent step in the relay. In fact, humans have a sufficiently sensitive somatosensory system to perceive the activation of a single tactile receptor in the hand (Gardner & Kandel, 2000).

Different features of an object are processed in parallel in different parts of the somatosensory cortex. For example, neurons in Brodmann's area 1 sense object size, having large receptive fields covering many fingers. Other cells, in area 2, respond best to moving stimuli and are sensitive to direction. One does not find this feature in the dorsal columns or in the thalamus. These higher-level processing cells also have larger receptive fields than the typical cells in the somatosensory cortex, often encompassing a number of fingers. These cells appear to respond preferentially when neighboring fingers are stimulated. This could indicate their participation in functions such as the grasping of objects.

It has been found that the receptive fields of neurons in the somatosensory cortex are not fixed in size. Both injury and experience can change their dimensions considerably. The implications of these studies are considered in the motor learning sections of this book.

Somatosensory cortex also has descending connections to the thalamus, dorsal column nucleus, and the spinal cord, and thus has the ability to modulate ascending information coming through these structures.

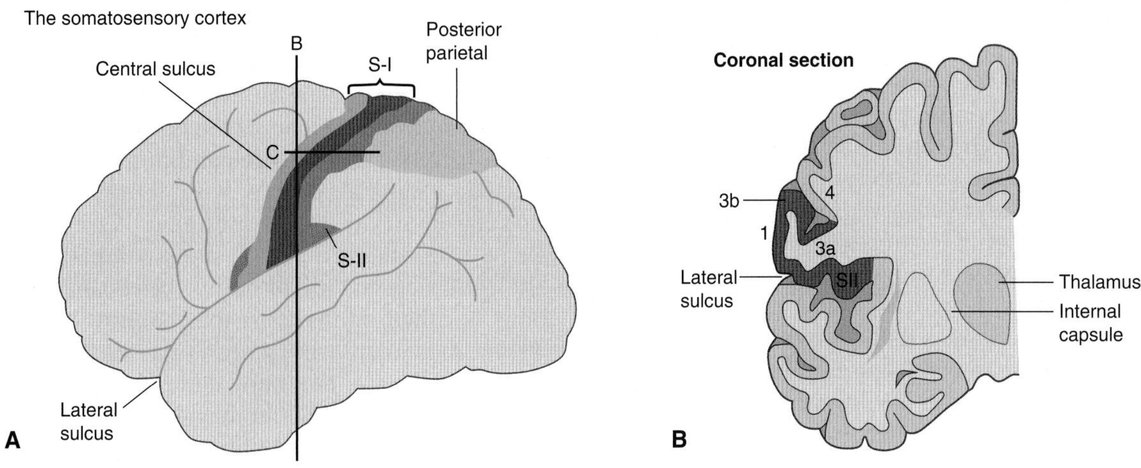

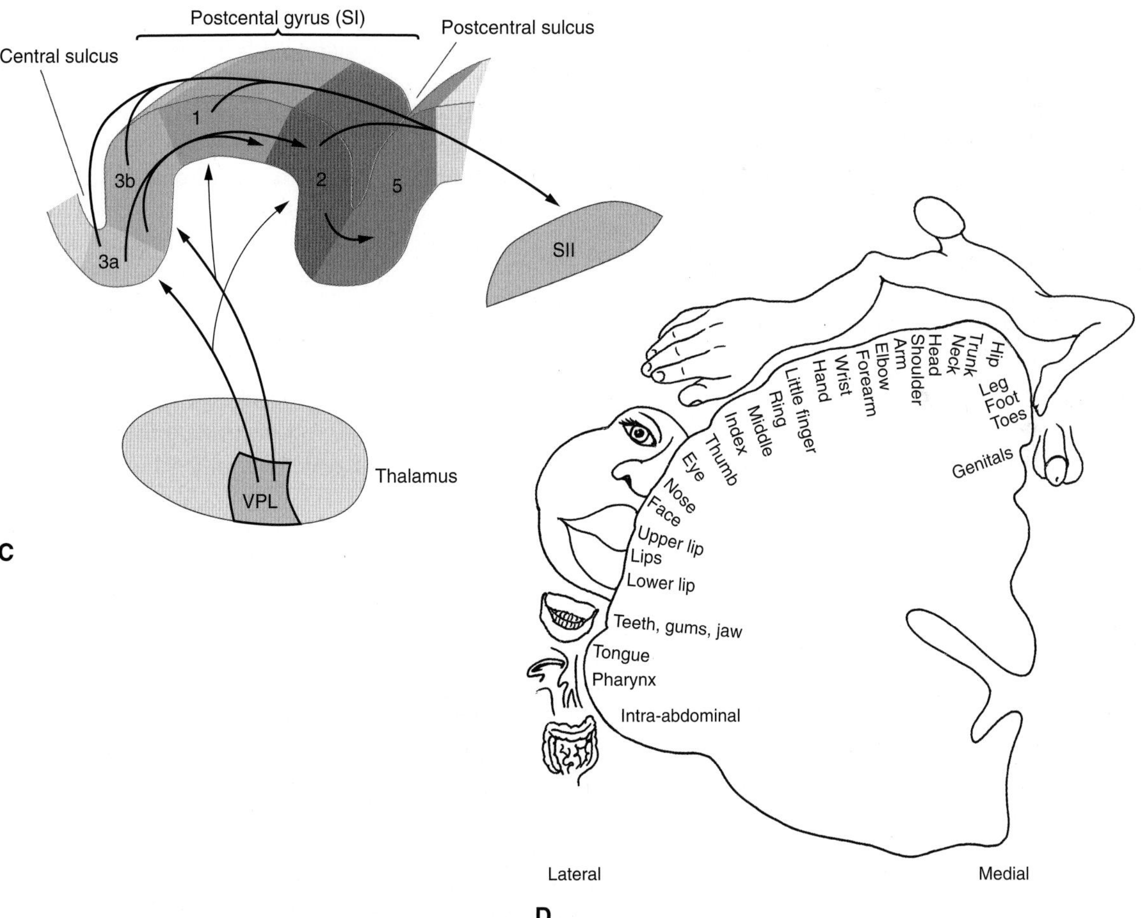

FIGURE 3.8 Somatosensory cortex and association areas. A, Located in the parietal lobe, the somatosensory cortex contains three major divisions: the primary (SI) and secondary (SII) somatosensory cortices and the posterior parietal cortex. B, Coronal section showing the location of Brodmann's areas 1, 2, 3a, and 3b within SI. C, Diagram showing the input to SI from the thalamus, internal connections within SI, and output to SII. D, Sensory homunculus showing the somatic sensory projections from the body surface. VPL = ventral posterolateral nucleus. (Adapted from Kandel ER, Schwartz JH, Jessell TM, eds. Principles of neuroscience, 3rd ed. New York: Elsevier, 1991:368, 372.)

Association Cortices

It is in the many association cortices that we begin to see the transition from perception to action. It is here, too, that we see the interplay between cognitive and perceptual processing. The association cortices, found in parietal, temporal, and occipital lobes, include centers for higher-level sensory processing and higher-level abstract cognitive processing. The locations of these various areas are shown in Figure 3.9.

Within the parietal, temporal, and occipital cortices are association areas that are hypothesized to link information from several senses. Brodmann's area 5 of the parietal cortex is a thin strip posterior to the postcentral gyrus. After intermodality processing has taken place within area SI, outputs are sent to area 5, which integrates information between body parts. Area 5 connects to area 7 of the parietal lobe. Area 7 also receives processed visual information. Thus, area 7 combines eye–limb processing in most visually triggered or guided activities.

Lesions in Brodmann's area 5 or 7 in humans and other animals cause problems with learning skills that use information regarding the position of the body in space. In addition, certain cells in these areas are activated during visually guided movements, with their activity becoming more intense when the animal attends to the movement. These findings support the hypothesis that the parietal lobe participates in processes involving attention to the position of and manipulation of objects in space.

These experimental results are further supported by observations of patients with damage to the parietal lobes. Deficits in these patients include problems with body image and perception of spatial relations, which may be very important in both postural control and voluntary movements. Clearly, lesions to this area do not simply reduce the ability to perceive information coming in from one part of the body; in addition, they can affect the ability to interpret this information.

For example, people with lesions in the right angular gyrus (the nondominant hemisphere), just behind Brodmann's area 7, show complete neglect of the contralateral side of body, objects, and drawings. This is called **agnosia,** or the inability to recognize. When their own arm or leg is passively moved into their visual field, they may claim that it is not theirs. In certain cases, patients may be totally unaware of the hemiplegia that accompanies the lesion and may thus desire to leave the hospital early since they are unaware that they have any problem (Kupfermann, 1991). Many of these same patients show problems when asked to copy drawn figures. They may make a drawing in which half of the object is missing. This is called "constructional apraxia." Larger lesions may cause the inability to operate and orient in space or the inability to perform complex sequential tasks.

When right-handed patients have lesions in the left angular gyrus (the dominant hemisphere), they show such symptoms as confusion between left and right; difficulty in naming their fingers, although they can sense touch; and difficulty in writing, although their motor and sensory functions are normal for the hands. Alternatively, when patients have lesions to both sides of these areas, they often have problems attending to visual stimuli, in using vision to grasp an object, and in making voluntary eye movements to a point in space (Kupfermann, 1991).

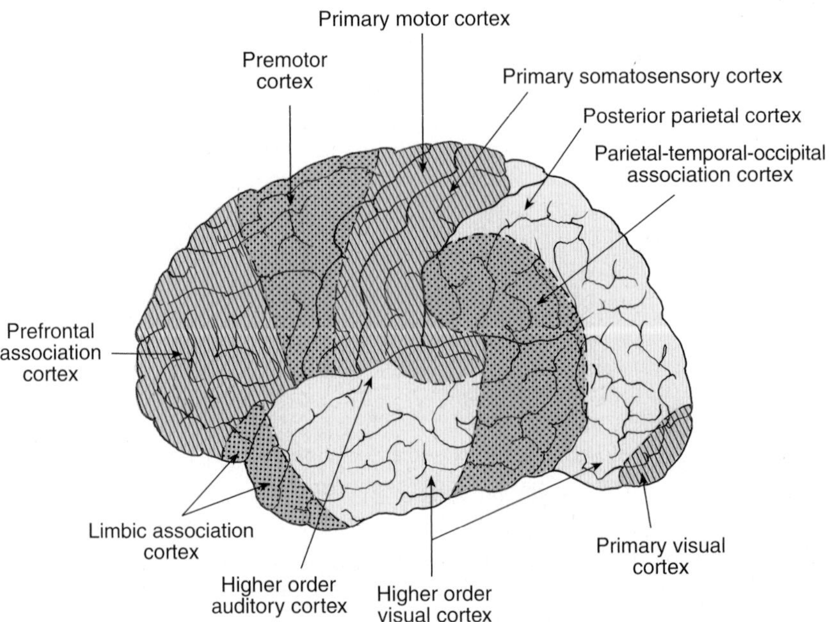

FIGURE 3.9 Locations of primary sensory areas, higher-level sensory association areas, and higher-level cognitive (abstract) association cortices. (Adapted from Kandel ER, Schwartz JH, Jessell TM, eds. Principles of neuroscience, 3rd ed. New York: Elsevier, 1991:825.)

We have just taken one sensory system, the somatosensory system, from the lowest to the highest level of the CNS hierarchy, going from the reception of signals in the periphery to the integration and interpretation of those signals relative to other sensory systems. We have also looked at how hierarchical and parallel distributed processing have contributed to the analysis of these signals. We are now going to look at a second sensory system, the visual system, in the same way.

Visual System

Vision serves motor control in a number of ways. Vision allows us to identify objects in space and to determine their movement. When vision plays this role, it is considered an exteroceptive sense. But vision also gives us information about where our bodies are in space, the relation of one body part to another, and the motion of our bodies. When vision plays this role, it is referred to as "visual proprioception," which means that it gives us information not only about the environment, but also about our own bodies. Later chapters show how vision plays a key role in the control of posture, locomotion, and manipulatory function. In the following sections, we consider the anatomy and physiology of the visual system to show how it supports these roles in motor control.

Peripheral Visual System

Photoreceptor Cells. Let us first look at an overall view of the eye. The eye is a great instrument, designed to focus the image of the world on the retina with high precision. As illustrated in Figure 3.10, light enters the eye through the cornea and is focused by the cornea and lens on the retina at the back of the eye. An interesting feature of the retina is that light must travel through all the layers of the eye and the neural layers of the retina before it hits the photoreceptors, which are at the back of the retina, facing away from the light source. Luckily, these layers are nearly transparent.

There are two types of photoreceptor cells: the *rods* and the *cones*. The cones are functional for vision in normal daylight and are responsible for color vision. The rods are responsible for vision at night, when the amount of light is very low and too weak to activate the cones. Right at the fovea, the rest of the layers are pushed aside so the cones can receive the light in its clearest form. The blind spot (where the optic nerve leaves the retina) has no photoreceptors, and therefore we are blind in this one part of the retina. Except for the fovea, there are 20 times more rods than cones in the retina. However, cones are more important than rods for normal vision, because their loss causes legal blindness, while total loss of rods causes only night blindness (Tessier-Lavigne, 2000).

Remember that sensory differentiation is a key aspect of sensory processing that supports motor control. To accomplish this, the visual system has to identify objects and determine whether they are moving. So how are *object identification* and *motion sense* accomplished in the visual system? There are two separate pathways to process them. We will follow these pathways from the retina all the way up to the visual cortex. We will see that *contrast sensitivity* is used in both pathways to accomplish the goals of object identification and motion sense. Contrast sensitivity enhances the edges of objects, giving us greater precision in perception. As in the somatosensory system, all three processes are used extensively in the visual system. This processing begins in the retina. So let us first look at the cells of the retina, so that we can understand how they work together to process information (Tessier-Lavigne, 2000).

Vertical Cells. In addition to the rods and cones, the retina contains *bipolar cells* and *ganglion cells,* which you might consider "vertical" cells, since they connect in series to one another but have no lateral connections (Fig. 3.10). For example, the rods and cones make direct synaptic contact with bipolar cells. The bipolar cells in turn connect to the ganglion cells. And the ganglion cells then relay visual information to the CNS by sending axons to the lateral geniculate nucleus and superior colliculus as well as to brainstem nuclei (Dowling, 1987; Tessier-Lavigne, 2000).

Horizontal Cells. There is another class of neurons in the retina, which we are calling "horizontal" cells. These neurons modulate the flow of information within the retina by connecting the "vertical" cells together laterally. These are called the *horizontal* and *amacrine cells*. The horizontal cells mediate interactions between the receptors and bipolar cells, while the amacrine cells mediate interactions between bipolar and ganglion cells. The horizontal cells and amacrine cells are critical for achieving contrast sensitivity. Although it may appear that there are complex interconnections between the receptor cells and other neurons before the final output of the ganglion cells is reached, the pathways and functions of the different classes of cells are straightforward.

Let us first look at the bipolar-cell pathway. There are two types of pathways that involve bipolar cells, a "direct" pathway and a "lateral" pathway. In the direct pathway, a cone, for example, makes a direct

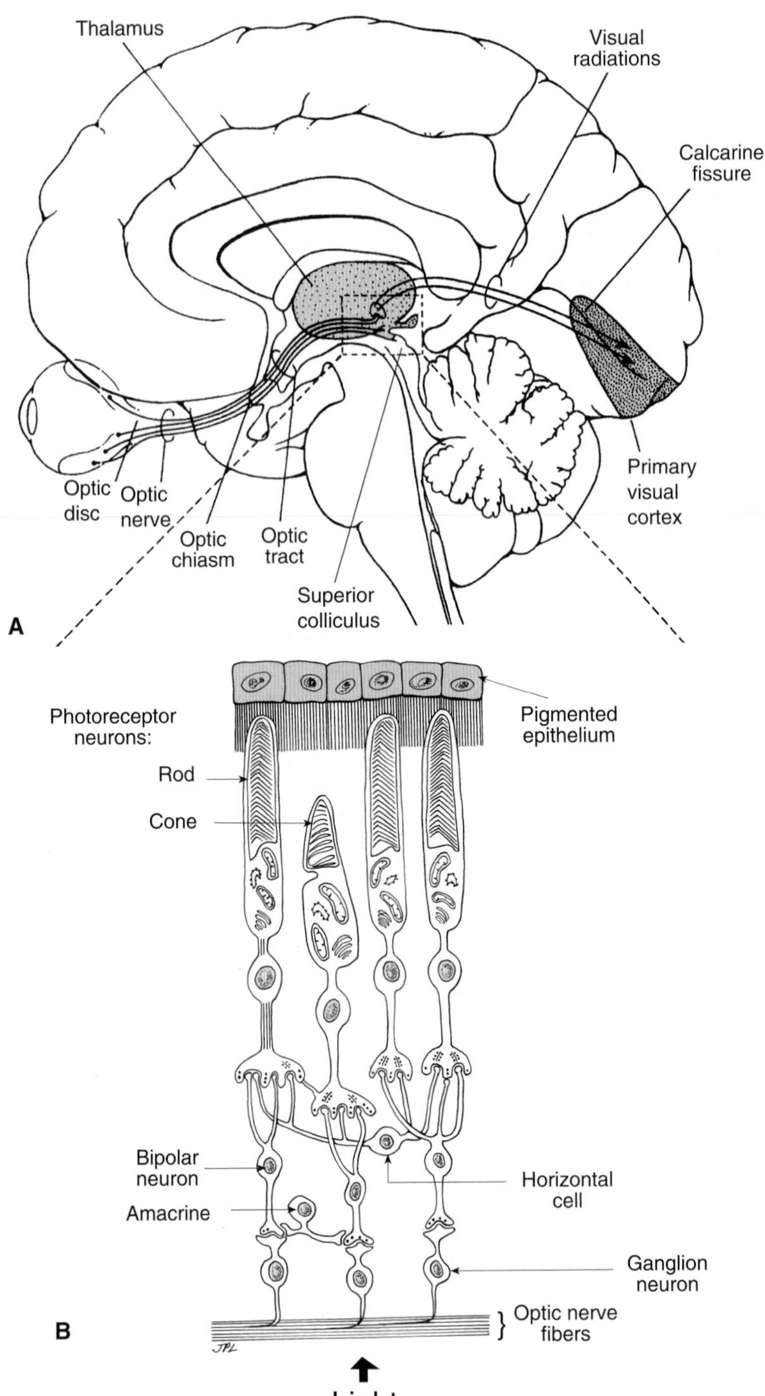

FIGURE 3.10 The eye, its relationship to the horizontal and vertical cells (inset), and the visual pathways from the retina to (1) the superior colliculus and (2) the thalamus and the primary visual cortex (area 17). (Adapted from Kandel ER, Schwartz JH, Jessell TM, eds. Principles of neuroscience, 3rd ed. New York: Elsevier, 1991:401, 415, 423.)

connection with a bipolar cell, which makes a direct connection with a ganglion cell. In the lateral pathway, activity of cones is transmitted to the ganglion cells lateral to them through horizontal cells or amacrine cells. Figure 3.10 shows these organizational possibilities (Dowling, 1987).

In the direct pathway, cones (or rods) connect directly to bipolar cells with either "on-center" or "off-center" receptive fields. The **receptive field** of a cell is the specific area of the retina to which the cell is sensitive, when that part of the retina is illuminated. The receptive field can be either excitatory or inhibitory, increasing or decreasing the cell's membrane potential. The receptive fields of bipolar cells (and ganglion cells) are circular. At the center of the retina, the receptive fields are small, while in the periphery receptive fields are large. The term *on-center* means that the cell has an excitatory central portion of the receptive field, with an inhibitory surrounding area. *Off-center* refers to the opposite case of an inhibitory center and excitatory surround (Dowling, 1987).

How do the cells take on their antagonistic surround characteristics? It appears that horizontal cells in the surround area of the bipolar-cell receptive field (RF) make connections onto cones in the center of the field. When light shines on the periphery of the receptive field, the horizontal cells inhibit the cones adjacent to them. Each type of bipolar cell then synapses with a corresponding type of ganglion cell: on-center and off-center, and makes excitatory connections with that ganglion cell.

On-center cells give very few action potentials in the dark, and they are activated when their RF is illuminated. When the periphery of the on-center cells' RF is illuminated, it inhibits the effect of stimulating the center. Off-center ganglion cells likewise show inhibition when light is applied to the center of their RF, and they fire at the fastest rate just after the light is turned off. They also are activated if light is applied only to the periphery of their RF.

Ganglion cells are also influenced by the activity of amacrine cells. Many of the amacrine cells function in a manner similar to that of horizontal cells, transmitting inhibitory inputs from nearby bipolar cells to the ganglion cell, increasing contrast sensitivity.

These two types of pathways (on- and off-center) for processing retinal information are two examples of *parallel distributed processing* of similar information within the nervous system. We talked about a similar *center-surround inhibition* in cutaneous-receptor receptive fields. What is the purpose of this type of inhibition? It appears to be very important in detecting contrasts between objects, rather than the absolute intensity of light produced or reflected by an object. This inhibition allows us to detect edges of objects very easily. It is very important in locomotion, when we are walking down stairs and need to see the edge of the step. It is also important in manipulatory function, in being able to determine the exact shape of an object for grasping.

The ganglion cells send their axons, via the optic nerve, to three different regions in the brain, the lateral geniculate nucleus, the pretectum, and the superior colliculus (Wurtz & Kandel, 2000a). Figure 3.10 shows connections to the lateral geniculate nucleus of the thalamus.

Central Visual Pathways

Lateral Geniculate Nucleus. To understand what parts of the retina and visual field are represented in these different areas of the brain, let us first discuss the configuration of the visual fields and hemiretina. The left half of the visual field projects on the nasal (medial—next to the nose) half of the retina of the left eye and the temporal (lateral) half of the retina of the right eye. The right visual field projects on the nasal half of the retina of the right eye and the temporal half of the retina of the left eye (Wurtz & Kandel, 2000a).

Thus, the optic nerves from the left and right eyes leave the retina at the optic disk, in the back. They travel to the optic chiasm, where the nerves from each eye come together, and axons from the nasal side of the eyes cross, while those from the temporal side do not cross. At this point, the optic nerve becomes the optic tract. Because of this resorting of the optic nerves, the left optic tract has a map of the right visual field. This is similar to what we found for the somatosensory system, in which information from the opposite side of the body was represented in the thalamus and cortex.

One of the targets of cells in the optic tract is the lateral geniculate nucleus (LGN) of the thalamus. The LGN has six layers of cells, which map the contralateral visual field. The ganglion cells from different areas project onto specific points in the LGN, but just as we find for somatosensory maps of the body, certain areas are represented much more strongly than others. The fovea of the retina, which we use for high-acuity vision, is represented to a far greater degree than the peripheral area. Each layer of the LGN gets input from only one eye. The first two layers (most ventral) are the *magnocellular* (large cell) layers, and layers four through six are called the *parvocellular* (small cell) layers. The projection cells of each layer send axons to the visual cortex (Wurtz & Kandel, 2000a).

The receptive fields of neurons in the LGN are very similar to those found in the ganglion cells of the retina. There are separate on-center and off-center receptive field pathways. The magnocellular layers appear to be involved in the analysis of movement of the visual image (they have high temporal resolution, detecting fast pattern changes), and the coarse details of an object (they have low spatial resolution), with almost no response to color, while the parvocellular layers function in color vision and a more detailed structural analysis (high spatial resolution and low temporal resolution). Thus, magnocellular layers will be more important in motor functions such as balance control, for which movement of the visual field gives us information about our body sway, and in reaching for moving objects. The parvocellular layers will be more important in the final phases of reaching for an object, when we need to grasp it accurately.

Amazingly, only 10 to 20% of the inputs to the LGN come from the retina, with the rest coming from the cortex and reticular formation of the brainstem. These are feedback circuits, probably modulating the type of information moving from the retina to higher centers. This suggests that one of the most important aspects of sensory processing is choosing the inputs that are most important for an individual to attend to in a given moment and that each individual may have very different perceptions of a given event according to the sensory inputs their system allowed to move to higher perceptual centers (Wurtz & Kandel, 2000a).

Superior Colliculus. Ganglion-cell axons in the optic tract also terminate in the *superior colliculus* (in addition to indirect visual inputs coming from the visual cortex). The superior colliculus is located posterior to the thalamus, in the roof of the midbrain, as shown in Figure 3.10. It has been hypothesized that the superior colliculus maps the visual space around us in terms of not only visual, but also auditory and somatosensory cues. The three sensory maps in the superior colliculus are different from those seen in the sensory cortex. Body areas here are not mapped in terms of density of receptor cells in a particular area, but in terms of their relationship to the retina. Areas close to the retina (the nose) are given more representation than areas far away (the hand). For any part of the body, the visual, auditory, and somatosensory maps are aligned, in the different layers of the colliculus. This means that when a friend greets you as they bicycle by, the superior colliculus neurons will be activated, representing a particular spatial location within the visual field through which the friend is moving, and these same neurons in the superior colliculus will also be activated when their voice is in the same spatial location (Wurtz & Kandel, 2000a).

In addition to these three maps, located in the upper and middle of the seven layers of the colliculus, there is a motor map in the deeper layers of the colliculus. Through these output neurons, the colliculus controls saccadic eye movements that cause the eye to move toward a specific stimulus. The superior colliculus then sends outputs to: (a) regions of the brainstem that control eye movements; (b) the tectospinal tract, mediating the reflex control of the neck and head; and (c) the tectopontine tract, which projects to the cerebellum, for further processing of eye–head control.

Pretectal Region. Ganglion cells also terminate in the *pretectal* region, which is just anterior to the superior colliculus. The pretectal region is an important visual reflex center involved in pupillary eye reflexes, in which the pupil constricts in response to light shining on the retina.

Primary Visual Cortex

From the LGN, axons project to the *primary visual cortex* (V1, also called "striate cortex") to Brodmann's area 17, which is in the occipital lobe (Fig. 3.10). The inputs from the two eyes alternate throughout the striate cortex, producing what are called "ocular dominance columns." Output cells from primary visual cortex (V1) then project to Brodmann's area 18 (V2). From area 18 neurons project to medial temporal (MT) cortex (Brodmann's area 19) to inferotemporal cortex (Brodmann's areas 20 and 21) and posterior parietal cortex (Brodmann's area 7). In addition, outputs go to the superior colliculus and also project back to the LGN (feedback control). The primary visual cortex contains a topographic map of the retina. In addition, there are six other representations of the retina in the occipital lobe alone.

The receptive fields of cells in the visual cortex are not circular anymore, but linear: the light must be in the shape of a line, a bar, or an edge to excite them. These cells are classified as *simple* or *complex cells*. Simple cells respond to bars, with an excitatory center and an inhibitory surround, or vice versa. They also have a specific axis of orientation, for which the bar is most effective in exciting the cell. All axes of orientation for all parts of the retina are represented in the visual cortex. Results of experiments by Hubel and Wiesel (1959, 1962) suggest that this bar-shaped receptive field is created from many geniculate neurons with partially overlapping circular receptive fields in one line, converging onto a simple cortical cell. It has been suggested that complex cells have convergent input from many simple cells. Thus, their receptive fields are larger than simple cells, and have a critical axis of orientation. For many complex cells, the most useful stimulus is movement across the field.

The specific changes in the orientation axis across columns are interlaced with the presence of cells responding to color stimuli, organized in cylindrical shapes, known as "blobs."

In summary, we see that the visual cortex is divided into orientation columns, with each column consisting of cells with one axis of orientation, blobs, which are activated more by color than by orientation, and ocular dominance columns receiving input from the left versus the right eye. Hubel and Wiesel used the name *hypercolumn* to describe these sets of columns from one part of the retina, including color inputs and all orientation angles for the two eyes (Hubel & Wiesel, 1959, 1962).

These hypercolumns are connected horizontally to other columns with the same response properties, integrating visual inputs over broader areas of cortex. Depending on the inputs from these other areas, a cell's axis of orientation may change, showing the effect of context on a cell's output. Thus, the context in which a feature is embedded modulates the cell's response to that feature (McGuire et al., 1991).

Higher-Order Visual Cortex

Central visual processing pathways continue on to include cells in the primary visual cortex, located in the occipital lobe, and cells in the higher-order visual cortices, located in the temporal and parietal cortex as well. Higher-order cortices are involved in the integration of somatosensory and visual information underlying spatial orientation, an essential part of all actions. This interaction between visual and somatosensory inputs within higher-order association cortices was discussed in the somatosensory section of this chapter.

The cells within the visual pathways contribute to a *hierarchy* within the visual system, with each level of the hierarchy increasing the visual abstraction (Hubel, 1988). In addition, Mishkin and Ungerleider (1982) have proposed a model of two visual systems, with *parallel pathways* through which visual information is processed. It has been proposed that these two pathways can be traced back to two main subdivisions of retinal ganglion cells, one of which synapses on the magnocellular layers (processing movement, depth, and coarse detail—processing "where") and the other on the parvocellular layers (processing fine detail, contrast, contours, and color—processing "what") of the LGN (Livingstone & Hubel, 1988; Wurtz & Kandel, 2000b).

One of these pathways, called the "dorsal stream" terminates finally in the posterior parietal region. The second pathway, the "ventral stream" terminates in the inferotemporal cortex. The authors noted that monkeys with lesions in the inferotemporal cortex were very impaired in visual pattern discrimination and recognition, but less impaired in solving tasks involving spatial visual cues. The opposite pattern of results was seen for monkeys with posterior parietal lesions (Milner et al., 1977; Ungerleider & Brody, 1977).

How do we sense motion? The magnocellular pathway continues to areas MT (middle temporal) and MST (medial superior temporal) and the visual motor area of the parietal lobe (the dorsal stream). In area MT, the activity in the neurons is related to the velocity and movement direction of objects. This information is then further processed in area MST for visual perception, pursuit eye movements, and guiding the movements of the body through space. Area MST has also been implicated in the processing of global motion or "optic flow," which plays a role in posture and balance control, giving information on an individual's movement through space (Duffy & Wurtz, 1997).

Object vision, which depends on the ventral pathway to the inferior temporal lobe, includes separate subregions sensitive to different object characteristics. Experiments recording from neurons in the monkey have shown that cells in visual cortex area 2 (V2) analyze object contours, in a further level of abstraction beyond that of V1 in the visual hierarchy. Cells in V4 respond to color and form. A further abstraction occurs in the inferior temporal cortex, where cells have large receptive fields that recognize the same feature anywhere in the visual field, thus allowing us to recognize the same object wherever it is situated in space. Finally, some cells in this area respond only to specific complex inputs, such as faces or hands (Wurtz & Kandel, 2000b).

There is also interesting clinical evidence to support the existence of these parallel processing pathways. There is a perceptual deficit called "movement agnosia," which occurs after damage to the MT or MST region of the cortex, which are part of the "dorsal stream." Patients show a specific loss of motion perception without any other perceptual problems. Other patients with damage to areas of the "ventral stream" lose color vision (achromatopsia) and the ability to identify forms (Wurtz & Kandel, 2000b).

Research by Goodale and Milner (Goodale & Milner, 1992; Goodale et al., 1991) suggests that there may be other functions for the dorsal and ventral streams. They suggest that the visual projection to the parietal cortex provides action-relevant information about the structure and orientation of objects and not just about their position. They also propose that projections to the ventral temporal lobe may provide our conscious visual perceptual experience.

Observations that support this model involve the fact that most neurons in the dorsal stream area show both sensory-related and movement-related activity (Andersen, 1987). In addition, patients with optic ataxia (due to lesions in the parietal areas) have problems not only with reaching in the right direction, but also with positioning their fingers or adjusting the orientation of their hand when reaching toward an object. They also have trouble adjusting their grasp to reflect the size of the object they are picking up. Goodale and colleagues note that damage to the parietal lobe can impair the ability of patients to use information about the size, shape, and orientation of an object to control the hand and fingers during a grasping movement, even though this same information can be used to identify and describe objects.

It is also interesting that the two cortical pathways are different with respect to their access to consciousness. One patient with "ventral stream" lesions had no conscious perception of the orientation or dimension of objects, but she could pick them up with great adeptness. Thus, it may be that information in the dorsal system can be processed without reaching conscious perception. As a result of their analysis of the above observations the authors propose that the ventral stream of projections plays a major role in the perceptual identification of objects, while the dorsal stream mediates the required sensorimotor transformations for visually guided actions directed at those objects (Goodale & Milner, 1992).

How do we take the information processed by these parallel pathways and organize it into a perceptual whole? This process by which the brain recombines information processed in its different regions is called the "binding problem." The recombination of this information appears to require attention, which may be mediated by subcortical structures such as the superior colliculus, as well as cortical areas, such as the posterior parietal and prefrontal cortex. It has been hypothesized that the CNS takes information related to color, size, distance, and orientation and organizes it into a "master map" of the image (Treisman, 1999). Our attentional systems allow us to focus on one small part of the master map as we identify objects or move through space.

One neural mechanism hypothesized to contribute to "binding" everything into one cohesive experience is that information from neural events in many different parts of the cortex (visual, auditory, kinesthetic, memory, etc.) is integrated by the cortex to produce perceptual binding through synchronizing their neural activation patterns, leaving all other neural activations nonsynchronized (Dehaene & Changeux, 2004; Roskies, 1999; Treisman, 1999). This creates a global neuronal workspace.

According to this hypothesis, multiple inputs compete for access to an attentional network, and those that "win" become the contents of conscious experience (Baars, 1993; Delacour, 1997). Behaviorally, the experimenter knows the contents that "won" because they are the pieces of information that a person is able to report on among the many pieces that might be shown to him or her in an experiment.

This theory divides the brain into two separate computational spaces: network processors and a global neuronal workspace. According to this theory there are many subcortical networks in the brain and also much of the cerebral cortex that can be considered to be like modular processing networks for particular types of information (e.g., motion processors or visual word-form processors). But in addition to these processing networks there is a special set of cerebral cortex neurons, the global workspace neurons, which have long-range axons and can send and receive information from modular processors in distant parts of the brain. The unconscious information from the modular processors would be temporarily made available (and therefore conscious) to the global workspace when these processors begin to fire in synchrony with these global neurons. This happens when the signals from the modular processes either becomes strong enough to "catch the attention" of the global neurons (a loud noise for example), or the material they are conveying matches the "interest patterns" that the global workspace deems significant (you shift your focus to something, so the sensory input connected with it suddenly becomes relevant to the processing mechanism of the global workspace). At any moment in time there would be a single global representation of workspace neurons and modular processors that are firing in synchrony and thus part of conscious awareness, with the rest of workspace neurons (neurons in the other processing modules) being inhibited (Woollacott, 2005).

Vestibular System

The vestibular system is sensitive to two types of information: the position of the head in space and sudden changes in the direction of movement of the head. Although we are not consciously aware of vestibular sensation, as we are of the other senses, vestibular inputs are important for the coordination of many motor responses, and these inputs help to stabilize the eyes and to maintain postural stability during stance and walking. Abnormalities within the vestibular system result in sensations such as dizziness or unsteadiness, which do reach our awareness, as well as problems with focusing our eyes and keeping our balance.

Like other sensory systems, the vestibular system can be divided into two parts, a peripheral and a central component. The peripheral component consists of the sensory receptors and eighth cranial nerve, while the central part consists of the four vestibular nuclei as well as the ascending and descending tracts.

Peripheral Receptors

Let us first look at the anatomy of the vestibular system (Fig. 3.11A). The vestibular system is part of the *membranous labyrinth* of the inner ear (right side of figure). The other part of the labyrinth is the *cochlea,* which is concerned with hearing. The membranous labyrinth consists of a continuous series of tubes and sacs located in the temporal bone of the skull. The membranous labyrinth is surrounded by a fluid called *perilymph* and filled with a fluid called *endolymph*. The endolymph has a density greater than water, giving it inertial characteristics that are important to the way the vestibular system functions. The vestibular portion of the labyrinth includes five receptors: three *semicircular canals,* the *utricle,* and the *saccule.*

Semicircular Canals. The semicircular canals function as angular accelerometers. They lie at right angles to each other on either side of the head and are named the anterior, posterior, and horizontal canals (Fig. 3.11). At least one pair is affected by any given angular acceleration of the head or body. The sensory endings of the semicircular canals are in the enlarged end of each canal, which is called the *ampulla,* near its junction with the utricle. Each ampulla has an *ampullary crest,* which contains the vestibular hair cells. The hair cells project upward into the *cupula* (Latin for "small inverted cup"), made of gelatinous material, and extending to the top of the ampulla, preventing movement of the endolymph past the cupula.

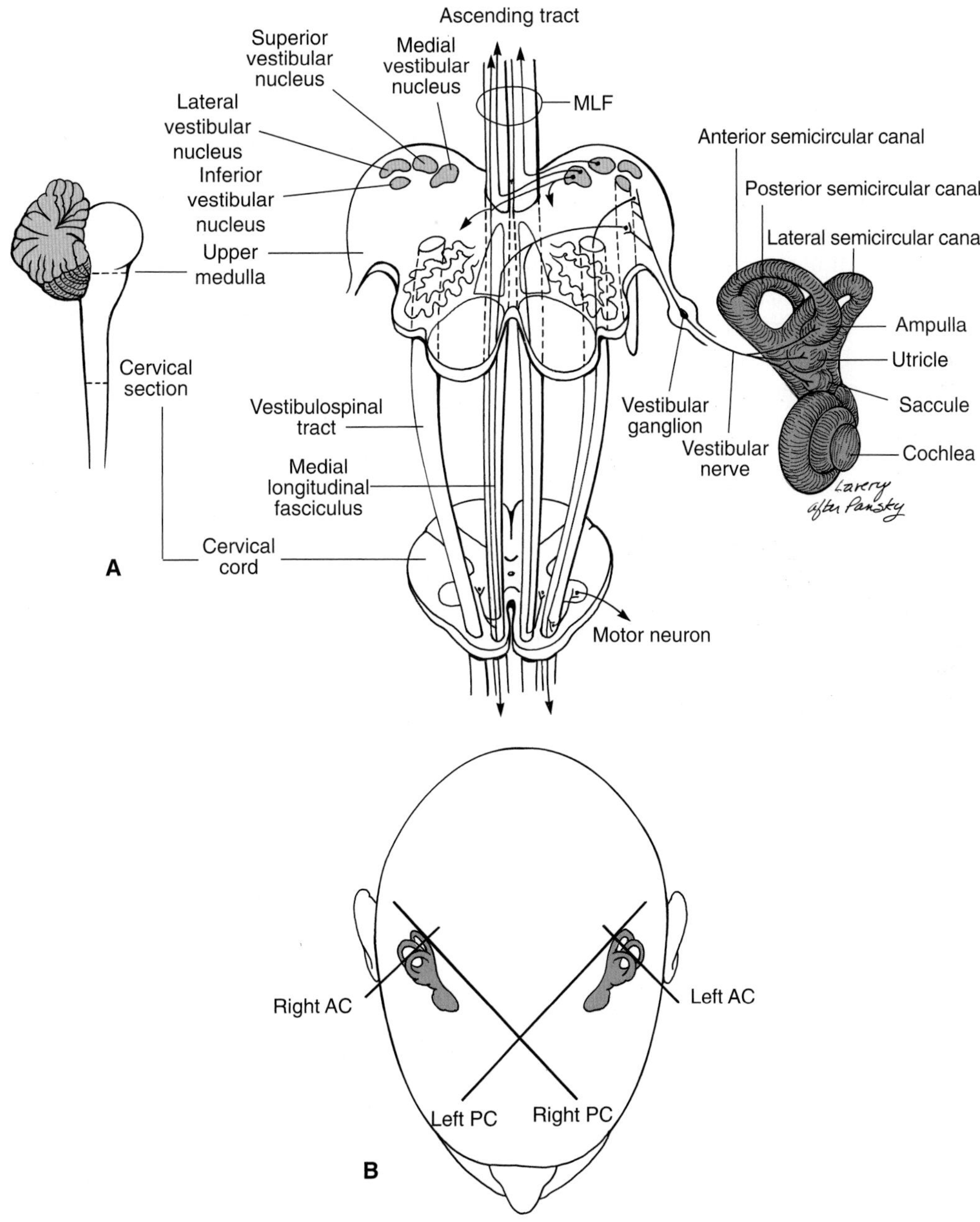

FIGURE 3.11 Vestibular system. A, Membranous labyrinth (otoliths and semicircular canals) and the central connections of the vestibular system. Shown are the ascending vestibular inputs to the oculomotor complex, important for stabilizing gaze, and the descending vestibulospinal system, important for posture and balance. B, The paired semicircular canals within the temporal bone of the skull. Lines show their orientation. AC = anterior canal; PC = posterior canal.

The hair cells are the vestibular receptors and are innervated by bipolar sensory neurons, which are part of the eighth nerve. Their cell bodies are located in the vestibular ganglion (Baloh, 1984; Goldberg & Hudspeth, 2000).

How do the semicircular canals signal head motion to the nervous system? When the head starts to rotate, initially the fluid in the canals does not move because of its inertial characteristics. As a result, the cupula, along with its hair cells, bends in the direction opposite to head movement. When head motion stops, the cupula and hair cells are deflected in the opposite direction, that is, the direction in which the head had been moving.

When the hair cells bend, they cause a change in the firing frequency of the nerve, depending on which way the hair cells are bent. For each hair cell, there is a *kinocilium* (the tallest tuft) and 40 to 70 *stereocilia,* which increase in length as they get closer to the kinocilium. Bending the hair cell toward the kinocilium causes a depolarization of the hair cell and an increase in the firing rate of the bipolar cells of the eighth nerve, and bending away causes hyperpolarization and a decrease in the firing rate of bipolar cells. At rest, the hair cells fire at 100 Hz, so they have a wide range of frequencies for modulation. Thus, increases or decreases in firing frequency of the neurons are possible because of this tonic resting discharge, which occurs in the absence of head motion (Baloh, 1984; Goldberg & Hudspeth, 2000).

Because canals on each side of the head are approximately parallel to one another, they work together in a reciprocal fashion. The two horizontal canals work together, while each anterior canal is paired with a posterior canal on the opposite side of the head, as shown in Figure 3.11B. When head motion occurs in a plane specific to a pair of canals, one canal will be excited, while its paired opposite canal will be hyperpolarized.

Thus, angular motion of the head, either horizontal or vertical, results in either an increase or decrease in hair-cell activity and an opposite change in the frequency of neuronal activity in paired canals. Receptors in the semicircular canal are very sensitive: they respond to angular accelerations of 0.1 degree per second^2, but do not respond to steady-state motion of the head. During prolonged motion of the head, the cupula returns to its resting position, and firing frequency in the neurons returns to its steady state.

Utricle and Saccule. The utricle and saccule provide information about body position with reference to the force of gravity and linear acceleration or movement of the head in a straight line. On the wall of these structures is a thickening where the epithelium contains hair cells. This area is called the *macula* (Latin for "spot") and is where the receptor cells are located. The hair cells project tufts or processes up into a gelatinous membrane, the *otolith organ* (Greek, from "lithos," meaning "stone"). The otolith organ has many calcium carbonate crystals called *otoconia,* or otoliths (Goldberg & Hudspeth, 2000).

The macula of the utricle lies in the horizontal plane when the head is held horizontally (normal position), so the otoliths rest upon it. But if the head is tilted, or accelerates, the hair cells are bent by the movement of the gelatinous mass. The macula of the saccule lies in the vertical plane when the head is positioned normally, so it responds selectively to vertically directed linear forces. As in the semicircular canals, hair cells in the otoliths respond to bending in a directional manner.

Central Connections

Vestibular Nuclei. Neurons from both the otoliths and the semicircular canals go through the eighth nerve and have their cell bodies in the vestibular ganglion (Scarpa's ganglion). The axons then enter the brain in the pons, and most go to the floor of the medulla, where the vestibular nuclei are located, as shown in Figure 3.11A, center. There are four nuclei in the complex: the *lateral vestibular nucleus* (Deiters'), the *medial vestibular nucleus,* the *superior vestibular nucleus,* and the *inferior,* or *descending, vestibular* nucleus. A certain portion of the vestibular sensory receptors goes directly to the cerebellum, the reticular formation, the thalamus, and the cerebral cortex.

The lateral vestibular nucleus receives input from the utricle, semicircular canals, cerebellum, and spinal cord. The output contributes to vestibulo-ocular tracts and to the lateral vestibulospinal tract, which activates antigravity muscles in the neck, trunk, and limbs.

Inputs to the medial and superior nuclei are from the semicircular canals. The outputs of the medial nucleus are to the medial vestibulospinal tract (MVST), with connections to the cervical spinal cord, controlling the neck muscles. The MVST plays an important role in coordinating interactions between head and eye movements. In addition, neurons from the medial and superior nuclei ascend to motor nuclei of the eye muscles and aid in stabilizing gaze during head motions.

The inputs to the inferior vestibular nucleus include neurons from the semicircular canals, utricle, saccule, and cerebellar vermis, while the outputs are part of the vestibulospinal tract and vestibuloreticular tracts.

Ascending information from the vestibular system to the oculomotor complex is responsible for the *vestibulo-ocular* reflex, which rotates the eyes opposite to head movement, allowing the gaze to remain steady on an image even when the head is moving.

Vestibular nystagmus is the rapid alternating movement of the eyes in response to continued rotation of the body. One can create vestibular nystagmus in a subject by rotating the person seated on a stool to the left: when the acceleration first begins, the eyes go slowly to the right, to keep the eyes on a single point in space. When the eyes reach the end of the orbit, they "reset" by moving rapidly to the left; then they move again slowly to the right.

This alternating slow movement of the eyes in the direction opposite head movement, and rapid resetting of the eyes in the direction of head movement, is called "nystagmus." It is a normal consequence of acceleration of the head. However, when nystagmus occurs without head movement it is usually an indication of dysfunction in the peripheral or central nervous system.

Postrotatory nystagmus is a reversal in the direction of nystagmus; it occurs when a person who is spinning stops abruptly. Postrotatory nystagmus has been used clinically to evaluate the function of the vestibular system.

The vestibular apparatus has both static and dynamic functions. The dynamic functions are controlled mainly by the semicircular canals, allowing us to sense head rotation and angular accelerations, and allowing the control of the eyes through the vestibulo-ocular reflexes. The static functions are controlled by the utricle and saccule, allowing us to monitor absolute position of the head in space, and are important in posture. (The utricle and saccule also detect linear acceleration, a dynamic function.)

ACTION SYSTEMS

The action system includes areas of the nervous system such as motor cortex, brainstem, cerebellum, and basal ganglia, which perform processing essential to the coordination of movement.

In our example presented in the beginning of this chapter, you are thirsty and want to pour some milk from the carton in front of you into a glass. We have already seen how sensory structures help you form the map of your body in space and locate the milk carton relative to your arm. Now you need to generate the movements that will allow you to pick up the carton and pour the milk. You will need a plan to move, you will need to specify specific muscles (both timing and force), and you will need a way to modify and refine the movement. So let us look at the structures that allow you to do that.

Motor Cortex

Primary Motor Cortex and Corticospinal Tract

The motor cortex is situated in the frontal lobe and consists of a number of different processing areas, including the *primary motor cortex* (MI) and two premotor cortical areas, including the *supplementary motor area* (SMA), (occasionally called MII), and the *premotor cortex,* shown in Figure 3.12A. These areas interact with sensory processing areas in the parietal lobe and also with basal ganglia and cerebellar areas to identify where we want to move, to plan the movement, and finally, to execute our actions (Krakauer & Ghez, 2000).

All three of these areas have their own somatotopic maps of the body, so if different regions are stimulated, different muscles and body parts move. The primary motor cortex (Brodmann's area 4) contains a very complex map of the body. Early experiments suggested a one-to-one correspondence between cells stimulated in the primary motor cortex and the activation of individual alpha motor neurons in the spinal cord; however, more recently it has been shown that the same muscles can be activated from several sites in the cortex, suggesting that neurons from several motor cortex areas project to the same muscle. In addition, it has been found that most stimuli from the primary motor cortex activate many muscles. However, stimulations tend to activate simple movements of single joints. In contrast, stimulation of neurons in the premotor areas typically activates multiple muscles at multiple joints, giving rise to more coordinated movements. The motor map, or motor homunculus (shown in Fig. 3.12B), is similar to the sensory map in the way it distorts the representations of the body. In both cases, the areas that require the most detailed control (the mouth, throat, and hand), allowing finely graded movements, are most highly represented (Penfield & Rassmussen, 1950).

Inputs to the motor areas come from the basal ganglia, the cerebellum, and sensory areas, including the periphery (via the thalamus), SI, and sensory association areas in the parietal lobe. Interestingly, MI neurons receive sensory inputs from their own muscles and also from the skin above the muscles. It has been suggested that this transcortical pathway might be used in parallel with the spinal reflex pathway to give additional force output in the muscles when an unexpected load is encountered during a movement. This pathway has also been hypothesized to be an important proprioceptive pathway functioning in postural control.

Outputs from the primary motor cortex contribute to the *corticospinal tract* (also called the *pyramidal tract*)

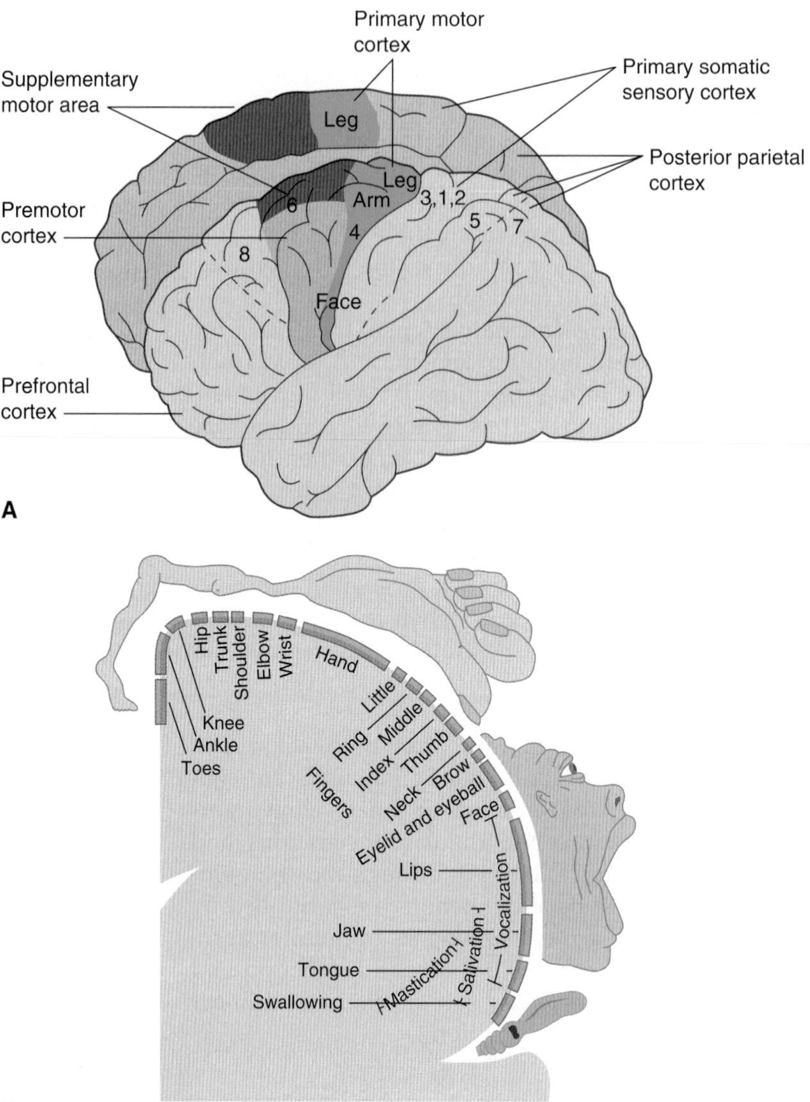

FIGURE 3.12 Motor cortex. A, Lateral view of the brain showing the location of the primary motor cortex, supplementary motor area, and premotor cortex. B, Motor homunculus. (Adapted from Kandel ER, Schwartz JH, Jessell TM, eds. Principles of neuroscience, 3rd ed. New York: Elsevier, 1991:610, 613.)

and often make excitatory monosynaptic connections onto alpha motor neurons, in addition to polysynaptic connections to gamma motor neurons, which control muscle spindle length. In addition to their monosynaptic connections, corticospinal neurons make many polysynaptic connections through interneurons within the spinal cord.

The corticospinal tract, shown in Figure 3.13, includes neurons from primary motor cortex (about 50%), and premotor areas including supplementary motor cortex, dorsal and ventral premotor cortex, and even somatosensory cortex. The fibers descend ipsilaterally from the cortex through the internal capsule, the midbrain, and the medulla. In the medulla, the fibers concentrate to form "pyramids," and near the junction of the medulla and the spinal cord, most (90%) cross to form the lateral corticospinal tract, controlling precise movements of the distal muscles of the limbs. The remaining 10% continue uncrossed to form the anterior (or ventral) corticospinal tract, controlling less precise movements of the proximal muscles of the limbs and trunk. The majority of the anterior corticospinal neurons cross just before they terminate in the ventral horn of the spinal cord. Most axons enter the ventral horn and terminate in the intermediate and ventral areas on interneurons and motor neurons.

What is the specific function of primary motor cortex and corticospinal tract in movement control? Evarts (1968) recorded the activity of corticospinal neurons in monkeys while they made wrist flexion and extension movements. He found that the firing rate of the corticospinal neurons codes: (a) the force

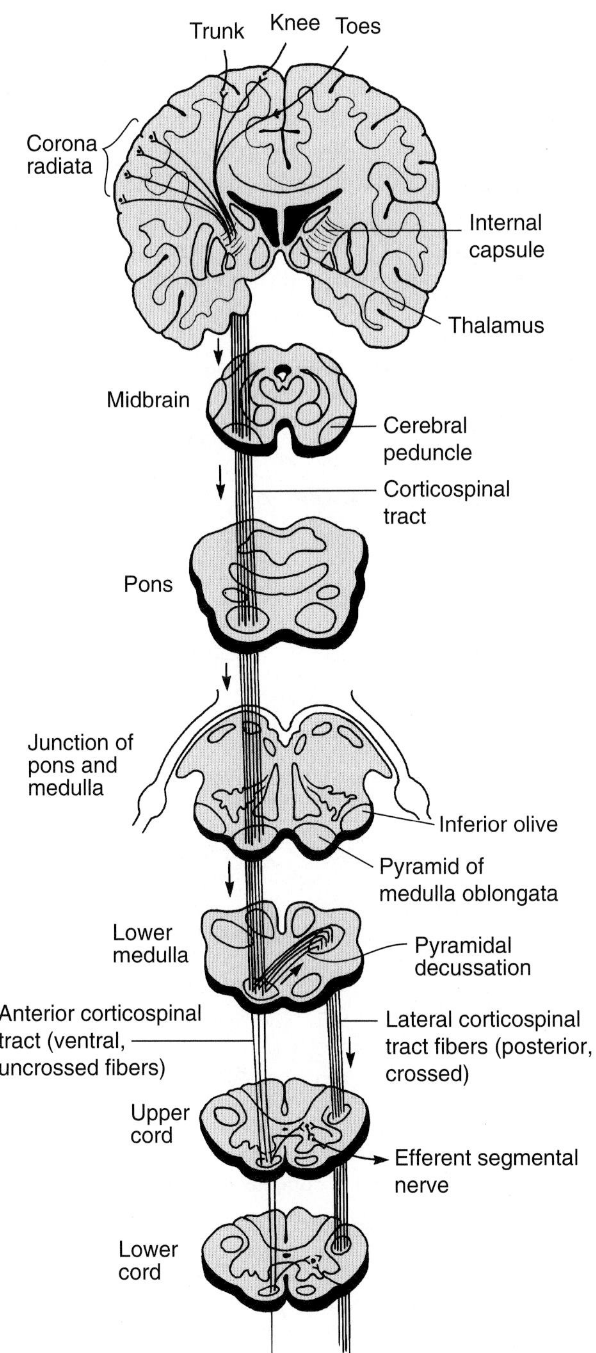

FIGURE 3.13 Pyramidal (corticospinal) tract, including lateral (crossed) and ventromedial (uncrossed) pathways.

used to move a limb, and (b) in some cases, the rate of change of force. Thus, both absolute force and the speed of a movement are controlled by the primary motor cortex.

Now, think about a typical movement that we make—reaching for the carton of milk, for example. How does the motor cortex encode the execution of such a complex movement? Georgopoulos et al. (1982) performed experiments in which a monkey made arm movements to many different targets around a central starting point. They found that there were specific movement directions for which each neuron was activated maximally, yet each responded for a wide range of movement directions. To explain how movements could be finely controlled when neurons are so broadly tuned, these researchers suggested that actions are controlled by a population of neurons. The activity of each of the neurons can be represented as a vector, whose length represents the degree of activity in any direction. The sum of the vectors of all the neurons would then predict the movement direction and amplitude.

If this is the case, does it mean that whenever we make a movement, for example, with our hand, the exact same neurons are activated in the primary motor cortex? No. It has been shown that specific neurons in the cortex, activated when we pick up an object, may remain totally silent when we make a similar movement, such as a gesture in anger. This is a very important point to understand because it implies that there are many parallel motor pathways for carrying out an action sequence, just as there are parallel pathways for sensory processing. Thus, simply by training a patient in one situation, we cannot automatically assume that the training will transfer to all other activities requiring the same set of muscles (Krakauer & Ghez, 2000).

Supplementary Motor and Premotor Areas

What are the functions of the supplementary motor area (SMA), and the premotor area? Each of these areas send projections to primary motor cortex and also to the spinal cord. Surprisingly, there are direct monosynaptic connections from premotor neurons to motor nuclei of the hand and proximal limb muscles, suggesting that these neurons can control movements separately from the primary cortex. In addition, these areas receive largely distinct inputs from the thalamus and other cortical areas. This suggests that they may have very different functions.

Each of these areas controls different aspects of motor planning and motor learning. Movements that are initiated internally are controlled primarily by the SMA. (In fact, the negative preparatory or Bereitschafts potential electroencephalogram recorded when subjects are getting ready to make a movement appears to be associated with activity in the SMA.) This area also contributes to activating the motor programs involved in learned sequences. The learning of sequences themselves also involves the presupplementary motor area. The presupplementary motor area is the rostral extension of the SMA. However, when sequences become overlearned with extensive training, the control of the movement sequence can be transferred to the primary motor cortex (Krakauer & Ghez, 2000).

Movements that are activated by external stimuli (e.g., a visual cue such as a traffic light changing from red to green) are controlled primarily by the lateral premotor area (dorsal and ventral premotor cortex). These areas control how stimuli are to be used to direct the action, specifically associating a given sensory event with a movement to be made. This is defined as associative learning (see Chapters 2 and 4 for more details). Monkeys that have lesions in this area are unable to learn new tasks involving associating a specific stimulus with a movement they are to make, although they can execute the movements without a problem.

Research by Mushiake et al. (1991) supports the hypothesis that premotor and supplementary motor areas differ in their activity depending on how the movement is initiated and guided. They found that premotor neurons were more active when a sequential task was visually guided, while supplementary motor area neurons were more active when the sequence was remembered and self-determined.

Previous researchers had proposed a hypothesis about the functional specialization of the SMA and PM based on different phylogenetic origins, with the SMA being specialized for controlling internally referenced motor output and the PM area specialized for control of externally referenced motor acts (Roland et al., 1980; Passingham, 1985). Studies also indicate that premotor lesions cause impairment of retrieval of movements in accordance with visual cues, while SMA lesions disrupt retrieval of self-initiated movements (Passingham, 1985; Passingham et al., 1989).

Interestingly, the supplementary motor area receives inputs from the putamen of the basal ganglia complex, while the premotor area receives inputs from the cerebellum. In Parkinson's disease there is massive depletion of dopamine in the putamen, and patients with Parkinson's disease have difficulty with self-initiating movements such as walking. Thus, Parkinson's disease may cause impaired input to the supplementary cortex, which results in bradykinesia or slowness in initiating movement (Marsden, 1989).

Works by Roland and others (Lang et al., 1990; Roland et al., 1980) have examined the role of the supplementary cortex in humans and have begun to clarify its functions. Roland et al. (1980) asked subjects to perform tasks ranging from very simple to complex movements, and while they were making the movements, the investigators assessed the amount of cerebral blood flow in different areas of the brain. (To measure blood flow, one injects short-lived radioactive tracer into the blood, then measures the radioactivity in different brain areas with detectors on the scalp.)

As shown in Figure 3.14, when subjects were asked to perform a simple task (simple repetitive movements of the index finger or pressing a spring between the thumb and index finger) the blood flow increase was only in primary motor and sensory cortex. In contrast, when they were asked to perform a complex task (a sequence of movements involving all

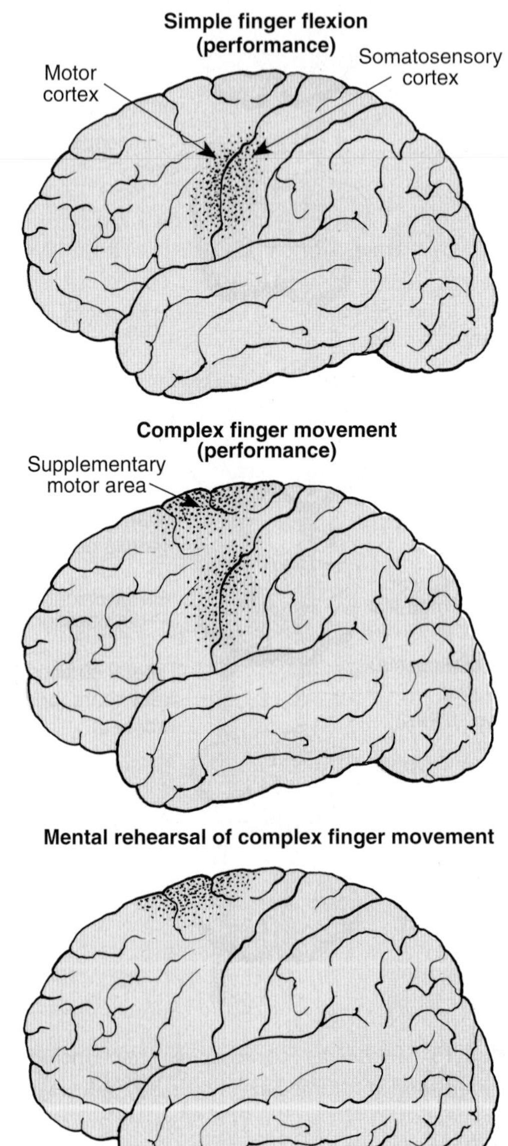

FIGURE 3.14 Changes in blood flow during different motor behaviors, indicating the areas of the motor cortex involved in the behavior. (Adapted with permission from Roland PE, Larsen B, Lassen NA, Skinhof E. Supplementary motor area and other cortical areas in organization of voluntary movements in man. J Neurophysiol 1980;43:118–136.)

four fingers, touching the thumb in different orders), subjects showed a blood flow increase in the supplementary motor area, bilaterally, and the primary motor and sensory areas. Finally, when they were asked to rehearse the task, but not perform it, the blood flow increase was only in the supplementary motor area, not the primary sensory or motor cortex. Roland et al. concluded that the supplementary area is active when a sequence of simple ballistic movements is planned. Thus, they proposed that it participates in the assembly of the central motor program or forms a motor subroutine.

Research suggests that two separate pathways from the parietal cortex to the premotor areas control reaching and grasping. The reaching pathway originates in the parieto-occipital area and terminates in the dorsal premotor area, with some neurons synapsing in other areas en route. This pathway uses visual information about object location in three-dimensional space to control the direction of reaching movements. The grasping pathway originates in the dorsal extrastriate area of the occipital cortex and terminates in the ventral premotor area, with relays to other areas. This pathway uses visual information about object characteristics (shape, size, etc.) to control hand shaping for grasping (Krakauer & Ghez, 2000).

Work by Rizzolatti and colleagues (1988) suggests an interesting function of the ventral premotor area (F5) in reaching. They recorded from single neurons in F5 in monkeys during reaching. They found that an important property of most (85%) of these neurons was their selectivity for different types of hand grip: precision grip (most common), finger prehension, and whole-hand prehension. Interestingly, precision grip neurons were activated only by small visual objects (Jeannerod et al., 1995; Taira et al., 1990).

Higher-Level Association Areas

Association Areas of the Frontal Regions

The association areas of the frontal regions (areas rostral to Brodmann's area 6) are important for motor planning and other cognitive behaviors. For example, these areas have been hypothesized to integrate sensory information and then select the appropriate motor response from the many possible responses (Fuster, 1989).

The prefrontal cortex may be divided into the principal sulcus and the prefrontal convexities. Experiments have indicated that the neurons of the principal sulcus are involved in the strategic planning of higher motor functions. For example, monkeys with lesions in this area had difficulty performing spatial tasks in which information had to be stored in working memory in order to guide future action. This area is densely interconnected with the posterior parietal areas. These areas are hypothesized to work closely together in spatial tasks that require attention.

Lesions in the prefrontal convexity, in contrast, cause problems in performing any kind of delayed response task. Animals with these lesions have problems with tasks for which they have to inhibit certain motor responses at specific moments. Lesions in adjacent areas cause problems with a monkey's ability to select from a variety of motor responses when they are given different sensory cues (Kupfermann, 1991).

Lesions in other prefrontal regions cause patients to have difficulty with changing strategies when they are asked to. Even when they are shown their errors, they fail to correct them.

Cerebellum

The cerebellum is considered one of three important brain areas contributing to coordination of movement, in addition to the motor cortex and basal ganglia. Yet despite its important role in the coordination of movement, the cerebellum does not play a primary role in either sensory or motor function. If the cerebellum is destroyed, we do not lose sensation or become paralyzed. However, lesions of the cerebellum do produce devastating changes in our ability to perform movements, from the very simple to the most elegant. The cerebellum receives afferent information from almost every sensory system, consistent with its role as a regulator of motor output (Ghez & Thatch, 2000; Ito, 1984).

How does the cerebellum adjust the output of the motor systems? Its function is related to its neuronal circuitry. Through this circuitry and its input and output connections, it appears to act as a comparator, a system that compensates for errors by comparing intention with performance.

The cerebellum's input and output connections are vital to its role as error detector, and they are summarized in Figure 3.15. It receives information from other modules of the brain related to the programming and execution of movements (corticopontine areas). This information is often referred to as "efference copy" or "corollary discharge" when it comes from the primary motor cortex, since it is hypothesized to be a direct copy of the motor cortex output to the spinal cord. The cerebellum also receives sensory feedback information (reafference) from the receptors about the movements as they are being made (spinal/trigeminal somatosensory inputs, visual, auditory, and vestibular inputs).

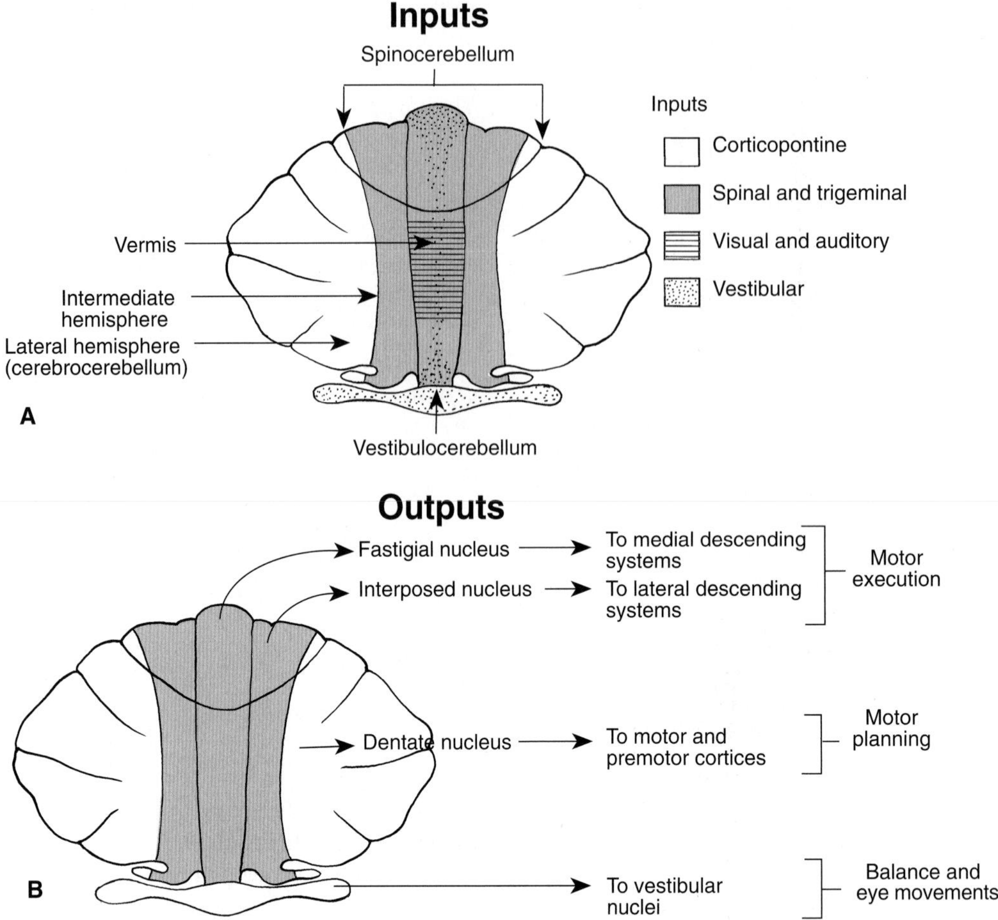

FIGURE 3.15 Basic anatomy of the cerebellum, including: A, its inputs; and B, its outputs. The white area represents the lateral cerebellum with inputs from the corticopontine systems. The shaded area represents the spinocerebellum with inputs from the spinal and trigeminal somatosensory systems. The stippled (visual and auditory) and lined (vestibular) areas receive inputs from other sensory systems. (Adapted from Ghez C. The cerebellum. In: Kandel ER, Schwartz JH, Jessell TM, eds. Principles of neuroscience, 3rd ed. New York: Elsevier, 1991:633.)

After processing this information, outputs (Fig. 3.15B) from the cerebellum go to the motor cortex and other systems within the brainstem to modulate their motor output. In addition to its role in motor control processes, research has also suggested that the cerebellum may have important nonmotor functions, including cognition, which will be discussed below (Fiez et al., 1992).

Anatomy of the Cerebellum

An understanding of the anatomy of the cerebellum is helpful in explaining its function. The cerebellum consists of an outer layer of gray matter (the cortex), internal white matter (input and output fibers), and three pairs of *deep nuclei:* the *fastigial nucleus,* the *interposed nucleus,* and the *dentate nucleus.* All the inputs to the cerebellum go first to one of these three deep cerebellar nuclei and then go on to the cortex. All the outputs of the cerebellum go back to the deep nuclei, before going on to the cerebral cortex or the brainstem (Ghez & Thatch 2000; Ito, 1984).

The cerebellum can be divided into three phylogenetic zones (see Fig. 3.15). The oldest zone corresponds to the flocculonodular lobe and is functionally related to the vestibular system. The phylogenetically more recent areas to develop are: (a) the *vermis* and *intermediate* part of the hemispheres and (b) the *lateral hemispheres,* respectively. These three parts of the cerebellum have distinct functions and distinct input–output connections, as you see in Figure 3.15.

Flocculonodular Lobe. The flocculonodular lobe, often referred to as the "vestibulocerebellum," receives inputs from both the visual system and the vestibular system, and its outputs return to the vestibular nuclei. It functions in the control of the axial muscles, which are used in equilibrium control. If a patient experiences dysfunction in this system, one observes an ataxic gait, wide-based stance and nystagmus.

Vermis and Intermediate Hemispheres. The vermis and intermediate hemispheres, often referred to as the "spinocerebellum," receive proprioceptive and cutaneous inputs from the spinal cord (via the spinocerebellar tracts), in addition to visual, vestibular, and auditory information. Researchers used to think that there were two maps of the complete body in the cerebellum, but now it has been shown that the maps are much more complex and can be divided into many smaller maps. This has been called "fractured somatotopy." These smaller maps appear to be related to functional activities; thus, in the rat, the mouth and paw receptive fields are positioned close together, possibly to contribute to the control of grooming behavior. Inputs to this part of the cerebellum go through the fastigial nucleus (vermis) and interposed nucleus (intermediate lobes) (Shambes et al., 1978).

There are four spinocerebellar tracts that relay information from the spinal cord to the cerebellum. Two tracts relay information from the arms and the neck and two relay information from the trunk and legs. Inputs are also from the spino-olivo-cerebellar tract, through the inferior olivary nucleus (climbing fibers). These inputs are important in learning and will be discussed later.

What are the output pathways of the spinocerebellum? The outputs go to the: (a) brainstem reticular formation, (b) vestibular nuclei, (c) thalamus and motor cortex, and (d) red nucleus in the midbrain.

What are the functions of the vermis and intermediate lobes (spinocerebellum)? First, they appear to function in the control of the actual execution of movement: they correct for deviations from an intended movement through comparing feedback from the spinal cord with the intended motor command. They also modulate muscle tone. This occurs through the continuous output of excitatory activity from the fastigial and interpositus nucleus, which modulates the activity of the gamma motor neurons to the muscle spindles. When there are lesions in these nuclei, there is a significant drop in muscle tone (hypotonia) (Ghez & Thatch, 2000).

Finally, the spinocerebellum is involved in feedforward mechanisms to regulate movements. This was discovered in experiments on monkeys in which the dentate and interposed nuclei of this part of the cerebellum were temporarily cooled while they were making precise elbow flexion movements (by activating the biceps muscle) back to a target after the arm was moved. When the cerebellar nuclei were cooled, the triceps muscle, used to keep the arm from overshooting its target, was no longer activated in a feedforward manner, but only in a feedback manner, after being stretched when the biceps moved the elbow too far (Ghez & Thatch, 2000; Vilis & Hore, 1980).

Lateral Hemispheres. The last part of the cerebellum, and the newest phylogenetically, is the lateral zone of the cerebellar hemispheres, often called the "cerebrocerebellum" (see Fig. 3.15). It has undergone a marked expansion in the course of human evolution, which has added many nonmotor functions to its repertoire. It receives inputs from the pontine nuclei in the brainstem, which relay information from wide areas of the cerebral cortex (sensory, motor, premotor, and posterior parietal). Its outputs are to the thalamus and then to the motor, premotor, and prefrontal cortex (Middleton & Strick, 1994).

What is the function of the lateral hemispheres? This part of the cerebellum appears to have a number of higher-level functions involving both motor and nonmotor skills. First, research suggests that it is involved in the planning or preparation of movement and the evaluation of sensory information for action as a part of the motor learning process. In contrast, the intermediate lobes function in movement execution and fine-tuning of ongoing movement via feedback information. It appears that the lateral hemispheres of the cerebellum participate in programming the motor cortex for the execution of movement. For example, lateral cerebellar lesions disrupt the timing of movements, so that joints are moved sequentially rather than simultaneously. This deficit is referred to as "decomposition of movement." During a reach-and-grasp movement, grasp formation begins during the transport phase. However, lesions of the cerebrocerebellum disrupt this coordination so that reaching and grasping occur sequentially instead of simultaneously. The cerebellar pathways are a part of many parallel pathways affecting the motor cortex.

Cerebellar Involvement in Nonmotor Tasks

In addition to its role in motor control processes, research has suggested that the lateral cerebellum may have important nonmotor functions, including cognition (Fiez et al., 1992). It is interesting to note that neuroanatomical experiments have shown projections from the lateral dentate nucleus of the cerebellum to frontal association areas known to be involved in higher-level cognitive processing (Middleton & Strick, 1994). These connections suggest that subjects do not have to make a movement to activate the cerebellum; research measuring cerebral blood flow has shown that there is an increase in cerebellar activity when subjects are asked only to imagine making a movement (Decety et al., 1990).

Ivry and Keele (1989) have shown that the cerebellum has important timing functions, with patients with cerebellar lesions showing problems in both timing production and perception. Patients with lateral hemisphere lesions showed errors in timing related to perceptual abilities, which researchers think may be related to a central clock-like mechanism. In contrast patients with intermediate-lobe lesions made errors related to movement execution.

Many parts of the cerebellum, including the lateral cerebellum seem to be important in both motor and nonmotor learning. The unique cellular circuitry of the cerebellum has been shown to be perfect for the long-term modification of motor responses, including simple types of learning, such as adaptation. Experiments have shown that as animals learn a new task, the climbing fiber (which detects movement error) changes the effectiveness of the synapse between the granule-cell parallel fiber and the Purkinje cells (the main output cells of the cerebellum) (Gilbert & Thatch, 1977).

This type of cerebellar learning also appears to occur in the vestibulo-ocular reflex (VOR) circuitry, which includes cerebellar pathways. The VOR keeps the eyes fixed on an object when the head turns. In experiments in which humans wore prismatic lenses that reversed the image on the eye, adaptation of the gain of the VOR occurred over time, with the size of the reflex progressively reducing and then reversing in direction. This modification of the reflex did not occur in patients with cerebellar lesions (Gonshor & Melville-Jones, 1976). The cerebellum may also contribute to associative learning, and specifically, classical conditioning, as lesions to the cerebellum constrain the ability of animals to acquire and retain the eye-blink reflex (Ghez & Thatch, 2000).

Studies have shown that the right lateral cerebellum becomes active when subjects read verbs aloud, but not when they read nouns, implying that something about the cognitive processing of verb generation requires the cerebellum, whereas the same processing of other words does not. Correlated with this, certain patients with cerebellar deficits also showed difficulty in these verb-generation tasks and in learning and performing a variety of tasks involving complex nonmotor (cognitive) cortical processing. This is the case even though scores on intelligence, language, "frontal function," and memory were normal. For example, patients showed problems in detecting errors they made in nonmotor as well as motor tasks. This implies that they had problems with both perception and production processes in higher-order analyses, including those involving language (Fiez et al., 1992).

Research on learning problems in patients with cerebellar lesions has shown that while they had normal scores on the Wechsler Memory Scale, they had problems with some types of learned responses. In particular, problems were found in recalling habits, defined as automatic responses learned through repetition. This is opposite to the learning problems seen in patients with severe amnesia (resulting from hippocampal and/or midline diencephalic damage), who do not learn tasks that rely on conscious recall of previous experience, but show normal improvement on a variety of skill-learning tasks that involve repetition (Squire, 1986; Fiez et al., 1992).

It is interesting to note that certain neurons in the dentate nucleus of the cerebellum are preferentially involved in the generation and/or guidance of movement based on visual cues. As mentioned earlier, these neurons project to the premotor areas of the cerebral cortex (Mushiake & Strick, 1993). Experiments have shown that patients with cerebellar deficits showed improved motor performance when their eyes were closed or when visual feedback was reduced. In fact, Sanes et al. (1988) noted that cerebellar tremor was greatest when patients used visual cues to guide movements.

Basal Ganglia

The basal ganglia complex consists of a set of nuclei at the base of the cerebral cortex, including the *putamen, caudate nucleus, globus pallidus, subthalamic nucleus,* and *substantia nigra. Basal* literally means "at the base," or in other words, "just below the cortex." As with patients with cerebellar lesions, patients with damage to the basal ganglia are not paralyzed, but have problems with the coordination of movement. Advancement in our understanding of the function of basal ganglia first came from clinicians, especially James Parkinson, who in 1817 first described Parkinson's disease as "the shaking palsy" (Cote & Crutcher, 1991).

The basal ganglia were once believed to be part of the extrapyramidal motor system, which was believed to act in parallel with the pyramidal system (the corticospinal tract) in movement control. Thus, clinicians defined pyramidal problems as relating to spasticity and paralysis, while extrapyramidal problems were defined as involuntary movements and rigidity. As we have seen in this chapter, this distinction is no longer valid, since many other brain systems also control movement. In addition, the pyramidal and extrapyramidal systems are not independent, but work together in controlling movements.

Anatomy of the Basal Ganglia

The major connections of the basal ganglia are summarized in Figure 3.16, including the major afferent

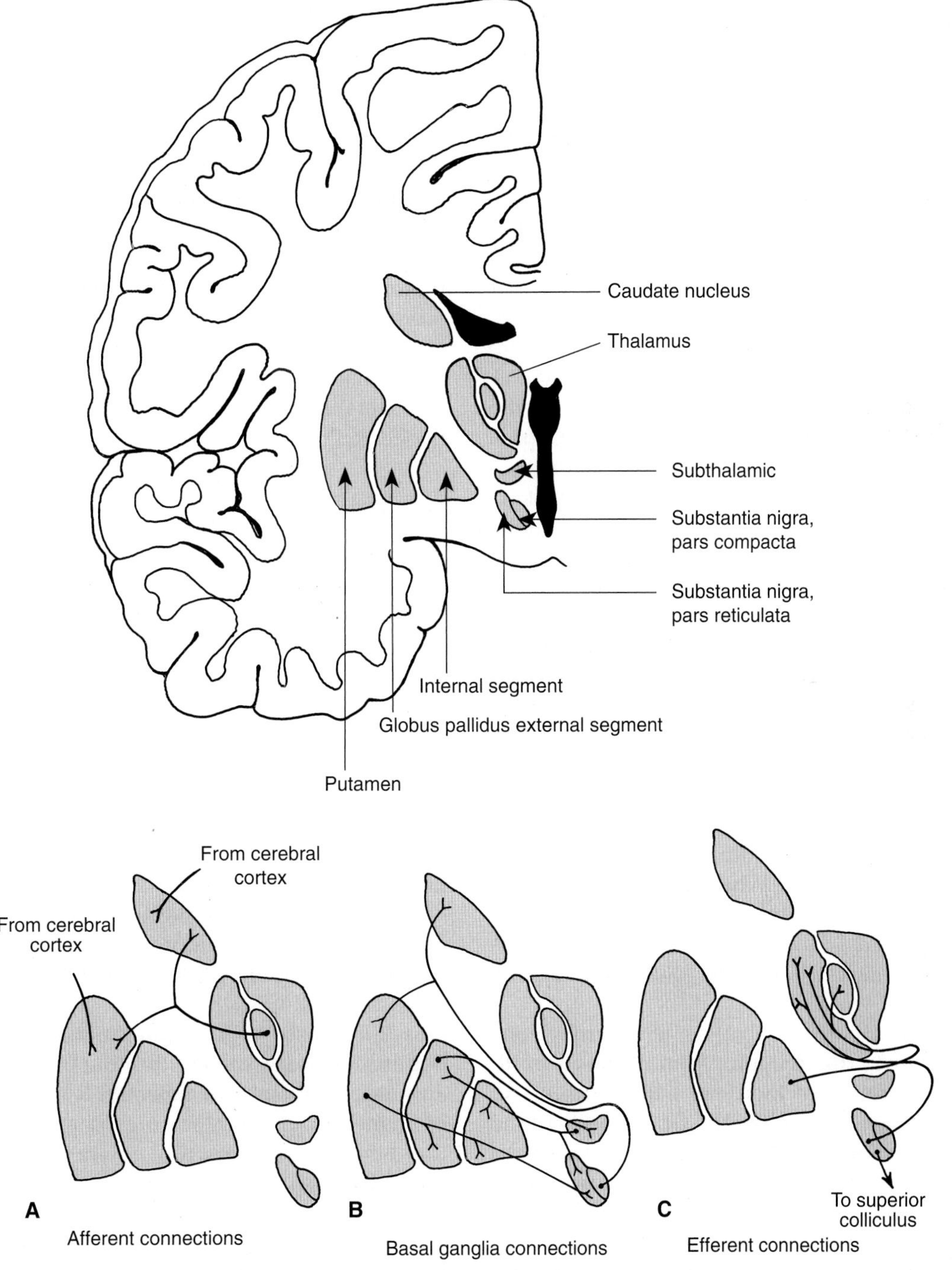

FIGURE 3.16 Top, Locations of the nuclei of the basal ganglia complex. Bottom, A, the major afferent; B, internal; and C, efferent connections of the basal ganglia. (Adapted from Cote L, Crutcher MD. The basal ganglia. In: Kandel ER, Schwartz JH, Jessell TM, eds. Principles of neuroscience. 3rd ed. New York: Elsevier, 1991:649.)

(Fig. 3.16A), internal (Fig. 3.16B), and efferent (Fig. 3.16C) connections. The main input nuclei of the basal ganglia complex are the caudate and the putamen. The caudate and the putamen develop from the same structure and are often discussed as a single unit, the *striatum*. Their primary inputs are from widespread areas of the neocortex, including sensory, motor, and association areas (Alexander & Crutcher, 1990).

The globus pallidus has two segments, internal and external (GPi and GPe), and is situated next to the putamen, while the substantia nigra is situated a little more caudally, in the midbrain, as shown in the top half of Figure 3.16. The internal segment of the globus pallidus (GPi) and the substantia nigra (SN) are the major output areas of the basal ganglia. Their outputs terminate in the prefrontal, supplementary, and premotor cortex areas, by way of the thalamus. The final nucleus, the subthalamic nucleus (STN), is situated just below the thalamus.

The connections within the basal ganglia are complex. The striatum receives direct excitatory cortical inputs and projects to the output nuclei of the basal ganglia (the GPi) and the substantia nigra pars reticulata (SNr) through two major projection systems, "direct" and "indirect" pathways (Nambu et al., 2002). The direct pathway begins with projections from the cortex to the striatum, which project monosynaptically to the GPi/SNr. The Gpi projects to the thalamus, which then projects back to the cortex. The connections from the cortex to the striatum are excitatory, while the connections from the striatum to the GPi and from the GPi to the thalamus are inhibitory. The connections from the thalamus back to the cortex are excitatory. How does activity in the direct pathway facilitate movement? The cortex excites the striatum, which then inhibits the GPi through the direct pathway. The GPi is normally tonically active and inhibitory to the thalamus. When the GPi is inhibited, this reduces the tonic inhibitory influence of the thalamus (this is called "disinhibition"), increasing excitatory drive to the cortex and reinforcing the desired movement.

The indirect pathway begins with projections from the cortex to the striatum, from the striatum to the external segment of the Gpe, which projects to the STN, and then to the Gpi. The Gpi projects to the thalamus, which projects back to the cortex. The projections from the striatum to the Gpe, and from GPe to STN are inhibitory, while the projections from the STN to the Gpi are excitatory. How does activity in the indirect pathway inhibit unwanted movement? Input from the cortex excites the striatum, which then inhibits Gpe. Since Gpe is inhibitory to the STN, the STN becomes more active and excites the Gpi. Increased activation of the Gpi inhibits the thalamus, and as a result the thalamus does not excite the cortex. In this way, activation of the indirect pathway by the striatum causes a relative inhibition of movement.

A third "hyperdirect" pathway has also been proposed, whereby the STN receives inputs from the cerebral cortex and, in turn, sends outputs to the GPi/SNr. The cortico-STN-pallidal "hyperdirect" pathway has a powerful excitatory effect on the output nuclei of the basal ganglia, which results in inhibition of large areas of the thalamus and cerebral cortex (Nambu et al., 2002).

The basal ganglia really consist of four different functional circuits that also include the thalamus and the cortex. These comprise the skeletomotor circuit (including the premotor cortex, supplementary motor cortex and primary motor cortex), the oculomotor circuit (including the frontal and supplementary eye fields of the cortex), the prefrontal circuits, and the limbic circuit. The existence of these different functional circuits explains the variety of movement disorders involving the dysfunction of basal ganglia (DeLong, 2000).

Role of the Basal Ganglia

The skeletomotor circuit contributes to both the preparation for and execution of movement. For example, it has been shown that many neurons in the premotor areas and in the basal ganglia skeletomotor circuitry show changes in activity after the presentation of a cue that gives information on a movement to be made later. The activity continues until the movement is made. This is referred to as "motor set." Other subsets of neurons in the skeletomotor circuitry show only movement-related responses, indicating that there are separate populations of neurons for these two functions (DeLong, 2000).

It has also been hypothesized that the circuitry of the basal ganglia may play a role in selectively activating some movements as it suppresses others (Alexander & Crutcher, 1990). Nambu and associates (2002) also propose that the direct, indirect, and hyperdirect pathways within the basal ganglia play an important role in selectively activating some movements while inhibiting others. They suggest that when a voluntary movement is about to be initiated by cortical mechanisms, a corollary signal is transmitted simultaneously from the motor cortex to the GPi through the cortico-STN-pallidal hyperdirect pathway. Activation of the GPi neurons results in the inhibition of large areas of the thalamus and cortex that are related to both the selected motor program and other competing programs. Another corollary signal is sent via the direct pathway to the GPi to inhibit a specific population of pallidal neurons in the center area, which disinhibit their targets and release only the selected motor program. Finally, the third corollary signal possibly through the indirect pathway reaches the GPi to activate neurons therein and causes inhibition of competing motor programs. Through this sequential information processing, only the selected motor program is initiated, executed, and terminated at the appropriate time, whereas other, competing, programs are inhibited.

The oculomotor circuit is involved in the control of saccadic eye movements. The prefrontal circuit and the limbic circuits are involved in nonmotor functions. The prefrontal circuits contribute to executive functions, including organizing behaviors using verbal skills in problem solving and mediating socially appropriate responses. Lesions in this area contribute to obsessive–compulsive disorder. The limbic circuit is involved in the control of motivated behavior (involving circuits for reinforcing stimuli for behaviors) and procedural learning.

Most disorders of the basal ganglia involve problems with action rather than perception. They may involve either hyperactivity/impulsivity (e.g., Huntington's disease or obsessive–compulsive disorder) or reduced activity and flat affect (e.g., Parkinson's disease, depression) (DeLong, 2000).

For example, certain diseases of the basal ganglia may produce poverty and slowness of movement and disorders of muscle tone and postural reflexes. Parkinson's disease symptoms include resting tremor, increased muscle tone or rigidity, and slowness in the initiation of movement (akinesia) as well as in the execution of movement (bradykinesia). The site of the lesion for Parkinson's disease is in the dopaminergic pathway from the substantia nigra to the striatum. The tremor and rigidity may be due to loss of inhibitory influences within the basal ganglia. On the other hand, other diseases of the basal ganglia produce involuntary movements (dyskinesia). For example, Huntington's disease characteristics include chorea and dementia. Symptoms appear to be caused by loss of cholinergic neurons and gamma aminobutyric acid (GABA)-ergic neurons in the striatum (Alexander & Crutcher, 1990; Cote & Crutcher, 1991).

What are the functional differences between the basal ganglia and the cerebellum? Research suggests that the basal ganglia may be particularly concerned with internally generated movements, while the cerebellum is involved in visually triggered and guided movements. For example, experiments have shown that in the internal globus pallidus, cells that project to the supplementary motor area are activated during internally generated movements (Mushiake & Strick, 1995). This is consistent with clinical data demonstrating that patients with Parkinson's disease have a great deal of difficulty with internally generated movements (Georgiou et al., 1993; Morris et al., 1996). It is interesting to note that patients with Parkinson's disease with frozen gait syndrome (difficulty initiating or maintaining gait) are able to use visual cues to improve their walking abilities. The above research suggests that this may be due to the use of alternative pathways from the cerebellum to trigger and guide the movements.

Mesencephalon and Brainstem

The nuclei and pathways from the mesencephalon and brainstem to the spinal cord mediate many aspects of motor control as part of descending pathways from the cerebral cortex, cerebellum, and basal ganglia. This includes the generation of locomotor rhythms, the regulation of postural tone, the integration of sensory information for posture and balance, as well as contributions to anticipatory postural control accompanying voluntary movements.

Stimulation of the mesencephalic locomotor region (and also the subthalamic locomotor region initiates locomotion and adjusts stepping movements). Signals from this system are relayed to the spinal cord central pattern generators for locomotion via the medial reticular formation and reticulospinal pathways (including the pontomedullary locomotor strip). These pathways and brainstem centers are shown in Figure 3.17A. The brainstem has important centers for controlling the facilitation and inhibition of muscle tone important for the control of posture. These muscle tone facilitatory and inhibitory systems within the brainstem are shown in Figure 3.17, A and B. It is interesting to note that when the brainstem reticular formation is inactivated by pharmacologic means, anticipatory postural adjustments that would normally be activated to stabilize a voluntary movement initiated through activation of the motor cortex are no longer activated. This indicates the importance of brainstem nuclei in anticipatory postural control.

Thus, as shown in Figure 3.18, basal ganglia–cortical–spinal pathways are important to the control of voluntary movements, while basal ganglia–brainstem–spinal cord pathways contribute to automatic control of movements such as locomotion and postural tone mainly via pathways originating in the substantia nigra.

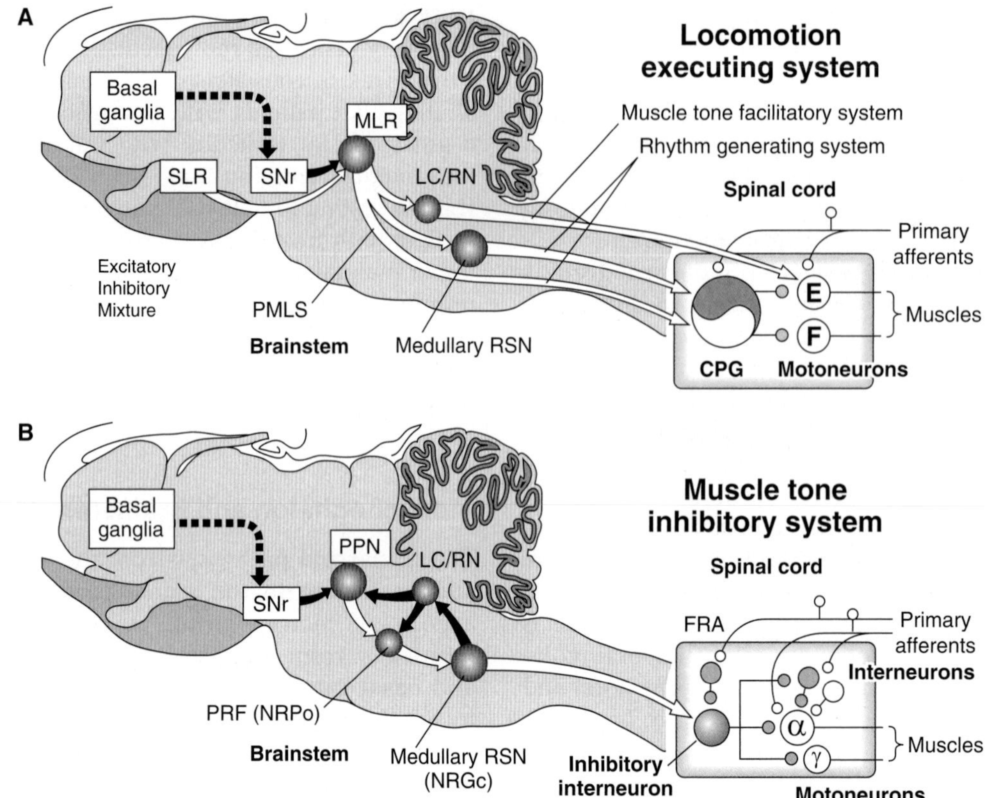

FIGURE 3.17 Important connections between the basal ganglia, brainstem, and spinal cord for regulation of locomotion and muscle tone. A, Circuitry involved in the locomotor executing systems, including the muscle tone facilitatory system and the rhythm-generating system, with its connections to the central pattern generators (CPGs) for locomotion in the spinal cord. B, Circuitry for the muscle tone inhibitory system. E = extensor motor neurons; F = flexor motor neurons; FRA = flexion reflex afferents; LC = locus coeruleus; MLR = mesencephalic locomotor region; NRGc = nucleus reticularis gigantocellularis; PMLS = pontomedullary locomotor strip; PPN = pedunculopontine tegmental nucleus; PRF = pontine reticular formation; RN = raphe nuclei; RSN = reticulospinal neuron; SLR = subthalamic locomotor region; SNr = substantia nigra. (Adapted with permission from Takakusaki K, Saitaoh K, Harada H, Kashiwayanagi M. Role of the basal ganglia-brainstem pathways in the control of motor behaviors. Neurosci Res 2004;50:141, Fig. 3.)

Figure 3.18 shows both the locomotor execution system and the muscle-tone facilitation and inhibition system pathways from the basal ganglia through the spinal motor neurons (Takakusaki et al., 2004).

Tracts for motor control that originate in the brainstem consist of the medial pathways (controlling posture and balance), including the vestibulospinal tract (discussed in the vestibular section of this chapter), the reticulospinal tract (discussed above), the tectospinal path (from the superior colliculus, and mediating head and eye movement), and the lateral pathways, controlling goal-directed movements, and including the rubrospinal pathway from the red nucleus. Figure 3.19 summarizes the major descending spinal tracts from both the cortex and the brainstem.

This concludes our review of the physiologic basis for motor control. In this chapter we have tried to show you the neural substrates for movement. This has involved a review of the perception and action systems and the higher level cognitive processes that play a part in their elaboration. We have tried to show the importance of both the hierarchical and distributed nature of these systems. The presentation of the perception and action systems separately is somewhat misleading. In real life, as movements are generated to accomplish tasks in varied environments, the boundaries between perception, action, and cognition are blurred.

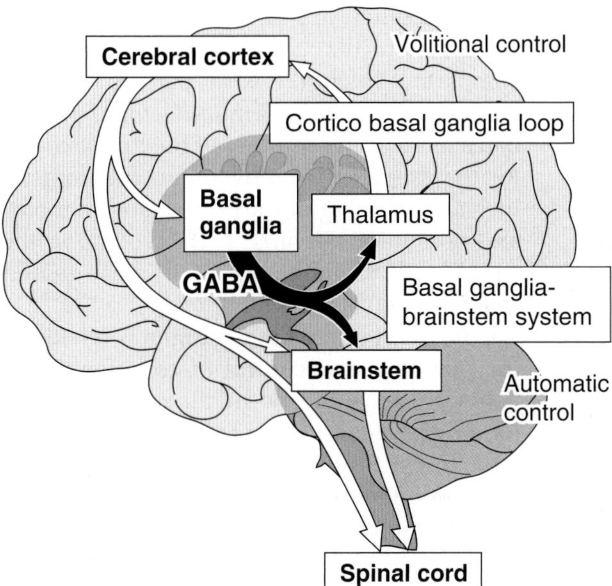

FIGURE 3.18 Hypothetical model for the control of movements by the basal ganglia, showing cortical–basal ganglia–spinal pathways important for volitional control, and basal ganglia–brainstem–spinal pathways important for automatic control of muscle tone and locomotion. (Adapted with permission from Takakusaki K, Saitaoh K, Harada H, Kashiwayanagi M. Role of the basal ganglia-brainstem pathways in the control of motor behaviors. Neurosci Res 2004;50:139, Fig. 1.)

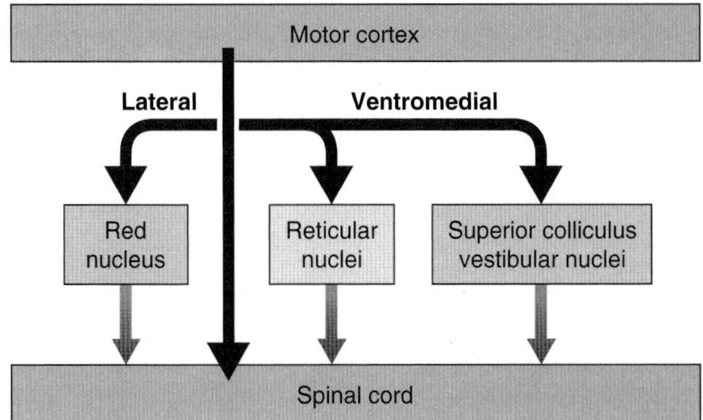

FIGURE 3.19 Summary diagram of the major descending tracts to the spinal cord, including the lateral corticospinal tract (from the motor cortex), the lateral rubrospinal tract (from the red nucleus), the ventromedial reticulospinal (from the reticular formation), the tectospinal tract (from the superior colliculus), and the vestibulospinal tract (from the vestibular nuclei).

SUMMARY

1. Movement control is achieved through the cooperative effort of many brain structures, which are organized both hierarchically and in parallel.
2. Sensory inputs perform many functions in the control of movement. They: (a) serve as the stimuli for reflexive movement organized in the spinal cord; (b) modulate the output of movement that results from the activity of pattern generators in the spinal cord; (c) modulate commands that originate in higher centers of the nervous system; and (d) contribute to the perception and control of movement through ascending pathways in much more complex ways.
3. In the somatosensory system, muscle spindles, Golgi tendon organs, joint receptors, and cutaneous receptors contribute to spinal reflex control, modulate spinal pattern generator output, modulate descending commands, and contribute to perception and control of movement through ascending pathways.
4. Vision: (a) allows us to identify objects in space and to determine their movement (exteroceptive sensation); and (b) gives us information about where our body is in space, about the relation of one body part to another, and about the motion of our body (visual proprioception).
5. The vestibular system is sensitive to two types of information: the position of the head in space and sudden changes in the direction of movement of the head.
6. As sensory information ascends to higher levels of processing, every level of the hierarchy has the ability to modulate the information coming into it from below, allowing higher centers to selectively tune (up or down) the information coming from lower centers.
7. Information from sensory receptors is increasingly processed as it ascends the neural hierarchy, enabling meaningful interpretation of the information. This is done by selectively enlarging the receptive field of each successively higher neuron.
8. The somatosensory and visual systems process incoming information to increase contrast sensitivity so that we can more easily identify and discriminate between different objects. This is done through lateral inhibition, in which the cell that is excited inhibits

the cells next to it, thus enhancing contrast between excited and nonexcited regions of the body or visual field.

9. There are also special cells within the somatosensory and visual systems that respond best to moving stimuli and are directionally sensitive.
10. In the association cortices we begin to see the transition from perception to action. The parietal lobe participates in processes involving attention to the position of and manipulation of objects in space.
11. The action system includes areas of the nervous system such as the motor cortex, the cerebellum, the basal ganglia, and brainstem.
12. The motor cortex interacts with sensory processing areas in the parietal lobe and also with basal ganglia and cerebellar areas to identify where we want to move, to plan the movement, and finally, to execute our actions.
13. The cerebellum appears to act as a comparator, a system that compensates for errors by comparing intention with performance. In addition, it modulates muscle tone, participates in the programming of the motor cortex for the execution of movement, and contributes to the timing of movement and to motor and nonmotor learning. It is involved in the control of visually triggered and guided movements.
14. The function of the basal ganglia is related to the planning and control of complex motor behavior, including modulating the central set for a movement and controlling self-initiated movements through outputs to premotor and supplementary motor areas. In addition, it may play a role in selectively activating some movements and suppressing others.

CHAPTER 4

PHYSIOLOGICAL BASIS OF MOTOR LEARNING AND RECOVERY OF FUNCTION

LEARNING OBJECTIVES

Following completion of this chapter, the reader will be able to:

1. Define plasticity and discuss its relationship to recovery of function.
2. Describe the neural mechanisms that underlie implicit forms of learning, including nonassociative, associative, and procedural learning.
3. Discuss the similarities and differences in neural mechanisms underlying explicit and declarative forms of learning.
4. Describe the neural mechanisms involved in the shift from implicit to explicit knowledge.
5. Describe the transient events that occur following central nervous system (CNS) pathology and discuss their contribution to early recovery of function.
6. Describe the different forms of synaptogenesis and discuss their role in recovery of function.
7. Summarize the changes in cortical reorganization that occur following injury, including changes in the affected and contralateral hemispheres.
8. Briefly describe some of the emerging strategies designed to enhance neural plasticity and optimize recovery of function.

INTRODUCTION

In Chapter 2 we defined *learning* as the process of acquiring knowledge about the world and *motor learning* as the process of the acquisition and/or modification of movement. We also mentioned that, just as motor control must be seen in light of the interaction between the individual, the task, and the environment, this also applies to motor learning.

In this chapter we extend our knowledge of the physiological basis of motor control to include motor learning. We show that the physiological basis for motor learning, like motor control, is typically distributed among many brain structures and processing levels, rather than being localized to a particular learning site of the brain. Likewise, the physiological basis for the recovery of function is similar to learning, in that recovery involves processes occurring throughout the nervous system and not just at the lesioned site. These processes have many properties in common with those occurring during learning.

This chapter focuses on the physiological basis of motor learning and recovery of function, showing the similarities and differences between these important functions. The material in this chapter builds on material presented in the chapters on the physiological basis of motor control and motor learning and recovery of function. Since we assume that the reader has a basic familiarity with the concepts presented in Chapters 2 and 3, these concepts will not be reviewed in this chapter.

Integral to a discussion of the physiological basis of motor learning are issues related to neural plasticity. A fundamental question addressed in this chapter is: What is the relationship between neural plasticity and motor learning? Specifically, we want to know how learning modifies the structure and function of neurons in the brain. Of equal concern is understanding the relationship between neural plasticity and recovery of function. Specifically, we want to know what changes in the structure and function of neurons underlie the recovery of function following injury.

We will also look at research that explores whether physiological plasticity associated with recovery of function is the same as or different from that involved with learning. Previous views have typically held that recovery of function and learning are served by different neural mechanisms. More recent physiological studies suggest that the same mechanisms of neural plasticity underlie both recovery of function and learning. Finally, in this chapter we consider how developmental processes modify the neural mechanisms underlying both learning and recovery of function. During development, synaptic connectivity develops and is fine-tuned during critical periods because of interacting environmental and genetic factors. Thus, developmental factors play a significant role in how plasticity manifests throughout life.

Defining Neural Plasticity

Plasticity is a general term describing the ability to show modification. Throughout this book we use the term *plasticity* in reference to mechanisms related to neural modifiability. Plasticity, or neural modifiability, may be seen as a continuum from short-term changes in the efficiency or strength of synaptic connections, to long-term structural changes in the organization and numbers of connections among neurons.

Learning also can be seen as a continuum of short-term to long-term changes in the ability to produce skilled actions. The gradual shift from short-term to long-term learning reflects a move along the continuum of neural modifiability, as increased synaptic efficiency gradually gives way to structural changes, which are the underpinning of long-term modification of behavior. This relationship is shown in Figure 4.1.

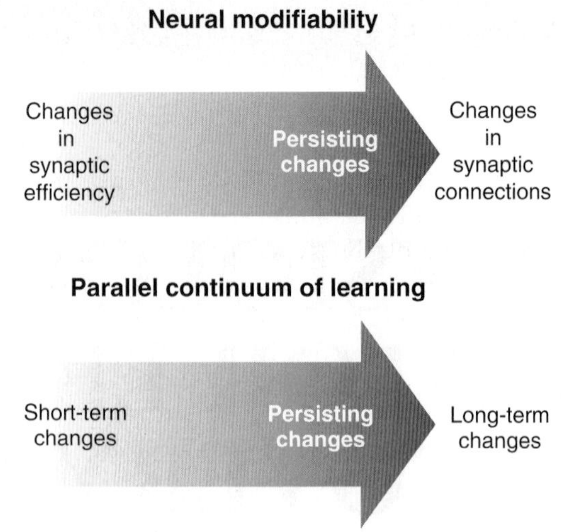

FIGURE 4.1 The gradual shift from short-term to long-term learning is reflected in a move along the continuum of neural modifiability. Short-term changes, associated with an increased synaptic efficiency, persist and gradually give way to structural changes, the underpinning of long-term learning.

Like learning, recovery of function can also be characterized by a continuum of changes from short-term functional changes that occur immediately following injury (like unmasking of existing but weak connections), to long-term structural changes such as remapping of the sensory or motor cortex.

Learning and Memory

Learning is defined as the acquisition of knowledge or ability; **memory** is the outcome of learning, including the retention and storage of that knowledge or ability (Kandel, 2000a). Learning reflects the *process* by which we acquire knowledge; memory is the *product* of that process. Memory storage is often divided into short- and long-term components. **Short-term memory** refers to *working* memory, which has a limited capacity for information and lasts for only a few moments. Short-term memory reflects a momentary attention to something, such as when we remember a phone number only long enough to dial it and then forget it.

Long-term memory is intimately related to the process of learning. Long-term memory can also be seen as a continuum. Initial stages of long-term memory formation reflect functional changes in the efficiency of synapses. Later stages of memory formation reflect structural changes in synaptic connections. These memories are less subject to disruption.

Localization of Learning and Memory

Are learning and memory localized in a specific brain structure? As noted in the previous chapter they are not. In fact, learning can occur in all parts of the brain. Learning and the storage of that learning, memory, appear to involve both parallel and hierarchical processing within the central nervous system (CNS). Even for relatively simple learning tasks, multiple parallel channels of information are used. In addition, the information can be stored in many different areas of the brain.

Apparently, mechanisms underlying learning and memory are the same whether the learning is occurring in fairly simple circuits or involves very complex circuits incorporating many aspects of the CNS hierarchy. Thus, current neuronal models of memory suggest that a memory consists of a pattern of changes in synaptic connections among networks of neurons distributed in many parts of the brain. It is interesting to note that in 1929, Lashley was the first to hypothesize that memory was stored throughout the nervous system (Lashley, 1929, 1950). In order to try to find the location of memory storage, he performed experiments in which he made lesions to many areas of the cortex of animals. To his surprise, he found that loss of memory abilities was not related to the site of the lesion but to the amount of cortex in which lesions were made.

This chapter describes the continuum of plasticity within the nervous system that represents learning, and specifically, motor learning. The processes underlying learning in the nervous system, as well as those that underlie recovery of function, are described. In later chapters these principles of plasticity related to learning and recovery of function are then applied to therapy settings.

PLASTICITY AND LEARNING

Many factors potentially modify synaptic connections. We are concerned in this chapter with activity-dependent modifications of synaptic connections, that is, both the transient and long-term modulation of synapses resulting from experience. Learning alters our capability for acting by changing both the effectiveness and anatomic connections of neural pathways. We discuss modifications of synaptic connections at both the cellular level and at the level of whole networks of neurons.

Plasticity and Nondeclarative (Implicit) Forms of Learning

Remember that in implicit forms of learning, especially nonassociative learning, the person is learning about the properties of a stimulus that is repeated. The learned suppression of a response to a nonnoxious stimulus is called "habituation." In contrast, an increased response to one stimulus that is consistently preceded by a noxious stimulus is called "sensitization." Keep in mind that nonassociative forms of learning can be short-term or long-term. What are the neural mechanisms underlying these simple forms of learning, and do the same neural mechanisms underlie both short- and long-term changes?

Habituation

Habituation was first studied by Sherrington, who found that the flexion reflex habituated with many stimulus repetitions. More recent research examining habituation in relatively simple networks of neurons in invertebrate animals has shown that habituation is related to a decrease in synaptic activity between sensory neurons and their connections to interneurons and motor neurons (Kandel, 2000a; Sherrington, 1906).

During habituation, there is a reduction in the amplitude of synaptic potentials (a decreased excitatory postsynaptic potential [EPSP]) produced by the sensory neuron on the interneuron and motor neuron. This short-term change in EPSP amplitude during habituation is illustrated in Figure 4.2, A and B. During initial stages of learning, the decreased size of the EPSP may last for only several minutes. With continued presentation of the stimulus, persisting changes in synaptic efficacy occur, representing longer-term memory for habituation.

During the course of learning, continued presentation of the stimulus results in structural changes in the sensory cells themselves. Structural changes include a decrease in the number of synaptic connections between the sensory neuron and interneurons and motor neurons, shown diagrammatically in Figure 4.2C. In addition, the number of active transmitting zones within existing connections decreases. As a result of these structural changes, habituation persists over weeks and months, representing long-term memory for habituation. Thus, the process of habituation does not involve specific memory storage neurons found in specialized parts of the CNS. Rather, memory (retention of habituation) results from a change in the neurons that are normal components of the response pathway.

Different synapses have different levels of adaptability. For example, some synapses show little change with high levels of activation, while others, especially synapses between sensory and motor neurons and some interneurons show large changes with a small amount of training. In addition, if the habituating

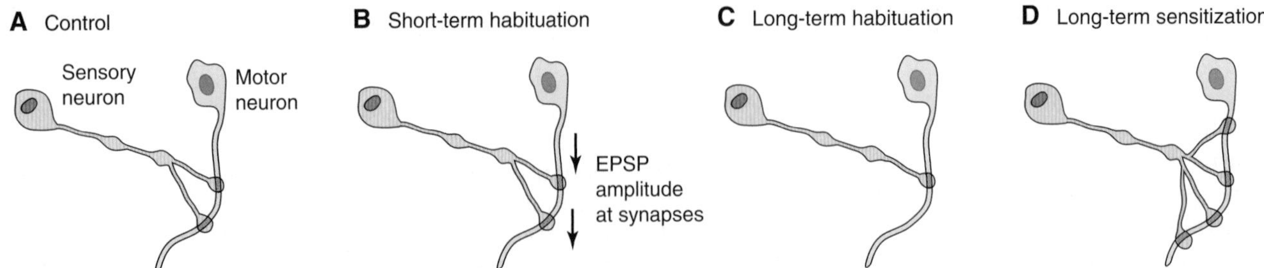

FIGURE 4.2 Neuronal modifications underlying short- and long-term nonassociative learning. A, Synapse prior to nonassociative learning. B, Short-term habituation results from a decrease in excitatory postsynaptic potential (EPSP) amplitude at the synapse between the sensory and motor neuron, but no change in the synaptic structure. C, Long-term habituation results in a decrease in the numbers of connections. D, Long-term sensitization results in an increase in the numbers of connections. (Adapted from Kandel ER. Cellular mechanisms of learning and the biological basis of individuality. In: Kandel ER, Schwartz JH, Jessell TM, eds. Principles of neuroscience, 3rd ed. New York: Elsevier, 1991:1009–1031.)

stimulus is massed without rest between sessions, there is a large short-term effect but very little long-term effect (Kandel, 2000a).

How might this research apply to intervention strategies used by therapists in the clinic? As we mentioned earlier, habituation exercises are given to patients who have certain types of inner ear disorders that result in reports of dizziness when they move their head in certain ways. When patients begin therapy, they may experience an initial decline in the intensity of their dizziness symptoms during the course of one session of exercise. But the next day, dizziness is back at the same level. Gradually, over days and weeks of practicing the exercises, the patient begins to see decreases in dizziness persist across sessions (Herdman, 2007; Shumway-Cook & Horak, 1990).

Application of Kandel's research to patients with inner ear disorders would suggest that initially with exercise there is a temporary decrease in the synaptic effectiveness of certain vestibular neurons and their connections, due to a decrease in the size of the EPSPs. With continued exercise, changes in synaptic effectiveness would become more permanent. In addition, structural changes, including a reduction in the number of vestibular neuron synapses connecting to interneurons, would occur. With the advent of structural changes, the decline in dizziness in response to the repeated head movement would persist, allowing the patient to discontinue the exercise without reexperiencing symptoms of dizziness. It is possible that if exercises were discontinued too soon, or practiced within a single session rather than over many separate sessions, structural changes in the sensory connections would not occur and dizziness symptoms would recur because of the absence of long-term structural changes underlying persisting habituation.

Sensitization

As we mentioned in Chapter 2, sensitization is caused by a strengthening of responses to potentially injurious stimuli. Sensitization may also be short- or long-term, and it may involve the exact set of synapses that show habituation. However, the mechanisms involved in sensitization are a little more complex than those involved in habituation. One way that sensitization may occur is by prolonging the action potential through changes in potassium conductance. This allows more transmitter to be released from the terminals, giving an increased EPSP. It also appears to improve the mobilization of transmitter, making it more available for release. Surprisingly, the same synapse can participate in both habituation and sensitization, with synaptic efficacy being depressed in one situation and enhanced in another, since the different types of learning use different cellular mechanisms (Kandel, 2000a).

Sensitization, like habituation, can be short- or long-term. Mechanisms for long-term memory of sensitization involve the same cells as short-term memory, but now reflect structural changes in these cells (Kandel & Schwartz, 1982; Sweatt & Kandel, 1989). Kandel (1989) has shown that in invertebrates short-term sensitization involves changes in preexisting protein structures, while long-term sensitization involves the synthesis of new protein. This synthesis of new protein at the synapse implies that long-term sensitization involves changes that are genetically influenced.

This genetic influence also encompasses the growth of new synaptic connections, as illustrated in Figure 4.2D. Animals who showed long-term sensitization were found to have twice as many synaptic terminals as untrained animals, increased dendrites in the postsynaptic cells, and an increase in the numbers of active zones at synaptic terminals, from 40 to 65% (Bailey & Chen, 1983).

In summary, the research on habituation and sensitization suggests that short-term and long-term memory may not be separate categories, but may be part of a single graded memory function. With sensitization, as with habituation, long-term memory and short-term memory involve change at the same synapses. While short-term changes reflect relatively temporary changes in synaptic effectiveness, structural changes are the hallmark of long-term memory (Kandel, 2000a).

Associative Learning

Remember that during associative learning a person learns to predict relationships, either relationships of one stimulus to another (*classical conditioning*), or the relationship of one's behavior to a consequence (*operant conditioning*). Through associative learning, we learn to form key relationships that help us adapt our actions to the environment.

Researchers examining the physiological basis for associative learning have found that it can take place through simple changes in synaptic efficiency without requiring complex learning networks. Associative learning, whether short-term or long-term, uses common cellular processes. Initially, when two neurons are active at the same time (i.e., in association), there is a modification of existing proteins within these two neurons that produces a change in synaptic efficiency. Long-term association results in the synthesis of new proteins and the subsequent formation of new synaptic connections between the neurons.

Classical Conditioning

During classical conditioning, an initially weak stimulus (the conditioned stimulus) becomes highly effective in producing a response when it becomes associated with another stronger stimulus (the unconditioned stimulus). It is similar to, although more complex than, sensitization. In fact, it may be that classical conditioning is simply an extension of the processes involved in sensitization.

Remember that in classical conditioning, timing is critical. When conditioned and unconditioned stimuli converge on the same neurons, facilitation occurs if the conditioned stimulus causes action potentials in the neurons just before (usually about 0.5 second) the unconditioned stimulus arrives. This is because action potentials allow Ca^+ to move into the presynaptic neuron and this Ca^+ activates special modulatory transmitters involved in classical conditioning. If the activity occurs after the unconditioned stimulus, Ca^+ is not released at the right time, and the stimulus has no effect (Abrams & Kandel, 1988; Kandel, 2000a).

Operant Conditioning

Although operant conditioning and classical conditioning may seem like two different processes, in fact, the laws that govern the two are similar, indicating that the same neural mechanisms may control them. In each type of conditioning, learning involves the development of predictive relationships. In classical conditioning, a specific stimulus predicts a specific response. In operant conditioning, we learn to predict the outcome of specific behaviors. However, the same cellular mechanisms that underlie classical conditioning are also responsible for operant conditioning.

Procedural Learning

Procedural learning is one of the more complex forms of nondeclarative or implicit learning. It includes the learning and execution of motor and nondeclarative cognitive skills, especially those involving sequences. It occurs only when a movement is performed by learners themselves through trial-and-error practice and within the context of actions that will be carried out in a normal setting.

It depends on a neural system distinct from that of explicit or declarative learning, described below. The implicit system underlying procedural learning is composed of a network of specific frontal (including sensorimotor cortex), basal-ganglion (tail of the caudate nucleus), parietal, and cerebellar structures. As will be noted in the next section on declarative learning, the neural pathways underlying the explicit system include frontal brain areas such as the anterior cingulate, prefrontal cortex (PFC), head of the caudate nucleus, hippocampus and other medial temporal lobe structures (Maddox & Ashby, 2004; Ullman, 2004).

The following experiments support the hypothesis that procedural learning involves the cerebellum and/or the motor cortex. Gilbert and Thatch (1977) examined the involvement of the cerebellum in a very simple form of procedural learning, involving increasing or decreasing the gain of a response when increased or decreased forces are required, a form of **adaptation**. You will recall that the cerebellum has two types of input fibers, the climbing fibers and the mossy fibers, and one type of output fiber, the Purkinje cells. Climbing fiber inputs to the Purkinje cells typically signal error and are important in the correction of ongoing movements. In contrast, mossy-fiber inputs to the Purkinje cells provide kinesthetic information about ongoing movements, important in the control of those movements. Figure 4.3B reviews the relationship of these fibers. It has been shown that the climbing-fiber inputs signaling error to the Purkinje cells may increase or decrease the strength of mossy-fiber synapses onto the same Purkinje cells. This produces a long-term change in Purkinje-cell output, which contributes to motor learning.

Gilbert and Thatch (1977) examined the role of the cerebellum in motor learning during experiments in which monkeys were trained to return a handle to a central position whenever it was moved to the left or right. During the sessions, they recorded the activity of Purkinje neurons in the arm area of the anterior lobe of the cerebellum. Once the task was learned and repeatedly performed in the same way, the arm movement was accompanied by predictable changes occurring primarily in mossy-fiber inputs reporting the kinesthetics of the movement, with occasional climbing-fiber input. Figure 4.3A1 shows the activity of the mossy fibers (simple spikes) and climbing fibers (complex spikes) during the wrist-flexion movements when the monkeys were moving against an expected force or load.

Then the experimenters modified the task, requiring the monkeys to use more force to return the handle to the original position. At first the animal was not able to return the handle in one simple movement. But gradually, the animal learned to respond correctly. During the first few trials of the new task, there was a sudden increase in activity in the climbing fibers, signaling the error, as shown in Figure 4.3A2.

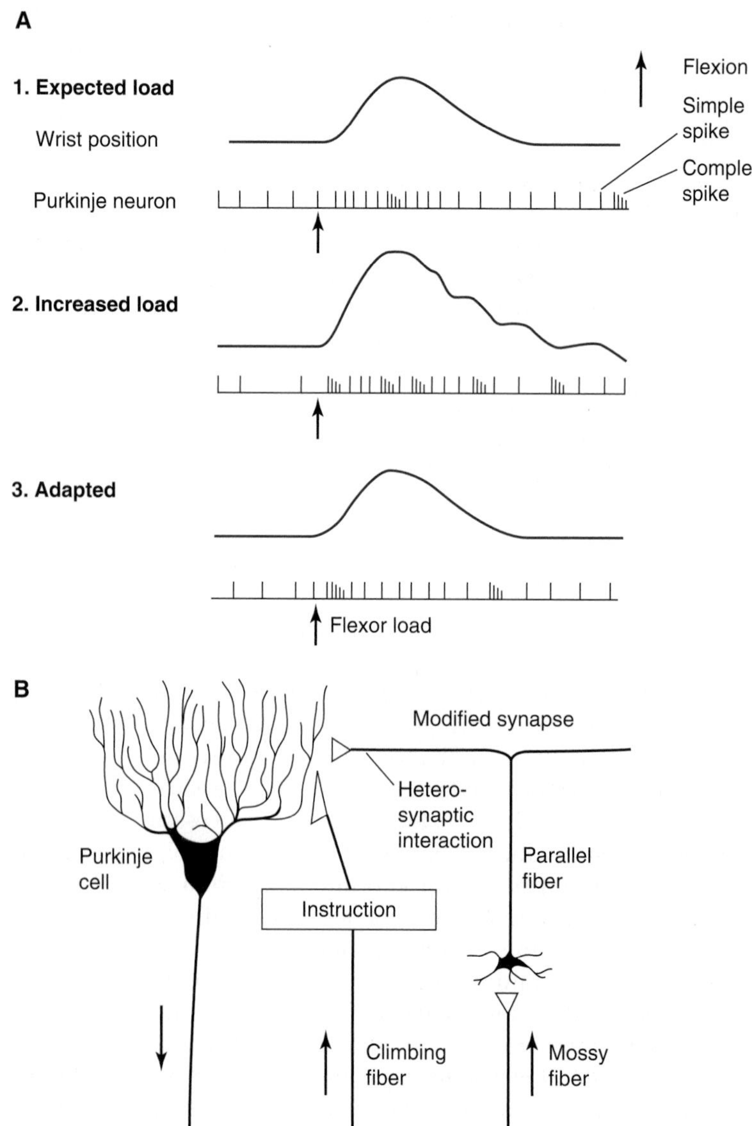

FIGURE 4.3 A, Activity of mossy fibers (simple spikes) and climbing fibers (complex spikes) during wrist flexion movements when monkeys were moving against: (1) an expected load; (2) an unexpectedly increased load; and (3) the increased load, after practice (adapted). Note that climbing-fiber (complex spike) activity increased with the increase in load, signaling error in returning the handle to its original position and reducing the efficiency of the mossy-fiber/Purkinje-cell synapse. After adaptation, the simple spike activity is reduced and complex spike activity is back to low levels. B, Cerebellum, showing the relationship between mossy-fiber input (via parallel fibers and climbing-fiber input important to learning). (Adapted from C. Ghez, The Cerebellum. In: Kandel ER, Schwartz JH, Jessell TM. Principles of neuroscience, 3rd ed. Norwalk, CT: Appleton & Lange, 1991:643.)

This increase in climbing-fiber activity was associated with a reduction in the efficiency of the mossy-fiber connections to the Purkinje cells. The reduction in Purkinje-cell output then was associated with an increase in force generation, allowing the monkey to complete the task successfully, as shown in Figure 4.3A3. Thus, it appears that changes in synaptic efficiency between these neurons in the cerebellum are an important link in the modification of movements through procedural learning.

This type of cerebellar learning may also occur in the vestibulo-ocular reflex circuitry, which includes cerebellar pathways. This reflex keeps the eyes fixed on an object when the head turns. In experiments in which humans wore prismatic lenses that reversed the image on the eye, the vestibulo-ocular reflex was reversed over time. This modification of the reflex, another form of adaptation, did not occur with cerebellar lesions (Melville-Jones & Mandl, 1983).

Plasticity and Declarative (Explicit) Forms of Learning

Remember that associative learning can also be thought of in terms of the type of knowledge acquired. *Nondeclarative learning* and specifically, *procedural learning* (resulting in implicit knowledge) refers to learning tasks that can be performed automatically without attention or conscious thought. In contrast, *declarative learning* (resulting in explicit knowledge) requires conscious processes such as awareness and attention, and results in knowledge that can be expressed consciously. Procedural learning is expressed through improved performance of the task learned, while declarative learning can be expressed in a form other than that in which it was learned. As noted above, the neural pathways underlying declarative or explicit learning include frontal brain areas such as the anterior cingulate, PFC, and head of the caudate nucleus as well as the medial temporal lobes and hippocampus.

Wilder Penfield, a neurosurgeon, was one of the first researchers to understand the important role of the temporal lobes in memory function. While performing temporal-lobe surgery in patients with epilepsy, he stimulated the temporal lobes of the conscious patients, in order to determine the location of the diseased versus the normal tissue. The patients experienced memories from the past as if they were happening again. For example, one patient heard music from an event long ago and saw the situation and felt the emotions that surrounded the singing of that music, with everything happening in real time (Penfield, 1958).

In humans, lesions in the temporal lobe of the cortex and the hippocampus may interfere with the laying down of declarative memory. A few patients have been studied after having the hippocampus and related temporal lobe areas removed because of epilepsy. After surgery, the patients were no longer able to acquire long-term declarative memories, although they remembered old memories. Their short-term memory was normal, but if their attention was distracted from an item held in short-term memory, they forgot it completely. However, skill learning was unaffected in these patients. They would often learn a complex task but be unable to remember the procedures that made up the task or the events surrounding learning the task (Milner, 1966). This work suggests that the temporal lobes and hippocampus may be important to establishing memory, but are not a part of the memory storage area.

The hippocampus, which is a subcortical structure, and part of the temporal lobe circuitry, is critical for declarative learning. Research has shown evidence of plastic changes in hippocampal neurons similar to those found in neural circuits of simpler animals when learning takes place.

Researchers have shown that pathways in the hippocampus show a facilitation that has been called **long-term potentiation (LTP)**, which is similar to the mechanisms causing sensitization (Bliss & Lomo, 1973). For example, in one region of the hippocampus, LTP occurs when a weak and an excitatory input arrive at the same region of a neuron's dendrite. The weak input will be enhanced if it is activated in association with the strong one. This process is shown in Figure 4.4, which shows the size of the response to the first stimulus and the response to the same stimulus after LTP was induced. LTP appears to

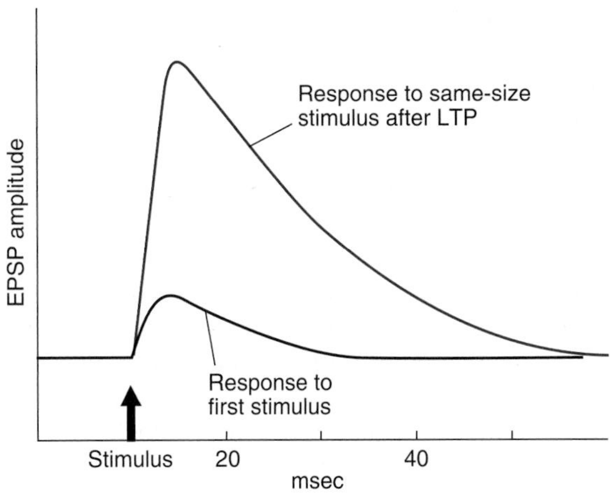

FIGURE 4.4 Cellular basis for long-term potentiation (LTP), showing small excitatory postsynaptic potentials (EPSPs) to first stimulus and large EPSPs to the same size stimulus after LTP.

require the simultaneous firing of both presynaptic and postsynaptic cells. After this occurs, LTP is maintained through an increase in presynaptic transmitter release.

There is both a short-term early phase to LTP (1 to 3 hour) that does not require protein synthesis and a longer late phase that lasts at least 24 hour and requires cAMP (cyclic adenosine monophosphate)-induced and CREB (cAMP-responsible element-binding protein)–mediated gene expression, accompanied by protein synthesis. The early phase involves a functional change, with no new synapses, while the late phase involves a structural change, involving new synaptic release sites (Kandel, 2000a).

In the 1970s it was discovered that the hippocampus codes a cognitive map of the spatial areas in which we move. The cells that code these spatial characteristics have been called "place cells," and each cell is activated optimally when an animal moves in a given part of its environment. In this way, the animal creates a place field, or an internal representation of the space in which it lives. These place fields are created very quickly (e.g., minutes) when they enter a new space and are often present for months. The same neurons may be active as part of different place fields, so they can be used in multiple maps (Kandel, 2000a; O'Keefe & Dostrovsky, 1971).

In order to determine whether LTP was important in forming place fields, scientists determined the ability of mice with genetic mutations affecting LTP to create place fields. They found that the two mutations only made the place fields fuzzier than normal, showing that LTP was not required for the basic sensory process of creating place fields. However, the place fields were no longer stable over time, suggesting that the mice had a long-term problem like patients with medial-temporal-lobe lesions (Kandel, 2000a).

In addition to being important for the formation of long-term memory of spatial maps, LTP within the hippocampus has also been shown to be critical for spatial memory (Kandel, 2000a). For example, Morris et al. (1986) performed an experiment in which rats swam a water maze to find a platform under the water. The water was made opaque in order to block the use of vision in finding the target. The rats were released in different parts of the maze and were required to use spatial cues related to the position of the walls to find the target. They also performed a nonspatial task in which the platform was above the water and the rat could simply use visual cues to swim to the target.

These experimenters showed that blocking special receptors (*N*-methyl-D-aspartate [NMDA] receptors) in hippocampal neurons caused the rats to fail to learn the spatial version of the task. This finding suggests that certain hippocampal neurons are involved in spatial learning through LTP. Mice with genetic mutations affecting NMDA receptors, which disrupted LTP, showed a profound deficit in spatial memory on the water maze. Animals with genetic deficits affecting only late LTP show normal learning and short-term memory, but have defective long-term memory (Kandel, 2000a).

In comparing the results of experiments on short- and long-term learning, it is noteworthy that simple forms of nondeclarative implicit learning involving habituation or sensitization have much in common with complex declarative explicit learning, although different brain structures may be involved. Both show a short-term memory phase involving only functional changes in synaptic output, followed by a long-term memory phase involving structural changes in synapses. In both implicit and explicit learning, long-term changes are activated by cAMP-responsive genes and the CREB gene expression, which are accompanied by protein synthesis and new synapses (Bailey & Kandel, 2004).

Motor Cortex Contributions to Procedural Learning and the Shift from Implicit to Explicit Knowledge

Pascual-Leone and colleagues (1994) have shown that modulation of motor cortex outputs occurs when explicit knowledge is associated with improved motor performance. In addition, they have now explored the changes in motor cortical outputs when implicit knowledge is transformed into explicit knowledge.

They used a sequential-finger-movement task, in which the subject sat in front of the computer with a response pad with four buttons, to be pressed by the four fingers of the hand. When a number was displayed on the screen, the subject was to press the appropriate button as quickly as possible. A group of experimental subjects was given a repeating sequence of cues, but not told of the repetitive nature. Their performance was compared with that of a control group given a random sequence. Subjects were asked whether the sequence was random or repeating at the end of each block of 10 repetitions of the sequence.

Pascual-Leone et al. (1994) found that during the course of learning the sequence of finger-movement reaction times became shorter and the cortical maps representing the finger muscles involved in the movement became progressively larger (measured by transcranial magnetic stimulation). After four blocks of trials, reaction time was significantly shorter and peak amplitudes and sizes of the cortical outputs to the muscles were significantly higher. At this point, all subjects knew that the sequences were not random, but did not yet know the entire sequence. The maps of cortical output to the muscles continued to enlarge until the subjects attained explicit knowledge of the sequence (six to nine blocks). At this point, the maps returned to baseline size within three additional blocks of trials, as subjects also began to anticipate the cues for the finger presses. The authors suggest that after explicit learning of a sequence the contribution of the motor cortex is attenuated and other brain structures begin to assume a more active role in task execution (Pascual-Leone et al., 1994).

Complex Forms of Motor Learning

Motor learning includes both simple forms, such as both instrumental and classical conditioning, as well as more complex forms involving the acquisition of skilled movements. Asanuma and Keller (1991) have begun to examine the neural mechanisms underlying these more complex motor skills. In an initial study, they noted that removal of the somatosensory cortex in monkeys did not produce overt motor deficits in previously learned motor skills, but it did slow the learning of new motor skills. They hypothesized that one mechanism underlying motor learning involved LTP of specific cells in the motor cortex by cells in the somatosensory cortex. In order to test this hypothesis, they stimulated cells in the somatosensory cortex. Whenever they saw short-latency EPSPs in the motor cortex cells, they gave a tetanic stimulus through the somatosensory cortex electrode (50 Hz, 5 second). They found that the amplitude of the EPSPs was increased to about twice control levels. This supports the idea that repeated practice of a motor skill results in improved synaptic efficiency between the sensory and motor cortices.

These results seemed to contradict the fact that somatosensory cortex lesions did not appear to affect the performance of previously learned skills. To explain this apparent contradiction, the authors hypothesized that during learning, changes in the sensorimotor cortical pathways also increase the efficiency of the thalamocortical pathways that are coactivated during the learning process. Thus, with training, these alternative pathways could take over activation of the motor cortex. Subsequent experiments found that after repeated practice, the efficiency of the thalamic input to the motor cortex was facilitated, and it remained so, even when sensorimotor cortical inputs were no longer activated (Asanuma & Keller, 1991). This could thus explain the lack of sensory input required in making movements after learning, since the somatosensory cortex could be bypassed and other pathways could take over.

When learning a new motor skill, a beginner tends to coactivate many muscles simultaneously, and then with practice, these less efficient contractions are eliminated and only the necessary muscles contract. Can LTP between the sensory and motor cortices explain this change with motor learning?

To answer this question, Asanuma and Keller (1991) carried out the following experiments. A cat was placed in a clear plastic box with a small opening in the front (Fig. 4.5). In front of the box, was a rotating beaker, in which a biscuit was placed. There was a gap between the beaker and the box, so the cat would drop the food unless it learned a new technique of supinating the wrist while picking up the food. Prior to training, the somatosensory cortex in one hemisphere was removed. Acquisition of the skill by the contralateral limb to the lesion was severely affected as compared with the control limb. After training, the

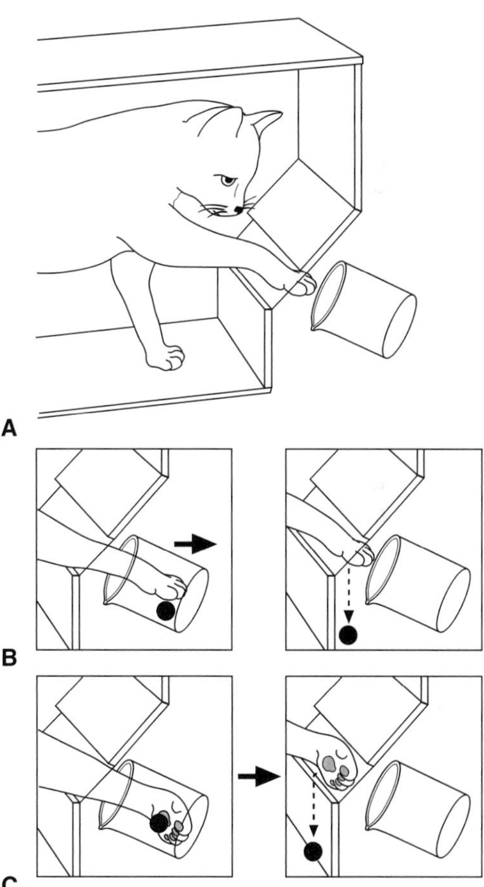

FIGURE 4.5 Paradigm used to study the role of the somatosensory cortex in learning complex motor skills in the cat. A, The cat reaches through a slit in a clear plastic training box to retrieve a food pellet placed in a rotating beaker. B, Untrained cats flex the paw and the pellet drops between the beaker and the box. C, Trained cats learn to supinate and flex the paw to retrieve the pellet (Adapted with permission from Asanuma H, Keller A. Neuronal mechanisms of motor learning in mammals. Neuroreport 1991;2:217–224.)

other somatosensory cortex was removed. Interestingly, the previously learned skill was not affected. This suggests that the somatosensory cortex participates in the learning of motor skills, through LTP, and that after learning, other areas, such as the thalamus, may take over.

Acquisition of Skill: The Shift to Automaticity

The development of a motor skill has been characterized as a shift toward automaticity (Fitts & Posner, 1967). One of the important steps on the road to becoming expert in a motor skill occurs when the individual can perform the movements in an apparently effortless and automatic fashion (Milton et al., 2004). Automation with skill development allows general attentional resources to become available for other tasks. Thus, as automaticity increases, it becomes easier to perform a second, attention-demanding task simultaneously. Many activities of daily living, such as speaking, writing, and pointing at a target, are examples of automatic skilled voluntary movements (Fitts & Posner, 1967). Neurological diseases affecting the control of movement frequently alter motor automaticity; thus, tasks that were previously performed automatically, that is, without exerting full attention, now require attentional resources.

A number of research studies have investigated the changes in neural activity associated with the shift to automaticity that occurs when learning a new movement skill in healthy adults (Floyer-Lea & Matthews, 2004; Poldrack et al., 2005; Wu et al., 2004a), and explored changes in activity patterns during learning in older adults (Wu & Hallet, 2005) and in persons with neurologic pathology (Wu & Hallet, 2008).

Floyer-Lea and Matthews (2004) used functional magnetic resonance imaging (fMRI) to examine changes in the level and pattern of brain activity in healthy young adults during short-term learning of a visuomotor skill. A separate experiment was carried on outside the fMRI to evaluate stages of development of automaticity; interference during dual-task performance of the visual tracking task (a serial subtraction task was the secondary task) was used to determine shifts in automaticity during learning. When a new level of automaticity was reached, subjects were again asked to perform the visual motor tracking task by itself in the fMRI. The study found two distinct, time-dependent patterns of functional changes in the brain associated with learning this task. The initial phase of learning, when performance of the task was more attentionally demanding, was associated with activity in widely distributed, predominantly cortical regions, including prefrontal, bilateral sensorimotor, and parietal cortices. Specifically, the dorsolateral prefrontal cortex, the caudate nucleus and the ipsilateral cerebellar hemisphere showed significant activity during initial stages of learning. There was a progressive decrease in neural activity in certain brain regions as performance improved and a shift in the pattern of brain activity. Later stages of learning were associated with a decrease in primary motor cortex, but an increase in activity in subcortical motor regions, including that of the cerebellar dentate nucleus, the thalamus, and the putamen. The authors suggest that motor-skill learning is associated with a progressive reduction of widely distributed activation in cortical regions responsible for executive functions, processing somatosensory feedback, and motor planning. Performance gains during early learning strongly rely on prefrontal–caudate interactions, while later learning improvements in performance involve increased activity in a subcortical circuit involving the thalamus, cerebellar nuclei, and basal ganglia as the task becomes more automatic.

Wu and Hallet (2005) also examined age-related changes in neural activity associated with the shift to automaticity during acquisition of a simple motor skill (sequence of 4 finger movements) and a more complex one (sequence of 12 finger movements) in healthy older adults as compared with younger adults. They found that older adults were able to achieve automaticity in both simple and more complex learning tasks, but required significantly more training than did the young adults. In addition, fMRI results showed that while the pattern of brain activity was similar between the two groups before and after training, significantly greater amounts of brain activity were necessary to achieve the same level of automaticity in older as compared with young adults. They suggest that older adults can achieve the same level of automaticity as young adults (albeit with more practice), but automaticity requires more brain activity in elders as compared with young adults. This may be one reason that older adults have difficulty with dual-task performance.

In a study using similar methods, Wu and Hallet (2005, 2008) studied neural correlates of dual-task performance in persons with Parkinson's disease (PD). They found that many of the individuals with PD were able to learn to perform simple tasks automatically; however, many were unable to perform complex tasks automatically, and thus, complex dual-task performance was impaired, even with extended practice. Results from the fMRI showed that for both groups, simple sequential movements activated similar brain regions before and after automaticity was achieved,

However, whereas normal subjects reduced brain activity at the automatic stage, the individuals with PD had greater activity in the cerebellum, premotor area, parietal cortex, precuneus, and prefrontal cortex as compared with normal subjects while performing automatic movements. The authors suggest that persons with PD require more brain activity to compensate for basal ganglia dysfunction in order to perform automatic movements.

This research suggests that the shift to automaticity during skill acquisition is associated with a reduction of brain activation in several regions, such as the cerebellar hemispheres, premotor area, and dorsolateral prefrontal cortex. In addition, there is some evidence that activity in specific regions like the basal ganglia increases with automaticity. Finally, aging and neurologic pathology can affect the ability of the brain to control movements automatically, and this can impair dual-task performance in these populations.

INJURY-INDUCED PLASTICITY AND RECOVERY OF FUNCTION

In the early part of this century, Ramon y Cajal performed experiments that suggested that growth was not possible in neurons in the adult mammalian CNS. In a paper written in 1928, he said that when development was complete, the growth and regeneration of axons and dendrites was lost. He noted that in the adult brain, nervous system pathways were fixed and unmodifiable (Ramon y Cajal, 1928). This led to a view of the CNS as a static structure with rigid and unalterable connections (Gordon, 1987; Stein et al., 1995). This view persisted until the late 1960s and 1970s, when researchers began to discover growth and reorganization of neurons in the adult CNS after injury. This research has revealed that the brain is not structurally static but continuously changes in structure and function. Plasticity occurs at many levels, including the:

- Brain level (glial and vascular support)
- Network level (changes in patterns of neural activation and cortical remapping)
- Intercellular level (changes between neurons at the synaptic level, including synaptic sprouting)
- Intracellular level (mitochondrial and ribosomal function)
- Biochemical level (protein conformation, enzyme mobilization)
- Genetic level (transcription, translation, and posttranslation modifications)

A complete discussion of plasticity at all these levels is beyond the scope of this book. Instead we will focus primarily on intercellular (changes at the synaptic level) and network (cortical reorganization) levels.

Mechanisms underlying recovery of function after neural injury have been categorized as either restorative (direct) or compensatory (indirect) (Friel & Nudo, 1998). Direct mechanisms involve the resolution of temporary changes and recovery of the injured neural tissue itself. In addition, nearby neural tissue takes over identical neural functions to the original damaged tissue, resulting in restitution of function. In indirect, or compensatory, recovery completely different neural circuits enable the recovery of lost or impaired function. Compensatory neural reorganization can include both function-enabling and function-disabling plasticity. Examples of function-enabling plasticity include changes in cortical representation associated with forced-use paradigms that improve motor function. Examples of function-disabling plasticity include changes in cortical representation associated with disuse that reduce motor capabilities and phantom limb sensation after amputation that is attributed to cortical reorganization and sensory-disabling plasticity.

Injury to the CNS can affect neuronal function through direct damage to the neurons themselves. In addition, disruption of neuronal function can occur as the result of indirect effects of injuries that impair cerebral blood flow, control of the cerebrospinal fluid, or cerebral metabolism. As shown in Figure 4.6, whether the trauma occurs through a direct or an indirect mechanism, the effect on neuronal function can include: (a) interrupting axonal projections from areas injured (Fig. 4.6A); (b) denervation of the population of neurons innervated by the injured neurons (Fig. 4.6B); and (c) removing some neurons entirely (Fig. 4.6C) (Steward, 1989).

Aside from the loss of neurons damaged at the site of injury, the consequences of synaptic loss from these neurons produces a cascading degeneration along neuronal pathways, increasing the extent of neuronal disruption with time (Steward, 1989).

Early Transient Events That Depress Brain Function

Before discussing intercellular responses to CNS injury we will review other events that occur within the nervous system following injury that produce transient disruption of brain tissue not directly due to the injury. These events may contribute to initial loss of function, and their resolution produces early recovery of function.

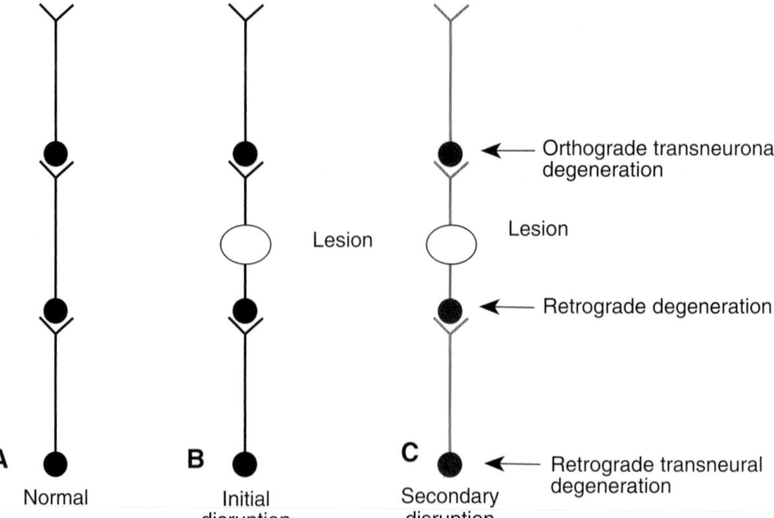

FIGURE 4.6 Secondary neuronal disruption that occurs as part of the cascade of events following neural injury. A, Normal neuronal function. B, Interruption of axonal projections from injured area. C, Secondary neuronal disruption.

Diaschisis

One of the first events following nervous system injury is diaschisis (Feeney, 1991). **Diaschisis** is a transient CNS disorder involving loss of function in a structurally intact brain area because of loss of input from an anatomically connected injured area of the brain (Feeney & Baron, 1986). The sudden functional depression of brain regions distant from the primary site of injury can be due to a reduction in blood flow and/or metabolism. Research using positron-emission tomographic (PET) scans (to measure blood flow to various parts of the brain, and thus infer neural activity) indicates that in many cases there is recovery of normal activity levels with time (Stein et al., 1995). It has been proposed that drugs such as amphetamines may promote recovery of function by acting to accelerate the resolution of diaschisis (Feeney et al., 1985).

Edema

Cerebral edema commonly follows brain injury. Cytotoxic cerebral edema involves the accumulation of intracellular fluid, whereas vasogenic edema entails leakage of proteins and fluid from damaged blood vessels. Cerebral edema can be local (i.e., adjacent to the primary injury site) or remote and produces a functional depression in brain tissue that is not part of the primary injury (Goldstein, 1993).

Edema at the site of neuronal injury may lead to a compression of axons and physiological blocking of neuronal conduction (Craik, 1992). Reduction of the edema would then restore a portion of the functional loss. This process is shown in Figure 4.7.

Intercellular Responses to Injury

Intercellular response to injury reflects the formation and regeneration of synapses (synaptogenesis).

Denervation Supersensitivity

Denervation supersensitivity can occur when neurons show a loss of input from another brain region. In this case, the postsynaptic membrane of a neuron becomes hyperactive to a released transmitter substance. For example, Parkinson's disease causes a loss of dopamine-producing neurons in the substantia nigra of the basal ganglia. In response to this disease-induced denervation, the postsynaptic target neurons in the striatum become hypersensitive to the dopamine that is released by the remaining substantia nigra neurons. This occurs through the postsynaptic cells forming more receptors to capture more dopamine. It is interesting that this denervation supersensitivity occurs only when at least 90% of the nerve fibers in the substantia nigra are gone. Thus, it occurs only when a critical number of neurons have been destroyed (Stein et al., 1995).

Unmasking of Silent Synapses

Recruitment of previously silent synapses also occurs during recovery of function. This suggests that structural synapses are present in many areas of the brain that may not normally be functional because of competition within neuronal pathways. However, experiential factors or lesions may lead to their being unmasked when they are released from these previous effects. Certain drugs, such as amphetamines,

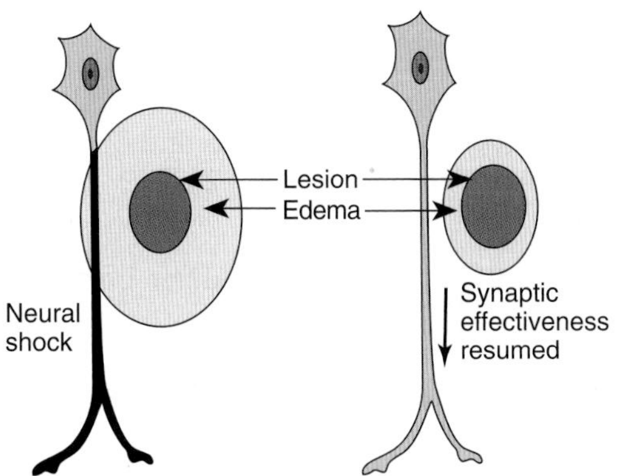

FIGURE 4.7 Recovery of synaptic effectiveness due to the resolution of edema, allowing nerve conduction to resume. (Adapted with permission from Craik RL. Recovery processes: maximizing function. In: Contemporary management of motor control problems. Proceedings of the II Step Conference. Alexandria, VA: American Physical Therapy Association, 1992:165–173.)

may promote recovery of function by facilitating unmasking (Goldstein, 1990).

Neural Regeneration (Regenerative Synaptogenesis)

Neural regeneration or **regenerative synaptogenesis** occurs when injured axons begin sprouting. An example of regenerative synaptogenesis is shown in Figure 4.8 (Held, 1987; Craik, 1992). Bjorklund, a neurologist from Sweden, was one of the first scientists to perform research that provided evidence that neural growth and regeneration were possible after brain damage. He and his colleagues made lesions in nigrostriatal pathways within the basal ganglia of rats, trying to simulate the degeneration of the pathway that occurs with Parkinson's disease. They then examined the brains with special histologic fluorescence techniques at different times after the lesions. They found that within 3 to 7 days, neurons had begun to grow across the cut area, and eventually reestablished their connections with their target neurons in the caudate nucleus of the basal ganglia (Bjorklund, 1994).

In addition, Albert Aguayo and colleagues from McGill University tried to determine why it is difficult for neurons to regenerate axons over long distances, as in the spinal cord. They hypothesized that one problem might be mechanical factors at the site of damage, so they created a "bridge" out of sciatic nerve to help the regenerating nerve fibers grow across the site of the lesion. In a series of experiments they showed that when they used a long sciatic nerve bridge between the spinal cord and the brainstem (the length of the

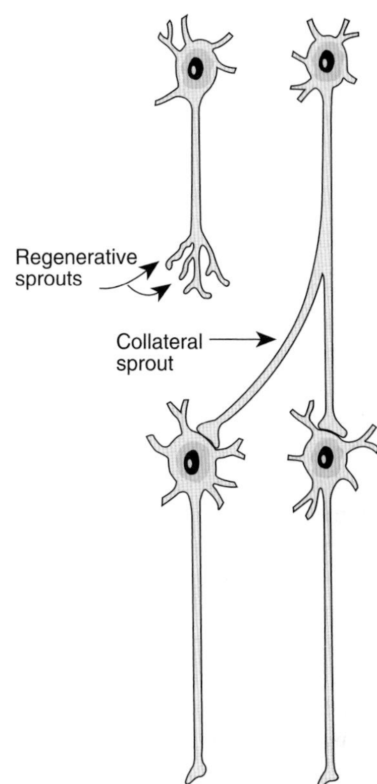

FIGURE 4.8 Regenerative and reactive synaptogenesis in related neurons following injury. (Adapted from Held JM. Recovery of function after brain damage: theoretical implications for therapeutic intervention. In: Carr JH, Shepherd RB, Gordon F, et al., eds. Movement sciences: foundations for physical therapy in rehabilitation. Rockville, MD: Aspen Systems, 1987:155–177.)

bridge lay outside the spinal cord, with the ends inserted into the spinal cord or the brainstem), both brainstem and spinal cord neurons did grow over distances of about 3 cm in the adult rat. However, their penetration into the nervous system was only about 2 mm. In another set of experiments, they showed that a portion of the retinal neurons (about 10%) could also grow across a sciatic nerve bridge into the superior colliculus and make connections in the appropriate layers. When they recorded from these neurons while shining light on the retina, they found that they did respond, although not completely normally (Aguayo et al., 1996).

Although the previous work was performed on rats, other experiments have shown that human adult retinal nerve cells can also be induced to regenerate in vitro. Stein et al. (1995) note that, although this work may be promising, it is not yet clear whether regenerative growth will really help patients with lesions and whether it will lead to a return of previous behaviors and remain functional throughout the lifetime of the patient. Can postinjury reorganizational processes be manipulated to facilitate CNS reorganization? These and other questions have critical importance for basic scientists and clinicians involved in the rehabilitation of patients with brain injuries.

Collateral Sprouting (Reactive Synaptogenesis)

Collateral sprouting, or **reactive synaptogenesis**, may occur when neighboring normal axons sprout to innervate synaptic sites that were previously activated by the injured axons. Typically, the axons that begin to sprout belong to the same neural system that originally innervated the synaptic sites. Steward (1989), working with rats, decided to determine whether collateral sprouting could occur in the entorhinal–hippocampal circuitry, which is involved in short-term memory. He showed that when lesions were made in the entorhinal cortex on one side of the brain, fibers from the intact entorhinal cortex on the opposite side of the brain sprouted branches that crossed over and innervated the hippocampal sites damaged by the lesion. The new connections were similar in organization to the original ones. Steward (1989) and Stein et al. (1995) also noted that the time for the fibers to sprout and make connections was about the same as the time for the return of the behaviors used to indicate the return of short-term memory.

Previous research had suggested that early recovery was due to resolution of temporary factors interfering with neural function, such as diaschisis and reduction of edema, and that later recovery was due to plastic changes involving synaptic modulation and cortical reorganization. More recently, it has been documented that plastic changes, including synaptic potentiation, pruning, and sprouting, and dendritic arborization occur within milliseconds to hours following injury (Zucker & Regehr, 2002).

Changes in Cortical Maps after Lesions and during Recovery of Function

There is a growing body of evidence demonstrating that cortical representation of the body is continuously modified in healthy adults in response to activity, behavior, and skill acquisition. Cortical reorganization also occurs after a peripheral injury (such as amputation) or CNS injury (such as stroke or traumatic brain injury). Research on cortical reorganization following neural injury suggests that a focal lesion opens a window of increased plasticity in the CNS. This early lesion–induced cortical hyperexcitability facilitates cortical plasticity (Ward & Cohen, 2004). Of particular interest to professionals in neurologic rehabilitation is the research on activity-dependent changes in structure and function that occur following injury.

If you are unfamiliar with the technology used to study neural plasticity during recovery of function, See Technology Tool 4.1 for a brief review of some of these methods.

Remapping following Peripheral Lesions

What have researchers learned about how cortical maps change during recovery of function? When the median nerve (which innervates the radial part of the

TECHNOLOGY TOOL 4-1 Methods Used to Study Neural Plasticity

Many methods have evolved to assist researchers in studying neural plasticity and cortical reorganization underlying the recovery of function following CSN injury, including neuroimaging techniques with different temporal and spatial resolution. Positron-emission tomography (PET) has a temporal resolution of minutes, while the resolution of functional magnetic resonance imaging (fMRI) is seconds and the resolution using magnetoencephalography (MEG) is milliseconds, allowing researchers to determine where and when activation starts and to track its temporal spread to other brain regions (Johansson, 2004). Transcranial magnetic stimulation (TMS) is another noninvasive method for studying brain function. A pulsed magnetic field creates a current flow in the brain and can temporarily excite or inhibit synaptic efficiency and alter brain function (Hallet, 2000). Motor evoked potentials (MEPs) are recorded and used to determine changes in representation and excitability of the motor system. (Chen et al., 2002). For example a researcher may use TMS to activate pyramidal-tract neurons and record the MEP amplitude of muscles proximal to the amputation to determine the extent of cortical reorganization that occurs following amputation. PET scans, which plot regional cerebral blood flow and infer the level of neural activity from the level of blood flow to specific brain areas, can be used to examine changes in activation patterns following injury.

glabrous [nonhairy] regions of the hand) of the monkey is severed, one might expect that corresponding parts of the somatosensory cortex would become silent, since there would be no input coming into them. In studies examining this issue, Merzenich and colleagues (1983a, b) found that immediately after the lesion, much of the deprived cortex did not respond to light cutaneous stimulation, but over the next days and weeks, the neurons began to respond again. Now they responded when the hairy dorsal surface was stimulated.

When experiments were performed to test the mapping of the cortex after surgery, it was found that neighboring maps had expanded their receptive fields to cover much of the denervated region. These representations increased even further in the weeks following denervation (Merzenich et al., 1983a, b). Since the extent of the reorganization of cortex was a few millimeters, it was assumed that it occurred because of the increased responsiveness of existing, previously weak connections.

However, if nerves to matching parts of the back and front of the hand were cut, there were zones of cortex that remained unresponsive even months after the lesion (Garraghty et al., 1994; Kaas et al., 1997). These studies support the proposal that the reactivation of the cortex was due to the increased responsiveness of weak inputs from neighboring areas, and if the denervation exceeded a certain distance, silent areas would remain (Kaas et al., 1997).

Other related work suggests that there can be reactivation of cortex in areas that are too large to be explained by the strengthening of existing connections. For example, Taub (1976) showed that at least 12 years after a dorsal rhizotomy to eliminate sensory input from the arm of a monkey, the somatosensory cortex had been completely reactivated by remaining inputs, mainly from the face. Since this area covered more than 10 mm of Brodmann's area 3b, it was too large to have occurred through the increased effectiveness of previously weak connections. Thus, new connections had formed somewhere in the nervous system.

To determine where these connections occurred, Florence and Kaas (1995) studied the reorganization of the spinal cord, brainstem, and cortex in monkeys with a history of amputation of the hand or forearm. They found that the central termination of the nerves that had not been injured by the amputation had sprouted into territories of the spinal cord and brainstem that were no longer in use because of the amputation. They believed that the expansion of the arm representation in the cortex after amputation was due to the growth of axons that relayed information about the arms into the parts of the spinal cord and brainstem previously occupied by the hand. Thus, the researchers hypothesized that the key to the large-scale reorganization following amputations and dorsal-root damage is due to sensory neuron loss and the creation of space in the spinal cord and cuneate nucleus, allowing new growth that leads to reactivation of cortex (Kaas et al., 1997).

In humans, reorganization of the somatosensory and motor systems also occurs following amputation. Researchers used transcranial magnetic stimulation to map motor responses of different muscles activated by cortical areas. They found that muscles proximal to the amputation showed evoked potentials that were larger than those of the equivalent muscles on the opposite side of the body. These muscles were also activated at lower stimulation levels and over a wider area of cortex than those on the opposite side (Cohen et al., 1991, 1993; Lee & van Donkelaar, 1995). Researchers have found that stimulation of the face and upper body in patients who have had their upper limbs amputated can elicit phantom-limb sensation, suggesting that after upper-limb amputation, the somatosensory representation of the face and upper body expanded to occupy the arm and hand area (Chen et al., 2002; Ramachandran et al., 1992). The extent of shift in cortical representation correlated with the amount of phantom sensation (Chen et al., 2002). This research demonstrates that alterations in cortical mapping occur following peripheral-nerve lesions or amputation.

Remapping following Central Lesions

In addition to peripheral injury, damage to central neural structures also results in alterations to cortical maps and changes in neural activation patterns. Focal damage to the CNS can increase the capacity for structural and functional changes within the CNS, such as happens in development during critical periods (Ward & Cohen, 2004). Researchers are examining the relationship between cortical reorganization and recovery of function using longitudinal studies to understand processes associated with complete versus incomplete recovery of function. In addition, studies are exploring how neural plasticity following injury can be enhanced through various manipulations, including environmental modifications, behavioral training, and pharmacology. Studies on recovery of function and cortical reorganization have used both animal models and studies of humans recovering from neurologic injury such as stroke and traumatic brain injury.

Reorganization Of The Affected Hemisphere During Recovery Of Function. Motor recovery following damage to the primary motor cortex may be mediated by other cortical areas in the damaged hemisphere, through the use of either redundant pathways or new regions that take over the function of the damaged area (Chen et al., 2002; Nudo, 2006, 2007). Jenkins and Merzernich (1987) were some of the earliest scientists to suggest that reorganization of cortical representation after brain injury could be a model for the basis for recovery from cortical lesions. They performed a study in the monkey, in which they made ablations in the sensory cortex area representing one of the fingers. They found that skin surfaces originally represented in the ablated area were now represented in the nearby intact somatosensory areas. Studies of human subjects with infarcts in the internal capsule have shown that recovery of hand function was associated with a ventral extension of the hand area of the cortex into the area normally controlled by the face (Weiller et al., 1993). In another study, Pons et al. (1988) selectively removed the hand area of primary somatosensory cortex (SI), which is the input to the secondary somatosensory area (SII). They found that the hand areas of SII no longer responded to cutaneous stimulation of the hand, but after a number of weeks of recovery the area became responsive to light touch of the foot. These results demonstrate that the nervous system is capable of reorganization following central as well as peripheral lesions.

Damage to primary motor areas also results in reorganization of neural activity during recovery of function. Primary motor cortex lesions result in activation of secondary motor areas, including premotor and supplementary motor cortex as well as the cingulate cortex. Thus, recovery of function related to small lesions to the internal capsule may be mediated by undamaged parallel motor pathways (Alexander & Crutcher, 1990; Chen et al., 2002; Fries et al., 1993; Lee & van Donkelaar, 1995; Strick, 1988).

Is activation of secondary motor areas associated with good recovery of function following stroke? Longitudinal studies using neural imaging technology to study the relationship between reorganized neural activation patterns and levels of recovery of function following stroke are beginning to answer this question. These studies support findings that after damage to primary motor cortex there is recruitment of secondary motor regions as described above. However, among individuals demonstrating good motor recovery, these initial patterns of overactivation in secondary motor regions are replaced by focused and more normal activation patterns. Normalization of activation patterns is associated with better motor recovery, while continued activation of secondary areas appears to be associated with less than optimal recovery of function (Ward et al., 2003).

There is also evidence that adjacent cortex takes over the function of damaged areas. For example, following stroke recovered hand movements were associated with activation of motor cortex that extended into the face area, suggesting that the hand representation shifted toward the face area (Weiller et al., 1993).

Contributions of Ipsilateral (Uncrossed) Motor Pathways To Recovery Of Function. Do uncrossed pathways play an important role in recovery of function? This appears to be the case in many patients. For example, a complete cerebral hemisphere was removed in certain patients to control intractable epilepsy, but no significant hemiplegia was seen. This unusual occurrence may have been due to the fact that the hemisphere had been abnormal since early childhood, and thus there had been many years during which the ipsilateral hemisphere could gradually take over control of the limbs (Lee & van Donkelaar, 1995).

Weiller et al. (1992) used PET scans to examine ipsilateral motor activity in patients who had a capsular infarct and eventually recovered from the resulting paresis. The patients were asked to sequentially touch their thumbs to the different fingers of the same hand, while regional blood flow was measured. The investigators found that in control subjects and for the unaffected hand of the patients, the contralateral motor cortex and premotor areas were active during the task. But when the previously paretic hand was used, both ipsilateral and contralateral motor areas showed increased blood flow, indicating that ipsilateral pathways were now contributing to the control of this movement (Weiller et al., 1993). However, the role of contralesional primary motor cortex (motor cortex in the side opposite to the affected cortex) to the recovery of function is not clear. Although researchers have demonstrated activation of contralesional primary motor cortex during hand movements on the paretic side, disruption of this activity using transcranial magnetic stimulation did not impair hand movements. There is also some evidence that recruitment of contralesional primary motor cortex can impede recovery through increased intracortical inhibition (Hummel et al., 2005; Ward & Cohen, 2004).

Cerebellar Contributions to Recovery from Cortical Injury. New longitudinal studies have reported the importance of cerebellar activation to motor recovery after lesions to the primary motor cortex, with the cerebellar hemisphere opposite to the damaged corticospinal tract appearing to have a more important role (Small et al., 2002). These studies suggest that the role of the cerebellum in recovery of function may be related to its role in motor learning.

Specifically, the cerebellum is thought to play a role in the improvement of motor performance through the establishment of automatic motor skills. The timing of cerebellar activation beginning at 2 or 3 months after stroke and persisting for 6 months, supports the hypothesis that its role in recovery is through learning. Further support for the role of the cerebellum in recovery of function following neural injury is from research showing that new cerebellar cortical synapses are associated with complex skill learning but not with gross motor activation in the absence of learning (Kleim et al., 1997, 1998).

Cross-Modality Plasticity. *Cross-modality plasticity* refers to the idea that when deprived of its usual input, the part of the cortex normally responsive to that input may now be responsive to inputs from other sensory modalities (Chen et al., 2002). Cross-modality plasticity has been most often studied in the visual system. The visual system projects to the visual cortex, while the auditory system projects to the auditory cortex. Experiments in ferrets by Sur et al. (1990) have shown that retinal cells may be induced to project into the medial geniculate nucleus, which projects onto the auditory cortex. When this occurs, the primary auditory cortex also responds to visual stimulation, with both orientation- and direction-selective neurons. Other researchers have performed similar experiments to induce visual neurons to project onto the somatosensory thalamus, and they have then found somatosensory cells responding to visual stimulation. This suggested that the different primary sensory areas had many characteristics in common, which allowed sensory inputs from one modality to activate cortical areas of others. However, although these new connections were functional, there were many abnormalities, indicating that prior specification had already occurred in these primary cortical areas (Sur et al., 1990). In humans, Braille readers have expanded sensory and motor representation for the reading finger, again showing that cortical representations are dynamically modulated based on learning and experience (Donoghue 1995; Pascual-Leone et al., 1993).

Neuroimaging research has shown task-dependent activation of the occipital cortex during tactile-, auditory-, memory-, and language-related neural processing in subjects blind from an early age. Both PET and fMRI studies have shown that auditory spatial processing and auditory motion occurs over the same areas that would normally process visual spatial and visual motion information in sighted individuals, suggesting that areas keep their function and neural coding abilities when a new modality takes over cortical areas. It has also been shown that there is a functional dissociation between a ventral "What" stream for the processing of object shape and a dorsal "Where" stream for the processing of space for auditory stimuli treated in the occipital cortex of blind subjects. There has been considerable debate about the extent of plastic changes that can occur in the cortex of subjects blinded later in life. It has now been shown that these individuals do show altered functioning of their deafferented visual cortices. However, the extent of plasticity and the regions recruited for auditory tasks is affected by the age of onset (Collignon et al., 2009).

Behavioral and cortical reorganization can also occur in visually normal individuals when deprived of vision for short periods. For example Pascua-Leone et al. (2005) showed a significant increase in occipital responses to sounds in sighted subjects blindfolded for 5 days, while Lewald (2007) showed reversible improvements in accuracy during sound localization after 90 minutes of blindfolding, a smaller but similar effect to those seen in blind subjects. How could this occur in such a short period of time. It has been shown that even in sighted individuals there is involvement of visual cortex in the processing of sounds (Collignon et al., 2008).

Strategies to Enhance Neural Plasticity and Cortical Reorganization

These studies have demonstrated the incredible plasticity of the nervous system and have shown the importance of this plasticity to the recovery of function following neural injury. Even more exciting is research exploring the effect of strategies to enhance neural plasticity and drive CNS reorganization in order to optimize recovery.

Effect of Training

Studies by Merzenich and colleagues looked at the effect of experience on reorganization of somatotopic maps in normal monkeys (Jenkins et al., 1990). In one experiment, monkeys were able to reach for food by using a strategy that involved use of their middle fingers only. After considerable experience with this task, the monkeys' cortical map showed an area for the middle fingers that was significantly larger than normal. This reorganization in somatosensory cortex resulting from training is shown in Figure 4.9. Later experiments found that once a new task is learned, there are certain aspects of central mapping changes that persist for long periods (Nudo, 2006; 2007; Nudo et al., 1996).

Research is also helping to clarify the optimal timing and intensity of training to maximize neural

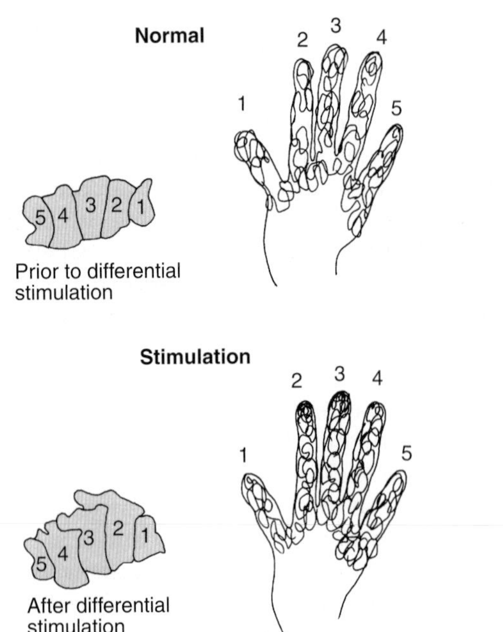

FIGURE 4.9 Training causes an expansion of cortical representation. (Adapted with permission from Jenkins WM, Merzenich MM, Och MT, Allard T, Guic-Robles E. Functional reorganization of primary somatosensory cortex in adult owl monkeys after behaviorally controlled tactile stimulation. J Neurophysiol 1990;63:82–104.)

plasticity. Not all forms of training appear to induce cortical reorganization. In animal models, skill learning was associated with cortical reorganization; however, strength training was not (Maldonado et al., 2008; Remple et al., 2001). Exercise affected angiogenesis but did not alter movement representation in the rat cortex (Kleim and Jones, 2008; Kleim et al., 2002). Early and intense forced motor behavior led to undesirable neurodegeneration in vulnerable neural tissue (Kozlowski et al., 1996; Schallert et al., 2000). However, training in combination with other interventions, such as pharmacologic treatment or neural transplantation, improved outcomes beyond that associated with an individual intervention (Dobrossy & Dunnett, 2001).

Cortical stimulation is also being used to facilitate motor recovery. Researchers have shown that noninvasive cortical stimulation enhances the effects of motor training on cortical plasticity in healthy adults (Antal et al., 2004; Bütefisch et al., 2004; Nitsche et al., 2003). Does cortical stimulation enhance function following a stroke? Stimulation of the contralateral intact hemisphere has been used to decrease cortical activity, reducing abnormal inhibition of the affected hemisphere by the intact hemisphere (Kobayashi et al., 2004). Hummel and colleagues (2005) examined the effects of cortical stimulation on hand function in individuals with chronic stroke. They examined performance of paretic hand function using the Jebsen–Taylor hand-function test (JTT) before and during cortical stimulation of the affected hemisphere. Performance on the JTT improved by about 12% during stimulation, and improved hand function persisted for about 25 minutes after stimulation ended.

While noninvasive cortical stimulation applied during or shortly before skill training has been shown to enhance motor learning, cortical stimulation given after training reduced the training-dependent increases in cortical excitability (Rosenkranz et al., 2000). It has been suggested that synchronizing training with stimulation improves performance because the behavioral signals driving plasticity during training are augmented by the presence of the extra stimulation. In contrast, when stimulation is applied outside the training experience, it disrupts the memory consolidation process and may induce plasticity that is not shaped by behavioral signals and is, therefore, detrimental to performance (Kleim and Jones, 2008).

What do all these studies tell us? They suggest that we have multiple pathways innervating any given part of the sensory or motor cortex, with only the dominant pathway showing functional activity. However, when a lesion occurs in one pathway, the less dominant pathway may immediately show functional connections. This leads us to the conclusion that even in adults, cortical maps are very dynamic. There appears to be use-dependent competition among neurons for synaptic connections. Thus, when one area becomes inactive, a neighboring area can take over its former targets and put them to functional use.

These experiments also suggest that our sensory and motor maps in the cortex are constantly changing in accordance with the amount to which they are activated by peripheral inputs. Since each of us has been brought up in a different environment and has practiced very different types of motor skills, the maps of each of our brains are unique and constantly changing as a result of these experiences.

Clinical Implications

What are the clinical implications of this research? First, it can help us to understand some of the neural changes that occur following injury. For example, following the neural lesion, cortical maps will demonstrate both: (a) immediate reorganization, due to the unmasking of previously nonfunctional synaptic connections from neighboring areas; and (b) a longer-term change, in which neighboring inputs to the areas take over the parts of the map that were previously occupied by damaged or destroyed cells.

Second, it tells us that experience is very important in shaping cortical maps. Thus, if we leave patients without rehabilitation training for many weeks or months, their brains will show changes in organization, reflecting disuse, which will be most detrimental to these patients. However, the good news is that training appears to make a difference no matter when it is given, since the brain continues to be plastic throughout our lives.

Visual prosthetic implants have been used to aid vision in blind individuals. However, it has been shown that the loss of visual abilities following early blindness and the recruitment of occipital regions by nonvisual inputs may actually interfere with the reacquisition of visual function using the prosthetic implant. For example, research has shown that persons who had recovered their sight still had robust responses to auditory stimulation in their visual cortex many years after regaining their sight (Collignon et al., 2009; Saenz et al., 2008).

Based on an extensive review of relevant research on activity-dependent neural plasticity, Kleim and Jones (2008) suggested 10 principles that potentially impact neurorehabilitation practices. These principles are summarized in Table 4.1. Principle 1, "use it or lose it," suggests that neural circuits not actively engaged in task performance for an extended period of time begin to degrade. In contrast, training can protect neurons and networks that would otherwise be lost after the injury (This refers to principle 2, "use it and improve it"). Principle 3, specificity, indicates that while practice associated with acquisition of a novel or reacquisition of a lost skill is associated with changes in motor cortex, repetition of a movement already learned is not. Research suggests that specific forms of neural plasticity are dependent upon specific kinds of experience. Neural plasticity is facilitated during practice related to acquisition of skill, not just repetition of an already learned or non-relevant movement.

Principle 4 reflects the importance of repetition to neural reorganization. Repetition of a newly learned (or relearned) behavior is required to induce lasting neural changes, making repetition an important principle in neurorehabilitation. Kleim and Jones (2008) suggest that repetition of a skilled movement is needed to obtain a level of brain reorganization sufficient to allow the patient to continue to use the affected function outside of therapy and to maintain and make further functional gains. Closely related to repetition, is Principle 5, "intensity." Training must be sufficiently intense to stimulate experience-dependent neural plasticity. This also requires that training be progressively modified to match the dynamic and changing skill level of the patient, thus maintaining a level of training intensity that ensures continued

TABLE 4.1 Principles of Experience-Dependent Plasticity

Principle	Description
1. Use it or lose it	Failure to drive specific brain functions can lead to functional degradation.
2. Use it and improve it	Training that drives a specific brain function can lead to an enhancement of that function.
3. Specificity	The nature of the training experience dictates the nature of the plasticity.
4. Repetition matters	Induction of plasticity requires sufficient repetition.
5. Intensity matters	Induction of plasticity requires sufficient training intensity.
6. Time matters	Different forms of plasticity occur at different times during training.
7. Salience matters	The training experience must be sufficiently salient to induce plasticity.
8. Age matters	Training-induced plasticity occurs more readily in younger brains.
9. Transference	Plasticity in response to one training experience can enhance the acquisition of similar behaviors.
10. Interference	Plasticity in response to one experience can interfere with the acquisition of other behaviors.

Adapted from Kleim JA, Jones TA. Principles of experience-dependent neural plasticity: implications for rehabilitation after brain damage. J Speech Lang Hear Res 2008;51:S225–S239.

neural adaptation throughout recovery and rehabilitation. However, the effect of intensity of training may be dependent on the timing of that intervention.

The Very Early Constraint-Induced Movement during Stroke Rehabilitation (VECTORS) study compared recovery of arm function recovery in a population of acute (within 14 days after stroke) patients with stroke in response to three types of training: (constraint induced movement therapy (CIMT) (2 hours task-specific training, 6 hours per day constraint of the noninvolved hand), conventional training (2 hours traditional occupational therapy) and a high-intensity dose of CIMT (3 hours shaping, 90% waking hours constraint of noninvolved hand) (Dromerick et al., 2009). Recovery of arm function measures using the Action Research Arm Test (ARAT) at 90 days after randomization was best in the groups receiving CIMT and conventional therapy, with no difference between the two. Most surprising was the finding that the group that received the high intensity CIMT training had the poorest arm function at 90 days. Thus, the VECTORS study did not support the hypothesis that more intense therapy in the acute stage would lead to better outcomes. Instead a *higher dose* of CIMT was associated with *less motor recovery,* at least in the acute stage of recovery (Dromerick et al., 2009). This study reminds us that the benefits of using a highly intense training schedule may vary depending on where the patient is in the recovery process. In early recovery, less may actually be more.

Principle 6, "time matters," reflects the fact that neural plasticity underlying learning and recovery of function is a process, with later types of plasticity often dependent on those that occur earlier in the process. For example, during motor skill training, gene expression precedes synapse formation, which in turn precedes motor map reorganization (Kleim & Jones, 2008). The importance of time in the recovery process is also supported by research demonstrating that specific types of interventions may be more or less effective depending on the time at which they are introduced. For example, Biernaskie et al. (2004) found that a 5-week period of rehabilitation initiated 30 days after cerebral infarcts was far less effective in improving functional outcome and in promoting growth of cortical dendrites than the same regimen initiated 5 days after infarct. However, as reported in Principle 5, the VECTORS study suggests that the intensity of training may need to be modified based on timing.

Principle 7 states that "salience matters"; in order to maximize activity-dependent neural plasticity, training must be functionally relevant and significant to the individual. For an activity to be salient, it must reflect an activity that the person wants to do (Hadders-Algra & Gramsberg, 2007; Kleim & Jones, 2008). Simply repeating an activity that is not functionally relevant will not induce neural plasticity and reorganization after brain damage; instead activity related to plasticity has to be salient, that is, make some sense to the person being trained. Thus, the desire and motivation of the patient to do a task increases the likelihood for neural adaptation associated with task-specific training.

Experience-dependent synaptic potentiation, synaptogenesis, and cortical-map reorganization are all reduced with aging, suggesting support for Principle 8, that "age matters" when it comes to activity dependent neural plasticity (Kleim & Jones, 2008). However, researchers have shown that the aging brain demonstrates experience-dependent reorganization, though brain changes may be less profound and/or slower to occur than those observed in younger brains (Kleim & Jones, 2008).

Principle 9, transference, refers to the ability of plasticity within one set of neural circuits to promote concurrent or subsequent plasticity in other circuits (Principle 9: Plasticity in response to one training experience can enhance the acquisition of similar behaviors.) (Kleim & Jones, 2008). In contrast, principle 10, interference, refers to the possibility of plasticity within a given neural circuitry impeding the induction of new, or expression of existing, plasticity within the same or other circuitry, which can impair learning (Principle 10: Plasticity in response to one experience can interfere with the acquisition of other behaviors.). Noninvasive cortical stimulation has been shown to improve plasticity in some instances (transference) but impede plasticity (interference) in others. For example, noninvasive cortical stimulation applied during or shortly before skill training may enhance motor learning (Bütefisch et al., 2004; Floel & Cohen, 2006), while transcranial direct current stimulation given after training reduced the training-dependent increases in cortical excitability (Rosenkranz et al., 2000). Synchronizing training with stimulation improves performance because the behavioral signals driving plasticity during training are augmented by the presence of the extra stimulation. In contrast, when stimulation is applied outside the training experience, it disrupts the memory consolidation process and may induce plasticity that is not shaped by behavioral signals and is, therefore, detrimental to performance.

Research indicates that neural plasticity is the basis for both motor learning in the intact brain and relearning in the damaged brain. Principles derived from research on activity-dependent neural plasticity can inform and guide the application of interventions designed to facilitate neural adaptation and promote the recovery of function in patients with impaired motor control.

SUMMARY

The research on the neurophysiological basis for learning, memory, and recovery of function covered in this chapter suggests the following important principles:

1. The brain is incredibly plastic, and it has great capacity to change; this includes not just the immature brain but also the mature adult brain.
2. The most important way in which the environment changes behavior in humans is through learning.
3. CNS structural changes occur because of the interaction between both genetic and experiential factors.
4. A key factor in experience is the concept of active competition, and this may be summed up in the phrase "the squeaky wheel gets the oil," or in this case, it gets the new synaptic connections. This concept is applicable from simple circuits to complex neural pathways.
5. Research suggests that short-term and long-term memory may not be separate categories, but may be part of a single graded memory function involving the same synapses.
6. Short-term changes reflect relatively temporary changes in synaptic effectiveness; structural changes are the hallmark of long-term memory.
7. Scientists believe that the circuits involved in the storage of procedural and declarative learning are different, with procedural memory involving cerebellar circuitry and declarative memory involving temporal-lobe circuitry.
8. Principles derived from research on activity-dependent neural plasticity can inform and guide rehabilitation practices to promote neural adaptation and functional recovery in patients with impaired motor control.

CHAPTER 5

CONSTRAINTS ON MOTOR CONTROL: AN OVERVIEW OF NEUROLOGIC IMPAIRMENTS

LEARNING OBJECTIVES

Following completion of this chapter, the reader will be able to:

1. Define the following terms used to classify impairments associated with central nervous system (CNS) pathology: signs versus symptoms, positive versus negative symptoms, primary versus secondary effects.
2. Define and describe impairments associated with pathophysiology of the motor cortex, including motor weakness (paresis), abnormal muscle tone (spasticity), and coordination problems, including abnormal synergies of movement. Discuss methods for assessing and treating these impairments.
3. Compare and contrast impairments in persons with pathology in the cerebellum versus the basal ganglia. Discuss the assessment and treatment of impairments associated with these subcortical structures, including abnormal muscle tone, tremor, and coordination problems affecting the timing and scaling of muscle activity.
4. Discuss the relationship between secondary musculoskeletal impairments and primary neuromuscular impairments; describe the management of musculoskeletal impairments in persons with neurologic pathology.
5. Review the effects of neural pathology on sensory systems; discuss clinical methods for assessing somatosensory, visual, and vestibular problems; and briefly review methods for treating sensory impairments.
6. Discuss the effect of neural pathology on explicit and implicit motor learning, and describe the relevance of this information to therapeutic strategies for teaching recovery of functional motor skills.

INTRODUCTION: SIGNS AND SYMPTOMS OF PATHOPHYSIOLOGY OF MOTOR CONTROL

Clinical treatment of the patient with motor control problems requires both knowledge and skill. Part of an essential knowledge base in treating patients with movement problems is understanding the physiology and pathophysiology of motor control. This information enables the therapist to form initial assumptions regarding the pattern of impairments likely to be found in patients with a specific neural pathology. In addition, understanding the impairments constraining movement helps the clinician to form initial assumptions regarding the probable functional limitations that will be found.

The formation of initial hypotheses regarding likely impairments and functional limitations guides the selection of appropriate tests and measures that are used to examine initial assumptions relative to a specific patient. Through examination procedures, the clinician determines the impairments and functional limitations in a specific patient. This then leads to the selection of interventions appropriate to that patient.

Since movement arises from the interaction of multiple processes, including those related to sensory/perceptual, cognitive, and action or motor systems, pathology within any of the systems will result in impairments that potentially constrain functional movement. A comprehensive discussion of the pathophysiology of motor control and learning is beyond the scope of this chapter. Instead, the purpose of this chapter is to introduce the topic of pathophysiology of motor control, presenting an overview of impairments associated with pathology in sensory/perceptual, action, and cognitive systems important to motor control. This chapter on pathophysiology parallels the organization of Chapter 3, which covers the physiology of normal motor control. Pathology within a specific part of the CNS produces characteristic impairments; however, because of the interacting nature of the CNS, impairments associated with pathology in other parts of the CNS may occur. For example, pathophysiology of the basal ganglia, specifically the substantia nigra, results in primary motor impairments, including bradykinesia, rigidity, and tremor. However, because of the complex loops between the basal ganglia and the cerebral cortex, other types of impairments, such as impaired cognition, may also accompany basal ganglia pathology.

We begin with a discussion of issues related to classifying or categorizing impairments in persons with neurologic pathology. We then present an overview of impairments associated with pathophysiology within the action systems, sensory/perceptual systems, and cognitive systems. A discussion of impairments in each of these systems is accompanied by a brief description of common approaches to clinical examination and treatment. In later chapters, we discuss in more detail the effects of these impairments on the specific functions of postural control, mobility, and reach and grasp behavior. We conclude the chapter with a summary of the constellation of impairments likely to be found in our four case studies.

Classifying Impairments Associated with CNS Lesions

Signs versus Symptoms

Brain pathology produces a unique pattern of behavioral signs and symptoms associated with the destruction of specific neuronal populations. Signs of neurologic dysfunction represent objective findings of pathology that can be determined by physical examination (e.g., the presence of nystagmus suggests that a patient has a vestibular disorder). In contrast, symptoms are subjective reports associated with pathology that are perceived by the patient, but may not necessarily be objectively documented on examination. Dizziness is a common symptom associated with vestibular pathology.

Positive versus Negative Signs and Symptoms

Hughlings Jackson described upper motor neuron lesions as damage to cortical and subcortical structures producing motor dyscontrol because of either: (1) the release of abnormal behaviors, called "positive symptoms"; and/or (2) the loss of normal behaviors, called "negative symptoms" (Foerster, 1977). Positive symptoms might include the presence of abnormal reflexes such as the extensor plantar (or Babinski) reflex or hyperactive stretch reflexes resulting in spasticity. Paresis, the loss of descending control of lower motor neurons, is an example of a negative symptom. In the rehabilitation environment, attempts to understand functional deficits in the patient with neurologic pathology often emphasize positive symptoms, such as increased muscle tone, at the expense of negative symptoms, such as loss of strength (Gordon, 1987; Katz & Rymer, 1989).

Primary versus Secondary Effects

CNS lesions can result in a wide variety of primary impairments affecting motor (neuromuscular), sensory/perceptual, and/or cognitive/behavioral systems. In addition to primary impairments such as paralysis or spasticity, secondary effects also contribute to motor control problems in the person with neurologic dysfunction. Secondary impairments do not result from the CNS lesion directly, but rather develop as a result of the original problem (Schenkman, 1990). For example, as shown in Figure 5.1, an upper motor neuron lesion results in primary impairments of paresis and spasticity. These impairments limit movement capabilities in the patient, and this immobility may result in the development of a secondary musculoskeletal impairment, such as changes in the structure

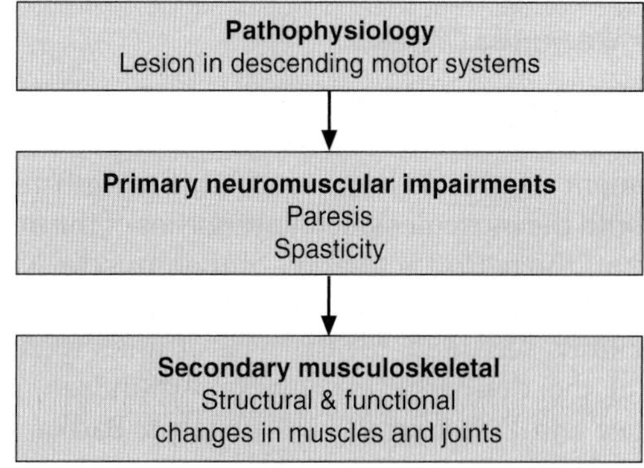

FIGURE 5.1 Pathophysiology within the CNS can result in both primary impairments and secondary impairments. For example, a CNS lesion produces primary neuromuscular impairments such as paresis and spasticity. These impairments, which limit movement, can result in the development of secondary musculoskeletal system impairments, such as changes in the structure and function of muscles and joints, which further constrain the person's ability to move.

and function of muscles, muscle contractures, and decreased joint range of motion, which further constrain the person's ability to move.

With this overview of methods for classifying impairments associated with CNS lesions, we can now turn our attention to the heart of this chapter, an overview of the pathophysiological basis for deficits in motor control in the patient with neurologic pathology. We begin with impairments resulting from pathology within the action systems, including both primary neural and secondary musculoskeletal impairments. This is followed by a discussion of impairments in sensory/perceptual systems. We then discuss cognitive impairments associated with pathology in specific association cortices in the frontal and parietal regions. We end the chapter with a summary of the impairments in a select group of patient case studies.

IMPAIRMENTS IN THE ACTION SYSTEMS

The action system includes areas of the nervous system such as motor cortex, cerebellum, and basal ganglia, which perform processing essential to the control of movement.

Motor Cortex Deficits

Pathophysiology of the motor cortex results in a wide range of neuromuscular impairments that constrain functional movement in the person with neurologic dysfunction.

Motor Weakness (Paresis)

Strength is defined as the ability to generate sufficient tension in a muscle for the purposes of posture and movement (Smidt & Rogers, 1982). Strength results from both the musculoskeletal properties of the muscle itself and the neural activation of that muscle. Neural aspects of force production reflect: (a) the number of motor units recruited, (b) the type of units recruited, and (c) the discharge frequency (Amundsen, 1990; Buchner and DeLateur, 1991; Duncan & Badke, 1987; Rogers, 1991).

Weakness is defined as an inability to generate normal levels of force; it is a major impairment of motor function in many patients with upper motor neuron lesions. Depending on the extent of the lesion, weakness in the patient with a cerebral cortex lesion can vary in severity from total or severe loss of muscle activity, called "paralysis" or "plegia," to mild or partial loss of muscle activity, called "paresis." Paralysis or paresis is defined as decreased voluntary motor unit recruitment, and reflects an inability or difficulty in recruiting skeletal motor units to generate torque or movement; it is one component of the upper motor neuron syndrome (Gracies, 2005a, b). Paresis results from a lesion within descending motor pathways, which interferes with the central excitatory drive to the motor units (Ghez, 1991). This results in an inability to recruit and/or modulate the motor neurons, leading to a loss of movement. Paresis and plegia are often referred to by their distribution: hemiplegia (or hemiparesis) is weakness affecting one side of the body, paraplegia affects the lower extremities, and tetraplegia affects all four limbs.

Many studies have documented problems in motor unit recruitment and discharge behavior in patients with cerebral cortex lesions and resultant hemiparesis (Frascarelli et al., 1998; Yan et al., 1998a, b). Reduced descending drive is associated with a failure to recruit high-threshold motor units and a reduced ability to modulate or increase motor unit discharge rate when trying to increase voluntary force (Gracies, 2005a, b). These changes are more apparent in the distal than in the proximal muscles (Frascarelli et al., 1998). Reduced excitatory input to the spinal motor neurons significantly reduces maximal voluntary power, since the main factor in determining power developed by a muscle is the number of motor units recruited (Gracies, 2005a, b; Petit et al., 2003).

Prolonged paresis, a primary neuromuscular impairment, also produces peripheral changes in the muscle, discussed in later sections of this chapter.

Abnormal Synergies

Pathology within the CNS can produce problems in activating and sequencing appropriate muscles for functional tasks, which results in the production of unnecessary movements in joints and muscles not directly involved in a functional movement task. Lesions to the corticospinal centers can lead to loss of the ability to recruit a limited number of muscles controlling movement and the ability to control individual joints. The result is the emergence of mass patterns of movement, often referred to as "abnormal synergies."

In the rehabilitation literature, the term *synergy* has often been used to describe abnormal or disordered motor control (Bobath, 1990; Brunnstrom, 1970). Abnormal synergies are stereotypical patterns of movement that cannot be changed or adapted to changes in task or environmental demands. Abnormal synergies, also called "abnormal patterns" or "mass patterns of movement," reflect a lack of fractionation, defined as the ability to move a single joint without simultaneously generating movements in other joints. Because muscles in an abnormal synergy are so strongly linked, movement outside the fixed pattern is often not possible (O'Sullivan & Schmitz, 2001).

Twitchell's 1951 classic paper described the role of synergies as part of the stepwise sequence of motor recovery following stroke. He suggested that stroke recovery begins with an initial areflexic flaccid paralysis; reflexes then return and become hyperactive, spasticity develops, and voluntary movement appears first as stereotyped flexor and extensor muscle synergies. As recovery continues voluntary movement out of synergies emerges, and finally the ability to move normally returns. Twitchell described the process of recovery proceeding from proximal to distal, with flexor movements occurring first in the upper extremity and extensor movements occurring first in the lower extremity. In both the arm and the leg, the return of reflexes precedes the recovery of voluntary movement; however, recovery could stop at any stage. The flexion synergy of the upper extremity, shown in Figure 5.2, is characterized by: scapular retraction and elevation, shoulder abduction and external rotation, elbow flexion, forearm supination, and wrist and finger flexion. The extensor synergy in the lower extremity involves hip extension, adduction and internal rotation, knee extension, ankle plantar flexion and inversion, and toe plantar flexion. Similar to Twitchell, Brunnstrom (1970) described six stages in the process of stroke recovery, including the emergence and dissolution of abnormal synergies. Table 5.1 compares the stages of recovery from stroke as described by Twitchell and Brunnstrom. There is some evidence to suggest that abnormal synergies result from the recruitment of brainstem centers, such as rubrospinal centers, associated with reduction in the recruitment of corticospinal descending controls.

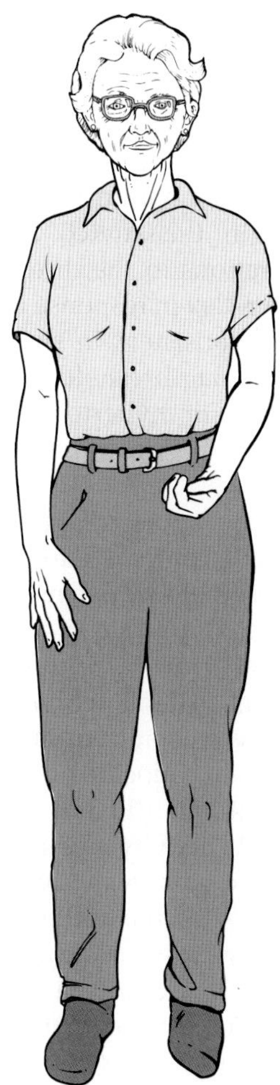

FIGURE 5.2 Flexion synergy of the upper extremity.

Coactivation

Coactivation of agonist and antagonist muscles during functional movements has been observed in many adults and children with pathophysiology in a wide variety of motor systems, including motor cortex, basal ganglia, and cerebellum (Crenna et al., 1994; Knutsson & Richards, 1979; Nashner et al., 1983). Coactivation is also present in the early stages of learning a skilled movement in neurologically intact adults and children. In addition, it is found during the early stages of postural development in healthy infants and children just learning to balance. The finding that coactivation is a common characteristic of unskilled early stages of learning in healthy neurologically intact individuals suggests that coactivation is not necessarily a result of impairment of function, but represents a potentially primary, perhaps primitive or unrefined, form of coordination.

Abnormal Muscle Tone—Spasticity

Muscle tone is characterized by a muscle's resistance to passive stretch, and a certain level of tone is typical in normal muscles. On the upper end of the tone spectrum (Fig. 5.3) is hypertonicity, manifested by spasticity or rigidity. At the other end are disorders of hypotonicity. The presence of abnormalities of muscle tone in persons with CNS pathology is well known. However, the exact contributions of abnormalities of muscle tone to functional deficits are not well understood.

Spasticity is defined as "a motor disorder characterized by a velocity-dependent increase in tonic stretch reflexes (muscle tone) with exaggerated tendon jerks, resulting from hyperexcitability of the stretch reflex, and is one component of the upper motor neuron syndrome" (Lance, 1980, p. 485). In this chapter we typically use the term *lesion in the descending motor systems* in place of *upper motor neuron lesion*. A lesion

TABLE 5.1 A Comparison of the Stages of Recovery from Stroke as Described by Twitchell (1951) and Brunnstrom (1970)

Twitchell (1951)	Brunnstrom (1970)
Flaccid Paralysis with areflexia	Stage 1: Flaccid paralysis
Reflex activity returns/spasticity develops	Stage 2: Development of minimal movement in synergies
Voluntary movement in stereotyped flexor (upper extremity) and extensor (lower extremity) synergies; spasticity is at maximal level	Stage 3: Voluntary movement synergy-dependent
Voluntary movement with breaking up of synergies; spasticity reducing	Stage 4: Some movements out of synergy
Normal voluntary movement with normal speed and dexterity/slight hyperactivity of tendon reflexes	Stage 5: Movements almost independent of synergies
	Stage 6: Normal movement with normal speed

Adapted from Crow JL, Harmeling-van der Wel BC. Hierarchical properties of the motor function sections of the Fugl-Meyer Assessment Scale for people after stroke: a retrospective study. Phys Ther 2008;88:1556, Figure 1, with permission of the American Physical Therapy Association.

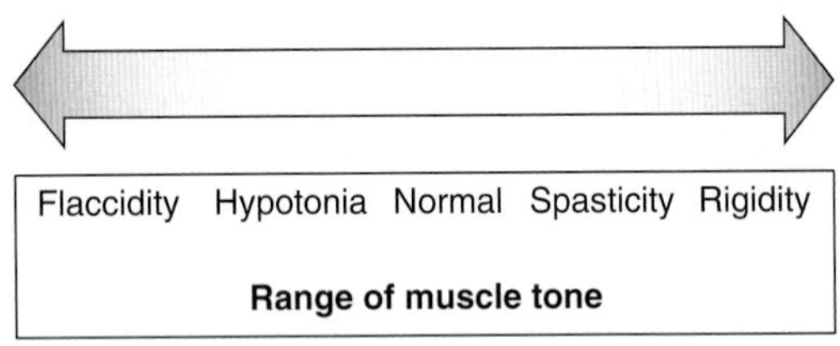

FIGURE 5.3 Continuum of muscle tone. The center of the graph illustrates the range of normal muscle tone. A decrease in muscle tone compared with normal is referred to as "hypotonia." In contrast, an increase in muscle tone compared with normal is referred to as "hypertonia," and manifests as either spasticity or rigidity.

in the descending motor systems could reflect pathology in the pyramidal tract or other nearby descending motor pathways such as the corticoreticulospinal tract. Damage to these tracts results in increased alpha motor neuron excitability, with a resulting increase in muscle tone (enhanced tonic stretch reflex activity) and exaggerated tendon jerks (phasic stretch reflexes) (Mayer, 1997).

Understanding spasticity is difficult in part because the term is used clinically to cover a wide range of abnormal behaviors. It is used to describe: (a) hyperactive stretch reflexes, (b) abnormal posturing of the limbs, (c) excessive coactivation of antagonist muscles, (d) associated movements, (e) clonus, and (f) stereotyped movement synergies. Thus, the one word *spasticity* is used to describe many abnormal behaviors often seen in patients with CNS pathology.

A key sign of spasticity is a velocity-dependent increase in resistance of a muscle or muscle group to passive stretch. The predominant hypothesis regarding the neural mechanism underlying spasticity is that it is due to changes in descending activity that result in abnormalities within the segmental stretch reflex. Disorders in the stretch reflex mechanism could reflect alterations in the threshold and/or the gain of the stretch reflex in response to stretch. Several studies have been consistent in showing changes in the set point, or angular threshold, of the stretch reflex in muscles with spastic hypertonus (Katz & Rymer, 1989; Latash et al, 1998; Powers et al., 1989; Thilmann et al., 1991).

Rymer and colleagues (Katz & Rymer, 1989; Powers et al., 1989) compared torque at the elbow joint during imposed elbow extension using a ramp-and-hold stimulus, at a range of velocities, between normal subjects and subjects with spastic hemiparesis. They found that patients with elbow flexor spasticity had high levels of electromyographic (EMG) activity at movement velocities of 112 degrees/sec. Normal healthy subjects did not exhibit substantial stretch evoked EMG activity at this velocity. Surprisingly, stretch reflex gain was comparable between the two groups. This led the authors to conclude that enhanced EMG activity in spastic muscles in response to imposed stretch was due to a decrease in stretch reflex threshold rather than an increase in gain.

Thilmann and colleagues (1991) compared muscle response to passively imposed stretch (elbow extension) in patients with hemiparesis following a stroke of the middle cerebral artery. Responses of the normal control subjects are shown in Figure 5.4A. Each trace is the rectified and averaged biceps EMG responses obtained from 10 displacements at velocities from 35 to 300 degrees/sec. The joint position traces are shown in the center of the figure. Half the normal subjects showed a reflex response at 200 degrees/sec; in the remainder, no reflex response was found even at the highest velocities. In contrast, the patients with spastic hemiparesis showed an early reflex response to displacements at velocities as low as 110 degrees/sec, along with a velocity-dependent increase in stretch reflex responsiveness, as shown in Figure 5.4B. Thus, in response to imposed stretch, there was both an early activation of the muscle and a prolonged activation of the muscle that lasted as long as the displacement was applied. The results from these experiments suggest that spasticity is related to both a decrease in stretch reflex threshold and persisting reflex hyperexcitability.

What is the neural basis for abnormal stretch reflex activity? It has been proposed that enhanced stretch reflex activity can occur because the alpha motor neuron pool at the segmental level is hyperexcitable, the amount of excitatory afferent input elicited by muscle stretch is increased, or both. Hyperexcitability of the alpha motor neuron pool can be due to a loss of descending inhibitory input, postsynaptic denervation supersensitivity, shortening of the motor neuron dendrites, or collateral sprouting of the dorsal-root afferents (Mayer et al., 1997; Noth, 1991).

Although we have greater understanding of the neural mechanisms underlying spastic hypertonicity, there is still no agreement on the role of spasticity in the loss of functional performance (Rymer & Katz, 1994). It has been suggested that spasticity limits a patient's ability to move quickly, since activation of the stretch reflex is velocity-dependent. While excessive activation of the stretch reflex mechanism in an antagonist muscle could serve to prevent lengthening of that muscle during a shortening contraction of the agonist, researchers have shown that it is inadequate recruitment of agonist motor neurons, not increased activity in the antagonist, that is the primary basis for disorders

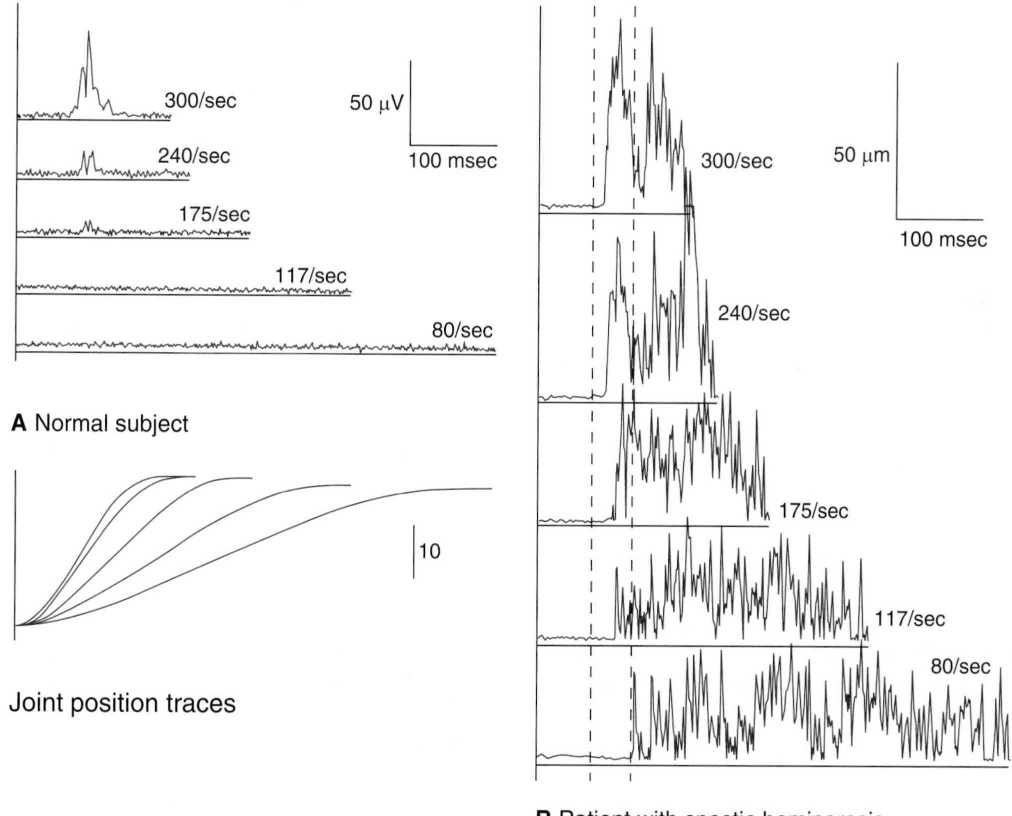

FIGURE 5.4 A comparison of EMG activity of the biceps brachii muscle in response to imposed elbow extension (30 degrees) at five different velocities ranging from 80 degrees/sec to 300 degrees/sec, in a normal control subject (A) and a person with spastic paresis of the left arm due to a middle cerebral artery stroke (B), showing the velocity-dependent activation of muscle. (Adapted with permission from Thilmann AF, Fellows SJ, Garms E. The mechanism of spastic muscle hypertonus. Brain 1991;114:237.)

of motor control following a CNS lesion (Bohannon & Andrews, 1990; Dietz et al., 1991; Gowland et al., 1992; McLellan, 1973; Sahrmann & Norton, 1977; Tang & Rymer, 1981). Thus, other problems, such as inability to recruit motor neurons (paresis), abnormal reciprocal inhibition between agonist and antagonist, and impaired coordination of muscle synergists may be more disabling in relation to motor control than simple hypertonicity (Katz & Rymer, 1994).

This research has tremendous implications for clinical practice. It suggests that treatment practices directed primarily at reducing spastic hypertonicity as the major focus in regaining motor control may have limited impact on helping patients regain functional independence. This is because loss of functional independence is often the result of many factors that limit the recovery of motor control and is not limited to the presence of abnormal muscle tone. Some of those factors include problems within the coordination of synergistic muscles activated in response to instability.

Clinical Examination of Motor Cortex Impairments

Motor Weakness. Can strength impairments be measured reliably in a person with a CNS lesion? Traditionally, clinicians believed that measuring strength in individuals with CNS pathology was not appropriate. This was based on the assumption that the primary impairment affecting functional performance was not weakness, but spasticity. In addition, strength training in the person with a CNS lesion was considered contraindicated, since it was believed that strength training would increase tone problems (Bobath, 1990; Davies, 1985). In more recent years there has been an increased emphasis on the examination of strength in persons with cerebral cortex lesions. In addition, researchers have begun to examine assumptions related to the positive and negative effects of strength training in the individual with a cerebral cortex lesion (Powell et al., 1999; Smith et al., 1999; Wiley & Damiano, 1998). This newer research reflects the growing awareness that paresis (a negative sign) is as important a factor in impaired functional performance as spasticity (a positive sign) (Andrews & Bohannon, 2000; Bohannon & Walsh, 1992; Katz & Rymer, 1989).

Strength can be measured under three conditions: isometrically, isotonically, or isokinetically (Buchner & DeLateur, 1991). However, in the clinic, the most common approach is to examine isometric or isokinetic strength during a shortening contraction (Amundsen, 1990). Manual muscle testing is the most common clinical approach to testing strength. This test assesses a subject's ability to move a body segment through its range of motion against gravity, or against externally applied resistance (Andrews, 1991). An ordinal scale is used to grade strength from 0 (no contraction) to 5 (full movement against gravity and maximal resistance). A limitation of manual muscle testing is that it does not examine the ability of a muscle to participate in a functional movement pattern.

An alternative approach to quantifying strength incorporates the use of handheld dynamometers, which provide an objective indication of muscle-group strength (Andrews, 1991; Bohannon, 1990). Handheld dynamometers are used to measure the force required to "break" the position held by the patient against resistance applied by the examiner. Finally, muscle performance can be tested dynamically through the use of instrumented isokinetic systems. Isokinetic testing assesses power, or the ability to generate force throughout the range of motion, at different speeds and over several repetitions (Wilk, 1990). Using these methods, researchers have begun to document the intensity and distribution of strength impairments in persons with CNS lesions. Results from these studies are beginning to challenge long-held clinical assumptions regarding strength deficits in the person with CNS pathology. For example, Andrews and Bohannon (2000) quantified the distribution of strength impairments following stroke in 48 patients with acute stroke. The strength of eight muscles was assessed bilaterally using a handheld dynamometer. Strength was impaired on both sides of the body, suggesting the bilateral effects of a cerebral cortex lesion. Interestingly, distal muscles were less impaired than proximal muscles on the nonparetic side, and extensor muscle activity was less affected than flexor activity bilaterally. The authors conclude that with few exceptions their results do not support common clinical assumptions about the distribution of strength impairments following stroke.

Many studies are now showing the bilateral effects of ipsilateral lesions of the cerebral cortex (Hermsdorfer et al., 1999; Marque et al., 1997; Winstein & Pohl, 1995). For example, Marque et al. (1997) used a handheld dynamometer, an isokinetic dynamometer, finger tapping, and a nine-hole peg test to examine motor impairments in ipsilateral extremities in 15 patients with acute stroke. They found significant motor impairments in the side ipsilateral to the lesion at 20 days after stroke. These impairments had almost completely resolved by 90 days after stroke.

Wiley and Damiano (1998) compared strength profiles in lower-extremity muscles in 30 children with cerebral palsy (CP) (15 children with spastic diplegia and 15 with spastic hemiplegia) with 16 age-matched peers. Using a handheld dynamometer, they quantified isometric strength in major lower-extremity muscle groups bilaterally. The results of

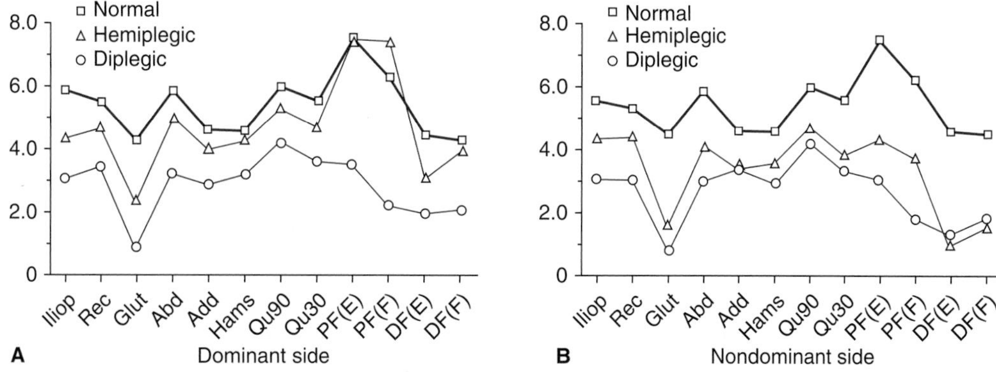

FIGURE 5.5 A comparison of strength profiles in lower-extremity muscles (normalized to body weight) in children with spastic hemiplegia and diplegia and age-matched peers ("normal"). Strength in the muscles of the dominant side is shown in A, and the nondominant side in B. (Adapted with permission from Wiley ME, Damiano DL. Lower-extremity strength profiles in spastic cerebral palsy. Dev Med Child Neurol 1998;40:104.)

this study are summarized in Figure 5.5, A and B, which compare strength values normalized by body weight in the three groups of children, across a variety of muscles, as shown along the x-axis. Significant results from the study included: (a) children with CP were weaker than age-matched peers in all muscles tested; (b) the children with hemiplegia showed significant weakness on both the involved and noninvolved limbs; (c) weakness was greater in the distal muscles as compared with proximal muscles; and (d) hip flexors and ankle plantar flexors were stronger than their antagonist muscles. In trying to explain the basis for weakness in these children, the authors collected EMG data during strength testing on several of their subjects. These data are shown in Figure 5.6, A and B. Shown are the rectified EMG recordings of the agonist and antagonist muscles during a strength test in a normally developing 8-year-old (Fig. 5.6A) and a child with CP. When asked to maximally contract her hamstrings, the normally developing child shows a phasic burst of activity in the left hamstrings with no activation of the antagonist quadriceps. Similarly, a maximal contraction of the quadriceps (Fig. 5.6B) is not associated with activation of the antagonist hamstrings. In contrast, when the child with cerebral palsy is asked to activate the quadriceps (Fig. 5.6D), there is a concomitant activation of the antagonist hamstrings. Interestingly, there is poor activation of the hamstring muscle when this child is trying to activate it for a maximal contraction (Fig. 5.6C). Thus, the studies suggest that weakness in children with CP appears to have both a neurophysiological and a biomechanical basis.

Abnormal Synergies. Clinical evaluation of the presence of abnormal synergies of movement most often involves the observation and description of the resting posture of the arm and leg. In addition, the patient is asked to perform volitional movements, and the quality and nature of those movements with reference to the presence of synergies is described.

The Fugl-Meyer Assessment (FMA) is a stroke specific test of impairments designed to evaluate recovery in the patient with post stroke hemiplegia (Fugl-Meyer, et al., 1975; Gladstone et al., 2002). The test is based on Twitchell's description of the natural history of motor recovery following stroke and Brunnstrom's stages of motor recovery, and was designed as a measure of neurologic recovery at the impairment level (Gladstone et al. 2002; Poole & Whitney, 1988). The scale is organized into five domains: motor function in the upper and lower extremities, sensory functioning including light touch and joint position sense, balance, joint range of motion, and joint pain. Items are scored using a 3-point ordinal scale, where 0 = cannot perform, 1 = performs partially, and 2 = performs fully. Motor scores range from 0 (hemiplegia) to 100 (normal motor performance) points, with 66 points for the upper extremity and 34 points for the lower extremity. Training in the correct administration of the FMA is recommended; the test takes approximately 30 minutes to administer.

The psychometric properties of the FMA, particularly the Motor Subscale, have been studied extensively and shown to have good reliability (Duncan et al., 1983; Sanford et al, 1993). Several studies have established construct validity with measures of performance of activities of daily living (Fugl-Meyer et al., 1975; Wood-Dauphinee et al., 1990) and other measures of arm and hand function in stroke (De Weerdt & Harrison, 1985; Malouin et al., 1994; Rabadi & Rabadi, 2006; van der Lee et al., 2001). Rasch analysis of the upper-extremity subscale has suggested removal of the three reflex items, leaving a

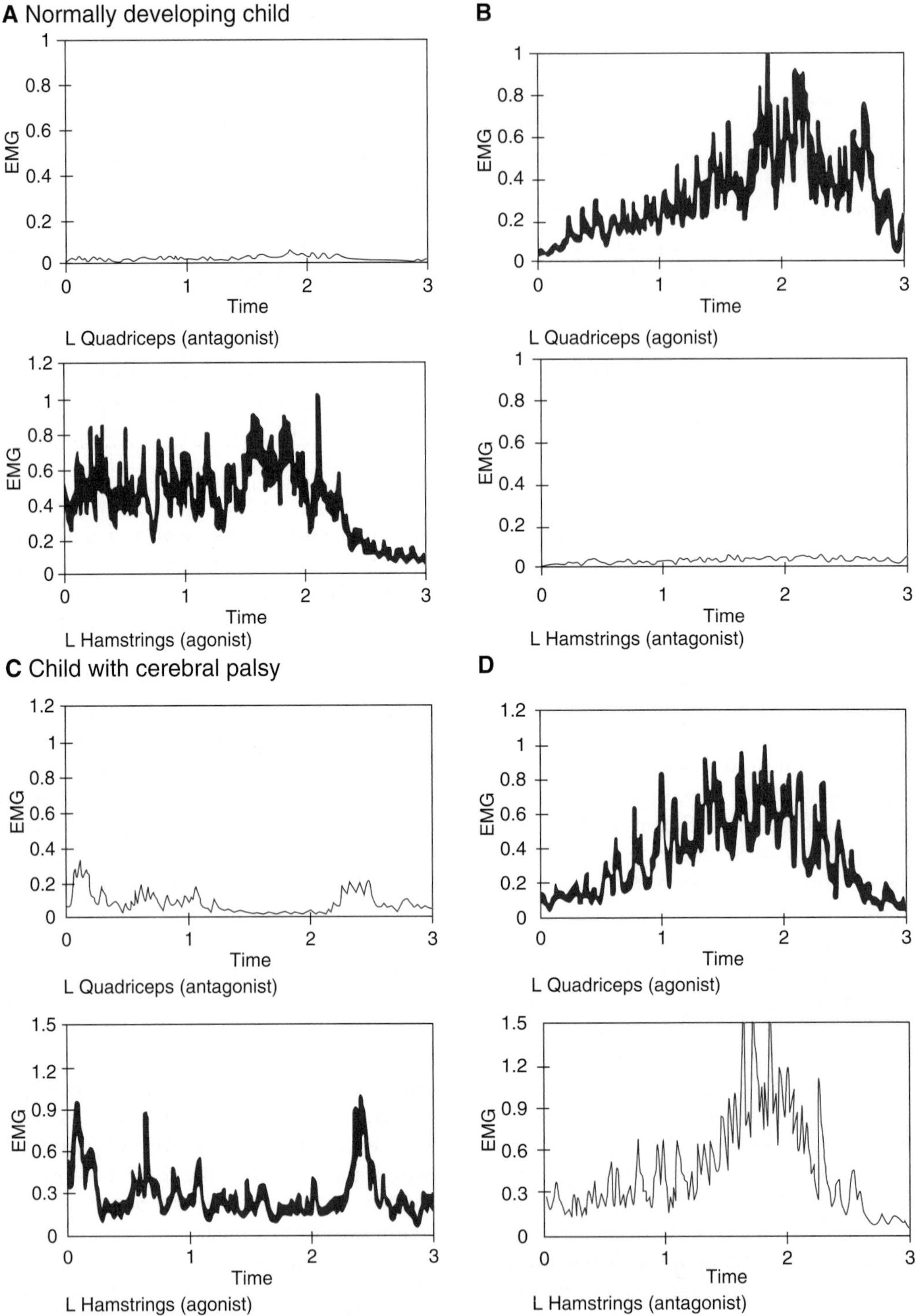

FIGURE 5.6 Rectified integrated EMG activity of the agonist and antagonist muscles in a normally developing 8-year-old child during isometric strength test of the left hamstrings (A) and quadriceps (B). EMG activity in the same set of muscles in an 8-year-old child with spastic cerebral palsy (C, D). (Adapted with permission from Wiley ME, Damiano DL. Lower-extremity strength profiles in spastic cerebral palsy. Dev Med Child Neurol 1998;40:105.)

30-item unidimensional measure of volitional movement (Woodbury et al., 2007). In addition, research has described and validated a short form of the Motor Scale (Hsieh et al., 2007). Other research examining the hierarchical properties of the Fugl-Meyer Motor Scale has suggested that it can be administered in a shortened manner and a summary score used (Crow et al., 2008).

Spasticity. Both clinical scales and instrumented measures have been developed to evaluate muscle tone. Muscle tone is assessed clinically by describing a muscle's resistance to passive stretch. Subjective rating scales, such as the modified Ashworth scale (MAS) shown in Assessment Tool 5.1, are often used to describe alterations in muscle tone (Bohannon & Smith, 1987; Snow et al., 1990). The Ashworth scale has been shown to have good interrater and intrarater reliability in patients with stroke (Brashear et al., 2002; Gregson et al., 1999), but its reliability in children with cerebral palsy was poor to moderate (Mutlu et al., 2008). In addition, questions have been raised as to the validity and psychometric properties of both the Ashworth and the modified Ashworth scale (Damiano et al., 2002; Haugh et al., 2006; Johnson, 2002; Patrick & Ada, 2006; Scholtes et al., 2006). Johnson points out that the addition of the 1+ to the scoring system raises questions as to whether it is now an ordinal scale, since it is not clear that the distances between 1 and 1+, and 1+ and 2 are equal and hierarchical in nature (Johnson, 2002). In addition, since soft-tissue changes associated with muscle contractures in spastic muscles also contribute to resistance to passive movement, resistance felt to passive movements cannot be attributed solely to spasticity (Haugh et al., 2006; Patrick & Ada, 2006; Scholtes et al., 2006). Gracies (2005a, b) suggests that to assess muscle stiffness accurately, the muscle should be stretched no more than once, if possible, as subsequent stretches reduce stiffness by 20 to 60% as compared with the initial stretch. In addition, it is important that the muscle is at rest, as muscle contraction will also contribute to increased resistance to stretch.

Behavioral indicators of spasticity can include a change in the resting position of a limb or the presence of characteristic movement patterns. Thus, careful observation of the patient at rest and while moving is essential. Table 5.2 summarizes common behavioral manifestations seen in patients with lesions in the descending motor system and suggests the probable spastic muscles producing the behavior (Mayer et al., 1997).

The pendulum or drop test, first reported by Wartenberg in the early 1950s, is a clinical method for assessing hypertonicity in the lower extremities (Wartenberg, 1951). In this test, the patient sits (or is supine) with legs dangling over the edge of a table. As shown in Figure 5.7, the relaxed leg is passively straightened and released so the leg swings by gravity alone. In subjects with normal muscle tone, the leg flexes to about 70 degrees and oscillates back and forth in a pendular motion about six times. In a patient with quadriceps or hamstrings spasticity, the leg may not reach vertical and swings with fewer repetitions than a noninvolved leg. Leg motion can be quantified using isokinetic exercise equipment, an electrogoniometer, or computerized video equipment that measures leg kinematics (Stillman & McMeeken, 1995). The drop test has been shown to be a relatively simple, reliable, and practical objective measure of abnormal muscle tone (Brown, 1993; Katz et al., 1992). Measures of spasticity, whether clinical or instrumented, are not always good predictors of motor performance and disability, suggesting the importance of other factors.

There is considerable discussion and disagreement among clinicians and researchers alike as to the validity, reliability, and clinical utility of various methods used to measure spasticity (see reviews by Scholtes et al., 2006; Burridge et al., 2005; Pandyan et al., 2001; Platz et al., 2005; Wood et al., 2005). Often methods appropriate for use by researchers are not useful to clinicians; thus, at this time it is difficult to identify a best practice related to the assessment of abnormalities of muscle tone.

Assessment Tool 5-1

Modified Ashworth Scale for Grading Abnormal Tone

0 = No increase in muscle tone

1 = Slight increase in muscle tone, manifested by a slight catch and release or by minimal resistance at the end of the range of motion when the affected part is moved in flexion or extension

1+ = Slight increase in muscle tone, manifested by a catch, followed by minimal resistance throughout the remainder (less than half) of the range of motion

2 = More marked increase in muscle tone, passive movement difficult

3 = Considerable increase in muscle tone, passive movement difficult

4 = Affected part(s) rigid in flexion or extension

Adapted from Bohannon RW, Smith MB. Interrater reliability of a modified Ashworth scale of muscle spasticity. Phys Ther 1987;67:206, with permission of the American Physical Therapy Association.

Treatment of Motor Cortex Impairments

Strategies To Improve Recruitment Of Paretic Muscles. Biofeedback and functional electrical stimulation are interventions typically used to assist patients in recruiting paretic muscles for functional activities. For example, electrical stimulation of the peroneal nerve is commonly performed in patients with hemiplegia to improve control over the anterior tibialis muscle during a voluntary contraction or during gait. Functional electrical stimulation (FES) has been used to improve recruitment of paretic upper-extremity

TABLE 5.2 Behavioral Observations in Patients with CNS Lesions that Produce Spasticity

Below are the common patterns of deformity seen in the upper motor neuron syndrome and the muscles that may contribute to each deformity. The weak muscles involved in each are also identified, but it should be remembered that these are unlikely to contribute to deformity even when spastic and therefore may not be candidates for chemodenervation. It must also be noted that not all listed muscles will be involved in any particular patient; strong agonists may counterbalance a spastic antagonist, and all muscles crossing a joint contribute to the net force across it. The bolded items reflect the behavior the person observed; the nonbold items are the muscles that are active and likely contributing to the pattern of movement.

The Upper Limbs	
The Adducted/Internally Rotated Shoulder	**The Flexed Wrist**
Pectoralis major	Flexor carpi radialis and brevis
Latissimus dorsi	Extrinsic finger flexors
Teres major	**The Clenched Fist**
Subscapularis	Various muscle slips of FDP
The Flexed Elbow	Various muscle slips of FDS
Brachioradialis	**The Intrinsic Plus Hand**
Biceps	Dorsal interossei
Brachialis	**The Thumb-in-Palm Deformity**
The Pronated Forearm	Adductor pollicis
Pronator quadratus	Thenar group
Pronator teres	Flexor pollicis longus
The Lower Limbs	
The Equinovarus Foot	**The Flexed Knee (with curled toes or claw toes)**
	Medial hamstrings
Medial gastrocnemius	Lateral hamstrings
Lateral hamstrings	Quadriceps
Soleus	Gastrocnemius
Tibialis posterior	**Adducted thighs**
Tibialis anterior	Adductor longus
Extensor hallucis longus	Adductor magnus
Long toe flexors	Gracilis
Peroneus longus	Iliopsoas (weak)
The Valgus Foot	Pectineus (weak)
Peroneus longus and brevis	**The Flexed Hip**
Gastrocnemius	Rectus femoris
Soleus	Iliopsoas
Tibialis anterior (weak)	Pectineus
Long toe flexors (weak)	Adductors longus

(continued)

TABLE 5.2 Behavioral Observations in Patients with CNS Lesions that Produce Spasticity

Striatal Toe (hitchhiker's great toe)	Adductor brevis (weak)
Extensor hallucis longus	Gluteus maximus (weak)
The Stiff (extended) Knee	
Gluteus maximus	
Rectus femoris	
Vastus lateralis	
Vastus medialis	
Vastus intermedius	
Hamstrings	
Gastrocnemius	
Iliopsoas (weak)	

FDP = flexor digitorum profundus; FDS = flexor digitorum superficialis.

Reprinted with permission from Mayer NH, Esquenazi A, Childers MK. Common patterns of clinical motor dysfunction. Muscle Nerve 1997;6;S21.

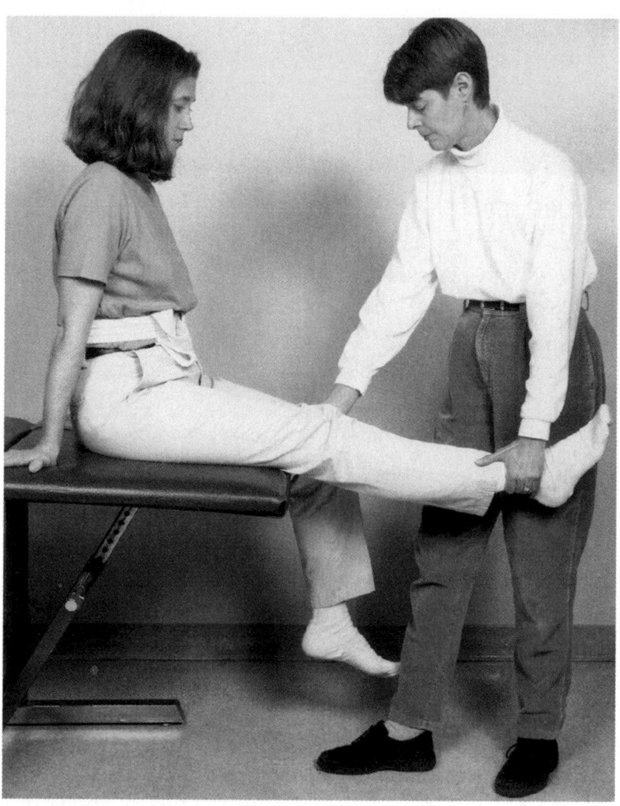

FIGURE 5.7 The pendulum test for spasticity in the lower extremity. The leg is passively extended then released so it swings by gravity alone. A reduction in the number of oscillations is indicative of spasticity.

muscles following stroke. Powell et al. (1999) used FES of the wrist extensors in 60 patients with hemiparesis 2 to 4 weeks after stroke. Subjects were randomly assigned to a control group who received standard treatment or to an experimental group who received standard treatment in addition to FES of the wrist extensors (30 minutes 3 times a day for 8 weeks). They found that the FES group had significantly greater isometric strength of the wrist extensors as compared with the control group, suggesting that FES is a viable therapeutic intervention to improve strength in wrist extensors in patients after stroke.

Case reports have been published on the integration of FES into functional task training of the upper extremity following stroke (Brown et al., 2000; Sullivan & Hedman, 2004). Sullivan & Hedman (2004) used a combination of sensory amplitude electrical stimulation and FES to improve upper limb function in a 67-year-old man 5 years after stroke. Sensory stimulation over the hemiparetic wrist extensors (electrical stimulation [10 seconds on and 10 seconds off] that was perceived but resulted in no observable or palpable muscle contraction) was carried out for 2 hours per day. FES was delivered to the wrist extensors while the patient practiced a lifting task for 15 minutes twice a day (Fig. 5.8). After 18 weeks of home exercise that included six physical therapy home visits there was a significant improvement on scores on the Action Research Arm Test (Fig. 5.9) and the Stroke Rehabilitation Assessment of Movement (STREAM).

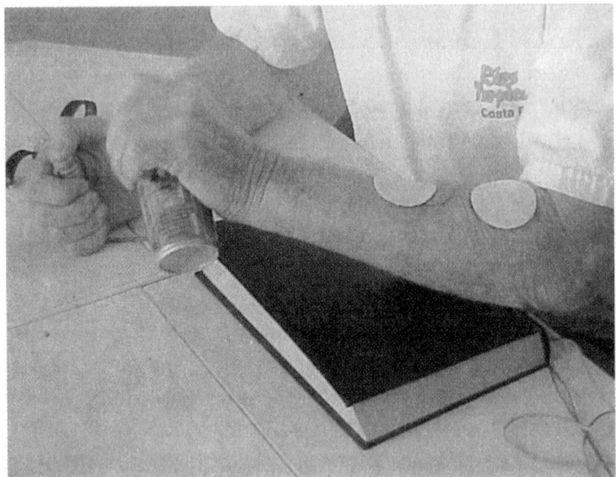

FIGURE 5.8 Use of neuromuscular electrical stimulation to facilitate recruitment of paretic muscles during a functional lifting task following stroke. (Adapted from Sullivan JE, Hedman LD. A home program of sensory and neuromuscular electrical stimulation with upper limb task practice in a patient 5 years after stroke. Phys Ther 2004;84:1049, with permission of the American Physical Therapy Association. This material is copyrighted, and any further reproduction or distribution requires written permission from APTA.)

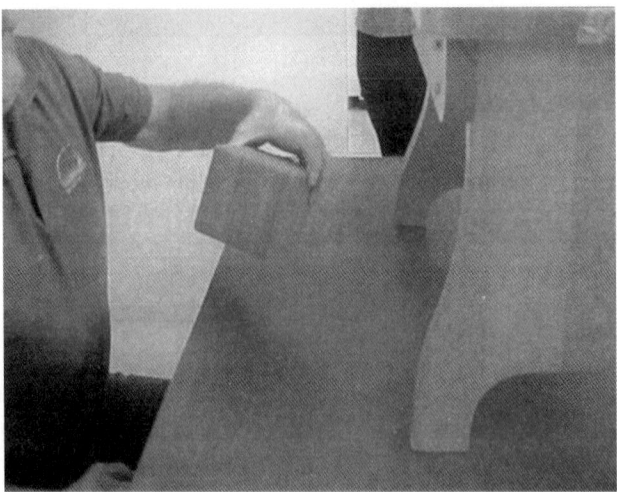

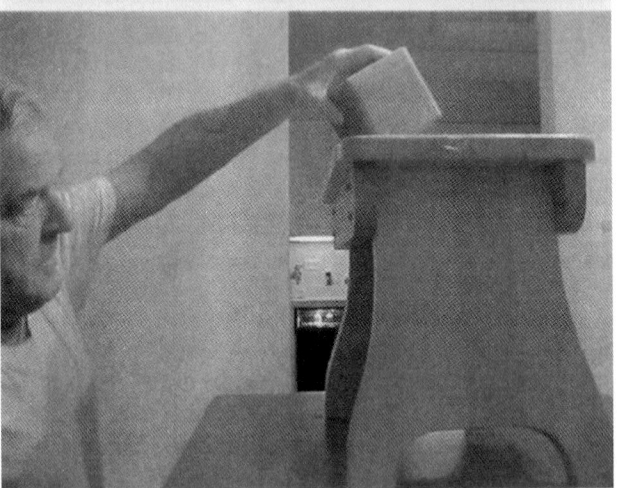

FIGURE 5.9 Effect of 18 weeks of FES on the Action Research Arm Test. A, When the person attempts to lift a block, the wrist remains flexed. B, Following FES treatment, the person lifts a block with the wrist in neutral position. (Adapted from Sullivan JE, Hedman LD. A home program of sensory and neuromuscular electrical stimulation with upper limb task practice in a person 5 years post stroke. Phys Ther 2004;84:1051, with permission of the American Physical Therapy Association. This material is copyrighted, and any further reproduction or distribution requires written permission from APTA.)

In addition, the patient reported improved functional ability to button clothing, use a knife and fork, and tie fishing knots (Sullivan & Hedman, 2004).

Several researchers have suggested the use of bimanual training to improve the recovery of paretic-limb function. The rationale for this approach is based on interlimb coordination studies by Kelso et al. (1981), who demonstrated that when the two hands perform identical tasks, there is a tight phasic relationship observed in which one limb "entrains" the other, causing them to function as a unit. Kelso also found that when the two limbs are performing asymmetric tasks, the limb performing the more difficult task has an impact on the limb performing the easier task. This has also been found for the performance of bilateral movements in patients with stroke hemiparesis. Following hemiparetic stroke, bilateral movement tasks resulted in slowed movement times in the nonhemiparetic limb (Lewis & Byblow, 2004; Rice & Newell, 2001, 2004) and improved movement characteristics (specifically, smoother kinetic profiles) in the hemiparetic limb (Rose & Winstein 2004). Rose and Winstein (2004) suggest that in addition to the bimanual requirement, other task requirements may be important to enhancing paretic-limb function. For example, they found an increase in peak velocity in the paretic limb of subjects with stroke during asymmetric rapid aiming tasks when the paretic limb aimed at a far target.

Task-specific effects were also reported by Lewis and Byblow (2004), who found that movement tasks involving proximal muscles benefited most from bilateral training. Research on the use of bimanual training to improve paretic-limb function is limited, and results have been mixed. A more complete review of this topic is presented in Rose and Winstein (2004) and in Chapter 19.

Treatment of Impaired Strength. The shift in emphasis on the functional significance of impaired strength in patients with CNS lesions has led to a growing stress on strength training in these patients. Techniques to improve strength can focus on generating force to move a body segment or, alternatively, on generating force to resist a movement. Progressive resistive exercises are commonly used to increase strength within individual muscles.

Isokinetic equipment can also be used to improve a patient's ability to generate force throughout the range of motion, at different speeds of motion, and through repeated efforts within individual and groups of muscles (Duncan & Badke, 1987). There have been numerous articles examining the effects of strength training in various patient groups. In addition, there are several good review articles on strength training in persons with cerebral palsy (Dodd et al., 2002; Mockford & Caulton, 2008; Scianni et al., 2009) and stroke (Morris et al., 2004; Riolo & Fisher, 2003). These reviews suggest fairly strong evidence related to the effect of strength training on improving muscle strength; however, the evidence for improving functional activities including gait was less compelling.

Treatment of Spasticity. A number of therapeutic interventions have been developed to manage spasticity, including pharmacologic, surgical, and physical treatments. The type of treatment chosen will depend on a number of factors, including the distribution, severity, and chronicity of spasticity (Ward, 2002). For example, mild spasticity may be treated with a combination of therapeutic exercise, splinting, orthotics, and oral medication. In contrast, severe spasticity may require chemodenervation (nerve blocks or injection with botulinum toxin) and/or surgery to reduce contracture and improve motor control (Gormley et al., 1997; Ward, 2002).

Pharmacologic Treatments. Medications have been shown to be effective in the management of spasticity, but the mechanisms and anatomical site of action of antispasticity drugs is not well understood (Abbruzzese, 2002; Gallichio, 2004; Gracies et al., 1997a, b; Satkunam, 2003). Table 5.3 summarizes the efficacy of antispasticity drugs in specific patient populations. Table 5.4 summarizes the potential side effects of these medications. A relatively new approach to treating severe spasticity is the continuous intrathecal application of baclofen via an implantable pump.

Surgical Management. The surgical treatment of spasticity has been aimed at four different levels: the brain, the spinal cord, peripheral nerves, and muscles (Chambers, 1997). Because spasticity is only one symptom of lesions to motor cortex neurons, its elimination or reduction may not alleviate functional movement problems because of the continued effect of remaining impairments. Table 5.5 summarizes some of the common surgical techniques used to treat spasticity. The table summarizes the procedure and the target (e.g., brain, spinal cord, peripheral nerves, or muscle). Discussion of the efficacy of surgical interventions for the treatment of spasticity and other movement disorders is beyond the scope of this chapter.

Physical Management. Considerable effort has been directed at developing physical therapeutic techniques to alter muscle tone in patients with neurologic impairments. Various approaches have been devised to manage problems in abnormal muscle tone; some are based on neurophysiological rationales, while others are biomechanically based (Richardson, 2002). Neurophysiological approaches use techniques designed to alter muscle tone by changing the background level of activity in the motor neuron pool of the muscle. As the background level of activity in the motor neuron pool increases, so does the likelihood that the muscle will respond to any incoming stimulus, whether from the periphery or as part of a descending command. The opposite is also true; as background levels of activity decrease, the muscle is less likely to be activated. What techniques can be used to alter the background activity of motor neuron pools and thereby influence muscle tone?

Neurophysiological approaches, including the use of sensory stimulation techniques (sensory modalities), have traditionally been used to facilitate or inhibit muscle tone, depending on the type of stimulus and how it is applied. However, the research to support the efficacy of these techniques in altering muscle tone in patients with neural pathology is lacking. Many therapists use ice to increase muscle tone in patients with hypotonia. Alternatively, prolonged icing is considered inhibitory and is used to decrease hypertonia. Vibrators have also been used to either facilitate or inhibit activity in a muscle. High-frequency vibration tends to facilitate muscle activity, while low-frequency vibration inhibits muscle activity levels (Bishop, 1974, 1975). In the same way, a quick stretch to a muscle facilitates activation of the muscle through the stretch reflex.

Techniques, such as approximation, that activate joint receptors have also been used to facilitate muscle activity in patients with neurologic impairments. Joint approximation involves compressing a joint either manually or through the application of weights. Manual techniques that apply traction to a joint are also used to facilitate muscle activity (Voss et al., 1985).

Biomechanical approaches to managing hypertonicity focus on altering muscle length through prolonged stretching (manually or through the use of casts, splints, or orthoses). A systematic review by Bovend'Eerdt and colleagues (2008) suggested that the clinical benefit of stretching for spasticity is uncertain; while research supported the immediate effects of a

TABLE 5.3 Pharmacologic Treatment of Spasticity Using Centrally Acting Drugs, and Effectiveness in Various Patient Populations*

	MS	SCI	Stroke	TBI	CP	Comments
Dantrolene fragile	+	+	++		+	Strength unimportant, cognitively
Baclofen (oral)	++	+	+/–			
Tizanidine	++	+	+			
Diazepam	+	+	+/–		+	Night administration
Clorazepate	+		+			
Ketazolam		+		+	+	
Clonazepam	+?					Night administration
Piracetam improved					+	Hand function and ambulation
Progabide		+				
Clonidine		+?				
Cyproheptadine	+?	+?				
Thymoxamine (IV)	+	+				Preparation for PT sessions?
Orphenadrine (IV)		+				Flexor reflexes reduced
Baclofen (intrathecal)	+	+		+?	+?	

\+ The antispastic efficacy and tolerance of the drug in the condition indicated have been established in a double-blind protocol.

++ The antispastic efficacy and tolerance of the drug in the condition indicated have been demonstrated to be greater than one of the standard drugs in double-blind comparative studies (e.g., baclofen ++ versus diazepam + in MS).

+/– The overall improvement was mitigated in the double-blind trials in which the drug was analyzed, usually because of bothersome side effects, while the antispastic efficacy was good.

+? Open trials have been promising, but the efficacy has not been established in a double-blind protocol.

An empty box means that the drug has not been investigated to our knowledge in the condition indicated in the column.

* We indicate important features of the drugs that may relate to the patient population in which they seem most appropriate (e.g., dantrolene), to the most adequate timing of administration (e.g., diazepam, clonazepam), or to a particular feature in their efficacy (e.g., thymoxamine, orphenadrine).

CP = cerebral palsy; MS = multiple sclerosis; PT = physical therapy; SCI = spinal cord injury; TBI = traumatic brain injury.

Reprinted with permission from Gracies JM, Elovic E, McGuire J, Simpson D. Traditional pharmacological treatments for spasticity. Part II. General and regional treatments. Muscle Nerve 1997;6:S93.

single stretching session, the functional benefits and long-term consequences of stretching were unclear. Uncertainty regarding the benefits of stretching was in part due to the diversity of research methods used, making comparisons across studies difficult.

Casts, splints, and orthoses have been used to manage hypertonia, maintain or increase the passive range of motion, and improve function in patients with neural pathology. Mortenson and Eng (2003) did a systematic review and graded the evidence for the use of casts in these three areas. They concluded that the evidence did support the use of casts for improving passive range of motion, but more research was needed to determine the efficacy of casts in managing muscle tone and improving functional outcomes.

Altering a patient's position has also been suggested as a technique that can be used to alter muscle tone. The use of positioning has been argued from both neurophysiological and biomechanical perspectives. Biomechanically, positioning patients is used to improve muscle length. A neurophysiological rationale for positioning patients is based on the assumption

TABLE 5.4 Side Effects of Drugs Commonly Used to Treat Spasticity

	Decreased Ambulation Speed	Muscle Weakness	Sedation	Others	Precautions
Dantrolene	+	+		Hepatotoxicity	Monitor liver functions
Baclofen (oral)	+	+	+	Difficulty in seizure control	
Tizanidine		+/–	+	Dry mouth, liver function	Monitor liver function
Diazepam	+		++	Cognitive	
Clorazepate			+/–		
Ketazolam			+		
Clonazepam			++		
Piracetam				Nausea	
Progabide		0	+	Hepatotoxicity	Monitor liver function
Clonidine				Depression, hypotension	Blood pressure monitoring
Cyproheptadine		+	+	Dry mouth	
Thymoxamine (IV)				Risk of hypotension	
Orphenadrine (IV)		0	0		
Baclofen (intrathecal)	+	+	+	Seizure control Pump dysfunction	

+ The side effect has been demonstrated as statistically more frequent with the drug than with placebo in double-blind protocols.

++ A major problem

+/– A minor problem

0 The side effect has been looked for but has not been more frequent than with placebo at the doses used in double-blind protocols.

An empty box means that the side effect has not been investigated with a double-blind protocol.

Reprinted with permission from Gracies JM, Elovic E, McGuire J, Simpson D. Traditional pharmacological treatments for spasticity. Part II. General and regional treatments. Muscle Nerve 1997;6:S96.

that placing patients in certain positions will alter the distribution of muscle (and postural) tone, primarily through the changes in reflex activity. For example, it has been suggested that placing a patient in the supine position will facilitate extensor tone, while flexor tone is facilitated when the patient is prone, because of the presence of released tonic labyrinthine reflexes in the patient with lesions to motor cortex neurons. The use of a side-lying position is often suggested as an approach to inhibiting the effects of the asymmetrical tonic neck reflex on muscle tone, facilitating bilateral symmetrical activities (Bobath & Bobath, 1984).

Effect of Strength Training on Spasticity. Finally, researchers have begun to investigate whether strength training does in fact increase spasticity in affected muscles. Teixeira-Salmela et al. (1999) examined these effects in subjects with chronic (>9 months) stroke after a 10-week (3 days/wk) program consisting of warm-up, aerobic exercise, lower-extremity muscle strengthening, and a cooldown. Changes in peak isokinetic torque production of the major muscle groups in the paretic lower limb, quadriceps and ankle plantar flexor spasticity, gait speed, and the rate of stair climbing were examined before and after

TABLE 5.5 Surgical Procedures Used in the Treatment of Spasticity

Procedure	Target	Results
Stereotactic encephalotomy	Globus pallidus	Variable to poor
	Ventrolateral thalamic	
	nuclei	
	Cerebellum	
Cerebellar stimulation	Cerebellum	Poor
Longitudinal myelotomy	Conus medullaris	Variable
Cervical posterior rhizotomy	C1–C3	Slight improvements
		Significant potential for complications
Selective posterior rhizotomy	Selected roots of L2–S2	Variable, encouraging
Neurectomy	Involved nerves	Variable, high recurrence, possibility of permanent, painful dysesthesias
Tendon lengthening, release or transfer	Contracted or spastic muscle	Variable but generally effective

Reprinted with permission from Chambers HG. The surgical treatment of spasticity. Muscle and Nerve 1997;6:S122.

training. The researchers found a significant improvement in strength in the affected muscle groups, as well as an increase in gait speed and rate of stair climbing after training. Improvements in strength were not associated with an increase in either quadriceps or ankle plantar flexor spasticity.

Damiano and Abel (1998) also investigated the effects of strength training in a group of adolescents with various forms of spastic cerebral palsy. They found that training significantly improved strength in the affected muscles without increasing the severity of spasticity. Ross and Engsberg (2002) examined the relationship between spasticity and strength in 60 individuals with spastic diplegia cerebral palsy (mean age, 12 years; range, 2 to 38) and 50 individuals without disability (mean age, 12 years; range, 4 to 36). They measured spasticity using a KinCom dynamometer that stretched the knee flexors and ankle plantar flexors at different speeds and recorded resistive torques. The strength of the knee flexors/extensors and ankle dorsiflexor/plantar flexors was also measured using the KinCom to measure maximum contraction through the range of motion at a speed of 10 degrees/sec. The group with cerebral palsy was significantly weaker and had greater resistance torques (spasticity) compared with the nondisabled group. There was no relationship between spasticity and strength within a muscle group; in addition, there was no correlation between spasticity of one muscle (agonist) and strength of the opposing (antagonist) muscle. Results of the study agree with other studies reporting muscle weakness in individuals with cerebral palsy, showing that the amount of weakness is not necessarily related to the amount of spasticity present (Giuliani, 1991).

In summary, research is now documenting the contribution of impaired strength to functional limitations in patients with CNS lesions. This has led to a growing awareness of the need to examine and document weakness in the patient with CNS pathology. In addition, training programs appear to be effective in improving strength without increasing spasticity.

Impairments Associated with Subcortical Pathology

Impairments Associated with Cerebellar Pathology

Disorders of the cerebellum result in distinctive symptoms and signs, described by Babinski in 1899 and Gordon Holmes in the 1920s and 1930s (Kandel et al., 2000). Holmes grouped signs and symptoms of cerebellar pathology into three categories: (a) hypotonia;

(b) ataxia or dyscoordination of voluntary movement; and (c) action or intention tremor.

However, lesions to specific sites within the cerebellum result in specific impairments. For example, lesions of the vermis and fastigial nuclei produce disturbances in the control of axial and trunk muscles affecting postural control and balance and characteristic speech deficits. In contrast, damage to the intermediate cerebellum or interposed nuclei produce action tremor in the limbs, while disorders in the lateral cerebellar hemispheres primarily cause delays in initiating movement and in impaired control of multijoint movements.

Hypotonia. We previously described deficits related to increased tone, specifically spasticity, associated with motor cortex deficits. At the other end of the tone spectrum is hypotonicity, defined as a reduction in the stiffness of a muscle to lengthening. Hypotonia is characteristically associated with deficits in the cerebellum; however, hypotonicity is described in many different kinds of patients, including those with spinocerebellar lesions (Ghez, 1991), and in many developmentally delayed children, such as children with Down syndrome (Shumway-Cook and Woollacott, 1985b). Hypotonia in patients with cerebellar pathology is often associated with pendular reflexes. In patients with cerebellar disease, a knee-jerk response to a brief tendon tap may result in prolonged oscillations of the leg (Kandel et al., 2000).

Coordination Problems Associated with Cerebellar Pathology. Problems in the coordination of movements are considered a hallmark of pathology within the cerebellum. Coordinated movement involves multiple joints and muscles that are activated at the appropriate time and with the correct amount of force so that smooth, efficient, and accurate movement occurs. Thus, the essence of coordination is the sequencing, timing, and grading of the activation of multiple muscle groups. Because of the synergistic nature of coordination, the capacity to generate force in an isolated muscle does not predict the ability of that muscle to work in concert with others in a task-specific way (Giuliani, 1991).

In healthy individuals, movements involving more than one joint are associated with movement trajectories that are straight and smooth and have bell-shaped velocity profiles (Hogan et al., 1987). In contrast, movement trajectories in patients with cerebellar pathology are often uneven and lack a bell-shaped profile because of the loss of coordinated coupling between synergistic muscles and joints. Cerebellar dyscoordination can manifest in a number of ways, including delays in the onset of movements (delayed reaction time), errors in the range and direction of movement (called "dysmetria"), and an inability to sustain regular rhythmic movements (called "dysdiadochokinesia"). These deficits are illustrated in Figure 5.10. Cerebellar lesions disrupt the timing and scaling of movements across multiple joints. Instead of movement occurring smoothly across multiple joints, patients with cerebellar pathology demonstrate movement trajectories that are characterized by decomposition (e.g., moving one joint at a time) (Bastian et al., 1996). It has been suggested that in patients with cerebellar pathology, decomposition may be a strategy used to compensate for impaired multijoint control. Since single-joint control appears to be better than multijoint control, patients with cerebellar lesions may decompose movements into sequential movement at individual joints as a strategy to minimize the impact of multijoint dyscoordination.

Patients with cerebellar pathology often have difficulty terminating a movement, which can manifest as an inability to stop a movement, but also as inability to change the direction of a movement. Difficulty terminating a movement can result from an inability to control appropriate forces of the agonist at the end of a movement (Sahrmann & Norton, 1977) or inadequate timing and force generation in the antagonist muscle, necessary to "brake" a movement. Problems terminating a movement can manifest as difficulties in checking or halting a movement, resulting in a "rebound" phenomenon. Rebound phenomena can be seen as involuntary movements of a limb when resistance to an isometric contraction is suddenly removed (Fredericks & Saladin, 1996).

In addition to appropriate timing of muscle activation, coordinated functional movement requires the scaling, or grading, of forces appropriate to the metrics of the task. *Dysmetria* is traditionally defined as problems in judging the distance or range of a movement (Schmitz, 2001). It has also been defined with reference to the ability to scale forces appropriately to task requirements (Horak et al., 1988). *Hypometria* is underestimation of the required force or range of movement, while *hypermetria* is overestimation of the force or range of movement needed for a specific task. Inability to scale or grade forces appropriately can be seen as undershooting or overshooting in tasks such as reaching or pointing. Dysmetria is commonly found in patients with cerebellar lesions (Bastian et al., 1996; Hore et al., 1991).

While dyscoordination is a symptom of cerebellar function, it can also be associated with pathology in other neural structures. For example, dyscoordination is also found with lesions in the motor cortex and basal ganglia, as well as in patients with proprioceptive

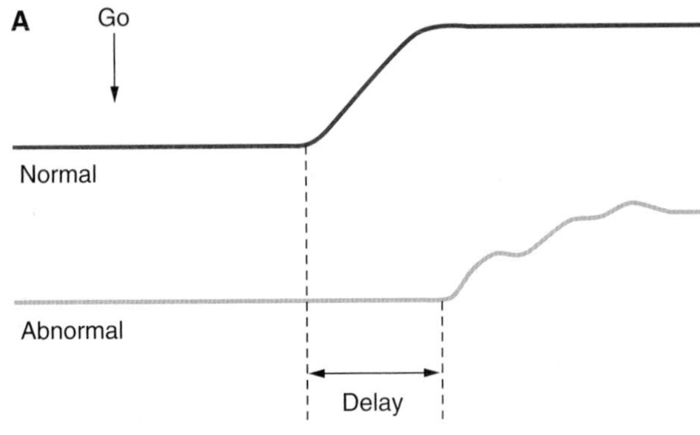

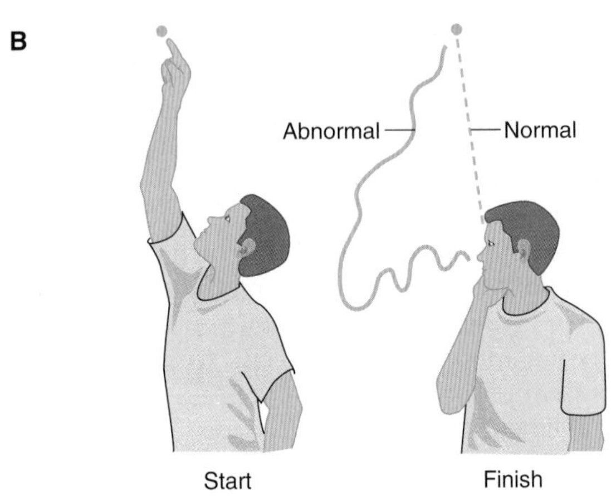

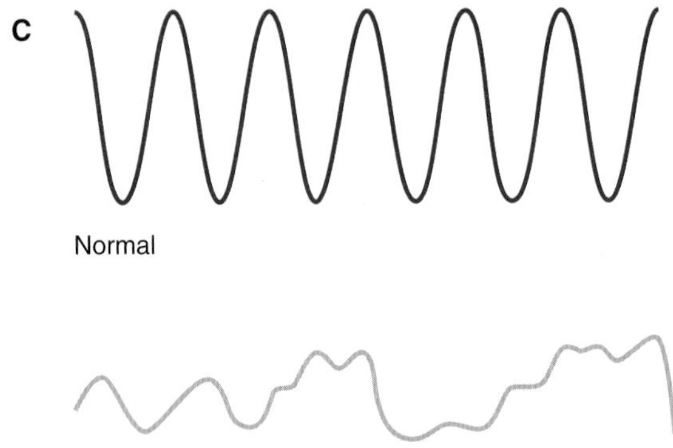

FIGURE 5.10 Movement deficits observed in persons with cerebellar disease. Delay in the onset of movement following the signal to "go" can be seen in the bottom trace as compared with the normal reaction time shown in the upper trace (A). Dysmetria, a disorder in the range and direction of movement is seen when the person is asked to move his arm from the target to his nose. Intention tremor can be seen when the arm approaches the nose (B). Dysdiadochokinesia, an irregular pattern of alternating movement, can be seen in the abnormal position trace made when the person with cerebellar pathology alternately pronates and supinates the forearm, compared with a normal position trace (C). (Adapted from Kandel ER, Schwartz JH, Jessell TM, eds. Principles of neuroscience, 3rd ed. New York: Elsevier, 1991:849, Figure 42.16.)

impairments. In addition, since coordinated functional movement requires both biomechanical and neuromuscular systems, peripheral factors including alterations in the viscoelastic properties of the muscles and tendons, can contribute to the loss of coordinated functional movement (Giuliani, 1991).

Intention Tremor. *Tremor* is defined as a rhythmic, involuntary oscillatory movement of a body part (Deuschl et al., 1998). The Movement Disorder Society has suggested a classification system for tremor disorder based on clinical features, including the conditions during which tremor occurs (Deuschl et al., 1998). *Intention tremor* is tremor that occurs during the performance of a voluntary movement, and is characteristic of pathology of the cerebellum and its afferent or efferent pathways. Intention tremor has a frequency range of less than 5 Hz and is most marked at the end of a movement, when the patient attempts to brake a movement.

Impaired Error Correction Affecting Motor Learning. The cerebellum plays a critical role in error correction, an essential part of motor learning. Within the cerebellum, internal feedback signals reporting intended movements are compared with external feedback signals that report actual movement. The cerebellum generates a corrective signal used in feedforward control to reduce errors in subsequent movements. Dysmetria and intention tremor result from disruption of feedforward mechanisms involving the cerebellum. Cerebellar lesions affecting error detection also contribute to motor learning deficits. Thus, in addition to their role in the control of movement, cerebellar structures also are important in practice-dependent motor adaptation and learning in many different systems (Morton & Bastian, 2004, 2007). Damage to the cerebellum affects the extent and rate at which individuals adapt movements to new contexts (Morton & Bastian, 2004, 2007). This suggests that the training of individuals with cerebellar pathology may require a longer duration or intensity of practice to improve motor function.

Basal Ganglia Pathology

Pathology in the basal ganglia can result in either diminished movement, often called "hypokinetic disorders," of which Parkinson's disease is the best example, or hyperkinetic disorders such as Huntington's disease, which are characterized by excessive movement. Because of complex connections with the cerebral cortex, damage to the basal ganglia is also associated with cognitive and behavioral disturbances.

Hypokinetic Disorders: Parkinson's Disease. Parkinson's disease (PD), a hypokinetic disorder of the basal ganglia, was first described by James Parkinson in 1817 (Kandel et al., 2000). Cardinal signs of PD include paucity of spontaneous movement (akinesia), voluntary movements that are slow and reduced in amplitude (bradykinesia), increased muscle tone (rigidity), and a resting tremor. Also characteristic of PD are flexed posture and impaired balance and gait. PD results from degeneration of dopaminergic neurons in the substantia nigra pars compacta.

Bradykinesia and Akinesia. In patients with PD, coordination problems can be seen in functional tasks such as handwriting and are reportedly caused by a reduced capability for coordinating wrist and finger movements (Teulings et al., 1997). Impairments in coordination result from disruptions to the timing, selection, and scaling of movements. *Bradykinesia* is defined as slowed movement time, which is the time taken to execute a task-specific movement once it has been initiated. While bradykinesia is characteristic of pathology in the basal ganglia, delayed movement time is a commonly reported impairment associated with a wide variety of neural pathologies. Longer movement times have been reported in patients with hemiparesis following stroke (Levin et al., 1993; Levin,1996), in patients with PD (Teulings et al., 1997), in children with various forms of cerebral palsy (Steenbergen et al., 1998), and in patients with cerebellar dysfunction (Van Donkelaar & Lee, 1994). Persons with PD also demonstrate hypokinesia, defined as movements that are decreased in amplitude and akinesia, or the reduced ability to initiate movement (Gordon et al., 1997; Horak, 1990).

Rigidity. Like spasticity, rigidity is characterized by a heightened resistance to passive movement of the limb, but it is independent of the velocity of stretch. Rigidity may be the result of hyperactivity in the fusimotor system (Noth, 1991). Rigidity tends to be predominant in flexor muscles of the trunk and limbs and results in numerous functional limitations, including difficulty with bed mobility, transfers, postural control, gait, speech, and eating. There are two types of rigidity, lead pipe and cogwheel. Lead pipe rigidity is characterized by a constant resistance to movement throughout the entire range of motion. Cogwheel rigidity is characterized by alternating episodes of resistance and relaxation, so-called catches, as the extremity is passively moved through its range of motion.

Resting Tremor. Resting tremor is a characteristic impairment associated with PD. It is defined as tremor that occurs in a body part that is not voluntarily activated and is supported against gravity. The amplitude of resting tremor increases during mental stress or during movements of another body part (especially the movements involved in walking). Action tremor is any tremor that is produced by voluntary contraction of muscle, including postural, isometric, and kinetic tremor (including intention tremor). Postural tremor is present when voluntarily maintaining a position against gravity. Kinetic tremor occurs during a voluntary movement and can vary from a simple kinetic tremor (not target-related) to an intention tremor (those occurring during a target-directed movement). A complete discussion of this complex topic is provided in reviews by Deuschl et al. (1998) and Hallett (1998).

Hyperkinetic Disorders. Hyperkinetic disorders of the basal ganglia, such as Huntington's disease and hemiballismus, are characterized by excessive and involuntary movements and decreased muscle tone (hypotonia). Involuntary movements may take several forms, including slow, writhing movements (athetosis), jerky random movements (chorea), large violent proximal limb movements (ballism), or more sustained abnormal posture and slower movements with cocontraction of agonist and antagonist muscles (dystonia).

Choreiform and Athetoid Movements. Chorea or choreiform movements are involuntary, rapid, irregular, and jerky movements that result from basal ganglia lesions. Chorea is one type of dyskinesia that is often observed as a side effect of antiparkinsonian medications in people with PD. Choreiform dyskinesias typically emerge after prolonged use of antiparkinsonian medications, and are typically observed at the peak or at the end of a dose of antiparkinsonian medications. Athetosis, or athetoid movement, consists of slow involuntary writhing and twisting movements, usually involving the upper extremities more than the lower extremities; however, they may also involve the neck, face, and tongue. Athetosis is a clinical feature of some forms of cerebral palsy.

Dystonia. The term *dystonia* was first used in 1911 by the neurologist Hermann Oppenheim (cited in Marsden & Quinn, 1990). *Dystonia* is defined as "a syndrome dominated by sustained muscle contractions, frequently causing twisting and repetitive movements of abnormal postures" (Fahn et al., 1987). The abnormal movements associated with dystonia are diverse, and range from slow athetotic to quick myoclonic dystonia (Fahn et al, 1987).

Dystonic movements are often characterized by cocontraction of agonist and antagonist muscles (Hallett, 1993; Rothwell, 1995-1996). Dystonia is thought to be a disorder of the basal ganglia, because patients with secondary dystonia often have lesions in the basal ganglia, particularly the putamen (Hallett, 1993; Marsden & Quinn, 1990). However, the pathophysiology of primary idiopathic dystonia is still unclear. Animal models have identified abnormalities not only in the basal ganglia, but in the thalamus, cerebellum, and brainstem. It is likely that the biochemical dysfunction varies depending on the subtype of dystonia (see Richter & Loscher, 1998, for a review of this topic).

Types of dystonia are classified according to cause, age at onset, and distribution of abnormal movement. Focal dystonia involves a single body region (e.g., torticollis or writer's cramp). Segmental dystonia involves two or more adjoining body regions (e.g., neck and arm, trunk and leg). Hemidystonia involves the arm and leg on one side of the body. Multifocal dystonia involves two or more nonadjoining body regions. Generalized dystonia involves the whole body (Fahn et al., 1987).

Dystonia is often divided into two categories, idiopathic (or primary) dystonia, which occurs in the absence of other lesions within the CNS, and symptomatic (or secondary) dystonia, which occurs in conjunction with other neurologic diseases (such as multiple sclerosis) or acquired brain lesions (e.g., head injury). About two thirds of the individuals affected have idiopathic dystonia (Kramer et al., 1994). There is no cure for dystonia, and treatment is largely aimed at reducing symptoms. Relaxation exercises are often used, since dystonia is exacerbated by stressful situations. Five to 10 percent of patients with idiopathic dystonia are responsive to levodopa, a medication commonly used to treat PD. Anticholinergic drugs have also been used successfully in the treatment of dystonia. Finally, botulinum toxin A, injected locally into the affected muscle, has been used to treat focal dystonias (Fahn & Marsden, 1987; Marsden & Quinn, 1990).

Clinical Examination of Cerebellar and Basal Ganglia Impairments

Examination of Coordination. The most common approach to examining coordination is to observe patients performing functional movements and noting the characteristics of the movements used. Does the patient have difficulty initiating or terminating the functional movement? Is the movement slow? Is the movement trajectory smooth and fluid or jerky? More formal tests of coordination have been proposed and are divided into nonequilibrium and equilibrium subcategories (Schmitz, 2001). Equilibrium tests of coordination generally reflect the coordination of multijoint movements for posture and gait and will be discussed in later chapters. Nonequilibrium tests are summarized in Table 5.6, and are often used to indicate specific pathology within the cerebellum (Schmitz, 2001). Performance is graded subjectively using the following ordinal scale: 5, normal; 4, minimal impairment; 3, moderate impairment; 2, severe impairment; 1, cannot perform.

Examination of Involuntary Movements. Involuntary movements, including tremor, are identified primarily through systematic clinical observation describing the body parts affected and the conditions under which tremor is activated. For example, a clinician might observe whether a tremor is resting versus

TABLE 5.6 Nonequilibrium Tests of Coordination

1. Finger to nose	The shoulder is abducted to 90 degrees with the elbow extended. The patient is asked to bring the tip of the index finger to the tip of the nose. Alterations may be made in the initial starting position to assess performance from different planes of motion.
2. Finger to therapist's	The patient and therapist sit opposite each other. The therapist's index finger is held in front of finger the patient. The patient is asked to touch the tip of the index finger to the therapist's index finger. The position of the therapist's finger may be altered during testing to assess ability to change distance, direction, and force of movement.
3. Finger to finger	Both shoulders are abducted to 90 degrees with the elbows extended. The patient is asked to bring both hands toward the midline and approximate the index fingers from opposing hands.
4. Alternate nose to finger	The patient alternately touches the tip of the nose and the tip of the therapist's finger with the index finger. The position of the therapist's finger may be altered during testing to assess ability to change distance, direction, and force of movement.

(continued)

TABLE 5.6 Nonequilibrium Tests of Coordination

5. Finger opposition	The patient touches the tip of the thumb to the tip of each finger in sequence. Speed may be gradually increased.
6. Mass grasp	An alternation is made between opening and closing fist (from finger flexion to full extension). Speed may be gradually increased.
7. Pronation/ supination	With elbows flexed to 90 degrees and held close to body, the patient alternately turns the palms up and down. This test also may be performed with shoulders flexed to 90 degrees and elbows extended. Speed may be gradually increased. The ability to reverse movements between opposing muscle groups can be assessed in many joints. Examples include active alternation between flexion and extension of the knee, ankle, elbow, fingers, and so forth.
8. Rebound test	The patient is positioned with the elbow flexed. The therapist applies sufficient manual resistance to produce an isometric contraction of biceps. Resistance is suddenly released. Normally, the opposing muscle group (triceps) will contract and check movement of the limb. Many other muscle groups can be tested for this phenomenon, such as the shoulder abductors or flexors, elbow extensors, and so forth.
9. Tapping (hand)	With the elbow flexed and the forearm pronated, the patient is asked to tap the hand on the knee.
10. Tapping (foot)	The patient is asked to tap the ball of one foot on the floor without raising the knee; heel maintains contact with floor.
11. Pointing and past pointing	The patient and therapist are opposite each other, either sitting or standing. Both patient and therapist bring shoulders to a horizontal position of 90 degrees of flexion with elbows extended. Index fingers are touching or the patient's finger may rest lightly on the therapist's. The patient is asked to fully flex the shoulder (fingers will be pointing toward ceiling) and then return to the horizontal position such that index fingers will again approximate. Both arms should be tested, either separately or simultaneously. A normal response consists of an accurate return to the starting position. In an abnormal response, there is typically a past pointing, or movement beyond the target. Several variations to this test included movements in other directions such as toward 90 degrees of shoulder abduction or toward 0 degrees of shoulder flexion (fingers will point toward floor). Following each movement, the patient is asked to return to the initial horizontal starting position.
12. Alternate heel to knee; heel to toe	From a supine position, the patient is asked to touch the knee and big toe alternately with the heel of the opposite extremity.
13. Toe to examiner's finger	From a supine position, the patient is instructed to touch the great toe to the examiner's finger.
	The position of the finger may be altered during testing to assess ability to change distance, direction, and force of movement.
14. Heel on shin	From a supine position, the heel of one foot is slid up and down the shin of the opposite lower extremity.
15. Drawing a circle	The patient draws an imaginary circle in the air with either upper or lower extremity (a table or or the floor alone may be used). This also may be done using a figure-eight pattern. This test may be performed in the supine position for lower extremity assessment.
16. Fixation or position holding	Upper extremity: The patient holds arms horizontally in front. Lower extremity: The patient is asked to hold the knee in an extended position.

Tests should be performed first with eyes open and then with eyes closed. Abnormal responses include a gradual deviation from the "hold" position and/or a diminished quality of response with vision occluded. Unless otherwise indicated, tests are performed with the patient in a sitting position.

Reprinted with permission from Schmitz TJ. Coordination assessment. In: O'Sullivan S, Schmitz TM, eds. Physical rehabilitation: assessment and treatment, 4th ed. Philadelphia: FA Davis, 2001: p 212.

associated with activity (action tremor). The intensity of the tremor can be graded on an ordinal scale. Conditions that increase versus decrease the severity of tremor are also noted.

Treatment of Cerebellar and Basal Ganglia Impairments

Treatment of Coordination Problems. There are many therapeutic techniques used to treat coordination problems in patients with neurologic deficits. Some techniques can be considered "general" approaches to dyscoordination, while others more specifically target problems in timing, sequencing, or grading synergistic muscle activity.

General Techniques. Probably the most frequently used technique to improve coordinated movement is repetition and practice of a functional task-specific movement. Since the requirement for accuracy creates increasing demands for coordination, therapists can select functional tasks with increasing accuracy demands when training the patient. To assist the patient in recognizing errors in performance of coordinated movement, the therapist can provide feedback (either knowledge of results or knowledge of performance). Remember from Chapter 2 that intermittent feedback facilitates learning better than constant feedback.

Use of weight-bearing activities has also been recommended for improving coordinated action in the lower extremities. In addition to functional movements, therapists often have patients practice nonfunctional movements to improve coordination. Examples of nonfunctional movements are rapid alternating movements, reciprocal movements of the hands or feet, and tracing shapes and numbers, such as a figure 8, with a limb.

Timing Problems. A number of different therapeutic strategies can have an impact on timing components (reaction time, movement time, and termination time) of functional movement. Practicing a functional movement under externally imposed time constraints is one approach. For example, having a patient perform functional movements to music or in time with a metronome can be used to influence the timing of movement. Timing a patient while he or she performs a functional task and using the time taken to complete the task as external feedback (knowledge of results) is another approach. Verbal, visual, or manual feedback regarding speed of performance can also be used. Sensory stimulation such as brisk icing or tapping to facilitate recruitment of motor neurons may improve reaction time. Although these are common techniques used by therapists to treat coordination problems, few if any of these techniques have been subjected to experimental testing.

Scaling Problems. Scaling problems represent an inability to grade forces appropriately to the demands of the task. Treatment focuses on having patients practice a wide variety of tasks that require precise grading of force and providing external feedback through knowledge of results and/or performance. Functional movements performed quickly will require less precision of force control than those performed slowly. In addition, functional tasks demanding a high degree of accuracy require more precise grading of forces than those demanding limited accuracy. For example, moving to a large target will require less force control than moving to a small target. Picking up a paper cup full of water will require more precision than lifting a paper cup that is empty. Therapeutic interventions directed at remediating coordination problems during tasks related to postural control, mobility, and upper-extremity functions are presented in sections of the book related to these functions.

Treatment of Involuntary Movements. Rehabilitation strategies for treating involuntary movement focus primarily on strategies to compensate for the movement, rather than on changing the movement itself. For example, since increased effort tends to magnify involuntary movements, patients can be taught to perform functional movements with reduced effort. Patients often tend to develop compensatory strategies on their own, such as walking with hands in pockets, or grasping objects to decrease resting tremor.

Weight bearing and approximation have been recommended as a method to increase joint stability in patients with chorea or athetosis. Distal fixation is another method used to control involuntary movements and can be achieved by providing external handholds on wheelchairs, lap boards, or desks (Figure 5.11). The use of limb weighting in the management of involuntary movement is somewhat controversial. Application of a weight to the distal portion of a limb segment increases the overall mass of the limb and results in reduced motion. However, there is some evidence that limb motion is worse when the weight is removed.

Secondary Musculoskeletal Impairments

In the patient with CNS lesions, musculoskeletal disorders develop most often secondary to the primary lesion. Since physical activity is necessary to the maintenance of both muscle and the bony skeleton,

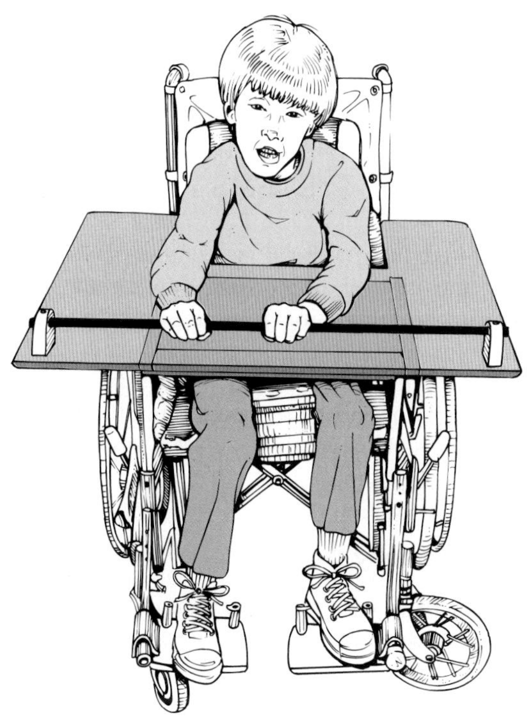

FIGURE 5.11 A horizontal dowel on a lapboard is used for distal fixation to control athetoid movements. (Adapted with permission from Kandel ER, Schwartz JH, Jessell TM, eds. Principles of neuroscience, 4th ed. New York: McGraw-Hill, 2000:544.)

the absence of physical activity associated with neurologic pathology can lead to a wide range of musculoskeletal problems, including muscle atrophy and deconditioning, contractures, degenerative joint disease, and osteoporosis (Fredericks & Saladin, 1996).

Spasticity, a primary neuromuscular impairment, changes the physical properties of the muscle and other tissues (Lieber et al., 2004). Biopsy studies have shown increased fiber-size variability in spastic muscles (Ito et al., 1996) and changes in the amount and composition of extracellular matrix material (Lieber et al., 2003). There is conflicting information from studies examining fiber-type distribution in spasticity, with some reporting an increase in type I fibers (Dietz et al., 1986; Ito et al., 1996), and others reporting an increased percentage of type II fibers (Sjostrom et al., 1980).

Individuals with spastic muscles present with increased joint stiffness, which is the basis for Lance's (Lance, 1980) classic definition of spasticity as a "velocity dependent resistance to stretch." While the common explanation of this increased stiffness is that it is due to abnormalities in the stretch reflex (e.g., increased gain or threshold), there are three mechanisms that contribute to total stiffness, resulting in resistance to passive stretch, including passive muscle stiffness, neurally mediated reflex stiffness, and active muscle stiffness. Sinkjaer and Magnussen (1994) reported an increased total stiffness in the spastic leg of patients with hemiparesis as compared with the nonspastic (control) leg. They found a significant increase in the intrinsic stiffness component, suggesting a change in the passive mechanical properties of the muscle of the spastic limb as compared with the nonspastic limb. Surprisingly, their study did not show an increase in reflex stiffness between the spastic and nonspastic limbs. In contrast, Mirbagheri et al. (2001) showed a change in both intrinsic muscle stiffness and reflex gain in spastic muscles of patients with spinal cord injury as compared with muscles of noninjured controls. Researchers analyzing gait in children with cerebral palsy have found that increased tension in the gastrocnemius muscle is not always associated with increased muscle activity in that muscle, supporting the concept that spastic patterns of movement are partly due to changes in intrinsic muscle characteristics (Berger et al., 1984a).

Paresis, another primary neuromuscular impairment, also results in underlying structural changes to the muscle, which will vary according to whether the paretic muscles are positioned in a shortened or a lengthened position. Positioning a paretic muscle in a shortened position results in muscle unloading (a reduction in longitudinal tension), which is the first step in muscle contracture (Gracies, 2005a, b). Muscle unloading results in loss of muscle mass (atrophy), cross-sectional area, loss of sarcomeres (shortening), an accumulation of connective tissues, and an increase in fat deposits in the tendons (Gracies, 2005a,b). Reduced extensibility in the shortened muscle means that any lengthening force will be transmitted more easily to the muscle spindles, contributing to increased stretch sensitivity in the paretic muscles (Gioux & Petit, 1993). Immobilization of a muscle at a shortened range also results in changes in the joint, including proliferation of connective tissue into the joint space, adherence of connective tissue to cartilage surfaces, atrophy of the cartilage, and disorganization of ligament alignment (Liebesman & Carafelli, 1994). Immobilization also results in a reduction in bone mineralization leading to regional osteoporosis (Alzghoul et al., 2004).

Paretic muscles positioned in a lengthened position have less muscle atrophy (Dupont Salter et al., 2003) and an increased number of sarcomeres in series as compared with those positioned in a shortened position (Gracies, 2005a,b). Researchers have also examined the effects of paresis and immobilization on motor unit type. Animal research suggests that with immobilization, muscles composed predominantly of type I fibers (e.g., low-threshold, slow-twitch, fatigue-resistant) such as the soleus muscle, take on properties of type II muscles (high-threshold, fast-twitch, fatigue-sensitive) (Booth, 1982; Gracies, 2005a, b). However, immobilization of fast muscles such as the gastrocnemius or mixed type I and II muscles (anterior tibialis) appear to shift toward slow-unit behavior (Petit et al., 2003) with atrophy of type II fibers (Powers & Rymer, 1988).

In humans with spastic hemiplegia, a new type of motor unit characterized by slow-twitch contraction times and increased fatigability (slow-fatigable units) appears (Young & Mayer, 1982). There appears to be preferential type II fiber atrophy and a predominance of type I fibers in fast muscles such as the gastrocnemius (Dietz et al., 1986) and mixed muscles such as the anterior tibialis (Toffola et al., 2001). Several researchers have documented musculoskeletal changes in the nonparetic limbs associated with decreased use after stroke. Significant weakness in the unaffected leg develops as early as the first week after stroke (Harris et al., 2001). In addition to weakness, dexterity and coordination problems are reported in chronic stroke (Desrosiers et al., 1996).These studies demonstrate that primary neuromuscular impairments resulting from CNS pathology are also associated with adaptation in the peripheral musculoskeletal system, and these musculoskeletal changes significantly constrain functional movements in patients.

Examination and Treatment of Musculoskeletal Impairments

Examination of the musculoskeletal system includes evaluation of range of motion, flexibility, strength, and alignment. This chapter does not discuss techniques for assessing the musculoskeletal system in depth; instead, the reader is urged to consult other textbooks (Kendall & McCreary, 1983; Kessler & Hertling, 1983; Magee, 1987; Saunders, 1991).

Musculoskeletal problems can be treated using traditional physical therapy techniques, including heat, ultrasound, massage, and biofeedback. Passive range-of-motion exercises are used to improve joint mobility and muscle flexibility. Progressive resistive exercises are used to improve muscle strength. Manual therapies focus on regaining passive range of motion and joint play. Proprioceptive neuromuscular facilitation (PNF) techniques (such as contract and relax) can be used to treat musculoskeletal problems such as contractures. Finally, plaster casts and splints are used to passively increase range of motion and flexibility in patients with neurologic impairments. For an in-depth discussion of treatment of this important area of musculoskeletal impairments, the reader is referred to the other sources cited above.

IMPAIRMENTS IN SENSORY/ PERCEPTUAL SYSTEMS

As discussed in Chapter 3, sensation plays multiple roles in the control of normal movement. Thus, it should not be surprising that sensory deficits are a major factor contributing to motor control problems in patients with CNS lesions. The type of sensory problem will depend on the location of the lesion (i.e., where in the sensory pathway the lesion is) as well as the size of the lesion.

Somatosensory Deficits

Remember from Chapter 3 that somatosensory information ascends to the cerebral cortex via two systems, the dorsal column–medial lemniscal (DC-ML) system and the anterolateral system. Lesions of the medial lemniscal system will result in loss of discriminative touch, including light touch, and kinesthetic sense. In contrast, lesions in the lateral spinothalamic tract affect pain sensibility and the ability to detect thermal changes, in addition to more coarse touch and kinesthetic discrimination. As discussed in Chapter 3, the primary somotosensory cortex (SI) is important for cross-modality sensory processing critical to normal coordination of movements in space. Cross-modality sensory processing provides information about the body's position in space relative to the environment and the position of one body segment relative to another. Lesions of the somatosensory cortex lead to loss of discriminative sensations such as proprioception, two-point discrimination, stereognosis, and localization of touch. Effects are contralateral to the side of the lesion. Since outputs from SI go to the parietal lobe (Brodmann's areas 5 and 7), lesions in these areas cause problems when learning skills that use information regarding the position of the body in space. Disorders in spatial relationships are discussed in more detail in a later section of this chapter.

Examination and Treatment of Somatosensory Impairments

Evaluation of somatosensation is complex, and many methods have been suggested. Sensory testing can vary from simple screening tests to complex assessment of the type and distribution of sensory function. Fess (1990) has described a hierarchy of sensory functioning. Detection, defined as the ability to distinguish a single point stimulus from background stimulation, is the lowest level of the hierarchy. Discrimination, the ability to distinguish the difference between stimulus a and stimulus b, is next. Quantification, the ability to organize tactile stimuli according to degree (e.g., roughness or weight) is the next level. Finally, recognition, the ability to recognize objects by touch, is the highest level.

Sensory tests associated with these levels within the hierarchy are summarized in Table 5.7. Fess's hierarchy suggests that it may not be necessary to test every sensory modality in a patient. If the patient is able to discriminate stimuli, sensory-detection tests need not be performed. In addition, researchers have shown a high correlation among sensory tests, so that results from one test (such as two-point discrimination) can be used to predict results on other tests, such as finger proprioception (Moberg, 1991). Thus, it may be possible to select a sample of sensory tests to predict overall somatosensory functioning.

Results from sensory testing can be interpreted in relationship to established norms, expected performance based on anatomy and pathology, or in comparison to noninvolved areas. The relationship between sensory loss and function, however, is not clear. Dellon and Kallman (1983) found that tests that best predict hand function are static and moving two-point discrimination tests.

Often, clinicians tend to view sensory impairments such as loss of limb position sense or somatosensory deficits leading to decreased object recognition, as being permanent or not modifiable by treatment. However, a number of interesting studies suggest that treatment can affect the patient's ability to process sensory stimuli. Based on some studies examining the reorganization of the somatosensory cortex in primates (Merzenich et al., 1983a, b), which were discussed in Chapter 4, a number of researchers have developed structured sensory reeducation programs to improve the patient's ability to discriminate and interpret sensory information (Carey et al., 1993; Dannenbaum & Dykes, 1988; DeJersey, 1979). The goal of these interventions is to improve a patient's ability to detect and process information in the environment and thereby improve motor performance. Suggestions for retraining sensory discrimination are presented in more detail in Chapter 19, which outlines methods for retraining upper-extremity control.

Visual Deficits

As discussed in Chapter 3, vision gives us information on the position and movement of objects in space (vision as an exteroceptive sense) as well as the position and movement of our own bodies (visual proprioception). As was true for the somatosensory system, disorders of the visual system will vary according to the location of the lesion (Fig. 5.12). Impairments to vision are usually described with reference to the visual-field deficit. A common visual problem following unilateral damage to the cerebral cortex is homonymous hemianopsia, or the loss of visual information for one hemifield. Further information on impairments associated with pathology within different parts of the visual system can be found in Chapter 3.

Examination and Treatment of Visual Deficits

Visual testing includes information on visual acuity, depth perception, visual fields, and oculomotor control. Visual acuity can be tested directly or determined via self-report. Depth perception is critical for functional skills such as mobility or driving. It can be tested by holding two identical objects at eye level and moving one in relation to the other, asking the patient to indicate which is closer (Quintana, 1995). Visual field deficits are identified using the Visual Field Confrontation Test. The patient is told to look forward at the therapist, who sits in front of the patient. The patient is asked to indicate when he or she detects a visual stimulus (often the therapist's finger) presented in the periphery; all four visual quadrants are tested. Oculomotor tests examine the control of eye movements. These are discussed in Chapter 19, under examination of visual regard, a component of reach and grasp.

Vestibular Deficits

The vestibular system provides sensory information regarding head movements and position with reference to gravity. Vestibular afferent information is used for gaze stabilization, posture and balance, and it contributes to our conscious sense of orientation in space. Thus, pathology within the vestibular system can produce problems related to: (a) gaze stabilization, including blurred vision or oscillopsia (oscillating vision) due to the disruption of the vestibulo-ocular reflex; (b) posture and balance; and (c) vertigo or dizziness (Herdman, 2007; Shumway-Cook & Horak, 1989, 1990).

The term *dizziness* is often used by patients to describe a variety of sensations, including spinning (referred to as "vertigo"), rocking, tilting, unsteadiness, and light-headedness. The specific types of symptoms found depend on the type and location of pathology within the vestibular system.

Examination and Treatment of Vestibular Deficits

Examination of vestibular function includes tests of gaze stabilization, posture and balance control, and dizziness. Treatment varies, depending on the underlying cause. Specific procedures for assessing

TABLE 5.7 A Summary of Methods for Testing Somatosensation*

Sensory Modality	Stimulus	Response	Score
Discriminative Touch			
Touch awareness	Light touch to skin with cotton ball	With vision occluded, patient says "yes" or signals when stimulus is felt.	% of correct responses out of total (e.g., 50% correct touches felt)
Touch localization	Lightly touch skin with cotton ball or monofilament number 4.17.	With vision occluded, patient points to location of touch.	Record error in accuracy of location.
Bilateral touch (sensory extinction)	Touch patient on one vs. both sides of the body with fingertips.	With vision occluded, patient says "one" or "two" to indicate number of stimuli felt.	Record presence of sensory extinction.
Touch pressure threshold	Use range of Semmes-Weinstein monofilaments.	With vision occluded, patient indicates when he or she feels stimulus.	Score the number of the thinnest filament felt (normal is perception of filament 2.83).
Two-point discrimination	Using two paper clips, apply the two points to the skin; start 5 m apart; gradually bring points together.	Patient responds "one," "two" or "can't tell."	Percentage of correct responses out of total
Proprioception			
Vibration	Apply tuning fork or vibrometer to skin.	Patient indicates when he or she feels stimulus.	Percentage of correct responses out of total
Joint position	Passively position joint in flexion or extension.	With vision occluded, patient mimics position with contralateral limb	Percentage of correct responses out of total
Joint motion	Passively move the joint into flexion or extension.	With vision occluded, patient reports whether joint is bending or straightening.	Percentage of correct responses out of total
Stereognosis	Place a series of small objects in patient's hand.	Patient names object (may manipulate object first).	Percentage of correct responses out of total
Pain			
Pain: Sharp/dull	Randomly apply sharp and blunt end of safety pin to skin.	With vision occluded, patient indicates "sharp" or "dull."	Percentage of correct responses out of total
Temperature			
Temperature	Apply cold (40°F) or hot (115°F) to patient's skin	Patient indicates "hot" or "cold."	Percentage of correct responses out of total

*Based on material from Bentzel K. Evaluation of sensation. In: Trombly CA, ed. Occupational therapy for physical dysfunction, 4th ed. Baltimore: Williams & Wilkins, 1995.

gaze stabilization are discussed in Chapter 19, while those for assessing posture and balance are presented in Chapter 11. Thus, the following section gives a brief overview of the examination and treatment of dizziness.

Examination begins with taking a careful history to determine the patient's perceptions of whether dizziness is constant or provoked and the situations or conditions that stimulate dizziness. The Vertigo Positions and Movement Test (Shumway-Cook & Horak, 1990)

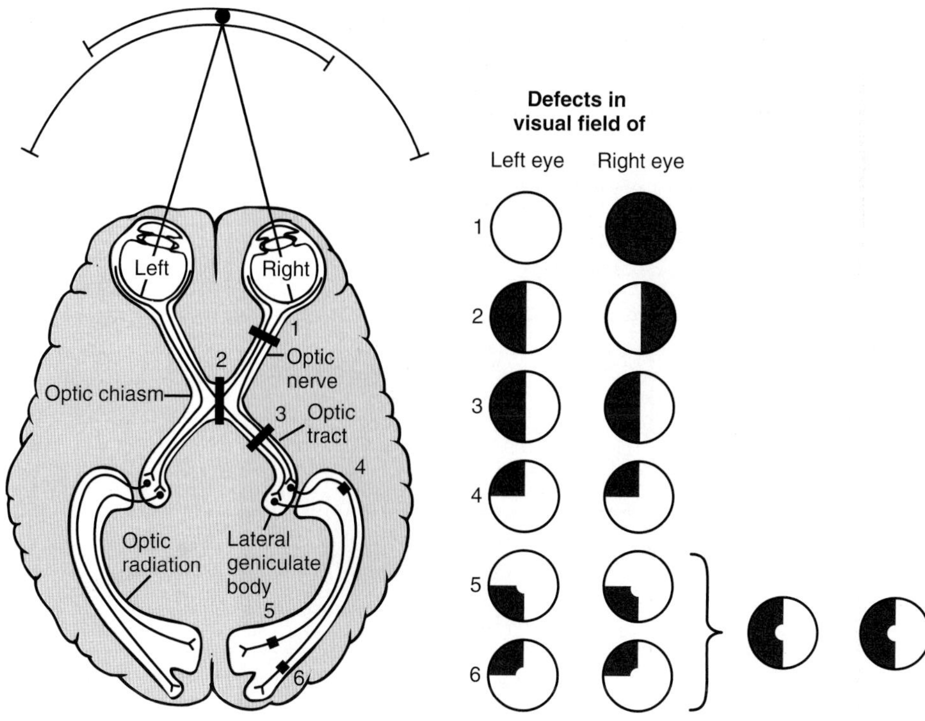

FIGURE 5.12 Visual deficits produced by lesions at various locations in the visual system.

examines the intensity and duration of dizziness in response to movement and/or positional changes of the head while sitting, standing, and walking. The patient is asked to rate the intensity of dizziness on a scale of 0 (no dizziness) to 10 (severe dizziness). In addition, the duration of symptoms is timed and recorded, as are the presence of nystagmus and autonomic nervous system symptoms including nausea, sweating, and pallor. The Dix–Hallpike maneuver (Fig. 5.13) is used to test for posterior semicircular canal benign paroxysmal positional vertigo (BPPV). BPPV is the most common cause of vertigo (Fetter, 2000). Most often, patients describe a spinning vertigo associated with head positions involving rapid extension of the neck (such as looking up into a high shelf) or when lying down and rolling to the affected side. Key to the diagnosis of BPPV is the Dix–Hallpike maneuver. In response to this rapid position change, the patient describes vertigo lasting from 30 seconds to 1 minute, and tortional nystagmus in the direction of the downward ear is present. The pathophysiology of BPPV is thought to be displacement of otoconia into the posterior semicircular canals (SCC). For a detailed description of examination of dizziness, the reader is referred to other sources (Herdman, 2007; Shumway-Cook & Horak, 1989, 1990).

Treatment of vestibular pathology, referred to as "vestibular rehabilitation," uses exercises to treat symptoms of dizziness and imbalance that result from pathology within the vestibular system. Since there are many potential causes of dizziness, including metabolic disturbances, side effects of medication, cardiovascular problems, such as orthostatic hypotension, and pathology within peripheral or central vestibular structures, it is essential that the therapist know the underlying diagnosis prior to beginning an exercise-based approach.

The type of exercise used to treat dizziness depends on the specific type of pathology causing the dizziness. Vertigo secondary to posterior SCC BPPV is most often treated with a repositioning maneuver designed to mechanically move displaced otoconia from the semicircular canal(s) (Herdman, 2007). This procedure is shown in Figure 5.14, A to E.

In contrast to treatment of positional vertigo, dizziness associated with asymmetric vestibular loss is treated with habituation exercises. The patient is instructed to repeat the position or movements that provoke dizziness 5 to 10 times in a row, two to three times per day. Exercises are progressive in nature. The patient begins with fairly simple exercises, such as horizontal head movements in the seated position, and progresses to more difficult tasks, such as horizontal head movements integrated into gait. This approach is discussed in more detail elsewhere (Herdman, 2007; Shumway-Cook & Horak, 1989, 1990).

Perceptual Impairments

Body Image/Scheme Disorders Associated with Parietal and Temporal Lobe Lesions

Patients with damage to the parietal lobes demonstrate a variety of deficiencies related to body image and perception of spatial relations. Lesions to the

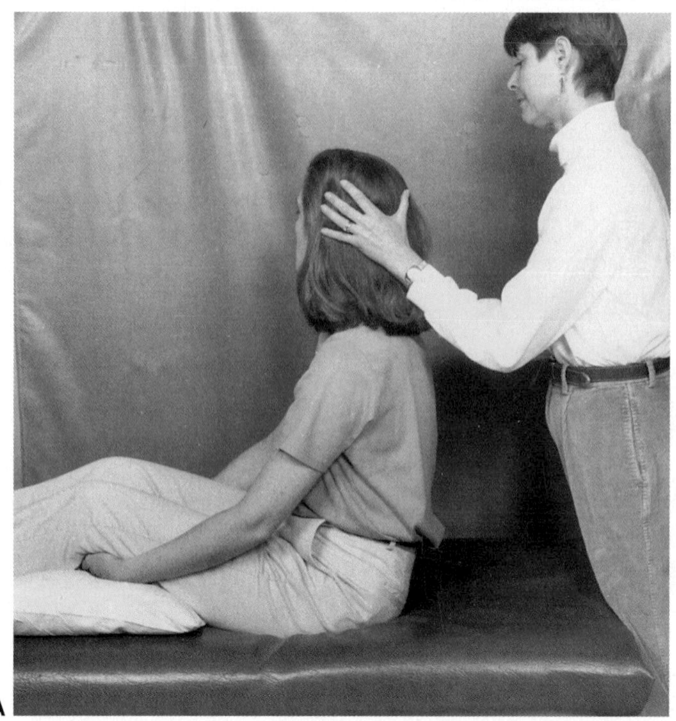

A

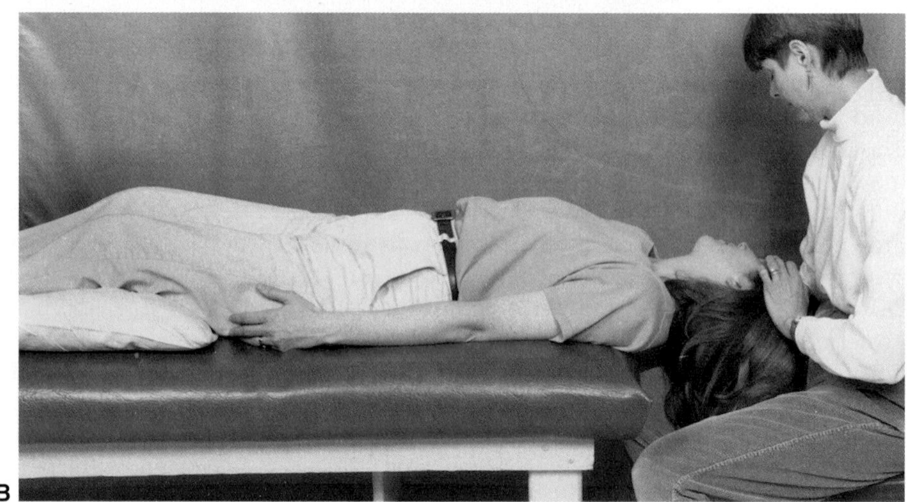

B

FIGURE 5.13 The Dix–Hallpike position, a specific test for benign paroxysmal positional vertigo. The test is begun with the patient in the seated position (A). The person is quickly assisted into a position in which the head is hanging off the edge of the supporting surface (B).

parietal lobe do not simply reduce the ability to perceive information coming in from one part of the body, they affect the ability to interpret this information.

Body scheme is the awareness of body parts and their relationship to one another and the environment. Many patients with neurologic dysfunction have problems with impaired body image, including somatagnosia (lack of awareness of the body structure and the relationship of body parts to one another) unilateral spatial neglect, right–left discrimination, finger agnosia, and anosognosia (denial of the presence or severity of one's paralysis). Assessment of body-image problems includes asking patients to identify body parts—their own and others'. The goal of treatment is to improve the patient's awareness of his or her own body. A number of treatment approaches have been suggested to accomplish this, including the use of controlled tactile stimulation and/or developmental activities; however, there is no research to document the effectiveness of treatment strategies for improving body image and scheme disorders.

Unilateral neglect, also referred to as "hemi-inattention" and "hemispatial neglect," is the inability to perceive and integrate stimuli on one side of the body. Neglect is related to damage to the temporoparietal junction and posterior parietal cortex and can manifest as a lack of attention to the left side of space in the visual, auditory, proprioceptive, and olfactory domains. Neglect is similar to a related but separate condition known as "extinction." Following

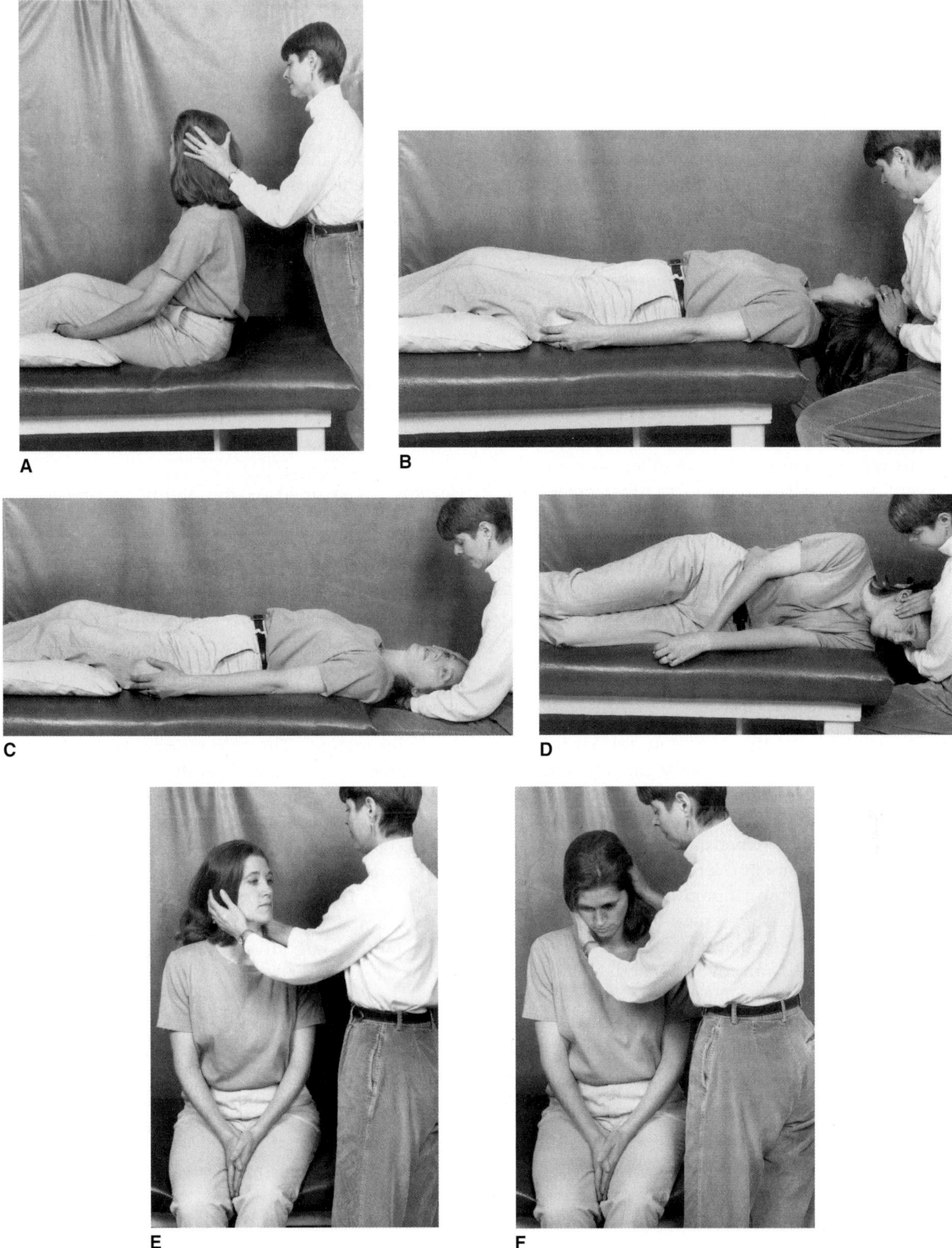

FIGURE 5.14 The canalith repositioning maneuver for treatment of benign paroxysmal positional vertigo. Each position is held for 1 to 2 minutes, or until nystagmus and vertigo subside. The first two positions (A and B) are the same as those found in the Dix–Hallpike maneuver. In position 3 (C), the head is moved into the opposite Dix–Hallpike position. In position 4, the person rolls to the side-lying position, nose down (D); in position 5, the person is brought to the sitting position, with the head turned to 45 degrees from midline (E), and finally the head is dropped into a flexed position (F) and held there for 2 minutes.

right-hemisphere damage, a patient with extinction can correctly identify an object in left space if it is the only object present. However, when presented with objects in both the right and left spaces, a patient with extinction will report only the object on the right.

Assessment of unilateral neglect usually relies on observation of the patient performing functional tasks. The disorder may manifest functionally as eating food on one half of the plate, shaving one side of the face, or walking into objects present in the involved side. Treatment strategies suggested for unilateral neglect include teaching patients scanning strategies, use of sensory stimulation to increase awareness, or modifying the environment to accommodate the impairment (Quintana, 1995).

Spatial Relation Disorders

Problems with spatial relations manifest as difficulty in perceiving oneself in relation to other objects, or other objects in relation to oneself (Quintana, 1995). Spatial-relation problems can include topographic disorientation (an inability to remember the relationship of one place to another), figure ground perception problems (the inability to distinguish foreground from background), and problems with position in space, including understanding concepts such as over, under, front, and back.

Examination may be done through observation of functional skills, or through more formal testing. Both adaptive and remedial strategies are used in treatment (Neistadt, 1990). An adaptive treatment approach attempts to circumvent the problem by teaching the patient compensatory strategies or by changing the environment (Neistadt, 1990). An adaptive strategy for retraining topographic disorientation would be to practice using a map to find one's way around. In contrast, remedial treatment strategies are those that attempt to improve the underlying cognitive functions leading to the deficit. In the case of topographic disorientation, remedial treatment strategies would focus on having the patient practice with mazes (Borst & Peterson, 1993). A good overview of treatment of cognitive deficits may be found in a review by Quintana (1995).

Apraxia

Apraxia is the inability to carry out purposeful movement in the presence of intact sensation, movement, and coordination (Quintana, 1995). There are five types of apraxia: verbal, buccofacial, limb, constructional, and dressing. Two types of limb apraxia have been described: ideomotor and ideational apraxia. In ideomotor apraxia, movement may occur automatically but cannot be performed on command. In ideational apraxia purposeful movement is not possible either automatically or on command (O'Sullivan & Schmitz, 2001).

Apraxia is generally found in patients with left-sided brain damage. Assessment of apraxia can be through either informal methods, such as observation of the patient performing functional tasks, or more formal methods, using standardized tests such as the Sensory Integration and Praxis Test (Ayres, 1989). Treatment of apraxia focuses on practicing functional tasks, such as activities of daily living or nonfunctional tasks that are designed to improve sequencing of skills.

DEFICITS RELATED TO PATHOLOGY IN THE FRONTAL PARIETAL ASSOCIATION AREAS

Cognition is defined as the ability to process, sort, retrieve and manipulate information (Prigatano & Fordyce, 1986). Perception is the integration of sensory impressions into psychologically meaningful information (Lezak, 1976). Intact sensation is a necessary prerequisite for perception. Thus, patients with primary sensory impairments will of necessity have some cognitive/perceptual problems.

Normally functioning cognitive and perceptual systems are critical to successful interaction with the environment. Thus, impairments in these systems affect the patient's ability to move effectively and efficiently about their environment. In addition, cognitive and perceptual deficits are a major factor in lack of progress in many patients who have sustained a neurologic injury (Bernspang et al, 1989; Sea et al., 1993; Titus et al., 1991; Warburg, 1994). Because of their impact on functional movement behavior, understanding cognitive and perceptual impairments is critical to therapists engaged in retraining functional movement in patients with neurologic deficits. This is, however, a highly complex area of study, which can be only briefly reviewed here. Table 5.8 provides a summary of cognitive and perceptual impairments. For further discussion of this subject, readers are referred to other sources (Perry & Hodges, 1999; Quintana, 1995; Warburg, 1994).

Cognitive Impairments

Cognitive impairments include deficits affecting memory, attention, and executive functions. Evaluation of cognitive deficits is usually carried out by a psychologist using psychometric tests. A complete discussion of this important topic is beyond the scope of this book.

TABLE 5.8 Cognitive/Perceptual Deficits

Deficit	Definition	Functions Effects
Perceptual Impairments		
Body scheme	Awareness of body parts, position of body in relationship to environment	Difficulty dressing, unsafe transfers
Right–left discrimination	Ability to understand concepts of right and left	Difficulty with dressing, transfers, mobility, following directions that include right/left
Body-part identification	Ability to identify body parts of self and others	Incorrect response to instructions to move a body part
Anosognosia	Unawareness or denial of deficits	Unsafe in functional activities
Unilateral neglect	Neglect of one side of body or extrapersonal space	Activities of daily living limited to one half of body, transfers and mobility unsafe
Position in space	Ability to understand concepts like over, under, around, above, and below	Difficulty with mobility, following directions that include these terms
Spatial relations	Ability to perceive self in relation to other objects	Transfers and mobility unsafe
Topographic orientation	Ability to find one's way from one place to another	Mobility unsafe
Figure ground perception	Ability to distinguish foreground from background	Unable to find objects in cluttered drawing
Limb apraxia	Inability to carry out purposeful movement in the presence of intact sensation	ADL affected due to difficulty in using objects.
Constructional apraxia	Deficit in constructional activities	ADL apraxia
Dressing apraxia	Inability to dress oneself	Puts clothing on incorrectly
Cognitive Impairments		
Attention	Ability to focus on a specific stimulus without being distracted	Inability to follow direction
Orientation	Knowledge related to person, place, and time	Disoriented
Memory	Registration, encoding, storage, recall, and retrieval of information	Appears disoriented, will forget names, schedules etc., decreased ability to learn
Problem solving	The ability to manipulate a fund of knowledge and apply this information to new or unfamiliar situations	Difficulty with ADL, socially inappropriate, inability to recognize threats to safety

ADL = activities of daily living.

Adapted with permission from Quintana LA. Evaluation of perception and cognition. In: Trombly CA, ed. Occupational therapy for physical dysfunction, 4th ed. Baltimore: Williams & Wilkins, 1995.

Attention

Attention is the ability to focus on a specific stimulus without being distracted. Attention is multidimensional, and has been subdivided into multiple factors, including: (a) focused attention (ability to respond to specific stimuli), (b) sustained attention (the ability to sustain attention over a period of time), (c) selective attention (ability to focus attention in the presence of distracting stimuli), (d) alternating attention (ability to shift focus of attention from one task to another), and (e) divided attention (ability to respond simultaneously to multiple tasks). Specific tests have been developed to examine these different aspects of attention. For example, the Random Letter Test is used as a test of sustained attention, while the Stroop test is used for testing selective attention, and the Trail Making Test parts A and B are used to examine the ability to alternate attention between two tasks (Sohlberg & Mateer, 1989).

Orientation

The term *orientation* is used in several different contexts. In a cognitive context, it has been used to refer to an understanding of people, place, time, and situation. Used in a postural context, the term refers to the ability to maintain a position in space with reference to a specific sensory reference. In the context of cognitive function, orientation to person, place, and time is usually determined by asking the patient questions such as "How old are you?" "What is your full name?" "What is today's date?" "What day is it today?" "Where are you?" and "Do you know why you are here?"

A more formal measurement of mental status may be done by using either the Mini–Mental State Exam (Folstein et al., 1975) or the Short Portable Mental Status Questionnaire (Pfeiffer, 1975). The Mini–Mental State Exam is shown in Assessment Tool 5.2.

Assessment Tool 5-2

The Mini–Mental State Exam

1. What is the date today?
2. What day of the week is it?
3. What is the name of this place?
4. What is your telephone number? Or What is your address?
5. How old are you?
6. When were you born?
7. Who is the President of the United States now?
8. Who was the President before him?
9. What was your mother's maiden name?
10. Subtract 3 from 20 and keep subtracting 3 from each new number, all the way down. (20, 17, 14, 11, 8, 5, 2)

Scoring

Total number of errors_____

0 = Oriented at all times (0–2 errors on test)

1 = Mild intellectual impairment (3–4 errors)

2 = Moderate intellectual impairment (5–7 errors)

3 = Severe intellectual impairment (8–10 errors)

Memory

Like attention, memory is a complex concept involving many facets. Memory is the ability to process, store, and retrieve information. After brain injury, deficits in both short-term memory (STM) and long-term memory (LTM) have been reported. Assessment of STM and LTM involves asking patients to remember four words and then testing their immediate recall and their recall after 5, 10, and 30 minutes (Strub & Black, 1977).

Explicit and Implicit Motor Learning

Therapists rely on both implicit (repetition of movement to promote learning) and explicit (instructions on how to perform a task) motor learning strategies to guide recovery of motor skills in patients with CNS pathology. Understanding the effect of CNS pathology on explicit and implicit learning is very important because of its impact on the therapeutic interventions we use when assisting patients to acquire functional motor skills.

Several studies have explored the effect of unilateral CNS pathology on implicit and explicit learning, with varied results. Explicit learning is impaired in patients with medial temporal lobe damage; however, implicit learning is retained (Reber & Squire, 1998). Lesions in the prefrontal cortex appear to impair both implicit and explicit learning of visuomotor sequencing tasks (Beldarrain et al., 2002). Patients with middle cerebral artery (MCA) stroke affecting the sensorimotor cortex appear to retain the capacity for implicit motor sequence learning (Boyd & Winstein, 2001; Pohl et al., 2001; Winstein et al., 1999), as do patients with cerebellar lesions (Boyd & Winstein, 2003). This research underscores the concept that the neural systems underlying implicit and explicit memory and learning are anatomically separate, and therefore the effects of CNS pathology on learning is in part lesion-dependent. In addition, because control of implicit learning is distributed among many brain structures, the research suggests that no single lesion completely eliminates the capacity for implicit learning (Boyd & Winstein, 2003).

Does providing explicit information improve implicit learning of a motor skill? It is generally assumed by therapists that it does, so we routinely provide explicit instructions to patients while they are practicing a motor skill. However, results from current research examining the effect of explicit instructions on implicit learning suggest a need to reexamine these assumptions. A number of studies have examined the effect of explicit instructions on implicit motor skill learning in patients with various CNS pathologies. Boyd and Winstein (2003) examined this in 10 patients with MCA stroke affecting the sensorimotor cortex and 10 nonimpaired controls.

Some of the results of this study are shown in Figure 5.15. This study found that implicit learning did occur in the patients with MCA stroke. Similar to the control group, the subjects with stroke (shown in Fig. 5.15B) reduced reaction time over the 3 days of practicing the repeated sequence motor task (reaction time did not change when practicing a random-sequence motor task). This figure also shows the differential effects of explicit instruction on implicit learning in the two groups. Explicit instruction improved implicit learning in the control group (Fig. 5.15A, steeper drop in reaction time in the control subjects who received explicit instructions [solid line] compared with those who did not [dashed line]).

In contrast, explicit instruction had a detrimental effect on learning in the subjects with stroke. This can be seen in Figure 5.15B, which shows that the subjects with stroke who received explicit information (solid line) had less improvement in reaction time compared with subjects with stroke who did not receive explicit information (dashed line). The finding that explicit instruction impairs implicit learning was also found for patients with basal ganglia stroke (Pohl & Winstein, 2004). In contrast, in patients with cerebellar stroke, explicit instruction improved implicit learning (Molinari et al., 1997). These results suggest that the impact of explicit instruction on implicit learning depends on a number of factors, including the type, timing, and meaningfulness of instructions, as well as the location of CNS pathology.

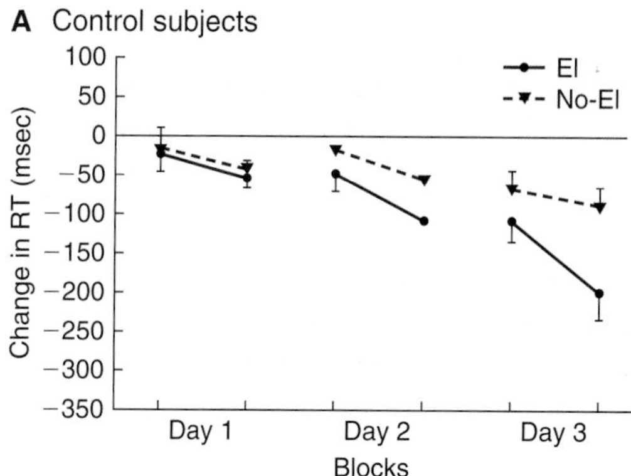

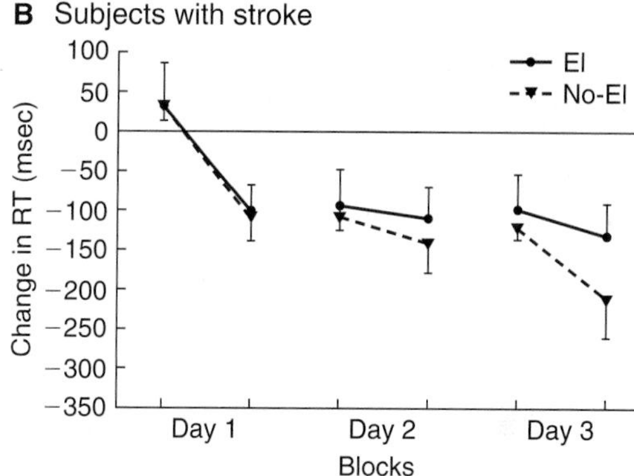

FIGURE 5.15 Effect of explicit instructions on implicit motor sequence learning in persons with stroke. Both control subjects (A) and subjects with stroke (B) demonstrate implicit learning, as indicated by a change in reaction time (RT) over the 3 days of practicing an implicit motor sequence task. Explicit instruction (EI) improved implicit learning in the control subjects who receive it (shown by the solid lines) compared to subjects who did not receive it (shown by the dashed lines). In contrast, subjects with stroke who received explicit instructions (solid line) had less improvement in reaction time as compared with subjects who did not receive it (dashed line), suggesting that explicit instruction impeded implicit learning after stroke. (Adapted from Boyd LA, Winstein CJ. Impact of explicit information on implicit motor sequence learning following middle cerebral artery stroke. Phys Ther 2003;83:983, with permission of the American Physical Therapy Association. This material is copyrighted, and any further reproduction or distribution requires written permission from APTA.)

Arousal/Level of Consciousness

Alertness is a basic arousal process allowing the patient to respond to stimuli in the environment. The Rancho Los Amigos scale is probably the most well known approach to quantifying level of consciousness in the patient with neurologic impairments. This scale is shown in Assessment Tool 5.3. Assessment of level of consciousness, arousal, or state is an essential part of assessing motor control, since motor behavior is very dependent on arousal level (Duncan & Badke, 1987).

Treatment of Cognitive Impairments

Many patients with CNS lesions demonstrate significant cognitive impairments that affect the patient's ability to participate fully in a retraining program.

Assessment Tool 5-3

Rancho Los Amigos Scale of Level of Consciousness

I. No response: unresponsive to any stimulus.

II. Generalized response: limited, inconsistent, nonpurposeful responses, often to pain only.

III. Localized response: purposeful responses; may follow simple commands; may focus on presented object.

IV. Confused, agitated: heightened state of activity; confusion, disorientation; aggressive behavior; unable to do self-care; unaware of present events; agitation appears related to internal confusion.

V. Confused, inappropriate: nonagitated; appears alert; responds to commands; distractible; does not concentrate on task; agitated response to external stimuli; verbally inappropriate; does not learn new information.

VI. Confused, appropriate: good directed behavior; needs cueing; can relearn old skills as activities of daily living (ADLs); serious memory problems; some awareness of self and others.

VII. Automatic, appropriate: appears appropriate, oriented; frequently robot-like in daily routine; minimal or absent confusion; shallow recall; increased awareness of self, interaction in environment; lacks insight into condition; decreased judgment and problem-solving; lacks realistic planning for future.

VIII. Purposeful, appropriate: alert, oriented; recalls and integrates past events; learns new activities and can continue without supervision; independent in home and living skills; capable of driving; defects in stress tolerance, judgment, abstract reasoning persist; many function at reduced levels in society.

(Reprinted with permission from Adult Brain Injury Service, Rancho Los Amigo Medical Center, Downy, CA.)

With this in mind, Figure 5.16 provides a few suggestions for modifying treatment strategies when working with a patient who has cognitive problems.

Cognitive problems are quite common in patients with CNS lesions. Cognitive problems can include an altered level of consciousness, change in mental status, and deficits in learning, memory, attention, and information processing. Behavioral problems are also common, and may include apathy, aggression, low frustration tolerance, emotional lability, and loss of behavioral inhibition, resulting in impulsivity.

A CASE STUDY APPROACH TO UNDERSTANDING NEUROLOGIC DISORDERS

As therapists, we do not treat a diagnosis; we treat underlying impairments and functional problems that result from neurologic pathology. Nonetheless, an important part of clinical decision making regarding the choice of appropriate tests and measures as well as therapeutic techniques is understanding what impairments are likely to manifest in patients with a certain diagnosis. The following section uses case studies to present impairments commonly associated with specific diagnoses.

Jean J.: Impairments Associated with Cerebral Vascular Accident

Jean J is an 82-year-old woman who has had a stroke. Stroke, or cerebral vascular accident (CVA), is defined as a sudden, focal, neurologic deficit resulting from disruption to the blood supply in the brain that persists for at least 24 hours. Transient ischemic attacks (TIAs) result from the temporary interruption of blood supply, with symptoms lasting less than 24 hours. There are two main categories of brain damage: ischemia (a lack of blood flow) and hemorrhage (release of blood into the extravascular space).

The impairments resulting from a stroke are numerous, and will vary depending on the site and extent of vascular damage. Jean J has had a middle cerebral artery stroke in the left cerebral hemisphere. Her neuromuscular impairments include right-sided weakness (paresis), abnormal muscle tone (spasticity), abnormal coordination (characterized by abnormal synergies of movement) and an inability to activate muscles in isolation, so-called lack of fractionation of movement. She has sensory and perceptual impairments, including deficits in somatosensation and proprioception. While she does not, many persons with stroke have impaired vision, specifically homonymous hemianopsia.

Cognitive/behavioral deficits depend on the side of the lesion. Patients such as Jean, with a left-sided CVA (resultant right hemiparesis) often have difficulty processing information, and they tend to be depressed, anxious, cautious, and uncertain. In contrast, patients who have had a right-sided CVA and resultant left hemiparesis, are often impulsive and

1. Reduce confusion—make sure the task goal is clear to the patient.
2. Improve motivation—work on tasks that are relevant and important to the patient.
3. Encourage consistency of performance—be consistent in your goals and reinforce only those behaviors that are compatible with those goals.
4. Reduce confusion—use simple, clear, and concise instructions.
5. Improve attention—accentuate perceptual cues that are essential to the task, and minimize the number of irrelevant stimuli in the environment.
6. Improve problem-solving ability—begin with relatively simple tasks, and gradually increase the complexity of the task demands.
7. Encourage declarative as well as procedural learning—have a patient verbally and/or mentally rehearse sequences when performing a task.
8. Seek a moderate level of arousal to optimize learning—moderate the sensory stimulation in the environment; agitated patients require decreased intensity of stimulation (soft voice, low lights, slow touch) to reduce arousal levels; stuporous patients require increased intensity of stimulation (use brisk, loud commands, fast movements; work in a vertical position).
9. Provide increased levels of supervision, especially during the early stages of retraining.
10. Recognize that progress may be slower when working with patients who have cognitive impairments.

FIGURE 5.16 Strategies for modifying treatment to accommodate a cognitive impairment.

unrealistic regarding their own abilities. They tend to deny problems (anosognosia), which can lead to poor judgment and safety issues. Jean J's neuromuscular impairments that restrict motion have led to the development of a variety of musculoskeletal impairments, including muscle tightness and contractures (limiting range of motion) in both her upper and lower extremities. Because of the location of her stroke, Jean J has retained the capacity for implicit motor learning; however, explicit instructions limit her implicit learning of motor skills.

Mike M.: Impairments Associated with Parkinson's Disease

Mike M has Parkinson's disease (PD), a slowly progressing disorder of the basal ganglia resulting from degeneration of the nigrostriatal pathway. His primary neuromuscular impairments include rigidity, bradykinesia, resting and postural tremor, and impairments of postural control and gait. Bradykinesia manifests as slowed voluntary movement, decreased arm swing, slow and shuffling gait, and difficulty in initiating or changing the direction of a movement. Mike M demonstrates other common signs of PD, including festinating gait (small shuffling steps), stooped posture, poor balance, and a mask-like facial expression.

Though not present in Mike, many persons with PD develop cognitive impairments ranging from minimal involvement to severe depression and global dementia. Because PD results in a gradual and progressive loss of movement, Mike M has developed secondary musculoskeletal impairments that significantly affect functional performance. Like Jean J, implicit learning capacity is likely to be present in Mike M; however, he, too, may find that explicit information limits his ability for implicit learning.

John C.: Impairments Associated with Cerebellar Degeneration

John C is an 33-year-old with spinocerebellar ataxia type 2, a genetic disorder causing slow degeneration of the cerebellum. As reported by Gordon Holmes in the 1920s and 1930s (Kandel et al., 2000), disorders of the cerebellum result in three principal deficits: hypotonia, ataxia, and action tremor; all are present in John. Ataxia is a problem executing coordinated movement and is characterized by dysmetria (errors in the metrics of movement), dysdiadochokinesia (inability to sustain a regular alternating rhythmic movement), and dyssynergia (errors in the timing of multijoint movements). In general, lesions in the cerebellum result in impairments ipsilateral to the lesion; however, the specific constellation of impairments depends on what part of the cerebellum is affected. Implicit learning capacity is intact in John C, and he will benefit from explicit instructions while practicing implicit learning tasks.

Thomas: Impairments Associated with Spastic Diplegia Cerebral Palsy

Thomas is a 7-year-old with a spastic diplegia form of cerebral palsy. Cerebral palsy (CP) is a nonprogressive disorder that results from prenatal or perinatal damage to the CNS. The site and extent of damage to the developing CNS determines the continuum of impairments seen in a patient diagnosed with CP. Classification is based on the type of motor disorder found and the extremities involved. Spastic cerebral palsy (hemiplegia, diplegia, and quadriplegia) represents 50 to 60% of the cases, and results from damage to the cerebral cortex and the corticospinal tract. Because Thomas has spastic diplegia, his impairments affect his lower extremities more than his upper extremities. His neuromuscular impairments include hypertonicity (spasticity), hyperreflexia, abnormal reflexes, weakness, and impaired coordination as well as poor postural control and gait. In addition to his primary neuromuscular impairments he has developed secondary musculoskeletal impairments (particularly in the lower extremities). He has mild sensory deficits, particularly affecting somatosensory and proprioceptive systems. Finally, though he does not, many children with CP have cognitive deficits, including attention and learning problems.

SUMMARY

1. Knowledge regarding both the physiology and pathophysiology of motor control is essential to examining and treating the patient with movement problems. This knowledge enables the therapist to form initial assumptions regarding the types of functional problems and underlying impairments likely to be present in a particular patient, thus guiding the selection of appropriate tests and measurements, as well as suitable intervention methods.
2. Brain injury produces a unique pattern of behavioral signs and symptoms associated with the destruction of specific neuronal populations. Hughlings Jackson divided abnormal behaviors associated with CNS lesions into either positive signs and symptoms (i.e., the presence of abnormal behaviors) or negative signs and symptoms (i.e., the loss of normal behaviors). In the rehabilitation environment, emphasis is often placed on positive signs and symptoms (such as abnormalities of muscle tonus) at the expense of negative signs and symptoms (such as loss of strength) when attempting to understand performance deficits in persons with a neurologic dysfunction.
3. Pathophysiology within the action system including the motor cortex and subcortical structures such as the cerebellum, and basal ganglia, result in a wide range of impairments affecting the control of movement.
4. Impairments associated with pathophysiology of the motor cortex include motor weakness (paresis), abnormal muscle tone (spasticity), and coordination problems including abnormal synergies of movement.
5. Pathophysiology of subcortical structures, such as the cerebellum and basal ganglia produce a range of impairments including abnormal muscle tone, tremor, and problems with the timing and scaling of muscle activity significantly affecting the coordination of movement.
6. In the person with neurologic pathology, musculoskeletal impairments develop secondary to neuromuscular impairments, but they can significantly constrain functional movement.
7. Sensory deficits are a major factor contributing to motor dyscontrol in persons with CNS lesions. Sensory deficits can result in a disruption of sensory information in somatosensory, visual, or vestibular systems.
8. Perceptual problems such as impaired body image and spatial relationship disorders also constrain functional movement in a person with brain pathology.
9. Cognitive problems, common in persons with CNS pathology, can include altered level of consciousness, change in mental status, and deficits in learning, memory, attention, and information processing. Behavioral problems, also common, include apathy, aggression, low frustration tolerance, emotional lability, and loss of behavioral inhibition, resulting in impulsivity.
10. Explicit and implicit learning and memory are differentially affected by CNS pathology because of their different anatomical substrates. In addition, the effect of providing explicit information on implicit learning of motor skills will also vary depending on the type and timing of instruction and the location of neural pathology.

CHAPTER 6

A CONCEPTUAL FRAMEWORK FOR CLINICAL PRACTICE

LEARNING OBJECTIVES

Following completion of this chapter, the reader will be able to:

1. Discuss the relationship between a conceptual framework and clinical practice.
2. Discuss each element in the American Physical Therapy Association's patient management process.
3. Describe components of the World Health Organization's International Classification of Functioning, Disability, and Health (ICF); discuss the similarities and differences between the ICF model and the Nagi model of disablement.
4. Define a hypothesis and describe how hypotheses are used in research versus clinical practice.
5. Define evidence-based practice and discuss the concept of levels of evidence.
6. Describe a task-oriented approach to examination and intervention.
7. Discuss factors that have an impact on the selection of tests and measures used to examine a patient with a movement disorder.
8. Describe the goal of treatment focused on recovery of function versus compensation; discuss factors that should be considered when choosing each approach.

INTRODUCTION

Clinicians responsible for retraining movement in a patient with neurologic impairments are faced with an overwhelming number of decisions. What is the most appropriate way to examine my patient? How much time should be spent on documenting functional ability versus evaluating underlying impairments leading to dysfunction? What criteria should I use in deciding what the priority problems are? How do I establish goals that are realistic and meaningful? What is the best approach to intervention and the most effective way to structure my therapy sessions? What are the most appropriate outcomes for evaluating the effects of intervention?

These questions reflect the critical need for a conceptual framework for clinical practice. A conceptual framework is a logical structure that helps the clinician organize clinical practices into a cohesive and comprehensive plan. It provides a context in which information is gathered and interpreted (Campbell, 2006; Darrah et al., 2006; Schenkman et al., 2006; Trombly, 1995). A conceptual framework influences clinical practice in several ways. It influences decisions about what to measure during the examination of the patient, the selection of intervention strategies, and the conclusions drawn regarding the intervention process. It provides the clinician with guidelines for how to proceed through the clinical intervention process (Campbell, 2006; Darrah et al., 2006; Schenkman et al., 2006; Trombly, 1995). The growing recognition of the importance of conceptual frameworks to clinical practice is seen in the increasing number of publications related to this topic (Campbell, 2006; Darrah et al., 2006; Rothstein et al., 2003; Schenkman et al., 2006). As was true for theories of motor control, each model represents an individual's perspective on the relative importance and usefulness of specific elements to their practice. There is no consensus on the best framework across all forms of practice.

The purposes of this chapter are to consider elements that contribute to a conceptual framework we find useful for guiding clinical practice and to describe a conceptual framework for retraining the patient with movement disorders, which we call a "task-oriented approach." A task-oriented approach is used in later chapters as the framework for retraining posture, mobility, and upper-extremity control in a patient with a neurologic deficit.

COMPONENTS OF A CONCEPTUAL FRAMEWORK FOR CLINICAL PRACTICE

While there are potentially many concepts that contribute to a conceptual framework for practice, we have identified five, including:

1. A model of practice, which outlines a method for gathering information and developing a plan of care consistent with the goals, problems and needs of the patient;
2. A model of function and disability, which describes a framework for examining the effects of a health condition on the individual and enables the clinician to identify the patient's strengths and limitations critical in developing a plan of care;
3. Hypothesis-oriented clinical practice, which provides the means to test assumptions about the nature and cause of motor control problems systematically;
4. Principles of motor control and motor learning, which help us to understand both the cause and nature of normal and abnormal movement, as well as assumptions about how movement skills are learned or relearned.
5. Evidence-based clinical practice, an approach to clinical practice that stresses the importance of integrating best research evidence with clinical expertise and patient values (Sackett et al., 1996).

The following sections describe each of these important components in detail.

Models of Practice

Mrs. Jean J is an 82-year-old woman who had a cerebral vascular accident (CVA) approximately 6 years ago. The CVA has produced motor dyscontrol in her right side. She has a resultant right hemiparesis, decreased sensation in the right upper and lower extremities, and associated right neglect. She has good language skills, but she tends to be impulsive. During her acute phase, she was referred to inpatient rehabilitation for management of the sequelae from her stroke.

Mike M is a 59-year-old man who was diagnosed with Parkinson's disease approximately 10 years ago. He lives in his own home with his wife, who is in relatively good health. His balance and walking have become increasingly worse, as has his ability to assist in bed mobility and transfers. He is beginning to fall when walking. They are referred for therapy to try to improve Mr. M's balance and mobility skills, reduce his risk for falls, and improve his independence in transfer abilities.

John C is a 33-year-old with a diagnosis of spinocerebellar degeneration, a genetic disorder affecting the cerebellum and resulting in severe ataxia. In addition, John has significant cognitive impairments, including attention and memory problems. He has significant instability when standing and walking, and has had several falls. Though independent, he has difficulty with his activities of daily living (ADLs) including dressing, cooking and grooming, because of dysmetria and dyscoordination.

Thomas L is a 7-year-old who was born with cerebral palsy and has moderate spastic diplegia. He has been in an early-intervention program since he was 4 months old. He has recently moved into a new area, and is referred for a continuation of his therapy to improve posture, mobility, and upper-extremity skills.

This diverse group of patients is typical of those referred to therapy for motor control problems affecting their ability to move and carry out ADLs. Can the same approach used to examine motor control in a man with Parkinson's disease be appropriate for a 33-year-old man with cerebellar degeneration? Can the same approach to intervention used with an 82-year-old woman with impaired balance following a stroke be used to habilitate mobility in a 7-year-old child with cerebral palsy?

As you will see, the answer to these questions is yes. Despite the diversity of these patients, the *process* used to gather information and design an intervention program is similar for all patients. Thus, while each patient's motor control problems and therapeutic solutions may be different, the process used to identify those problems and solutions will be consistent across patients.

American Physical Therapy Association Model of Practice

The American Physical Therapy Association (APTA) in its publication "Guide to Physical Therapist Practice" (APTA, 2003) has described a process for managing patient/client care. The APTA's patient-oriented management process is composed of five elements, including examination, evaluation, diagnosis, prognosis, and intervention. These elements are shown in Figure 6.1.

Examination. Examination is the process of obtaining data necessary to form a diagnosis, prognosis, and plan of care. There are three parts to the examination process: taking a history, reviewing relevant systems, and performing appropriate tests and measurements.

History. Information related to the patient's current and past health can be gathered directly from the patient, family, or caregiver; from medical records; and from other health care professionals. The types of data that might be generated from a patient history include general demographics (e.g., age, race, sex), current conditions and history of conditions (specific concerns expressed by patient/family/caregiver), living environment, growth and developmental history (if appropriate), family history, health status, social history (e.g., family and caregiver resources, cultural beliefs, social support), occupation/employment, functional status, and activity level (current and prior level of function with respect to self-care and home management (e.g., activities of daily living (ADL) and independent activities of daily living (IADL)). Also included in the history is a list of medications and relevant lab and diagnostic tests from other medical specialties (APTA, 2003, pp. S34–S37).

Interviewing the patient and/or the patient's family can be a critical part of the examination process. The interview is the first step in establishing a good

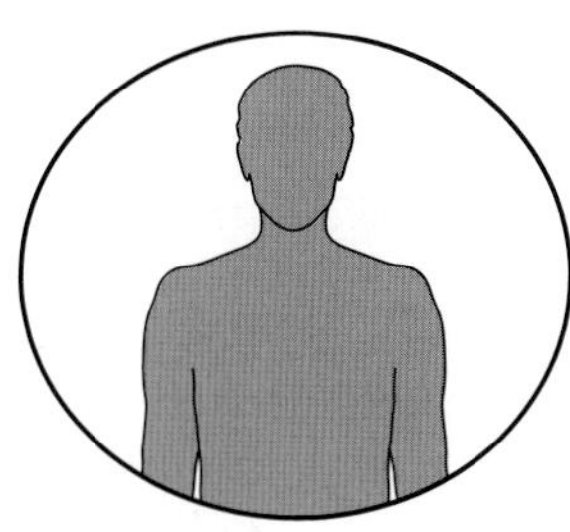

FIGURE 6.1 The patient/client treatment process suggested by the American Physical Therapy Association. (Adapted with permission from American Physical Therapy Association. Guide to physical therapist practice. Alexandria, VA: American Physical Therapy Association, 2003:1–4.)

rapport between the patient and the therapist. The interview is used to gather information on the patient's goals, expectations, and motivation, a central feature of a patient-oriented approach to clinical practice. The interview process also allows the therapist insight into the patient's level of understanding regarding his or her medical condition and the therapeutic process. Information on previous and current health behaviors, including exercise habits, is also critical information when planning intervention.

Systems Review. The examination also includes a brief review of the relevant systems in order to help direct the selection of specific tests and measurements and to assist in determining diagnosis and prognosis. A review of the systems includes a brief determination of the anatomical and/or physiological status of the cardiopulmonary, integumentary, musculoskeletal, and neuromuscular systems. It also includes a brief examination of the patient's communication ability, cognition, language, and learning style.

Tests and Measurements. The last part of the examination process includes the performance of specific tests and measurements that provide the clinician with insight into specific impairments and functional limitations that restrict the patient's ability to participate in the roles and activities that are important to his or her life. This aspect of the examination process will be discussed in more detail in later sections of this chapter.

Evaluation. The next step in APTA's patient/client management process is evaluation, defined as the process of making clinical judgments based on the data gathered during the examination. Factors that have an impact on the evaluation include not just clinical findings related to tests and measurements, but the extent of loss of function, social considerations, overall physical function, and health status. The evaluation reflects the severity and duration of the current problem, the presence of coexisting conditions or diseases, as well as the stability of the condition.

Diagnosis. The next step in the management process is determining a physical therapy diagnosis. A diagnosis is a label that identifies the impact of a condition on the function at both the level of a system (e.g., the movement system) and the level of the whole person (APTA, 2003). The physical therapy diagnosis encompasses the signs and symptoms, syndromes, and categories of problems that are used to guide the therapist in determining the most appropriate intervention. The term *diagnosis* as it relates to the profession of physical therapy is distinguished from a diagnosis made by physicians. Sahrmann (1988, p. 1705) proposed the following definition of a physical therapy diagnosis: "Diagnosis is a term that names the primary dysfunction toward which the physical therapist directs treatment. The dysfunction is identified by the physical therapist based on information obtained from the history, signs, symptoms, examination and tests the therapist performs or requests." The physical therapy diagnosis allows the clinician to name and classify clusters of signs and symptoms that will potentially benefit from physical therapy treatment (Rose, 1989). Thus, the purpose of a physical therapy diagnosis is to direct treatment. It allows the identification of specific problems that will likely respond successfully to a specific treatment.

Prognosis and Plan of Care. The fourth stage in APTA's management process includes determining a patient's prognosis and plan of care. A prognosis includes both the level of functional independence the patient is expected to achieve following intervention and the expected amount of time required to get to that level. A part of prognosis is determining intermediate levels of function that will be accomplished during the course of therapy. At this point in the management process the therapist establishes a plan of care, which includes anticipated goals and outcomes, interventions, and expected duration and frequency of interventions needed to achieve established goals and outcomes. In addition, a plan of care includes information related to discharge planning, including criteria for discharge, appropriate follow-up, and referral following discharge from Physical Therapy (APTA, 2003).

The *Guide to Physical Therapy Practice* defines anticipated goals and outcomes as "the intended results of patient/client management that indicate the changes in impairment, functional limitations and disabilities and the changes in health, well being and fitness needs that are expected as the result of implementing the plan of care. The anticipated goals and expected outcomes also address risk reduction, prevention, impact on societal resources and patient/client satisfaction. The anticipated goals and expected outcomes in the plan should be measurable and time limited" (APTA, 2003, p. S38).

Expected outcomes reflect the therapist's professional judgment about the likely level of function the patient will achieve, while goals may be used to measure progress toward expected outcomes (Quinn & Gordon, 2003). In a patient-oriented approach to clinical practice, goal-setting is a collaborative process involving the therapist, the patient (and family as appropriate), and often other health care professionals. Patient-centered goals—that is, goals that are relevant to the patient's desires—are important in ensuring successful outcomes (Payton et al., 1990; Quinn & Gordon, 2003).

Therapists are frequently asked to establish both short- and long-term goals for therapy. Short-term goals are those expected to be achieved in a reasonably short time, with the amount of time varying depending on where the patient is receiving care. For example, short-term goals in a rehabilitation program may be defined weekly; alternatively, short-term goals in an outpatient program may be defined monthly.

Long-term goals define the patient's expected level of performance at the end of the intervention process. Long-term goals are often expressed relative to functional gains, such as: (a) amount of independence; (b) supervision, or level of assistance required to carry out a task; or (c) in relationship to the equipment or environmental adaptation needed to perform the task. Quinn and Gordon (2003) have proposed an alternative approach to describing goals for intervention. They suggest writing goals and outcomes at three different levels: disability goals, functional goals, and impairment goals. Disability goals indicate outcomes related to recovery of participation in the specific roles and activities important to the patient. Functional goals reflect recovery of performance of important functional tasks and activities of daily living. Finally, impairment goals express changes in underlying impairments contributing to functional limitations; thus, these goals should be linked to a relevant functional goal (Quinn & Gordon, 2003).

Writing effective goals is facilitated by the use of a structure that guides the therapist in generating objective, measurable, patient-centered goals. The "ABCDE" structure shown in Figure 6.2 is based on five essential components of an effective goal (Quinn & Gordon, 2003). The first component is the actor (A), the individual who will accomplish the goal; the second is the behavior (B) or action that will be performed; the third component is the condition (C) under which the behavior will be performed; the fourth is the degree (D), quantifying the level of performance; and the fifth is the expected time frame (E) in which the goal is to be achieved.

Essential Components of a Well-Written Functional Goal-ABCDE

Actor
- Who will carry out the activity
- Usually the patient, occasionally family member or other caregiver
- e.g., "Patient will . . ." or "Patient's wife will . . ."

Behavior
- Description of the activity (in understandable terminology)
- E.g., ". . . will walk . . ." or ". . . will transfer . . ." or ". . . will put on shirt . . ."

Condition
- Circumstances under which the behavior is carried out
- Must include all essential elements of performance (e.g., assistive devices, environmental context)
- E.g., ". . . in hospital corridor with quad cane . . ."

Degree
- Quantitative specification of performance
- Examples of quantification: rate of success or failure, degree or level of assistance, time required, distance, number of repetitions, heart rate at end of activity, etc.
- ". . . 8/10 times successfully . . ." or ". . . in 4 minutes . . ." or ". . . three blocks . . ." or ". . . 500 feet . . ." or ". . . with increase of heart rate to no more than 110 beats/min . . ."
- Qualitative aspects of performance: "with effective toe clearance" "while maintaining proper body mechanics"

Expected Time
- How long it will it take to reach goal
- Stated in days, weeks, months, or, alternatively, number of visits
- E.g., ". . . within 2 weeks . . ." or ". . . within 3 therapy sessions . . ."

FIGURE 6.2 Five components of effective clinical goals and outcomes. (Adapted from Quinn L, Gordon J. Functional outcomes: documentation for rehabilitation. Philadelphia: Saunders, 2003:104, Figure 9.1.)

Intervention. The last step in APTA's management process is intervention. *Intervention* is the purposeful and skilled interaction of the therapist with the patient. It includes: (1) coordination, communication, and documentation; (2) patient/client-related instructions; and (3) procedural interventions (APTA, 2001). Intervention is the heart of the plan of care and, as shown in Figure 6.3, can include many different types of procedures.

While a model of practice gives you a broad framework for proceeding through the therapeutic process, it does not provide details regarding how each step should be implemented. It does not provide answers to critical questions such as: How shall I measure the effect of disease or injury on my patient? Toward what goals should I direct my intervention? In what order should problems be tackled? A model of functioning and disablement can help to answer these questions.

Models of Functioning and Disability

Models of functioning and disability suggest a framework for structuring the effects of a health condition on aspects of function in an individual. The term *disablement* is a global one that refers to the impact of disease on human functioning at many different levels (Jette, 1994). As health care professionals, we deal with the consequences of disease, injury, and congenital abnormalities on the health and functioning of individuals (Rothstein, 1994). The goal of therapeutic intervention is to maximize function and thereby minimize disability; however, in order to accomplish this goal we need to understand the effects of a health condition on the ability of an individual to function and participate in activities and roles that are important to them.

A number of theoretical frameworks have been proposed to describe the effect of a health condition on the functioning of an individual. These models can

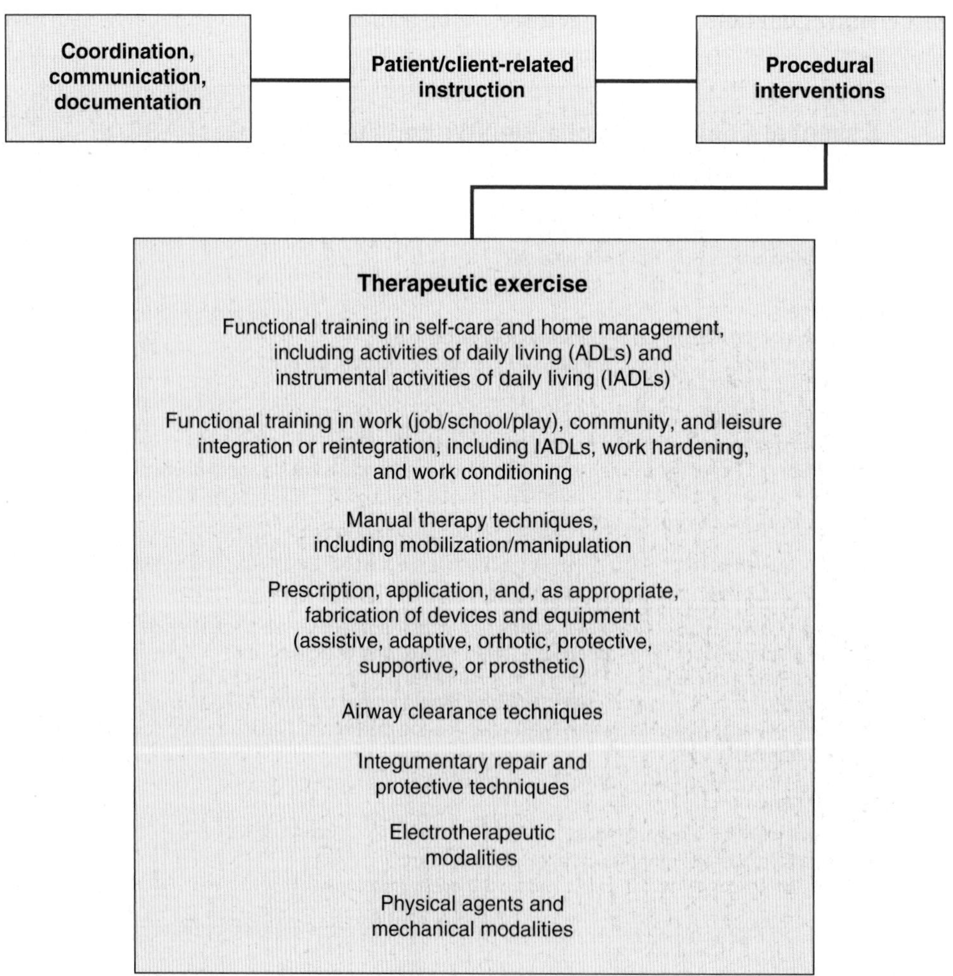

FIGURE 6.3 Components of physical therapy intervention. (Adapted with permission from American Physical Therapy Association. Guide to physical therapist practice, 2003:S98, Figure 1.)

be used as a framework for organizing and interpreting examination data and developing a comprehensive plan for intervention.

World Health Organization Model

The International Classification of Functioning, Disability, and Health (known as the ICF) is a framework proposed by the World Health Organization for describing health and health-related states (WHO, 2001). It provides a standard language and framework to describe how people with a health condition function in their daily lives. The new ICF is a major revision of the original International Classification of Impairments, Disabilities, and Handicaps (ICIDH) proposed in 1980 (WHO, 1980). In addition, the ICF is a significant departure from models of disablement proposed by Nagi and the National Center for Medical Rehabilitation Research (NCMRR) (described below).

In 2001, the 191 Member States of the World Health Organization (WHO) agreed to adopt the ICF as the basis for the scientific standardization of data on health and disability worldwide. In June 2008, the APTA House of Delegates officially endorsed and adopted the WHO's International Classification of Functioning, Disability and Heath.

The ICF model, shown in Figure 6.4, classifies factors that have an impact on human functioning (and its restrictions) into two major parts, each of which has two components. Part 1, functioning and disability, includes the components of body functions/structures and activities and participation. Part 2, contextual factors, includes the components of environmental factors and personal factors. Each component can be expressed in either positive (functioning) or negative (disability) terms.

Within Part 1, body functions include both physiological and psychological functions of the body, while body structures include anatomical parts of the body. The negative expression of these concepts is impairment, defined as a significant deviation or loss in body function or structure. Activity is defined as the execution of a task or action by an individual and thus represents the individual perspective of function. Participation reflects involvement in a life situation, and represents a societal perspective of functioning (WHO, 2001). Activity limitations and restricted participation are the negative aspects of these concepts.

The WHO lists nine domains of activities and participation, including learning and applying knowledge, general tasks and demands, communication, mobility, self-care, domestic life, interpersonal interactions and relationships, major life areas, and community, social, and civic life, many of which can be considered as both an activity and a reflection of participation. For example, mobility is both an activity (a task the individual performs) and a component of participation (societal perspective of moving around to different locations and using transportation).

The terms *performance* and *capacity* are used to describe behavior of the individual in the nine domains. The performance qualifier describes what the individual does in his or her current environment, that is, within the actual context in which they live (WHO, 2001, p. 15). In contrast, the capacity qualifier describes the highest probable level of functioning a person could achieve in an environment adjusted to the ability of that person. Thus, *capacity* quantifies ability in a standard or uniform environment, in contrast to *performance,* which quantifies ability in the current environment.

Part 2 of the ICF model identifies contextual factors, both environmental and personal, that can modify and influence the affect of a health condition on functioning of the individual. Personal factors can include those such as age, education, socioeconomic status, and presence of other comorbidities. Other examples include lifestyle and health behaviors such as exercise and diet; psychosocial attributes such as positive affect, prayer, and self-efficacy; and the ability to adapt to and accommodate potential limitations (WHO, 2001; Verbrugge & Jette, 1994).

Environmental factors are external to the individual and include physical, social, and attitudinal factors. These factors can have an impact at the level of the individual, reflecting the immediate environment in which the person is living, or at the societal level, reflecting social agencies, services, laws, and regulations as well as attitudes and cultural values.

Environmental factors can have either a positive (enhancing function/participation) or negative (limiting function/participation) effect. Environmental factors are critical because disability emerges from a complex relationship between factors in the individual and external factors reflecting the circumstances in which the person is living (WHO, 2001, p. 17). Some environments facilitate functioning and reduce disability, while others restrict functioning and increase disability. Thus, determination of disability cannot be made solely by factors intrinsic to the individual; demands of the environment must be considered in the disabling process (Patla & Shumway-Cook, 1999). For example, a person who has limited walking ability due to a stroke may be less disabled in a flat geographical location such as Chicago than in a hilly location such as San Francisco. A person with limited visual acuity may be able to function independently in daylight hours, but show disability when light levels are

<table>
<tr><th></th><th colspan="2">Part 1: Functioning and disability</th><th colspan="2">Part 2: Contextual factors</th></tr>
<tr><td>Components</td><td>Body functions and structures</td><td>Activities and participation</td><td>Environmental factors</td><td>Personal factors</td></tr>
<tr><td>Domains</td><td>Body functions
Body structures</td><td>Life areas (tasks, actions)</td><td>External influences on functioning and disability</td><td>Internal influences on functioning and disability</td></tr>
<tr><td>Constructs</td><td>Change in body functions (physiologic)

Change in body structures (anatomic)</td><td>Capacity
Executing tasks in a standard environment

Performance
Executing tasks in the current environment</td><td>Facilitating or hindering impact of features of the physical, social, and attitudinal world</td><td>Impact of attributes of the person</td></tr>
<tr><td rowspan="2">Positive aspect</td><td>Functional and structural integrity</td><td>Activities
Participation</td><td rowspan="2">Facilitators</td><td rowspan="2">Not applicable</td></tr>
<tr><td colspan="2">Functioning</td></tr>
<tr><td rowspan="2">Negative aspect</td><td>Impairment</td><td>Activity limitation
Participation restriction</td><td rowspan="2">Barriers/ hindrances</td><td rowspan="2">Not applicable</td></tr>
<tr><td colspan="2">Disability</td></tr>
</table>

FIGURE 6.4 International Classification of Functioning and Disability. (Adapted from World Health Organization. International Classification Functioning, Disability and Health [ICF]. Geneva: World Health Organization, 2001:11, Table 1.)

low. Thus, the environment and characteristics of the individual conjointly determine disability.

In summary, the ICF provides a framework for examining the components of functioning that are impacted by a health condition. It is a tool that enables the collection of data as to how an individual with a health condition functions in his or her daily life, taking into consideration both environmental context and personal factors. It was developed and tested for cross-cultural applicability in over 40 countries, providing a common global framework for organizing and communicating information on human functioning (WHO, 2001).

Nagi Model

Saad Nagi, a sociologist, developed the Nagi model. This model contains four levels of dysfunction (Jette, 1989; Nagi, 1965). The first level, pathology, represents a description of the disease or injury process at the organ level. The second level, impairment, includes psychological, physiological, or anatomical problems related to structure or function, such as decreased strength or range of motion (ROM), or the presence of spastic hemiplegia. Impairments can be either the direct result of pathology, such as limited ROM in a joint associated with osteoarthritis, or indirectly associated with pathology, such as cardiopulmonary deconditioning secondary to inactivity (Jette, 1994). Functional limitations reflect an inability of the individual to perform a task or activity in the way it is usually done. Functional limitations describe a patient's problems with reference to specific tasks independent of their purpose—that is, standing, walking, climbing, or reaching. Functional limitations can contribute to disability, which reflects the impact of disease on the behavior or the person in desired roles and activities in society. Thus, Nagi considers functional limitations to be attributes of the individual, while disability is determined by looking at the individual in relationship to society. Disability (the inverse of participation in the ICF model, is expressed as a limited ability to carry out expected tasks and activities of daily living and social roles (such as wife, mother, and therapist). Disability in activities of daily living are often separated into limitations in basic and instrumental activities of daily living (ADL and IADL). ADLs include bathing, dressing, transferring from bed to chair, using the toilet, and eating (Keith et al., 1987). IADLs are complex tasks necessary for independent living in the community. IADLs include shopping, food preparation, housekeeping, doing laundry, using transportation, taking medications, handling finances, and using the telephone (Lawton, 1971). A modification to the Nagi model of disablement was proposed by the National Center for Medical Rehabilitation Research (NCMRR). The NCMRR's model of disablement adds a fifth concept, that of societal limitation, to the Nagi model. Societal limitations are restrictions that arise because of social policies and/or barriers that limit individuals' abilities to fulfill their expected roles (Jette, 1994). Often societal limitations reflect problems in access and attitude—that is, access within the environment and negative attitudes encountered within society.

Restricted participation (disability in the Nagi model) has both a personal and a societal impact, since it is inability to participate, not disease per se, that determines the need for support services, long-term care and institutionalization, and ultimately the quality of a person's life (Guralnik et al., 1989). Limited participation affects the quality of life of the individual, but the concomitant increases in health care utilization and need for long-term care makes this a societal issue as well.

Posture, Balance, and Gait: Functional Activity or Underlying Impairments?

It is often not clear where postural control, balance, and gait fit into the various levels described by models of functioning and disablement. Some clinicians classify them as functional activities, while others suggest that they are underlying "multisystem," or composite, impairments. Perhaps some of the confusion stems from the fact that models of disablement have taken a continuum of effects and broken them down into arbitrary levels, which may not have clear-cut boundaries. For example, functional limitations have been defined as limitations of tasks performed by the individual independent of the environment in which they are performed. However, as we have discussed in earlier chapters, the central nervous system (CNS) takes into consideration factors within the environment when it organizes functional behaviors. Thus, it is not possible to evaluate function independently of any environmental influence.

Posture, balance, and gait are controlled by multiple systems, and thus do not easily fit into the impairment category. However, it is difficult to define balance as a "functional task" in the same way that standing, walking, or reaching are considered functional tasks. Rather, posture and balance are part of the many systems that contribute to the performance of these functional tasks. We suggest that the essential issue is not at what level postural control is placed (e.g., body structure and function vs. activity), but rather that it be included in our understanding of the impact of disease on the individual.

Clinical Implications

Models of function and disability provide a conceptual framework for examining the effect of a health condition on the individual. They provide a common language for communicating information, and they improve our ability to be understood by both clinicians and nonclinicians. How do these models assist a clinician in formulating a clinical plan for intervention? Before continuing, complete Lab Activity 6.1.

Clinicians are involved in identifying and documenting the effects of a health condition on body structure and function (impairments), as well as activities and participation (functional limitations and restricted participation) (Campbell, 2006; Jette, 1994; Schenkman et al., 2006). During the examination, clinicians identify and document the sensory, motor, and cognitive impairments that potentially constrain functional abilities and limit participation. These impairments can be the direct result of the neurologic lesion (e.g., weakness) or the indirect effect of another impairment (such as the development of contractures in the weak and immobile patient). Examination also includes the identification and documentation of limitations in functional activities (tasks performed by the individual), for example, the ability to walk, transfer, reach for, and manipulate objects. The clinician also examines the effect of a health condition on the individual's ability to participate in the necessary activities and roles of his or her daily life (referred to as a disability level examination in the Nagi model). Finally, a comprehensive examination includes a description of the contextual factors (personal and environmental) that also influence functioning and disability in the individual.

The process of identifying functional problems and their underlying cause(s) is not always easy. Most

LAB ACTIVITY 6-1

Objective: To apply the ICF framework to a patient with neurologic pathology.

Procedure: Select one or more of the case studies presented at the beginning of this chapter. Use the ICF framework to describe the effect of pathology on this individual.

Assignment:

1. Define the health condition of the disease or injury.
2. Make a list of the probable impairments (limitations in body structure and function) associated with this disease.
3. How will limitations in body structure and function change as the patient moves from an acute to a chronic condition?
4. What functional activities are likely to be affected given the range of impairments? What may be spared?
5. What will this patient's level of participation be?
6. Will this person be restricted (disabled) in the roles and activities in which he or she is able to participate?
7. Consider how contextual factors impact this case. What are the personal factors that influence the effect of this health condition on function in this patient? What environmental factors are likely to influence the patient's functioning?

CNS pathology affects multiple systems, resulting in a diverse set of impairments. This means that functional problems in a patient with a neurologic deficit are often associated with many possible causes. How does a therapist establish a link between impairment and functional limitations? Which impairments are critical to loss of function? Which impairments should be treated, and in what order? What is the most efficacious approach to intervention? Hypothesis-driven clinical practice can assist the clinician in answering some of these questions (Rothstein & Echternach, 1986).

Hypothesis-Oriented Clinical Practice

What is a hypothesis, and how do we use it in the clinic? A **hypothesis** can be defined as a proposal to explain certain facts. In clinical practice, a hypothesis can be considered one possible explanation of the cause or causes of a patient's problem (Platt, 1964; Rothstein et al., 2003; Rothstein & Echternach, 1986). To a great extent, the hypotheses generated reflect the theories a clinician has about the cause and nature of function and dysfunction in patients with neurologic disease (Shepard, 1991). As noted in Chapter 1, there are many theories of motor control that present varying views on the nature and cause of movement. As a result, there can be many different hypotheses about the underlying cause(s) of motor control problems in patients with neurologic dysfunction.

Clarifying the cause(s) of functional movement problems requires the clinician to: (a) generate several alternative hypotheses about the potential cause(s); (b) determine the crucial test(s) and their expected outcomes that would rule out one or more of the hypotheses; (c) carry out the tests; and (d) continue the process of generating and testing hypotheses, refining one's understanding of the cause(s) of the problem (Platt, 1964). Hypothesis testing can be used to explain factors associated with functional limitations and restricted participation.

For example, Mrs. Jean J, who has a right hemiplegia secondary to a CVA, is referred for balance retraining because of recurrent falls. During the course of your evaluation, you observe that she is unable to stand safely while performing functional tasks, and has a tendency to fall primarily backward (a functional-level problem). Your knowledge of normal postural control suggests the importance of the ankle muscles during the recovery of stance balance. You generate three hypotheses regarding possible impairments that could explain why she is falling backward: (a) weak anterior tibialis muscle, (b) shortened gastrocnemius, and (c) a problem coordinating the anterior tibialis muscle within a postural response synergy. What clinical tests can be used to distinguish among these hypotheses? Strength testing indicates Mrs. J is able to voluntarily generate force, thus weakening support for the first hypothesis. ROM tests suggest normal passive range of motion at the ankle, weakening support for the second hypothesis. In response to the nudge test (a brief displacement in the backward direction), Mrs. J does not perform dorsiflexion of the foot of the hemiplegic leg. The inability to achieve dorsiflexion of the foot, even though the capacity to generate force voluntarily is present, suggests support for the third hypothesis.

If it were available, surface electromyography could be used to investigate further whether the anterior tibialis muscle is activated as part of a postural synergy responding to backward instability.

The generation and testing of hypotheses are an important part of clinical practice. However, there is a difference between hypothesis testing in a research laboratory versus in a clinic. In the laboratory, it is often possible to set up a carefully controlled experiment that will test the hypothesis. The outcome is a "clean result," that is, a result that accepts one hypothesis and rejects the alternative hypothesis. In contrast, in the clinic, we are often unable to get a clean result. Clinical tests are often not sufficiently sensitive and specific to differentiate clearly between two hypotheses. Rather, they indicate the likelihood for the origin of the problem. For example, in the case presented above, passive ROM tests may not be a valid way of predicting the active range of a muscle during dynamic activities. In addition, manual muscle testing may not be a valid way to predict the patient's ability to generate force in that muscle when performing a functional activity such as walking.

Despite the limitations of clinical tests in providing clean results, the generation, testing, and revision of alternative hypotheses is an important part of clinical care. Hypothesis generation assists the clinician in determining the relationship between functional limitations and underlying impairments. We treat the impairments that relate directly to functional limitations and are within the scope of treatments available to us (Rothstein et al., 2003; Rothstein & Echternach, 1989).

Theories of Motor Control and Learning

The fourth element that contributes to a comprehensive conceptual framework for clinical practice is our understanding of the neural basis for movement control and learning underlying the (re)acquisition of skill. As discussed in Chapters 1 and 2, theories of motor control and learning have led to the development of clinical practices that apply assumptions from these theories to improving the control of movement. Thus, the approach a clinician chooses when examining and treating a patient with movement disorders is based in part on both implicit and explicit assumptions associated with an underlying theory of motor control and motor learning (Gordon, 1987; Horak, 1991; Woollacott & Shumway-Cook, 1990). In this book we use the term *systems theory* of motor control as part of our framework for clinical practice. In this theory, movement results from the dynamic interplay between multiple systems that are organized around a behavioral goal and constrained by the environment. Clinical practices related to retraining patients with motor control problems are constantly changing, in part to reflect new views on the physiological basis of motor control and motor learning. As new models evolve, clinical practices are modified to reflect emerging concepts related to how the brain controls movement, factors affecting neural reorganization, plasticity, and motor learning underlying the (re)acquisition of skilled movement following injury. Thus, a conceptual framework for structuring clinical practice must be dynamic, changing in response to new scientific theories about motor control and learning.

Evidence-Based Clinical Practice

Evidence-based practice (EBP) is a philosophical approach to clinical practice that integrates the best available research, clinician expertise, and client characteristics (Jette et al., 2003; Sackett et al., 1996). As defined by Sackett et al. (1996, p. 71), evidence-based medicine is "the conscientious, explicit, and judicious use of current best evidence in making decisions about the care of individual patients. The practice of evidence-based medicine means integrating individual clinical expertise with the best available external clinical evidence from systematic research." Sackett et al. define *best available research,* as clinically relevant research from both basic and clinical sciences that increase the accuracy and precision of diagnostic tests, prognostic markers, and the efficacy and safety of therapeutic, rehabilitation, and preventive interventions. EBP reflects a shift from clinical practices based on the opinions of authorities to an emphasis on data-based, clinically relevant studies and research (Jette et al., 2003). In EBP, a comprehensive review of relevant research from *both* basic and clinical science contributes to the foundation of evidence for clinical practice.

Research can provide the underlying evidence critical to the clinical decision-making process. Basic research on the physiology and pathophysiology of motor control can provide the evidence base for clinical hypotheses about the underlying cause(s) of impairments, functional limitations, and restricted participation in a patient with a specific diagnosis. This research can also assist in the generation of hypotheses regarding the prognosis for the patient. Research on the psychometric properties of tests and measures, including validity, reliability, sensitivity, and responsiveness in different patient populations can provide the clinician guidance when choosing appropriate tests and measures to evaluate a patient with a specific diagnosis. Finally, research on the relative effects of different therapeutic interventions provides the evidence base for choosing an intervention and determining both the appropriate dose and expected response of an intervention in a specific patient. Thus, evidence-based medicine is the integration of relevant research, clinician expertise, and patient preference into the decision-making process and is critical in ensuring that clinical practice is consistent with the evolving research basis for the field.

Applying a Conceptual Framework to Clinical Practice

How do these elements work together to provide a comprehensive framework for clinical practice? Theories of motor control and learning provide a framework of assumptions regarding the nature and cause of normal and abnormal movements, as well as factors affecting motor learning and recovery of function. A model of practice identifies the steps to follow during the course of clinical intervention, including examination, identification of goals and outcomes, and establishment of a plan for intervention to achieve them. A model of health-related function and disability provides a systematic way to examine the diverse effects of a health condition on the individual. It provides a common way of thinking and communicating information regarding underlying components of health and function in patients with motor control problems. Hypothesis-oriented practice helps us to explore the association between a health condition and components of functioning, including impairments of body structure and function, and limitations and restrictions in domains of activities and participation. This allows us to develop an intervention program that takes into consideration both the resources and the constraints on health and functioning of the individual. Evidence-based clinical practice reinforces the importance of integrating the best research evidence from both basic and applied clinical sciences, with clinical expertise and the goals and values of each individual patient.

The remaining section of this chapter discusses how these concepts are integrated into a "task-oriented" approach to patient treatment. In later chapters, we will show the specific application of this approach to retraining posture, mobility, and upper-extremity function in the patient with neurologic dysfunction.

TASK-ORIENTED APPROACH TO EXAMINATION

A task-oriented approach to clinical practice uses a multifaceted approach to clinical management of motor control problems in patients with CNS pathology. A task-oriented approach, integrated with the ICF framework examines behavior at a number of different levels, including: (1) evaluation of functional activities and participation, (2) a description of the strategies used to accomplish functional skills, and (3) quantification of the underlying sensory, motor, and cognitive impairments (limitations in underlying body structure and function) that constrain performance of functional activities and restrict participation. In addition, a task-oriented approach recognizes the importance of contextual factors, including personal and environmental features that affect how an individual functions. Since there is no single test or measure that allows one to collect information on all these components, clinicians are required to assemble a battery of tests and measures, enabling them to document problems at all levels of analysis.

Examination of Functional Activities and Participation

Examination of activities and participation looks at the ability of the individual to perform essential tasks and activities in a standard (clinical) environment (referred to in the ICF as "measurement of capacity") and the person's actual environment (referred to in the ICF as "measurement of performance"). Evaluation of functional activities and participation can use either self-report (or proxy report) or observation of the individual performing the test, also referred to as "performance-based measures." Performance-based measures examine the patient's ability to perform functional tasks, while interview measures rely on the patient's (or a proxy's) report of his or her ability to perform functional activities and engage in all aspects of participation. Researchers have found a high correlation between self-report and performance-based measures, suggesting that self-report can be a valid way to examine functional activities and participation. Self-reported measures can be used when a patient is temporarily unable to perform certain activities (such as asking a patient who has had a recent hip fracture to report on his or her previous independence in ADLs).

Measuring Participation—Function in a Social and Physical Context

An important aspect of examination of patients with motor control problems is examining the effect of a health condition within the context of the person's life, referred to as participation in the ICF framework. Limitations in functional activities are defined by the individual's capacity to do specific tasks and activities in a standardized environment, while participation is defined with reference to behavior in a social and physical context (Nagi, 1991; WHO, 2001). Measuring participation and its inverse, disability, is often difficult because of a lack of both a clear operational definition and valid methods of measurement (Jette, 2003; Yorkston et al., 2008). In addition, the concept of participation includes complex tasks, often performed with others and strongly influenced by environmental factors (Jette, 2003; Yorkston et al., 2008).

Participation has both objective and subjective dimensions. Traditional measures of participation and disability often focus on the objective dimension, quantifying frequency of participation or level of independence in performing activities of daily living (either basic or instrumental). For example, the Late Life Function and Disability Instrument (Jette et al., 2002; Haley et al., 2002) is an example of a measure designed to quantify activities (functional limitations) and participation (disability) as distinct dimensions. An example of a measure of disability that could be used with children is the Pediatric Evaluation of Disability Inventory (Haley et al., 1992).

A second approach to measuring participation focuses on the subjective dimension in which individuals themselves report their opinions and feelings about their actual level of participation relative to their desired level of participation. For example, the Children's Assessment of Participation and Enjoyment (CAPE) and its companion measure, Preferences for Activities of Children (PAC) measures participation in children ages 6 to 21 years (King et al., 2004; Law et al., 2006). The CAPE is a 55-item measure of six dimensions of participation (diversity, intensity, where, with whom, enjoyment and preference), with three levels of scoring: (i) overall participation scores; (ii) domain scores reflecting participation in formal (i.e., organized or structured activities) and informal activities; and (iii) scores in five types of activities (recreational, active physical, social, skill-based and self-improvement). The CAPE has been shown to have good reliability (King et al., 2004; Law et al., 2006) and construct validity (King et al., 2006).

Several researchers have found a low association between objective and subjective measures of participation (Brown et al., 2004; Johnston et al., 2002, 2005; Yorkston et al., 2008; Robinson et al., 2010). Researchers have found that frequency of participation in functional activities has only a slight relationship with perceived satisfaction and significance of these activities, suggesting that significance and satisfaction cannot be inferred from objective measures of frequency of participation. Thus, objective measures of participation must be supplemented by subjective measures that reflect an insider perspective.

Clinical Measures of Function

When measuring the ability to perform functional activities, clinicians have a wide variety of measures from which to choose, with more measures emerging in the clinical literature. Tests and measures can be task-, age-, or diagnosis-specific.

Task-Specific Tests and Measures. Some tests limit their focus to specific tasks such as balance, mobility, or upper-extremity control. Examples of these types of tools include the Berg Balance Test (Berg, 1993), the Performance Oriented Mobility Assessment (Tinetti, 1986), and the Erhardt Test of Manipulatory Skills (Erhardt, 1982). These tests have been developed to provide clinicians with a clearer picture of the patient's functional skills related to a limited set of tasks the clinician will be directly involved in retraining. These task-specific tests will be covered in later chapters, which discuss retraining posture and balance, mobility, and upper-extremity functions.

Age-Specific Tests and Measures. Age-specific tests and measures have also been created. There are a number of tests available for examining pediatric patients, including the Gross Motor Function Measure (Russell et al., 1993), the Test of Infant Motor Performance (Campbell et al., 1995; Kolobe et al., 2004); the Peabody Developmental Motor Scales (Folio & Fewell, 1983), the Bayley Scales of Infant Development (Bayley, 1969), and the Pediatric Evaluation of Disability Index (Feldman et al., 1990). The Bruininks–Oseretsky test is often used for examining motor function in older school-aged children (Bruininks, 1978). At the other end of the age range are tests designed specifically for a geriatric population. Examples of these tests include the Performance Oriented Mobility Assessment (Tinetti, 1986), the Functional Reach Test (Duncan et al., 1990), and the Physical Performance and Mobility Examination (Lemsky et al., 1991). In addition, pediatric versions of many tests developed for adults are now available, for example, the Functional Reach (Bartlett & Birmingham, 2003; Gan et al., 2008), the Berg Balance Test (Gan et al., 2008; Kembhavi et al., 2002), the Clinical Test for Sensory Interaction in Balance (Gagnon et al., 2006; Richardson et al., 1992) and the Timed Up and Go (Gan et al., 2008; Williams et al., 2005).

Diagnosis-Specific Tests and Measures. A number of tools have been developed to examine functional limitations and underlying impairments in specific patient populations. The most prevalent of this type of tool relates to examining function following stroke. Examples of these include the Motor Assessment

Scale for Stroke Patients (Carr & Shepherd, 1983), the Fugl-Meyer test (Fugl-Meyer et al., 1975), the Motor Assessment in Hemiplegia (Brunnstrom, 1966), and the Stroke Rehabilitation Assessment of Movement (Stream) (Ahmed et al., 2003; Daley et al., 1999). Scales have been developed to evaluate the severity of symptoms associated with Parkinson's disease, including the Unified Parkinson's Disease Rating Scale (Hoehn & Yahr, 1967) and the Schwab Classification of Parkinson Progression (Schwab, 1960), and the Expanded Disability Status Scale for persons with Multiple Sclerosis (Kurtzke, 1983).

Choosing Appropriate Tests and Measures. As you can see, a large number of tests and measures are available from which to choose. How does a clinician decide what tool to use? A number of factors can be considered when choosing an instrument. Patient-related factors such as age and diagnosis should be considered. Level of function in your patient population must also be considered in order to avoid floor or ceiling affects. Floor effects result when a test is chosen that is too difficult for the patient population; thus, scores are all uniformly too low. Alternatively, a test that is too easy will result in scores that are all uniformly too high, thus creating a ceiling effect.

Test-related factors should also be considered when choosing a clinical test or measure. The purpose of the examination and the ability of a test to accomplish that purpose is an important factor to consider when choosing a test or measure. An examination can serve different purposes; it can be used to discriminate, evaluate, or predict (Campbell, 1991; Ketelaar et al., 1998). Discriminative measures are used to distinguish individuals who have a particular problem from those who do not. For example, the Up and Go Test (Podsiadlo & Richardson, 1991) determines the relative risk for functional dependence in older adults. Based on results from this test, an older adult could be classified as being in a low-risk or a high-risk group. Another example is the Berg Balance Test, which has been found useful in discriminating, elders who are prone to falling from those who are not (Muir et al., 2008; Shumway-Cook et al., 1997a, b).

An evaluative measure is used to measure change over time or after treatment. The Gross Motor Function Measure is a standardized observational instrument developed to measure change in gross motor function over time in children with cerebral palsy (Russell et al., 1993). A predictive measure classifies people based on future status. The Bleck scale predicts ambulation in 7-year-olds using postural and reflex activity evaluated at a preschool age (Bleck, 1975). Results from the Walk and Talk test are predictive of future falls in a population of institutionalized elders (Lundin-Olsson, 1997). Often therapists choose a test or measure based on personal preference rather than for theoretical reasons (Ketelaar et al., 1998). This can result in problems. For example, your intent as a therapist may be to measure change following your intervention. If you select a measure designed primarily to discriminate among people, you may find no significant difference in preintervention and postintervention scores, not because your patient has not responded to your treatment, but because you have chosen a test that may not be sensitive to change.

Psychometric properties such as reliability, validity, sensitivity, and specificity will vary from test to test. Reliability reflects the dependability or consistency of a test, that is, its ability to measure accurately and predictably without variation when no true change has occurred (Dobkin, 1996). Consistency is reflected through both intrarater and interrater reliability. Intrarater reliability indicates a high degree of correlation when performance is measured by the same therapist over repeated applications of the test; interrater reliability indicates a high degree of agreement among multiple raters. If more than one therapist is to examine a patient over time, interrater reliability is critical to accurate data collection (Guccione, 1991).

Validity of a test is a complex concept that reflects the degree to which an instrument measures what it purports to measure (Dobkin, 1996). There are many aspects to validity. **Content validity** is often determined by a panel of experts who determine whether the instrument measures all dimensions of a particular function. **Face validity** indicates the degree to which the instrument measures what it is supposed to measure. **Construct validity** indicates the degree to which the instrument behaves as hypothesized (Dobkin, 1996). **Concurrent validity** is the degree to which the instrument agrees with other instruments that are measuring the same factors. Finally, both sensitivity and specificity are important attributes of an instrument. **Sensitivity** is the degree to which a diagnostic test detects a disorder or dysfunction when it is present. In contrast, **specificity** reflects the ability of a test to rule out a disorder or dysfunction when it is not present.

Unfortunately, the reliability, validity, sensitivity, and specificity of many of the tests used in the clinic are not published. This makes it difficult to judge the quality of the instrument and raises questions regarding the value of the data collected with untested instruments.

Finally, *resource-related* factors may be considered when choosing a test. Consideration must be given to the skill and level of training of the therapists giving the test. Many standardized tests require that therapists be trained to give the test with an established level of proficiency. This requires time and resources that a facility may not be willing to provide. The amount of time available for examination as well as available space and equipment also need to be considered.

Limitations of Functional Tests and Measures. There are a number of limitations inherent in clinical measures of function. While functional measures will allow a therapist to document functional status (e.g., level of independence associated with performing specific functional tasks and activities), they do not provide information as to why the patient is dependent in performing functional skills. Thus, functional tests will not allow the therapist to test hypotheses about the cause of motor dysfunction.

Therapists retraining patients with movement disorders are concerned about not just the degree to which patients can carry out a task, but also about how they perform the task. Functional measures in general are limited to providing information on the former, but rarely the latter. Finally, clinical measures of function are limited to evaluating performance at one instant in time, under a fairly limited, and often relatively ideal, set of circumstances. Results from a functional-based examination do not always predict participation, that is, performance in the home or community environment. For example, because a patient can walk safely and independently with a cane in the clinic does not necessarily mean the patient can (or will) walk safely and independently in a cluttered, poorly lit home environment.

Despite these limitations, clinical measures of function enable the clinician to document a patient's functional status and are an important part of justifying therapy to the patient, the patient's family, and third-party insurers.

Examination at the Strategy Level

Examination at the strategy level is a qualitative approach to measuring function activities, since it examines the strategies used to perform functional tasks. The term *strategy* is not limited to the evaluation of the movement pattern used to accomplish a task, but includes how the person organizes sensory and perceptual information necessary to performing a task in various environments.

Why is it important for clinicians to examine the strategies a patient uses when performing a functional task? One answer is that the strategies used to perform a task largely determine the level of performance. According to Welford (1982), a psychologist from England, performance depends on four factors. The first relates to the demands of the task and the person's desire for particular standards of achievement. The second relates to the capacities, both mental and physical, that a person brings to the task. The third relates to the strategies that the person uses to meet the demands of the task, while the fourth relates to the ability to choose the most efficient strategy for a given task.

Note that two of the four factors relate to strategies, emphasizing their importance in determining our level of performance. Thus, the strategies we use relate the demands of the task to our capacity to perform it. If we choose poor strategies, and the task is difficult, we may reach the limits of our capacities well before we have met the demands of the task. In contrast, inefficient strategies may still be effective in carrying out simple, less demanding tasks. As the capacity to perform a task declines either because of age or disease, we may be unable to meet its demands unless we use alternative strategies to maintain performance levels.

For example, as a young adult you rise quickly out of a chair without the need to use your arms. You rely on the ability to generate momentum, using movements of your trunk then your legs to rise from the sitting position. As you age, strength may slowly decline without affecting your ability to use this strategy for getting up. But at some threshold, the loss of strength means that you are no longer able to get up using your once-effective momentum strategy. Instead, you begin to use your arms to get up, thereby maintaining the functional ability to rise from a chair, albeit with a new strategy. Thus, in an individual with a neurologic deficit, maintaining functional independence depends on the capacity of that individual to meet the demands of the task in a particular environment. When impairments limit the capacity to use well-learned strategies, the patient must learn new ways to accomplish functional tasks despite these limitations.

Limitations to a Strategy Examination of Function

Clinicians are hampered in their ability to examine sensory, motor, and cognitive strategies used to perform daily tasks because methods for examining these strategies are just being developed. Only limited information exists defining sensory, motor, and cognitive strategies in neurologically intact subjects. In addition, we know very little about how compensatory strategies develop as a result of neurologic impairments.

Researchers have begun to quantify movement strategies used in functional tasks such as gait, stance postural control, and other mobility skills such as moving from sitting to standing, from a supine to a prone position, and from a supine to a standing position. Clinical tools to examine movement strategies have grown out of these analyses. An example is the use of observational gait analysis to define the movement strategies used during ambulation.

Examining Impairments of Body Structure and Function

Finally, examination at the third level focuses on identifying the impairments that potentially constrain functional movement skills. This requires examination of impairments within individual sensory, motor, and cognitive systems contributing to movement control, as well as multisystem impairments of posture, balance, and gait. Examination of the motor system includes both the neuromuscular and musculoskeletal systems. Since perception is essential to action, examination of sensory and perceptual abilities in the control of movement is necessary. And since task-specific movement is performed within the context of intent and motivation, cognitive aspects of motor control, including mental status, attention, motivation, and emotional considerations must be examined.

In summary, a task-oriented approach to examination is directed at answering the following questions:

1. To what degree can the patient perform functional tasks?
2. How do functional limitations restrict the patient's ability to participate in appropriate social roles and activities of daily living (disablement)?
3. What strategies are used to perform functional tasks, and are those strategies adapted to changing task and environmental conditions?
4. What is the constellation of impairments that constrains how the patient performs the task, and can these impairments be changed through intervention?
5. Is the patient functioning at an optimal level given the current set of impairments, or can therapy improve either the strategies being used to accomplish functional tasks or the underlying impairments?

Once the examination is completed, the clinician can translate information gained through examination into a list of patient problems that reflect functional limitations and associated areas of disablement and underlying impairments constraining function. From this comprehensive list, the therapist and patient identify the most critical problems, which will become the focus for initial intervention strategies. Thus, a list of short- and long-term treatment goals is established and a specific treatment plan is formulated for each of the problems identified.

TASK-ORIENTED APPROACH TO INTERVENTION

A task-oriented approach to establishing a comprehensive plan of care includes intervention strategies designed to achieve the following goals derived from the examination:

1. Resolve, reduce, or prevent impairments in body structure and function;
2. Develop effective and efficient task-specific strategies for accomplishing functional task goals; and
3. Adapt functional goal-oriented strategies to changing task and environmental conditions in order to maximize participation and minimize disablement.

These goals are not approached sequentially, but rather, concurrently. Thus, a clinician may use intervention strategies designed to focus on one or more of the aforementioned goals within the same therapy session. For example, when retraining mobility in a patient who has had a stroke, the clinician may use therapeutic techniques to: (a) decrease the effect of spasticity and abnormal synergies on functional movement (impairments in body structure and function), (b) improve weight-bearing on the involved leg during the stance phase of gait, to produce a more symmetrical gait pattern (strategy-level intervention), (c) practice walking a distance of 100 ft on a level surface in the clinic (improved performance of a functional activity), and (d) practice walking from the clinic to the car, crossing uneven surfaces while engaged in a conversation (participation-oriented intervention).

Recovery versus Compensation

A question that frequently arises during the course of rehabilitating the patient with a CNS lesion regards how much emphasis should be placed on promoting recovery of normal strategies versus teaching compensatory strategies for performing a task. Recovery of normal strategies for function is defined as the returning capability of the individual to perform a task using mechanisms previously used. Compensatory strategies can be defined as atypical approaches to meeting the requirements of the task using alternative mechanisms not typically used, for example, standing with the weight shifted to the nonparetic leg

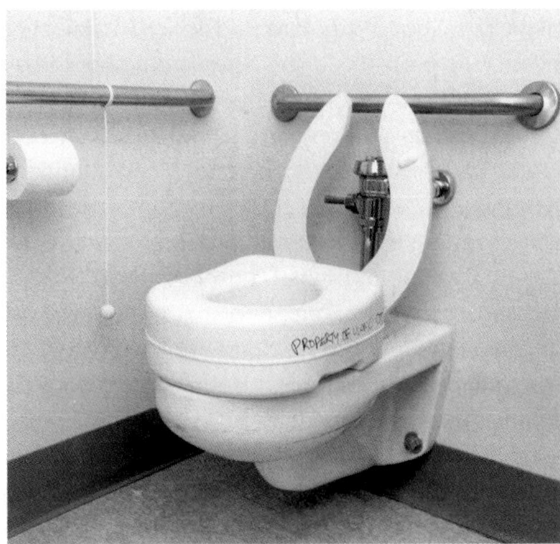

FIGURE 6.5 Changing the environment to accommodate functional limitations—bars around a toilet to facilitate transfers.

following a stroke. Compensatory strategies can also reflect modifications to the environment that simplify the demands of the task itself. For example, as shown in Figure 6.5, grab bars may be installed to assist a patient in transferring onto and off of the toilet.

When to facilitate normal strategies versus compensatory strategies is not easy to determine and will vary from patient to patient. Often, the criterion used to determine when compensatory strategies should be taught is time. That is, in the patient with an acute injury, emphasis is on recovery of normal function, while in the patient with a chronic condition, the emphasis shifts to maximizing function through compensatory strategies.

We have found it helpful in the decision-making process to consider the nature of the impairments themselves in determining whether normal versus compensatory strategies should be taught. Compensatory strategies will be needed in the case of permanent, unchanging impairments, regardless of whether the patient has an acute or a chronic condition. An example would be teaching a patient with a permanent loss of vestibular function to rely on alternative vision and somatosensory cues for maintaining balance during functional tasks, or teaching a patient with a complete spinal cord lesion to become independent in ADLs using compensatory strategies. Alternatively, if impairments are temporary and changeable (either through natural recovery or in response to therapy), the emphasis would be on remediating impairments and recovery of normal strategies for action.

A problem arises when it is not known whether impairments will resolve. For example, in the patient with an acute CVA whose affected extremities are flaccid, it is often not possible to predict whether the patient will remain flaccid or regain control over affected extremities. In this case, the clinician may revert to a time-based decision-making process, working toward recovery of normal strategies in the acute stage, and switching to a compensatory focus in the chronic stage.

SUMMARY

1. The conceptual framework for clinical practice presented in this chapter is built on five key elements: (a) a model of practice that establishes the steps for intervention; (b) hypothesis-oriented practice, which provides a process for testing assumptions regarding the nature and cause of motor control problems; (c) a model of functioning and disability that examines the constituents of health and the effects of disease on the individual; (d) theories of motor control and learning that suggests essential elements to examine and treat; and (e) evidence-based practice, which emphasizes the integration of research evidence, clinical expertise and patient characteristics in clinical practice.
2. The APTA model of practice is a five-step process including: (a) examination, (b) evaluation, (c) diagnosis, (d) prognosis, and (e) intervention.
3. A model of functioning and disability provides a system for examining the effects of a health condition on functioning in the individual. Functioning and its inverse, disablement, and can be used as a framework for organizing and interpreting examination data.
4. During the course of clinical intervention, the clinician will be required to generate multiple hypotheses, proposing possible explanations regarding the problem and its cause(s), and must investigate these hypotheses through observation, tests, and measurement.
5. A theory of motor control contributes assumptions regarding the nature and control of movement, movement disorders, and treatment, while theories of motor learning identify factors critical to the (re)acquisition of functional movement skills.
6. A task-oriented approach examines the effect of a health condition at many levels, including the ability and strategies used to perform functional tasks and activities, the extent to which limitations in performance of functional activities restricts participation in social

and environmental contexts, and the underlying impairments in body structure and function, including sensory, motor and cognitive impairments.

7. A task-oriented approach to intervention focuses on: (a) resolving or preventing impairments, (b) developing effective task-specific strategies, and (c) adapting functional goal-oriented tasks to changing environmental conditions, thus maximizing participation and minimizing disablement.

ANSWERS TO LAB ACTIVITY ASSIGNMENTS

Lab Activity 6-1

If you selected the case study on stroke, the following answers to this lab activity apply.

1. Health condition: Cerebrovascular accident
2. Limitations in body structure and function (impairments): could include problems in the neural control of force (paresis), abnormal muscle tone, decreased coordination, sensory loss, impaired balance and gait, problems with cognition including impaired memory, judgment, and attention.
3. Over time a patient with stroke may improve his or her ability to generate and control muscle forces (decrease in paresis); however, abnormal muscle tone may get worse (increased spasticity). Persisting inactivity and increased tone may result in the development of secondary musculoskeletal problems such as ankle-joint limitations or wrist and hand flexor tightness.
4. The patient may have difficulty with functional activities and tasks such as reaching, standing, walking, transfers, and bimanual activities.
5. During the initial phase of their recovery patients may be restricted in participating in most activities and roles important to them. With improvements in underlying structure and function, and recovery of functional abilities, participation will increase.

PART II

POSTURAL CONTROL

The ability to control our body's position in space is fundamental to everything we do.

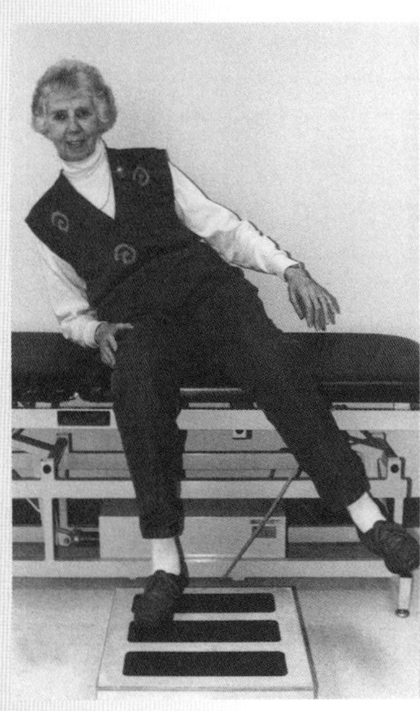

CHAPTER 7

NORMAL POSTURAL CONTROL

LEARNING OBJECTIVES

Following completion of this chapter, the reader will be able to:

1. Define postural control, distinguish between postural orientation and stability, and describe a dynamic definition of limits of stability.
2. Describe the action components of postural control, being able to define strategies and synergies and how they change according to task and environmental demands.
3. Describe perception systems in postural control, including the role of individual senses, current theories for sensory organization, and how sensory organization is adapted to changing task and environmental demands.
4. Define anticipatory postural control and describe the ways that it aids voluntary movement control.
5. Describe the attentional demands of postural control and the implications of this for maintaining stability in multitask situations.

INTRODUCTION

While few clinicians would argue the importance of posture and balance to independence in activities such as sitting, standing, and walking, there is no universal definition of posture and balance, or agreement on the neural mechanisms underlying the control of these functions.

Over the past several decades, research into posture and balance control and their disorders has shifted and broadened. The very definitions of posture and balance, as well as our understanding of the underlying neural mechanisms, has changed, and will continue to change, in response to emerging research in the field.

As noted in Chapter 1, postural control, like all aspects of motor control, emerges from an interaction of the individual with the task and the environment (Fig. 7.1). The ability to control our body's position in space emerges from a complex interaction of musculoskeletal and neural systems, collectively referred to as the "postural control system."

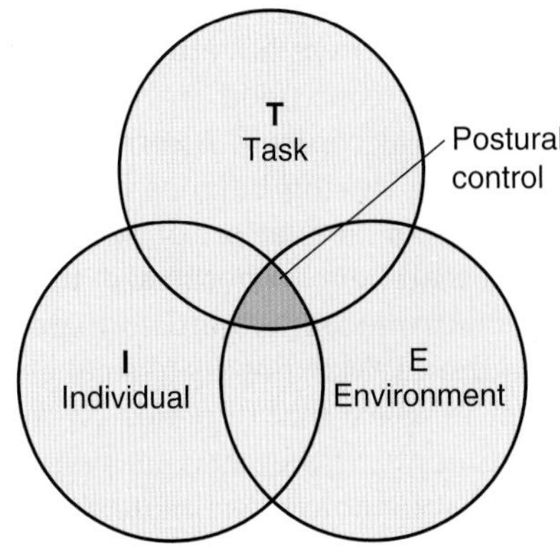

FIGURE 7.1 Postural actions emerge from an interaction of the individual, the task with its inherent postural demands, and the environmental constraints on postural actions.

Defining Postural Control

To understand postural control in the individual, we must understand the task of postural control and examine the effect of the environment on that task.

Postural control involves controlling the body's position in space for the dual purposes of stability and orientation. **Postural orientation** is defined as the ability to maintain an appropriate relationship between the body segments, and between the body and the environment for a task (Horak & Macpherson, 1996). The term *posture* is often used to describe both biomechanical alignment of the body and the orientation of the body to the environment. We use the term *postural orientation* to include both of these concepts. For most functional tasks, we maintain a vertical orientation of the body. In the process of establishing a vertical orientation, we use multiple sensory references, including gravity (the vestibular system), the interrelationship of different body segments, the relationship of our body to the support surface (somatosensory system), and the relationship of our body to objects in our environment (visual system).

Postural stability, also referred to as *balance,* is the ability to control the center of mass in relationship to the base of support. The **center of mass (COM)** is defined as a point that is at the center of the total body mass, which is determined by finding the weighted average of the COM of each body segment. It has been hypothesized that the COM is the key variable that is controlled by the postural control system. The vertical projection of the COM is defined as the **center of gravity (COG).** The **base of support (BOS)** is defined as the area of the body that is in contact with the support surface. While researchers often talk about stability as controlling the COM relative to the BOS, they often mean controlling the vertical projection of the COM, the COG, relative to the BOS. In this book we often use COM and COG interchangeably.

What evidence do we have that the COM is the key variable being controlled by the nervous system during postural control? Alternatively, the key variable controlled during balance could be control of joint positions or activation of specific muscles. While most researchers hypothesize that it is the COM that is controlled, it is hard to experimentally verify this, as the COM is not a physical entity but is a virtual point in space that depends on the position of all body segments. If the nervous system controls the COM, it must be able to estimate the position of the COM using information from the various sensory receptors (Scholz et al., 2007). In order to determine whether the COM was the primary variable controlled by the nervous system during postural control, Scholz and colleagues (2007) used a new analysis tool, the Uncontrolled Manifold (UCM) approach. The UCM approach to studying movement control is discussed in more detail in the Technology Tool 7.1. Using this approach, these researchers showed that when recovering from a loss of balance, subjects tend to reestablish the preperturbation COM position rather than the preperturbation joint configuration. This finding supports the hypothesis that the key variable controlled by the central nervous system (CNS) during postural control is the COM (Scholz et al., 2007).

What is the center of pressure (COP), and what is its role in stability? As will be discussed in more detail in later sections of this chapter, to ensure stability, the nervous system generates forces to control motion of the COM. The COP is the center of the distribution of the total force applied to the supporting surface. The COP moves continuously around the COM to keep the COM within the support base (Benda et al., 1994; Winter, 1990).

Several researchers have suggested that characterizing the relationship between the COM and the COP provides better insight into stability than either COP or COM alone (Corriveau et al., 2000, 2001; Winter, 1995). Stability is represented as the scalar distance between the COP and the COM at any given point in time. During quiet standing, the difference between the COP and the COM is proportional to the horizontal acceleration of the COM. The distance between the COP and the COM is proposed as the "error" signal that is detected and used to drive the postural control system during balance control. Thus, researchers have used the COP–COM interaction as an estimate of the efficacy of postural control.

Postural Control Requirements Vary with the Task and Environment

The ability to control our body's position in space is fundamental to everything we do. All tasks require postural control. That is, every task has an orientation component and a stability component. However, the stability and orientation requirements will vary with the task and the environment. Some tasks place importance on maintaining an appropriate orientation at the expense of stability. The successful blocking of a goal in soccer or catching a fly ball in baseball requires that the player always remain oriented with respect to the ball, sometimes falling to the ground in an effort to block a goal or to catch a ball. Thus, while postural control is a requirement that most tasks have in common, stability and orientation demands change with each task (Horak & Macpherson, 1996; Shumway-Cook & McCollum, 1990).

TECHNOLOGY TOOL 7-1 Uncontrolled Manifold Analysis of Movement Control

The Uncontrolled Manifold Analysis is a new approach to studying movement based on the early work of Georg Schöner (1995), with further developments by Scholz and Schöner (1999). It is based on a new approach to analyzing trial-to-trial variability on outputs of the nervous system. Thus, the UCM analysis can be applied to kinematic, force, EMG, COM, or any other type of data that contain variability. In this approach, variability is seen not as a sign of imperfection or noise in the output of the nervous system, but as an important component contributing to high level motor function. Schöner and Scholz developed a technical procedure, the method of the "uncontrolled manifold" (UCM), for testing whether aspects of trial-to-trial variability of individual components, called "elemental variables" (such as muscle activation levels, joint motion, or force output of individual joints contributing to performance), could actually stabilize or optimize particular higher-level performance variables (such as COM or total force output) (Latash et al., 2005).

For example, if you were to try to produce force using a single finger, variability in your force output (i.e., the standard deviation of the output) would increase nearly linearly with your total force output level. However, if you used two fingers, pressing down together to produce a certain level of total force, total force variability would be low at all levels of force production (Latash et al., 2002). This is because the force outputs of your individual fingers are not independent, but rather covary to keep the total force variability at low levels, even when there is an increase in total force output. These researchers have shown that individual variability has two components; one works to reduce overall variability and thus improves performance, while the other leads to a reduced ability to accomplish the task goal. Figure 7.2 (adapted from Latash et al., 2005) illustrates these two aspects of variability. In this figure, the task is to maintain a constant level of force output (either 5, 10, or 20 N). The dots represent the data from individual trials. The red dot illustrates that in this trial the participant accomplished the goal of maintaining a 20-N output by generating 12.5 N with the finger labeled F1 and 7.5 N with the finger labeled F2. The rest of the dots illustrate the forces used in each finger to achieve the task goal. As you can see, when the force output in one finger decreases, it is compensated for by an increase in the force output of the other finger. This

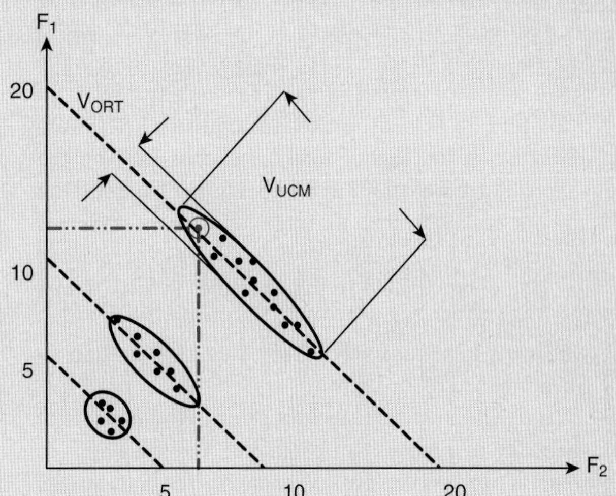

FIGURE 7.2 Hypothetical distribution of data points across many trials when an individual is asked to produce a certain level of total force by pressing on force sensors with two fingers. The three dashed lines correspond to the total forces of 5 N, 10 N, and 20 N. The red dot illustrates that in this trial the participant accomplished the goal of maintaining a 20 N output by generating 12.5 N with the finger labeled F1 and 7.5 N with the finger labeled F2. There are two aspects of variability: one aspect works to reduce overall variability and thus improves performance (V_{UCM}), while the other aspect leads to a reduced ability to accomplish the task goal (V_{ORT}). (Adapted from Latash ML, Krishnamoorthy V, Scholz JP, Zatsiorsky VM. Postural synergies and their development. Neural Plasticity 2005;12:122.)

force relationship between the two fingers can also be seen in the 5- and 10-N tasks, shown by the additional ellipses of data points. One component of variability is represented by the length of the data ellipse; you can see that this aspect of variability is aligned with the dotted lines. This component of variability (labeled as V_{UCM}) helps maintain low variability in the total force output, enabling the person to accomplish the task goal of maintaining a constant 20-N force output.

The other component of variability is orthogonal or perpendicular to the dotted line (labeled V_{ORT}), and actually leads to a reduced ability to accomplish the task goal of maintaining a constant force output. This is because the force output of one finger is not compensating for change in the force output of the other. Thus, if both fingers reduce their force at the same time, it would not allow the total force to stay constant, and total force would drop.

Thus, the first type of variability keeps the total force at the desired level, as required by the task, while the second leads to fluctuations in the total force, and a reduced ability to accomplish the task goal. Note in the figure that an increase in the total force output from 5 to 10 to 20 N leads to changes primarily in the variability along the axis of total force, thus keeping the variability of the total force virtually unchanged. The authors conclude that the nervous system organizes covariation of the individual finger forces (considered the elemental variable in this example) in such a way that their variability is primarily restricted to subspace within the total variability, which they call the "uncontrolled manifold," or UCM.

The UCM analysis uses four steps in the analysis of variability of a movement parameter. The first step is to select a task and a level of analysis. In our example, the task was to maintain a constant force output with two fingers. The level of analysis was the force output, including the force of each finger as well as the total force output. The second step is to select the elemental variable for this task; in our example, the elemental variable was the force output of the individual fingers. The third step is to generate a hypothesis about how covariation of the elemental variables will work to stabilize an important performance variable. In our example, the important performance variable is the task goal of maintaining a total force output as required by the task (e.g., 5,10, or 20 N). The researchers expected that the elemental variables (individual force output of each finger would covary in such a way as to ensure a stable force output that met the demands of the task). The fourth step is to create a matrix (this is called a "Jacobian matrix") that is used to show the effects of change in the elemental variables on the performance variable. In the fifth step, the null space of this matrix has to be computed. The null space is considered the UCM of this task, and represents space where the two elemental variables are compensating for one another. In the last step, an index of variability, representing both the V_{UCM} and the V_{ORT} variability is calculated. This allows researchers to quantify the relationship between these two types of variability. Thus, a strength of the UCM approach is that it allows testing different control hypotheses based on the same data set and produces indexes of variability of different performance variables. You can compute an index of the two components of variability. If the variability within the UCM is great with respect to the variability orthogonal to it (the variability that does not improve overall performance) then you can conclude that the performance variable is definitely stabilized by the elements contributing to its overall output (Latash et al., 2005).

The UCM analysis has been applied to a variety of tasks, including postural control. The UCM in postural control research has been used to help determine the variable that is primarily regulated by the nervous system in the control of balance (e.g., the COM). In addition, it has been used to examine different characteristics of muscle synergies used in the control of balance.

The task of sitting on a bench and reading has a postural orientation requirement of keeping the head and gaze stable and fixed on the reading material (Fig. 7.3A). The arms and hands maintain an appropriate task-specific orientation that allows the book to be held in the appropriate position in relationship to the head and eyes. The stability requirements of this task are lenient. Since the contact of the body with the bench back and seat provides a fairly large base of support, the primary postural control requirement is controlling the unsupported mass of the head with respect to the mass of the trunk.

In contrast, the task of standing and reading a book has roughly the same postural orientation requirement with respect to the head, eyes, arms, and book, but the stability requirement is considerably more stringent (Fig. 7.3B), as it involves controlling the COM (more accurately, the COG, which is the vertical projection of the COM) relative to a much smaller base of support defined by the two feet.

The stability demands in this task, standing and reading a book, become even more difficult if the person is standing on a moving bus, since the COM has to be controlled relative to a base of support that is moving in often unpredictable ways. In this case, the task demands vary from moment to moment, requiring constant adaptation of the postural system.

Postural control ensuring orientation and stability is also an essential part of mobility tasks in which the body is in motion, such as when walking (Fig. 7.3C). The task of controlling stability during walking is very different from the task of balance during stance (Winter et al., 1991). In walking, the COM (COG) does not stay within the support base of the feet, and thus the body is in a continuous state of imbalance. To prevent a fall, the swinging foot is placed ahead of and lateral to the

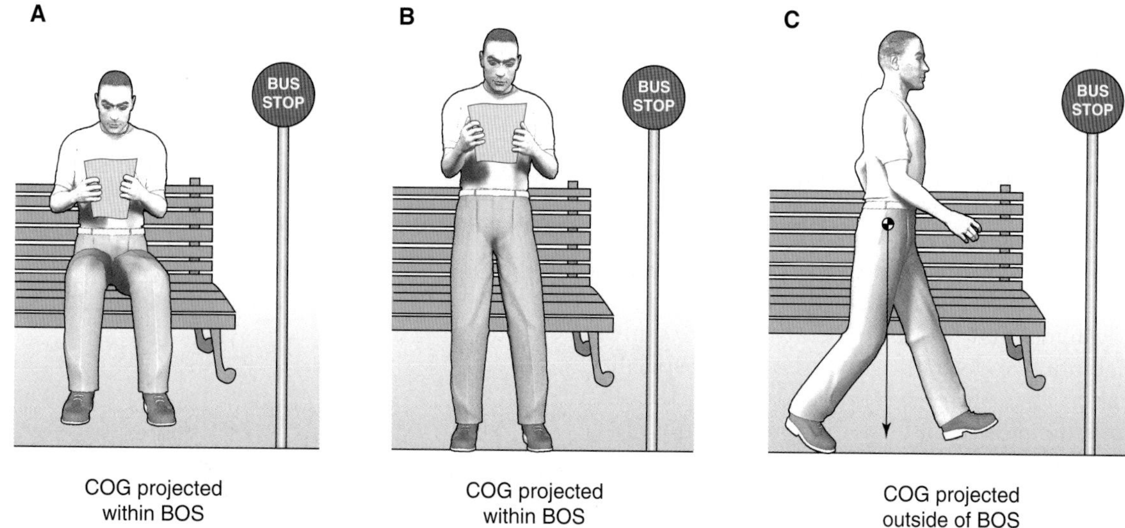

FIGURE 7.3 Stability requirements vary with the task. Stability when sitting and standing requires that the center of gravity (COG) be maintained within the base of support (BOS). A, Stability demands are low when sitting fully supported, since the BOS (the bench) is large. B, Stability demands increase in standing, since the COG must be maintained within a smaller BOS, defined by the feet. C, When walking, the COG often falls outside the BOS and is recaptured by placement of the swinging limb.

center of gravity as it moves forward, thus ensuring control of the COM relative to a moving BOS.

Thus, you can see that while these tasks demand postural control, the specific orientation and stability requirements vary according to the task and the environment. Because of this, the perception/action strategies used to accomplish postural control must adapt to varying task and environmental demands.

In this section of the book we will focus on research related to controlling postural orientation and stability while sitting or standing, and consider the applications of this research to the clinical treatment of patients with impaired postural control limiting the performance of activities in these positions. In the next section we will consider research related to the control of mobility, examining the control of stability and orientation within the context of tasks involving movement of the body.

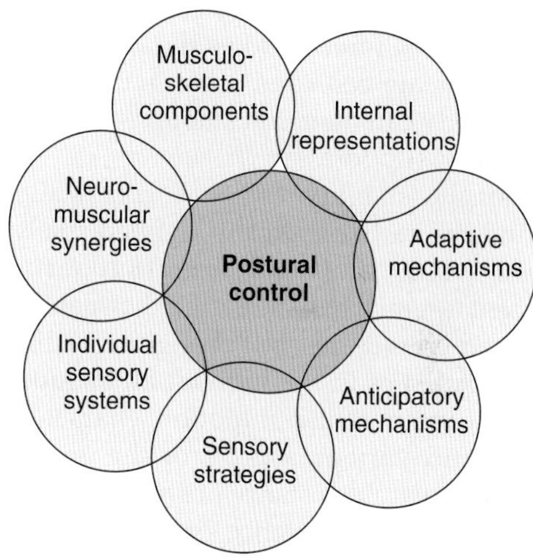

FIGURE 7.4 Conceptual model representing the many components of postural control that have been studied by researchers. Postural control is not regulated by a single system, but emerges from the interaction of many systems.

Defining Systems for Postural Control

Postural control for stability and orientation requires a complex interaction of musculoskeletal and neural systems, as shown in Figure 7.4. Musculoskeletal components include such things as joint range of motion, spinal flexibility, muscle properties, and biomechanical relationships among linked body segments.

Neural components essential to postural control include: (a) motor processes, which include organizing muscles throughout the body into neuromuscular synergies; (b) sensory/perceptual processes, involving the organization and integration of visual, vestibular, and somatosensory systems; and (c) higher-level processes essential for mapping sensation to action, and ensuring anticipatory and adaptive aspects of postural control.

In this book we refer to higher-level neural processes as cognitive influences on postural control. It is very important to understand, however, that the term *cognitive* as it is used here does not necessarily mean conscious control. Higher-level cognitive aspects of postural control are the basis for adaptive and anticipatory aspects of postural control. **Adaptive**

postural control involves modifying sensory and motor systems in response to changing task and environmental demands. Anticipatory aspects of postural control pretune sensory and motor systems for postural demands based on previous experience and learning. Other aspects of cognition that affect postural control include processes such as attention, motivation, and intent.

Thus, in a systems approach, postural control results from a complex interaction among many bodily systems that work cooperatively to control both orientation and stability of the body. The specific organization of postural systems is determined both by the functional task and the environment in which it is being performed.

STANCE POSTURAL CONTROL

How do the perception/action systems work together to control a stable standing position? As described earlier, when examined in relation to the control of quiet stance, *postural stability,* or *balance,* is defined as the ability to maintain the projected COM within the limits of the BOS, referred to as the "stability limits." Stability limits are considered the boundaries within which the body can maintain stability without changing the base of support.

Previously, stability limits during stance were conceptualized rather statically, defined solely by the physical characteristics of the base of support, the feet. More recent research has suggested that stability limits are not fixed boundaries, but change according to the task, characteristics in the individual, including such things as strength, range of motion, characteristics of the COM, and various aspects of the environment. While early research on stance postural control tended to emphasize the importance of the position of the COM relative to stability limits, more recent research has suggested that any understanding of stability must consider both the position and the velocity of the COM at any given moment (Pai et al., 2000). It is the interaction between these two variables, rather than just the position of the COM alone, that determines whether a person will be able to remain stable within his or her current base of support or be required to take a step or reach for support in order to regain stability.

Figure 7.5 illustrates this point. In this figure, three possible trajectories of the COM (combining velocity and displacement) in response to an external perturbation in standing are plotted. The shaded area indicates the region of the COM state space where stepping is predicted to be necessary. The initial position of the COM is indicated by the arrow and is about midfoot prior to the perturbation. In trajectory 1, the combined change of COM position and velocity remain small enough so that stability is recovered without a change in the base of support. In contrast, in trajectory 2, displacement and velocity are sufficient to move the COM beyond the stability boundary, necessitating a step to recover stability. Trajectory 3 also requires a step, not because the amplitude of displacement of the COM is great, but because the velocity is high, resulting in the need for a step to recover stability. For both trajectories 2 and 3, the final position of the COM is in front of the toe, indicating that a step has occurred (Pai et al., 2000).

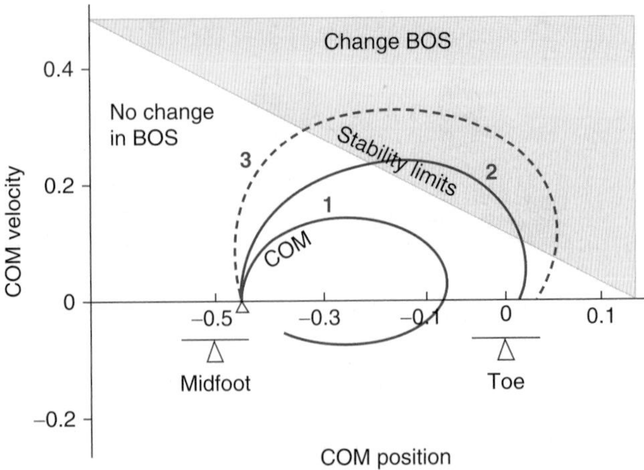

FIGURE 7.5 Interaction between COM motion (characterized by velocity on the *y*-axis and displacement on the x-axis) and type of response used to recover stability following an external perturbation. The shaded area indicates the region of the COM state space, where stepping is predicted to be necessary. Three possible trajectories of the COM in response to a perturbation are shown. In trajectory 1, the combined change of COM position and velocity remain small enough so the COM does not cross the stability boundary; thus, stability is recovered without a step. In contrast, in trajectory 2, COM displacement and velocity are sufficient to move the COM beyond the stability boundary, necessitating a step to recover stability. The step is reflected by a trajectory that stabilized at a point beyond the toe of the original base of support. Trajectory 3 also requires a step, but this is because the initial COM velocity is high, though the displacement was initially small. The model illustrates the importance of COM velocity, not just position, in determining strategies for recovery of stability. (Adapted with permission from Pai YC, Maki BE, Iqbal K, et al., Thresholds for step initiation induced by support surface translation: a dynamic center of mass model provides much better prediction than a static model. J Biomech 2000;33:390, Figure 3.)

Thus, many factors have an impact on how the COM is controlled relative to the stability limits of the body in stance, including both the velocity and the position of the COM. In addition, stability limits (the point at which a person will change the configuration of is or her base of support to achieve stability) are affected by many other factors, such as fear of falling and perception of safety (Pai et al., 2000).

Over the past decade, strategies underlying stance postural control have been widely studied. What do we mean by strategies for postural control? A strategy is a plan for action, an approach to organizing individual elements within a system into a collective structure. Some examples of strategies contributing to postural control include postural action strategies, which refers to the organization of movements appropriate for controlling the body's position in space. Sensory strategies are used to describe how sensory information from visual, somatosensory, and vestibular systems are organized for postural control. Sensorimotor strategies reflect the rules for coordinating sensory and motor aspects of postural control (Nashner, 1989). Researchers have begun to define attentional strategies for postural control. Attentional strategies determine the degree of attention given to a postural task when performing other tasks simultaneously (e.g., walking while talking to a friend) (see Woollacott & Shumway-Cook, 2002; and Fraizer & Mitra, 2008, for reviews of this area). We will begin by examining the action system's contribution to postural control, both when we are standing quietly and in response to perturbations to the COM.

Action Systems in Postural Control

Action systems underlying the control of posture include systems involved in higher-level planning (frontal cortex and motor cortex), coordination (brainstem and spinal networks coordinating muscle response synergies), and generation (motor neurons and muscles) of forces that produce movements effective in controlling the body's position in space.

Motor Control of Quiet Stance

What are the behavioral characteristics of quiet stance, and what is it that allows us to remain upright and stable when standing? Stability underlying sitting and/or standing quietly has often been called "static balance," because the base of support is not changing. However, this term is misleading, as postural control, even when sitting or standing quietly is quite dynamic.

Quiet stance is characterized by small amounts of spontaneous postural sway. A number of factors contribute to our stability in this situation. First, body alignment can minimize the effect of gravitational forces, which tend to pull us off center. Second, muscle tone keeps the body from collapsing in response to the pull of gravity. Three main factors contribute to our background muscle tone during quiet stance: (a) the intrinsic stiffness of the muscles themselves, (b) the background muscle tone, which exists normally in all muscles because of neural contributions, and (c) postural tone, the activation of antigravity muscles during quiet stance. In the following section we will look at these factors (Basmajian & Deluca, 1985; Kendall & McCreary, 1983; Roberts, 1979; Schenkman & Butler, 1992).

Alignment. In a perfectly aligned posture, shown in Figure 7.6, A and B, the vertical line of gravity falls in the midline between: (a) the mastoid process, (b) a point just in front of the shoulder joints, (c) the hip joints (or just behind), (d) a point just in front of the center of the knee joints, and (e) a point just in front of the ankle joints (Basmajian & Deluca, 1985). The ideal alignment in stance allows the body to be

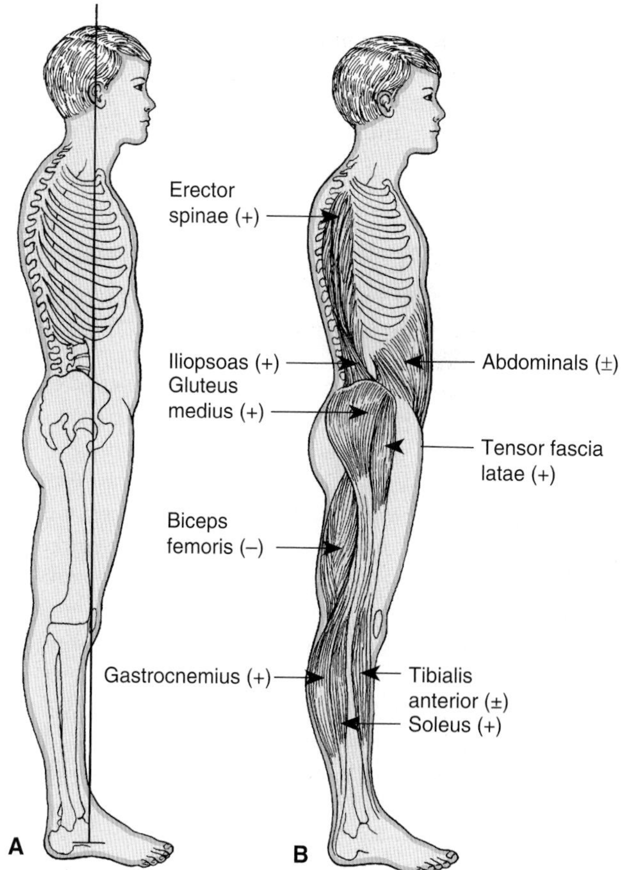

FIGURE 7.6 A, The ideal alignment in stance, requiring minimal muscular effort to sustain the vertical position. B, The muscles that are tonically active during the control of quiet stance. (Adapted with permission from Kendall FP, McCreary EK. Muscles: testing and function, 3rd ed. Baltimore: Williams & Wilkins, 1983:280.)

maintained in equilibrium with the least expenditure of internal energy.

Before we continue reviewing the research concerning postural control, be sure to review the information contained in the Technology boxes (pp. 163–169), which include a discussion of techniques for movement analysis at different levels of control, including electromyography (Technology Tool 7.2), kinematics (Technology Tool 7.3), and kinetics (Technology Tool 7.4).

Muscle Tone. What is muscle tone, and how does it help us to keep our balance? **Muscle tone** refers to the force with which a muscle resists being lengthened, that is, its stiffness (Basmajian & Deluca, 1985). Muscle tone is often tested clinically by passively extending and flexing a relaxed patient's limbs and feeling the resistance offered by the muscles. Both nonneural and neural mechanisms contribute to muscle tone or stiffness.

A certain level of muscle tone is present in a normal, conscious, and relaxed person. However, in the relaxed state no electrical activity is recorded in normal human skeletal muscle using electromyography (EMG). This has led researchers to argue that nonneural contributions to muscle tone are the result of small amounts of free calcium in the muscle fiber, which cause a low level of continuous recycling of cross-bridges (Hoyle, 1983).

There are also neural contributions to muscle tone or stiffness, associated with the activation of the stretch reflex, which resists lengthening of the muscle. The role of the stretch reflex as a contributor to normal muscle tone is fairly clear. The role of stretch reflexes in maintaining an upright stance position, however, is not. According to one theory, stretch reflexes play a feedback role during the maintenance of stance posture. Thus, this theory suggests that as we sway back and forth at the ankle while standing, the ankle muscles are stretched, activating the stretch reflex. This results in a reflex shortening of the muscle, and subsequent control of forward and backward sway. Researchers have shown that the gain of the spinal stretch reflex in the ankle muscles is quite low during stance, leading to doubts about the relevance of these stretch reflexes in the control of stance (Gurfinkel et al., 1974).

Postural Tone. When we stand upright, activity increases in antigravity postural muscles to counteract the force of gravity; this is referred to as **postural tone.** Sensory inputs from multiple systems are

TECHNOLOGY TOOL 7-2 Electromyography

Electromyography is a technique used for measuring the activity of muscles through electrodes placed on the surface of the skin, over the muscle to be recorded, or in the muscle itself. The output signal from the electrode (the electromyogram, or EMG) describes the output to the muscular system from the motor neuron pool. It provides the clinician with information about: (a) the identity of the muscles that are active during a movement, (b) the timing and relative intensity of muscle contraction, and (c) whether antagonistic or synergistic muscle activity is occurring. Surface electrodes are most often used; however, the ability of these electrodes to differentiate between the activity of neighboring muscles is not very effective.

The amplitude of the EMG signal is often interpreted as a rough measure of tension generated in the muscle. However, caution must be used when interpreting EMG amplitude measurements. There are many variables that can affect the amplitude of EMG signals, including how rapidly the muscle is changing length, resistance associated with cutaneous tissue and subcutaneous fat, and location of the electrode. Thus, generally, it is not accurate to compare absolute amplitudes of EMG activity of a muscle across subjects, or within the same subject across different days. Researchers who use EMG amplitude data to compare temporal and spatial patterns of muscle activity across subjects or within a subject on different days generally convert absolute amplitude measures to relative measures. For example, one can determine the ratio between the response amplitude (the area under the curve of EMG activity for a specified time period, called "integrated EMG," or IEMG) and the amplitude of a maximum voluntary contraction of that muscle. Alternatively, the ratio of IEMG for agonist and antagonist muscles at a joint can be determined. Likewise, the ratio of IEMG for synergistic muscles can be found. One can then examine how this ratio changes as a function of changing task or environmental conditions (Gronley & Perry, 1984; Winter, 1990).

TECHNOLOGY TOOL 7-3 Kinematic Analysis

Kinematic analysis is the description of the characteristics of an object's movement, including linear and angular displacements, velocities, and accelerations. Displacement data are usually gathered from the measurement of the position of markers placed over anatomic landmarks and reported relative to either an anatomic coordinate system (i.e., relative joint angle) or to an external spatial reference system. There are various ways to measure the kinematics of body movement. Goniometers, or electrical potentiometers, can be attached to a joint to measure a joint angle (a change in joint angle produces a proportional change in voltage). Accelerometers are usually force transducers that measure the reaction forces associated with acceleration of a body segment. The mass of the body is accelerated against a force transducer, producing a signal voltage proportional to the acceleration. Finally, imaging measurement techniques, including cinematography, videography, or optoelectronic systems, can be used to measure body movement. Optoelectronic systems require the subject to wear special infrared lights or reflective markers on each anatomic landmark; these lights are recorded by one or more cameras. The location of the light, or marker, is expressed in terms of *x*- and *y*-coordinates in a two-dimensional system, or *x*-, *y*-, and *z*-coordinates in a three-dimensional system. Output from these systems is expressed as changes in segment displacements, joint angles, velocities, or accelerations, and the data can be used to reconstruct the body's movement in space (Gronley & Perry, 1984; Winter, 1990).

TECHNOLOGY TOOL 7-4 Kinetic Analysis

Kinetic analysis refers to the analysis of the forces that cause movement, including both internal and external forces. Internal forces come from muscle activity, ligaments, or friction in the muscles and joints; external forces come from the ground or external loads. Kinetic analysis gives us insight into the forces contributing to movement. Force-measuring devices or force transducers are used to measure force, with output signals that are proportional to the applied force. Force plates measure ground-reaction forces, which are the forces under the area of the foot, from which center of pressure data are calculated. The term *center of gravity* (COG) of the body is not the same as the *center of pressure* (COP). The COG of the body is the net location of the center of mass in the vertical direction. COP is the location of the vertical ground reaction force on the force plate and is equal and opposite to all the downward-acting forces (Gronley & Perry, 1984; Winter, 1990).

critical to postural tone. Lesions of the dorsal (sensory) roots of the spinal cord reduce postural tone, indicating the importance of somatosensory inputs to postural tone. Activation of cutaneous inputs on the soles of the feet causes a placing reaction, which results in an automatic extension of the foot toward the support surface, thus increasing postural tone in extensor muscles. Somatosensory inputs from the neck activated by changes in head orientation can also influence the distribution of postural tone in the trunk and limbs. These have been referred to as the "tonic neck reflexes" (Ghez, 1991; Roberts, 1979). Inputs from the visual and vestibular systems also influence postural tone. Vestibular inputs, activated by a change in head orientation, alter the distribution of postural tone in the neck and limbs and have been referred to as the "vestibulocollic" and "vestibulospinal" reflexes (Massion & Woollacott, 2004).

In the clinical literature, much emphasis has been placed on the concept of postural tone as a major mechanism in supporting the body against gravity. In particular, many clinicians have suggested that postural tone in the trunk segment is the key element for control of normal postural stability in the erect position (Davies, 1985; Schenkman & Butler, 1989). How consistent is this assumption with EMG studies that have examined the muscles active in quiet stance?

Researchers have found that many muscles in the body are tonically active during quiet stance (Basmajian & Deluca, 1985). Some of these muscles are shown in Figure 7.6B, and include: (a) the soleus and gastrocnemius, because the line of gravity falls slightly in front of the knee and ankle; (b) the tibialis anterior, when the body sways in the backward direction; (c) the gluteus medius and tensor fasciae latae but not the gluteus maximus; (d) the iliopsoas, which prevents hyperextension of the hips, but not the hamstrings and quadriceps; and (e) the thoracic erector spinae in the trunk (along with intermittent activation of the abdominals), because the line of gravity falls in front of the spinal column. Research has suggested that appropriate activation of abdominal and other trunk muscles often discussed in relation to "core stability" is important for efficient postural control, including postural compensation for respiration-induced movement of the body (Hodges et al., 2002; Mok et al., 2004).

These studies suggest that muscles throughout the body are tonically active to maintain the body in a narrowly confined vertical position during quiet stance. Though the term *"static" postural control* may traditionally be used to describe postural control during quiet stance, you can see that control is actually dynamic. In fact, research suggests that postural control involves active sensory processing, with a constant mapping of perception to action, so that the postural system is able to calculate where the body is in space and can predict where it is going and what actions will be necessary to control this movement.

Movement Strategies during Quiet Stance

As you can see "quiet" stance is not quiet from the perspective of the neural control processes, since many mechanisms are active when we are standing up. Because quiet stance is characterized by body sway, passive skeletal alignment, in conjunction with muscle and postural tone are not enough; rather movement strategies are needed to maintain stability even when standing quietly. Traditionally, researchers studying stance postural control in humans have modeled the body as a single segment, with sway occurring around the ankles, approximating an inverted pendulum (including the legs, trunk and head). In this model, sway is controlled mainly by movement about the ankle joint. More recently, research has shown that control is more complex than this and that during quiet stance the body behaves more like a multilink pendulum (legs and trunk) with two coexisting modes of control (Creath et al., 2005). These modes of control could be described as an ankle strategy (in which both leg and trunk segments move in phase) when sway frequencies are low (<1 Hz) or a hip strategy (in which the leg and trunk segments move out of phase) when sway frequencies are higher (>1 Hz). Depending on conditions, the CNS can move back and forth between these control modes. Both are always present, but one may predominate depending on sensory information and task conditions. As you will see below, these two control strategies (ankle and hip modes of control) have also been described for recovery of perturbed stance. This suggests that quiet stance and perturbed stance are on the same continuum and use a common control strategy, rather than involving separate modes of control (Creath et al., 2005).

Movement Strategies during Perturbed Stance

Many research labs have studied the organization of movement strategies used to recover stability in response to brief displacements of the supporting surface, using a variety of moving platforms such as the one shown in Figure 7.7 (Allum & Pfaltz, 1985; Diener et al., 1982; Nashner, 1976). In addition, characteristic patterns of muscle activity, called "muscle synergies," which are associated with postural movement strategies used to recover stability in the sagittal plane, have been described (Horak & Nashner, 1986; Nashner, 1977; Nashner & Woollacott, 1979). Early researchers focused primarily on examining movement strategies for controlling forward and backward sway. Why? To answer this question for yourself, do Lab Activity 7.1.

As the lab exercise shows, no one stands absolutely still; instead, the body sways in small amounts, mostly

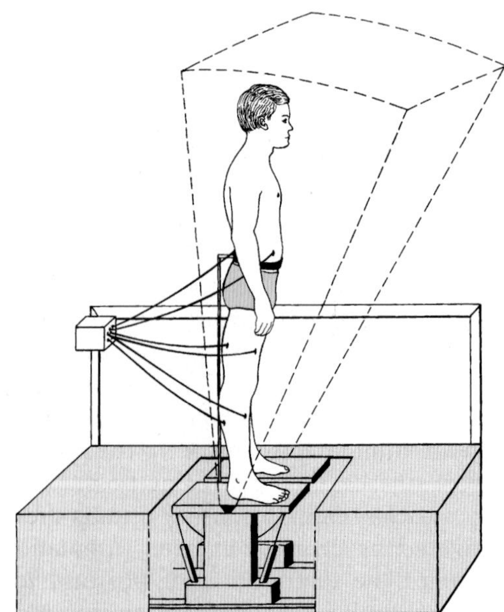

FIGURE 7.7 Moving platform posturography used to study postural control. (Adapted from Woollacott MH, Shumway-Cook A, Nashner LM. Aging and posture control: changes in sensory organization and muscular coordination. Int J Aging Hum Dev 1986;23:108.)

LAB ACTIVITY 7-1

Objective: To explore the motor strategies used for stance postural control

Procedure: With a partner, observe body movement in the following conditions:

1. Stand with your feet shoulder distance apart for 1 minute.
2. Try leaning forward and backward a little, then as far as you can without taking a step. Now lean so far forward or backward that you have to take a step.
3. Come up on your toes and do the same thing.
4. Put on a pair of ski boots (constraining ankle movement) and try swaying backward and forward.
5. Now have your partner place three fingers on your sternum and nudge you backward, first gently, and then with more force.

Assignment:

Write answers to the following questions, based on your observations of your and your partner's balance under the different conditions:

1. During quiet stance, did you stand perfectly still, or did you move very slightly? In which direction did you feel yourself swaying most?
2. During active sway, describe the movement strategies you used to control body sway.
3. Describe the movement strategies used when reacting to nudges from your partner.
4. Discuss how those strategies change as a function of: (a) size of base of support; (b) speed of movement; (c) where the center of mass was relative to the base of support (well inside, near edge, outside); and (d) when movement was constrained at the ankle (wearing ski boots).
5. List the muscles you think were active to control sway in these conditions. (a) What muscles did you feel working to keep you balanced when you swayed a little? (b) What muscles worked when you swayed further? (c) What happened when you leaned so far forward that your center of mass moved outside the base of support of your feet?

in the forward and backward direction. This is why researchers have concentrated primarily on understanding how normal adults maintain stability in the sagittal plane. However, in recent years, researchers have begun to focus on mechanisms underlying stability in other directions as well.

The specific movement patterns used to recover stability following displacement of the COM in the sagittal plane are selected by the central nervous system based on a number of factors, including characteristics of the perturbation (e.g., direction and magnitude), and biomechanical constraints, including musculoskeletal geometry and intersegmental dynamics of the individual's body (Kuo & Zajac, 1993). The patterns have been described as either: ankle, hip, and stepping strategies (illustrated in Figure 7.8) or, alternatively, fixed base of support and changing base of support (step or reach) strategies, depending on the research laboratory. Some researchers prefer the term *fixed base of support* strategy rather than terms such as *ankle* or *hip* because discrete strategies are usually not observed during balance recovery under normal slip conditions. Rather, subjects show a continuum of movements ranging from ankle through hip motion. In addition, as shown above for quiet stance, these two modes may both be present in postural control, with one dominating, depending on the sensory and task conditions.

These postural movement strategies are used in both feedback and feedforward control modes to maintain equilibrium in a number of circumstances. **Feedback control** refers to postural control that occurs in response to sensory feedback (visual, vestibular, or somatosensory) from an external perturbation. For example:

1. In response to external disturbances to equilibrium, such as when the support surface moves; and
2. During gait and in response to unexpected disruptions to the gait cycle, such as a trip or slip.

Feedforward control refers to postural responses that are made in anticipation of a voluntary movement that is potentially destabilizing in order to maintain stability during the movement. For example:

1. To prevent a disturbance to the system, for example, prior to a voluntary movement that is potentially destabilizing, such as when lifting a heavy object, or leaning over to pick up a heavy object; and
2. During volitional COM movements in stance.

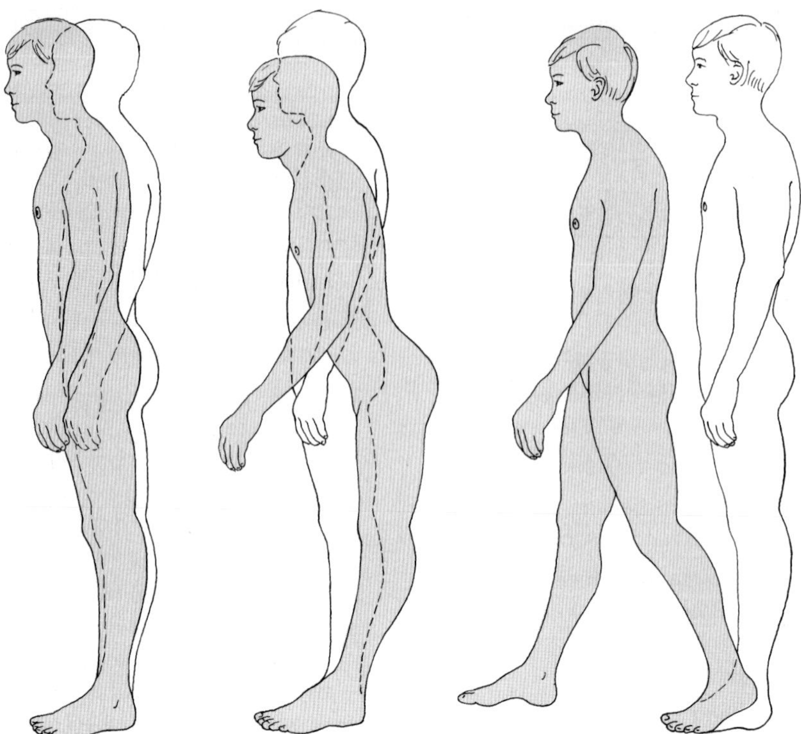

FIGURE 7.8 Three postural movement strategies used by normal adults for controlling upright sway. (Reprinted with permission from Shumway-Cook A, Horak F. Vestibular rehabilitation: an exercise approach to managing symptoms of vestibular dysfunction. Semin Hearing 1989;10:199.)

Early postural control research by Nashner and colleagues (Horak & Nashner, 1986; Nashner, 1977; Nashner et al., 1979; Nashner & Woollacott, 1979) explored muscle patterns that underlie movement strategies for balance. Results from postural control research in neurologically intact young adults suggest that the nervous system combines independent, though related, muscles into units called "muscle synergies." A **synergy** is defined as the functional coupling of groups of muscles that are constrained to act together as a unit; this simplifies the control demands on the CNS. It is important to keep in mind that while muscle synergies are important, they are only one of many motor mechanisms that affect outputs for postural control.

What are some of the muscle synergies underlying movement strategies critical for stance postural control? How do scientists know whether these neuromuscular responses are due to neural programs (i.e., synergies) or whether they are the result of independent stretch of the individual muscles at mechanically coupled joints? Are there different types of strategies and underlying muscle response synergies for anteroposterior stability versus mediolateral stability? In the following sections we examine strategies used for stabilization in multiple directions, including anteroposterior, mediolateral and also multidirectional planes of motion.

Anteroposterior Stability

Ankle Strategy. Traditionally, the ankle strategy and its related muscle synergy were among the first patterns for controlling upright sway to be identified. The ankle strategy restores the COM to a position of stability through body movement centered primarily about the ankle joints. Figure 7.9A shows the typical synergistic muscle activity and body movements associated with corrections for loss of balance in the forward direction. In this case, motion of the platform in the backward direction causes the subject to sway forward. Muscle activity begins at about 90 to 100 msec after perturbation onset in the gastrocnemius, followed by activation of the hamstrings 20 to 30 msec later, and finally by the activation of the paraspinal muscles (Nashner, 1977, 1989).

Activation of the gastrocnemius produces a plantar flexion torque that slows, then reverses, the body's forward motion. Activation of the hamstrings and paraspinal muscles maintains the hip and knees in an extended position. Without the synergistic activation of the hamstrings and paraspinal muscles, the indirect effect of the gastrocnemius ankle torque on proximal body segments would result in forward motion of the trunk mass relative to the lower extremities.

Figure 7.9B shows the synergistic muscle activity and body motions used when reestablishing stability

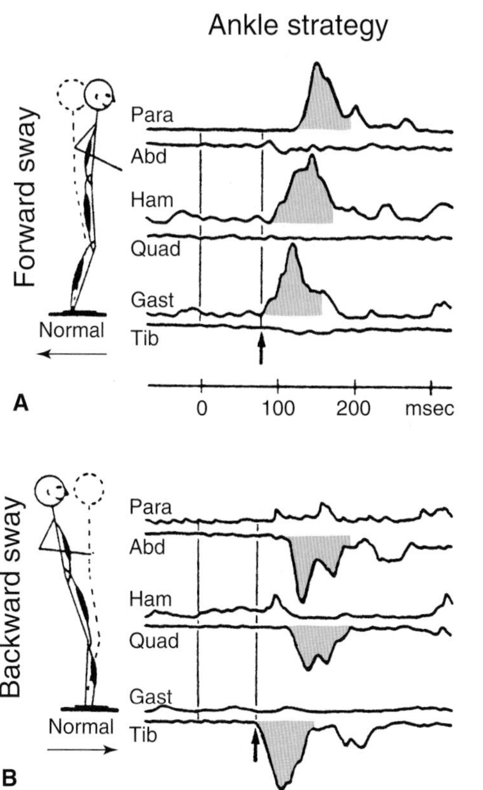

FIGURE 7.9 Muscle synergy and body motions associated with ankle strategy for controlling forward sway (A) and backward sway (B). (Reprinted with permission from Horak F, Nashner L. Central programming of postural movements: adaptation to altered support surface configurations. J Neurophysiol 1986;55:1372.)

in response to backward instability. Muscle activity begins in the distal muscle, the anterior tibialis, followed by activation of the quadriceps and abdominal muscles.

How do scientists know that the ankle, knee, and hip muscles are part of a neuromuscular synergy, instead of being activated in response to stretching of each individual joint? Some of the first experiments in postural control (Nashner, 1977; Nashner & Woollacott, 1979) provide some evidence for synergistic organization of muscles.

In these early experiments, the platform was rotated in a toes-up or toes-down direction. In a toes-up rotation, the platform motion provides stretch to the gastrocnemius muscle and dorsiflexion of the ankle, but these inputs are not associated with movements at the mechanically coupled knee and hip. The neuromuscular response that occurs in response to toes-up platform rotation includes activation of muscles at the ankle, knee, and hip joints, despite the fact that motion has occurred only at the ankle joint. Evidence from these experiments supports the hypothesis of a neurally programmed muscle synergy (Nashner, 1976, 1977; Nashner & Woollacott, 1979), including knee and hip muscles on the same side of the body as the stretched ankle muscle.

Since these responses to rotation are destabilizing, in order to regain balance, muscles on the opposite side of the body are activated. These responses have been hypothesized to be activated in response to visual and vestibular inputs (Allum & Pfalz, 1985) and are sometimes referred to as M3 responses, as opposed to an M1 response, that is, a monosynaptic stretch reflex, and the longer-latency stretch responses, which have been called M2 responses (Diener et al., 1982).

The ankle movement strategy described above appears to be used most commonly in situations in which the perturbation to equilibrium is small and the support surface is firm. Use of the ankle strategy requires intact range of motion and strength in the ankles. What happens if the perturbation to balance is large, or if we are in a situation in which we are unable to generate force using ankle joint muscles?

Hip Strategy. Scientists have identified another in-place strategy for controlling body sway, the hip movement strategy (Horak & Nashner, 1986). This strategy controls motion of the COM by producing large and rapid motion at the hip joints with antiphase rotations of the ankles (see Fig. 7.8).

Figure 7.10A shows the typical synergistic muscle activity associated with a hip strategy. Motion of the platform in the backward direction again causes the subject to sway forward. As shown in Figure 7.10A, the muscles that typically respond to forward sway when a subject is standing on a narrow beam are different from the muscles that become active in response to forward sway while standing on a flat surface. Muscle activity begins at about 90 to 100 msec after perturbation onset in the abdominal muscles, followed by activation of the quadriceps. Figure 7.10B shows the muscle pattern and body motions associated with the hip strategy, correcting for backward sway.

Horak and Nashner (1986) suggest that the hip strategy is used to restore equilibrium in response to larger, faster perturbations or when the support surface is compliant or smaller than the feet—for example, when standing on a beam. As mentioned above, researchers have noted more recently that there is actually a continuum of movement strategies ranging from pure ankle to ankle plus hip when individuals respond to perturbations of increasing amplitudes and velocities.

Stepping Strategy. When in-place strategies such as the ankle and hip strategy are insufficient to recover balance, a reach or a step is used to realign the base

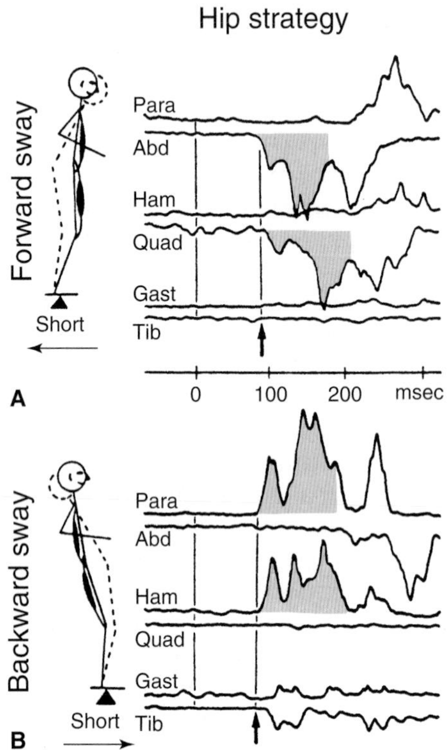

FIGURE 7.10 Muscle synergy and body motions associated with the hip strategy for controlling forward sway (A) and backward sway (B). (Reprinted with permission from Horak F, Nashner L. Central programming of postural movements: adaptation to altered support surface configurations. J Neurophysiol 1986;55:1372.)

of support under the COM (see Fig. 7.8). Initially, researchers believed that these changes in support strategies were used solely in response to perturbations that moved the COM outside the BOS (Horak, 1991; Nashner, 1989; Shumway-Cook & Horak, 1989). More recent research has found that in many conditions, stepping and/or reaching occurs even when the COM is well within the BOS (Brown et al., 1999; McIlroy & Maki, 1993).

Maki has noted that most research studies examining recovery of stability after a threat to standing balance have discouraged stepping responses, with instructions to subjects to refrain from stepping unless absolutely necessary. This may encourage subjects to use other strategies, such as the hip strategy. In order to determine whether this is the case, McIlroy and Maki (1993) studied the relationship between the prevalence of stepping responses and the instructions given to the subject. They noted that early automatic postural responses were recorded in ankle muscles in all trials, whether they resulted in stepping or not. They found that the frequency of stepping showed a trend to be higher in unconstrained (no specific instructions given) versus constrained (keep feet in place) conditions. However, no significant effects were found. This raises questions as to whether instructions to the subject play a role in the type of movement strategy used to recover stability following perturbation.

Emerging Concepts in the Neural Control of Synergies

While early research suggested that the ankle, hip, and stepping strategies and their associated muscular synergies were discrete entities, in which a sensory input would trigger a group of muscle synergists controlled as a single unit (Horak & Nashner, 1986), more recent research is challenging these views on the organization and control of muscle synergies used to control posture. Researchers are examining the extent to which during postural control, the nervous system stores and selects from a discrete group of preprogrammed postural strategies (as originally proposed by Nashner, Horak and others), or alternatively dynamically activates individual muscles using multiple sensory inputs and continuous feedback control. Research laboratories have used an experimental paradigm in which they gradually increased platform perturbation magnitudes and examined the muscle and torque output to determine whether responses appeared to be selected from preprogrammed postural strategies, through continuous feedback control of individual joints, or a combination of these two control strategies.

Runge et al. (1999) found that as platform velocities gradually increase from 10 cm/sec up to as much as 55 to 80 cm/sec, subjects do not simply shift from using forces primarily at the ankles at the low velocities to forces primarily at the hip for higher velocities. Instead, they continue to increase forces applied at the ankle, and then begin to add in forces at the hip at a certain critical threshold. The specific point at which a person begins to add hip forces varies from subject to subject, with some subjects using primarily forces at the ankle for most perturbation velocities. Pure hip strategies, previously identified using EMG patterns when subjects responded to postural perturbations while standing on a narrow support surface (Horak & Nashner, 1986), were never observed in subjects perturbed while standing on a flat surface, regardless of the size or speed of the perturbation. EMG records also showed that when trunk abdominal muscle activation occurred, correlated with trunk flexion, ankle muscle activity remained (Jensen et al., 1996; Runge et al., 1999). Figure 7.11 illustrates the combination of ankle and hip muscles seen in response to platform perturbations of increasing size. Muscle responses (surface EMGs) are shown in Figure 7.11A, while the accompanying joint torques are shown in Figure 7.11B. Runge's

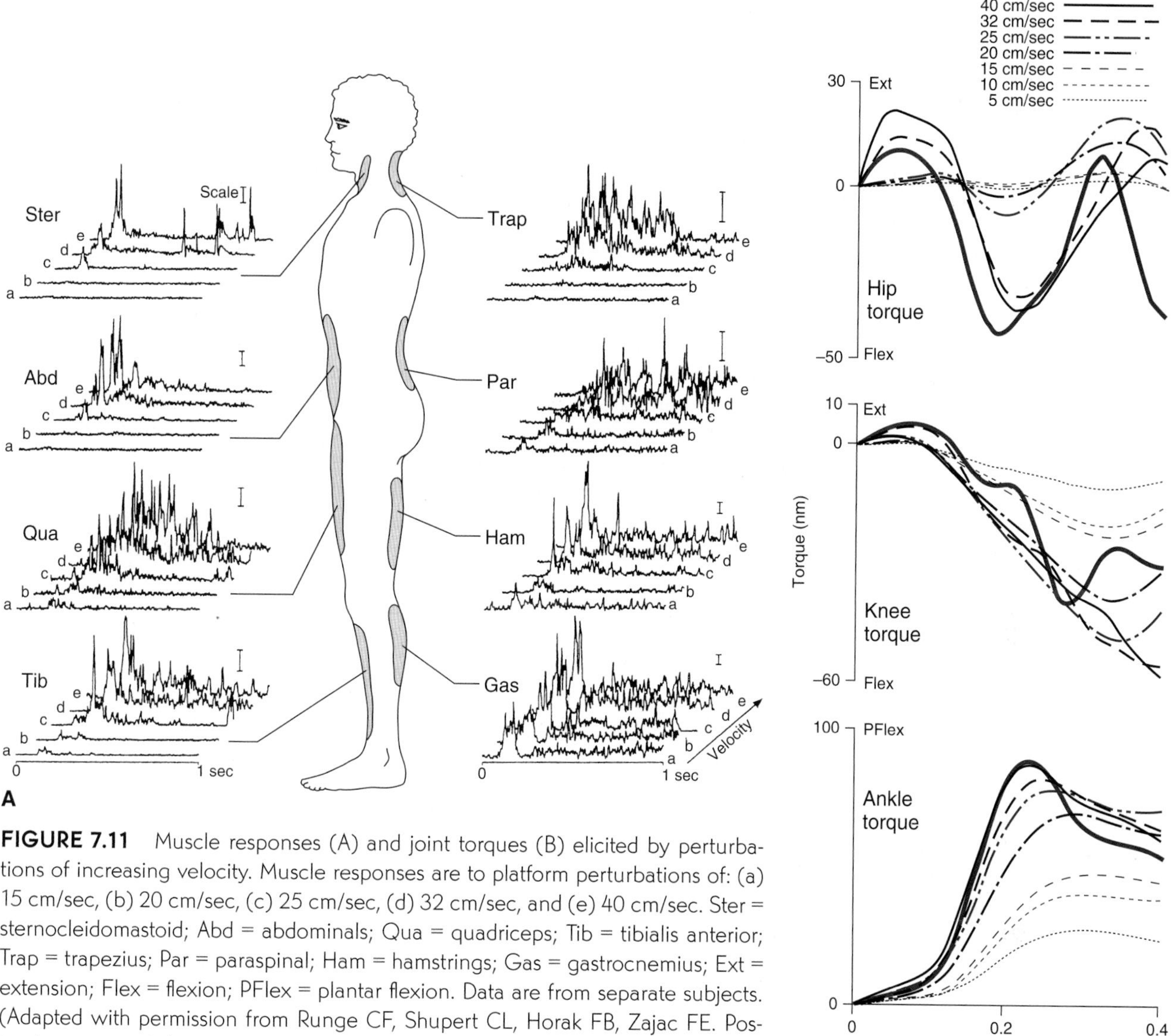

FIGURE 7.11 Muscle responses (A) and joint torques (B) elicited by perturbations of increasing velocity. Muscle responses are to platform perturbations of: (a) 15 cm/sec, (b) 20 cm/sec, (c) 25 cm/sec, (d) 32 cm/sec, and (e) 40 cm/sec. Ster = sternocleidomastoid; Abd = abdominals; Qua = quadriceps; Tib = tibialis anterior; Trap = trapezius; Par = paraspinal; Ham = hamstrings; Gas = gastrocnemius; Ext = extension; Flex = flexion; PFlex = plantar flexion. Data are from separate subjects. (Adapted with permission from Runge CF, Shupert CL, Horak FB, Zajac FE. Postural strategies defined by joint torques. Gait Posture 1999;10:161–170.)

research does not support the concept that ankle and hip strategies are distinct and separately controlled, as increasing platform perturbation magnitudes show that subjects do not switch between two distinct strategies but tend to blend movements in a more continuous manner.

Park et al. (2004) confirmed results by Runge et al. (1999) and suggested that this gradual scaling of postural muscle activity in response to perturbations of increasing magnitudes, suggested a model of postural control best represented by a *feedback control system* (Park et al., 2004) rather than a control process of selected preprogrammed responses. Further research (Welch & Ting, 2008) has also supported a feedback model to explain muscle response characteristics to support-surface translations.

As mentioned in Chapter 1, Latash et al. (2005) have proposed a new definition of the term *synergy*, as a neural organization of a multi-element system (e.g., muscles) that: (1) organizes sharing of a task among a set of elemental variables (e.g., muscles); and (2) ensures covariation among elemental variables with the purpose of stabilizing performance variables (e.g., COM in posture control). An elemental variable is defined as the smallest variable that can be used to describe a system of interest at a selected level of analysis. It could be the rotation of joints or muscle activation patterns, for example. They have analyzed the efficiency of synergy output in contributing to accurate performance by looking at the variability of each unit (e.g., each muscle or joint angle change) and how its variability contributes to the total force output. According to this definition of synergies, a certain portion of variability contributes to stabilizing the performance variable, such as the COP; the remaining variability is not related to improving stability of performance. They have used UCM analysis to measure these two types of variability and their relative contributions to performance output of a synergy. Refer to the Technology Tool 7.1 box on page 163 for an explanation of UCM analysis.

This research has confirmed the existence of what the authors call "muscle modes" and others call synergies that control COP shifts when an individual sways forward or backward while standing (Krishnamoorthy et al., 2003). They used principal component analysis (PCA) to identify the muscle modes, or synergies, used to produce COP shifts. They showed that the gains of the muscle outputs covaried across trials so that the effects of their variation on the COP shift compensated for each other. These results fit with the new definition of synergy that was proposed by Latash et al. (2005).

These results support the understanding that the nervous system may use both types (preprogrammed and continuous feedback) of control strategies in postural control. While it is true that groups of muscles appear to be constrained to act together as muscle synergies, during postural control (supported by the research of Latash and colleagues [2005] as well as Horak & Nashner [1986] and others [Torres-Oviedo et al., 2006]), there appears to be support for an additive effect of continuous feedback control of individual muscles and joints (research by Runge et al. [1999], Park et al. [2004], and Welch & Ting [2008]).

Mediolateral Stability. Early research on postural response strategies explored stability only in the anteroposterior (AP) direction. More recent research has revealed that alternative strategies are used to recover stability in the mediolateral (ML) direction. This is because the alignment of body segments and muscles requires the activation of forces at different joints and in different directions to recover stability. For example, in the lower limb, very little ML movement is possible at the ankle and knee joints. Thus, the hip joint is the lower limb joint that is primarily used when recovering stability in the ML direction.

A number of researchers (Day et al., 1993; Kapteyn, 1973; Rozendal, 1986; Winter et al., 1996) have proposed that in contrast to AP postural control, ML control of balance occurs primarily at the hip and trunk, rather than at the ankle. They have noted that the primary ML motion of the body is lateral movement at the pelvis, which requires adduction of one leg and abduction of the other. With narrow stance widths there is also motion at the ankle joint; however, this is minimal with stance widths wider than 8 cm (Day et al., 1993).

Winter and colleagues (1993, 1996) have examined the AP and ML components of balance during quiet stance. They noted that with ML sway, the loading and unloading of the left and right side look like mirror images, with the weight unloaded from one side being taken up by the other. In addition, ML movements that occur during quiet stance show a descending response organization, with head movements occurring first, followed by hip movements (20-msec latency) and then ankle movements (40-msec latency). Head movements occur in the direction opposite to those at the hip and ankle (Lekhel et al., 1994).

Correlated with these biomechanical changes are specific muscle responses to control lateral sway. A number of laboratories have shown that the hip abductor (gluteus medius and tensor fascia latae) and adductor muscle groups are activated in the control of the loading and unloading of the two legs with ML sway (Maki et al., 1994b; Winter et al., 1993, 1996; Horak & Moore, 1989). In contrast to AP muscle response patterns, which are organized in a distal to proximal manner, ML muscle patterns are organized in a proximal-to-distal direction, with hip muscles being activated before ankle muscles (Horak & Moore, 1989).

Multidirectional Stability. Much of the research cited above suggests that a limited number of synergies may contribute to posture control, specifically synergies compensating for AP and ML sway. However, it is alternatively possible that there is a continuum of response patterns that control stability in the 360-degree continuum of possible perturbation directions. To determine whether this was the case, Macpherson performed experiments in which she perturbed cats in 16 different directions, around a 360-degree continuum. She noted that in response to ML perturbations causing loading of one hindlimb and unloading of the other, the hip abductors of the loaded limb were activated, while in response to AP perturbations the hip flexors and extensors were activated (Macpherson, 1988). By increasing the range of directions used to study muscle activation patterns, it became apparent that traditional concepts related to the organization of synergies would have to be revised. The complex muscle response patterns observed by perturbing cats in multiple (16) directions could no longer be explained by the traditional concept of separate synergies, each with a unique group of muscles, used to control balance in each of the cardinal directions of sway (e.g., anterior synergy, posterior synergy, medial synergy, and lateral synergy).

Newer methods of analysis using computational techniques suggested a new way of thinking about synergies (Ting & Macpherson, 2004; Torres-Oviedo et al., 2006; Torres-Oviedo & Ting, 2007). There are two differences between the traditional way of viewing synergies and the new one that is associated with computational analysis. According to the traditional view of synergies, shown in Figure 7.12, top, each muscle belongs to only one synergy and muscles within a synergy are activated equally. Thus, for example, the gluteus muscle (labeled GLUT) is part of synergy 1, but not 2 or 3, while the posterior semimembranosus (labeled SEMP) is part of synergy 3, but not 1 or 2. The problem with this approach was that the EMG tuning curves of different muscles in a synergy were not aligned (i.e., they were not equally activated in the same perturbation regions), suggesting that this synergy definition was not completely accurate. According to the new view of synergies, shown in the lower portion of Figure 7.12, each muscle can belong to more than one synergy, as for example SEMP, which is now part of synergies 1, 2, and 3. Within a synergy an individual muscle has a unique or fixed weighting factor that represents the level of activation of that muscle within the synergy. This activation level is shown in Figure 7.12 as varying from 0 (not active at all) to 1 (very active). Thus, in our example, SEMP is least active in synergy 1 (close to 0) and most active in synergy 2 (close to 1) and moderately active in synergy 3. The total activity of a muscle in response to a perturbation is determined by simultaneous activation of multiple synergies incorporating that muscle, and the relative weighting factor of that muscle within those synergies.

A number of studies (Ting & Macpherson; 2005; Torres-Oviedo et al., 2006; Torres-Oviedo & Ting, 2007) have now shown in both humans and cats that a limited number of synergies (five to six) are sufficient to explain muscle activity across all perturbation directions. Their concept of the synergy control structure is shown in Figure 7.13. At the top of the schematic is the COM controller, which specifies the

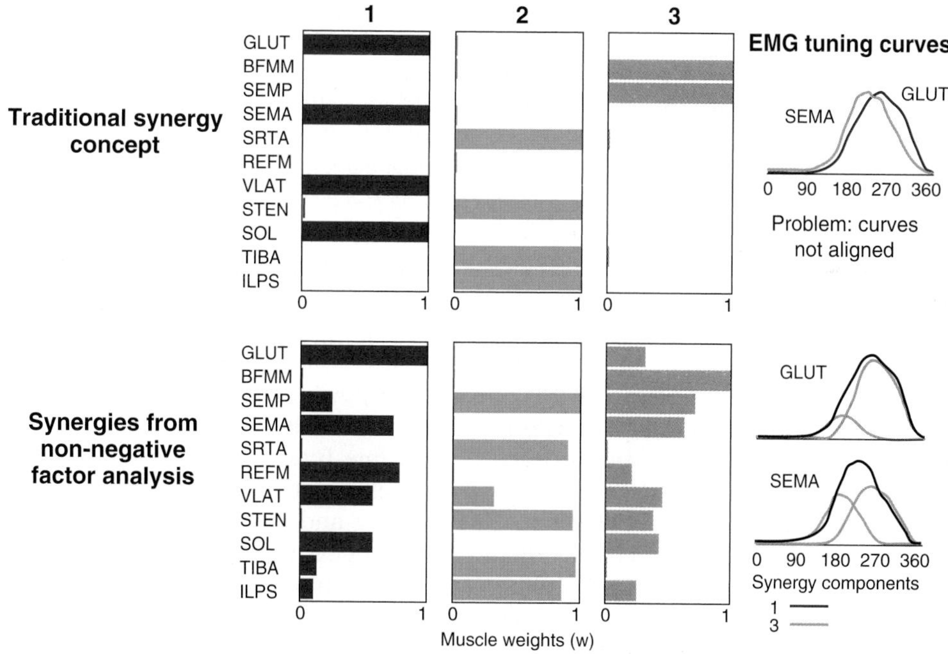

FIGURE 7.12 Top, Traditional view of synergies. Shown are three hypothetical synergies with different sets of muscles in each synergy. Each muscle belongs to only one synergy and muscles within a synergy are activated equally. The tuning curves for two muscles show that the two muscles are not equally activated in the same perturbation regions, thus showing lack of experimental support for this concept. Bottom, New view of synergies, from nonnegative factor analysis. Shown are three hypothetical synergies, with each muscle capable of belonging to more than one synergy. Within a synergy an individual muscle has a unique or fixed weighting factor that represents the level of activation of that muscle within the synergy. The total activity of a muscle in response to a perturbation is determined by simultaneous activation of multiple synergies incorporating that muscle, and the relative weighting factor of that muscle within those synergies. GLUT = gluteus medius; BFMM = biceps femoris middle head; SEMP = posterior semimembranosus; SEMA = anterior semimembranosus; SRTA = anterior sartorius; REFM = rectus femoris; VLAT = vastus lateralis; STEN = semitendinosus; SOL = soleus; TIBA = tibialis anterior; ILPS = iliopsoas. (From personal archives of Jane McPherson.)

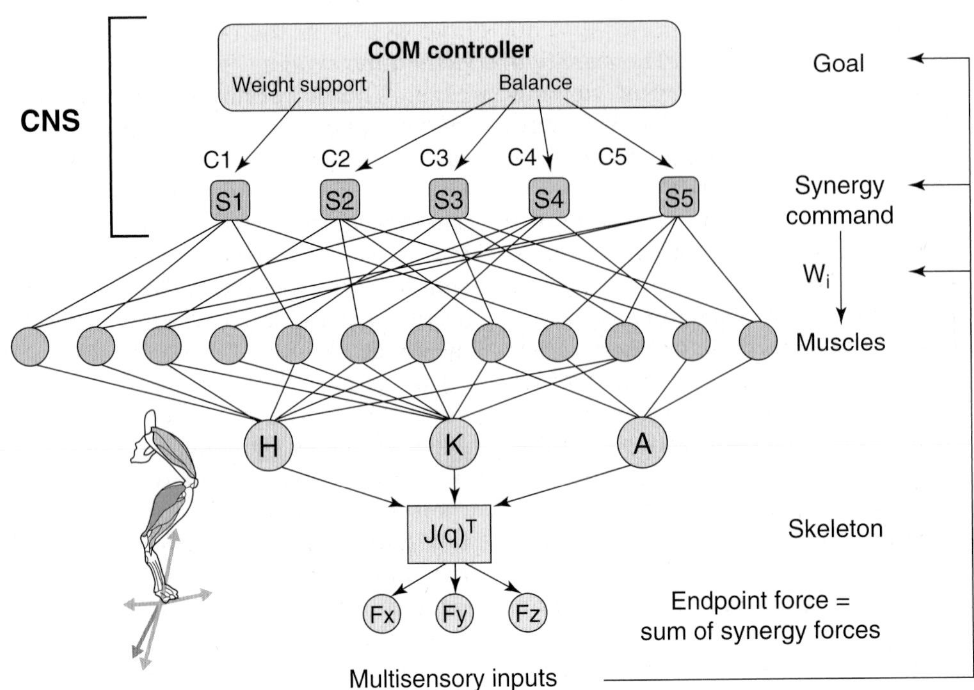

FIGURE 7.13 Synergy control structure. At the top of the schematic is the COM controller, which specifies the twin goals of postural control weight support and balance. One synergy (S1) is activated (C1) for weight support during quiet stance. The other four synergies (S2–S5) are activated in varying amounts in order to control balance in response to instability in different directions. Each synergy activates a specific set of muscles in a fixed amount. Activation of these muscles causes torques at the hip (H), knee (K), and ankle (A) joints. The combined torques from the three joints then create an endpoint force ($J(q)^T$) between the foot and the floor, which serves to control balance (position and motion of the COM). Multisensory inputs, (bottom of the figure) are responsible for giving feedback to the COM controller regarding the body's position in space, so that appropriate synergies can be activated. W_i = weighting of each muscle in synergy; Fx, Fy, Fz = forces in the *x*-,*y*-, and *z*-axes.

twin goals of postural control weight support and balance. In both cats and humans, one synergy (S1) is activated (C1) for weight support during quiet stance. The other synergies (S2 through S5 for the cat) are activated in varying amounts in order to control balance in response to instability in different directions. The support synergy (S1) is inhibited when the other synergies (S2 through S5) are actively controlling the COM, but is recruited again if the limb is near maximal loading.

Each synergy activates a specific set of muscles in a fixed amount. Activation of these muscles causes torques at the hip, knee, and ankle joints. The combined torques from the three joints then create an end-point force between the foot and the floor, which serves to control balance (position and motion of the COM). Each synergy produces a specific and unique direction of end-point force and the combined activation of several synergies produces the summed, or net, force between foot and floor. Multisensory inputs, shown at the bottom of the figure are responsible for giving feedback to the COM controller regarding the body's position in space, so that appropriate synergies can be activated. Finally, these researchers found that the same functional muscle synergies were used to control balance across a wide range of postural tasks.

Ting and colleagues have found that in humans there appear to be six synergy groupings, not five as in the cat; the composition and timing of two of these muscle response synergies are consistent with the hip and ankle strategies previously identified by other researchers (Torres-Oviedo & Ting, 2007). In addition, a number of subjects used a "knee" strategy synergy, a balance strategy previously reported by researchers in response to support surface rotations (Allum et al., 2003). They also found that more complex motor patterns (e.g., the combination of hip and ankle strategies in either the sagittal or the frontal plane) could be generated by adding different muscle synergies together.

What are the implications of this research reporting the presence of fixed synergies activated during postural adjustments, to the model of postural control as a feedback process and not as triggered motor patterns? Torres-Oviedo and Ting (2007) suggest that each muscle synergy (which is characterized by a fixed pattern of muscle activity) could nonetheless be modulated by continuous feedback signals; thus, different combinations of synergies are continuously activated in a feedback manner to create context-specific postural adjustments.

In summary, the research examining multidirectional postural control is consistent with the findings from sagittal-plane postural control research. The central nervous system appears to use two types of control strategies for recovery of stability, activation of different combinations of preprogrammed synergies and continuous feedback control of individual muscles and joints.

Clinical Applications of Research on Motor Strategies for Postural Control

So what are the clinical implications of the research on the neural control of movement strategies in both quiet and perturbed stance? Researchers have shown that two control strategies are important in the control of motor strategies for postural control, a preprogrammed synergy mechanism and a continuous feedback system. It is possible that neural pathology could interrupt one of these systems (e.g., loss of preprogrammed synergies) but not the other (feedback control). Further research is needed to identify clinical strategies that would distinguish between these two problems, so that focused interventions could be created.

In addition, since both quiet stance and recovery from perturbations use common control mechanisms, it is possible that training in one context (e.g., quiet stance) may transfer to improved movement control in the other context (e.g., recovery of perturbed stance). Finally, since we appear to continuously modulate and add multiple synergies depending on contextual factors, it will be important not to limit training to the activation of a single synergy (e.g., ankle vs. hip vs. step) but to create conditions in which strategies are continuously modulated. For example, Creath et al. (2005) report that use of an ankle strategy (legs and trunk moving in phase) is predominant when standing on a firm surface; however, there is a shift to using a hip strategy (legs and trunk out of phase) when standing on a foam surface.

Adapting Motor Strategies

Postural control under changing task and environmental conditions requires that we modify how we move when maintaining stability in response to new demands. *Adaptation* is a term that reflects the ability to modify behavior in response to new task demands. Several studies have examined how individuals adapt movement strategies to changing task and environmental conditions. These studies suggest that subjects without neural pathology can shift relatively quickly from one postural movement strategy to another. For example, when asked to stand on a narrow beam while experiencing AP platform displacements, most subjects shifted from an ankle to a hip strategy within 5 to 15 trials, and when returned to a normal support surface, they shifted back to an ankle strategy within 6 trials. During the transition from one strategy to the next, subjects used complex movement strategies that were combinations of the pure strategies (Horak & Nashner, 1986).

Research has shown that we are constantly modulating the amplitudes of our postural responses, fine-tuning them to the context. For example, Woollacott and colleagues (1988) examined the responses of adults to repeated translational platform movements and found that with repeated exposure to the movements, the subjects swayed less and showed smaller-amplitude postural responses. Thus, with repeated exposure to a given postural task, subjects refine their response characteristics to optimize response efficiency.

Neural Subsystems Controlling Postural Orientation and Stability

Do different neural subsystems control postural orientation and stability? Research comparing postural control in normal cats versus cats with the spinal cord transected (referred to as "spinalized') has contributed a partial answer to this question (Macpherson et al., 1997). Spinalized cats are able to regain normal orientation, including full weight support and appropriate horizontal orientation of the trunk, and a semiflexed posture of the hindlimbs, with training (Lovely et al., 1986). The pattern of ground reaction forces are normal, although the amplitude is lower. Thus, it appears that the spinal neural circuitry by itself is able to activate extensor muscles tonically for appropriate antigravity support, ensuring postural orientation of the four limbs (Macpherson et al., 1997).

However, the control of postural stability in the chronic spinalized cat is greatly diminished. These animals do not show lateral stability, although they can support their own weight. They also do not show their normal pattern of EMG activation, with a complete absence of flexor activation when a limb is unloaded, unlike the responses seen in normal cats. Extensor muscles still show responses to balance perturbations, but with much smaller amplitudes than normal. It is also interesting that most muscles are no longer modulated in relation to vertical force, except those tonically active for weight support. Thus, it appears that postural stability is not organized at the spinal level, but is controlled by higher centers, such as the brainstem (including the vestibular nuclei) and cerebellum (Macpherson et al., 1997; Macpherson & Fung, 1999).

Research on brainstem nuclei contributing to postural control has shown that these centers are active in the regulation of postural tone, the integration of sensory information for posture and balance, as well as contributing to anticipatory postural control accompanying voluntary movements. For example, the brainstem has important centers for controlling the facilitation (through raphe-spinal and cerulospinal tracts) and inhibition of muscle tone (the pedunculopontine tegmental nucleus in the mesopontine tegmentum and the reticulospinal tract) important for the control of posture. These muscle-tone facilitatory and inhibitory systems within the brainstem are shown in Figure 3.18. Stapley and Drew (2009) have also shown that pontomedullary reticular formation neurons in the brainstem of the cat discharge strongly in response to support surface perturbations, suggesting that nuclei in the brainstem contribute to the restoration of equilibrium following a balance threat. It is also important to note that when the brainstem reticular formation is inactivated by pharmacologic means, anticipatory postural adjustments that would normally be activated to stabilize a voluntary movement initiated through activation of the motor cortex, are no longer activated. This indicates the importance of brainstem nuclei in anticipatory postural control (Takakusaki et al., 2004).

In addition, research on postural control in patients with pathology in the basal ganglia and cerebellum, discussed in detail in Chapter 10, is increasing our understanding of the contributions of these neural structures to postural control. The cerebellum is known to control adaptation of postural responses—that is, the ability to modify postural muscle response amplitudes in response to changing environmental and task conditions. The basal ganglia are involved in the control of postural set—that is, the ability to quickly change muscle patterns in response to changing task and environmental conditions. When all systems are intact, the individual shows adaptable postural control and is able to meet the goals of stability and orientation in any environment. Figure 7.14 summarizes the hypothesized contributions of the brain and spinal cord systems discussed above to postural control.

In summary, we know that the ability to generate and apply forces in a coordinated way to control the body's position in space is an essential part of the action component of postural control. We know the CNS must activate synergistic muscles at mechanically related joints to ensure that forces generated at one joint for balance control do not produce instability elsewhere in the body. We believe that the CNS internally represents the body's position in space with reference to behavioral strategies that are effective in controlling that movement; however, it is not clear whether these behavioral strategies are internally represented as muscle synergies, movement strategies, or force strategies. We also know the contributions of a variety of motor subsystems to posture control, including the spinal cord, the brainstem, the basal ganglia, the cerebellum, and higher cortical centers.

Perceptual Systems in Postural Control

Effective postural control requires more than the ability to generate and apply forces for controlling the body's position in space. In order to know *when* and *how* to apply restoring forces, the CNS must have an accurate picture of *where* the body is in space and whether it is stationary or in motion. How does the CNS accomplish this?

Senses Contributing to Postural Control

The CNS must organize information from sensory receptors throughout the body before it can determine the body's position in space. Normally, peripheral inputs from visual, somatosensory (proprioceptive, cutaneous, and joint receptors), and vestibular systems are available to detect the body's position and movement in space with respect to gravity and the environment. Each sense provides the CNS with specific information about position and motion of the body; thus, each sense provides a different *frame of reference* for postural control (Gurfinkel & Levick, 1991; Hirschfeld, 1992).

Visual inputs provide information regarding the position and motion of the head with respect to surrounding objects as well as a reference for verticality, since many things that surround us, like windows and doors, are aligned vertically. In addition, the visual system reports motion of the head, since as your head moves forward, surrounding objects move in the opposite direction. Visual inputs include both peripheral visual information and foveal information, although there is some evidence to suggest that a peripheral (or a large visual field) stimulus is more important for controlling posture (Paillard, 1987).

Visual inputs are an important source of information for postural control, but are they absolutely necessary? No, since most of us can keep our balance when

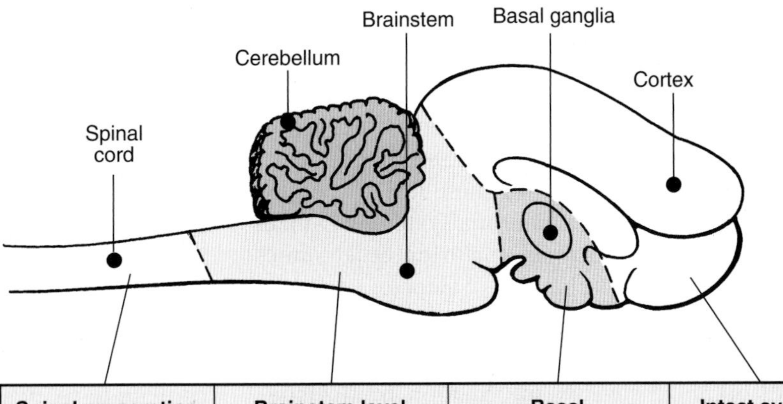

Spinal preparation	Brainstem level	Basal ganglia/cerebellum	Intact system
Ground reaction forces for orientation present though diminished Tonically active extensor muscle for antigravity support for postural orientation No lateral stability Somatosensory contributions to postural control	Controls level of postural tone in combination with cerebellum Circuits for automatic postural synergies (hypothesized) Vestibular contributions to postural control	*Cerebellum* Control of adaptation — abilities to modify postural muscle amplitude in response to changing task and environmental conditions *Basal ganglia* Control of postural set—ability to quickly change muscle patterns in response to changing task and environmental conditions	Adaptable postural control system to meet the goals of stability and orientation in any environment Visual contribution to postural control

FIGURE 7.14 The hypothesized contributions of various neural systems to postural control.

we close our eyes or when we are in a dark room. In addition, visual inputs are not always an accurate source of orientation information about *self-motion*. If you are sitting in your car at a stoplight and the car next to you moves, what do you do? You quickly put your foot on the brake. In this situation, visual inputs signal *motion,* which the brain initially interprets as self-motion; in other words, *my car is rolling.* The brain therefore sends out signals to the motor neurons of the leg and foot, so you step on the brake to *stop* the motion. Thus, the brain may misinterpret visual information. The visual system has difficulty distinguishing between object motion, referred to as "exocentric motion," and self-motion, referred to as "egocentric motion."

The somatosensory system provides the CNS with position and motion information about the body with reference to supporting surfaces. In addition, somatosensory inputs throughout the body report information about the relationship of body segments to one another. Under normal circumstances, when standing on a firm, flat surface, somatosensory receptors provide information about the position and movement of your body with respect to a horizontal surface. However, if you are standing on a surface that is moving relative to you (e.g., a boat) or on a surface that is not horizontal (such as a ramp), it is not appropriate to establish a vertical orientation with reference to the surface, since under these conditions it is not a stable reference. In these situations, somatosensory inputs reporting the position of the body relative to the support surface are not helpful.

Information from the vestibular system is also a powerful source of information for postural control. The vestibular system provides the CNS with information about the position and movement of the head with respect to gravity and inertial forces, providing a *gravito-inertial* frame of reference for postural control. Vestibular signals alone cannot provide the CNS with a true picture of how the body is moving in space. For example, the CNS cannot distinguish between a simple head nod (movement of the head relative to a stable trunk) and a forward bend (movement of the head in conjunction with a moving trunk) using vestibular inputs alone (Horak & Shupert, 1994).

Central Integration: Combining and Adapting Senses for Postural Control

Since postural demands during quiet stance are different from those during perturbations to stance or during locomotion, it is likely that sensory information is organized differently for these tasks. The next sections compare how the nervous system organizes and adapts sensory information during quiet stance and in response to perturbations in stance.

Sensory Strategies During Quiet Stance. How does the CNS organize sensory information from visual, somatosensory, and vestibular systems for postural control? Many studies examining the effect of vision on quiet stance have examined the amplitude of sway with eyes open versus eyes closed, and have found that there is a significant increase in sway in normal subjects with eyes closed. Thus, it has been proposed that while vision is not absolutely necessary to the control of quiet stance, it does actively contribute to balance control during quiet stance (Edwards, 1946; Lee & Lishman, 1975; Paulus et al., 1984). The ratio of body sway during eyes-open and eyes-closed conditions has been referred to as the "Romberg quotient," and is frequently used as a measure of stability in the clinic (Romberg, 1853).

Several researchers have examined the role of visual inputs to stance postural control using continuous and transient visual motion cues in people of different ages (Brandt et al., 1976; Butterworth & Hicks, 1977; Butterworth & Pope, 1983; Lee & Lishman, 1975; Sundermier et al., 1996). The first experiments of this type were performed by David Lee and his colleagues from Edinburgh, Scotland, using a novel paradigm in which subjects stood in a room that had a fixed floor, but with walls and a ceiling that could be moved forward or backward, creating the illusion of sway in the opposite direction (Lee & Lishman, 1975). The moving room can be used to create slow oscillations, simulating visual cues during quiet stance sway, or an abrupt perturbation to the visual field, simulating an unexpected loss of balance. If very small continuous room oscillations are used, neurologically intact adults begin to sway with the room's oscillations, thus showing that visual inputs have an important influence on postural control of adults during quiet stance. Young children and older adults show more sway in response to room oscillations than adults, probably because of reduced ability to process information from the feet and ankles and thus a greater reliance on visual cues for balance (Lee & Aronson, 1974; Sundermier et al., 1996). When adults were exposed to similar oscillations while balancing across a narrow beam, the influence of visual cues was higher (closer to those of children and older adults), indicating that a more difficult balancing task is associated with higher reliance on visual cues (Lee & Lishman, 1975).

In addition to vision, somatosensory inputs from the feet in contact with the surface appear to be important for quiet stance postural control. In fact, several studies have shown that reduction of afferent input from the lower limb due to vascular ischemia, anesthesia, or cooling causes an increase in COP motion during quiet stance (Asai et al., 1994; Diener et al., 1984; Magnusson et al., 1990). But it appears that somatosensory inputs from all parts of the body contribute to postural control and body orientation during quiet stance (Andersson & Magnusson, 2002; Kavounoudias et al., 1999; Roll & Roll, 1988). Studies by the French scientist Roll and his colleagues used minivibrators to excite eye, neck, and ankle muscles as well as forefoot cutaneous areas and explored the contributions of proprioceptive inputs from these muscles to postural control during quiet stance (Kavounoudias et al., 1999, 2001; Roll & Roll, 1988). They found that vibration applied to the eye muscles of a standing subject with eyes closed produced body sway, with sway direction depending on the muscle vibrated. Body sway also was produced by applying vibration to the sternocleidomastoid muscles of the neck or the soleus muscles of the leg. When forefoot areas of the foot soles or ankle flexor (tibialis anterior) muscles were vibrated, subjects swayed backward or forward, respectively, When these muscles and/or sole areas were vibrated simultaneously, the effects were additive, with no clear domination of one proprioceptive or cutaneous influence over another. Other studies showed that ankle muscle responses activated by posterior neck vibration occurred in the tibialis anterior within 70 to 100 msec of the onset of vibration, showing the effect of neck receptor activation on whole body sway (Andersson & Magnusson, 2002).

Jeka and Lackner (1994, 1995) have shown that lightly touching a fingertip to a stable surface reduces postural sway in subjects standing on one leg or in a heel-to-toe stance. They measured mediolateral COP under three different fingertip-contact conditions: no contact, touch contact (up to 1 N or 100 *g* force) or force contact (as much force as desired). They found that sway was highest in the no-contact condition and was reduced equally in the light-contact and force-contact conditions, even though fingertip contact was about 10 times higher in the force-contact condition. From calculations, they showed that contact forces of 0.4 N predicted a 2 to 3% reduction in sway; however, touch contact caused a 50 to 60% reduction. They showed that the additional stabilization provided by light-touch contact is due to forces generated by muscles far away from the fingertip (legs and trunk) guided by sensory information from cutaneous receptors in the fingertip and proprioceptive information about arm position (Jeka, 1997). Results from all of these studies demonstrate that somatosensory information from all parts of the body plays an important role in the maintenance of postural control and body orientation in quiet stance.

What can we conclude from all of these studies? They suggest that in healthy young adults, when all three senses are present, they each contribute to postural control during quiet stance.

Sensory Strategies During Perturbed Stance. How do visual, vestibular, and somatosensory inputs contribute to postural control during recovery from a transient perturbation to balance? Let us look at some of the research examining this question.

Moving rooms, as we just described, have also been used to examine the contribution of visual inputs to recovery from transient perturbations. When abrupt room movements are made, young children (1-year-olds) compensate for this illusory loss of balance with motor responses designed to restore the vertical position. However, since there is no actual body sway, only the illusion of sway, motor responses have a destabilizing effect, causing the infants to stagger or fall in the direction of the room movement (Lee & Aronson, 1974; Lee & Lishman, 1975). This indicates that vision may be a dominant input in compensating for transient perturbations in infants first learning to stand.

Interestingly, older children and adults typically do not show large sway responses to these movements, indicating that in adults, vision does not appear to play an important role in compensating for transient perturbations.

Muscle response latencies to visual cues signaling perturbations to balance are quite slow, on the order of 200 msec, in contrast to the somatosensory responses, which are activated at 80 to 100 msec (Dietz et al., 1991; Nashner & Woollacott, 1979). Because somatosensory responses to support-surface translations appear to be much faster than those triggered by vision, researchers have suggested that the nervous system preferentially relies on somatosensory inputs for controlling body sway when imbalance is caused by rapid displacements of the supporting surface.

What is the relative contribution of the vestibular system to postural responses to support surface perturbations? Experiments by Dietz and his colleagues (Dietz et al., 1991, 1994; Horak et al., 1994) indicate that the contribution of the vestibular system is much smaller than that of somatosensory inputs. In these experiments, the onset latency and amplitude of muscle responses were compared for two different types of perturbations of stance: (a) the support surface was moved forward or backward, stimulating somatosensory inputs; and (b) a forward or backward displacement of a load (2 kg) attached to the head was applied, stimulating the vestibular system (the response was absent in patients with vestibular deficits). For comparable accelerations, muscle responses to vestibular signals were about 10 times smaller than the somatosensory responses induced by the displacement of the feet. This suggests that vestibular inputs may play only a minor role in recovery of postural control when the support surface is displaced horizontally.

However, under certain conditions, vestibular and visual inputs are important in controlling responses to transient perturbations. For example, when the support surface is rotated toes-upward, stretching and activating the gastrocnemius muscle, this response is destabilizing, pulling the body backward. Allum, a researcher from Switzerland, has shown that the subsequent compensatory response in the tibialis anterior muscle, used to restore balance, is activated by the visual and vestibular systems when the eyes are open. When the eyes are closed, it is primarily (80%) activated by the vestibular semicircular canals (Allum & Pfaltz, 1985).

In a study comparing bilateral peripheral vestibular loss in humans on postural responses to multidirectional surface rotations in the sagittal (AP or pitch) and ML (roll) planes, Carpenter et al. (2001) showed that vestibular influences are earlier for the sagittal plane and are directed to leg muscles, whereas ML control is later and focused on trunk muscles. This correlates with other experiments using platform translations that showed that AP perturbations activate primarily leg muscles at early onset times while ML translations activate primarily trunk and hip muscles (Henry et al., 1998; Nashner, 1977).

The organization of sensory information for postural control in response to other types of perturbations appears to involve complex interactions among the different sensory modalities. Horak et al. (2001) examined how the vestibular and somatosensory systems interact to control posture when the head and body are displaced. In this study individuals were given different combinations of head and support surface perturbations and resulting postural muscle response characteristics were analyzed. The authors found that when head and support surface perturbations were presented close in time (10–50 msec apart) the onset of muscle contraction for somatosensory-evoked responses to body displacement (platform perturbations) was longer and vestibular-evoked responses (head displacements) were absent or of low amplitude. The authors concluded that integration of vestibular and somatosensory information for postural control is a complex process with common shared circuitry between the vestibulospinal and somatosensory-spinal pathways (Horak et al., 2001).

These studies suggest that similar to quiet stance, all three sensory inputs are important in the recovery of stability following an unexpected perturbation. However, the relative contribution of individual senses appears to depend on many factors, including the processing speed within each sensory system. For example, early postural responses to transient horizontal perturbations to stance may rely heavily on somatosensory inputs, because of their fast processing speed. However, vision and vestibular inputs, which have slower processing speeds, do contribute to early responses, albeit to a much lesser degree. Vision and vestibular inputs may be more important, however, in later aspects of the postural response.

Adapting the Organization of Sensory Inputs to Changes in Context. We live in a constantly changing environment. Adapting how we use the senses for postural control is a critical aspect of maintaining stability in a wide variety of environments, and has been studied by several researchers. There are two hypotheses describing the process by which the CNS organizes sensory information for postural orientation. In the intermodal theory of sensory orientation, all three senses contribute equally to postural orientation at all times. It is only through the interaction of all three senses that the CNS is able to maintain appropriate postural orientation. In contrast to this theory is the sensory weighting model, which suggests that the CNS modifies the weight, or importance, of a sensory input depending on its relative accuracy as a sensory input for orientation. In this model, the CNS has to resolve sensory conflicts (situations in which there is disagreement among sensory inputs) by changing the relative weight of a sensory input to postural control.

Intermodal Theory of Sensory Organization. Stoffregen and Riccio (1988) used an ecological approach to describe how sensory information is used for orientation. They suggest that information critical for postural orientation is gained through the interaction of the different sensory systems. The organization of sensory information for postural orientation is based on lawful relationships between patterns of sensory stimulation and properties of the environment, and these lawful relationships are called "invariants." Invariants describe intermodal relationships across perceptual systems. In this view, there is never sensory conflict; rather, all the senses provide information that increases specificity in control and perception. There is no relative weighting of sensory information; rather, orientation emerges from an interaction of all three senses. They use a triangle to illustrate this concept of intermodal organization. It is the relationship among three lines that makes a triangle; you understand a triangle only by understanding the relationship of the three lines to one another. Similarly, it is the relationship of the three senses to one another, intermodal information, that provides the CNS with the essential information for postural orientation.

Sensory Weighting Hypothesis. In contrast to the intermodal theory is the sensory weighting theory, which suggests that the postural control system is able to reweight sensory inputs in order to optimize stance in altered sensory environments (Oie et al., 2002). The sensory weighting hypothesis predicts that each sense provides a unique contribution to postural control. In addition, the sensory weighting hypothesis predicts that changes in postural responses in different sensory conditions are due to changes in sensory weights. Sensory weighting implies that the "gain" of a sensory input will depend on its accuracy as a reference for body motion. For example, as vision becomes less reliable as an indicator of self-motion, the visual input will be weighted less heavily and somatosensory cues will be weighted more heavily. In contexts in which touch becomes a less reliable indicator of self-motion, the visual inputs are weighted more heavily. The sensory weighting hypothesis is supported by a number of researchers (Jeka & Lackner, 1994, 1995; Kuo et al., 1998; Nashner, 1976, 1982). This research suggests that sensory strategies, that is, the relative weight given to a sense, vary as a function of age, task, and environment.

One approach to investigating how the CNS adapts multiple sensory inputs for postural control was developed by Nashner and coworkers. This approach uses a moving platform with a moving visual surround (Nashner, 1976, 1982). A simplified version of Nashner's protocol was developed by Shumway-Cook and Horak (1986) to examine the role of sensory interaction in balance.

In Nashner's protocol, body sway is measured while the subject stands quietly under six different conditions that alter the availability and accuracy of visual and somatosensory inputs for postural orientation. In conditions 1 to 3, the subject stands on a normal surface with eyes open (1), with eyes closed (2), or within a box-like enclosure that moves in the same direction and speed as the person sways, giving the visual illusion that they are not moving. Conditions 4 to 6 are identical to 1 to 3 except that the support surface now rotates with body sway as well. These conditions are shown in Figure 7.15.

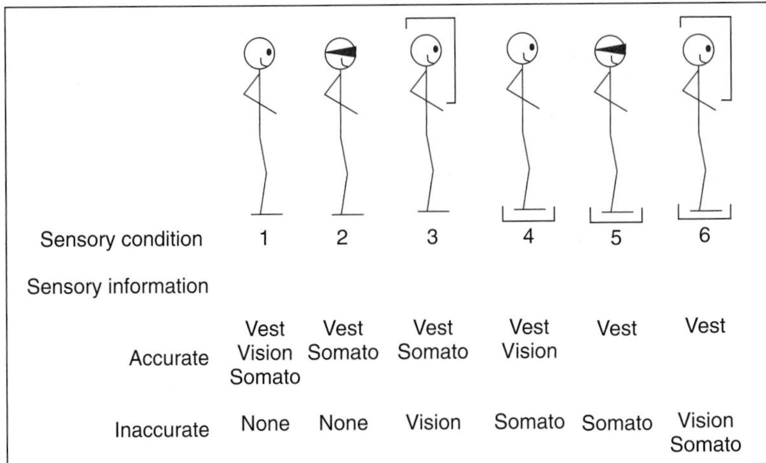

FIGURE 7.15 The six sensory conditions used to test how people adapt the senses to changing sensory conditions during the maintenance of stance. (Adapted from Horak F, Shumway-Cook A, Black FO. Are vestibular deficits responsible for developmental disorders in children? Insights Otolaryngol 1988;3:2.)

Differences in the amount of body sway in the different conditions are used to determine a subject's ability to adapt sensory information for postural control. Several studies have examined the performance of normal subjects when sensory inputs for postural control are varied (Jeka et al., 2000; Nashner, 1982; Peterka, 2002; Peterka & Black, 1990; Peterka & Loughlin, 2004; Woollacott et al., 1986). In general, these studies have shown that adults and children over the age of 7 easily maintain balance under all six conditions.

Average differences in body sway across the six sensory conditions within a large group of neurologically intact adults are shown in Figure 7.16. Adults sway the least in the conditions in which support-surface orientation inputs are accurately reporting the body's position in space relative to the surface regardless of the availability and accuracy of visual inputs (conditions 1, 2, and 3). When support-surface information is no longer available as an accurate source of orientation information, adults begin to sway more. The greatest amount of sway is seen in conditions 5 and 6, in which only one accurate set of inputs, the vestibular inputs, is available to mediate postural control (Peterka & Black, 1990). The application of this concept can be found in Lab Activity 7.2.

Further support for the sensory (re)weighting hypothesis comes from work by Oie et al. (2002). The authors systematically changed the amplitudes of both visual and somatosensory inputs used for balance during a quiet-stance task. They found that the gain of COM displacement systematically changed with a change in the amplitude of each of the sensory inputs. In addition, there was much interdependency between the two stimuli. Thus, changes in the COM

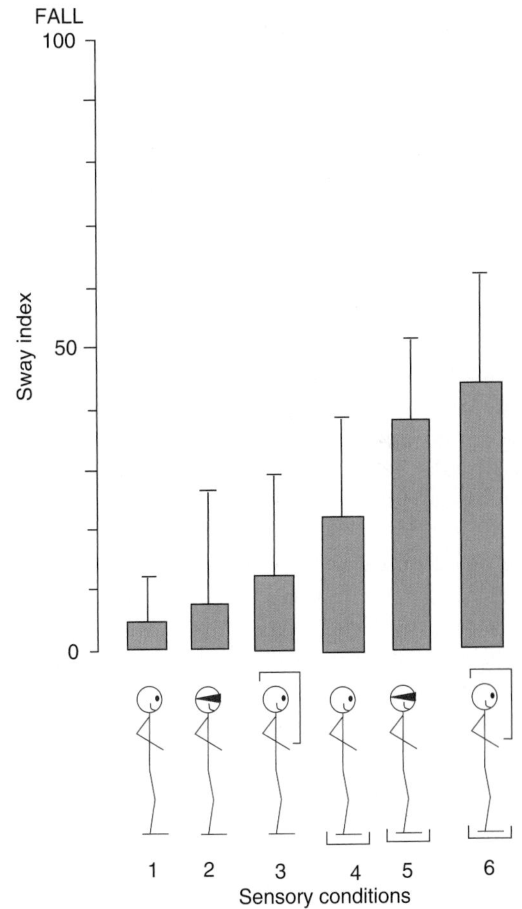

FIGURE 7.16 Body sway in healthy young adults in the six sensory conditions used to test sensory adaptation during stance postural control. RMS = root mean square. (Adapted from Woollacott MH, Shumway-Cook A, Nashner L. Aging and posture control: changes in sensory organization and muscular coordination. Int J Aging Hum Dev 1986;23:108.)

LAB ACTIVITY 7-2

Objective: To examine central organization and adaptation of sensory inputs to stance postural control.

Procedures: This lab REQUIRES a partner (for safety). Equipment needed is a stopwatch, an 18-by-18-by-3-in. piece of medium-density foam and a meter stick mounted horizontally on the wall at shoulder height, next to your partner. You will be measuring maximum sway in a forward/backward direction during a 20-sec period of quiet stance in four conditions. In condition 1, your partner should stand on a firm surface (e.g., linoleum or wood) with feet together, hands on hips, and eyes open. Record the maximum shoulder displacement in the forward and backward direction. In condition 2, stand as above, but with eyes closed. Record displacement. In condition 3, the subject should stand with feet together on the foam, with eyes open. Record displacement. In condition 4, stand on the foam with eyes closed. There is an increased risk for loss of balance in this condition, so be sure to stand close and guard your partner well. Record displacement.

Assignment

1. For each condition, make a list of the sensory cues that are available for postural control. Compare sway using your displacement measures across all conditions.
2. How does sway vary as a function of available sensory cues?
3. How do your results compare with Woollacott et al.'s (1986) results (conditions 1, 2, 4, and 5), found in Figure 7.16?

displacement in response to visual input change were in part dependent on how somatosensory input amplitudes were changing. In addition to supporting the concept of sensory weighting, Oie et al.'s work also suggests that sensory processing for postural control under changing task conditions is highly complex (Oie et al., 2001, 2002).

Finally, research by Peterka (2002) also demonstrated this task specific shift in how sensory information is used for postural control, providing evidence for the sensory reweighting hypothesis. In their experiments, they examined the relative contribution of somatosensory and vestibular inputs to the control of balance and orientation by measuring body sway while blindfolded subjects stood quietly on a surface that rotated continuously up and down by varying amounts, up to 8 degrees in magnitude. They tested both healthy young adults and people with loss of vestibular function. Figure 7.17 summarizes their findings; the graph on the left compares body sway measures relative to vertical, which is expressed as root mean square (RMS) sway in degrees. The dashed line plots the situation in which body sway and platform sway are exactly comparable. In the healthy participant (red trace) body sway and platform sway were equal for low-amplitude stimuli of less than 2 degrees, suggesting that this participant oriented the body axis relative to the support surface using somatosensory information. At larger amplitudes of surface rotation the healthy participant maintained a more vertical posture, minimizing body sway, suggesting that he or she was relying more on vestibular and less on somatosensory inputs for postural control.

In contrast to the healthy participant, when the blindfolded participant with loss of vestibular function (gray trace) stood on the rotating platform, the participant oriented the body axis to the surface and maintained balance during small-amplitude platform rotations (relying on somatosensory inputs for postural control), but could not maintain balance on the large-amplitude tilts. Lacking visual (blindfold) and vestibular inputs, the participant persisted in orienting the body axis to the surface (relying on somatosensory inputs for balance), but this was not effective in the face of large-amplitude platform tilts, resulting in imbalance and falls. The graph on the right illustrates this shift in the dominance of a specific sense with a shift in conditions. During the control of balance, the influence of somatosensory information decreases while the influence of vestibular information increases with increasing platform tilt; thus, body sway is minimized as participants shift and orient to gravitational vertical rather than the support surface.

This research suggests a number of things about how the CNS organizes and adapts sensory information for postural control. It supports the concept of hierarchical weighting of sensory inputs for postural control based on their relative accuracy in reporting the body's position and movements in space. In environments in which a sense is not providing optimal or accurate information regarding the body's position, the weight given to that sense as a source of orientation is reduced, while the weight of other more accurate senses is increased. Because of the redundancy of senses available for orientation and

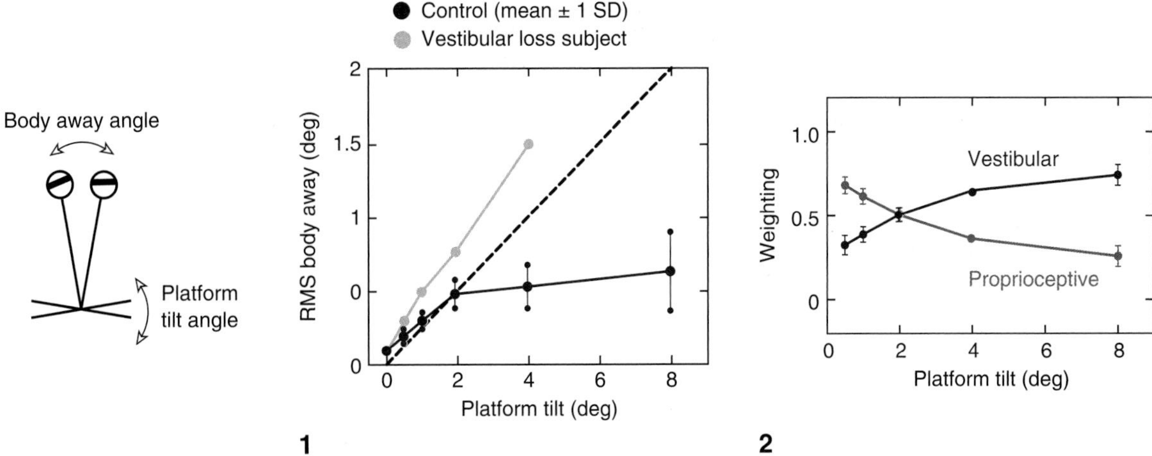

FIGURE 7.17 An experiment to illustrate the dynamic use of sensory information under varying conditions. In this experiment, human subjects stood blindfolded on a platform that rotated continuously in the toes-up—toes-down direction at amplitudes of up to 8 degrees peak-to-peak. 1. Body sway angle was measured relative to gravitational vertical during platform tilt and expressed as root mean square (RMS) sway in degrees in the graph on the left. The dashed line indicates equal platform and body sway; for example, for a platform tilt of 8 degrees peak-to-peak, an equal amount of body sway would be 2 degrees RMS. In control subjects (red trace) the body and platform sway were equal for small platform tilts up to 2 degrees, suggesting that people normally use somatosensory information to remain perpendicular to the platform (minimizing changes in ankle angle). With larger platform tilts, body sway does not increase; instead people rely on vestibular inputs and orient to gravitational vertical. In contrast, the person with vestibular loss (gray trace) sways with the platform at small platform tilts, but is unable to maintain balance at platform tilts above 4 degrees. 2. In control subjects, the influence of proprioceptive input decreases while that of vestibular input increases with increasing platform tilt. At higher tilt amplitudes, the greater influence of vestibular input minimizes the degree of body sway away from gravitational vertical. (Adapted from Peterka RJ. Sensorimotor integration in human postural control. J Neurophysiol 2002;88:1102, Figure 4.)

the ability of the CNS to modify the relative importance of any one sense for postural control, individuals are able to maintain stability in a variety of environments.

Adapting Senses When Learning a New Task

Thus far, we have talked about adapting sensory information in environments in which it is not appropriate to use a particular sense for postural control. A similar adaptation or change in the primary senses used for postural control appears to occur during the process of learning new motor skills. Lee and Lishman (1975) found increased reliance on visual inputs when adults were just learning a task. As the task became more automatic, there appeared to be a decrease in the relative importance of visual inputs for postural control and increased reliance on somatosensory inputs.

It has been suggested that adults recovering from a neurologic lesion also rely predominantly on vision during the early part of the recovery process. As motor skills, including postural control, are regained, patients become less reliant on vision, and are more able to use somatosensory inputs (Mulder et al., 1993).

Clinical Applications of Research on Sensory Organizational Aspects of Postural Control

As you can see from this review of the research on sensory aspects of postural control, the ability to organize and select appropriate sensory inputs is an important aspect of maintaining stability under changing task and environmental contexts. As discussed in Chapter 10, instability can result from not only the loss of an individual sensory input important to postural control (e.g., loss of vision or somatosensory inputs), but also from an inability to effectively organize and select sensory inputs appropriate to the task and environmental context. Balance rehabilitation must include clinical strategies for assessing both the integrity of individual sensory systems and the ability to organize sensory inputs for balance control. Clinical strategies for improving balance should include not only activities to improve the organization of muscle activity, but also the way in which sensory information is used for balance control. In the case when a specific sensory input is permanently lost (e.g., loss of vestibular inputs following head injury or some types of medications), activities that promote the reliance on alternative senses such as vision and somatosensory inputs can be used. Other strategies that promote the appropriate organization and selection of sensory inputs can be used when the problem is the context-specific organization of sensory inputs.

Anticipatory Postural Control

Did you ever pick up a box expecting it to be heavy and find it to be light? The fact that you lifted the box higher than you expected shows that your CNS preprogrammed force based on anticipation of what the task required. Based on previous experience with lifting other boxes of similar and different shapes and weights, the CNS forms a representation of what perception/action systems are needed to accomplish this task. It pretunes these systems for the task. Our mistakes are evidence that the CNS uses anticipatory processes in controlling action.

Perform Lab Activity 7.3. What you may notice through this lab experience is that you are able to use anticipatory postural adjustments when you are lifting the book out of your own hand, so that your hand does not involuntarily move upward, while you cannot use these adjustments when someone else is lifting the same book from your hand.

Research on the importance of anticipatory aspects of postural control began in the 1960s, when scientists in Russia first began to explore the way we use posture in an anticipatory manner to steady the execution of our skilled movements. In a paper published in 1967, Belen'kii, Gurfinkel, and Paltsev noted that when a standing adult is asked to raise the arm, both postural (leg and trunk) and prime mover (arm) muscles were activated. They observed that the postural muscle activation patterns could be divided into two parts. The first was a preparatory phase, in which postural muscles were activated more than 50 msec in advance of the prime mover muscles, to compensate in advance for the destabilizing effects of the movement. The second was a compensatory phase, in which the postural muscles were again activated after the prime movers, in a feedback manner, to stabilize the body further. They found that the sequence of postural muscles activated, and thus the manner of preparing for the movement, was specific to the task.

After it was discovered that postural responses involved in feedback control of posture were organized into distinct synergies (Nashner, 1977), an important question was raised: Are the synergies used in feedback postural control the same synergies that are used in anticipatory postural control? To answer this question, Cordo and Nashner (1982) performed experiments in which they asked standing subjects to forcefully push or pull on a handle, in a reaction-time task. They found that the same postural response synergies used in standing balance control were activated in an anticipatory fashion before the arm movements.

LAB ACTIVITY 7-3

Objective: To explore the use of anticipatory postural adjustments in a lifting task.

Procedure: Work with a partner. Tape a ruler vertically to the wall near where you are standing. Stand with your arm outstretched, at about waist height, palm up. Place a heavy book on your outstretched palm and have your partner note the vertical position of your hand on the ruler. Now, have your partner lift the book off that hand. Have your partner note the movement of your hand when he or she lifts the book. Reposition the book. Now, lift the book off your own hand with your opposite hand. Have your partner note the movement of your hand in this condition.

Assignment

Answer the following questions.

1. What did the hand holding the book do when your partner lifted the book? Was it steady? Or did it move upward as the book was lifted off?
2. How much did it move?
3. What happened when you lifted the book yourself? Was it steady? How much did it move?
4. In which of these two conditions is there evidence for anticipatory postural adjustments?
5. What was necessary for the anticipatory postural adjustment to occur?
6. How do your results compare with those of Hugon et al. (1982), explained below?

For example, when a person is asked to pull on a handle, first the gastrocnemius, hamstrings, and trunk extensors are activated and then the prime mover, the biceps of the arm, is activated.

One feature of postural adjustments associated with movement is their adaptability to the conditions of the task. In Cordo and Nashner's (1982) experiment, when the subjects leaned forward against a horizontal bar at chest height, the leg postural adjustments were reduced or disappeared. Thus, there is an immediate preselection of the postural muscles as a function of their ability to contribute appropriate support. Researchers refer to this preselection of tuning of sensorimotor systems for upcoming events as "central set." **Central set** refers to a state of the nervous system that is influenced or determined by the context of a task. In the previous example, leaning against a horizontal bar changed the context under which balance recovery would occur. This change in context was associated with a change in central set, such that certain muscles were selected in advance based on their ability to contribute to balance recovery in light of the new conditions. Change in central set enables the nervous system to optimize postural responses quickly under new conditions (Chong et al., 2000; Horak, 1996).

Although we usually think of anticipatory adjustments in terms of activating postural muscles in advance of a skilled movement, we also use anticipation when scaling the amplitude of postural adjustments to perturbations to balance. The amplitude of the muscle response is related to our expectations regarding the size or amplitude of the upcoming perturbation.

Horak et al. (1989a) examined the influence of prior experience and central set on the characteristics of postural adjustments by giving subjects platform perturbations under the following conditions: (a) serial versus random conditions, (b) expected versus unexpected conditions, and (c) practiced versus unpracticed conditions. They found that expectation played a large factor in modulating the amplitude of postural responses. For example, subjects overresponded when they expected a larger perturbation than they received and underresponded when they expected a smaller one.

Practice also caused a reduction in postural response magnitude and in the amplitude of antagonist muscle responses. However, central set did not affect EMG onset latencies. The authors noted that when different perturbations were presented in random order, all scaling disappeared. Evidently, scaling of postural responses is based on our anticipation of what is needed in a given situation.

It is important to realize that anticipatory postural adjustments are not isolated to tasks we perform while standing. Scientists from France and Switzerland, Hugon, Massion, and Wiesendanger (1982), first made this discovery in experiments in which they measured the EMGs of the biceps of both the left and right arms during a modification of the task just mentioned in Lab Activity 7.3. In this case, either the subject or the experimenter lifted a 1-kg weight from the subject's forearm (Fig. 7.18). They found that in the active unloading of the arm by the subject, there was preparatory biceps muscle inhibition to keep the arm from moving upward when it was unloaded. The anticipatory reduction in the biceps EMG of the arm holding the load was time-locked with the onset of the activation of the biceps of the lifting arm. This reduction was not observed in the passive unloading condition.

How are these anticipatory postural adjustments associated with movements organized by the CNS? Animal experiments performed by Massion and his colleagues looked at this question at the neural circuitry level (Massion, 1979). They trained animals to perform a leg-lifting task that required the animal to activate postural muscles simultaneously in the other three legs when it lifted the prime mover leg. They found that they could also directly stimulate the motor cortex or the red nucleus in the area of the forelimb flexors and produce the leg-lifting movement. When they did this, the movement was always accompanied by a postural adjustment in the other limbs, initiated in a feedforward manner. They hypothesized that the postural adjustments are organized at the bulbospinal (brainstem) level and that the pyramidal tract (from the motor cortex) activates these pathways as it sends descending commands to the prime mover muscle. Massion suggested that, while the basic mechanisms for postural adjustments could be organized at this level, they appear to be modulated by several other parts of the nervous system, including the cerebellum.

Visual Contributions to Anticipatory or Proactive Control

Visual inputs can influence postural control both reactively, as discussed above, and in an anticipatory manner. For example, visual cues about the configuration of the environment can determine the strategies that are used to respond to a slip or trip. To determine the proactive contributions of vision to balance-recovery experiments were performed in which young adults walked into a room and then were instructed to use a handrail to recover balance in response to a platform translation (movement of the feet was blocked). Liquid crystal goggles were used to occlude vision during response initiation, just after the platform movement onset (Ghafouri et al., 2004). Results showed that

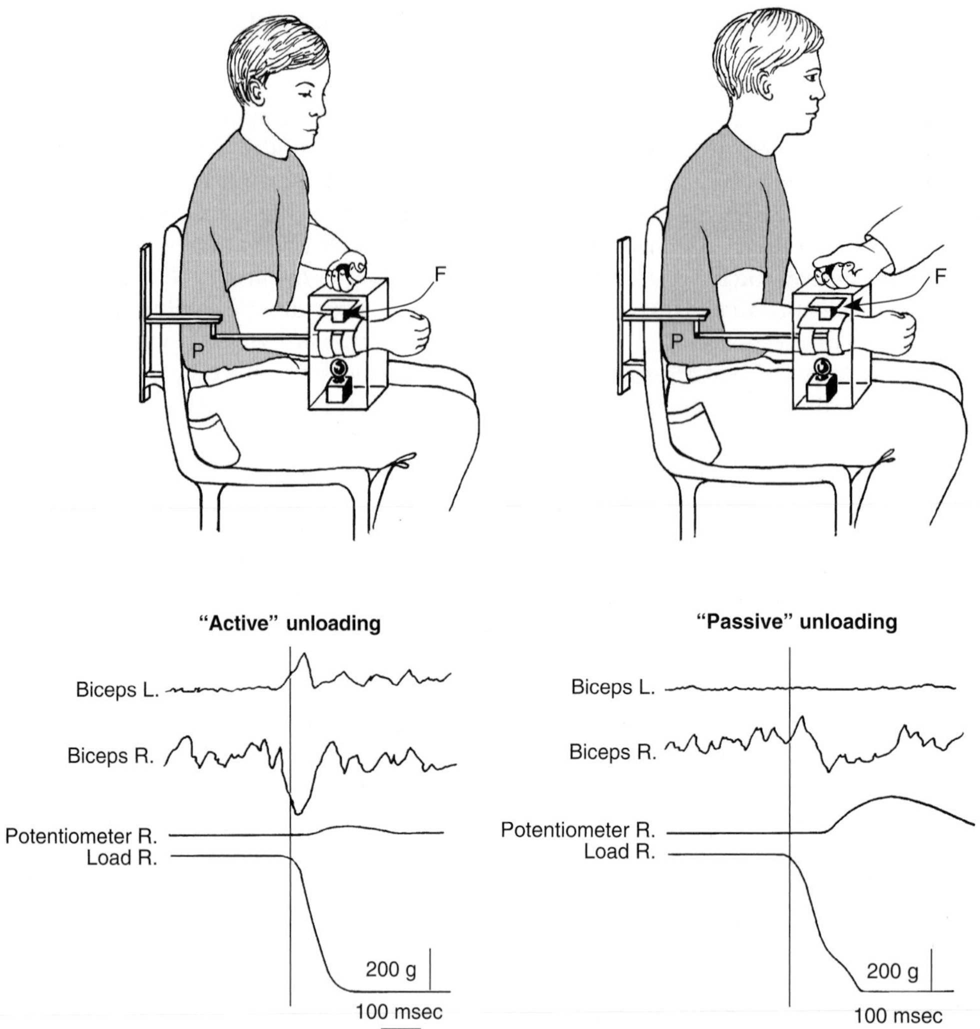

FIGURE 7.18 Experiments examining anticipatory postural activity associated with lifting a weight from a subject's arm. (Adapted from Hugon M, Massion J, Wiesendanger M. Anticipatory postural changes induced by active unloading and comparison with passive unloading in man. Pflugers Arch 1982;393:292–296.)

the initial grasping trajectory was not affected by visual occlusion, indicating that information about the location of the railing was obtained prior to the perturbation onset, probably through the creation of an egocentric spatial map created upon entering the room. This thus ensures very rapid and accurate response onsets to unexpected balance threats.

Clinical Applications of Research on Anticipatory Postural Control

As researchers identify the factors that determine the necessity for anticipatory postural control, this information can be used in a therapeutic environment to facilitate anticipatory control of posture during voluntary movements. Research has shown that behavioral context and speed of the focal movement affect anticipatory aspects of postural control. When subjects are told to move as fast as possible, versus at a comfortable speed, postural responses tend to be earlier and more reliably activated (Horak et al., 1984; Lee et al., 1987). This suggests that asking patients who are having difficulty activating postural muscles in advance of voluntary movement to move quickly may facilitate the activation of postural muscle activity. Researchers have shown that the weight of the load to be moved also influences anticipatory postural muscle activity (Bouisset & Zattara, 1981; Horak et al., 1984). The heavier the load, the more likely it is to engender instability and thus an anticipatory postural response. Therefore, asking patients to move heavier objects at faster speeds increases the likelihood that anticipatory postural adjustments will accompany movements. Activation of lower-limb muscles tends to precede that of prime-mover muscles in tasks that require raising an arm or pulling or pushing on an object.

Research has shown that when support is given during performance of a voluntary task, there is a reduction in anticipatory postural activity. For example, when pulling a lever while steadying yourself with your other arm, the first muscles activated are in the arm used to steady yourself. However, when doing the same task with no upper-limb support, leg muscles are activated first (Marsden et al., 1977). This means that if external support is provided to the patient who is having difficulty activating postural muscles in advance of prime movers, functional arm movements are likely to improve. Gradually removing the available support while functional arm movements are practiced may facilitate the activation of anticipatory postural activity. Finally, the degree of practice has also been shown to influence the timing of anticipatory postural adjustments. Dancers have been shown to activate anticipatory postural adjustments in a leg-lifting task significantly earlier than nondancers (Brauer, 1998; Mouchnino et al., 1992). This suggests the possibility that practicing tasks that require anticipatory postural activity may increase the efficacy of this component of postural control over time. More research is needed to see whether these results could be applied to training anticipatory control in patients with neurologic pathology.

Cognitive Systems in Postural Control

Since normal postural control occurs automatically, without conscious effort, it was traditionally assumed that few attentional resources were needed when controlling balance. However, research examining changes in postural control during the performance of another attentionally demanding task, referred to as dual-task interference, has suggested that there are significant attentional requirements for postural control. In addition, it appears that attentional requirements are not constant, but vary depending on the postural task, on the age of the individual, and on the individual's balance abilities (Woollacott & Shumway-Cook, 2002).

Before discussing dual-task research examining the attentional requirements of postural control it is necessary to introduce concepts related to attentional processing from psychology. There are two primary theories to explain interference between two tasks that are performed at the same time. The first, capacity theory, considers dual-task interference to result from the sharing of a limited set of information processing (i.e., attentional) resources. In this case, when processing demands of the two combined tasks exceed attentional capacity, reduced performance is observed on one or both tasks. The second, bottleneck theory, hypothesizes the sequential nature of the dual-task process and proposes that there is competition between tasks for stimulus encoding, identification, or response selection. In this case, it is proposed that the nervous system delays information-processing operations on one task in favor of operations on the prioritized task, which causes impaired performance on the nonprioritized task (Fraizer & Mitra, 2008; Neumann, 1984; Shumway-Cook & Woollacott, 2000; Wickens, 1989).

Research methods for studying attention and posture control use dual-task paradigms in which postural task (often considered the primary task) and a secondary cognitive task are performed together. A decrease in performance on either task suggests interference (either due to limited resources or to task competition within a processing bottleneck) between the processes controlling the two tasks, and therefore the amount of attentional resources that are shared (Kerr et al., 1985).

Kerr and colleagues (1985) performed the first research to demonstrate the attentional demands of stance postural control. They hypothesized that a difficult balance task would interfere with a spatial (visual) memory but not a verbal memory task, because postural control is assumed to involve visual/spatial processing. The visual/spatial cognitive task was the Brooks spatial memory task, which involved placing numbers in imagined matrices and then remembering the position of these numbers. The nonspatial verbal memory task involved remembering similar sentences. They found that performing the memory task with the concurrent balance task caused an increase in the number of errors in the spatial but not the nonspatial memory task and that there was no significant difference in postural sway during the performance of either cognitive task. They concluded that postural control in young adults is attentionally demanding; however, not all cognitive tasks interact with postural control processing in the same way. It could be hypothesized that this was due to the postural and visual spatial task competing for the same visual processing channels (bottleneck theory).

A study by Lajoie et al. (1993) determined that attentional demands vary as a function of the type of postural task being performed. They asked young adults to perform an auditory reaction-time task while sitting, standing with a normal versus a reduced base of support, and during walking (single- vs. double-support phase). They found that reaction times were fastest for sitting and slowed for the standing (slower in narrow stance than normal stance) and walking (slower for single-support phase compared with double support) tasks. They concluded that as the demand for stability increases, there is a concomitant increase in attentional resources used by the postural control system, competing for limited attentional resources (capacity theory).

The performance of a secondary task does not always have a detrimental effect on postural control. Stoffregen et al. (2000) showed that when individuals were asked to fixate on a visual target and perform a visual task (counting the frequency of letters in a block of text) they showed less sway than when inspecting a blank target. In addition, focusing on a near target caused sway to be reduced relative to focusing on a distant target. In this case, postural control is enhanced, not reduced, during the performance of a secondary task. The authors conclude that postural control is organized as part of an integrated perception/action system and can be modified to facilitate the performance of other tasks.

Similar to the results of Stoffregen and colleagues, other researchers have shown that adding a variety of secondary tasks can reduce both stance sway and sway variability in young adults, and offer other possible explanations for these findings (Huxhold et al., 2006; Riley et al., 2005; Vuillerme & Nafati, 2007). For example, Huxhold et al. (2006) showed that when young adults were asked to perform a secondary task (working memory task, in which they had to remember numbers presented 1, 2, or 3 items back in an auditory recording) while standing with feet shoulder width apart, they showed reduced postural sway in the dual-task condition. The authors proposed that improvements in postural control under these dual-task conditions was due to the possibility that directing subjects' attention to a highly automatic process like postural control may actually reduce the efficacy of postural mechanisms, and that directing attention toward a secondary task may actually improve the automaticity and efficacy of the postural-control processes. Other researchers have proposed that reduced sway in a dual-task setting may be due to heightened arousal when performing a secondary task, causing improved performance (Andersson et al., 2002). It is interesting that though these effects are typically present in young adults, they are only present in older or balance-impaired individuals when performing a very simple cognitive task; with increased cognitive task difficulty, postural sway and variability increases in older and balance-impaired populations (Huxhold et al., 2006).

These experiments suggest that postural control is attentionally demanding in young adults and that some secondary tasks can increase postural sway (often interpreted as interference with postural control), but others decrease sway (often interpreted as improved postural control). In addition, in healthy young adults, attentional effects are small unless you increase the difficulty of the postural-control task or, alternatively, ask subjects to perform more complex secondary tasks. As will be discussed in later chapters, the attentional demands associated with postural control appear to be different in older adults with balance impairments and individuals with neurologic impairment.

Clinical Implications of Research on Cognitive Aspects of Postural Control

This research reminds us that the attentional demands of postural control are very dynamic and depend on many factors. In healthy young adults, postural control is automatic, that is, relatively low in attentional demands, but can increase as postural-task complexity increases. Many patients with neurologic pathology demonstrate impaired dual task performance. This could be the result of either impaired balance control and subsequent loss of automaticity or deficits in attentional processing. Clinical strategies are needed to effectively distinguish between these two possibilities, so that appropriate interventions can be created.

SEATED POSTURAL CONTROL

The maintenance of postural control in the seated position has not been studied to the extent that stance postural control has. However, many scientists believe that concepts important for stance postural control will be shown to be equally valid for understanding postural control in sitting.

Forssberg and Hirshfeld (1994) compared postural responses elicited by platform translations versus rotations in subjects seated with the legs extended forward. The authors noted that forward platform movements causing the body to sway backward elicited well-organized, consistent responses in the quadriceps, abdominal, and neck flexor muscles at 63 ± 12 msec, 74 ± 21 msec, and 77 ± 10 msec, respectively. Similar responses were elicited by legs-up rotations. However, in response to backward platform perturbations, causing forward sway, smaller and more variable responses were elicited in the trunk and neck extensor muscles. These differences reflect the asymmetry of the stability limits during sitting.

The authors suggest that the postural control system sets a threshold for activation of postural responses according to an internal representation of the body, including the relationship between the center of gravity and the support surface. Since the rotational and translational perturbations caused very different head movements, but very similar muscle response patterns, the authors conclude that somatosensory inputs from the backward rotation of the pelvis trigger the postural response synergies in sitting.

Experiments have also been performed to examine the characteristics of anticipatory postural adjustments used in reaching for an object while sitting (Moore et al., 1992). Researchers found that increased reach distance and decreased support were associated with earlier, larger postural adjustments. It has also been shown that leg muscles are consistently active during anticipatory postural adjustments in advance of voluntary reaching while sitting (Shepherd et al., 1993).

SUMMARY

1. The task of postural control involves controlling the body's position in space for: (a) stability, defined as controlling the center of body mass relative to the base of support, and (b) orientation, defined as the ability to maintain an appropriate relationship between the body segments, and between the body and the environment for a task.
2. A number of factors contribute to postural control during quiet stance (so-called steady-state or static balance), including: (a) body alignment, which minimizes the effect of gravitational forces, (b) muscle tone, and (c) postural tone, which keeps the body from collapsing in response to the pull of gravity.
3. When quiet stance is perturbed, the recovery of stability requires movement strategies that are effective in controlling the center of mass relative to the base of support.
4. Movement patterns used to recover stance balance from sagittal-plane instability are referred to as ankle, hip, and suspensory/or stepping strategies. Normal subjects can shift relatively quickly from one postural movement strategy to another.
5. The CNS activates synergistic muscles at mechanically related joints, possibly to ensure that forces generated at one joint for balance control do not produce instability elsewhere in the body.
6. Inputs from visual, somatosensory (proprioceptive, cutaneous, and joint receptors), and vestibular systems are important sources of information about the body's position and movement in space with respect to gravity and the environment. Each sense provides the CNS with a different kind of information about position and motion of the body; thus, each sense provides a different frame of reference for postural control.
7. In adults, all three senses contribute to postural control during quiet stance; in contrast, in response to transient perturbations, adults tend to rely on somatosensory inputs, while young children rely more heavily on visual inputs.
8. Because of the redundancy of senses available for orientation and the ability of the CNS to modify the importance of any one sense for postural control, individuals are able to maintain stability in a variety of environments.
9. Postural adjustments are also activated before voluntary movements to minimize potential disturbances to balance that the movement may cause. This is called "anticipatory postural control."
10. Postural control requires attentional processing, and thus can reduce the performance of a second task performed simultaneously. In addition, complex secondary tasks can, in some cases, reduce the performance of a concurrently performed postural task. However, attention to some secondary tasks improves postural control, either through improving the automaticity of postural control, through increased arousal, or through the use of reduced postural sway to support the efficiency of performance of the suprapostural task.
11. The maintenance of postural control in the seated position has not been studied in depth. However, many scientists believe that concepts important for stance postural control will be shown to be equally valid for postural control in sitting.

ANSWERS TO LAB ACTIVITY ASSIGNMENTS

Lab Activity 7-1

1. You probably moved slightly, since it is rare to stand perfectly still. You also would typically move most in the anteroposterior direction, but there would also be a certain amount of mediolateral sway.
2. Movement would be at the ankle for small amounts of anteroposterior sway; movements would be about the hip when swaying close to your stability limits.
3. The toes came up when responding to the light nudge, indicating that the tibialis anterior muscle was activated; you probably took a step backward in response to a harder nudge.

4. (a) It would be easier to balance using an ankle strategy with a larger base of support; (b) harder to recover from a faster movement; (c) hardest to respond with an ankle movement when the COM was already close to the edge of the base of support; a person tends to use a hip or stepping strategy; and (d) could not use ankle strategy, so would shift to movement about the hips.
5. (a) One would use predominantly ankle muscles for anteroposterior sway, hip muscles for mediolateral sway. (b) Hip muscles. (c) Took a step.

Lab Activity 7-2

1. **Condition 1:** Firm surface (e.g., linoleum or wood) with feet together, hands on hips, and eyes open. Sensory cues available: vision, vestibular, somatosensory.
   Shoulder displacement amplitude: low levels.
   Condition 2: Eyes closed, firm surface: Sensory cues available: somatosensory, vestibular.
   Shoulder displacement amplitude: slightly higher.
   Condition 3: Feet together on the foam, with eyes open. Sensory cues available: vision, vestibular, distorted somatosensory.
   Shoulder displacement amplitude: higher than in conditions 1 and 2.
   Condition 4: Feet together on foam with eyes closed. Sensory cues available: vestibular, distorted somatosensory.
   Shoulder displacement amplitude: highest of the four conditions.
2. It becomes larger as sensory cues are removed or made less accurate.
3. They should be similar in relative amplitude for the same four conditions.

Lab Activity 7-3

1. It moved upward.
2. This will vary depending on the person: if a person is very relaxed, the hand may move more, if the person is very stiff, it may move less.
3. It was nearly steady, moving very little, if at all.
4. The second.
5. The lifting of the book must be internally generated rather than externally generated.
6. They are similar: when his subject lifts the weight the arm does not move, due to anticipatory inhibition of the biceps muscle, but when someone else lifts the weight, the arm moves up, as there is no anticipatory inhibition of biceps.

CHAPTER 8

DEVELOPMENT OF POSTURAL CONTROL

LEARNING OBJECTIVES

Following completion of this chapter, the reader will be able to:

1. Describe the reflex/hierarchical theory of postural control and the specific reflexes and reactions that are hypothesized to contribute to the development of postural control according to this view.
2. Describe the systems approach to the study of balance development and the systems that are considered critical for the emergence of balance control from this perspective.
3. Discuss the development of head, trunk, and stance postural control from a systems perspective, describing the research showing the contributions of sensory, motor, and higher-level adaptive systems to the emergence of steady state, reactive, and proactive control underlying these different developmental stages of postural control.
4. Discuss the research on the validity of reflex/hierarchical theory to balance development and compare predictions of the reflex/hierarchical and systems theories regarding the origins of the emergence of head, trunk, and stance balance.

INTRODUCTION

During the early years of life, children develop an incredible repertoire of skills, including crawling, independent walking and running, climbing, eye–hand coordination, and the manipulation of objects in a variety of ways. The emergence of all these skills requires the development of postural activity to support the primary movement.

To understand the emergence of mobility and manipulatory skills in children, therapists need to understand the postural substrate for these skills. Similarly, understanding the best therapeutic approach for a child with difficulties in walking or reaching skills requires the knowledge of any limitations in their postural abilities. Understanding the basis for postural development, then, is the first step in determining the best therapeutic approach for improving related skills.

This chapter discusses the research on the development of postural control and how it contributes to the emergence of stability and mobility skills. Later chapters consider the implications of this research when assessing and treating postural control in nontypical populations.

Postural Control and Development

Let's first look at some of the evidence showing that postural control is a critical part of motor development. Research on early development has shown that the simultaneous development of the postural, locomotor, and manipulative systems is essential to the emergence and refinement of skills in all these areas. In a neonate, when the chaotic movements of the head that regularly disturb the infant's seated balance are stabilized, movements and behaviors normally seen in more mature infants emerge (Amiel-Tison &

Grenier, 1980). For example, as shown in Figure 8.1, when the clinician stabilizes the head of a newborn, he or she may begin to attend to the clinician, reach for objects, and maintain his or her arms at the sides, with the fingers open, suggesting inhibition of the grasp and Moro reflexes.

These results support the concept that an immature postural system is a limiting factor or a constraint on the emergence of other behaviors, such as coordinated arm and hand movements, as well as the inhibition of reflexes. It has also been suggested that delayed or abnormal development of the postural system may also constrain a child's ability to develop independence in mobility and manipulatory skills.

Motor Milestones and Emerging Postural Control

The development of postural control has traditionally been associated with a predictable sequence of motor behaviors, referred to as "motor milestones." Some of the major motor milestones in development are shown in Figure 8.2. They include crawling, sitting, creeping, pull-to-stand, independent stance, and walking. The sequence and timing of the emergence of these motor milestones has been well described by several developmental researchers.

In 1946, Arnold Gesell, a pediatrician, described the emergence of general patterns of behavior in the first few years of life. He noted the general direction of behavioral development as moving from head to foot, and proximally to distally within segments. Thus, he formulated the law of developmental direction (Gesell, 1946). In addition, Gesell portrayed development as a spiraling hierarchy. He suggested that the development of skilled behavior does not follow a strict linear sequence, always advancing, constantly improving with time and maturity. Instead, Gesell believed that development is much more dynamic in nature and seems to be characterized by alternating advancement and regression in the ability to perform skills.

Gesell gave the example of children learning to crawl and then creep. Initially, in learning to crawl, the child uses a primarily symmetrical arm pattern, eventually switching to a more complex alternating arm pattern as the skill of crawling is perfected. When the child first begins to creep, there is a return to the symmetrical arm pattern. Eventually, as creeping becomes perfected, the emergence of an alternating arm pattern occurs. Thus, as children progress to each new stage in the development of a skill, they may appear to regress to an earlier form of the behavior as new, more mature and adaptive, versions of these skills emerge.

Most of the traditional assessment scales created to evaluate the emergence of motor behaviors use developmental norms established by McGraw (1932) and Gesell. Using these scales, the therapist evaluates the performance of the infant or child on functional skills that require postural control. These skills include sitting, standing, walking unsupported, reaching forward, and moving from a sitting to a standing position. Examples of developmental tests and measures include the Gross Motor Function Measure (GMFM) (Russell et al., 1993), the Peabody Developmental Motor Scales (Folio & Fewell, 1983), the Bayley Scales of Infant Development (Bayley, 1969), and the Movement Assessment of Infants (Chandler et al., 1980). These and other tests follow normal development and are used to identify children at risk for developmental problems.

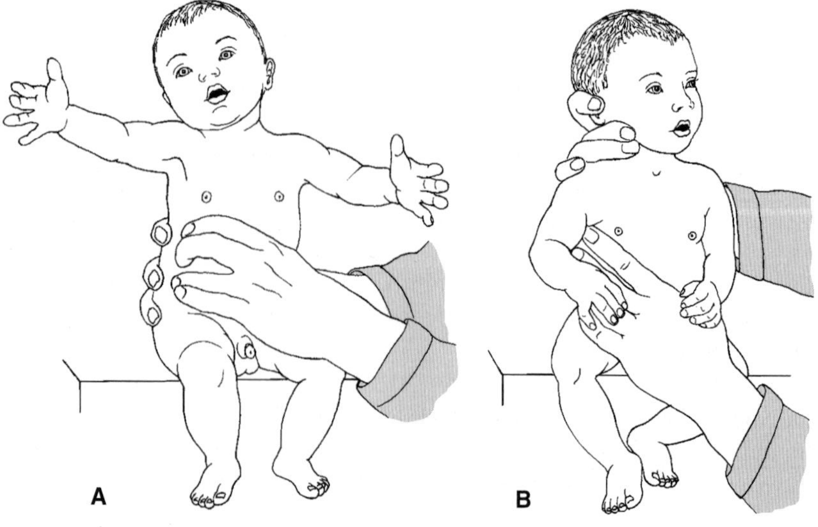

FIGURE 8.1 Stabilizing the head in a neonate can produce dramatic changes in behavior. A, Uncontrolled movements of the head produce a Moro response. B, External support to the child's head and trunk results in more mature behaviors, including attending to people and objects, and even reaching. (Adapted from Amiel-Tison C, Grenier A. Evaluation neurologique du nouveau-né et du nourrisson. [Neurological evaluation of the human infant.] New York: Masson, 1980:82).

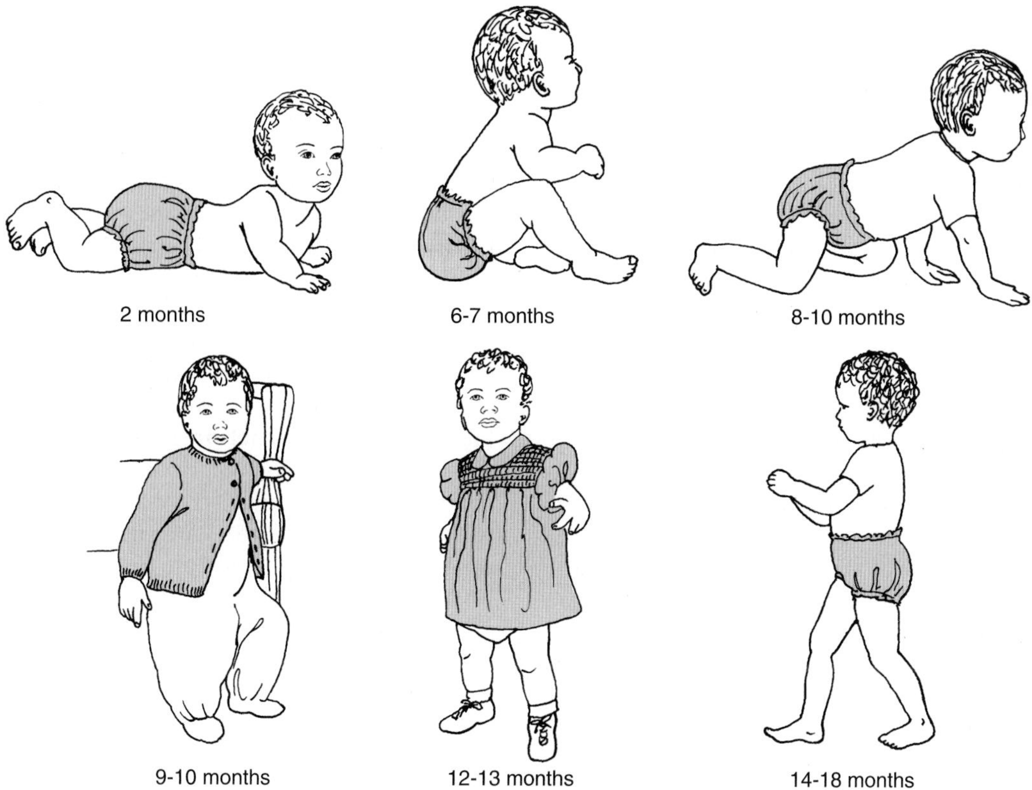

FIGURE 8.2 Motor milestones that emerge with the development of postural control, including crawling (2 months), sitting (6–7 months), creeping (8–10 months), pull-to-stand (9–10 months), independent stance (12–13 months), and walking (14–18 months). (Adapted from Shumway-Cook A, Woollacott M. Theoretical issues in assessing postural control. In: Wilhelm I, ed. Physical therapy assessment in early infancy. New York: Churchill Livingstone, 1993:163.)

THEORIES OF DEVELOPING POSTURAL CONTROL

What is the basis for the development of postural control underlying this predictable sequence of motor behaviors? Several theories of child development try to relate neural structure and behavior in developing infants. Classic theories of child development place great importance on a reflex substrate for the emergence of mature human behavior patterns. This means that in the normal child the emergence of posture and movement control is dependent on the appearance and subsequent integration of reflexes. According to these theories, the appearance and disappearance of these reflexes reflect the increasing maturity of cortical structures that inhibit and integrate reflexes controlled at lower levels within the central nervous system (CNS) into more functional postural and voluntary motor responses (see Fig. 1.5). This classic theory has been referred to as a reflex/hierarchical theory (Horak & Shumway-Cook, 1990; Woollacott & Shumway-Cook, 1990).

Alternatively, more recent theories of motor control, such as the dynamic systems and ecological theories, have suggested that postural control emerges from a complex interaction of musculo-skeletal and neural systems collectively referred to as the "postural control system." The organization of elements within the postural control system is determined by both the task and the environment. Systems theory does not deny the existence of reflexes, but considers them as only one of many influences on the control of posture and movement.

Let's briefly review the reflexes that have been associated with the emergence of postural control.

Reflex-Hierarchical Theory of Postural Control

Postural reflexes were studied in the early part of 20th century by investigators such as Magnus (1926), DeKleijn (1923), Rademaker (1924), and Schaltenbrand (1928). In this early work, researchers selectively produced lesions in different parts of the CNS and examined an animal's capacity to orient. Magnus and associates took the animal down to what they referred to as the "zero condition," a condition in which no postural reflex activity could be elicited. Subsequent animals received selective lesions, leaving systematically greater and greater amounts of the CNS intact. In this way, Magnus identified individually and collectively all the reflexes that worked cooperatively to maintain postural orientation in various types of animals.

Postural reflexes in animals were classified by Magnus as local static reactions, segmental static reactions, general static reactions, and righting reactions. **Local static reactions** stiffen the animal's limb for support of body weight against gravity. **Segmental static reactions** involve more than one body segment and include the flexor withdrawal reflex and the crossed extensor reflex. **General static reactions**, called "attitudinal reflexes," involve changes in position of the whole body in response to changes in head position. Finally, Magnus described a series of five **righting reactions**, which allowed the animal to assume or resume a species-specific orientation of the body with respect to its environment.

Postural Reflexes in Human Development

Many researchers have tried to document accurately the time frame for the appearance and disappearance of postural reflexes in normal children, with widely varying results. There is little agreement on the presence and time course of these reflexes, or on the significance of these reflexes to normal and abnormal development (Claverie et al., 1973).

Attitudinal Reflexes. According to the reflex theory of postural control, tonic attitudinal reflexes produce persisting changes in body posture that result from a change in head position, and include: (a) the asymmetric tonic neck reflex (ATNR), (b) the symmetric tonic neck reflex (STNR) (shown in Figure 8.3A), and (c) the tonic labyrinthine reflex (TLR) (Milani-Comparetti & Gidoni, 1967). The ATNR produces extension in the face arm, and flexion in the skull arm when the head is turned. The STNR results in flexion in the upper extremities and extension in the lower extremities when the head is flexed; however, when the head is extended, the upper extremities extend while the lower extremities flex.

Righting Reactions. According to a reflex/hierarchical model, the interaction of five righting reactions produces orientation of the head in space and orientation of the body in relationship to the head and ground. Righting reactions are considered automatic reactions that enable a person to assume the normal standing position and maintain stability when changing positions (Barnes et al., 1978). Three righting reactions (Fig. 8.3B) orient the head in space, and include: (a) the **optical righting reaction**, which contributes to the reflex orientation of the head using visual inputs; (b) the **labyrinthine righting reaction**, which orients the head to an upright vertical position in response to vestibular signals (Ornitz, 1983; Peiper, 1963); and (c) the **body-on-head righting reaction,** which orients the head in response to proprioceptive and tactile signals from the body in contact with a supporting surface. The **Landau reaction** combines the effects of all three head-righting reactions (Cupps et al., 1976). Two reflexes interact to keep the body oriented with respect to the head and the surface. The **neck-on-body righting reaction** (Fig. 8.3C) orients the body in response to cervical afferents, which report changes in the position of the head and neck. The **body-on-body righting reaction,** shown in Figure 8.3C, right, keeps the body oriented with respect to the ground, regardless of the position of the head.

Balance and Protective Reactions. According to reflex/hierarchical theory, balance emerges in association with a sequentially organized series of equilibrium reactions, including the **tilting reactions** (Fig. 8.3D), used for controlling the center of gravity in response to a tilting surface; the **parachute,** or **protective, responses** (Fig. 8.3E), which protect the body from injury during a fall; and the staggering reactions (sideways stepping), a response to instability in the lateral direction.

Figure 8.19 summarizes the times of appearance of postural reflexes purported to underlie the emergence of postural control in children.

Role of Reflexes in Development

What is the role of reflexes in motor development? Scientists do not know for sure; as a result, the role of reflexes in motor control is controversial. Many theorists believe that reflexes form the substrate for normal motor control. For example, it has been suggested that the asymmetric tonic neck reflex is part of the developmental process of eye–hand coordination since movement of the head (and eyes) brings the hand within view (Coryell & Henderson, 1979; Gesell, 1954). However, another study showed no relationship between reaching behavior and the presence or absence of this reflex in a group of infants 2 to 4 months old (Larson et al., 1990). The neck-on-body and body-on-body righting reactions are reported to be the basis for rolling in infants; the persistence of the immature form of

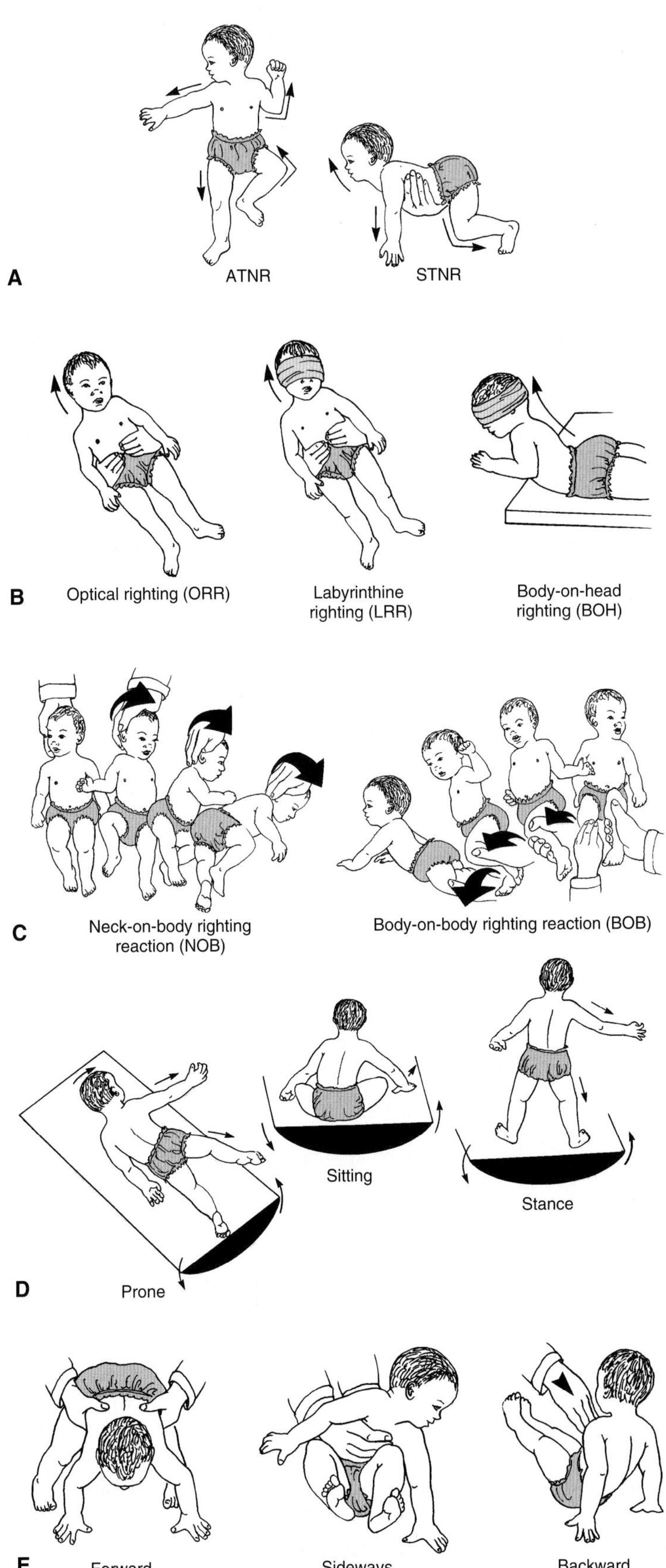

FIGURE 8.3 A, Attitudinal reflexes. Left, The ATNR reflex: extension in the face arm, and flexion in the skull arm when the head is turned. Right, The STNR reflex: head flexion causes flexion of the upper extremities and extension of the lower extremities; head extension causes extension in the upper extremities and flexion in the lower extremities. B, Righting reactions that orient the head. Left, The optical righting reaction orients the head to visual vertical. Center, The labyrinthine righting reaction orients the head in response to vestibular signals signaling vertical. Right, The body-on-head righting reaction uses tactile and neck proprioceptive information to orient the head to vertical. C, Righting reactions of the body. Shown are the mature form of (L), the neck-on-body righting reaction (left) and the body-on-body righting reaction (right). D, Tilting reactions. Tilting responses are purported to emerge first in prone (left), then supine (not shown), then sitting (center), then emerge in all fours (not shown), and finally, standing (right). E, Protective reactions. These reactions protect the body from injury resulting from a fall, and develop first in the forward direction (left), then sideways (center), and then backward (right). (Adapted from Barnes MR, Crutchfield CA, Heriza CB. The neurophysiological basis of patient treatment. Morgantown, WV: Stokesville, 1978:222.)

rolling at 4 months of age is purported to be predictive of CNS pathology, including cerebral palsy (Campbell & Wilhelm, 1985). However, the role of these reflexes in more mature rolling patterns has been questioned (VanSant, 1990). Clearly, there is considerable uncertainty about the contribution of reflex testing in clarifying the basis for normal and abnormal development in children.

New Models of Development

Many of the newer theories of motor control presented in Chapter 1 have associated theories of motor development. These newer theories are consistent in suggesting that development involves much more than the maturation of reflexes within the CNS. Development is a complex process, with new behaviors and skills emerging from an interaction of the child (and the maturing nervous and musculoskeletal system) with the environment.

With this framework, the emergence of postural control is likewise ascribed to complex interactions between neural and musculoskeletal systems. These include (see Fig. 7.3):

1. Changes in the musculoskeletal system, including development of muscle strength and changes in relative mass of the different body segments;
2. Development or construction of the coordinative structures or neuromuscular response synergies used in maintaining balance;
3. Development of individual sensory systems, including somatosensory, visual, or vestibular systems;
4. Development of sensory strategies for organizing these multiple inputs;
5. Development of internal representations important in the mapping of perception to action; and
6. Development of adaptive and anticipatory mechanisms that allow children to modify the way they sense and move for postural control (Woollacott, 1989).

An important part of interpreting senses and coordinating actions for postural control is the presence of an internal representation or body schema providing a postural frame of reference. It has been hypothesized that this postural frame of reference is used as a comparison for incoming sensory inputs, as an essential part of interpreting self-motion, and to calibrate motor actions (Gurfinkel & Levik, 1978).

Development of sensory and motor aspects of postural control has been hypothesized to involve the capacity to build up appropriate internal representations related to posture that reflect the rules for organizing sensory inputs and coordinating them with motor actions. For example, as the child gains experience moving in a gravity environment, sensory/motor maps would develop. These maps would relate actions to incoming sensory inputs from visual, somatosensory, and vestibular systems. In this way, rules for moving would develop and be reflected in altered synaptic relationships. Thus, researchers argue, the path from sensation to motor actions proceeds via an internal representational structure or body schema (Gurfinkel & Levik, 1978; Hirschfeld, 1992).

Examination Based on Newer Models

According to these newer theories, examination of early motor development includes examining both emerging behavioral motor milestones and the supporting systems for that behavior such as postural control. In addition, examination must occur within the context of different tasks and environments. The child's capacity to anticipate and adapt to a changing environment, as evidenced by variability of performance, is also included in an analysis of development. The ability to adapt how we sense and how we move is a critical part of normal development; as a result, it is as crucial to assess as the acquisition of stereotypical motor milestones.

Since different systems affecting postural control develop at different rates, it is important to understand which components are rate limiting at each developmental stage, or conversely, which ones push the system to a new level of function when they have matured. According to newer models of development, finding the connection between critical postural components and development ultimately guides the clinician in determining which systems should be examined and how the contribution of these systems changes at various developmental stages. It also allows the clinician to determine appropriate interventions specific to the system that is dysfunctional.

DEVELOPMENT OF POSTURAL CONTROL: A SYSTEMS PERSPECTIVE

Since Gesell's original studies in 1946 describing the cephalocaudal nature of development, many researchers have found exceptions to some of his general developmental rules. For example, some studies have found that infants show control of the legs in kicking and supported walking behaviors well before they can control their head and trunk in space (Forssberg, 1985; Thelen et al., 1989). However, in the area of balance and postural control, it does appear as if development follows a cephalocaudal sequence.

General Movements in Infants

Heinz Prechtl (1986), a researcher and physician from the Netherlands, has studied the general movements that are part of the spontaneous repertoire of infants from fetal development through the end of the first 6 months of life, when intentional and antigravity movements become more predominant. He has noted that these general movements are complex, involving the whole body (arm, leg, neck, and trunk movements in variable sequences), and occur often. They appear to have a gradual beginning and ending, and vary in intensity and velocity, showing coordination and fluidity. Also found in normally developing infants are so-called fidgety movements, small movements of the neck, trunk, and limbs performed at medium speed. These are the predominant movement patterns seen in awake typically developing 3-to-5-month-olds. His research also indicates that when the nervous system is impaired, movements become monotonous and poorly differentiated. In fact, two specific changes in the movement patterns have been reliably shown to predict a later diagnosis of cerebral palsy. These include: (1) cramped-synchronized general movements (lacking a normal fluid character) and (2) absence of general movements of a fidgety character (Einspieler & Prechtl, 2005).

Prechtl also used ultrasound techniques to study the spontaneous postural behavior of infants during prenatal development. He observed spontaneous postural changes and described several different motor patterns responsible for these changes. Positional changes occurred as often as 20 times per hour in the first half of pregnancy, but decreased in later pregnancy, perhaps because of space restriction.

Emerging Head Control

Motor Coordination

Prechtl and colleagues also observed spontaneous head control in neonates and noted that infants had very poor postural or antigravity control at birth. They hypothesized that this could be due either to lack of muscle strength (a musculoskeletal constraint) or, alternatively, to lack of maturity of the motor processes controlling posture of the head and neck at this age (motor coordination constraint). To test this, they examined spontaneous head movements using both electromyographic (EMG) and video recordings to determine whether coordinated muscle activity was present. They found no organized patterns of muscle activity that appeared to counteract the force of gravity on any consistent basis. This finding suggests that the lack of head control in newborns is not solely the result of a lack of strength, but also results from a lack of organized muscle activity (Schloon et al., 1976).

Experiments examining infants' development of reactive balance control have been performed in many labs (Harbourne et al., 1993; Hedberg et al., 2005; Hirschfeld & Forssberg, 1994; Woollacott et al., 1987). Figure 8.4 shows a typical experimental paradigm for the examination of reactive balance development in

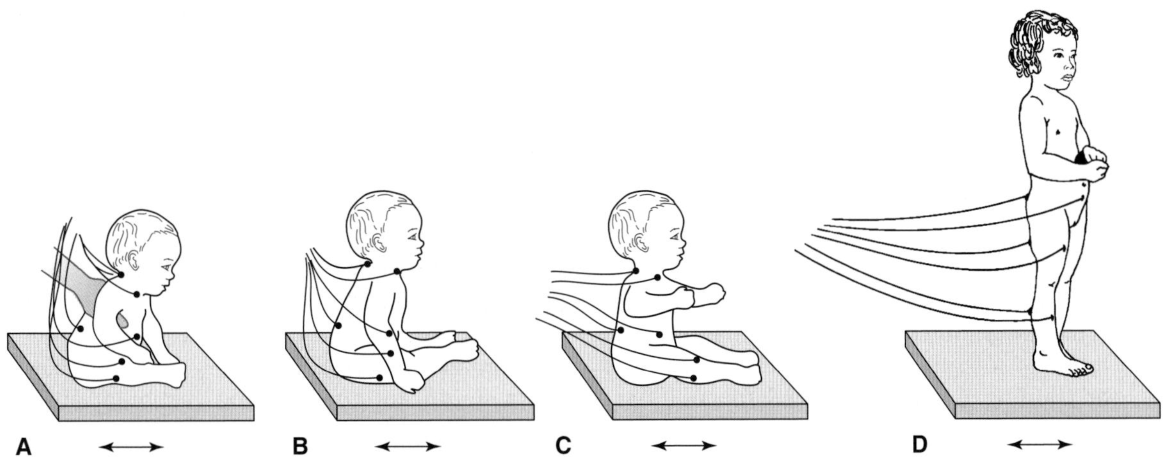

FIGURE 8.4 Moving platform posturography used to study postural response patterns in infants in response to a moving surface in various stages of sitting. A, Stage 1, holding up head with trunk support. B, Stage 2, propping on arms during sitting or sitting independently for brief periods. C, Stage 3, sitting independently without falling. D, Standing. (Adapted from Harbourne RT, Stergiou N. Nonlinear analysis of the development of sitting postural control. Dev Psychobiol 2003;42:368.)

infants of varying developmental levels. Infants are placed on the platform with surface electrodes used to record muscle responses in the neck, trunk, and legs. Infants who are unable to sit independently are given support by the experimenter before the perturbation as needed. They are released just after the platform begins to move in order to examine unsupported balance control. This figure shows infants of four levels of balance ability: stage 1, sitting holding up the head but requiring trunk support (4–5 months); stage 2, propping the arms during sitting or sitting independently for brief periods (5–6 months); stage 3, sitting independently without falling (6–8 months); and independent stance (12+ months).

To examine the development of infants' responses to perturbations of balance, Hedberg et al. (2005) placed infants from 1 to 10 months of age on a platform that could be moved forward or backward. They found that infants at 1 month of age showed direction-specific responses in the neck flexors in 28 to 30% of the trials, increasing to 55% at 4 and 5 months of age. Time of onset of muscle contraction varied greatly in the 1-month-olds, from 45 to 447 msec in the neck flexors. The median time of contraction onset was reduced from 238 msec at 1 month to 147 msec at 5 months of age. In neck extensor muscles, direction-specific responses were present in 70% of trials at 1 month and remained at this level through 5 months. A drop in postural response probability was found between 1 and 3 months of age, before rising again at 4 months. The authors suggest that this might be because these pathways not being used substantially during prone and supine behaviors during these early months of life (Hedberg et al., 2004, 2005).

This research suggests that the emergence of direction-specific postural responses in neck muscles underlying reactive balance control begins to occur in infants as young as 1 month of age, although responses are present in only 28 to 30% of trials across infants for neck flexors. A drop in response rate during the first 3 months of life may be due to lack of experience using reactive postural control in early behavior.

Sensory Contributions

Babies as young as 60 hours old are able to orient themselves toward a source of visual stimulation, and they can follow a moving object by correctly orienting the head (Bullinger, 1981; Bullinger & Jouen, 1983). These orientation movements appear to be part of a global form of postural control involving the head and entire body.

When do visually controlled postural adjustments become available to the infant? To examine visual contributions to the control of head movements, Jouen and colleagues (Jouen, 1993; Jouen et al., 2000) examined the capability of neonates to make responses to visual stimuli giving the illusion of a postural perturbation. Three-day-old infants were placed between two video screens that showed pseudo-random patterns of dots moving either forward or backward at varying velocities. Postural responses were measured with a pressure-sensitive pillow behind the infant's head. The neonates made postural adjustments of the head in response to the optical flow; for example, when the visual patterns moved backward, the infants appeared to perceive forward sway of the head, because they moved the head backward, as if to compensate. The magnitude of their responses was directly correlated with velocity. This suggests that: (1) the subcortical neural networks that contribute to visual proprioceptive control of posture are functional at birth and (2) learning is not required for the emergence of optic flow sensitivity, although experience and self-produced movement may be important for visual/postural coupling (Jouen et al., 2000).

It is interesting to note that blind infants show a clear delay in head control at 2 months of age, including a lack of the normal calibration by the visual system onto the proprioceptive and vestibular systems. Although these infants show early visual/motor coordination (coordinated eye–head scanning and head orienting, probably controlled by the superior colliculus), it disappears after a few weeks, showing the importance of this type of experience for the normal development of postural control (Prechtl et al., 2001).

Research has also examined the early development of sensory contributions to antigravity responses in infants. In these experiments, infants 2.5 or 5 months old were placed in a chair that could be tilted 25 degrees to the right or left. During some trials, a red wool ball was placed in the visual field to catch the infant's attention (Jouen, 1984, 1990). The infants showed an antigravity response (keeping the head from falling to the side to which the baby was tilted) that improved with developmental level, with the older infants dropping the head less than the younger infants. Interestingly, when the wool ball was placed in the visual field, both age groups tilted the head less, with the effect being strongest in the younger group. The authors conclude that vision has a significant effect on the vestibular antigravity response in infants and that the response improves with age. However, in this paradigm it is difficult to determine whether the improvement is due to enhanced neck muscle strength, somatosensory/motor processing in neck muscles, or vestibular/motor processing.

Emergence of Independent Sitting

As infants begin to sit independently, and thus develop trunk control, they must learn to master the control of spontaneous background sway of both the head and the trunk and to respond to perturbations of balance. This requires the coordination of sensory/motor information relating two body segments (the head and the trunk) together in the control of posture. Are the rules newborns used regarding sensory/motor relationships for head postural control already available for controlling trunk musculature, or do they need to be learned with experience in sitting? As you will see in the research discussed below, it appears as though there may be both innate components of control, available in the newborn, and emergent aspects of control, resulting from the infant interacting with the environment in a dynamic way.

Motor Coordination

Static Balance Control. The emergence of independent sitting is characterized by the infant's ability to control spontaneous sway sufficiently to remain upright. This occurs at approximately 6 to 8 months of age (Butterworth & Cicchetti, 1978). Research on the emergence of static balance control during sitting supports the hypothesis that postural development of the head and trunk is an emergent dynamic skill.

In studies on the development of control of static balance in sitting Harbourne & Stergiou (2003) used methods from nonlinear dynamics to analyze the complexity (level of predictability) and dimensionality (degrees of freedom) of center of pressure (COP) data across three stages of sitting development, stage 1 (defined as the time when infants were able to hold up the head and upper trunk, but not sit independently; age range, 4–5.5 months), stage 2 (infants able to sit independently briefly, i.e., 10–30 sec, or prop themselves on their arms; age range, 5–6.5 months), and stage 3 (independent sitting, but not yet crawling; age range, 6–8 months). They found that there was a high complexity and dimensionality in stage 1 sitting that decreased as children reached stage 2 sitting, indicating a reduction in the degrees of freedom of movement and possibly homing in on a strategy for trunk control. This is often found when individuals are learning a new skill. They then found that dimensionality increased from stage 2 to stage 3, indicating a subsequent increase in degrees of freedom of trunk/head movement, as infants mastered sitting skills and increased their adaptability and flexibility in postural control. This research suggests that the development of sitting postural control is a dynamic process in which the infant gradually learns to control the degrees of freedom involved in head/trunk control through three stages of the development of sitting balance.

Though the trunk has traditionally been modeled as a single segment when postural development has been studied in infants, the trunk is clearly made up of multiple spinal subunits, controlled by a combination of muscles. Saavedra and Woollacott (in press) have asked how infants solve the problem of learning to sit upright and whether we can determine a specific sequence of changes in the control of spinal segments during this process. In a longitudinal study of infants from 3 to 9 months of age, they examined steady-state postural control at four levels of support (under the arms, midribs, waist, and hips) and found that control of the trunk in sitting develops gradually, in a top-down manner, between 3 (no control) and 9 (functional control) months of age. They found that control developed gradually, with four different stages present in most infants (no control, attempts to initiate upright sitting, partial control with large range of body sway, and functional control with minimal sway). This is shown in Figure 8.5 for the development of hip control. The figure shows the sway of the trunk at each of the stages of control, with the circle showing the base of support circumference at the level of the hips. Note that at stage 1, the child simply collapses forward and cannot recover sitting balance. At stage 2, the infant attempts to initiate balance, but continually loses balance either forward or backward. At stage 3, he can stay upright but is "wobbly" and leans forward, while in stage 4, he shows controlled sitting balance. Histograms showing the amount of time spent at various positions in the anteroposterior plane (vertical bar is midline) also show this shift from no control through functional control, across time. Data from an adult are shown at the right of the figure, for comparison.

Reactive Balance Control. Does reactive balance control for sitting develop at the same time as voluntary sitting control, or is it available earlier? Results of experiments (Harbourne et al., 1993; Hedberg et al., 2005; Hirschfeld and Forssberg, 1994; Woollacott et al., 1987) suggest that reactive balance control in the trunk appears to be available to a limited extent in infants well before sitting develops (as early as 1 month of age) and continues to develop through the onset of independent sitting. Thus, there may be innate components available at birth, which are refined with practice.

The study by Hedberg et al. (2005) discussed above for reactive head control also examined the development of reactive sitting balance, including measurements of trunk and leg muscle responses

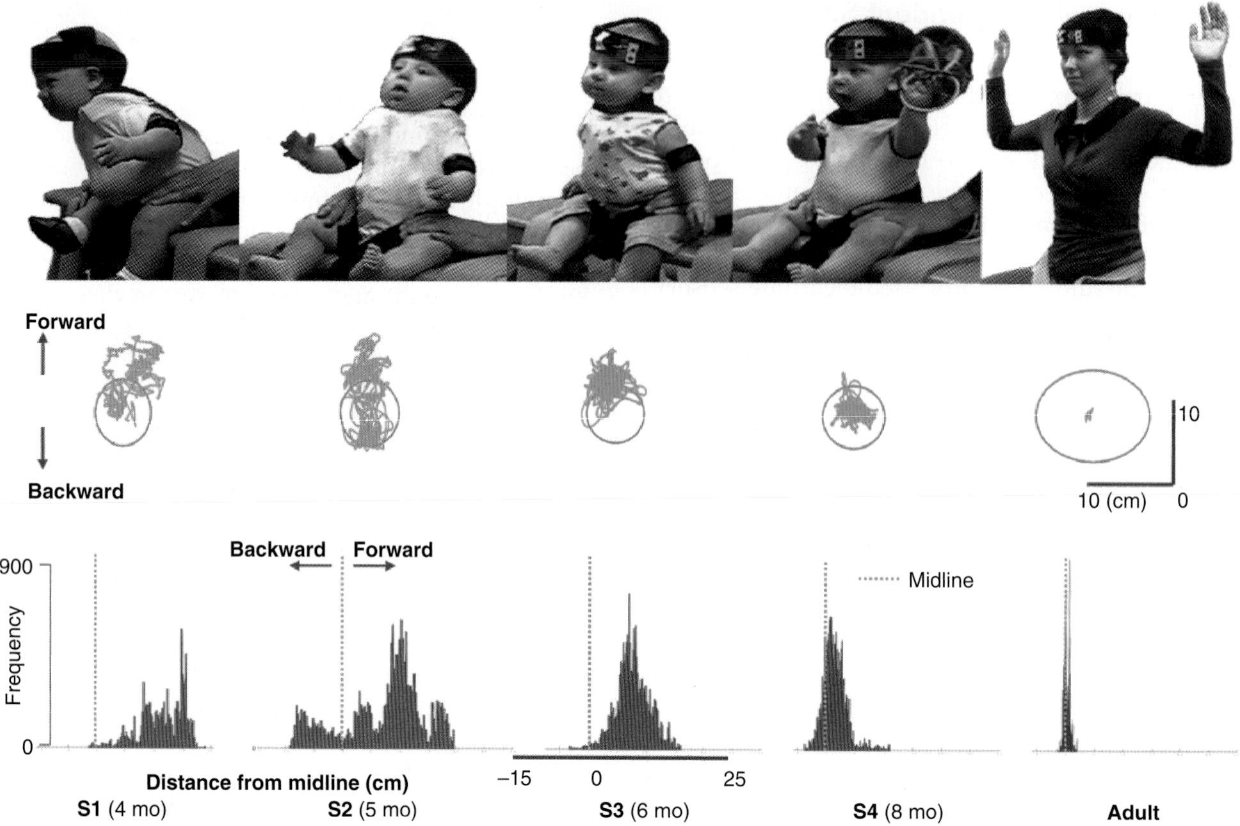

FIGURE 8.5 Photos of a child showing the four stages involved in mastering hip control, along with an adult with full control. The circles immediately below the photographs indicate the base of support circumference at the level of the hips and the sway of the trunk in relation to this base of support circumference during the period of data collection. Note that at stage 1 (far left), the child simply collapses forward and cannot recover sitting balance. At stage 2, the infant attempts to initiate balance, but continually loses balance either forward or backward. At stage 3, he can stay upright but is "wobbly" and leans forward, while in stage 4, he shows controlled sitting balance. However, sway is still higher than for the adult (far right). At the bottom of the figure are shown histograms indicating the amount of time spent at various positions in the anteroposterior plane (vertical bar is midline) for each stage of hip control development. Data for the adult are shown on the right (Data from Saavedra S, Woollacott MH. Contributions of spinal segments to trunk postural control during typical development. Dev Med Child Neurol 2009;51(Suppl. 5):82).

during recovery from balance threats while sitting. The authors showed that in response to perturbations causing backward sway, infants activated abdominal (flexor) muscles in about 10% of trials and trunk extensor muscles in about 30% of the trials at 1 month of age. Although this shows some limited capability of reactive balance for sitting at 1 month, response probability was subsequently reduced from 2 to 4 months of age, with direction specificity of reactive postural control also disappearing. Directional specificity returned again at 5 months. Time of contraction onset for these muscles was variable and slow at 1 month of age, indicating the limited nature of reactive control. At 1 to 2 months, median abdominal onsets were 150 to 200 msec, slowing to 296 msec at 3 months, before decreasing to 134 msec at 7 to 10 months. Extensor muscles of the trunk showed slightly faster contraction onsets, being reduced from 180 msec at 1 to 2 months to 88 msec at 5 months. Similar results were found for contributions of leg muscles to balance recovery to seated perturbations, although direction-specific activity did not even emerge until about 2 months of age. Figure 8.6 shows the probability of seeing complete response patterns (all three flexor or extensor muscles) to forward and backward translations in children from 1 to 10 months of age. Note that complete responses are present at low probabilities at 1 month, then diminish further in probability through 3 months, and finally begin to increase again at 4 to 5 months of age.

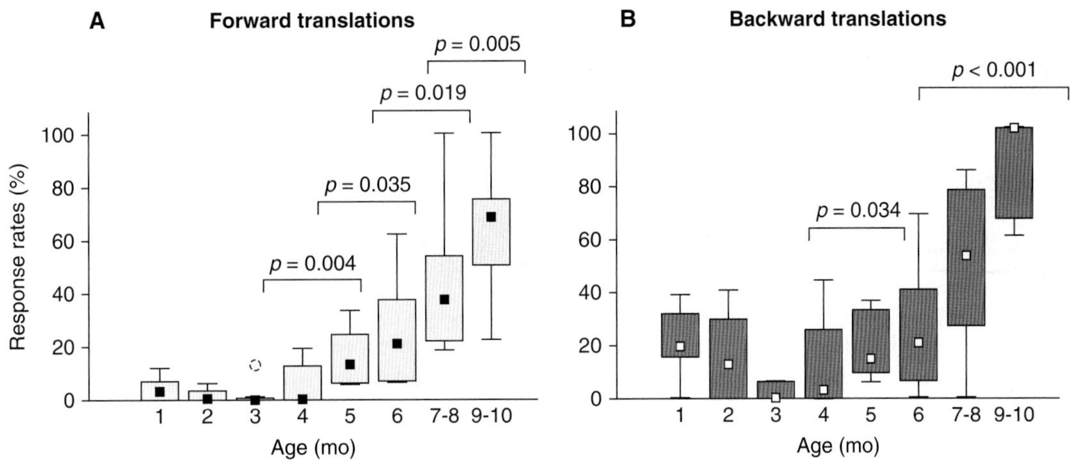

FIGURE 8.6 Response rates of complete EMG patterns (from neck, trunk, and leg muscles) during seated perturbations for children from 1 through 10 months of age. A, Responses to forward translations. B, Responses to backward translations. Vertical bars show ranges, rectangular boxes show interquartile ranges, and small squares show median values for each group. Open boxes indicate responses of the three flexor muscles (neck, trunk, and hip), while filled boxes indicate extensor muscles (neck, trunk, and hip). The *p* values show significantly different distributions of response rates across age groups. (Reprinted with permission from Hedberg, A, Carlberg EB, Forssberg H, Hadders-Algra M. Development of postural adjustments in sitting position during the first half year of life. Dev Med Child Neurol 2005;47:318.)

Hedberg et al. (2005) examined the relationship between spontaneous motor behavior and direction-specific responses to perturbations and found that there was no correlation between the two until 4 months of age. At this point, correlations occurred between postural activity and backward pelvis tilt, the ability of the hands to touch the lower legs, and the ability to turn into the prone position.

Hirschfeld and Forssberg (1994) showed that platform movements causing backward sway give much stronger and less variable postural muscle response synergies than those causing forward sway. This may be caused by the larger base of postural support in the forward direction in seated infants (Hirschfeld & Forssberg, 1994). In this study, infants too young to sit independently (5–7 months) responded with only one to two muscles for most forward perturbations, with all three anterior muscles (neck flexors, rectus abdominus, and rectus femoris) being activated in 25% of the trials. By the time infants were independent sitters (7–8 months), all three muscles were activated in 100% of the trials. These results also suggest that response synergies are being shaped during the months prior to the emergence of independent sitting and are organized appropriately in all trials by the time infants are able to sit independently.

This research suggests that by 1 month, postural response synergies are present; however, they are highly variable and present in only a small percentage of trials. Paradoxically, they appear less frequently in infants at 3 to 4 months of age (Hedberg et al., 2005; Woollacott et al., 1987), then reappear with greater frequency and refinement as the child learns to sit independently. Thus, these early more variable synergies may be considered precursors to later more refined postural synergies underlying the development of seated postural control.

Sensory Contributions

Early research investigated the role of vision in seated postural control by examining the response of infants at different stages in the development of independent sitting to visual stimuli, giving the illusion of a postural perturbation (the moving-room paradigm) (Butterworth & Hicks, 1977; Butterworth & Pope, 1983). Infants with relatively little experience in sitting independently showed a complete loss of balance in response to the visual stimulation (a single ramp stimulus); with increasing experience in sitting, the response amplitude declined. This implies that newly sitting infants rely heavily on visual inputs when controlling sway and that this dependence decreases with increasing experience in independent sitting, as infants rely more on somatosensory inputs.

Experiments by Bertenthal and colleagues (1997) have also examined the responses of infants to visual cues using continuous oscillations, as they mastered independent sitting. In this study, infants 5 to 13 months old sat on a child's bicycle seat (with a back) in a room that continuously oscillated at a variety of speeds and amplitudes. The postural responses were measured with a force plate under the bicycle seat. They noted that even 5-month-old infants who were not yet sitting independently showed some entrainment to the driving frequency of the moving visual stimuli; however, this response became more consistent with age and experience. They concluded that during the process of learning to sit independently infants are learning to scale or map visual sensory information to their postural activity.

Other studies have examined sensory contributions to the emergence of independent sitting balance using support-surface perturbations that activate all three senses, rather than just vision alone. Woollacott and coworkers (1987) studied muscle patterns in the head and trunk in response to platform perturbations in seated infants with and without vision. They found that taking away visual stimuli did not change the muscle activation patterns in response to a moving platform. They concluded that somatosensory and vestibular systems are capable of eliciting postural actions in isolation from vision in infants first learning to sit.

In an effort to understand the relationship among vestibular and visual inputs reporting head motion, and proprioceptive inputs from the trunk, Hirschfeld and Forssberg (1994) performed experiments in which head orientation was systematically varied in seated infants undergoing platform perturbations. Coordinated muscle activity stabilizing the trunk did not change regardless of how the head was oriented. This suggests that in the seated position, postural responses to perturbations are largely controlled by somatosensory inputs at the hip joints, not by vestibular or visual stimulation.

These studies suggest that infants appear to have a crude map of relationships between sensory inputs and the neck, trunk, and leg muscles for sitting postural control by 1 month of age; this appears to go through a reduction in expression until 4 months, possibly because of a lack of practice with reactive postural control in the prone and supine positions. It then gradually matures with the continued development of independent sitting control.

Modifiability of Postural Responses

What is the effect of practice on the emergence of postural responses? Hadders-Algra and colleagues (1996) examined the effect of training on the development of postural adjustments in infants who were not yet sitting independently (they used parents to train the infants at home [5 minutes, three times a day for 3 months]). The training consisted of toy presentation to the side or semibackward at the infant's limits of stability. When comparing EMG responses to platform perturbations pretraining versus posttraining they found that the trained infants (as compared with nontrained controls) showed a higher probability of complete responses to perturbations and increased response modulation at higher perturbation velocities, along with decreased pelvic displacement. There were no changes in muscle-response onset latencies.

These data give support for the development of similar types of postural training programs in children with motor delays. Studies are currently being conducted in our own labs to determine whether postural training programs are effective in children with cerebral palsy.

Transition to Independent Stance

Motor Coordination

Development of Quiet Stance. The postural demands of quiet sitting and stance balance are very different. During the process of learning to stand independently, infants must learn to: (a) balance within significantly reduced stability limits compared to those used during sitting, (b) control many additional degrees of freedom, as they add the coordination of the leg and thigh segments to those of the trunk and head, and recalibrate sensorimotor representations for postural control to include the thigh, shank, and foot for balance to create an improved internal model for postural control of independent stance. As we mentioned above, research suggests that an important part of transitions in development of new behaviors is the recalibration of the sensorimotor systems. One would expect that the sesnsorimotor coupling calibration that occurred with the development of head control, would need to be extended and recalibrated with the development of sitting and then again in the development of standing.

Chen et al. (2007) examined whether infants' sitting postural control changed during the transition to independent walking. They longitudinally assessed infants' postural sway monthly from the onset of sitting through the 9th month of independent walking while they sat on a saddle-shaped chair positioned on a force plate, as shown in Figure 8.7. It was hypothesized that the transition to bipedal locomotion would be associated with decreases in the stability of sitting posture, suggesting a recalibration or tuning of a generalized internal representation for the sensorimotor control of sway. When data across the 11 months were compared, sway amplitude, variability, area, and velocity of COP trajectory showed a peak just before or at the onset of walking, as shown in Figure 8.8, and at this point peak sway was greater than at any other

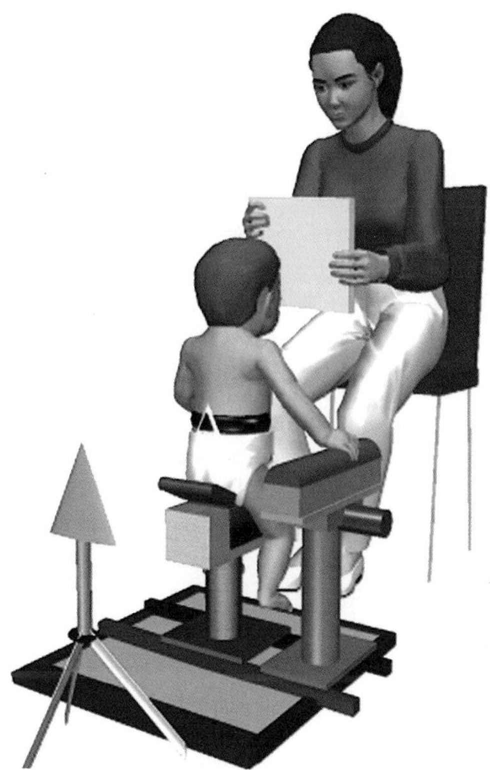

FIGURE 8.7 The infant sits independently on a saddle-shaped chair attached to the force platform in either the no-touch condition or in the touch condition (pictured), in which he/she places the hand on the touchpad. The experimenter sits in front of the infant to keep attention on the task. (Reprinted with permission from Chen LC, Metcalfe JS, Jeka JJ, Clark JE. Two steps forward and one back: learning to walk affects infants' sitting posture. Infant Behav Dev 2007;30:19.)

stage. The authors conclude that this transient disruption in sitting posture results from a process involving recalibration of the infants' internal model for the sensorimotor control of posture as they practice the newly emerging bipedal behavior of independent walking.

In a second longitudinal study of infants of the same age range, Chen et al. (2008) recorded similar periods of unperturbed independent stance on the same force plate, in order to determine the effect of walking experience on COP excursion, velocity, and frequency variables during independent stance. They noted that quiet stance posture is usually characterized as having two components, a slow drift and a fast damped oscillatory component. The fast oscillatory component is hypothesized to be due to the control dynamics of the inverted pendulum oscillation properties of body sway and is responsible for most of the sway variance, while the slower components are hypothesized to be due to errors in postural state and their correction. As shown in Figure 8.9, results suggest that early development of upright postural control involves changes in these rate-related characteristics of sway rather than in a progressive attenuation of postural sway. The figure shows that with increased stance and walking experience, infants' upright postural sway develops toward a lower frequency and a slower and less variable velocity, more similar to that of adults. The authors conclude that these changes in standing posture reflect changes in "how" the infant is swaying (lower frequency/less variable) than how much the infant is swaying.

These results of no significant reduction in sway as infants gain more experience in upright standing and walking is different from that found in previous studies showing age-related decreases in sway variability in older children (i.e., 2–14 years old) (Riach & Hayes, 1987). What might explain the lack of reduction in sway in early development of stance and walking? The authors propose that infants first learning to walk combine two mechanisms or strategies that underly the control of postural sway: the first is exploratory and the second is performatory (Newell, 1991; Reed 1982; Riley et al., 1997). Exploratory postural sway investigates the sensorimotor work space for posture control to create sensory information for refining sensorimotor relationships underlying postural control; performatory postural sway, on the other hand, uses sensory information to control posture. It is suggested that for infants who have not yet formed a reliable sensorimotor relationship for postural control, it is important to explore the sensorimotor workspace for postural control. This helps them to gain sensory information for calibrating the sensorimotor relationship for postural control and creating a strong sensorimotor representation. Thus, it is possible that the exploratory behavior of these infants may mask any improvements in control of sway magnitude. In addition, it is possible that it would require a larger time scale (about 1 yr) for developmental changes in postural sway attenuation to be consistently observed (Chen et al., 2008).

Role of Strength. Several researchers have suggested that a primary rate-limiting factor for the emergence of independent walking is the development of sufficient muscle strength to support the body during static balance and walking (Thelen & Fisher, 1982). Can leg-muscle strength be tested in the infant to determine whether this is the case?

Researchers have shown that by 6 months of age infants are capable of producing forces well beyond their own body weight (Roncesvalles & Jensen, 1993). These experiments suggest that the ability to support weight against the force of gravity in the standing position occurs well before the emergence

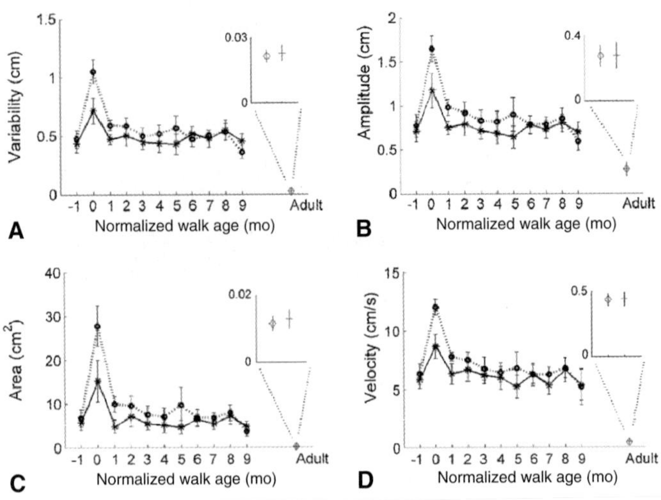

FIGURE 8.8 Resultant COP sway was derived from mediolateral and anteroposteiror COP. Resultant COP sway: (A) variability (cm), (B) amplitude (cm), (C) area of 90% ellipse (cm^2), and (D) velocity (cm/sec) across normalized walk ages and touch conditions. Infants' postural sway was presented as means ±SE. Adults' averaged postural sway was presented for comparison (·) infant no-touch; (*) infant touch; (♦) adult no-touch; (+) adult touch. Note the difference in scale between infants and adults. (Reprinted with permission from Chen LC, Metcalfe JS, Jeka JJ, Clark JE. Two steps forward and one back: learning to walk affects infants' sitting posture. Infant Behav Dev 2007;30:22.)

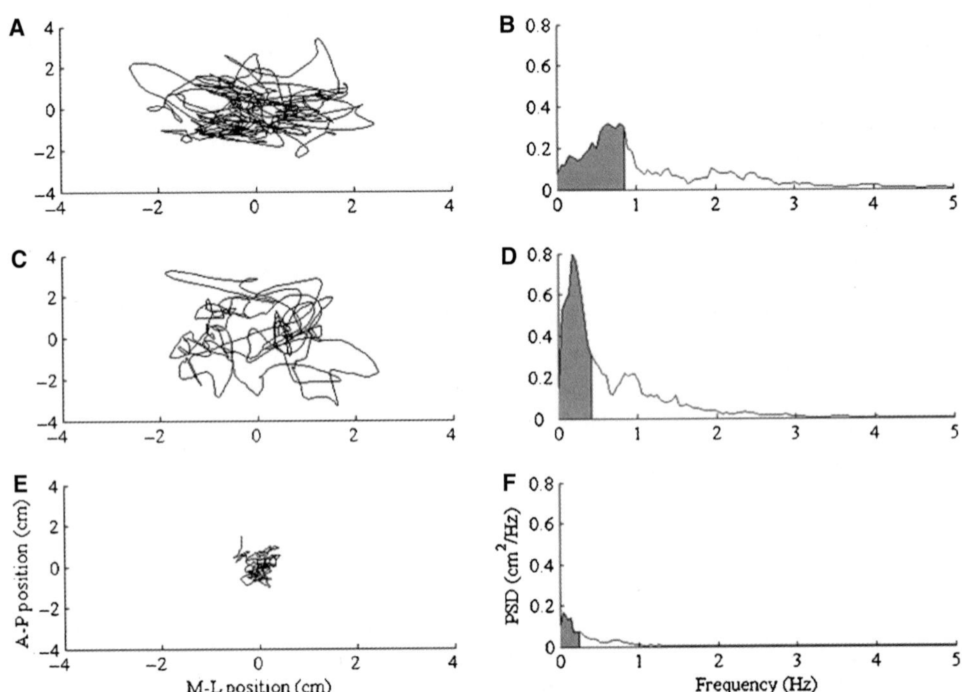

FIGURE 8.9 Exemplar of CP trajectories and power spectrum for: A and B, an infant at 1 month after beginning to walk; C and D, the same infant at 8 months after beginning to walk; and E and F, an adult. The *gray area* represents the spectral bandwidth in which 50% power of the frequency spectrum was accumulated. (Reprinted with permission from Chen LC, Metcalfe JS, Chang TY, et al. The development of infant upright posture: sway less or sway differently? Exp Brain Res 2008;186:298.)

of independent stance, so it is probably not the major constraint to emerging stance postural control in infants.

Reactive Balance: Development of Muscle Synergies. How do postural response synergies compensating for perturbations to balance begin to emerge in the newly standing infant? Longitudinal studies have explored the emergence of postural response synergies in infants from ages 2 to 18 months, during the transition to independent stance (Sveistrup & Woollacott, 1996; Woollacott & Sveistrup, 1992). As shown in Figure 8.4D, infants stood (with varying degrees of support, which are not shown) on the moving platform while EMGs were used to record muscle activity in the leg and trunk in response to loss of balance.

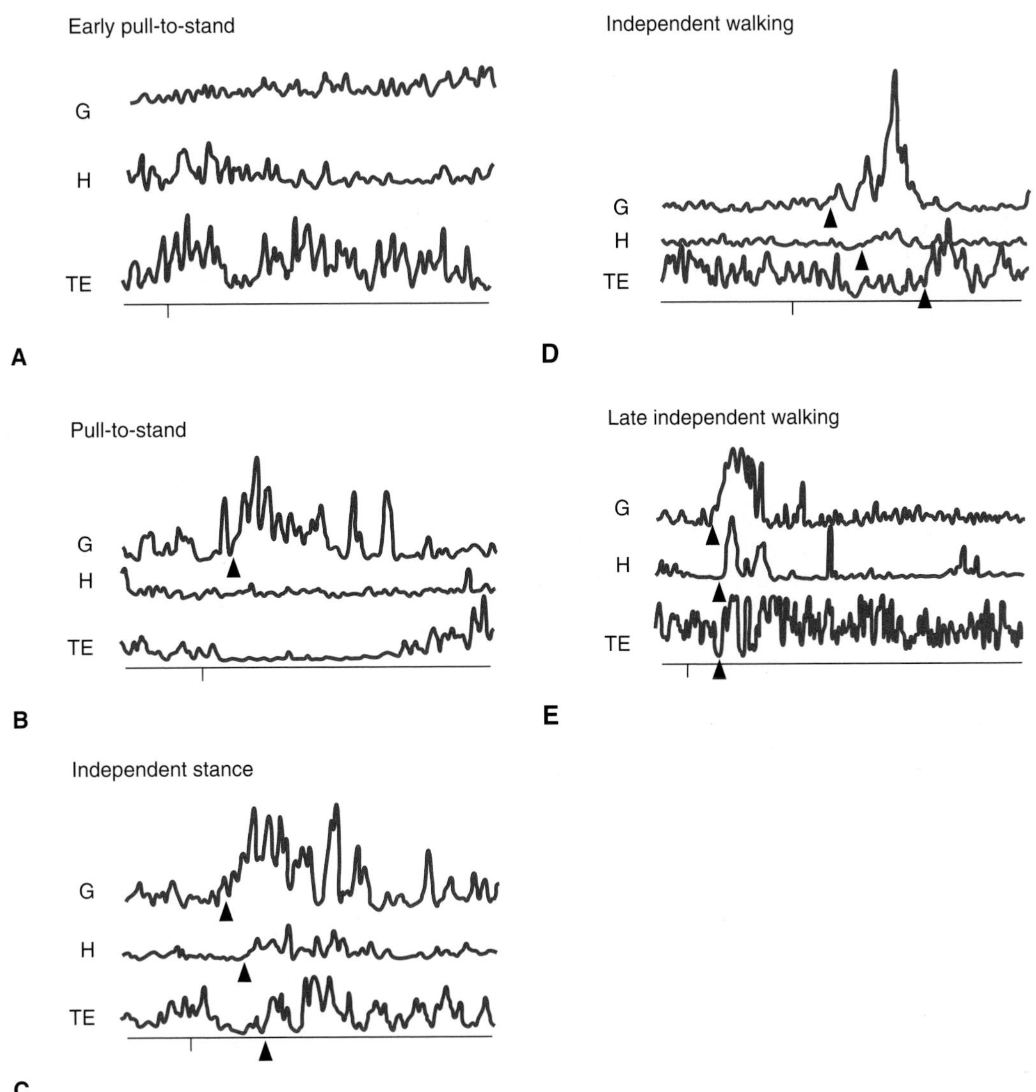

FIGURE 8.10 Responses from one child during the emergence of coordinated muscle activity in the leg and trunk muscles in response to platform perturbations in: A, Early pull-to-stand; B, Pull-to-stand; C, Independent stance; and D and E, Independent walking and late independent walking. Note that there was no response in early pull-to-stand, and responses gradually developed at subsequent behavioral levels. G = gastrocnemius; H = hamstrings; TE = trunk extensors. The vertical line under the TE muscle indicates the onset of platform movement. Arrows indicate the onset of muscle responses. Each trace corresponds to a 1-sec recording. (Adapted with permission from Sveistrup H, Woollacott MH. Longitudinal development of the automatic postural response in infants. J Motor Behav 1996;28:63.)

Figure 8.10 shows EMG responses from one child during the emergence of coordinated muscle activity in the leg and trunk muscles in response to a fall backward. Infants tested at 2 to 6 months of age, before the onset of pull-to-stand behavior and often during the beginning of pull-to-stand behavior, did not show coordinated muscle response organization in response to threats to balance (Fig. 8.10A). As pull-to-stand behavior progressed (7–9 months), the infants began to show directionally appropriate responses in their ankle muscles (Fig. 8.10B). As pull-to-stand skills improved, muscles in the thigh segment were added, and a consistent distal-to-proximal sequence began to emerge during late pull-to-stand and independent stance and walking (9–11 months) (Fig. 8.10C–E); at this point, trunk muscles were consistently activated, resulting in a complete synergy. Figure 8.11 shows the gradual shift in percentage of trials in which a one- or two-muscle response versus a three-muscle response was found as children moved from pre–pull-to-stand to independent walking. Note the gradual addition of muscles to the synergy with experience and development.

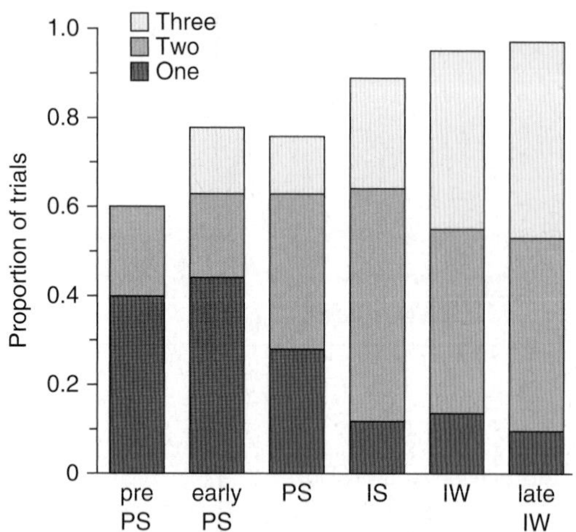

FIGURE 8.11 Proportion of trials with responses recorded in one, two, or three muscles following the platform perturbation, in each of the stages of stance development. PS = pull-to-stand; IS = independent stance; IW = independent walking. (Adapted with permission from Sveistrup H, Woollacott MH. Longitudinal development of the automatic postural response in infants. J Motor Behav 1996;28:67.)

Sensory Contributions

Once an infant learns how to organize synergistic muscles for controlling stance in association with one sense, will this automatically transfer to other senses reporting sway? This may not always be the case. It appears that vision maps to muscles controlling stance posture by at least 5 to 6 months, prior to somatosensory system mapping, and long before the infant has much experience in the standing position (Foster et al., 1996). This suggests that the infant has to reassemble the synergies when somatosensory inputs are mapped for stance postural control.

EMG responses and sway patterns in response to visual flow created by a moving room were examined in infants and children of varying ages and abilities and compared with those of young adults (Foster et al., 1996). Figure 8.12 shows an example of an infant positioned in a moving room. The child's sway was recorded through one-way glass with a video camera mounted outside the room, and muscle responses were recorded from the legs and hips. Infants who were unable to stand independently were supported about the hip by their parents.

Children as young as 5 months of age swayed in response to room movements; sway amplitudes increased in the pull-to-stand stage, peaked in the independent walkers, and dropped to low levels of sway in experienced walkers (Foster et al., 1996). Sway responses were associated with clear patterns of muscle responses that pulled the child in the direction of the visual stimulus.

These experiments suggest that the visual system will elicit organized postural responses in standing infants at an earlier time than the somatosensory system and that the somatosensory system develops postural synergies separately in association with somatosensory inputs signaling sway.

Other studies using the moving-room paradigm have shown that directionally appropriate postural responses to peripheral (side-wall) optic flow were much stronger in infants with experience in self-produced locomotion. Those without this experience needed global optic flow to generate appropriate responses (Higgins et al., 1996).

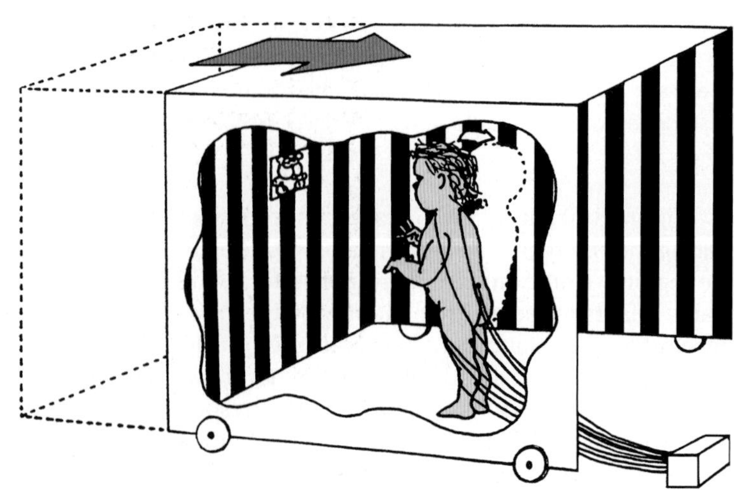

FIGURE 8.12 Diagram showing the moving-room paradigm used to examine the development of visual contributions to postural control. When the room moves toward the child, he or she perceives forward sway and responds by swaying backward. (Reprinted with permission from Sveistrup H, Woollacott MH. Systems contributing to the emergence and maturation of stability in postnatal development. In: Savelsbergh GJP, ed. The development of coordination in infancy. Amsterdam: Elsevier, 1993:324.)

Development of Adaptive Capability

To determine whether higher-level adaptive processes are available to infants during pull-to-stand behavior, independent stance, and early walking, the ability of the infants to attenuate postural responses to the visual flow created by the moving room was monitored (Foster et al., 1996). None of the infants in any of these behavioral categories was able to adapt inappropriate postural responses to low levels, over five trials. The researchers concluded that higher-level adaptive processes related to postural control have not yet matured by the time of emergence of independent walking.

When does the ability to adapt responses to changes in support-surface characteristics emerge? A study examined the ability of infants during their first year of walking (13–14 months old) to adapt to altered support-surface conditions, including high friction (high-friction plastic), low friction (Formica coated with baby oil), and foam surfaces as well as standing crosswise on a narrow beam (Stoffregen et al., 1997). The children had two poles available to hold to help with balance. It is interesting to note that the greatest amount of time spent in free standing was on the high-friction surface, with minimal hand support used. As the surfaces became more compliant (foam) or lower friction (baby oil), pole holding increased substantially, with a concomitant drop in free standing. Finally, it was impossible for the infants to stand crosswise on the beam while standing independently. Since standing crosswise on a beam requires active control of the hips, rather than purely control of ankle movements, this suggests that this adaptive ability to use the hips in balance is not mastered in infants during their first year of walking.

Previous research on adults has shown that increasing the size of a balance threat will often elicit a hip strategy (activated by abdominal muscle activity), rather than an ankle strategy, as the center of mass (COM) nears the edges of the base of support. In order to determine when the ability to control the hips during balance recovery emerges, researchers (Roncesvalles et al., 2003; Woollacott et al., 1998) gave children from new walkers (10–17 months) through hoppers (2–3 year), gallopers (4–6 year), and skippers (7–10 year) increasing magnitudes of balance threats in order to elicit a hip strategy if it was available in these children. They found that hip-dominated responses were present in the walkers with only 3 to 6 months of walking experience. However, these responses were passively activated, with minimal abdominal activity used. It was not until the children reached 7 to 10 years of age (skippers) that they began to show consistent active control of the strategy with high levels of abdominal muscle activity.

Effect of Practice: Modifiability of Postural Responses

To determine whether experience is important in the development of postural response characteristics in infants learning to stand, postural responses were compared in two groups of infants in the pull-to-stand stage of balance development (Sveistrup & Woollacott, 1997). One group of infants was given extensive experience with platform perturbations, receiving 300 perturbations over 3 days. The second (control) group of infants did not receive this training.

Infants who had extensive experience on the platform were more likely to activate postural muscle responses, and these responses were better organized. Figure 8.13 shows the probability of seeing a response in tibialis anterior, quadriceps, and abdominal muscles in response to platform movements causing backward sway, both before and after training. Note that the probability of seeing a response in all three muscles was significantly increased. However, onset latencies of postural responses did not change.

These results suggest that experience may influence the strength of the connections between the

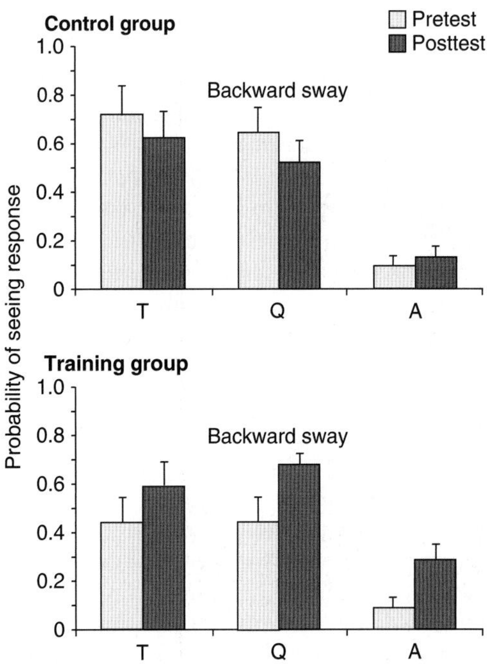

FIGURE 8.13 Probability of seeing a response in tibialis anterior (T), quadriceps (Q), and abdominal (A) muscles in response to platform movements causing backward sway, both before and after 3 days of balance training. Note that the probability of seeing a response in all three muscles was significantly increased. (Adapted with permission from Sveistrup H, Woollacott M. Can practice modify the developing automatic postural response? Exp Brain Res 1997;114:41.)

sensory and motor pathways controlling balance, thus increasing the probability of producing postural responses. However, the lack of a training effect on muscle response latency suggests that neural maturation may be a rate-limiting factor in latency reduction with development. It is probable that the myelination of nervous system pathways responsible for reducing latencies of postural responses during development is not affected by training.

Relating Reflex to Systems Theory

Differences in focus between reflex/hierarchical and systems models make it difficult to relate findings examining the emergence of independent stance. Reflex/hierarchical theory distinguishes the righting reactions underlying orientation from the tilting and postural fixation reactions essential to the emergence of balance, suggesting that different neural mechanisms are involved in these two functions. Researchers studying tilting and postural fixation reactions have examined neither the importance of individual sensory systems to these reactions nor their capability for adaptation.

Systems-based research suggests that the time course for emerging stability behaviors is different in each of the sensory systems. Visual inputs relating the body's position in space map to muscular actions controlling the body's position during stance earlier than do inputs from the somatosensory system. It is not yet known how early vestibular inputs map to stance postural actions. Results from systems-based studies suggest that, for the most part, experience within a specific posture is important for sensory information signaling the body's position in space to be mapped to muscular actions, which control the body's position in space.

Refinement of Stance Control

Up until now, we have examined changes within the postural control system in the first 12 months of life that contribute to the emergence of sitting and stance. Researchers have found that postural control is essentially adult-like by 10 to 12 years of age. What are the key changes that contribute to this refinement of postural control? It appears that the emergence of adult levels of control occurs at different times for different aspects of postural control.

Musculoskeletal System: Changes in Body Morphology

Are children inherently more stable than adults? Children are shorter and therefore closer to the ground. Does their height make balancing an easier task? Anyone who has watched a fearless young child ski down a steep slope with relative ease, falling and bouncing back up, might assume that their task is easier. They don't have as far to fall! It turns out that while children are shorter than adults, they are proportioned differently. Children are top-heavy. The relative size of the head, in comparison to the lower extremities, places the center of mass at about T12 in the child, as compared with L5–S1 in the adult. Because of their shorter height, and the difference in the location of their center of mass, children sway at a faster rate than adults. Thus, the task of static balance is slightly more difficult, since the body is moving at a faster rate during imbalance. However, after 7 years of age, there is no correlation between structural growth of the human body (body height, body mass, and age) and sway during normal quiet stance (Lebiedowska & Syczewska, 2000; Zeller, 1964).

Motor Coordination

Refinement of Quiet Stance. How is the control of spontaneous sway during quiet stance refined as children develop beyond early independent stance? A number of studies have examined refinement in spontaneous sway with development (e.g., from 2 to 14 years of age) and have shown that both the amplitude and the frequency of postural sway decreased during this period (Hayes & Riach, 1989; Kirshenbaum et al., 2001; Taguchi & Tada, 1988). Young children used a high-velocity balance strategy, making large, fast corrections of the COP as they attempted to maintain their COM within their base of support, while at around 8 to 9 years of age they show shorter excursions and more accurate control (Riach & Starkes, 1994).

Research also shows considerable variability in sway amplitude in the young children. This variance became systematically lower with age and with the children's improved balance. Effects of eye closure were represented by the Romberg quotient (eyes-closed sway expressed as a percentage of eyes-open sway), giving an indication of the contributions of vision to balance during quiet stance. Very low Romberg quotients were recorded for the youngest children who completed the task (4-year-olds), with values of less than 100%. This indicates that these children were swaying more with eyes open than with eyes closed (Hayes & Riach, 1989). Spontaneous sway in children reaches adult levels by 9 to 12 years of age for eyes-open conditions and at 12 to 15 years of age for eyes-closed conditions. Sway velocity also decreased with age, reaching adult levels at 12 to 15 years of age (Taguchi & Tada, 1988).

Research using nonlinear analysis techniques (correlation dimension and complexity, described above) to examine changes in balance control during quiet stance has shown that 3-year-old children show a decreased COP dimensionality and complexity, indicating that they are using restricted degrees of freedom in balance during quiet stance. Five-year-olds showed significantly increased dimensionality and complexity of their COP path, similar to that of adults, indicating that they have more control and adaptability in their balance abilities during quiet stance (Newell, 1997).

Refinement of Reactive Postural Control. Refinement of compensatory balance adjustments in children 15 months to 10 years of age has been studied by several researchers using a movable platform to examine changes in postural control (Berger et al., 1985; Forssberg & Nashner, 1982; Hass et al., 1986; Shumway-Cook & Woollacott, 1985). Research has shown that compensatory postural responses of young children (15 months of age) are more variable and slower than those of adults (Forssberg & Nashner, 1982). These slower muscle responses and the more rapid rates of sway acceleration observed in young children cause sway amplitudes (in response to balance threats) that are bigger and often more oscillatory than those of older children and adults.

Even children of 1.5 to 3 years of age generally produce well-organized muscle responses to postural perturbations while standing (Shumway-Cook & Woollacott, 1985; Forssberg & Nashner, 1982). However, the amplitudes of these responses are larger, and the latencies and durations of these responses are longer than those of adults. Other studies have also found a longer duration of postural responses in young children and have also noted the activation of monosynaptic stretch reflexes in young children in response to platform perturbations. These responses disappear as the children mature (Berger et al., 1985; Hass et al., 1986).

Surprisingly, postural responses in children 4 to 6 years of age are, in general, slower and more variable than those found in children 15 months to 3 years old, those 7 to 10 years old, or adults, suggesting an apparent regression in the postural response organization. Figure 8.14 compares EMG responses in the four age groups.

In these studies, by 7 to 10 years of age, postural responses were basically like those in adults. There were no significant differences in onset latency, variability, or temporal coordination between muscles within the leg synergy between this age group and adults (Shumway-Cook & Woollacott, 1985).

Why are postural actions so much more variable in 4-to-6-year-old children? It may be significant that the variability in response parameters of 4-to-6-year-old children occurs during a period of disproportionate growth with respect to critical changes in body form. It has been suggested that discontinuous changes seen in the development of many skills, including postural control may be the result of critical dimension changes in the body of the growing child (Kugler et al., 1982). The system would remain stable until dimensional changes reached a point at which previous motor programs were no longer highly effective. At that point, the system would undergo a period of transition marked by instability and variability, and then a new plateau of stability.

Research analyzing the movements of different segments of the body, in response to platform perturbations in both children and adults (Woollacott et al., 1988), has shown that the kinematics of passive body movements caused by platform translations are very similar in the 4-to-6-year-olds, 7-to-9-year-olds, and adults. Thus, it is more probable that changes in response latencies and variability seen in 4-to-6-year-olds represent developmental changes in the nervous system itself.

In addition to looking at the development of reactive balance control from a neurophysiological perspective, one can look at it from a biomechanical perspective, examining the development of forces used to recover from balance threats. More recent work has used kinetics to examine the refinement in the development of force capabilities in children from 9 months to 10 years of age, as they recover from balance threats (Roncesvalles et al., 2001). In examining COP trajectories used to recover from balance threats, it was noted that children just learning to stand and walk were the slowest to recover stability (about 2 sec) with COP trajectories more than twice as large as those of the older children (7-to-10-year-olds, 1.1 sec). Why was this the case? Examination of the torque profiles at the ankle, knee, and hip showed that, in contrast to older children and adults, who rapidly generated large torques, the younger children (standers and walkers, 9–23 months of age) used multiple torque adjustments before regaining control. Figure 8.15 shows torque profiles of children from 9 to 13 months (new standers), 14 to 23 months (advanced walkers), 2 to 3 years (runners/jumpers), 4 to 6 years (gallopers), and 7 to 10 years (skippers). Note that there are at least three bursts of torque production at the ankle, knee, and hip in the stander and walker, while this is reduced to two bursts and then one burst in the older age groups. The youngest age groups tended to overshoot and undershoot torque requirements, with many torque reversals.

These data support the previous work found on refinement of balance strategies using neurophysiological and kinematic measures (Forssberg &

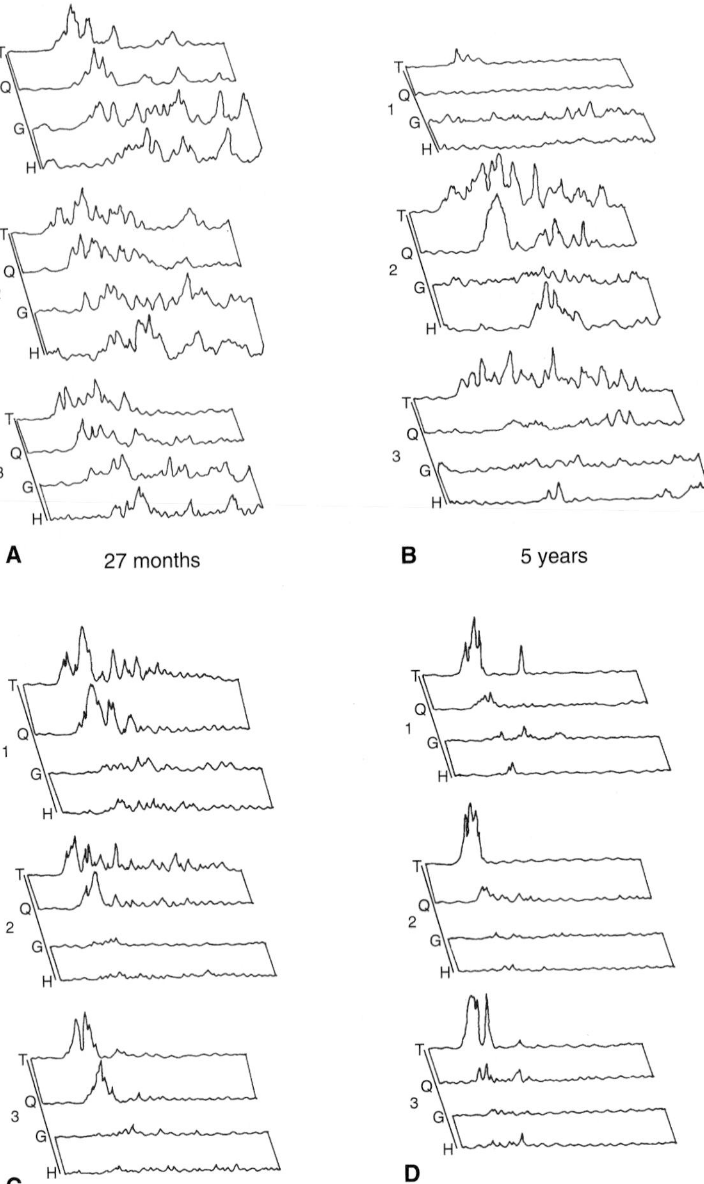

FIGURE 8.14 A comparison of muscle activation patterns in leg and trunk muscles in response to forward platform perturbations causing backward sway in children from four age groups. Three successive responses to platform perturbations are shown for each child. Platform perturbation started at the onset of the EMG recording. Recording is 600 msec. T = tibialis anterior; Q = quadriceps; G = gastrocnemius; H = hamstrings. (Reprinted with permission from Shumway-Cook A, Woollacott M. The growth of stability: postural control from a developmental perspective. J Mot Behav 1985;17:136.)

Nashner, 1982; Shumway-Cook & Woollacott, 1985) that showed that children 1 to 3 years of age exhibited large and oscillatory sway excursions, while response patterns were gradually refined and became similar to those of adults by 7 to 10 years of age.

Development of Sensory Adaptation

Postural control is characterized by the ability to adapt how we use sensory information about the position and movement of the body in space to changing task and environmental conditions. How does the CNS learn to interpret information from vision, vestibular, and somatosensory receptors and relate it to postural actions? One theory is that children and adults learn to reweight sensory inputs under changing sensory conditions in order to primarily rely on inputs that are giving accurate information within the environmental context. For example, if visual information from the environment gives the illusion of sway when the individual is actually remaining steady, then the CNS would reduce the reliance on vision and rely primarily on somatosensory and vestibular inputs.

We have already described evidence from moving-room experiments suggesting that the visual system plays a predominant role in the development of postural actions. That is, visual inputs reporting the body's position in space appear to be mapped to

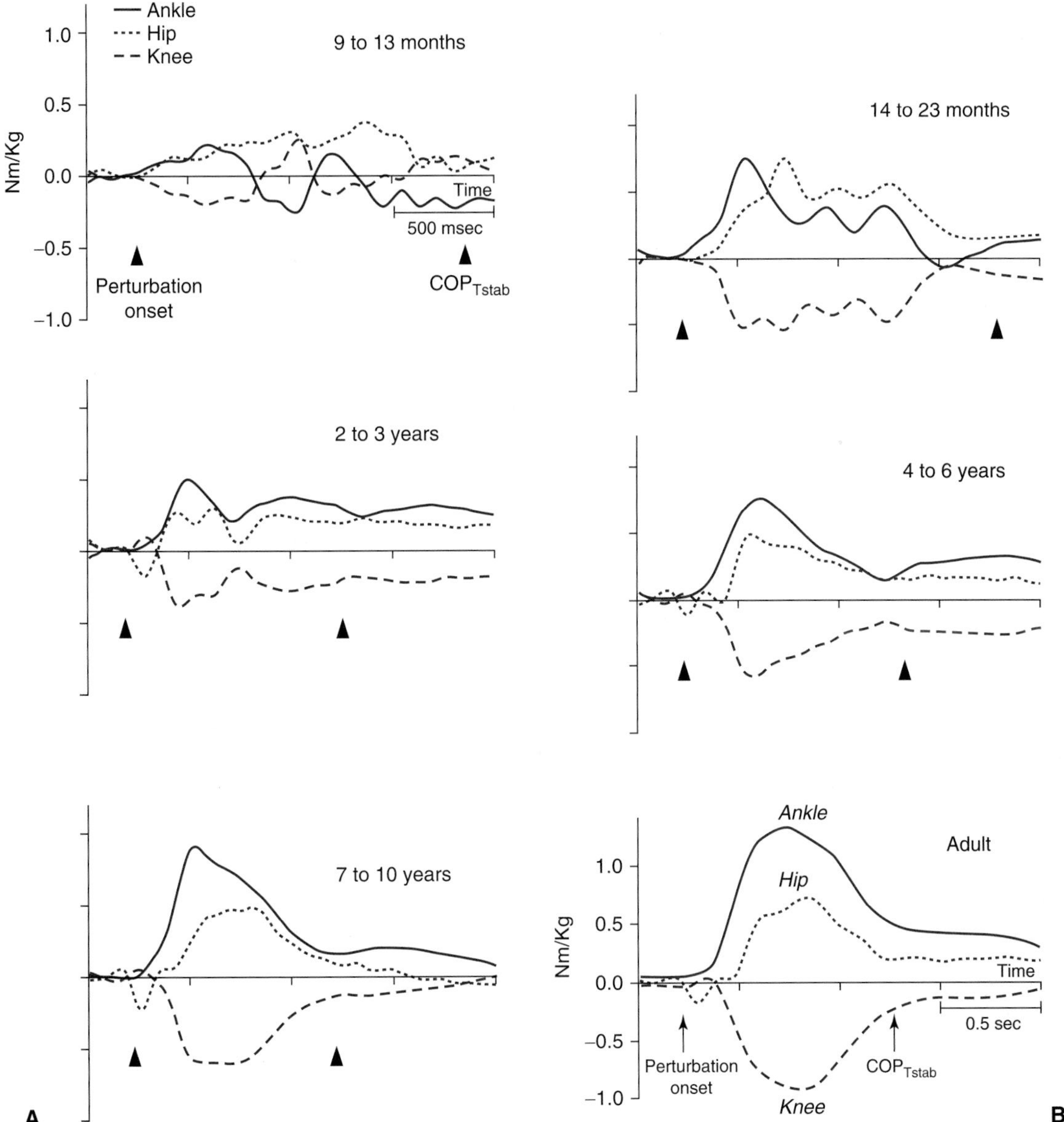

FIGURE 8.15 Torque profiles of children from 9 to 13 months (new standers), 14 to 23 months (advanced walkers), 2 to 3 years (runners/jumpers), 4 to 6 years (gallopers), and 7 to 10 years (skippers) in response to backward platform movements causing forward sway. Note that there are at least three bursts of torque production at the ankle, knee, and hip in the stander and walker, while this is reduced to two bursts and then one burst in the older age groups. The onset of perturbation and recovery of balance are marked by arrowheads. The ankle and hip torques are extensor (positive) and responsible for returning the COM to its resting range. Knee torque was flexor, counterbalancing the extensor torques generated at ankle and hip. Muscle torques were normalized to body mass, and all graphs were plotted on the same scale. The time scale is 500 msec. Nm/kg = Newton meters/kilogram; COP_{Tstab} = time to stabilization of COP.

muscular actions earlier than inputs from other sensory systems. In young children, the invariant use of visual inputs for postural control can sometimes mask the capability of other senses to activate postural actions. Results from the experiments in which children balanced without visual inputs suggest that in certain age groups, postural actions activated by other sensory inputs can be better organized than those associated with vision.

Moving-platform posturography in conjunction with a moving visual surround has also been used to examine the development of intersensory integration and the ability to reweight sensory inputs for postural control. The platform protocols used to study the organization and selection of senses for postural control were described in detail Chapter 7.

The development of sensory adaptation in children ages 2 to 14 years of age has been studied by a number of investigators using this protocol (Ferber-Viart et al., 2007; Forssberg & Nashner, 1982; Foudriat et al., 1993; Shumway-Cook & Woollacott, 1985). The results of the combined studies suggest that 1.5-to-3-year-olds sway more than older children and adults, even when all three sensory inputs are present (condition 1). Performance continues to improve slightly across all age groups through 14 years of age. With eyes closed (condition 2), children's stability did not significantly decrease further, in the youngest age groups (Forssberg & Nashner, 1982); however, other studies using children 4 and older have shown slight decreases in stability in most age groups either with eyes closed or the visual surround stabilized (conditions 2 and 3). Stability in these conditions improves through 14 years of age, as shown in Figure 8.16.

Reducing the accuracy of somatosensory information for postural control by rotating the platform surface in correlation with the infants' sway, reducing reliable ankle-joint inputs (condition 4), further reduced the stability of all age groups substantially. Finally, when children closed their eyes (condition 5) or balanced in the support surface and visual surround sway referenced conditions (condition 6) stability continued to decrease, especially in the youngest age groups (Fig. 8.16).

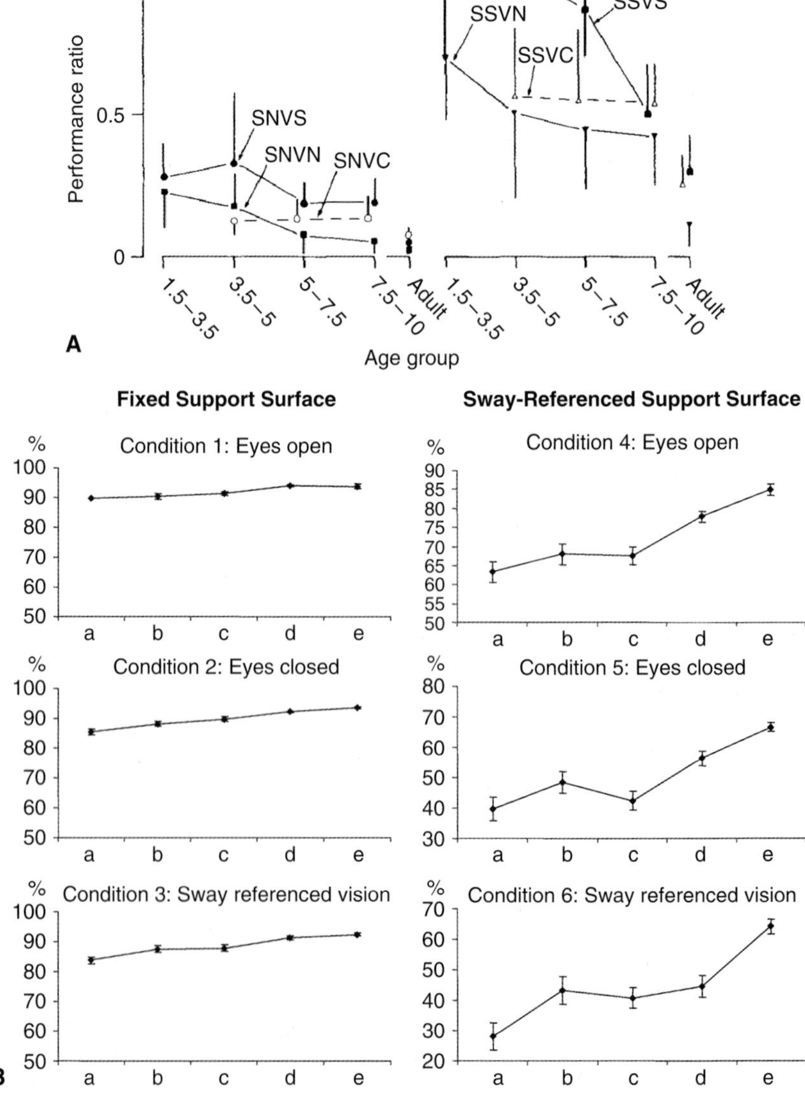

FIGURE 8.16 A, Average (±SD) performance ratios of different age groups of children standing under the six different conditions of the Sensory Orientation Test (SOT): on the left side with fixed support surface and eyes open (SNVN), eyes closed (SNVC), and the visual surface stabilized (SNVS); on the right side with support surface stabilized and eyes open (SSVN), eyes closed (SSVC), and the visual surface also stabilized (SSVS) (On the x-axis, 1 is equal to a fall and 0 is equal to perfect stability with no sway) (Reprinted with permission from Forssberg H, Nashner L. Ontogenetic development of postural control in man: adaptation to altered support and visual conditions during stance. J Neurosci 1982;2:549.) B, SOT Equilibrium scores for each group (a: 6–8, b: 8–10, c: 10–12, d: 12–14, and e: 20-yr-olds) in both normal surface (Left) and sway referenced (Right) platform trials (On the x-axis, 100% is equal to perfect stability and 0 is equal to a fall.). (From Ferber-Viart C, Ionescu E, Morlet T, Froehlich P, Dubreuil C. Balance in healthy individuals assessed with Equitest: maturation and normative data for children and young adults. Int J Pediatr Otorhinolaryngol. 2007;71:1043–1044.)

These results suggest that children under 7 to 8 years of age are unable to balance efficiently when both somatosensory and visual cues are removed, leaving only vestibular cues to control stability. In addition, children younger than 7 to 8 years of age show a reduced ability to adapt senses for postural control appropriately when one (or more) of these senses is inaccurately reporting body orientation information.

Another way of examining the development of the ability to adapt to changing sensory inputs is to put children into a context in which they perceive simultaneous small-amplitude somatosensory movement (of a movable bar they touch with a finger) and visual environmental movement (of a visual scene in front of them), as shown in Figure 8.17. In the experimental protocol, the amplitude of these movements is varied independently across different conditions. The experimenters then measure body sway amplitude relative to each stimulus amplitude in order to determine touch gain and vision gain, that is, the manner in which children weight these sensory inputs as they attempt to balance under the different conditions (Bair et al., 2007).

Bair et al. (2007) asked children 4 to 10 years of age to perform this task. They observed that children could reweight responses to multisensory inputs as early as 4 years of age. They define *intramodal reweighting* as, for example, the dependence of visual system gain on visual movement amplitude; and they define *inter-modal reweighting* as the dependence of visual system gain on touch bar movement amplitude. They found that intramodal reweighting was present in 4-year-old children; however, intermodal reweighting was observed only in the older children (10 years). With older age, children showed an increase in the amount of reweighting, suggesting better adaptation to changing sensory conditions. Thus, these results add elegantly to the previous results of others using the Sensory Organization Test, to show that the development of multisensory reweighting is present at 4 years of age and contributes to more stable and flexible control of upright stance.

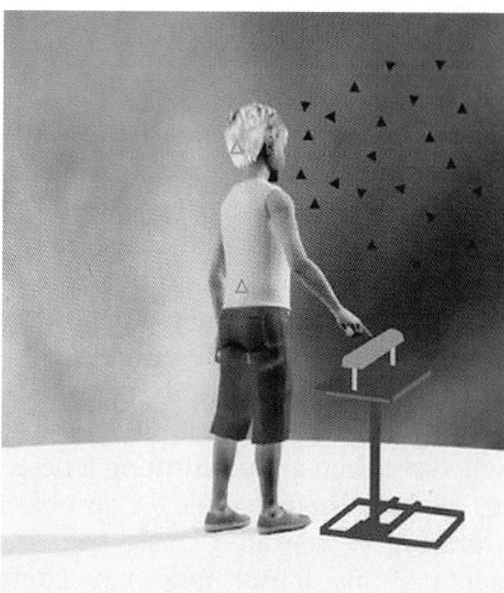

FIGURE 8.17 Experimental setup in which a child is performing the multisensory posture task (room illumination not dimmed for illustrative purposes; fewer dots are plotted for a clear view of child's posture. (Reprinted with permission from Bair WN, Kiemel T, Jeka JJ, Clark JE. Development of multisensory reweighting for posture control in children. Exp Brain Res 2007;183:437.)

Refinement of Anticipatory Postural Control

Skilled movement has both postural and voluntary components; the postural component establishes a stabilizing framework that supports the second component, that of the primary movement (Gahery & Massion, 1981). Without this supporting postural framework, skilled action deteriorates, as seen in patients with a variety of motor problems. The development of reaching in seated infants shows changes that parallel postural development. Later sections of this book detail the development of manipulatory function.

Infants as young as 9 months of age show activation of the postural muscles of the trunk in advance of most, but not all, reaching movements. In one study, infants 9 months of age were balanced on the thigh of a parent, with support only at the hip, while toys were presented to them, as shown in Figure 8.18A (von Hofsten & Woollacott, 1989). By 9 months of age, when infants were able to sit independently and were showing relatively mature reaching movements; they were also showing advance activation of postural muscles to stabilize voluntary movements in the seated position. Figure 8.18B shows the activation of trunk muscles before the anterior deltoid during a forward reach.

Van der Fits et al. (1999) examined the longitudinal development of anticipatory postural control while seated infants from 3 to 6 months of age reached for a toy. They found that postural muscle activation accompanied spontaneous and goal-directed arm movements before the onset of successful reaching at 4 to 5 months of age. During goal-directed arm movements, postural responses were direction-specific and were predominantly in the neck extensor muscles. As age increased and successful reaching increased, the amount of postural activity decreased (possibly because of increased postural stability in sitting), although it continued to improve in organization.

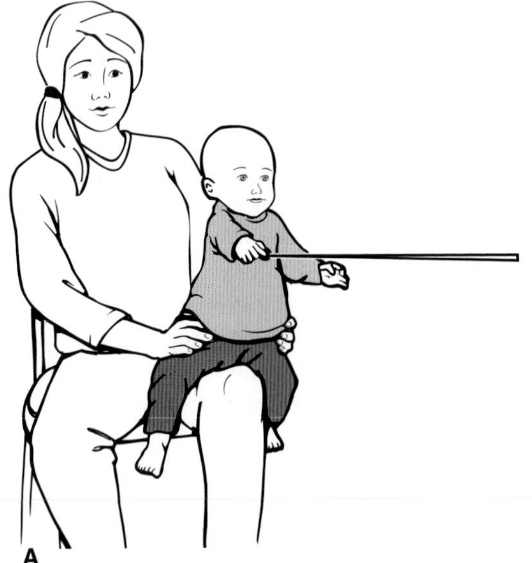

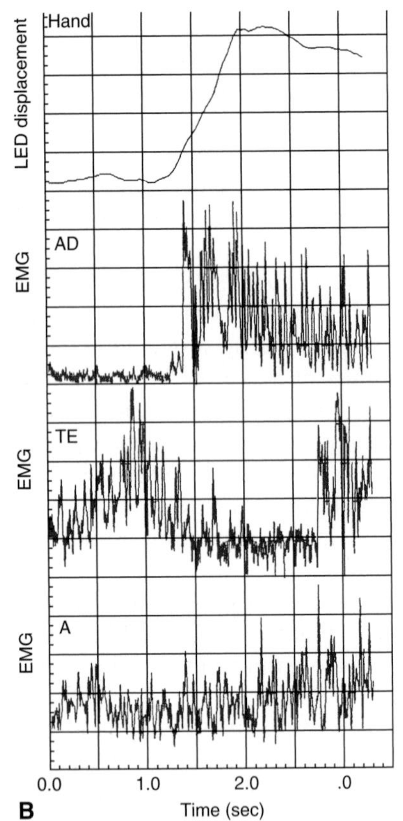

FIGURE 8.18 A, Experimental setup for a study of anticipatory postural control during reaching movements. A, The infant was balanced on the thigh of a parent, with support only at the hip, while toys on the end of a wood rod were moved toward the infant (Hofsten & Woollacott, 1989). B, EMG response of the postural muscle, the trunk extensor (TE) and the arm muscle, the anterior deltoid (AD) during a forward reach. Note that the TE is activated in advance of the AD. A = abdominal muscle; LED = light-emitting diode attached to the toy.

In standing, children as young as 10 months old are able to activate postural muscles in advance of arm movements (Forssberg & Nashner, 1982; Witherington et al., 2002). In a cross-sectional study examining the development of preparatory postural control during standing in infants from 10 to 17 months of age, standing infants were asked to open a cabinet drawer to retrieve a toy while a force resisting the pull was applied to the drawer. Results showed that both timing and the proportion of trials involving anticipatory postural activity in the gastrocnemius before the biceps was activated (to pull the drawer open) progressively improved from 10 to 17 months. At 10 to 11 months (infants were just beginning to stand independently), anticipatory activity was present, but highly inconsistent. By 13 months, as they gained experience walking, infants began to show consistent anticipatory postural activity. After the onset of independent walking, over half of the infants' pulls involved anticipatory adjustment in the gastrocnemius muscle within 240 msec of pull onset. However, the ability of the infants to deal with different external resistances during the drawer pull (adaptational abilities) did not occur until about 15 months of age (Witherington et al., 2002).

By 4 to 6 years of age, anticipatory postural adjustments preceding arm movements while standing are essentially mature (Nashner et al., 1983; Woollacott & Shumway-Cook, 1986).

Cognitive Systems in Postural Development

As we mentioned in Chapter 7, postural control requires attentional resources, with additional resources required with increasing postural task complexity. Since many activities that children perform have both a postural and a cognitive component, it is possible that performance on the postural task, the cognitive task, or both will deteriorate if the attentional capacity of the child is exceeded while performing the two tasks. For example, in the academic setting, when children are performing a postural task (standing, walking, or reaching for an object) while also performing a cognitive task, the attentional requirements of the motor task may compete for processing resources within the limited attentional capacity of the child.

In order to determine whether there are changing attentional demands of postural control during development, researchers asked children of two different age levels (4 to 6 years and 7 to 13 years) and adults to perform postural tasks both alone and in combination with a cognitive task (a visual memory task, in which they had to hold in memory a set of colored squares and then determine whether a new set of squares was the same as the set they had seen 5 seconds earlier). They then examined the extent to which performance on either the postural or cognitive task decreased during simultaneous dual-task performance. Although the cognitive task was calibrated so that all groups showed the same accuracy on the task when they performed it alone (the different groups had to remember different numbers of squares), the adults and older children were 2.5 and 1.7 times more likely to have greater accuracy on the cognitive task than the younger children when performing a demanding postural task (the modified Romberg task) at the same time. In addition, the younger children showed greater increases in postural instability (greater COP velocity) than the older children and adults when they were asked to balance in the tandem Romberg task simultaneously with the cognitive task (Reilly et al., 2008a). This suggests that the postural demands of younger children tax their attentional resources more than for older children, and this may affect both their postural and cognitive performance in dual-task situations.

Olivier et al. (2007) have also shown decreased abilities of children (7 years of age) to perform cognitive tasks (modified Stroop task) while simultaneously performing postural tasks of varying levels of complexity (quiet stance vs. standing with an ankle vibrator attached to the Achilles tendon to activate muscle spindle reflexes and thus cause a perturbation to postural sway). They found that in the ankle vibration perturbation condition that the sway was significantly higher for the children while performing the cognitive task. In adults there was no effect of cognitive task on mean velocity of COP. Interestingly, as the cognitive task difficulty increased, sway decreased slightly in the 7-year-old group and the adults. The authors interpret this to mean that the children adopt a different postural strategy, which gives more stability, under more complex cognitive task conditions. At first this type of behavior may seem counterintuitive, as the children are showing more stability under more complex cognitive task conditions. However, this type of behavior has also been seen in some other experiments under certain dual-task conditions. This increased performance has been hypothesized to be due to a number of possible factors, including the possibility of increased arousal, anchoring vision more consistently to the visual task, or shifting attention from the task of postural control to another task, thus allowing the task to be more automatic. These authors showed in a second study that children from 4 to 11 years of age were more

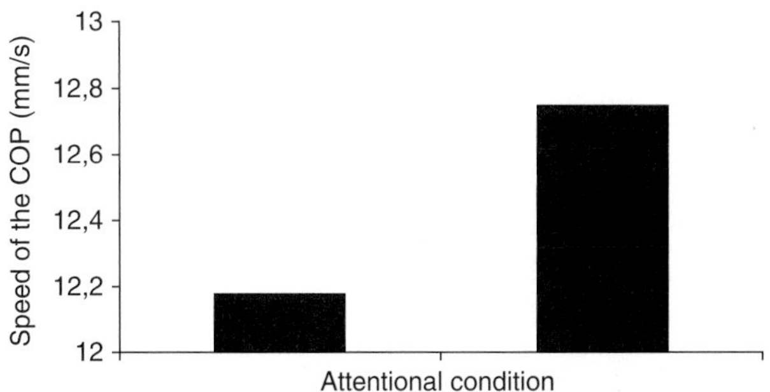

FIGURE 8.19 Mean and standard deviation for the speed (mm/sec) of the COP as a function of attentional condition (without (L) and with (R) attention focused on the posture) for all age groups. (Source: Olivier I, Palluel E, Nougier V. Effects of attentional focus on postural sway in children and adults. Exp Brain Res. 2008;185:343)

stable when looking at a video (without instruction about posture) as compared with looking at a cross at the center of the TV screen with the instruction to remain as stable as possible (Fig. 8.19). This lends support to the automaticity hypothesis as one important contributor to improved postural sway under certain dual-task conditions.

This research has described some of the critical refinements in the components of the postural control system that occur between 10 months and 13 years of age. Changes in the motor components involve changes in body morphology as well as refinement of the muscular response synergies, including: (1) a decrease in onset latencies, (2) improvement in the timing and amplitude of muscle responses, and (3) a decrease in the variability of muscle responses. Refinements in postural motor behavior are associated with a decrease in sway velocity and a reduction of oscillatory sway behavior.

Refinements in the sensory aspects of postural control include a shift from predominance of visual control of balance to a somatosensory control of balance by age 3. The ability to adapt senses for postural control appropriately when one or more of these senses is inaccurately reporting body orientation information and the ability to perform both postural and cognitive tasks in dual-task situations is reduced in children under 7.

Figure 8.20 summarizes the emergence of postural control from a systems perspective. By comparing Figures 8.20 and 8.21, you can see the similarities and differences between this model and the reflex/hierarchical model in describing the emergence of posture control in neurologically intact children. The application of these concepts can be found in Lab Activity 8.1.

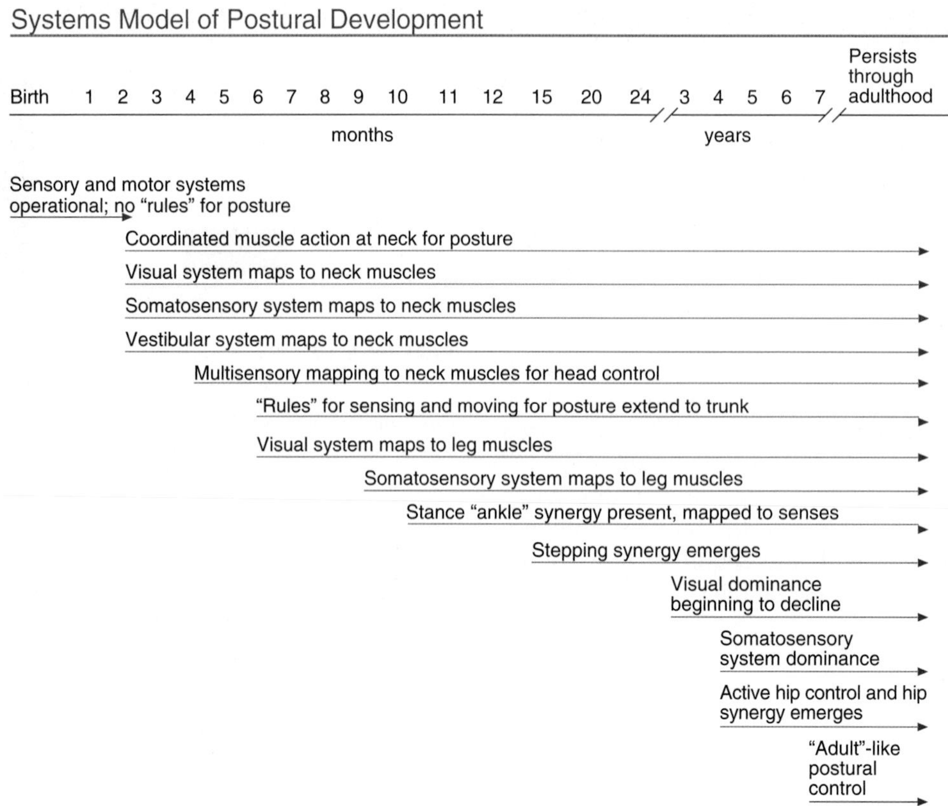

FIGURE 8.20 A systems model of postural development showing the emergence of critical stages in the development of postural control.

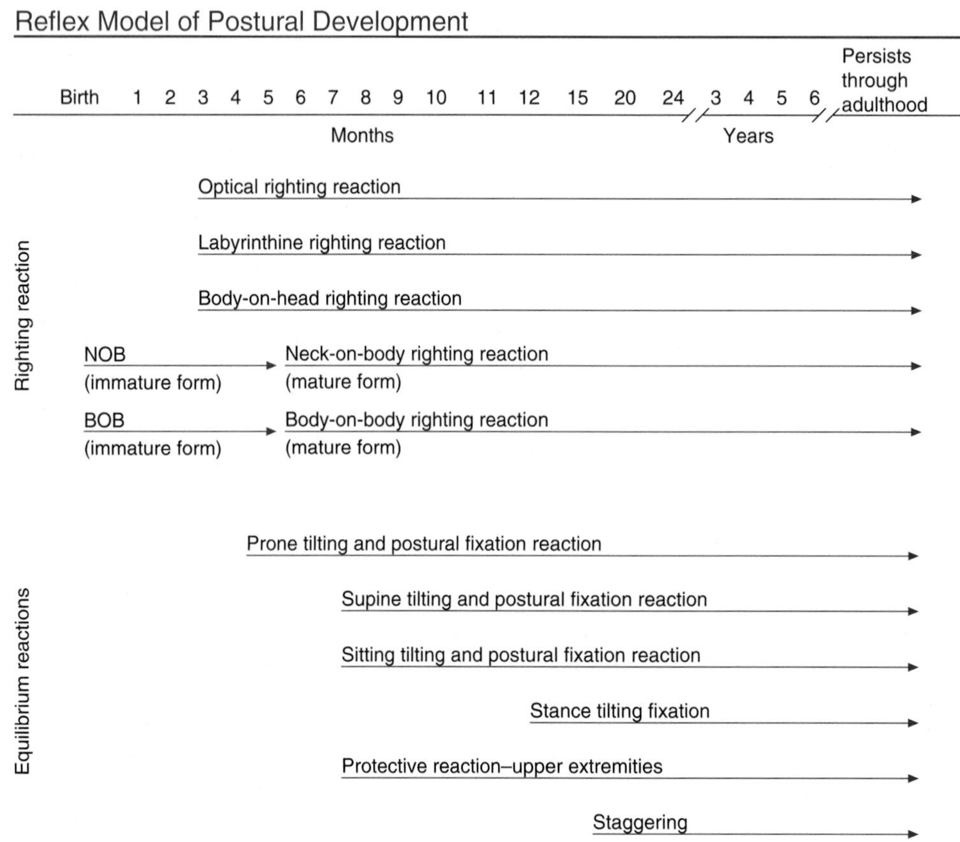

FIGURE 8.21 Reflex model of postural development.

LAB ACTIVITY 8-1

Objective: To explore both reflex/hierarchical and systems methods for evaluating balance development

Procedure: Test one or two infants of the following ages: 1–2 months, 4–6 months, 8–9 months, 18 months.

A. Motor Milestones

1. Make a list of the major motor milestones observed in each child at the varying ages.

B. Reflex/Hierarchy

Test for the presence of the following reflexes in each infant:

1. Asymmetric tonic neck reflex
2. Symmetric tonic neck reflex
3. Optical righting
4. Landau
5. Tilting reactions (prone, sitting, stance [when possible])
6. Postural fixation reactions (prone, sitting, stance [when possible])
7. Protective reactions (forward, sideways, backward)

C. Systems

Test each infant under the following postural conditions:

Steady-state postural control:

1. Vertical suspension: Hold the infants vertically with feet in contact with the supporting system. You will have to provide varying amounts of support to the infant, depending on the age. For infants who are able to stand, observe spontaneous sway in standing.
2. Sitting: Sitting quietly (supported as needed), check spontaneous sway of head and trunk.

Reactive balance:

1. Vertical suspension: Tip each child gently to the right, to the left, forward, and backward. Observe the ability to right the head, bringing it back to vertical.
2. Sitting: For infants able to sit with minimal support, give the infant a gentle nudge on the sternum, while they are sitting. Note their responses. Could they control the neck? Trunk?
3. Standing: Repeat the gentle nudge, again observe response. Could they control and recover stability?

D. Sensory dominance

Twirl a large cardboard wheel in front of the infants. How do they respond posturally to this visual stimulus?

Assignment

Write answers to the following questions, based on your observations of the infants' responses:

1. Reflexes: (a) In which children (what ages) were each of the reflexes present? (b) Did your observations coincide with those of Figure 8.21?
2. Systems: (a) What were the differences in control of quiet stance and reactive sway in the children? (b) What postural responses did you detect to a visual stimulus?
3. Did your observations coincide with those of Figure 8.20? For example, when did you see coordinated muscle action at the neck for posture? When did the visual system begin to map to neck muscles? At what age were they able to respond to sternum nudges when sitting? (When did rules for sensory/motor mapping extend to trunk?) At what age were they able to respond to sternum nudges when standing? (When did rules for sensory/motor mapping extend to leg posture control?)

SUMMARY

1. The development of postural control is an essential aspect of the development of skilled actions, like locomotion and manipulation.
2. Consistent with Gesell's developmental principles, postural development appears to be characterized by a cephalocaudal progression of control.
3. The emergence of postural control can be characterized by both the presence of limited innate components of reactive control and the subsequent development of more refined rules that relate sensory inputs reporting the body's position with respect to the environment, to motor actions that control the body's position.
   a. Control begins in the head segment. The first sense that is mapped to head control appears to be vision.
   b. As infants begin to sit independently, they learn to coordinate sensory/motor information relating the head and trunk segments, extending the sensorimotor rules for head postural control to trunk muscles.

   c. The mapping of individual senses to action may precede the mapping of multiple senses to action, thus creating internal neural representations necessary for coordinated postural abilities.
4. Anticipatory, or proactive, postural control, which provides a supportive framework for skilled movements, develops in parallel with reactive postural control.
5. Adaptive capabilities that allow a child to modify sensory and motor strategies to changing task and environmental conditions develops later. Experience in using sensory and motor strategies for posture may play a role in the development of adaptive capacities.
6. The development of postural control is best characterized as the continuous development of multiple sensory and motor systems, which manifests behaviorally in a discontinuous step-like progression of motor milestones. New strategies for sensing and moving can be associated with seeming regression in behavior as children incorporate new strategies into their repertoire for postural control.
7. Not all systems contributing to the emergence of postural control develop at the same rate. Rate-limiting components limit the pace at which an independent behavior emerges. Thus, the emergence of postural control must await the development of the slowest critical component.
8. Much debate has occurred in recent years over the relative merits of the reflex/hierarchical versus the systems models in explaining postural development. In many respects, the two models are consistent. Their differences include: (a) the reflex/hierarchical model views balance control from a reactive perspective, while the systems model stresses the importance of proactive, reactive, and adaptive aspects of the system, and (b) the reflex/hierarchical model tends to weight the role of CNS maturation more heavily than experience, while the systems model does not emphasize the role of one over the other.

ANSWERS TO LAB ACTIVITY ASSIGNMENTS

Lab Activity 8-1

1. (a) See Figure 8.21 for correct answers. (b) There may be children who show reflexes earlier or later than shown in the table, since development is variable.
2. (a) Refer to the text for ages when quiet stance and reactive balance emerge and are refined. Quiet stance control should emerge at about the time or slightly ahead of the time that reactive control is also being mastered. (b) The child should sway in the same direction as the visual motion.
3. Compare your results to Figure 8.20.

CHAPTER 9

AGING AND POSTURAL CONTROL

LEARNING OBJECTIVES

Following completion of this chapter, the reader will be able to:

1. Describe factors contributing to aging and discuss their implications for the rehabilitation of older adults.
2. Describe Spirduso's continuum of physical function and discuss factors contributing to the heterogeneity of aging.
3. Discuss the prevalence of falls in older adults and review intrinsic and extrinsic risk factors for falls among community-dwelling versus hospitalized older adults.
4. Describe age-related changes in the systems important to postural control, including both the musculoskeletal and neural systems.

INTRODUCTION

Why is it that George M, at the age of 90, is able to run marathons, while Lew N, at the age of 78, is in a nursing home, confined to a wheelchair, and unable to walk to the bathroom without assistance? Clearly, the answer to this question is complex. Many factors affect outcomes with respect to health and mobility. These factors contribute to the tremendous differences in abilities found among older adults.

This chapter does not describe all aspects of aging. Rather, the focus is on age-related changes that occur in systems critical to postural control. We review the research examining age-related changes in systems whose dysfunction may contribute to instability among older adults. Some introductory comments about research examining changes in older adults are important.

Factors Contributing to Aging

Although many studies have examined the process of aging and have shown a decline in a number of sensory and motor processes in many older adults, a surprising feature of most studies is the great heterogeneity in the aging process, with older adults of the same chronologic age showing physical function that ranges from the physically elite to the physically dependent and disabled (Aniansson et al., 1978; Duncan et al., 1993; Kosnik et al., 1988; Lewis & Bottomly, 1990; Sloane et al., 1989; Spirduso et al., 2005; Tinetti & Ginter, 1988). This has led to the understanding that there are many factors that contribute to health and longevity, including internal factors, such as genetics, and external factors, such as a person's lifestyle and the environment in which they live (Birren & Cunningham, 1985; Davies, 1987; Woollacott, 1989).

One set of theories on aging says that an important factor contributing to aging is DNA damage. For example, research has shown that the cells of our bodies undergo about 800 DNA lesions per hour, or 19,200 per cell per day (Lu et al., 2004; Vilenchik & Knudson, 2000). Though most of these lesions are repaired, there are some errors. Nonreplicating cells in the brain, muscle, and liver accumulate the most damage. Interestingly, the principal source of DNA damage leading to normal aging is reactive oxygen, from normal metabolism, and this is something that can be affected by diet and exercise. Specific genetically associated diseases, in which symptoms of aging occur early in life (Werner's syndrome, with a mean lifespan of 47 years, and progeria, with a mean lifespan of 13 years) are due to inherited defects in the enzyme that causes DNA repair, and thus offer support for this theory (Ly et al., 2000; Spirduso, et al., 2005). They suggest that the efficiency of DNA repair is a factor contributing to longevity, and in fact, DNA repair capacity is highly correlated with longevity in both humans and other animals (Burkle et al., 2005).

The second category includes factors contributing to longevity that are external to the organism and includes insults and damage caused by environmental factors such as radiation (causing genetic mutation), pollutants, bacteria/viruses, foods/toxins, and catastrophic insults that cause damage to the system and positive influences on longevity such as exercise. Interestingly, research indicates that genetic factors contribute about 20% to longevity, while health behaviors, including lifestyle, diet, exercise, and self-efficacy (a person's perception of their ability to succeed), contribute 80% (Bortz & Bortz, 1996).

However, a focus primarily on the first view, associated with genetic components as the main determinant of nervous system function with age, may create a rather pessimistic view of aging, since it suggests that functional loss is an invariant part of growing old. This type of reasoning can lead to self-limiting perceptions on the part of older individuals regarding what they can do (Tinetti et al., 1990). These self-limiting perceptions can be inadvertently reinforced by the medical professional, who may hold a limited view regarding what older adults can accomplish. For example, when assessing an older adult, a therapist may perceive that the patient's strength is good, considering the patient's age. As a result, a strength grade of 3 out of 5, which would never be accepted in a 30-year-old, is often accepted as normal in a 70-year-old.

In contrast, focus on secondary factors that contribute to longevity leads to a more optimistic view (Woollacott, 1989). In this model, one expects higher levels of function from the central nervous system (CNS) unless unexpected pathology occurs and if optimal experiential factors are present. Experiential factors involve leading a healthy and active life. Thus, when therapists with this perspective on aging evaluate an older person, they anticipate that function will be optimal. If a decline is detected in any area of the nervous system, this perspective will allow the therapist to work on rehabilitation strategies aimed at returning function toward that of a healthy young adult.

Interactions between Primary and Secondary Factors

Research is beginning to suggest that secondary or experiential factors have a profound effect on aging (Colman et al., 2009; van Praag, 2009; Wang et al., 2002). Secondary, or experiential, factors are more or less under our control. Some of these include nutrition, exercise, insults, and pathologies that affect our mind and body.

Scientists have shown that proper nutrition results in prolonged and healthier lives (Lee et al., 1993). Further, animal studies have shown that dietary restriction extends the life span (Colman et al., 2009). In addition, exercise programs have been shown to improve cardiovascular health, control obesity, and increase physical and mental function (Kramer et al., 2006). The resultant gains in aerobic power, muscle strength, and flexibility can improve biologic age by 10 to 20 years. This can result in delaying the age of dependency and increasing the quality of the remaining years of life (Fries, 2002; Wang et al., 2002). This knowledge that how we age is largely determined by how we live leads to an emphasis on preventive health care measures. It also has implications for rehabilitation. Therapists work to assist older patients who have experienced pathology to return to optimal lifestyles (Tinetti, 1986).

Thus, the factors that determine the health and mobility of George M versus Lew N are a combination of primary aging factors, primarily genetics, over which they have limited control, and secondary aging factors, primarily experiential, over which they have considerable control.

It also appears that aging, whether it is due to genetic or lifestyle factors, may not necessarily be characterized by an overall decline in function. Rather, decline may be limited to specific neural structures and functions. This is consistent with a major theme in this book, that function and dysfunction are not generalized, but emerge through the interaction of the capacities of the individual carrying out particular tasks within specific environmental contexts.

Heterogeneity of Aging

A review of the literature on aging shows that some studies report no change in function of the neural subsystems controlling posture and locomotion with age (Gabell & Nayak, 1984), while others show a severe decline in function in older adults (Imms & Edholm, 1981). How can there be such a discrepancy in studies reporting age-related changes in systems for posture and gait? This may be due to fundamental differences in the definition that researchers use in classifying an individual as elderly.

For example, some researchers have classified the elderly adult as anyone over 60 years of age. When no exclusionary criteria are used in the study of older adults, results can be very different from when researchers use restrictive criteria for including subjects for study. For example, a study on the effects of aging on walking ability selected a group of 71 subjects ranging in age from 60 to 99 years, using no exclusion criteria for possible pathology (Imms & Edholm, 1981). These researchers noted that the mean walking velocities for their older adults were slower than those reported in any previous studies.

In contrast, another study examined walking in healthy older adults. In this study, 1,187 individuals 65 years of age and older were screened to find 32 who were free of pathology, that is, who had no disorders of the musculoskeletal, neurologic, or cardiovascular systems or any previous history of falls (Gabell & Nayak, 1984). Interestingly, this study found no significant differences between their younger and older adult groups when comparing four parameters measuring the variability of gait. They thus concluded that an increase in variability in the gait cycle among older adults was not normal, but was always due to some pathology.

These types of results suggest that there is much heterogeneity among older adults. This amazing variability reminds us that it is important not to assume that physical capabilities decline in all older adults.

This continuum of function among older adults has been nicely described by Spirduso et al. (2005), who have illustrated the continuum of function found among older adults. This continuum is illustrated in Figure 9.1. At the high end of the continuum are older adults who are physically elite, who engage in competitive sports and are considered to undergo optimal aging. Moving down the continuum are older adults who are physically fit, that is, who engage in sports, games, and hobbies and who are capable of moderate physical work. Physically independent adults are also active, but engage in less physically demanding activities, such as golf or social dancing. Independence in all basic activities of daily living (BADLs) and instrumental activities of daily living (IADLs) is characteristic of this group. Adults in the physically frail group are usually independent in BADLs but are dependent in many IADLs. They are capable of light housekeeping, but often require assistance to continue living independently. Physically dependent adults are disabled; they are dependent in both BADLs and IADLs. They require full-time assistance or institutional care. Using this continuum you can see that George M. would fall at the upper end of the continuum, in the physically elite group, while Lew N, would fall at the lower end.

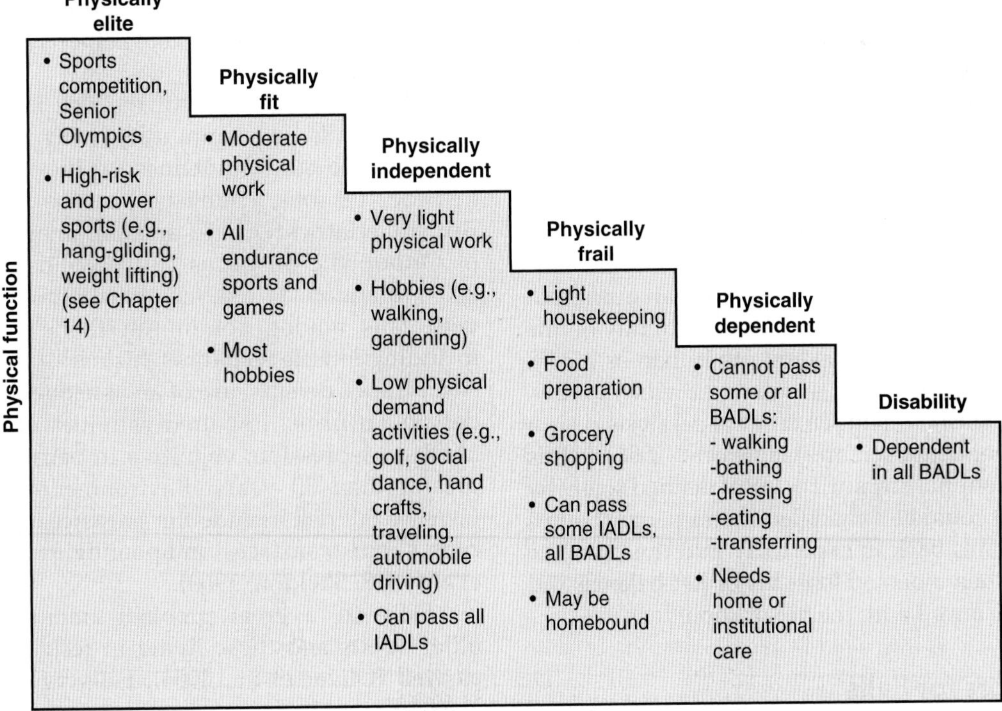

FIGURE 9.1 Continuum of physical function among older adults. (Adapted from Spirduso W, Francis K, MacRae PG. Physical dimensions of aging. Champaign IL: Human Kinetics, 2005:264, Figure 11.1.)

BEHAVIORAL INDICATORS OF INSTABILITY

Defining Falls

Before we can discuss falls and their causes in more detail, it is important to have a clear understanding of the definition of a fall and the different categories of falls that can be experienced. This knowledge allows the therapist to question patients more effectively regarding the frequency and nature of their falls, as well as offers a better understanding of the type of rehabilitative strategies appropriate for situations with a variety of types of balance risk. Falls are often defined differently in the clinic versus in the research environment. For example, in the clinic, a fall is often defined as a situation in which the older adult falls to the ground or is found lying on the ground. In addition, it is often defined as any unintended contact with a supporting surface, such as a chair, counter, or wall.

In the research environment, the safety of older adults is considered of utmost importance, and thus balance testing is typically done with a safety harness protecting the older adult from actual falls. In the laboratory, balance threats are often simulated by moving the support surface varying distances underneath the older adult. In the presence of small platform perturbations, a fall, or loss of balance, may be defined by movement of the center of mass outside the limits of the base of support, since this could result in a fall if a safety harness were not being used. However, it is important to remember that this definition could also include any situation in which the participant simply stepped in response to the balance threat, and still recovered stability, although with a different strategy than what might be used by a young adult.

Since the term *fall* is used in a variety of contexts it is important for clinicians to define their own meaning of the term when talking to patients about falls. One clinical definition used to define a fall is an event that results in a person coming to rest inadvertently on the ground or other lower level and other than as a consequence of the following: sustaining a violent blow; loss of consciousness; sudden onset of paralysis, as in a stroke; or an epileptic seizure (Hauer et al., 2006). In this definition, a supporting surface is not defined solely by the floor, but could be a chair (as when a person begins to rise and falls back unexpectedly into the chair) or a wall (as when a person loses his or her balance and staggers into a wall with the hip or shoulder).

Risk Factors for Falls

Statistics show that unintentional injuries are the fifth leading cause of death in the elderly (after cardiovascular disease, cancer, stroke and pulmonary disorders), and falls make up two-thirds of these deaths. Of significance, about three-fourths of the deaths from falls occur in people over 65 years (Ochs et al., 1985; Rubenstien, 2006). In addition, fall rates in persons 65 years of age or older are at least 33% per year in community-dwelling older adults, with women being found to fall more frequently than men (Campbell et al., 1981; Nevitt et al., 1989; Shumway-Cook et al., 2009). What factors contribute to these losses of balance? Many early studies on balance loss in the elderly expected to isolate a single cause of falls for a given older adult, such as vertigo, sensory neuropathy, or postural hypotension. In contrast, more current research indicates that many falls in the elderly have multiple contributing factors, including extrinsic environmental factors and intrinsic factors such as physiological, musculoskeletal, and psychosocial factors (Campbell et al., 1989; Lipsitz et al., 1991; Tinetti et al., 1986).

Perform Lab Activity 9.1 to explore issues related to determining fall risk. You may have discovered that when attempting to determine fall risk it is critical to know both the activity level and the risk of falls for the activity in which the person is engaged. Falls are not determined solely by factors within the individual (e.g., poor balance); falls emerge from an interaction of the individual performing specific tasks in certain environments. In fact, research shows that older adults (>75 years) tend to fall at home, while younger old adults (70–75 years) fall more frequently away from home (and suffer more serious injuries) (Shumway-Cook et al., 2009; Speechley & Tinetti, 1991; Tinetti et al., 1988).

Let us look at some of the risk factors contributing to falls in community-living older adults. According to the "Guidelines for Prevention of Falls in Older Persons," published by the American and British Geriatrics Societies and the American Academy of Orthopedic Surgeons (Rubenstein & Josephson, 2001), there are 11 risk factors commonly associated with falls among community-living older adults, including muscle weakness, history of falls, gait deficits, balance deficits, use of an assistive device, visual deficits, arthritis, impaired activities of daily living (ADLs), depression, cognitive impairment, and age greater than 80 years. Environmental factors that increase fall risk include the presence of stairs, throw rugs, slippery surfaces, and poor lighting (Rubenstein et al., 1988; Sheldon, 1960).

Falls are a great problem among hospitalized older adults and those living in residential facilities as well (Oliver et al., 2004). Falls by inpatients are associated with an increased duration of hospitalization and a greater chance of unplanned readmission or of discharge to residential or nursing home care

LAB ACTIVITY 9-1

Objective: To explore issues related to determining fall risk.

Procedure: Ask yourself how many times you have fallen in the past 12 months. Think about and list the activities you were performing at the time you fell. What were the environmental conditions like when you fell? What were the consequences of your falls? Were you injured? Since the fall, have you been afraid or reluctant to return to those activities? Now, find an older adult living within the community or within a residential facility like an assisted living retirement center or skilled nursing facility. Ask this older adult the same set of questions. What is their fall rate? What activities were they performing when they fell? What was the environment like? Were they injured, and what was the psychological consequence of the fall? Were they more fearful and reluctant to return to their prior level of activity?

Assignment

Write answers to the above questions and compare your responses to those of the older adult. What is the difference between your falls and those you would expect to see in 70-to-80-year-olds? What were the consequences?

(Bates et al., 1995). Are risk factors the same for older adults in hospital and residential facilities as for those living in the community? Many factors predictive of falls among elderly people in the community may not apply to hospital inpatients, for whom recovery from acute illness that is associated with changing mobility is more common. Since the occurrence of falls depends on patient characteristics and institutional characteristics, such as clinical and nursing practice, risk factors may be specific to particular hospital units (e.g., acute medical vs. inpatient rehabilitation) (Oliver et al., 1997). Many studies have examined risk factors for falls among hospitalized older adults, and they have consistently identified the following factors: gait instability, lower-extremity weakness, urinary incontinence/frequency or need for assistance in toileting, impaired cognition (agitation, confusion, or impaired judgment), history of falls, and the use of certain medications, in particular, centrally acting sedatives (Oliver et al., 2004).

The identification of factors predictive of falls in hospitalized elders has led to the development of a number of risk-factor assessment tools for use in hospitals and residential settings (see Oliver et al., 2004; Perell et al., 2001, for reviews of risk-assessment tools). Assessment Tool 9.1 is an example of one such tool, STRATIFY (St. Thomas's risk assessment tool in falling elderly inpatients), developed and validated by British researchers to predict falls in hospitalized elders. Among hospitalized elders, a risk score of 2 or more had a sensitivity of 93% and a specificity of 88% for predicting inpatient falls (Oliver et al., 1997).

Among older adults, fall risk is also high 1 to 6 months after discharge from the hospital. Several studies have examined postdischarge fall rates among older adults hospitalized for hip fracture. McKee et al.

Assessment Tool 9-1

STRATIFY

1. Did the patient present to hospital with a fall, or has he or she fallen on the ward since admission?

   (Yes = 1, No = 0)

DO YOU THINK THE PATIENT (QUESTIONS 2–5)

2. Is agitated?

   (Yes = 1, No = 0)

3. Is visually impaired to the extent that everyday function is affected?

   (Yes = 1, No = 0)

4. Is in need of especially frequent toileting?

   (Yes = 1, No = 0)

5. Has a transfer and mobility score of 3 or 4*?

   (Yes = 1, No = 0)

Total score

(range, 0–5) score ≥2 indicates an increased risk for falls

*Transfer score: 0 = unable, 1 = major help needed (one or two people, physical aids), 2 = minor help (verbal or physical), 3 = independent; mobility score: 0 = immobile, 1 = independent with aid of wheelchair, 2 = walks with help of one person, 3 = independent.

Reprinted with permission from Oliver D, Britton M, Seed P, et al. Development and evaluation of evidence based risk assessment tool (STRATIFY) to predict which elderly inpatients will fall: case-control and cohort studies. BMJ 1997;315:1049–1053.

(2002) followed 57 patients for 2 months and reported that 17.5% of those with a hip fracture went on to fall again. Colon-Emeric et al. (2000) reported that 19% of community-dwelling men and male veterans sustained a second hip or pelvic fracture within 1 year after the initial hip fracture. Shumway-Cook et al. (2005a) followed 90 older adults for 6 months after discharge for a fall-related hip fracture and reported that 53.3% of patients (48 of 90) reported one or more falls in the 6 months after hospitalization. Older adults who fell after discharge had significantly greater declines in independence in ADLs and lower performance on balance and mobility measures. These authors found that two factors—premorbid history of falls and use of a gait-assistive device (indicating impaired mobility)—predicted falls in the 6 months after discharge. The authors suggest that identification of older adults at risk for poor outcomes early in their hip fracture care could result in improved discharge planning. Specifically, older adults determined to be at risk for additional falls could be referred for further physical therapy after fracture healing for exercises specifically designed to improve balance and mobility function in order to reduce the risk for falls (Shumway-Cook et al., 2005).

Many studies have examined the physiological factors that contribute to a risk of falls (Campbell et al., 1989; Lipsitz et al., 1991; Lord et al., 1993; Maki et al., 1994a; Nevitt et al., 1989; Tinetti et al., 1988). The conclusions of these studies were that most falls in older adults involve multiple risk factors and that many of these factors may be remediated. The risk of falling increases with the number of risk factors. In a cohort of elderly persons living in the community, the risk for falling increased from 8% among those with no risk factors to 78% among those with four or more risk factors (Tinetti et al., 1988). Thus, it has been suggested that the clinician who is working with an older adult should determine both intrinsic and extrinsic factors associated with a particular fall and reduce or correct as many of these as possible (Lipsitz et al., 1991).

Studies examining intrinsic factors leading to falls have included examining the role of balance control. Several researchers, including Tinetti et al. from the United States, Berg et al. from Canada, and Mathias et al. from England, have measured functional skills related to balance in order to identify people at high risk for falls (Berg et al., 1989; Mathias et al., 1986; Speechley & Tinetti, 1990; Tinetti et al., 1986). Functional skills include sitting, standing and walking unsupported, standing and reaching forward, performing a 360-degree turn, and moving from a sitting to a standing position. A more recent approach to understanding balance function in the elderly examines specific variables relating to normal postural control and determines the extent to which deterioration in their function contributes to loss of stability and mobility in the elderly.

In the remaining sections of this chapter we examine the intrinsic factors related to balance problems in older adults from a systems perspective. We discuss changes in the motor system, the sensory systems, and higher-level adaptive and cognitive systems, as well as the use of anticipatory postural responses before making a voluntary movement. Studies on the ability of older adults to integrate balance adjustments into the step cycle are covered in the mobility section of this book.

AGE-RELATED CHANGES IN THE SYSTEMS OF POSTURAL CONTROL

In previous chapters, we discussed the many systems that contribute to postural control (see Fig. 7.3). What have researchers learned about how changes in these systems contribute to an increased likelihood for falls in the elderly?

Musculoskeletal System

Muscle Strength

Several researchers have reported changes in the musculoskeletal system in many older adults (Aniansson et al., 1986; Buchner & deLateur, 1991; Frontera et al., 2000; Narici et al., 2008). Strength, or the amount of force a muscle produces, declines with age. Lower-extremity muscle strength (defined as the amount of force produced during a single maximum contraction of a muscle) can be reduced by as much as 40% between the ages of 30 and 80 years (Aniansson et al., 1986). Longitudinal studies following muscle strength changes across 10 years in older adults (mean age at the start of the study, 60 years) showed a 12% to 17% loss of knee flexor and extensor strength over the two types of muscles. However, strength gains were also seen in some individuals, showing the heterogeneity of the aging process (Hughes et al., 2001). Muscle strength reduction is more severe in older nursing home residents with a history of falls (Whipple et al., 1987). In these subjects, the mean knee and ankle muscle strength was reduced twofold and fourfold, respectively, as compared with those with no history of falls.

Endurance, which is the capacity of the muscle to contract continuously at submaximal levels, also decreases with age. However, endurance is better preserved with age than is strength. As muscles age, they become smaller; this reduction in muscle mass is greater in the lower extremities than in the upper extremities (Medina, 1996). As muscle cells die, they are replaced with connective tissue and fat. A number of studies have examined the preferential loss of muscle fiber types with aging, with mixed results. There appears to be an age-related loss of both type I (slow-oxidative, used in activities such as postural control and long-distance running) and II (fast-twitch, used for sprinting, etc.) muscle fiber types. It used to be thought that with aging type II fast-twitch fibers may be lost at a faster rate than type I fibers (Timiras, 1994), but new evidence suggests that increasing numbers of muscle fibers simply become more of a blend of type I and type II, with characteristics of both (Anderson et al., 1999; Spirduso et al., 2005). Researchers have also shown that the number of motor units declines with age; there is a reduction in both large and small myelinated fibers. In addition, there are age-related changes at the neuromuscular junction (Medina, 1996).

Changes in skeletal muscle affect the functional capacity of the muscles. Maximum isometric force decreases, the muscles fatigue more rapidly, and the rate of tension development is slower. It appears that concentric contractions are more affected by age-related changes in the neuromuscular system than are eccentric contractions. Rapid-velocity contractions are more affected than slow-velocity contractions.

Researchers have shown that the association between strength and physical function is large, with over 20% of the variance in functional status explained by relative strength (Buchner & deLateur, 1991). In addition, lower-extremity lean muscle mass and reduced strength were strong independent predictors of severe functional impairment in older adults (Reid et al., 2008). Interestingly, muscle power has been found to be even more highly correlated with physical function than muscle strength, with power training being more effective than strength training for improving physical function in older adults with muscle weakness (Bean et al., 2003; Miszko et al., 2003).

However, the amount of strength or power needed for physical function is dependent on the task. For example, it has been suggested that the typical healthy 80-year-old woman is very near, if not at, the threshold value for quadriceps strength necessary to rise from a chair (Young, 1986). When strength falls below the threshold needed for a task, functional disability occurs.

Range of Motion

Decreased range of motion and loss of spinal flexibility in many older adults can lead to a characteristic flexed or stooped posture (Fig. 9.2) (Balzini et al., 2003; Katzman et al., 2007). Spinal flexibility shows the greatest decline with age, as compared with all other joints, and spinal extension shows the greatest decline, with 50% less extensor flexibility in 70-to-84-year-olds as compared with 20-to-29-year-olds (Einkauf et al., 1987; Katzman et al., 2007). This may be primarily a cause of the types of daily activities most often performed, with few activities requiring a backward extension (Spirduso et al., 2005). Loss of spinal flexibility can be associated with other changes in postural alignment, including a compensatory shift in the vertical displacement of the center of body mass backward toward the heels. Ankle-joint flexibility, critical for postural control, also declines by 50% in women and 35% in men between the ages of 55 and 85 (Vandervoort et al., 1992). Other conditions, such as arthritis, can lead to decreased range of motion in many joints throughout the body. In addition, pain may limit the functional range of motion of a particular joint (Horak et al., 1989). Increased kyphosis is associated with a decrease in spinal extensor muscle strength, as well as impaired balance, slower walking and stair climbing, a shorter functional reach, and decreased ADL performance (Balzini et al., 2003; Katzman et al., 2007).

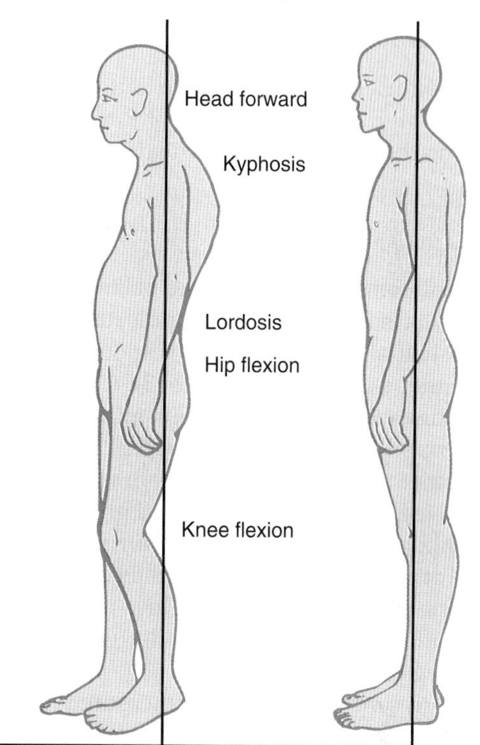

FIGURE 9.2 Comparison of postural alignment in a young versus an older adult. Changes in spinal flexibility can lead to a stooped or flexed posture in many elderly people. (Adapted with permission from Lewis C, Bottomley J. Musculoskeletal changes with age. In: Lewis C, ed. Aging: health care's challenge, 2nd ed. Philadelphia: FA Davis, 1990:146.)

Neuromuscular System

The neuromuscular system contributes to postural control through the coordination of forces effective in controlling the body's position in space.

Changes in Quiet Stance

Traditional methods for assessing balance function in older adults have used global indicators of balance control, such as determination of spontaneous sway during quiet stance (Sheldon, 1963). One of the earliest studies examined the extent to which subjects in age groups from 6 years through 80 years swayed during quiet stance. Subjects at both ends of the age spectrum (ages 6–14 and 50–80) had greater difficulty in minimizing spontaneous sway during quiet stance than the other age groups tested (Sheldon, 1963). This study tested a great variety of older adults, and did not try to limit subjects in the older groups to those who were free of pathology.

More recent studies have measured spontaneous sway in different age groups using stabilometry, or static force plates. One study examined 500 adults, aged 40 to 80 years, who were free of pathology, and found that postural sway increased with each decade of life. Thus, the greatest amount of spontaneous sway was seen in the 80-year-olds (Toupet et al., 1992). Similarly, a study examining spontaneous sway in older adults with and without a history of falls found a significant increase in sway even in healthy older adults as compared with young adults, with the greatest amount of sway found in older people with a recent history of falls (Shumway-Cook et al., 1997c). A number of studies that have examined spontaneous sway have found only small differences between young and older adults. For example Wolfson et al. (1992) found only a 3% (nonsignificant) difference between young adults (mean age [±SD], 35±12 years) and healthy older adults (76±5 years) who were relatively free of neurologic disease. Peterka and Black (1990–1991) also found no significant changes in anteroposterior postural sway in subjects from 7 to 81 years of age in eyes-open or eyes-closed conditions.

Another study, by Fernie and colleagues (1982), examined both sway amplitude and velocity in a population of institutionalized elderly and determined that sway velocity (but not amplitude) was significantly greater for those who fell one or more times in a year than for those who had not fallen. This implies that, in certain populations, velocity of sway may be more sensitive to balance problems than absolute sway.

If total magnitude or velocity of spontaneous sway or center-of-pressure (COP) displacement during a given period is seen as a clear measure of balance control, then according to a number of the studies cited above, one might conclude that there is a small decline in balance function in older adults. However, Patla et al. (1990) and others make the point that measures of spontaneous sway during normal quiet stance are not necessarily appropriate measures of balance dyscontrol, since older adults are not challenged by normal quiet stance balance and are thus typically well within their balance capacity. Patla notes that larger excursions of COP are generally interpreted as a reflection of a poor balance-control system, but that some older adults may use larger and higher-frequency excursions of COP to obtain more information about their posture from their sensory systems, while remaining well within their limits of stability (Patla et al., 1990). They suggest that static balance be assessed under challenging conditions such as tandem stance with eyes open versus closed.

Horak et al. (1992) also remind us that there are a variety of patients with neurologic disorders, such as Parkinson's disease, who have normal, or even reduced, sway in quiet stance. This may be due to the fact that they show increased stiffness or rigidity and this limits sway to a smaller area during quiet stance. This is one reason that measurement of sway with eyes open during normal quiet stance may not be the best way to evaluate balance dysfunction in older adults.

Another way of examining quiet-stance stability is to examine the spatial/temporal boundaries of postural instability. This can be done by measuring the COP trajectory in relation to estimated geometric stability boundaries (borders of the feet) or functional stability boundaries (COP movement during anteroposterior, lateral, and diagonal maximum sway efforts). In a study examining subjects from 60 to 96 years of age, it was shown that the ratio of the area of motion of the COP to the area of both geometric and functional stability boundary increased with age. Functional stability boundaries were much smaller than geometric boundaries, and became smaller with increasing age, suggesting that measures of stability limits using only foot boundaries may be inappropriate in older adults. A measure of virtual time to contact with the postural stability boundary also decreased with age, suggesting that older adults are at higher risk of instability that would necessitate taking a step or risking a fall (Slobounov et al., 1998).

Changes in Motor Strategies during Perturbed Stance

Is the older adult capable of activating muscle response synergies with appropriate timing, force, and muscle response organization when balance is threatened? Most research addresses this question by using a moving platform to provide an external threat to balance. Measures of balance control have included: (1) electromyography (EMG): postural muscle response characteristics (onset latency, duration, magnitude); (2) kinematics: changes in center of mass (COM) and joint angle during the balance threat and the recovery; and (3) kinetics: the forces (e.g., COP) applied by older adults to respond to the balance threat and recover stability. In the following pages we will summarize the studies that have examined changes in these variables that are correlated with aging and with falls.

Woollacott et al. (1986) performed one of the first studies to examine age-related changes in postural muscle response characteristics elicited when balance was threatened. They found that the muscle response organization of older adults (61–78 years) and younger adults (19–38 years) was generally similar, with responses being activated first in the stretched ankle muscle and radiating upward to the muscles of the thigh.

However, there were also differences between the two groups in certain response characteristics. The older adults showed significantly slower onset latencies in the ankle dorsiflexors in response to anterior platform movements, causing backward sway. This has been observed in other laboratories as well (Studenski et al., 1991). In addition, in some older adults, the muscle response organization was disrupted, with proximal muscles being activated before distal muscles. This response organization has also been seen in patients with CNS dysfunction (Nashner et al., 1983).

The older adult group also tended to coactivate the antagonist muscles along with the agonist muscles at a given joint significantly more often than the younger adults. Thus, many of the elderly people studied tended to stiffen the joints to a greater degree than young adults when compensating for sway perturbations.

Several labs have found that many older adults used a strategy involving hip movements rather than ankle movements significantly more often than young adults (Horak et al., 1989; Manchester et al., 1989). Hip movements are typically used by young adults when balancing on a short support surface that does not allow them to use ankle torque in compensating for sway. It has been hypothesized that this shift toward use of a hip strategy for balance control in older adults may be related to pathologic conditions such as ankle-muscle weakness or loss of peripheral sensory function. Horak et al. (1989) have suggested that in older adults, some falls, particularly those associated with slipping, may be the result of using a hip strategy in slippery conditions in which the surface cannot resist the sheer forces associated with the use of this strategy, for example, when on ice.

More recent studies have extended this research and have compared young adults with stable older adults and with older adults with balance problems (Chandler et al., 1990; Lin & Woollacott, 2002). Figure 9.3 summarizes some of the effects found in these studies. Figure 9.3A shows examples of responses (from individual trials) to anterior platform movements causing posterior sway in a young adult, a healthy older adult, and an older adult who had problems with balance and falls. Note that the onset latencies for the tibialis anterior and quadriceps postural muscles become progressively later for the

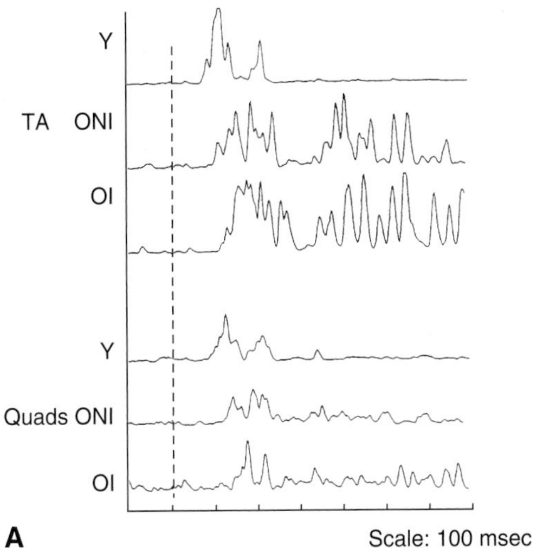

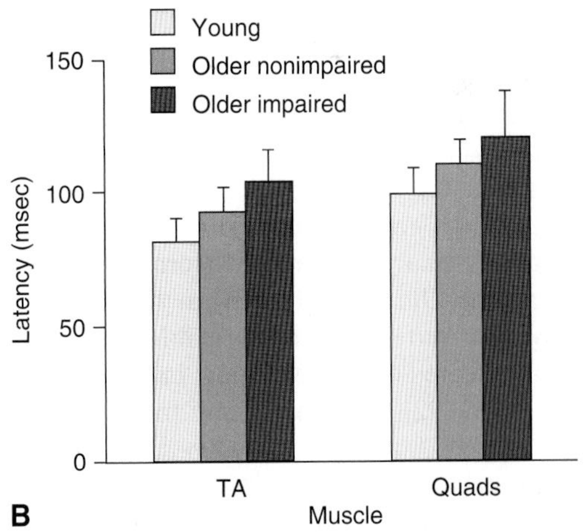

FIGURE 9.3 Changes in timing of muscle response synergies in the elderly. A, Examples of muscle responses to an anterior platform movement causing posterior sway in a young adult, a healthy older adult, and an older adult who had problems with balance and falls. Note that the onset latencies for the tibialis anterior (TA) and quadriceps (Q) postural muscles become progressively later for the stable and then the unstable older adults. B, Graphs showing mean response onset latencies for TA and Q in each subject group. ONI = older nonimpaired; OI = older impaired; Y = young.

stable and then the unstable older adults. Figure 9.3B shows the mean muscle onset latencies for all individuals in each group.

Adapting Movements to Changing Tasks and Environments

These early research studies provided information on age-related changes in responses to balance threats of a single size. It is possible that these changes in postural response characteristics in older adults are simply indications of deterioration in postural muscle response efficiency, as implied in the earlier literature. However, it is also possible that some of these changes may be due to the older adults using a different response strategy than that seen in young adults, as a way of adapting to certain constraints associated with aging, such as muscle weakness, reduced ankle-joint sensation, or joint stiffness. For example, it is possible that a shift toward the use of hip movements in balance control may be due to ankle-muscle weakness and the inability to generate large amounts of force at the ankle joint (Horak et al., 1989; Manchester et al., 1989). This might be seen more clearly as an older adult is subjected to larger balance threats that exceed his or her muscle response capacity at the ankle. In addition, older adults with balance problems may show more severe constraints within their neural and musculoskeletal systems and therefore show more limited response capacity.

In order to explore this question further, studies have examined the response characteristics of both well-balanced and less-stable older adults during balance threats of increasing magnitude and velocity, in order to simulate environmental situations with changing balance conditions (Lin & Woollacott, 2002, Lin et al., 2004). Young (mean [±SD] age, 25±4 years) and older adults were recruited from the community for the study. Older adults (mean age, 75±4 years) were divided into stable and unstable groups according to their scores on three clinical balance tests (Berg [Berg et al., 1992], Dynamic Gait Index [Shumway-Cook et al., 1997], and self-perceived balance ability). When comparing the fall history of the groups it was noted that the unstable older adults showed a mean of 0.63 fall in the past 6 months, while stable older adults showed only 0.06 in the past 6 months.

As one might expect, there were variations in the ability of stable and unstable older adults in their ability to respond effectively to balance threats of different magnitudes and velocities. For example, in response to small/slow forward perturbations, onset latencies across the three muscles tested (tibialis anterior [TA], quadriceps [Q], and abdominals [A]) were significantly delayed in both the stable and unstable older adults as compared with the young adults, but for the large/fast perturbations, only the unstable older adults showed delays as compared with the young adults. This suggests that the stable older adults had difficulty in sensing the onset of small/slow perturbations but were able to compensate adequately for larger scaling factors.

Could older adults increase muscle contraction amplitudes when perturbations were larger? The TA response of the unstable older adults was significantly lower than that of the stable and young adults for even smaller perturbations. In response to larger perturbations, both the stable older adults and unstable older adults showed significantly smaller responses than the young adults. This suggests that both older stable and unstable adults show a limited response capacity as compared with young adults, but this is not apparent in stable older adults until balance threats are large.

Were older adults using a higher percentage of maximal voluntary capacity in responding to balance threats? Lin and Woollacott (2002) compared postural response amplitudes during perturbations to amplitudes of a maximum voluntary gastrocnemius contraction. Figure 9.4 shows that for small perturbations, the young and stable older adults used similar amounts of maximum capacity (about 20%), but the unstable older adults used significantly more (almost 40%). As perturbation velocity increased to 40 cm/sec, the stable older adults also showed significantly larger amounts of maximum capacity utilization than the young adults.

How were these age-related changes in neuromuscular responses correlated with behavioral changes during balance recovery? For even very small/slow perturbation conditions that did not require a step, there were clear differences in strategies used by the groups. Both stable and unstable older adults used significantly less ankle-dominated responses and more hip-dominated responses than young adults. In addition, unstable older adults use alternative strategies such as bending at the knee and using the arms to balance. These differences were increased for faster perturbations, with older adults showing a significant percentage of stepping responses when young adults were still using in-place (ankle or hip) responses.

These differences can also be seen in the quantitative data showing COP changes in response to platform perturbations for young stable and unstable older adults. Figure 9.5 shows that when young adults were given a platform perturbation they efficiently returned the COP to a stable position, whereas the stable and unstable older adults each showed more COP oscillation before coming to a stable position, with the unstable group showing the largest excursion of the COP. This was accompanied by an increased time for

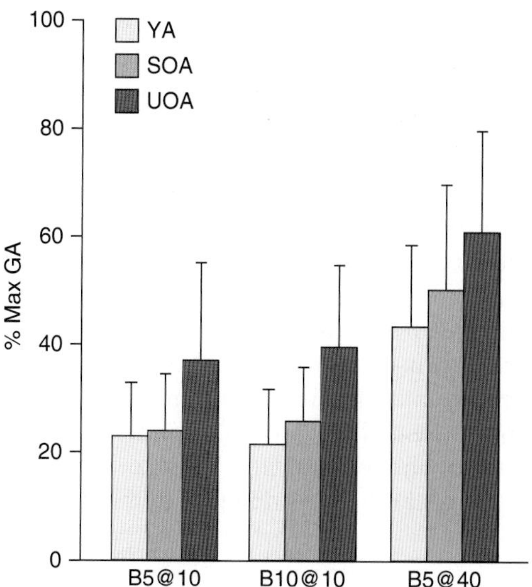

FIGURE 9.4 Comparison of postural response amplitudes (IEMG) of young stable adults (YA), stable older adults (SOA), and unstable older adults (UOA) for similar intervals when standing maximally on toes (maximum gastrocnemius capacity) versus when responding to balance threats of different sizes and velocities. Note that for small perturbations the young and stable older adults used similar amounts of maximum capacity (about 20%), but the unstable older adults used significantly more (almost 40%). As perturbation velocity increased to 40 cm/sec, the stable older adults also showed significantly larger amounts of maximum capacity utilization than the young adults. GA = gastrocnemius; B5 = backward perturbation at 5 cm/sec; B10 = backward perturbation at 10 cm/sec. (Adapted with permission from Lin S-I, Woollacott MH. Differentiating postural responses following dynamically changing balance threats in young adults, healthy older adults and unstable older adults: electromyography. J Mot Behav 2002;34:42, Figure 5.)

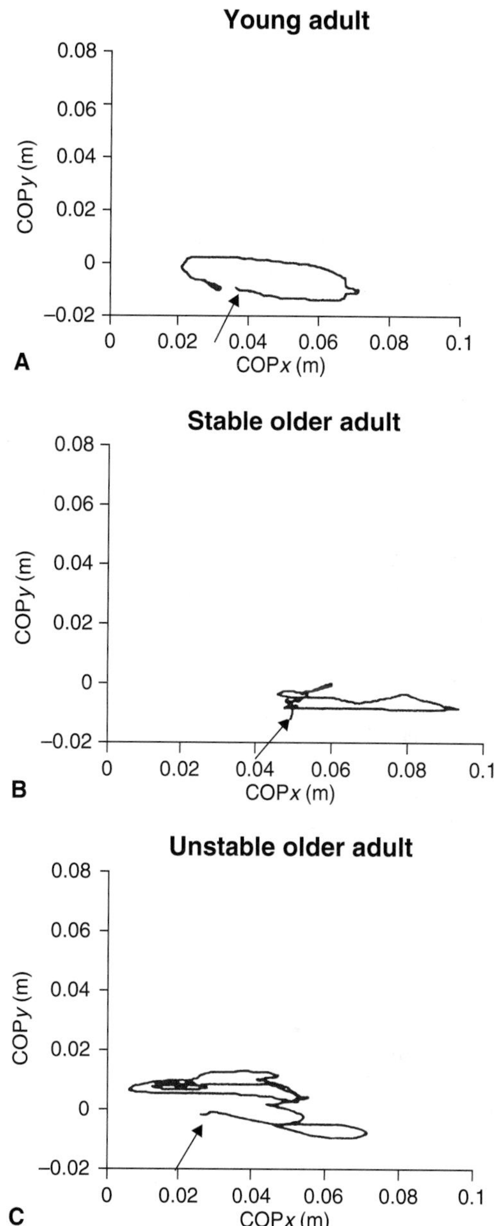

FIGURE 9.5 Graphs showing COP trajectory (in *x*- and *y*-coordinates) from perturbation onset to 2 sec after the perturbations for young stable and unstable older adults. The arrow indicates perturbation onset. Note that the COP trajectory shows much more movement within the 2-second period for unstable older adults. (Reprinted with permission from Lin S-I, Woollacott MH, Jensen J. Differentiating postural responses following dynamically changing balance threats in young adults, healthy older adults and unstable older adults: kinematics and kinetics. Aging Clin Exp Res 2004;16:373, Figure 4.)

the COP to come to stabilization. It is interesting that, in spite of the increases in these variables, there were no differences in peak COM displacements between the groups (Lin et al., 2004). This suggests that each group aimed at keeping a fairly low COM displacement, and when it went beyond this point, the older adults simply shifted strategies and took a step.

What might be the causes of these age-related changes in postural response characteristics to perturbations? Clinical tests showed that muscle strength was significantly lower for the unstable older adults than for the young and stable older adults for most muscles tested. In addition, the strength of the muscles tested was found to be significantly correlated with the scores of the three functional balance tests for almost all muscles tested. Other studies that have examined correlations between balance performance and sensory/motor system function have shown significant correlations between visual acuity, low vibrotactile thresholds, isometric muscle strength, and high psychomotor speed (reaction time and movement time) (Era et al., 1996; Kristinsdottir et al., 2001).

When do compensatory steps during balance recovery cause falls? Table 9.1 shows features of compensatory stepping and reaching reactions related to aging and increased fall risk (Maki & McIlroy, 2006). Note that taking one or more additional steps after the initial stepping response during recover is associated with both aging and fall risk. In addition, using a side-step sequence during recovery is associated with aging, but sustaining limb collisions during lateral stepping is associated with both aging and falls. Finally, slowed initiation and execution of reach and grasp movements is associated with both aging and falls. It is also important to note that holding a cane interferes with grasping a handrail during balance recovery (Bateni et al., 2004a,b). When subjects had either a cane or just a cane top, they seldom reached for a handrail, and when the rail was not contacted, balance was lost. This suggests that when we have something in our hands, the nervous system gives priority to that object rather than reaching to aid in balance.

In summary, these data suggest that older adults with and without balance problems show changes in the motor systems affecting postural control and that these can contribute significantly to an inability to maintain balance. Some of these motor system changes include: (1) muscle weakness; (2) impaired timing and organization among synergistic muscles activated in response to instability; and (3) limitations in the ability to adapt movements for balance in response to changing task and environmental demands.

TABLE 9.1 Features of Compensatory Stepping and Reaching Reactions Related to Ageing and Increased Falling Risk

Feature of the reaction		Significant association with: Ageing	Falling risk
Stepping reactions			
Takes one or more additional steps after the initial stepping reaction Follows a forward or backward stepping reaction with one or more lateral steps	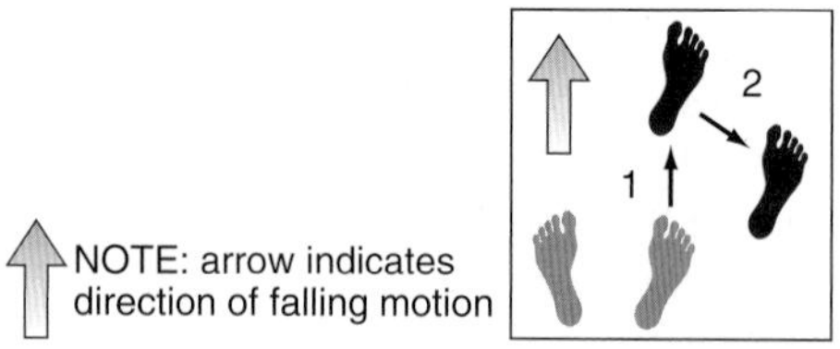 NOTE: arrow indicates direction of falling motion; 1; 2	Yes Yes	Yes (AP falls) Yes (ML falls)
Tends to use a side-step sequence (SSS), rather than a crossover step (COS) during lateral stepping reactions	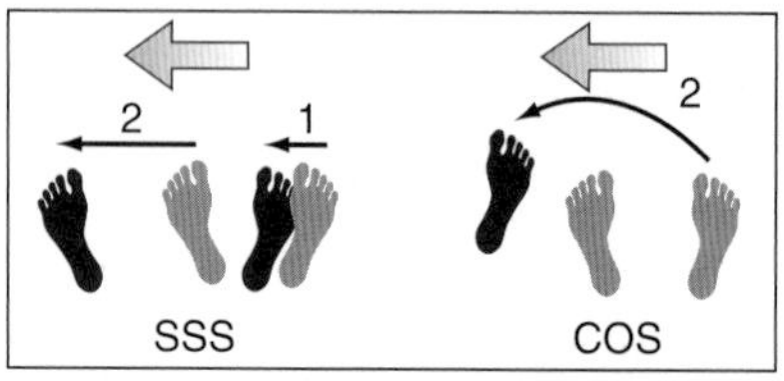 SSS (1, 2); COS (2)	Yes	No
Sustains limb collisions during lateral stepping reactions (during stance but particularly when walking in-place)	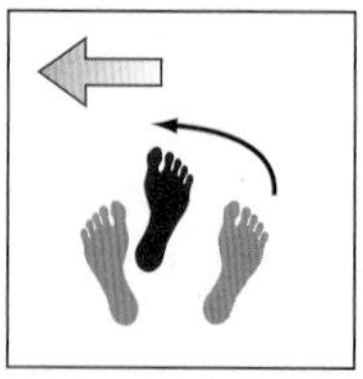	Yes	Yes (AP falls)
Reaching reactions			
Initiates arm movements despite instructions not to move the arms		Yes	Yes (AP falls)
Slowed initiation and execution of reach-to-grasp movements		Yes	Yes (all falls)

AP = anteroposterior; ML = mediolateral.

Adapted with permission from Maki BE, McIlroy WE. Control of rapid limb movements for balance recovery: age-related changes and implications for fall prevention. Age Ageing 2006;35-S2:ii14.

Sensory Systems

How do changes in the sensory systems important for posture and balance control contribute to declining stability as people age? The following sections review changes within individual sensory systems and then examine how these changes affect stability in quiet stance, as well as our ability to recover from loss of balance.

Changes in Individual Sensory Systems

Somatosensory. Studies have shown that *vibratory* sensation threshold at the great toe increases threefold by the age of 90 (Kenshalo, 1979). Vibratory thresholds in general increase more in the lower extremities than in the upper extremities. In fact, in some cases researchers reported an inability to record vibratory responses from the ankle, because many of the older subjects were not able to perceive sensation there (Whanger & Wang, 1974).

Many studies have shown that *tactile* sensitivity decreases with age, as measured by threshold to touch stimuli (Bruce, 1980; Kalisch et al., 2009). Researchers have documented a decline in fine touch and pressure/vibration sensation mediated by Meissner end organs and Pacinian corpuscles. Aging affects both the quantity and the quality of the Meissner and Pacinian corpuscles; however, it is thought that functional effects are determined primarily by the number of receptors lost. In addition to receptor loss, there is a decline of up to 30% of the sensory fibers innervating the peripheral receptors, causing peripheral neuropathy.

This peripheral neuropathy will cause increased reliance on other sensory systems, such as the visual and vestibular systems. Studies examining postural responses in patients with somatosensory deficits caused by peripheral neuropathy have shown significant delays in muscle response onset latencies in response to platform perturbations and an inability to modulate response amplitudes in relation to stimulus size. Figure 9.6A shows EMGs from a patient with peripheral neuropathy and a healthy subject in response to a platform perturbation. Figure 9.6B compares the onset latencies of muscles in the healthy subject with those of the subject with neuropathy. Note that EMGs from all recorded muscles slow equally (Inglis et al., 1994). Patients with multiple sclerosis show problems similar to those in patients with peripheral neuropathy (Jackson et al., 1995; Nelson et al., 1995).

In addition, osteoarthritis and accompanying reduced joint position sensitivity cause increased sway during quiet stance balance with either eyes open or closed in older adults. However, it does not affect reactive balance (McChesney & Woollacott, 2000).

Vision. Studies on the visual system show similar declines in function. Because of multiple changes within the structure of the eye itself, less light is transmitted to the retina; thus, the visual threshold (the

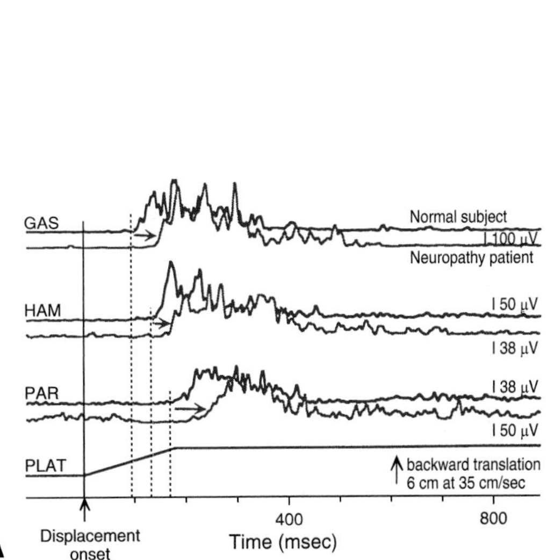

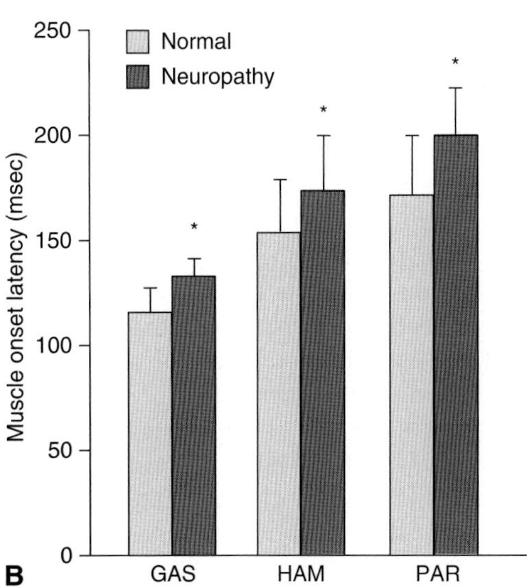

FIGURE 9.6 A, EMGs from the leg and trunk muscles of a patient with peripheral neuropathy and a healthy subject in response to a platform perturbation. Note that EMGs from all recorded muscles slow equally. GAS = gastrocnemius; HAM = hamstrings; PAR = paraspinal muscles; PLAT = platform displacement. B, Mean onset latencies for GAS, HAM, and PAR muscles in control subjects (Normal) versus patients with peripheral neuropathy. (Reprinted with permission from Inglis JT, Horak FB, Shupert CL, Rycewicz C. The importance of somatosensory information in triggering and scaling automatic postural responses in humans. Exp Brain Res 1994;101:161.)

minimum light needed to see an object) increases with age. In addition, there is typically a loss of visual field, a decline in visual acuity, and visual contrast sensitivity, which causes problems in contour and depth perception (Sturnieks et al., 2008). Loss of visual acuity can result from cataracts, macular degeneration, and loss of peripheral vision due to ischemic retinal or brain disease. These age-related changes in the visual system affect a broad range of functional skills, including postural control (Pastalan et al., 1973; Pitts, 1982). For example, a number of studies have indicated that age-related increases in sway during quiet stance become larger when visual cues are removed (eyes-closed condition) (Patla et al., 1990; Schultz et al., 1993; Sheldon, 1963; Wolfson et al., 1992). As mentioned in Chapter 8, one can test the influence of vision on balance control by creating the illusion of postural sway through visual flow generated by an experimental moving room. Normally, young adults show small amounts of sway in response to visual flow giving the illusion of sway. A study by Wade et al. (1995) comparing the effects of visual flow on postural responses (COP measurements) in older adults indicated that healthy older adults show increased sway as compared with young adults under these conditions. The authors suggest that this may be due to decreased somatosensory information available to older as compared with younger subjects.

A second study, by Sundermeier et al. (1996), compared the effects of visual flow on postural responses of young stable and unstable older adults. Figure 9.7A (left) shows the paradigm used. As the room moves forward (a), the subjects perceive that they are swaying backward (b) and sway forward (c) to compensate. Figure 9.7A (right) shows the COP responses of individuals in each group. As you can see, the unstable older adults showed significantly more reliance on the visual flow than the young or stable adults as measured by COP. In addition, they showed continuing COP oscillations after the room movements had stopped. The investigators also noted that the unstable older adults used higher levels of sheer forces when compensating for the simulated postural sway, thus suggesting greater use of hip strategies even in response to visual perturbations to posture. When analyzing muscle response characteristics to these room movements they found that when the room moved away from the subjects the unstable older adults used larger ankle dorsiflexor (TA) responses, which caused high amounts of sway in the forward direction (Fig. 9.7B).

In a similar study, Ring et al. (1988) used a visual image on a screen in front of subjects to create the illusion of movement toward the subject. In these "visual push" experiments, he noted that subjects who had recently fallen (within 2 weeks) and those who had fallen within the past year swayed significantly more than older adults (65–86 years of age) who had not fallen. He thus concluded that the visual push test might be capable of identifying older adults who are at risk for falls.

Vestibular. The vestibular system also shows a reduction in function, with a loss of 40% of the vestibular hair and nerve cells by 70 years of age and a 3% loss per decade of vestibular nucleus cells from 40 to 90 years (Rosenhall & Rubin, 1975).

One of the functions of the vestibular system is that of an absolute reference system with which the other systems (visual and somatosensory) may be compared and calibrated (Black & Nashner, 1985). The vestibular system would be especially important for balance control in situations of visual and somatosensory system conflict. A decline in vestibular function with age would cause this absolute reference system to be less reliable, and thus the nervous system would have difficulty dealing with conflicting information coming from the visual and somatosensory systems. This may be the reason that older adults with vestibular deficits have problems with dizziness and unsteadiness when they are in environments with conflicting visual and somatosensory inputs.

In addition to the vestibular system's function as an absolute reference system, vestibular inputs contribute to the amplitude of automatic postural adjustments to balance threats. Thus, older adults with vestibular deficits would show postural responses that were inappropriately small (Allum et al., 1994).

Dizziness, an additional consequence of some types of vestibular dysfunction, can also contribute to instability among older adults. **Dizziness** is a term used to describe the illusion of movement. It can encompass feelings of unsteadiness and imbalance, as well as feelings of faintness or the sense of being lightheaded. Dizziness can be a symptom of a variety of diseases, including those of the inner ear. Partial loss of vestibular function can lead to reports of dizziness, which can be a significant factor contributing to imbalance in the elderly. Degenerative processes within the otoliths of the vestibular system can produce positional vertigo and imbalance during walking.

Multisensory Deficit. **Multisensory deficit** is a term used to describe the loss of more than one sense important for balance and mobility functions (Brandt & Daroff, 1979). In many older people with multisensory deficits, the ability to compensate for the loss of one sense with alternative senses is not possible because of numerous impairments in all the sensory systems important for postural control.

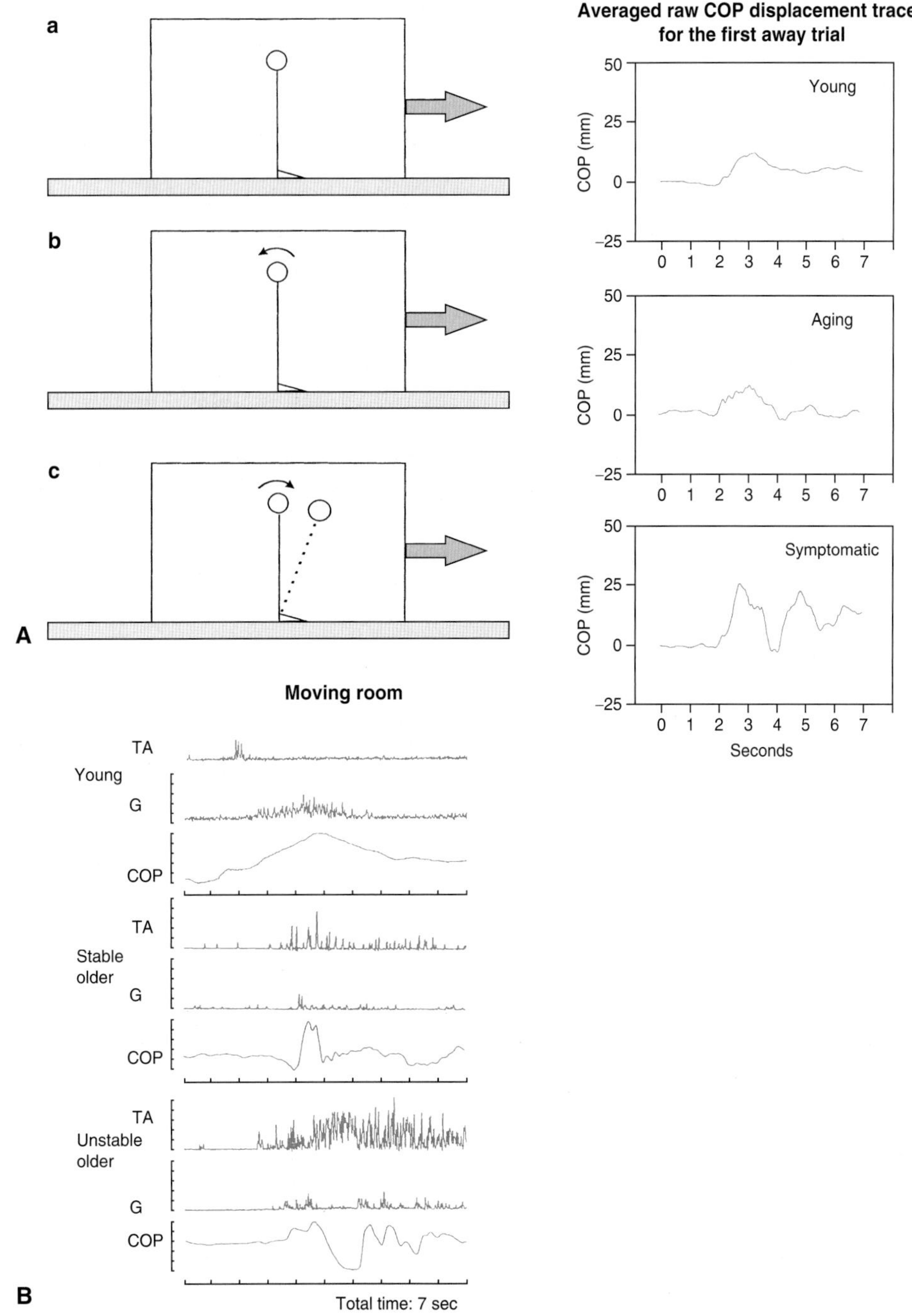

FIGURE 9.7 A, Left, Effect of moving room on subject's sway. Room moves forward (a) causing perception of backward sway (b) and active forward sway (c). Right, Plot of COP movement versus time for young, stable and unstable older adults in response to room movements. B, EMGs from tibialis anterior (TA) and gastrocnemius (G) in response to room movements. Note that responses were of much longer duration in the unstable older adults. (Adapted with permission from Sundermeier L, Woollacott M, Jensen J, Moore S. Postural sensitivity to visual flow in aging adults with and without balance problems. J Gerontol 1996;51:M49.)

Adapting Senses for Postural Control

In addition to showing declines in function within specific sensory systems, research from many labs has indicated that some older adults have more difficulty than younger adults in maintaining steadiness under conditions in which sensory information for postural control is severely reduced (Brandt & Daroff, 1979; Speers et al., 2002; Horak et al., 1989; Peterka & Black, 1990–1991; Teasdale et al., 1991; Toupet et al., 1992; Wolfson et al., 1985; Woollacott et al., 1986).

To understand the contribution of vision to the control of sway during quiet stance in older adults, researchers examined sway under altered visual conditions. When young people close their eyes, they show a slight increase in body sway, and this is also true for healthy older adults (Teasdale et al., 1991; Woollacott et al., 1986).

In addition, when their eyes are open, healthy older adults are often as steady as young adults when standing on a compliant surface, such as foam, a condition that reduces the effectiveness of somatosensory inputs reporting body sway. However, when healthy older adults are asked to stand on a compliant surface with their eyes closed, thus using vestibular inputs alone for controlling posture, sway significantly increases as compared with young adults (Teasdale et al., 1991).

Several studies have examined the ability of healthy older adults to adapt senses to changing conditions during quiet stance using posturography testing (Horak et al., 1989; Peterka and Black, 1990; Speers et al., 2002; Wolfson et al., 1985; Woollacott et al., 1986). Most studies found that healthy active older adults did not show significant differences from young adults in the amount of body sway (Fig. 9.8), except under conditions in which both ankle-joint inputs and visual inputs were distorted or absent (conditions 5 and 6). In one study, increased variability of shank and hip angles was found for older adults in conditions 2, 4, 5, and 6. The authors suggested that the increased sway in the older adults was due to their decreased ability to detect small movements of the platform (Speers et al., 2002).

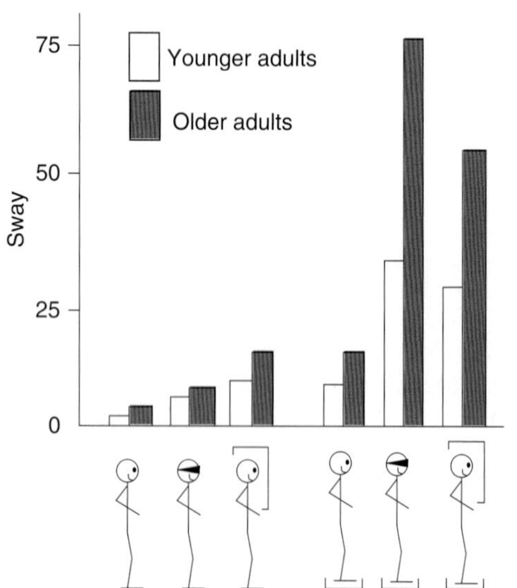

FIGURE 9.8 Comparison of body sway in the six sensory conditions in young versus active healthy elderly. (Adapted from Woollacott MH, Shumway-Cook A, Nashner LM. Aging and posture control: changes in sensory organization and muscular coordination. Int J Aging Hum Dev 1986;23:340.)

When both visual and somatosensory inputs for postural control were reduced (conditions 5 and 6), half of the older adults lost their balance on the first trial for these conditions and needed assistance. However, most of the older adults were able to maintain balance on the second trial within these two conditions. Thus, they were able to adapt senses for postural control, but only with practice in the condition (Woollacott et al., 1986).

These results suggest that healthy older adults do not sway significantly more than young people when there is a reduction in the availability or accuracy of a single sense for postural control. However, in contrast to young adults, reducing the availability of two senses appears to have a significant effect on postural steadiness in even apparently healthy older adults.

Are the changes summarized above the result of an inevitable decline in nervous system function, or are they the result of borderline pathology in specific subsystems contributing to postural function?

To determine whether evidence of borderline pathology existed in subjects who participated in a postural study and who considered themselves fit, active older adults, researchers gave each subject a neurologic exam and then correlated the existence of borderline pathology with performance on the balance tasks. Although all the older adults considered themselves to be healthy, a neurologist participating in the study found neural impairment, such as diminished deep tendon reflexes, mild peripheral-nerve deficits, distal weakness in the tibialis anterior and gastrocnemius muscles, and abnormal nystagmus in many adults in the population. Loss of balance in two subjects accounted for 58% of total losses of balance (Manchester et al., 1989).

These subjects had no history of neurologic impairment, but the neurologist diagnosed them as having borderline pathology of CNS origin. These results again suggest the importance of pathologies within specific subsystems contributing to imbalance in older adults, rather than a generalized decline in performance.

Other researchers have also studied the adaptation to changing sensory information during quiet stance in older adults (Horak et al., 1989). One group of older adults was active and healthy and had no history of falls (labeled "asymptomatic"). The second group was symptomatic for falling. Figure 9.9 illustrates some of the results of their study, showing that over 20% of the elderly (both symptomatic and asymptomatic) lost their balance when visual information was inaccurate for balance (condition 3), as

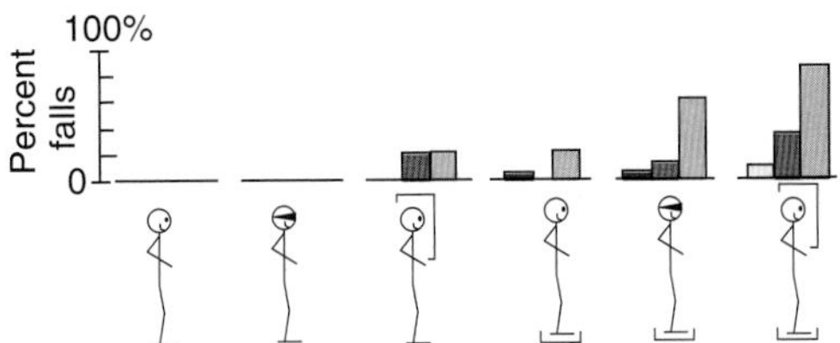

FIGURE 9.9 Comparison of number of falls in the six sensory conditions in young adults, elderly adults with no history of falling, and elderly adults with a history of falling. Open box = adults 20 to 39 years old; black box = adults >70 years old who had no history of falling; shaded box = adults >70 years old who had a history of falling. (Reprinted with permission from Horak F, Shupert C, Mirka A. Components of postural dyscontrol in the elderly: a review. Neurobiol Aging 1989;10:732.)

compared with none of the young subjects, ages 20 to 39. Forty percent of the asymptomatic elderly patients lost their balance under condition 6, when both visual and somatosensory information were inaccurately reporting body sway. By contrast, less than 10% of the healthy young adults fell under this condition. The symptomatic elderly had a larger percentage of falls in any condition that was sway-referenced, that is, with misleading somatosensory cues (conditions 4, 5, and 6).

This led researchers to conclude that the ability to select and weight alternative orientation references adaptively is a crucial factor contributing to postural dyscontrol in many older adults. This is especially true for those who are symptomatic for balance problems (Horak et al., 1989).

Another approach to studying adaptation of sensory systems involves the use of rotational movements of a platform. These experiments were described in more detail in earlier chapters. Results from platform-rotation studies with older adults found that 50% of the healthy older subjects lost their balance on the first trial. However, all but one of the subjects were able to maintain their balance on subsequent trials (Woollacott et al., 1986). This finding could suggest a slower ability to adapt postural control in this population.

A propensity for falls in the first trial of a new condition is a recurring finding in many studies examining postural control in older adults (Horak et al., 1989; Peterka and Black, 1990–1991; Teasdale et al., 1991; Woollacott et al., 1986). Perhaps this means that slowing occurs, rather than a total lack of adaptability, in many elderly people. A propensity to fall in new or novel situations could also be the result of impaired anticipatory mechanisms. Anticipatory processes related to postural control enable the selection of appropriate sensory and motor strategies needed for a particular task or environment.

Zettel et al. (2008) have explored whether there are age-related changes in the ability of older adults to use vision for clearing an obstacle during balance recovery. They found that older adults, like young adults rarely looked downward for obstacle clearance when they were also performing a second visual task, though they usually cleared the obstacle effectively. This suggests that both young and older adults use stored visual-spatial information, gained when they first enter a new environment, for stepping over obstacles.

Anticipatory Postural Abilities

Postural adjustments are often used in a proactive manner, to stabilize the body before making a voluntary movement. Adults in their 70s and 80s may begin to have more difficulty maneuvering in the world because they have lost some of their ability to integrate balance adjustments into ongoing voluntary movements such as lifting or carrying objects. Thus, it is important to study the effects of age on the ability to use postural responses proactively within the context of voluntary movements. It is under these dynamic conditions, including walking, lifting, and carrying objects, that most falls occur.

One of the first researchers to study age-related changes in anticipatory postural adjustments was Man'kovskii, from Russia (1980). He compared the characteristics of anticipatory postural responses and prime mover (voluntary) responses for young (19 to 29 years of age), medium old (60 to 69), and very old (90 to 99) adults who were asked to do the simple task of flexing one leg at the knee (prime mover response) while using the other leg for support (postural response), both at a comfortable and at a fast speed. Both the medium old adults and very old adults showed a slowing in both the postural (contralateral rectus femoris) and prime mover (ipsilateral biceps femoris) muscle response latencies for the movements at a comfortable speed, but this slowing did not result in an increased probability of losing balance. However, at the fast speeds, for both medium and very old adults: (a) the correlation between the postural and prime mover muscles decreased, and (b) there was a decrease in the time between the response onsets for postural and prime mover muscles. In the very old, postural and prime mover muscles were activated almost simultaneously. This inability to activate postural muscles far enough before the prime mover caused a loss of balance in many trials (Man'kovskii et al., 1980).

In Chapter 7, we mentioned that in the healthy young adult, the same postural response synergies that are activated during stance balance control are activated in an anticipatory manner before making a voluntary movement while standing. Thus, when a young adult is asked to pull on a handle, first the gastrocnemius is activated, followed by the hamstrings, trunk extensor, and then the prime mover muscle, the biceps of the arm. A slowing in onset latency or a disruption of the sequence of activation of these postural synergies could affect the ability of an older adult to make movements such as lifting objects.

Experiments were performed to explore age-related changes in the ability of older adults to activate postural muscle response synergies in an anticipatory manner (Frank et al., 1987; Inglin & Woollacott, 1988). In one study, standing young (mean age, 26 years) and older (mean age, 71 years) adults pushed or pulled on a handle that was adjusted to shoulder level, in response to a visual stimulus. Results of the study showed that the onset latencies of the postural muscles were significantly longer in the older adults than in the younger adults when they were activated in a complex reaction-time task. There were also large age-related increases in onset times for voluntary muscles. According to a systems perspective, this slowing in voluntary reaction time in older adults could be caused either by the need for advanced stabilization by the already delayed and weaker postural muscles or to slowing in the voluntary control system itself. Since the absolute differences in onset times between the young and the older adults were larger for the voluntary muscles than for the postural muscles, there may be a slowing in both systems in the older adult (Woollacott et al., 1988).

In a study of interactions between anticipatory and reactive postural control in a sit-to-stand task in older adults (Pai et al., 2003), older adults were given unexpected forward slips as they stood up from a chair. It was found that with repeated trials, the older adults made adaptive adjustments in advance (anticipatory control) to improve their stability. When exposed to both slip and nonslip trials the older adults began to select optimal movements that improved stability under both conditions. The authors suggest that these results can be explained if it assumed that an internal representation of COM stability limits guides the improvements in the anticipatory control of stability.

The results of these many studies suggest that many older adults have problems making anticipatory postural adjustments quickly and efficiently, especially without prior practice. This inability to stabilize the body in association with voluntary movement tasks such as lifting or carrying may be a major contributor to falls in many elderly people.

Cognitive Issues and Posture Control

Mrs. Eulalia H, who is 80 years old, normally has no problems with falls. She is walking down a busy sidewalk in the city, talking to a friend, while carrying a fragile piece of crystal she just bought at the department store. Suddenly, a dog runs in front of her. Will she be able to balance in this situation as well as she does when she is walking down a quiet street by herself?

Eulalia's friend, Mr. Shelby L, has within the past 6 months recovered from a series of serious falls. These falls have led to a loss of confidence and fear of falling, which has resulted in a reduction in his overall activity level and an unwillingness to leave the safety of his own home. Can fear of falling significantly affect how we perceive and move in relation to balance control?

Determining the answer to these and other questions related to the complex role of cognitive issues in postural control may be a key to understanding loss of balance in some older adults.

As we mentioned in the first part of this chapter, the capacity of an individual, the demands of a task, and the strategies the person uses to accomplish a task are important factors that contribute to the ability of a person to function in different environments. As individuals get older, their capacities to perform certain tasks such as balance control may be reduced as compared with their abilities at age 20, but they will still be able to function in normal situations, in which they can focus on the task. However, when they are faced with situations in which they are required to perform multiple tasks at once, such as the one just described, they may not have the attentional capacity to perform both tasks, as attentional or information-processing capacity and processing robustness is reduced with aging (Gilchrist et al., 2008; Li et al., 2004). Researchers are beginning to explore the question of how our attentional capacities affect our balance abilities in different environments (see Woollacott and Shumway-Cook, 2002, for a review).

If postural control does require attentional processing one might ask whether decreasing sensory information would demand more attention and whether older adults would have more difficulty than young adults under these circumstances.

Teasdale and his colleagues (1993) studied the balance (COP measurements) of young and older adults while sitting (control condition) versus standing with eyes open versus closed on a normal surface versus a foam surface. The foam surface was used to decrease sway-related somatosensory information available for balance control. They also measured reaction time (RT) on a secondary task, in which the subject pressed a button at the sound of an auditory cue. Figure 9.10 shows the RTs for the young versus older adults under the four conditions. Note that as sensory information decreased, RTs became significantly longer for both younger and older adults, but the effect

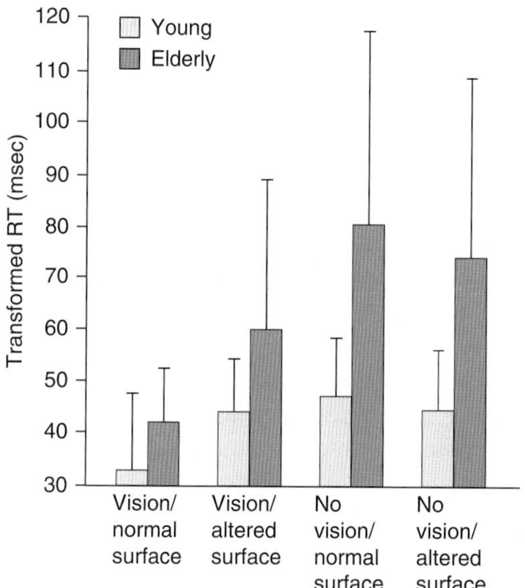

FIGURE 9.10 Reaction-time (RT) scores of young versus older adults for four sensory conditions. Note that as sensory information decreased, RTs became significantly longer for older adults as compared with young adults. This implies that the amount of attention is dependent on the degree of instability inherent in the task. (Adapted with permission from Teasdale N, Bard C, LaRue J, Fleury M. On the cognitive penetrability of postural control. Exp Aging Res 1993;19:8.)

was exaggerated in the older adults. This implies that the amount of attention is dependent on the degree of instability inherent in the task and that older adults require more attention to perform the postural task.

More recently Doumas et al. (2008) asked how older adults share dual-task costs when balancing under the six sensory conditions of the Sensory Organization test (described above), especially when sensory information from the different senses was in conflict or reduced. In this case, the cognitive task was the N-back task, in which participants continuously monitor a stream of numbers on a screen and must say the digit seen two or three cycles before (level of difficulty was chosen based on responses being 80% correct). They found that older adults on the stable surface had a 40% increase in sway in the dual-task condition, while the young adults did not. However, in the sway-referenced condition the postural performance in the single- and dual-task conditions were the same, with a 15% increase in costs for the cognitive task in the dual-task condition. Why was this the case? On the stable surface the older adults had the flexibility to increase their sway in the dual-task condition, as they diverted attention to the secondary task, as they were well within their stability limits. However, on the sway-referenced surface, they had high levels of sway, even in the single-task condition, and thus could not afford to divert attentional resources to the dual-task condition and increase sway, so instead, they diverted attention from the cognitive task and reduced the cognitive task performance. This shows the flexible nature of attentional resource allocation in healthy older adults.

How does performing an attentionally demanding task affect postural sway in healthy older adults versus those with a history of falling? A number of laboratories have examined this question (Redfern et al., 2001; Shumway-Cook et al., 1997c; Shumway-Cook & Woollacott, 2000). Shumway-Cook and colleagues (1997c) examined the ability of young adults, healthy older adults, and older adults with a history of, or recent recurrent episodes of, falling to perform postural tasks of varying difficulty (standing on a normal surface vs. foam) while performing cognitively demanding secondary tasks. They found that during the simultaneous performance of a postural and a cognitive task, there were decrements in performance in the postural stability measures rather than the cognitive measures for young adults, healthy older adults and balance-impaired older adults. It is interesting that differences between the young and healthy older adults became apparent only when task complexity was increased—either by adding the secondary task or by adding the more challenging postural condition. However, balance-impaired older adults showed problems even in less-complex-task conditions.

Interestingly, the task of reintegrating sensory information after it has been removed causes increased attentional demands in older adults. In a study in which visual and ankle proprioceptive inputs were removed or perturbed and suddenly reinserted, older adults showed a faster COP velocity than young adults when required to reintegrate proprioceptive inputs. This increased COP velocity in spite of the fact that there was increased availability of sensory information, suggests that for older adults, sensory reweighting requires additional attentional resources as compared with the young adult (Teasdale & Simoneau, 2001).

These experiments examined attentional constraints on older adults in quiet-stance situations, but it would also be important to know whether recovery from perturbations to stance requires more attention for older than for young adults, thus contributing to an increased likelihood of falls in these situations. To explore this, Brown et al. (1999) asked older and younger subjects to respond to unexpected platform displacements either with no secondary task or while performing a math task (count backward by threes). They found that attentional requirements for the recovery of balance are higher for older adults than for young adults. Performing a secondary task caused subjects to step earlier when using a stepping strategy. It is interesting to note that the postural muscle responses of the older adults were smaller when performing the secondary cognitive task. This may have been the reason the subjects were required to step earlier; their muscle responses were too small to use an in-place strategy (Rankin et al., 2000).

In a second study exploring the temporal dynamics of attention during postural perturbations in young versus older adults, Redfern et al. (2002) asked participants to perform a simple visual or auditory reaction-time task at different delays from the onset of a platform perturbation. They found that reaction time was slowed (more for auditory than for visual cues) both before and during the platform movement, particularly for the older adults; however, by 250 msec after the perturbation, the effects had disappeared.

This type of study was extended to compare the effects of a secondary task on balance recovery from a perturbation in balance-impaired older adults (Brauer et al., 2001, 2002). Results showed that balance-impaired older adults took a longer time to regain a stable posture in the dual-task condition than when responding to the postural task alone. When a compensatory step was required to regain balance, reaction

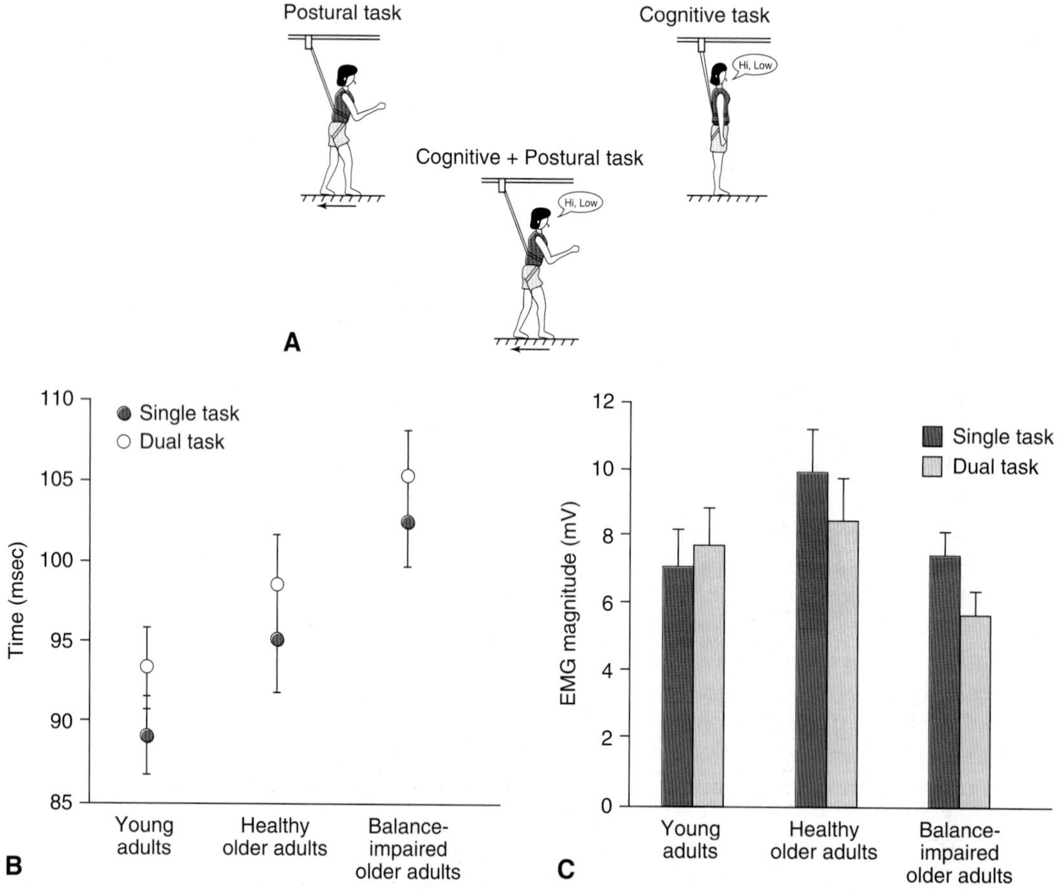

FIGURE 9.11 A, Single- and dual-task paradigms. Postural and cognitive task performance is measured in isolation ("postural task" and "cognitive task") and when performed simultaneously ("cognitive + postural task") and differences are compared between single- and dual-task conditions. B, Time of contraction onset for the gastrocnemius muscle for young, healthy adults and balance-impaired older, adults in the single- versus dual-task conditions. Note that all three groups show delays in the dual-task as compared with the single-task conditions, in addition to the delays in responses associated with age and balance impairment. C, Changes in muscle response (EMG) magnitude of the gastrocnemius muscle for the three subject groups in the single- and dual-task conditions. Note that the healthy and balance-impaired older adults show a reduction of response amplitude in the dual-task condition. (Reprinted with permission from Brauer SG, Woollacott M, Shumway-Cook A. The influence of a concurrent cognitive task on the compensatory stepping response to perturbations in balance-impaired and healthy elders. Gait Posture 2002;15:91, Figure 4.)

times were longer in all subjects than when recovering balance with an in-place strategy, and longer in balance-impaired older adults than in young adults (see Fig. 9.11A for a picture of the dual-task paradigm). The authors noted that this difference between young and balance-impaired older adults may have been related to prioritization of the two tasks, rather than to attentional demands, because the older adults completed the step before the reaction-time task, while the young adults performed both concurrently. Healthy older adults and balance-impaired adults also showed a delayed muscle response onset and reduced response amplitude when taking a compensatory step in the dual-task paradigm as compared with young adults. This is shown in panels B and C of Figure 9.11. Note that the time of onset of the gastrocnemius muscle response is delayed for young, healthy and balance-impaired older adults (B) and muscle response magnitude is reduced for both healthy and balance impaired older adults (C) in the dual-task condition.

Although many studies have explored the differences in postural performance between those with a history and those with no history of falling, very few have explored the effect of fear of falling on the control of balance. There is now experimental evidence that anxiety and fear of falling affect the performance of older adults on tests of balance control (Maki et al., 1991; Tinetti et al., 1990). As a result, older adults probably modulate strategies for postural control based on their perception of the level of postural threat. Thus, older adults who have a great deal of anxiety about falling related to poor perceptions regarding their level of balance skills will move in ways that reflect these perceptions. More work is needed to fully understand the relationship between fear of falling and postural control. Lab Activity 9.2 applies many concepts discussed in this chapter.

A CASE STUDY APPROACH TO UNDERSTANDING AGE-RELATED POSTURAL DISORDERS

Bonnie B is a 90-year-old woman with impaired balance resulting in multiple falls, two of which required hospitalization. Bonnie lives alone in an apartment; she has a home health aide who comes in three times a week for 4 hours to assist her with shopping, cooking, cleaning and laundry. Bonnie's main concerns relate to her declining balance. She is increasingly fearful because of her multiple falls.

Bonnie has a number of underlying sensory, motor, and cognitive impairments that contribute to her impaired balance. She has limited range of motion in her shoulders, hips, knees and ankles. She has reduced spinal flexibility that constrains her ability to rotate her trunk. She has reduced strength, in her arms and legs; is able to move against gravity but cannot take any additional resistance. She has age-related changes in vision and reduced somatosensory sensitivity. In addition, she has bilateral sensorineural hearing loss and a previous history of vertigo, due to partial loss of vestibular function. Bonnie has mild cognitive deficits affecting her memory and executive function.

These sensory, motor and cognitive impairments all contribute to impaired steady state balance. Bonnie is able to sit unsupported with her feet on the floor. She is able to stand unassisted, but requires close supervision when not using her walker, suggesting impaired steady-state balance in stance.

Bonnie has impaired reactive balance control using her arms to recover stability in response to both small and large perturbations. Researchers have shown that impaired reactive postural activity in older adults like Bonnie is due to slower muscle responses, changes in temporal coordination among proximal and distal muscles, and increased coactivation of agonist and antagonist muscle groups.

Bonnie has impaired sensory organization that contributes to her instability in certain environments. She is able to stand on a firm surface with her eyes open, a condition in which all three senses are available for balance control. When standing on a firm surface with her eyes closed, she shows increased sway and requires assistance. She is unable to stand on the foam surface with her eyes open or closed. This pattern suggests Bonnie has difficulty maintaining her balance when any sensory input for postural control is reduced. This is consistent with her complaints of loss of balance when walking on carpeted surfaces or in areas with low lighting levels. She must use a shower stool since she cannot maintain balance when taking a shower and closing her eyes to wash her hair.

Finally, Bonnie has significantly impaired proactive balance control, which reduces her ability to perform tasks such as leaning and reaching forward, or leaning over to pick up an object from the floor. She has had several falls in her apartment trying to pick up objects from the floor, and now uses an extended reacher. She is unable to step up or down without assistance even with her walker. Researchers have found delayed onset of anticipatory postural adjustments associated with voluntary movements in many older adults.

As you can see, many factors contribute to Bonnie's impaired balance control. Some of these factors reflect age related changes in the systems important to balance control. Others are less related to aging, and more related to her sedentary lifestyle. Balance

LAB ACTIVITY 9-2

Objective: Through the interview process, to explore the balance abilities of a healthy versus a balance-impaired older adult, and to define possible events that lead up to their current functional status.

Procedure: Find two older adults in your community whom you can interview, one who is very active and has good balance and the other with balance problems and a history of falling. In your interview ask the following questions:

1. What is your age?
2. Do you exercise regularly? If so, how much?
3. Have you had any medical problems that have affected your balance abilities?
4. Ask them to try standing in a tandem Romberg position (one foot in front of the other) for 20 seconds. Time their attempt.
5. Ask them to get up out of a chair, walk 10 feet, turn around and walk back, sitting down again in the chair. Using a watch with a second hand, determine the time taken for the task (timed Up-and-Go test).

Assignment

Write up an evaluation of each of the older adults, based on the following information:

1. Where do you think each of the people you interviewed would fit on Spirduso's (2005) scale: Physically Elite, Physically Fit, Physically Independent, Physically Frail, and Physically Dependent.
2. What do you think are their physiological ages as compared with their chronological ages?
3. Compare their performance on the static balance task and on the Up-and-Go test. How did each of them do when getting up out of the chair during the Up-and-Go test?
4. What do you think are factors contributing to their current balance status?

impairments significantly affect Bonnie's life. They reduce her independence and significantly increase her likelihood for future falls. Because she has had several fall-related injuries, she is very fearful of falling again, and is restricting her activity level because of this.

SUMMARY

1. Many scientists believe that factors contributing to aging can be considered either primary or secondary. Primary factors, such as genetics, contribute to the inevitable decline of neuronal function in a system. Secondary factors are experiential, and include nutrition, exercise, insults, and pathologies.
2. Researchers in all areas find much heterogeneity among older adults, suggesting that assumptions about declining physical capabilities cannot be generalized to all older adults.
3. Unintentional injuries are the fifth leading cause of death in the elderly, and falls make up two-thirds of these deaths. Falls in the elderly have multiple contributing factors, including intrinsic physiological and musculoskeletal factors and extrinsic environmental factors. Understanding the role of declining postural and balance abilities is a critical concern in helping to prevent falls among older adults.
4. Older adults typically show impaired reactive control with delays in the onsets of muscle responses and smaller response magnitudes, resulting in a longer time required to restabilize balance. Activation of postural responses during anticipatory or proactive balance control is often delayed, causing instability in performing tasks such as leg lifting or opening a door. In addition, when sensory inputs for balance control are reduced or distorted older adults have difficulty maintaining balance and sway excessively or lose balance.
5. Many factors can contribute to declining balance control in older adults who are symptomatic for imbalance and falls. Researchers have documented impairments in all of the systems contributing to balance control; however, there is no one predictable pattern that is characteristic of all elderly adults with a history of falling.

6. On a positive note, there are many older adults who have balance function that is equivalent to that of young people, suggesting that balance decline is not necessarily an inevitable result of aging. Experiential factors such as exercise can aid in the maintenance of good balance and decrease the likelihood for falls as people age.

ANSWERS TO LAB ACTIVITY ASSIGNMENTS

Lab Activity 9-1

Responses will differ, depending on the person interviewed.

Lab Activity 9-2

Results will differ, depending on the people interviewed.

CHAPTER 10

ABNORMAL POSTURAL CONTROL

LEARNING OBJECTIVES

Following completion of this chapter, the reader will be able to:

1. Summarize fall rates and risk factors for falls among persons with neurologic pathology.
2. Discuss changes to quiet stance in persons with neurologic pathology, and describe some of the factors contributing to impaired quiet stance.
3. Discuss the effects of neural pathology on postural movement strategies used to recover stability following an unexpected perturbation to quiet stance. Give examples of sequencing and timing problems that affect the coordination of postural motor responses; discuss the neural pathology likely to result in these types of problems.
4. Discuss two deficits affecting the ability to modify postural motor responses to changing task and environmental conditions; discuss the neural pathology likely to result in these types of problems.
5. Discuss the effect of different types of sensory problems on postural control, including loss of a sense and problems in organizing and selecting sensory inputs.
6. Describe the effect of impaired anticipatory postural control on voluntary movement; discuss the neural pathology likely to result in these types of problems.
7. Summarize postural control in persons with dementia.
8. Discuss components of impaired seated postural control in adults and children with neurologic pathology.

INTRODUCTION

Balance is critical to independence in activities of daily living. Impairments in postural control producing loss of stability have a profound impact on the daily life of individuals with neurologic pathology. The consequences of impaired stability include loss of functional independence, reduced or restricted participation in activities of daily living, and increased risk for falls.

Falls Following Neurologic Pathology

Falls are a major problem among persons with neurologic pathology, with prevalence varying by diagnosis and setting. The rate of falls among survivors of stroke ranges from 25% to 46%, and appears to be a problem at all stages in the recovery process (Ashburn et al., 2008; Divani et al., 2009; Nyberg & Gustafson, 1997; Teasell et al., 2002; Ugur et al., 2000). Falls following stroke vary by setting and acuity, from 36% among acute stroke survivors to 46% in chronic survivors of stroke living in the community (Divani et al., 2009; Kerse et al., 2008; Lamb et al., 2003; Nyberg & Gustafson, 1997). Approximately 15% of falls require medical attention (Divani et al., 2009), with a reported fourfold increase in the risk for hip fracture (Smith et al., 2001), due to an increased incidence of osteoporosis in both paretic and nonparetic limbs (Jorgensen et al., 2000; Poole et al., 2009; Ramnemark et al., 1999).

Falls are also a significant problem in Parkinson's disease (PD), with fall rates ranging from 40% to 68% (Ashburn et al., 2001; Bliem et al., 2001; Gray & Hildebrand, 2000; Wielinski et al., 2005; Wood et al., 2002; Woodford & Walker, 2005). In addition, fall rates are high among persons with multiple sclerosis (Cattaneo et al., 2002; Finlayson et al., 2006; Matsuda et al., 2009; Nilsagard et al., 2009a,b; Peterson et al., 2007, 2008). As was true for older adults, the majority of falls in persons with neurologic pathology are associated with mobility, occurring during walking, transfers, and stair climbing (Forster & Young, 1995; Lamb et al., 2003; Matsuda et al., 2009; Nilsagard et al., 2009a, b; Teasell et al., 2002).

Impaired balance has been found to be a major risk factor for falls among all patients with neurologic pathology, underscoring the importance of recovery of balance control in these patients (Ashburn et al., 2001; Bloem et al., 2001; Finlayson et al., 2006; Harris et al., 2005; Hyndman & Ashburn, 2003; Marchese et al., 2003; Matsuda et al., 2009; Nilsagaard et al., 2009a, b). In the therapeutic environment, the ability to retrain postural control to improve balance requires a conceptual framework that incorporates information on the physiological basis for normal postural control, as well as knowledge regarding the basis for instability.

Our understanding of the physiological basis for instability comes from research examining postural control in different categories of neurologic pathology, such as post-CVA (cerebral vascular accident) hemiparesis, traumatic brain injury, Parkinson's disease, multiple sclerosis, cerebellar disorders, and developmental disorders such as Down syndrome and cerebral palsy. This has led to an understanding of the different types of sensory, motor, and cognitive problems that contribute to instability. As we shall see, often the same type of postural control problem can manifest in a wide variety of neurologic disorders. For example, delayed onset of postural responses have been found in individuals with traumatic brain injury, in hemiplegia following CVA, and in children with different types of cerebral palsy, as well as those with Down syndrome.

We begin by exploring studies that have examined problems in the action systems of postural control affecting the ability to maintain balance in quiet stance (steady-state balance control), as well as the ability to recover stability following a perturbation while standing (reactive balance control) in persons with neurologic deficits. We will review studies exploring the effect of sensory/perceptual problems on postural control, and examine the effects of sensory and motor impairments on anticipatory aspects of stance postural control. Research examining the effects of cognitive problems on postural control will be reviewed, and finally we will examine research on the effect of neurologic pathology on seated postural control in both adults and children. The chapter will conclude with a summary of postural control problems in our case studies in order to provide an understanding of the types of problems found in people with different types of neurologic diagnoses.

PROBLEMS IN THE ACTION SYSTEMS

Problems in the action (motor) systems contributing to abnormal postural control include impairments in both neuromuscular and musculoskeletal systems. Many of the most common neuromuscular and musculoskeletal problems resulting from neurologic pathology were discussed in detail in Chapter 5, and thus will not be repeated here. The focus instead will be on problems affecting the ability to activate and coordinate muscle activity in order to maintain or recover stability in both quiet and perturbed stance.

Problems in Quiet Stance

Inability to maintain a stable standing position has enormous functional consequences for persons with neurologic pathology. Inability to assume and maintain a stable base from which to move often necessitates using the arms for support and balance, thus limiting the availability of the arms for functional tasks of daily living. In addition, impaired stance balance increases the risk for falls and injury. As discussed in Chapter 7, a number of factors contribute to our stability in quiet stance, including body alignment, muscle and postural tone, and movement strategies that control spontaneous sway and recovery from perturbations to stance stability.

Alignment

Alignment of the body refers to the relationship of body segments to one another, as well as to the position of the body with reference to gravity and the base of support. Alignment of body segments over the base of support determines to a great extent the effort required to support the body against gravity. In addition, alignment determines the constellation of movement strategies that will be effective in controlling posture. Changes in initial position or alignment are often characteristic of a person with a neurologic deficit. Abnormalities in alignment can reflect changes in the alignment of one body part to another or in alignment of the center of mass relative to the base of support.

The characteristically stooped posture of persons with Parkinson's disease (PD) is an example of changes in the alignment of body segments with respect to vertical. Stooped posture results from a forward trunk inclination and increased flexion at the hips and knees. Stooped posture in persons with PD may result from both neuromuscular impairments, such as flexor rigidity, as well as secondary musculoskeletal limitations, such as reduced trunk motion and spinal flexibility (Schenkman, 1990).

Children with cerebral palsy frequently show restricted range of motion in many joints, including the ankle, knee, and hip. Contractures of the hip, knee, and ankle muscles result in atypical postural alignment in sitting (Fig. 10.1A) and standing (Fig. 10.1B and 10.1C). Postural alignment influences how muscles are recruited and coordinated for recovery of stability. For example, in their study on postural control in children with spastic diplegia, Burtner and colleagues (1999) found that the children with spastic diplegia who maintained a crouched (flexed knees and hips) stance posture showed significant coactivation of leg and trunk muscles during recovery of balance following a perturbation. Interestingly, healthy children standing in a crouched position, mimicking the posture of the children with diplegia, used antagonistic muscles more often in response to platform perturbations, suggesting that the musculoskeletal constraints associated with standing in a crouched posture may play a significant role in the atypical postural muscle response patterns seen in children with spastic diplegia described in more detail in the section on impaired movement strategies during perturbed stance (Burtner et al., 1999; Woollacott et al., 1998).

Abnormal alignment can also be expressed as a change in the position of the body with reference to gravity and the base of support. For example, upright stance among individuals who have had a stroke is characterized by weight-bearing asymmetry (WBA), with more weight on the nonparetic leg (Duncan & Badke, 1987; Shumway-Cook et al., 1988). In addition, many persons with neurologic deficits stand with the center of mass displaced either forward or backward. For example, it has been reported that elderly persons with a fear of falling tend to stand in a forward lean posture, with the center of mass displaced anteriorly (Maki et al., 1991). However, persons with other types of postural deficits stand with the center of mass displaced posteriorly (Shumway-Cook & Horak, 1992). Changes in body alignment influence

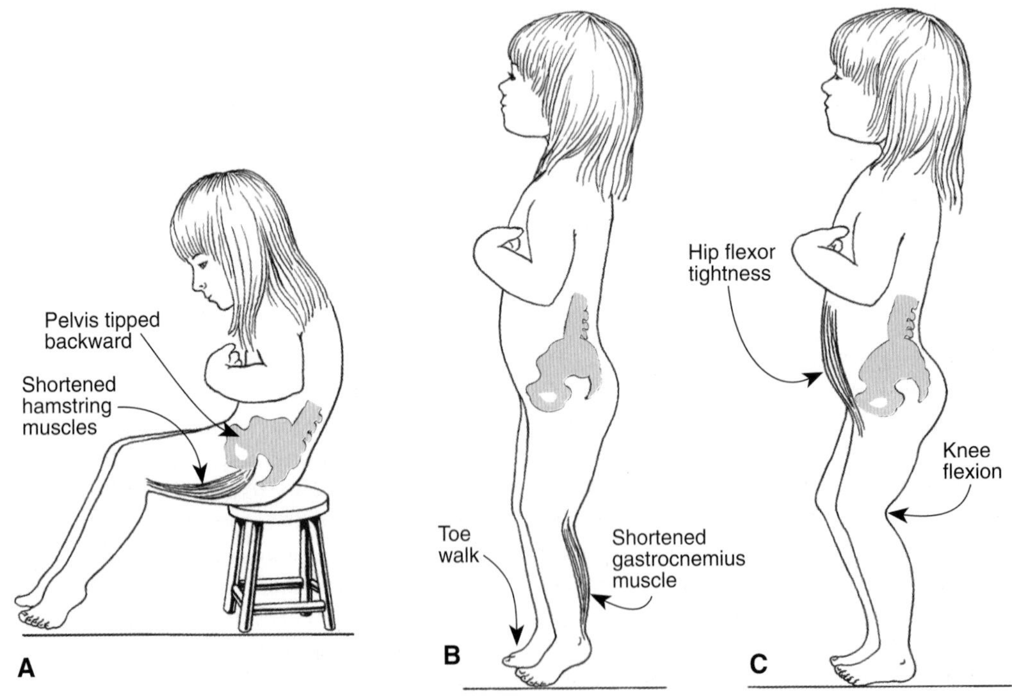

FIGURE 10.1 Atypical postures due to musculoskeletal impairments. A, Excessive posterior tilt of the pelvis in sitting accommodates shortened hamstrings. B, Shortening of the gastrocnemius muscle results in toe walk. C, Hip flexor tightness can result in tilting of the pelvis and flexion of the knee. (Adapted from Reimers J. Clinically based decision making for surgery. In: Sussman M, ed. The diplegic child. Rosemont, IL: American Academy of Orthopedic Surgeons, 1992:155, 156, 158.)

many aspects of postural control, including the characteristics of body sway in quiet stance and the way muscles are activated during recovery of stability following a perturbation.

Spontaneous Sway

One of the most common approaches to assessing stability during quiet stance is the use of single or dual force plates to quantify characteristics of the center of pressure (COP) excursion. While most studies use COP trajectories as an indicator of sway and thus a sign of postural stability, Patla and colleagues (2002) demonstrated that the changes in the COP may also be related to joint moments needed to maintain body alignment and prevent collapse of the body with respect to gravity.

Individuals with Parkinson's disease have abnormal postural sway in stance, including increased sway area and velocity (Rocchi et al., 2004). Increased mediolateral sway has been reported in several studies (Beuter et al., 2008; Viitasalo et al., 2002), while anteroposterior sway has been reported as comparable to normal in one study (Viitasalo et al, 2002) but increased in another (Rocchi et al., 2002). Rocchi and colleagues reported that treatment with levodopa increased postural sway abnormalities, while treatment with deep brain stimulation improved postural sway (Rocchi et al., 2004, 2006). In contrast, in a study on people in the early stages of PD, levodopa significantly reduced postural sway in quiet stance. Figure 10.2 illustrates changes in COP displacement in a person with PD off medication (A) and on medication (B).

Adults with Down syndrome (DS) had significantly higher sway velocity than control subjects in both eyes-open and eyes-closed conditions. Surprisingly, despite the presence of hypotonia, values of postural stiffness were higher than in control subjects and were related to increased sway velocity (Webber et al., 2004). The authors suggest that clinical measures of muscle tone, evaluated under passive conditions provide only limited information about the strategies used by the central nervous system (CNS) to control posture and movement. Among individuals with DS, increased stiffness may be a compensatory strategy to improve stability. Increased stiffness resulting from muscle cocontraction has been reported in individuals with DS (Aruin et al., 1996; Latash, 2000).

Pathology in different parts of the cerebellum may result in directionally specific increased postural sway (Dichgans & Fetter, 1993; Diener et al., 1984a, b; Mauritz et al., 1979; Sullivan et al., 2006). Several studies have reported that pathology in the spinocerebellar (upper vermal and intermediate) part of the anterior lobe results in predominantly anteroposterior body sway, with a frequency of about 3 Hz (Dichgans & Fetter, 1993; Diener et al., 1984a, b; Mauritz et al., 1979; Sullivan et al., 2006). Lesions of the lower (vestibulocerebellar) vermis are associated with increased omnidirectional postural sway, while lesions of spinocerebellar afferents (Friedreich's disease) are associated with a low frequency, large amplitude lateral sway pattern (Dichgans & Fetter, 1993; Diener et al., 1984a, b; Mauritz et al., 1979). Finally, among patients with anterior-lobe cerebellar pathology, postural sway was significantly increased in the absence of visual inputs, but reduced with additional orientation inputs from the somatosensory system (light finger tip touch) (Sullivan et al., 2006).

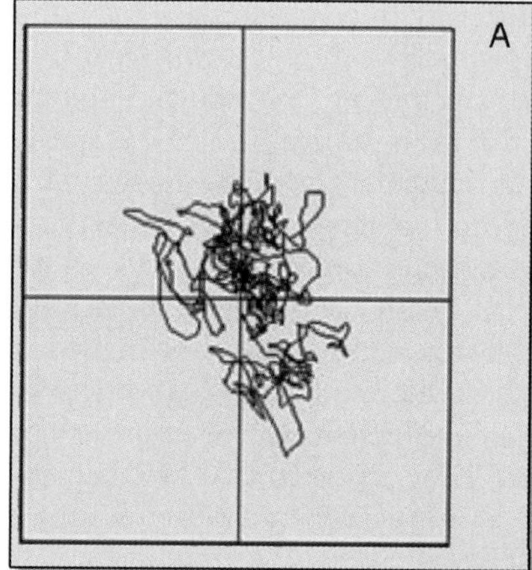

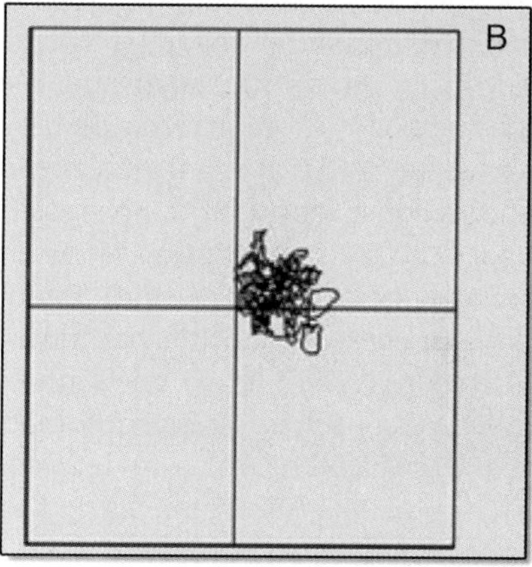

FIGURE 10.2 Changes in center of pressure during quiet stance in a person in the early stages of PD off levodopa medication (A) and on medication (B). (Adapted from Beuter A, Hernández R, Rigal R, et al. Postural sway and effect of levodopa in early Parkinson's disease. Can J Neurol Sci 2008;35:67.)

Liao and Hwang (2003) found increased sway in quiet stance in 15 children 5 to 12 years of age with cerebral palsy (CP; type not specified) and reported that postural stability in the eyes-closed condition was the best predictor of gross motor function. However, not all children with cerebral palsy may demonstrate abnormal postural sway in quiet stance. In a study of 23 ambulatory children and adolescents with spastic diplegia CP (5 to 18 years of age), the majority (14) had normal standing balance values (Rose et al., 2002).

Donker and colleagues (2007) used a dynamical analysis to examine the structure of COP trajectories in 10 children with CP and nine typically developing (TD) children in quiet stance with eyes open, eyes closed, and while performing a concurrent visual feedback task, which created a more external focus of attention. They reported that sway amplitude was larger and more regular in children with CP as compared with TD children. COP regularity is thought to be inversely related to the degree of automaticity in postural control (Donker et al., 2007; Roerdink et al., 2006). In addition, providing concurrent visual feedback, which created a more external focus on attention, decreased both the amount and the regularity of sway. This is consistent with the proposal by Wulf and colleagues (2001) that adopting an external focus of attention is beneficial when performing or learning a motor skill. In contrast, an internal focus of attention (e.g., directing attention to one's own body) is detrimental because it disrupts the automatic control of posture and movement (for a review, see Wulf & Prinz, 2001; see also, Wulf et al., 2001; McNevin & Wulf, 2002; McNevin et al., 2003).

Several researchers have quantified COP trajectories following stroke, reporting both asymmetrical and increased sway area in quiet stance (DiFabio & Badke, 1991; Genthon et al., 2008; Shumway-Cook et al., 1988). These studies have shown that many factors contribute to weight-bearing asymmetry following stroke, including motor weakness (Bohannon, 1990; Genthon et al., 2008), asymmetric muscular tone (Pérennou, 2005) and somatosensory deficits (DiFabio & Badke, 1991; Genthon et al., 2008). In addition, spatial cognitive disorders, such as impaired perceptions related to visual vertical, may also be involved (Barra et al., 2009; Bonan et al., 2006; Genthon et al., 2008).

Does asymmetrical stance alignment improve over time? A number of researchers have examined the recovery of stance postural control following stroke (De Haart et al., 2004; Geurts et al., 2005; Roerdink et al., 2009). De Haart et al. (2004) did a longitudinal follow-up of 30 patients after stroke to examine the contribution of paretic and nonparetic limbs to stance postural control. This study used two force plates to study COP under each limb separately at baseline (when patients were first able to stand for 30 seconds unsupported) then at 2, 4, 8, and 12 weeks later. Patients stood under three conditions, eyes open, eyes closed, and while performing a math task (dual-task condition). Early in recovery there was significant asymmetry in stance, with increased area and velocity in the nonparetic as compared with the paretic limb. Sway area and weight-bearing asymmetry both improved significantly with follow-up assessments; however the nonparetic limb continued to provide the majority of dynamic stabilization. The authors suggest that increased weight-bearing asymmetry and lateralized control (active control by the nonparetic limb) is an effective compensatory strategy for maintaining a stable stance position, particularly in patients with significant motor impairments. In addition, they suggest that rehabilitation strategies to reduce weight-bearing asymmetry in patients with severe motor impairments of the paretic limb may not be advisable, since this may be a reasonable compensatory strategy in the face of significant motor, sensory, and cognitive impairments.

Stability Limits

As discussed in Chapter 7, a main goal of the postural control system is to ensure stability by controlling the center of mass relative to functional stability limits. Stability limits are determined in part by the biomechanics of the body, but are also influenced by other factors, including subjective perceptions, postural control abilities, and environmental factors (Holbein & Redfern, 1997; Mancini et al., 2008). Functional limits of stability are often quantified by asking an individual to lean as far forward or backward as possible and recording the maximum COP excursion (Adkin et al., 2005; Bartolic et al., 2005; Mancini et al., 2008; Schieppati et al., 1994; van Wegen et al., 2001).

Reduced limits of stability as indicated by reduced COP excursion during voluntary leaning have been reported among minimally impaired adults with multiple sclerosis (Karst et al., 2005). Reduced functional limits of stability in the sagittal plane (as indicated by reduced maximum forward lean) have been reported in persons with PD (Adkin et al., 2005; Bartolic et al., 2005; Mancini et al., 2008; Schieppati et al., 1994; van Wegen et al., 2001). Individuals with PD reach their functional limits of stability more slowly than do age-matched controls, particularly in the backward direction (Mancini et al., 2008). The use of the drug levodopa improves functional limits of stability in subjects with PD but does not improve the anticipatory postural adjustments made prior to the forward lean (Mancini et al., 2008).

Several factors may contribute to reduced forward functional limits of stability in PD, including stooped posture (Bloem et al., 1999; Mancini et al., 2008), increased rigidity, and impaired postural preparation for the voluntary leans (Mancini et al., 2008). Several authors have suggested that forward voluntary leaning may be a good clinical measure of postural ability in PD, since it reflects composite effects of segment orientation, perceived postural stability, fear of falling, whole-body kinesthesia, and leg rigidity (Horak et al., 2009; Mancini et al., 2008).

As you can see, changes in quiet stance are complex, and they may be the direct result of motor and sensory/perceptual impairments affecting alignment, spontaneous sway, and perceived stability limits. In addition, changes in quiet stance may develop as part of a compensatory strategy. For example, the lateral shift in body alignment and asymmetric weight bearing seen in a person with hemiplegia may be due to perceptual impairments related to body scheme or alternatively a strategy that develops to compensate for motor impairments, such as weakness in the hemiparetic leg. Understanding these differences is important, since achieving a symmetrically aligned position may not be a reasonable goal for the person with hemiplegia until underlying impairments have resolved sufficiently to ensure that the hemiparetic leg will not collapse under the weight of the body.

Impaired Movement Strategies during Perturbed Stance

A number of researchers have begun to explore how neurologic deficits influence the coordination of postural muscle synergies (both in-place and stepping strategies) and affect the ability to recover stability following an unexpected perturbation. Problems affecting the coordination of muscle response synergies are classified into: (a) sequencing problems, (b) problems with the timely activation of postural responses, and (c) problems adapting postural activity to changing task and environmental demands.

Impaired In-Place Movement Strategies

Sequencing Problems. One of the earliest studies that reported information on motor coordination problems affecting stance postural control was one by Nashner and colleagues (1983) that examined postural control in children with different types of cerebral palsy. Ambulatory children (7 to 10 years of age) with different types of cerebral palsy stood on a platform that perturbed stance balance in the forward or backward direction. Electromyograms (EMGs) and ground reaction forces were used to examine the coordination of leg muscles responding to this induced sway. Figure 10.3 is an example of the EMG records from one of the children with spastic hemiplegia. Shown is muscle activity (gastrocnemius, hamstrings, anterior

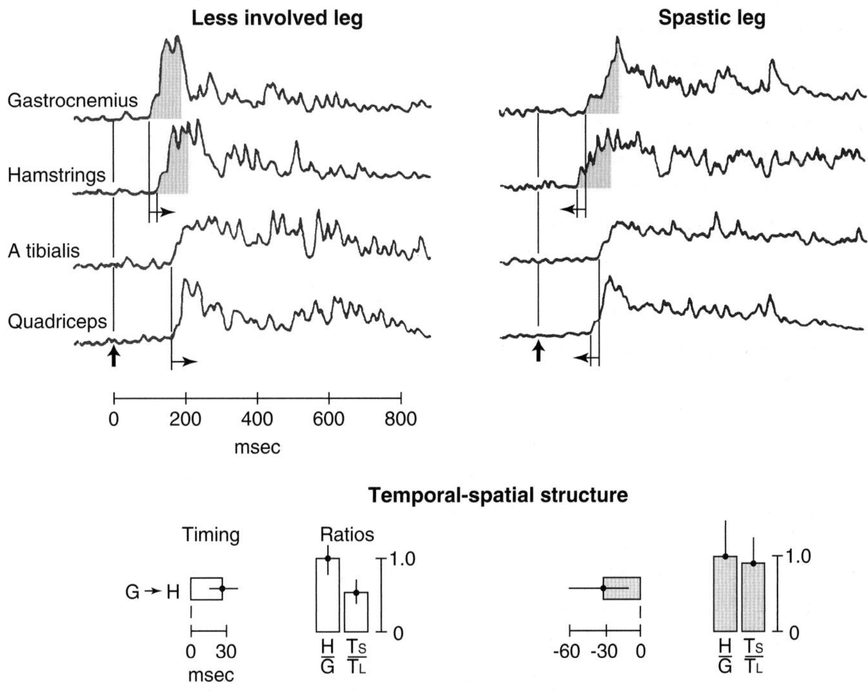

FIGURE 10.3 Abnormal sequencing of muscles in a child with hemiplegia responding to a backward translation of a moving platform. EMG recordings show an inappropriate activation of muscles responding to forward sway, with proximal muscles (hamstrings [H]) activated in advance of the so-called spastic distal muscles (gastrocnemius [G]). The upward arrow indicates the onset of platform movement. The horizontal arrows indicate the onset of muscle activity. T_L = anterior tibialis lengthening; T_S = anterior tibialis shortening. (Reprinted with permission from Nashner LM, Shumway-Cook A, Marin D. Stance posture control in select groups of children with cerebral palsy: deficits in sensory organization and muscular coordination. Exp Brain Res 1983;49:401.)

tibialis, and quadriceps) in both the spastic hemiplegic and nonhemiplegic legs in response to a backward platform perturbation producing forward sway. The sequencing of muscle activity in the nonhemiplegic leg (labeled "less involved") began in the gastrocnemius muscle at approximately 100 msec, followed 30 msec later by activation of the hamstrings muscle. In contrast, muscle activity in the spastic leg began first in the hamstrings, followed 30 to 50 msec later by activation of the gastrocnemius.

What is the consequence of changing the sequence in which muscles are activated when responding to a loss of balance? This can be seen in Figure 10.4, which presents the average torque, weight, and sway records for 10 trials of forward sway in this child. Abnormal sequencing of muscle activity in the hemiplegic leg (also labeled "left leg") resulted in significantly less torque than in the right leg. In addition, this pattern of muscle activity resulted in large lateral shifts of the body's center of mass, shown as the large oscillatory shifts in the weight record.

The delay in the activation of the gastrocnemius in the spastic leg was surprising for a number of reasons. On clinical examination, this child showed positive signs of spasticity in the gastrocnemius muscle, including increased stiffness in response to passive stretch, clonus, equinus gait, and lack of dorsiflexion at the ankle, in response to a backward displacement. Given these clinical findings, one might predict a hyperactive stretch response in the gastrocnemius when the child stood on the platform and swayed in the forward direction, as during forward sway the first muscle to be stretched is the gastrocnemius. But during forward sway, by imposing a stretch on the hyperactive gastrocnemius, the first muscles to respond were the hamstrings. The gastrocnemius muscle was slow to become active, and the amplitude of the muscle activity was low as compared with the uninvolved side. The finding of delayed activation of a stretched "spastic" muscle is consistent with the findings of other investigators, who have reported an inability to recruit and regulate the firing frequency of motor neurons in people with spastic hypertonia (Badke & DiFabio, 1990; Sahrmann & Norton, 1977).

The lack of an ascending (distal-to-proximal) pattern of muscle recruitment in response to perturbations to stance balance has also been reported in young children with spastic diplegia and limited walking experience (Burtner et al., 1999). In addition, these children, who often stand and walk on their toes, activated the antagonist tibialis anterior (TA) muscle before the gastrocnemius muscle in many trials. It is interesting that this is also the activation pattern seen in bipedal animals that stand on their toes. Thus, this pattern of activating the TA in response to backward

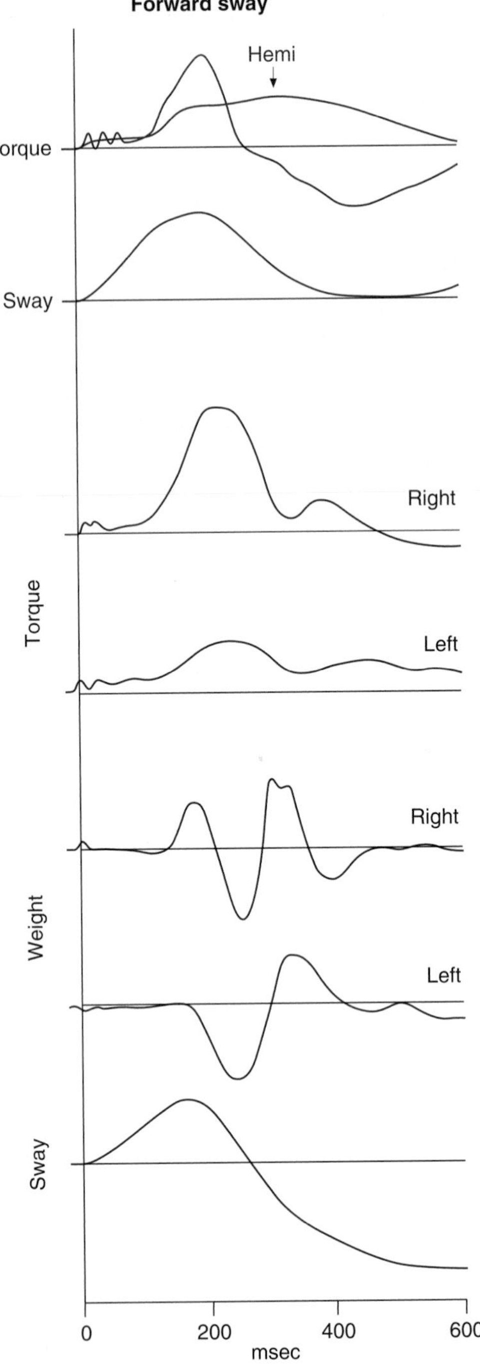

FIGURE 10.4 Illustration of the average torque, weight, and sway records for 10 trials of forward sway in a child with spastic hemiplegia. Abnormal sequencing of muscle activity in the left hemiplegic leg (Hemi) resulted in significantly less torque than in the right leg. In addition, this pattern of muscle activity resulted in large lateral shifts of the body's center of mass, shown as the large oscillatory shifts in the weight record. (Adapted with permission from Nashner LM, Shumway-Cook A, Marin D. Stance posture control in select groups of children with cerebral palsy: deficits in sensory organization and muscular coordination. Exp Brain Res 1983;49:401.)

displacements, causing forward sway, may be due to the varying stimulus characteristics created from an on-toes stance.

Brogren and colleagues (1996) also reported a disruption in the recruitment order of muscles responding to loss of balance in the seated position in children with the spastic diplegia form of CP. Neurologically intact children recruit muscles in a distal-to-proximal sequence, beginning with the muscles closest to the support surface. In contrast, as can be seen in Figure 10.5, children with spastic diplegia tended to recruit muscles in a proximal-to-distal sequence, that is, beginning at the neck and progressing downward. In addition, the children with spastic diplegia showed significant coactivation of muscles in the neck and hip, with antagonists being activated before agonists (similar to what was found by Burtner et al., 1999, for standing children).

What is the effect of constraining movement at a joint on the organization of muscle activity used to recover balance? Ankle–foot orthoses (AFOs) are often used by clinicians to control spasticity and prevent excessive plantar flexion. A variety of orthoses are used, including both solid AFOs, which do not allow movement at the ankle joint, and spiral or hinged AFOs, which allow a degree of dynamic ankle-joint movement. Burtner and colleagues (1999) examined the effects of solid versus dynamic AFOs on the coordination of muscles for postural control in both children with spastic diplegia and TD children. For both TD children and children with spastic diplegia, the percent of trials in which the ankle strategy was used was significantly reduced when balancing with the solid AFO compared to the no-AFO and dynamic-AFO conditions. Use of a solid AFO was associated with significantly delayed onset latency in the gastrocnemius muscle and a reduction in the frequency of the normal distal-to-proximal muscle response sequence. These results are shown in Figure 10.6, A and B, and suggest that the types of devices used to control position and motion at the ankles can have a significant impact on the sequencing and timing of muscles used for recovery of balance. AFOs that restrict motion at the ankle will reduce the participation of ankle-joint muscles in the control of stability, resulting in an increased use of hip and trunk muscles for balance control.

Sequencing problems can also manifest as abnormally long delays in the recruitment of proximal muscle synergists. This type of timing problem has been reported in children with Down syndrome (Shumway-Cook & Woollacott, 1985b) and in adults with traumatic brain injuries with focal cortical contusions (Shumway-Cook & Olmscheid, 1990). Delayed activation of proximal muscles following platform perturbations can be seen in Figure 10.7, which compares EMG responses in a child with Down syndrome to an age-matched normal child. In the normal child, proximal muscle delays were on the order of 36 msec,

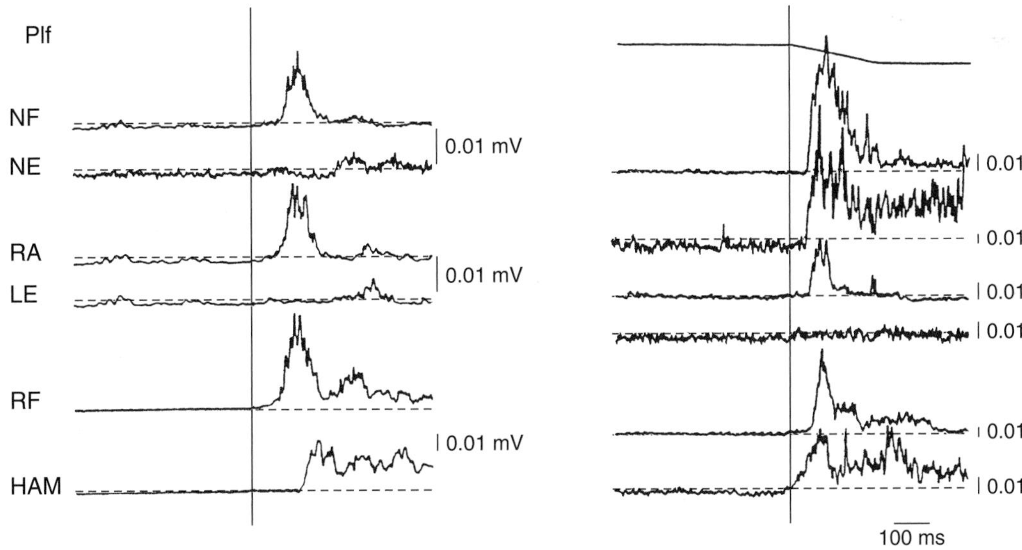

FIGURE 10.5 Comparison of EMG records from a control child (A) and a child with spastic diplegia (B). The sequencing of muscles in a child with spastic diplegia responding to a backward translation of a moving platform (Plf) while in the seated position is abnormal as compared with the muscles of the control child. EMG records show an inappropriate activation of muscles responding to forward sway, with proximal neck flexors and extensors (NF and NE) firing simultaneously with distal trunk (RA and LE) and leg (RF and HAM) muscles. (Reprinted with permission from Brogren E, Hadders-Algra M, Forssberg H. Postural control in children with spastic diplegia: muscle activity during perturbations in sitting. Dev Med Child Neurol 1998;38:381.)

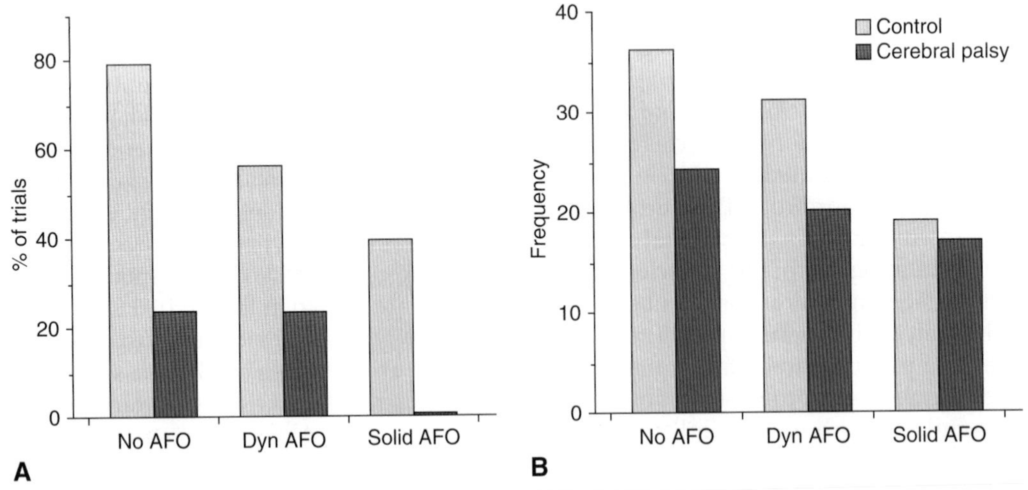

FIGURE 10.6 A, Percent of trials in which the ankle strategy was used in both control children and in children with cerebral palsy when wearing no AFO, a dynamic AFO, or a solid AFO. B, Frequency of observing the normal distal-to-proximal muscle response in both control children and those with cerebral palsy, in the no AFO condition compared with the dynamic and solid AFO conditions. Note that solid AFOs cause a reduction in both use of the ankle strategy and in distal-to-proximal response sequencing.

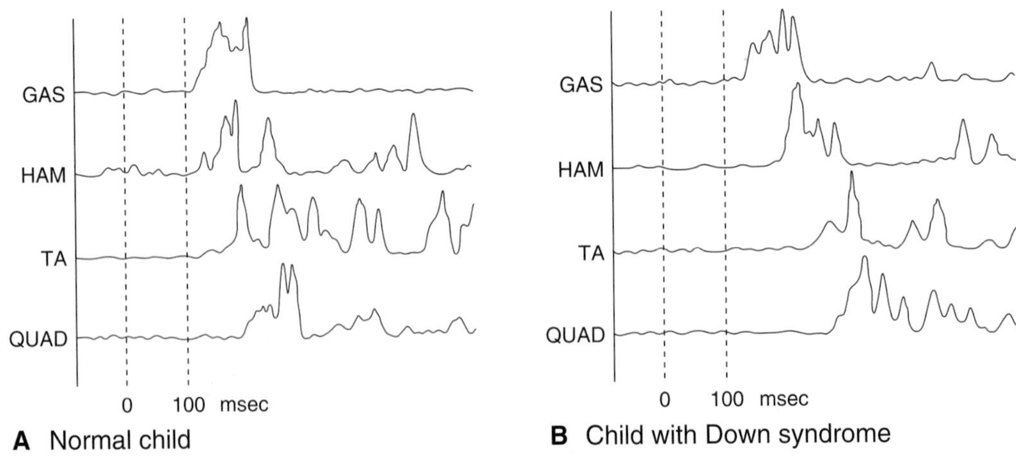

FIGURE 10.7 Comparison of EMG responses in a child with Down syndrome (B) with an age-matched typically developing child (A), illustrating the delay in proximal muscle activation during recovery of balance. In the typically developing child, proximal muscle delays were on the order of 36 msec, as compared with 60 to 80 msec in the child with Down syndrome. GAS = gastrocnemius; HAM = hamstrings; QUAD = quadriceps; TA = tibialis anterior. (Adapted with permission from Shumway-Cook A, Woollacott M. Postural control in the Down's syndrome child. Phys Ther 1985;9:1317.)

as compared with 60 to 80 msec in the child with Down syndrome (Shumway-Cook & Woollacott, 1985b). The biomechanical consequences of the delayed activation of the proximal muscles compared with the distal muscles include excessive motion at the knee and hip. This is because the timing of synergistic muscles is not efficient in controlling the indirect effects of forces generated at the ankle on more proximal joints.

Coactivation. The presence of coactivation is a common postural coordination strategy reported in both very young healthy children and a wide variety of people with neurologic deficits, including cerebral palsy (Crenna & Inverno, 1994; Nashner et al., 1983; Woollacott et al., 1998), CVA (Duncan & Badke, 1987), traumatic brain injury (Shumway-Cook & Olmscheid, 1991), Down syndrome (Shumway-Cook & Woollacott, 1985b), and Parkinson's disease (Dimitrova et al., 2004a; Horak et al., 1992). Coactivation is characterized by the simultaneous contraction of muscles on both anterior and posterior aspects of the body.

Coactivation in an individual with PD can be seen in Figure 10.8, which compares EMG responses in an elderly person without PD and an elderly person

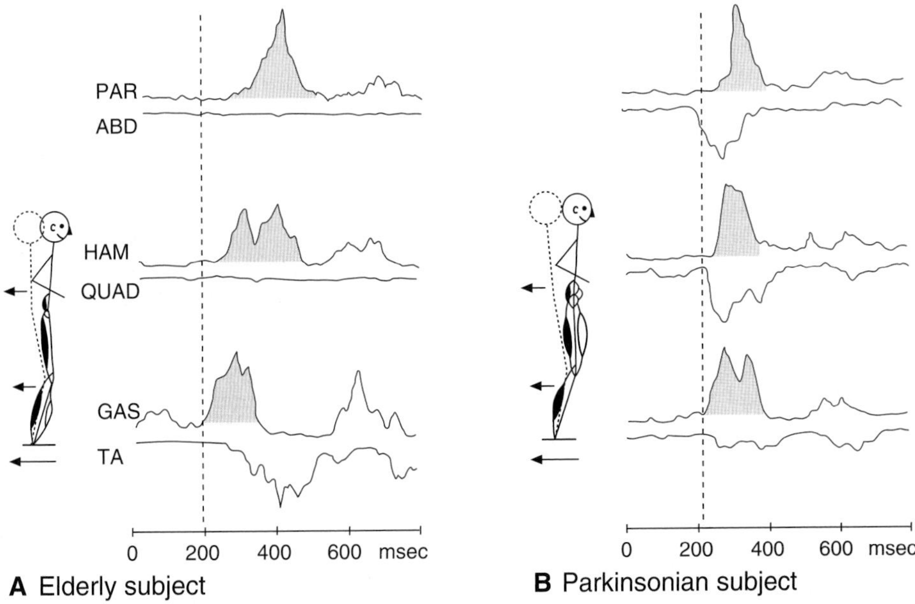

FIGURE 10.8 Comparison of muscle activation patterns in an elderly person without Parkinson's disease (A) and a person with PD (B), illustrating muscle activation patterns in response to forward sway. The person with PD coactivates antagonistic muscles around the hip and knee, while the elderly individual does not. Shown is the EMG response, and a schematic representation of the responses. ABD = abdominals; GAS = gastrocnemius; HAM = hamstring; PAR = paraspinals; QUAD = quadriceps; TA = tibialis anterior. (Adapted with permission from Horak FB, Nutt JG, Nashner LM. Postural inflexibility in Parkinsonian subjects. J Neurol Sci 1992;111:49, Figure 1, parts B and C.)

with PD. This activation of muscles on both sides of the joint results in a stiffening of the body, and is a very inefficient strategy for the recovery of balance (Horak et al., 1992). Carpenter et al. (2004) also reported increased coactivation in people with PD in response to multidirectional support-surface rotations. These results are not consistent with the classic work on PD by Purdue Martin (1967), who reported an absence of equilibrium and righting reactions in people with PD. The rigidity and loss of balance found during tilt tests suggested that equilibrium reactions were absent. However, placing EMG electrodes on the muscles of people with PD has allowed researchers to see that individuals with PD do indeed respond to disequilibrium, but the pattern of muscular activity used is ineffective in recovering balance.

Delayed Activation of Postural Responses. Researchers have also found that significant delays in the onset of postural responses can contribute to instability in persons with neurologic deficits. Muscle activity in response to platform perturbations (both horizontal translations and rotations) has been studied in persons with hemiplegia resulting from a CVA (Diener et al., 1984a, b; DiFabio et al., 1986; Ikai et al., 2003; Slijper et al., 2002). Researchers have reported deficits in the sequencing, timing, and amplitude of postural muscle activity in the paretic limb. Figure 10.9 shows

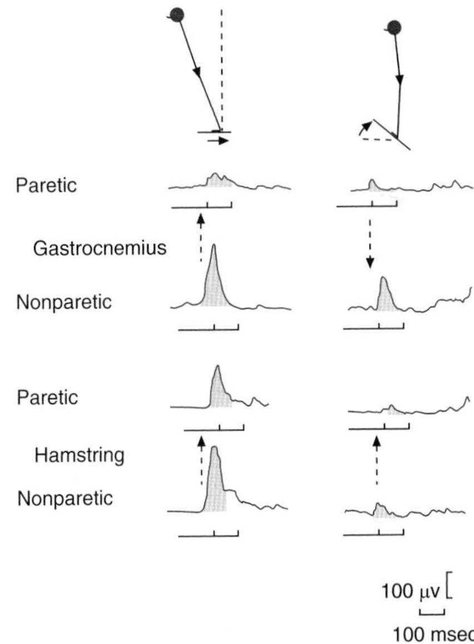

FIGURE 10.9 EMG responses in the gastrocnemius and hamstring muscles in paretic and nonparetic limbs of a person with hemiplegia following a CVA in response to a forward sway perturbation, and a toes-up rotational perturbation. Muscle responses in the paretic limb are slow and reduced in amplitude. (Adapted with permission from DiFabio RP, Badke MB, Duncan PW. Adapting human postural reflexes localized cerebrovascular lesion: analysis of bilateral long latency responses. Brain Res 1986;363:259.)

the EMG responses in the paretic and nonparetic legs of a person with hemiplegia in response to a forward sway perturbation (DiFabio et al., 1986). Onset latencies in the paretic distal muscles were significantly longer and smaller in amplitude than on the nonparetic side. Delays in the activation of distal muscles in the paretic limb were compensated for by early activation of proximal muscles in the nonparetic limb.

Following stroke, problems in the timing and organization of muscle activity during recovery from a perturbation can contribute to increased risk for falls. Marigold and Eng (2006) examined differences in body kinematics and postural muscle activity (surface EMGs) in 44 patients after they had had a stroke (11 fallers and 33 nonfallers) in response to forward and backward perturbations to stance. EMG analysis, shown in Figure 10.10, demonstrated that in the faller group, postural response in the paretic, but not the nonparetic limb, were slower and smaller in amplitude as compared with the nonfaller group (131 msec and 119 msec, respectively). In addition, in the faller group, the activation of the proximal synergist (the right femorus) was significantly delayed in both the paretic and nonparetic limbs as compared with the nonfallers, suggesting impaired intralimb coupling among muscle synergists.

Significant delays in the onset of postural activity have been reported in developmental abnormalities, including Down syndrome (Shumway-Cook & Woollacott, 1985b) and some forms of cerebral palsy (Nashner et al., 1983). This can be seen in Figure 10.11, which compares onset latencies to forward sway in healthy control children, children with Down syndrome, and children with cerebral palsy (spastic hemiplegia and ataxia).

Postural response latencies were significantly longer in persons with multiple sclerosis (MS) (average, 161±31 msec) as compared with control subjects (102±21 msec), with considerable asymmetry between the two legs, both of which were correlated to somatosensory conduction delays. The authors suggest that demyelination of the posterior columns of the spinal cord is the direct cause of the somatosensory conduction delays and that this causes delayed postural responses and imbalance in most people with MS (Cameron et al., 2008). These results also support the hypothesis that postural responses to surface translations are likely triggered by primary and/or secondary afferents from muscle spindles (Stapley et al., 2002).

Problems Modifying Postural Strategies. Normal postural control requires the ability to modify postural strategies in response to changing tasks and environmental demands. This includes the ability to modify

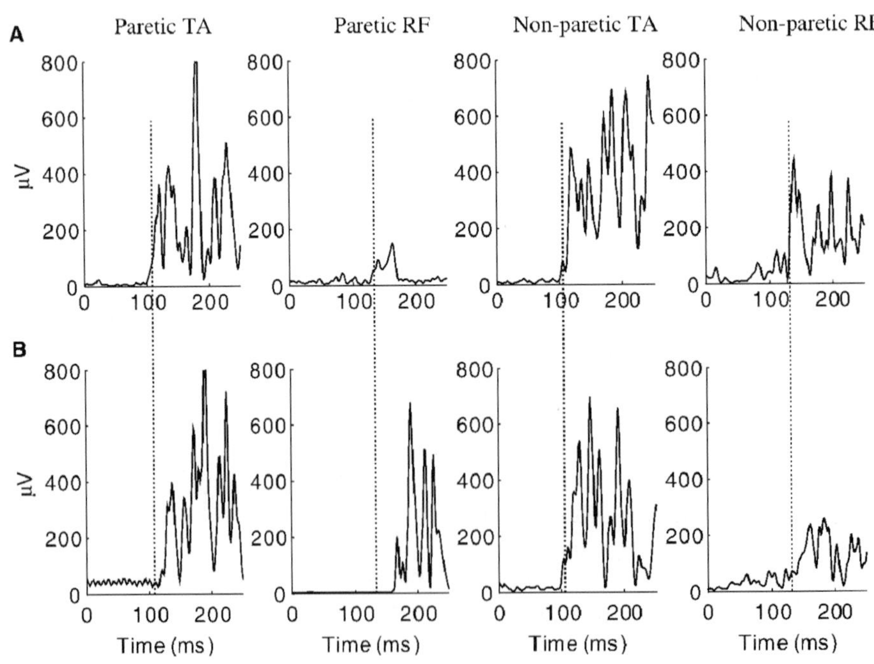

FIGURE 10.10 Differences in muscle activity in the paretic and nonparetic tibialis anterior (TA) and rectus femorus (RF) in response to a forward platform translation inducing backward sway in two subjects with stroke. In comparison to the nonfaller (A), the subject who fell had slower onset latencies in the paretic TA, and slower responses in both the paretic and nonparetic RF, suggesting poor intralimb coupling. (Adapted with permission from Marigold DS, Eng JJ. Altered timing of postural reflexes contributes to falling in persons with chronic stroke. Exp Brain Res 2006;171:454, Figure 3.)

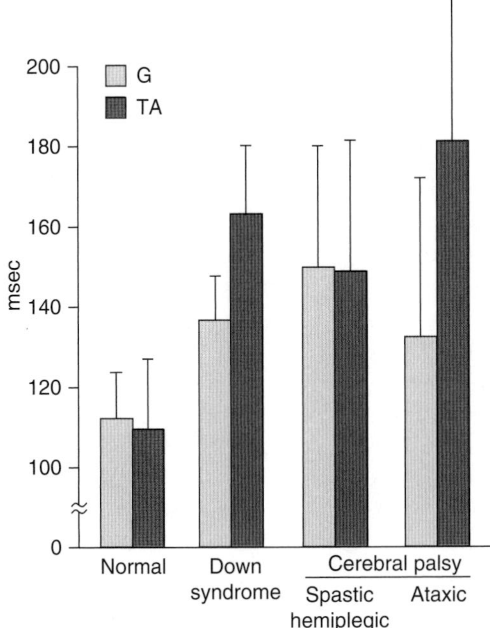

FIGURE 10.11 Onset of contraction of postural muscles to platform perturbations in typically developing children, children with Down syndrome, and children with cerebral palsy (spastic hemiplegic and ataxic). Onset of muscle contraction in the children with neurologic deficits is significantly slower than in the age-matched controls. G = gastrocnemius; TA = tibialis anterior.

postural activity with practice, referred to as "postural adaptation," and the ability to change the pattern of postural muscle activity quickly in response to changing task conditions, referred to as shifting central set (Chong et al., 2000; Horak, 1996). The inability to modify postural responses to changing task demands is a characteristic of many people with neurologic pathology.

Problems Adapting Motor Strategies. Maintaining balance requires that forces generated to control the body's position in space are appropriately scaled to the degree of instability. This means that a small perturbation to stability is met with an appropriately sized muscle response. Thus, force output must be appropriate to the amplitude of instability. Neurologically intact people use a combination of feedforward, or anticipatory, and feedback control mechanisms to scale forces needed for postural stability. Constraints on adaptation can be due to a variety of problems, including limitations in ability to increase the recruitment of agonist muscles in response to increasing perturbation size (strength problems) or problems in the ability to scale, or modulate, the amplitude of postural responses either up or down in response to different-sized perturbations to balance.

Researchers have found that children with CP have significant problems in adapting the amplitude of postural responses to perturbations of increasing distance and velocity (Roncesvalles et al., 2002). This reduced ability to adaptively increase the amplitude of the agonist muscle can be seen in Figure 10.12, which gives an example of muscle activity in a typically developing (TD) child and a child with CP in response to three levels of perturbation difficulty. While the TD child increased the amplitude of the gastrocnemius muscle in response to increasing perturbation size, the child with CP did not. These findings were consistent with research showing that maximum voluntary contraction levels for muscles in the lower extremities, and especially distal ankle joint muscles, are significantly lower in children with CP (Wiley & Damiano, 1998). This suggests that constraints on the ability to modulate the amplitude of muscle activity found in children with CP affect both the voluntary control system and the automatic postural response system (Roncesvalles et al., 2002).

Inability to grade or scale force output to perturbations of varying sizes has been reported in individuals with anterior cerebellar lesions (Horak & Diener, 1994; Horak et al., 1989a, 1990). Individuals with unilateral cerebellar pathology affecting the anterior lobe show hypermetric postural responses on the involved side of the body. Hypermetric postural responses are too large and are associated with excessive compensatory body sway in the direction opposite the initial direction of instability. Hypermetric balance responses can be seen in the video case study of John, who has spinocerebellar degeneration. An

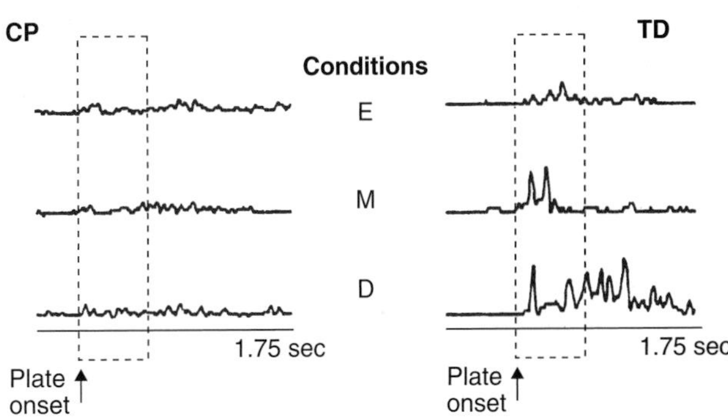

FIGURE 10.12 EMG from one child with cerebral palsy (CP) and one typically developing (TD) child, illustrating difficulty in adaptively increasing muscle activity in the gastrocnemius muscle to easy (E), moderate (M), and difficult (D) platform perturbations. (Adapted with permission from Roncesvalles MN, Woollacott MW, Burtner PA. Neural factors underlying reduced postural adaptability in children with cerebral palsy. NeuroReport 2002;13:2409, Figure 1.)

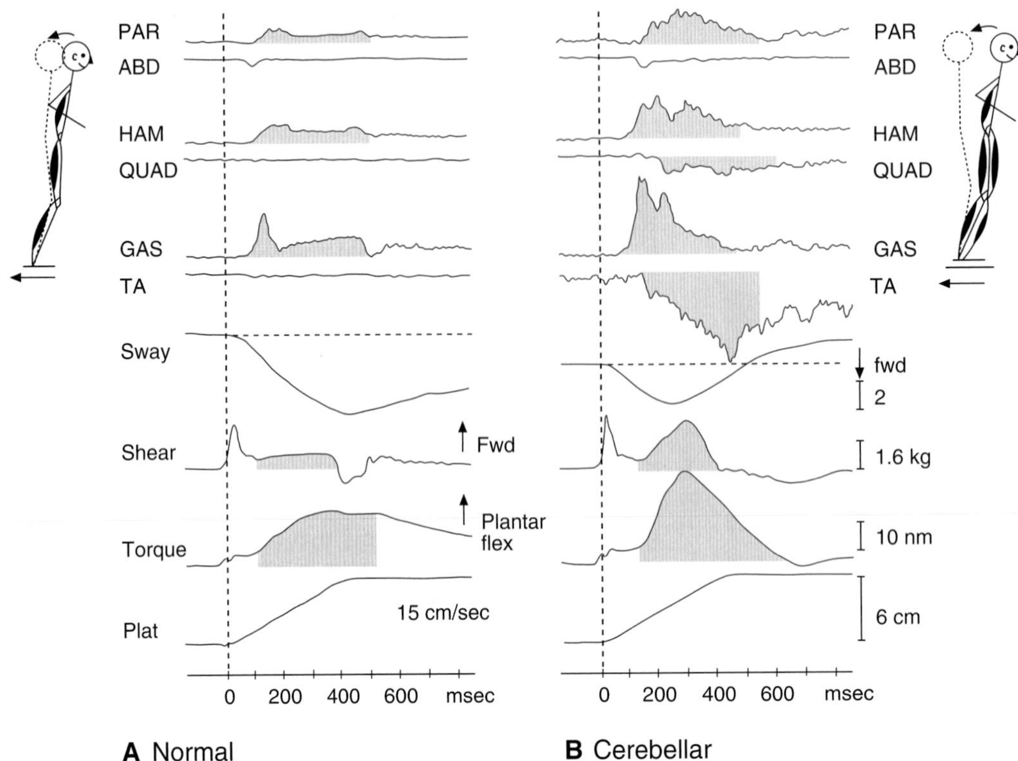

FIGURE 10.13 EMG activity in controls (A) versus persons with anterior-lobe cerebellar degeneration (B). Muscle responses of the person with cerebellar degeneration are hypermetric, that is, significantly larger in amplitude and longer in duration than in controls. ABD = abdominals; GAS = gastrocnemius; HAM = hamstring; PAR = paraspinals; QUAD = quadriceps; TA = tibialis anterior. (Adapted with permission from Horak FB, Diener HC. Cerebellar control of postural scaling and central set in stance. J Neurophysiol 1994;72:483.)

example of hypermetric postural responses found in people with anterior-lobe cerebellar damage is shown in Figure 10.13. EMG responses in people with cerebellar disease are larger in amplitude and longer in duration than those found in controls. An examination of the sway and torque records shown in Figure 10.13 shows that hypermetric muscle activity resulted in both excess torque and an overcorrection in sway during the recovery of stability (Horak & Diener, 1994). Hypermetric postural activity in persons with cerebellar pathology has also been reported in response to multidirectional perturbations (Kung et al., 2009). Finally, postural responses also appear to be larger than normal in persons with MS, possibly to compensate for their delayed onset of contraction. The larger postural responses seen in subjects with MS were similar to, but not as large as, the hypermetric postural responses seen in subjects with cerebellar ataxia (Cameron et al., 2008).

Impaired Central Set. Inability to change movement strategies quickly to adapt to changes in support-surface characteristics has been found in people with PD (Horak et al., 1992b). In this study, normal controls and a group of individuals with PD were asked to maintain stance balance in a variety of situations, including standing on a flat surface, standing with both feet on a narrow beam, and sitting on a stool with the feet unsupported. People in the control group were able to modify postural muscle responses quickly in response to changing task demands (Fig. 10.14A). In contrast, individuals with PD were unable to modify the complex movement strategy used in recovering balance while standing on a flat surface for use while standing on the beam or while seated, showing an inability to modify how they moved in response to changes in environmental and task demands (Fig. 10.14B). Researchers believe that these results suggest that the basal ganglia function to prime or set the nervous system to achieve its goal (Chong et al., 2000). Individuals with PD have difficulty changing from one movement set to another. A reduced ability to modify postural strategies in people with PD has also been shown in response to multidirectional surface perturbations and in response to changing stance width (Dimitrova et al., 2004a, 2004b; Horak et al., 2005).

The inability to modify postural activity in response to changing task and environmental

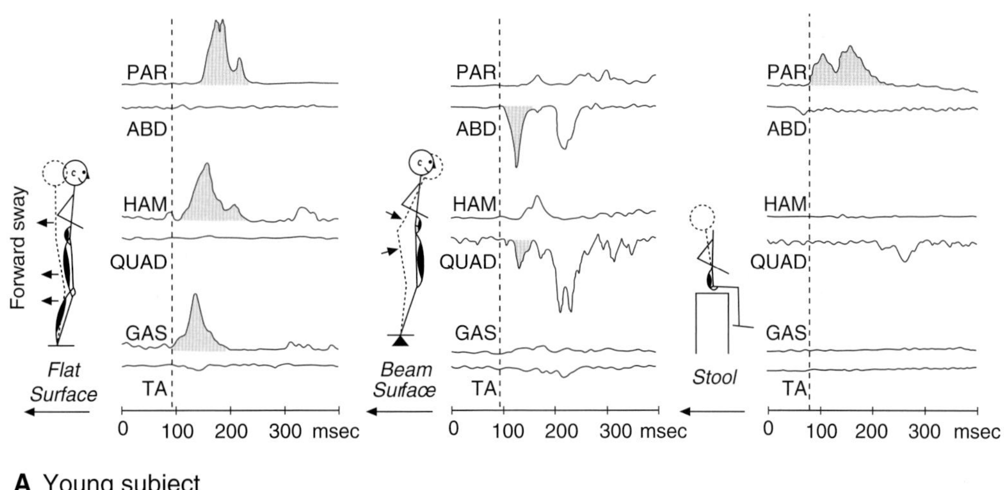

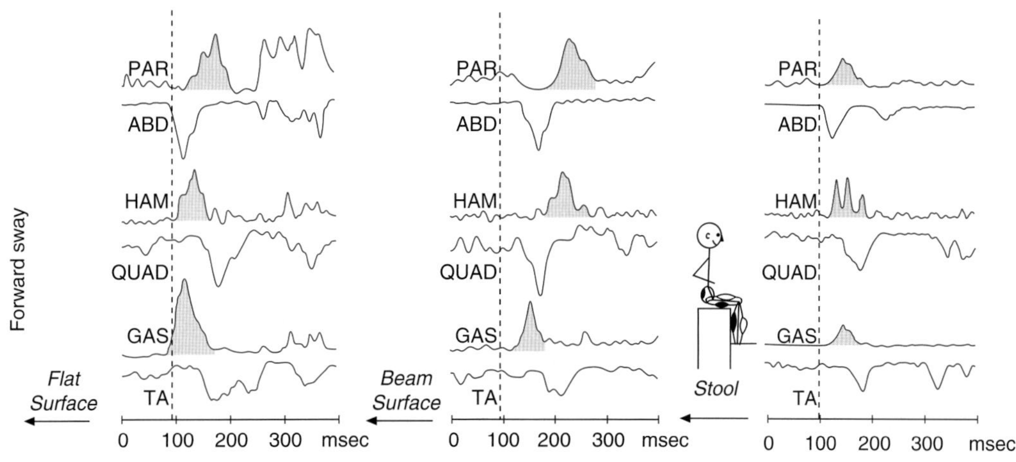

FIGURE 10.14 Normal and abnormal postural set changes. A, Normal modulation of muscle activity in response to perturbations producing forward sway under three different task conditions: standing on a flat surface, standing on a beam surface, and sitting on a stool. In contrast to a young subject in the control group (A), EMG patterns in a person with PD (B) revealed a complex strategy of muscle activity that did not change in response to task demands. ABD = abdominals; GAS = gastrocnemius; HAM = hamstring; PAR = paraspinals; QUAD = quadriceps; TA = tibialis anterior. (Adapted with permission from Horak FB, Nutt JG, Nashner LM. Postural inflexibility in Parkinsonian subjects. J Neurol Sci 1992;111:52.)

conditions is found in people with varying types of neural pathology, suggesting that mechanisms underlying postural flexibility are widely distributed among many neural structures.

Impaired Stepping Strategy

Very few researchers have studied the effect of neural pathology on the organization and timing of automatic stepping strategies used to recover from an unexpected perturbation. Much of the research related to stepping in patients with neurologic pathology has been done in the context of voluntary stepping and is covered in the section on gait initiation in Chapter 14, on abnormal mobility.

King and Horak (2008) examined lateral stepping strategies in persons with PD on and off medication. A movable force plate was used to elicit lateral steps in 13 participants with PD and 14 healthy controls. Participants with PD used a similar lateral stepping strategy to that of controls in response to lateral translations; however, a lack of an anticipatory lateral weight shift, and delayed onset reduced the effectiveness of the lateral stepping strategy, resulting in a significant number of falls among the group with PD. In addition, while the healthy controls tended to recover with a single lateral step, participants with PD took several small steps to recover. Though less frequent than the lateral step, both groups also used a crossover strategy to recover from the lateral perturbations;

however, this crossover strategy was frequently associated with falls in the PD group.

PROBLEMS IN THE SENSORY/ PERCEPTUAL SYSTEMS

Normal postural control requires: (1) the organization of sensory information from visual, somatosensory, and vestibular systems that provide information about the body's position and movement with respect to the environment, and (2) the coordination of sensory information with motor actions.

Sensory problems can disrupt postural control by: (1) affecting a person's ability to adapt sensory inputs to changes in task and environmental demands, and (2) preventing the development of accurate internal models of the body for postural control (Horak & Shupert, 1994).

Problems with Sensory Organization

Researchers examining the effect of neurologic injury on a person's ability to organize and select appropriate sensory inputs for postural control have focused primarily on the use of computerized force platforms in conjunction with moving visual surrounds, first developed by Nashner and colleagues (Black et al., 1988; Horak et al., 1990; Shumway-Cook et al., 1988). This approach, described in detail in the chapters on normal postural control, measures changes in body sway during stance in situations in which sensory information is reduced or made inaccurate for postural control. Alternatively, therapists have used compliant foam surfaces in conjunction with a visual dome to examine sensory adaptation in the clinic. This test, referred to as the Clinical Test for Sensory Interaction in Balance (CTSIB) measures the number of seconds (30 seconds maximum) a person can stand under six different sensory conditions (Horak, 1987; Shumway-Cook & Horak, 1986).

What is the effect of loss of a sensory input on postural control? It depends. Some important factors include: (a) the availability of other senses to detect the position of the body in space, (b) the availability of accurate orientation cues in the environment, and (c) the ability to correctly interpret and select sensory information for orientation (Shumway-Cook & Horak, 1992). Researchers are beginning to examine the extent to which persons with a loss of one sense can compensate by increasing the sensitivity of the remaining senses.

As shown in Figure 10.15, persons with loss of vestibular information for postural control may be stable under most conditions as long as alternative

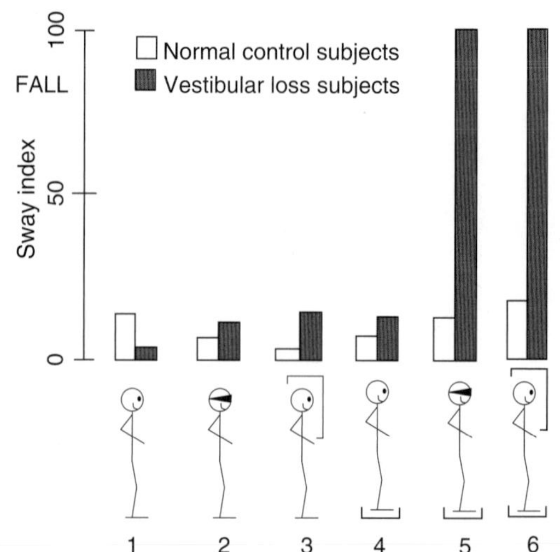

FIGURE 10.15 Comparison of body sway in the six sensory conditions in neurologically intact adults versus persons with loss of vestibular function. Results show that instability in persons with loss of vestibular function occurs only in conditions in which vision and somatosensory inputs are not available for postural control (conditions 5 and 6). (Source: Horak F, Nashner LM, Diener HC. Postural strategies associated with somatosensory and vestibular loss. Exp Brain Res 1990;82:418.)

sensory information from vision or the somatosensory systems is available for orientation. In situations in which vision and somatosensory inputs are reduced, leaving mainly vestibular inputs (the last two conditions in Fig. 10.15) for postural control, the person may experience sudden falls, indicated by the score of 100 on the sway index (Horak et al., 1990).

Functionally, persons with this type of postural dyscontrol might perform normally on most tests of balance as long as they are carried out in a well-lit environment and on a firm, flat surface. However, performance on balance tasks under ideal sensory conditions will not necessarily predict the person's likelihood for falls in more complex conditions, such as when getting up to go to the bathroom at night and negotiating a carpeted surface in the dark.

How does disruption of somatosensory information affect postural control? One might expect that a person with a sudden loss of somatosensory information could maintain stability as long as alternative information from vision and vestibular senses was available. Horak and colleagues (1990) examined this question by applying pressure cuffs to the ankles of normal adults and inflating them until cutaneous sensation in the feet and ankles was lost. As shown in Figure 10.16, neurologically intact persons were able to maintain balance on all sensory conditions, despite the loss of somatosensory cues from the feet and ankles,

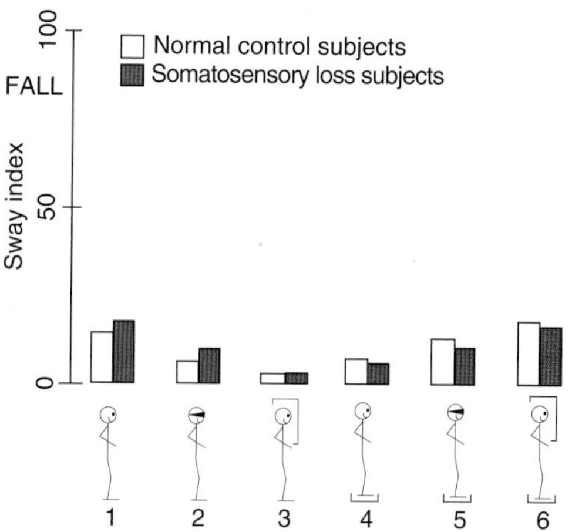

FIGURE 10.16 Body sway in the six sensory conditions in normal persons before use of pressure cuffs at the ankle and after subsequent temporary loss of cutaneous sensation with the use of pressure cuffs. Loss of somatosensory inputs did not affect the ability of these neurologically intact persons to maintain balance because of the availability of alternative senses and the capacity to adapt remaining senses to the changing demands. (Source: Horak F, Nashner LM, Diener HC. Postural strategies associated with somatosensory and vestibular loss. Exp Brain Res 1990; 82:418.)

as they always had an alternative sense (either vision or vestibular) available for orientation.

Jeka and colleagues (1996) studied the use of sensory cues for postural orientation in sighted and blind individuals. They were interested in understanding whether increasing haptic cues could improve postural orientation in blind individuals. Haptic perceptual cues involve both cutaneous receptors that provide information about surface properties (such as friction) and kinesthetic receptors that provide information about body movement and position. In sighted and blind individuals maintaining a tandem Romberg position, haptic cues were provided by contact with a cane. Touch contact with a slanted cane reduced postural sway more than did physically supportive forces with a perpendicular cane. This suggests that a hand-held cane provides haptic sensory cues with sufficient precision to improve postural stability substantially in blind individuals.

Providing additional sensory information for postural control through the use of haptic cues (fingertip touch to a supporting surface) has been found to improve postural stability in a number of persons with neurologic pathology, including those with cerebellar pathology (Sullivan et al., 2006), adults with Down syndrome (Gomes & Berela, 2007) and in persons with peripheral neuropathy due to long-standing diabetes (Dickstein et al., 2001, 2003). Researchers have also shown that somatosensory loss in persons with diabetic peripheral neuropathy was associated with an increased sensitivity to vestibular stimulation (Horak & Hlavacka, 2001). This type of sensory substitution mechanism is consistent with research showing an adaptive increase in somatosensory system input gain in persons with chronic loss of vestibular cues (Strupp et al., 1999).

In some cases, instability results from an inability to effectively organize and select appropriate sensory inputs for postural control. Sensory organization problems can manifest as an inflexible weighting of sensory information for orientation. This means that a person may depend heavily on one particular sense for postural control; for example, they may be either vision-dependent or somatosensory-system–dependent. When presented with a situation in which that sense is either not available or not accurately reporting self-motion, persons will continue to rely on the preferred sense, even though instability may be a consequence. For example, several studies have reported that following a stroke, there is an increased reliance on visual inputs for stance postural control in the early stages of recovery (Bonan et al., 2004; Geurts et al., 2005). Some have reported that over time, with recovery, there is a decreased reliance on visual inputs for stance postural control (De Haart et al., 2004), while others have reported that an increased reliance on vision persists (Laufer et al., 2005).

Patterns of sway associated with this type of sensory inflexibility are summarized in Figure 10.17.

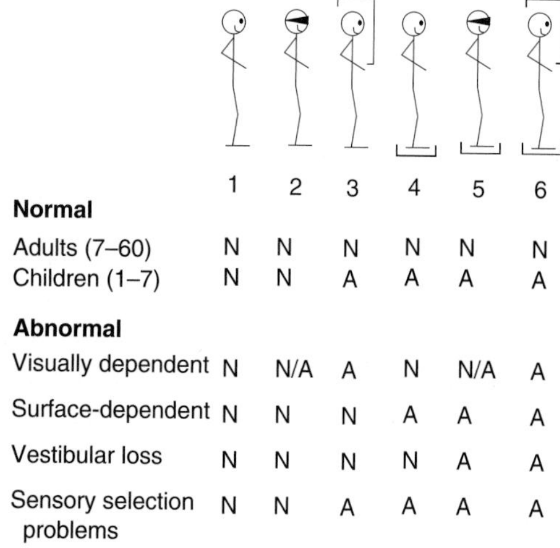

	1	2	3	4	5	6
Normal						
Adults (7–60)	N	N	N	N	N	N
Children (1–7)	N	N	A	A	A	A
Abnormal						
Visually dependent	N	N/A	A	N	N/A	A
Surface-dependent	N	N	N	A	A	A
Vestibular loss	N	N	N	N	A	A
Sensory selection problems	N	N	A	A	A	A

FIGURE 10.17 Classification scheme for identifying different problems related to organizing sensory information for stance postural control based on patterns of normal and abnormal sway in six sensory conditions used during dynamic posturography testing. A = abnormal sway; N = normal sway.

Persons who are dependent on visual information for postural control (referred to as "visually dependent" in Fig. 10.17) tend to show abnormally increased sway in any condition in which visual cues are reduced (such as standing with eyes closed) or made inaccurate (such as standing in the presence of visual motion in the environment) (Black & Nashner, 1984a, b).

Persons who demonstrate an inflexible use of somatosensory inputs for postural control (surface-dependent) become unstable in conditions in which surface inputs do not allow them to establish and maintain a vertical orientation (Horak & Shupert, 1994). This can be seen as excessive amounts of body sway in conditions 4, 5, and 6 (Fig. 10.17). Thus, when standing on a compliant surface, like sand or thick carpet; on a tilted surface, like a ramp; or on a moving surface, like a boat, the position of the ankle joint and other somatosensory and proprioceptive information from the feet and legs does not correlate well with the orientation of the rest of the body (Horak & Shupert, 1994). An overreliance on somatosensory inputs for postural control in these environments will result in instability.

Inability to appropriately select a sense for postural control in environments in which one or more orientation cues inaccurately report the body's position in space has been referred to as a "sensory selection problem" (Horak et al., 1988; Shumway-Cook et al., 1988). Persons with a sensory selection problem are often able to maintain balance in environments where sensory information for postural control is consistent; however, they are unable to maintain stability when there is incongruence among the senses. Persons with a sensory selection problem do not necessarily show a pattern of overreliance on any one sense, but rather appear to be unable to correctly select an accurate orientation reference; therefore, they are unstable in any environment in which a sensory orientation reference is not accurate. This is shown in Figure 10.17, where abnormal sway is seen in conditions 3, 4, 5, and 6.

Sensory selection problems have been reported in persons with stroke (Bensoussan et al., 2007; DiFabio & Badke, 1990; Marigold et al., 2004), following traumatic brain injury (Shumway-Cook & Olmscheid, 1990), and in children with developmental disorders, including cerebral palsy (Cherng et al., 1999; Nashner et al., 1983), Down syndrome (Shumway-Cook & Woollacott, 1985b), and learning disabilities (Shumway-Cook et al., 1988). In one of the earliest studies examining sensory organization for postural control following stroke, DiFabio and Badke (1991) used the clinical sensory organization test to examine the ability of persons with hemiplegia following stroke to maintain balance when sensory inputs for postural control were disrupted. As shown in Figure 10.18, persons with poststroke hemiparesis were able to maintain good stability, scoring 150 (30 seconds, 5 trials) when standing on a firm surface with eyes open. Changing the availability of visual information (no vision or dome) did not impair stance balance significantly as long as individuals had at least two sensory inputs (somatosensory and vestibular) to rely on. However, changing the availability of visual cues significantly affected stability when somatosensory inputs were reduced (conditions 5 and 6, standing on a compliant foam surface with eyes closed or while wearing the visual conflict dome).

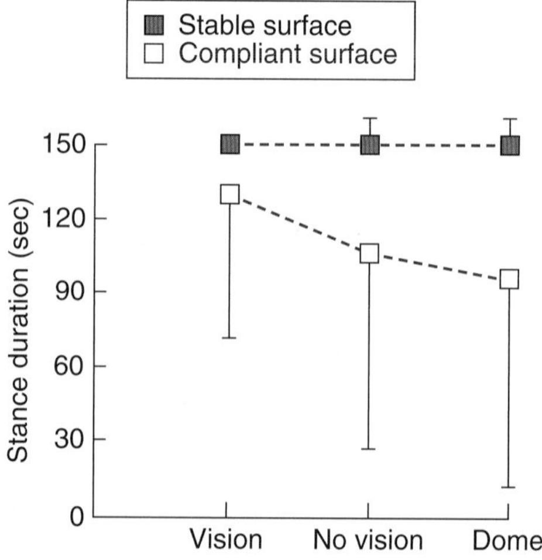

FIGURE 10.18 Mean stance duration scores for 10 persons with hemiplegia standing under six sensory conditions. Stability declines (as indicated by a decrease in the number of seconds able to stand) as sensory redundancy decreases (Reprinted with permission from DiFabio RP, Badke MB. Stance duration under sensory conflict conditions in patients with hemiplegia. Arch Phys Med Rehab 1991;72:294.)

Bensoussan et al. (2007) also examined the effect of altering sensory cues on sway in standing following stroke and reported that when standing on a firm surface with eyes open, sway did not differ between a group of 23 indivudals who had had a stroke and healthy age-matched controls. There were significant group differences, however, when patients stood with eyes closed. Similarly, Basford et al. (2003) reported that sway was not different between persons with traumatic brain injury as compared with age-matched controls when standing on a firm surface with eyes open; however, it was increased in more complex sensory conditions (conditions 4, 5, and 6) when somatosensory cues for balance were reduced.

Gatev et al. (1996) reported that participants with cerebellar pathology swayed more than control participants under all six sensory conditions, and most fell in conditions 5 and 6, when both visual and somatosensory inputs were reduced. The authors note that testing standing balance under altered sensory conditions had better sensitivity than normal stance testing (e.g., standing with eyes open or closed).

Cherng et al. (1999) reported that sway was not significantly different between children with spastic diplegia as compared with typically developing children when somatosensory information was reliable (fixed foot support), regardless of the visual conditions (conditions 1, 2, and 3 on the SOT test). In contrast, when somatosensory information was unreliable (compliant foot support), the difference in stance stability between the children with spastic diplegic cerebral palsy and their matched controls was significantly greater when the visual input was deprived (occluded) or unreliable (sway-referenced) than when it was reliable, suggesting the presence of sensory selection problems. Finally, sensory organization problems were reported in adults with multiple sclerosis (MS) (Cattaneo & Jonsdottir, 2009). Among persons with MS, there was no correlation between performance on the instrumented sensory organization tests and clinical measures of balance including the Berg Balance Test, Dynamic Gait Index, and the Activities-specific Balance Confidence scale, leading the authors to conclude that the tests assessed different aspects of balance control (Cattaneo & Jonsdottir, 2009).

Together these studies suggest a number of important clinical implications. First, pathology in widely distributed areas of the brain can disrupt the ability to organize and select sensory information essential to postural control. Functionally, sensory selection problems manifest as "context-specific" instability, defined as instability that is present in some environments but not in others. For example, a person with stroke or traumatic brain injury may be able to maintain balance in an environment in which sensory information is optimal (e.g., standing on a firm surface in a well-lit environment) but lose balance in an environment in which sensory conditions are less than optimal (e.g., standing on an incline or carpeted surface in low light conditions). This research also suggests that therapists must carefully consider the conditions under which balance is tested in persons with neurologic pathology. Since postural instability may not be readily apparent when a patient is tested in ideal or optimal sensory conditions (e.g., on a firm flat surface with eyes open), balance may need to be tested under more complex sensory conditions, such as when surface and or visual inputs for postural control are disrupted. Finally, sensory organization capability may not be readily identified using common clinical measures of balance that do not examine balance under altered sensory conditions. As discussed in more detail in the next chapter, different tests of balance measure different aspects of postural control.

LOSS OF ANTICIPATORY POSTURAL CONTROL

We have seen that an inability to adapt how we move and organize sensory information for postural control in response to changing task and environmental conditions can be a source of instability in many persons with neurologic impairments. Another source of postural dyscontrol is the loss of anticipatory processes that activate postural adjustments in advance of potentially destabilizing voluntary movements. Anticipatory postural activity is heavily dependent on previous experience and learning.

Inability to activate postural muscles in anticipation of voluntary arm movements has been described in many persons who are neurologically impaired, including individuals who have had a stroke (Horak et al., 1984; Slijper et al., 2002) or traumatic brain injury (Arce et al., 2004), children with cerebral palsy (Nashner et al., 1983; van der Heide et al., 2004), children with Down syndrome (Shumway-Cook & Woollacott, 1985b), and people with Parkinson's disease (Aruin et al., 1996; Latash et al., 1995; Rogers, 1990, 1991).

Problems in initiating postural muscle activity prior to voluntary muscle activity are present in children with spastic hemiplegia caused by cerebral palsy (Nashner et al., 1983; Zaino & McCoy, 2008). Figure 10.19 shows this lack of preparatory postural activity for the hemiparetic side, as compared with the normal (less involved) side in the children with cerebral palsy when they were asked to push or pull on a handle while standing. Onset of activity in postural muscles as indicated on EMG in the trunk and leg of the intact side preceded activity in the prime movers of the arm. In contrast, in the hemiparetic side, muscle activity in the arm preceded that in the postural muscles (Nashner et al., 1983).

Impaired anticipatory postural adjustments associated with a rapid upper-extremity movement in individuals who have had a stroke have been reported in several studies (Garland et al., 2003; Horak et al., 1984; Slijper et al., 2002). In a study involving 27 persons with acute stroke (34 to 84 years of age), Garland et al. (2003) recorded EMG activity from the legs and trunk during a rapid arm flexion movement immediately after stroke and 1 month after rehabilitation. Immediately after the stroke, there was a significant delay in the activation of the paretic hamstrings muscle during the arm raise task, indicating impaired anticipatory postural control. This can be seen in Figure 10.20A, which shows that the mean onset latency of the paretic hamstrings muscles (HAM_p)

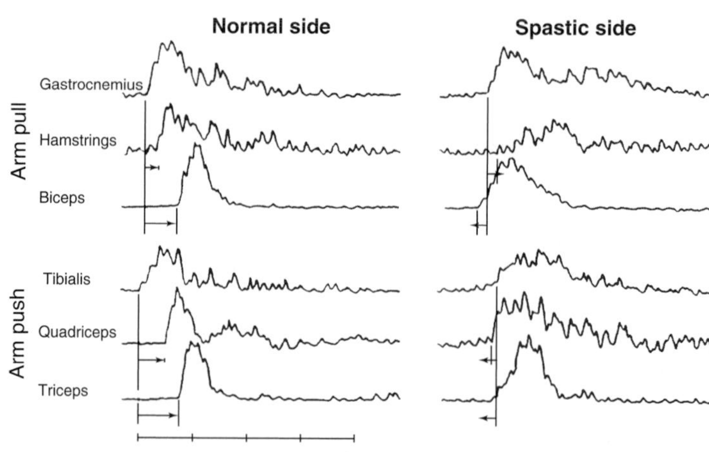

FIGURE 10.19 Normal and abnormal anticipatory postural control. EMG responses in arm (biceps/triceps) and leg (gastrocnemius/hamstrings and tibialis/quadriceps) muscles during a push or pull task in the normal versus the spastic side of a child with spastic hemiplegia. Muscle responses on the normal side show the activation of postural muscles in the leg in advance of the prime mover in the arm. In contrast, on the spastic side muscle activity in the arm precedes postural activity in the legs, resulting in instability (Reprinted with permission from Nashner LM, Shumway-Cook A, Marin O. Stance posture control in select groups of children with cerebral palsy: deficits in sensory organization and muscular coordination. Exp Brain Res 1983;49:401.)

occurred at the same time as the onset of arm movement (indicated by time 0). In contrast, the contraction onset of the nonparetic hamstrings (HAM_{NP}) was significantly earlier. After a month of rehabilitation, arm acceleration significantly increased. In addition, there was a significant decrease in the onset latency of both the paretic and nonparetic hamstrings muscles (open circles and filled circles, respectively). Recovery of anticipatory postural control was variable within the group, however. Ten of the individuals with stroke demonstrated an improved ability to recruit the paretic hamstrings muscles and showed no change in the nonparetic hamstrings activity. This pattern of recovery was called "true physiological recovery," as it is consistent with activity patterns used by neurologically intact adults. Twelve of the people with stroke showed a compensatory pattern of recovery. In these 12 people, improved arm acceleration was associated with early compensatory activation of the nonparetic hamstrings, with no significant improvement on the paretic side (Fig. 10.20b). Why do lesions in so many areas of the nervous system produce problems in anticipatory postural control? The circuitry underlying anticipatory postural control involves many neural structures, including supplementary motor cortex, basal ganglia, and the cerebellum. Thus, lesions in any one of these areas can disrupt critical pathways contributing to anticipatory postural control.

PROBLEMS IN COGNITIVE SYSTEMS

There is increasing evidence demonstrating the interacting effects of impaired cognition and postural control in persons with neurologic pathology. Research in this area is expanding rapidly, and includes studies related to the impact of cognitive load on postural stability in persons with neurologic pathology, as well as studies examining postural deficits in individuals with different forms of dementia, including Alzheimer's disease.

Impaired Postural Stability under Dual-Task Conditions

Inability to maintain balance while performing multiple tasks has been found in persons with various types of neurologic pathology. Morris and colleagues (2000) found that postural stability declined in persons with PD during the concurrent performance of a verbal cognitive task. Similar findings were also reported by Ashburn et al. (2000, 2001) and Marchese et al. (2003). Bloem et al. (2006) also reported impaired stability under dual-task conditions in persons with PD and suggested that individuals with PD use a "posture second" strategy, in which cognitive rather than balance tasks are prioritized under dual-task conditions.

Impaired dual-task performance has been shown following traumatic brain injury (Brauer et al., 2004) and stroke (Bensoussan et al., 2007; Cockburn et al., 2003; Hyndman et al., 2003; 2009). Bensoussan et al. (2007) reported increased sway under dual-task conditions, especially among stroke survivors with a history of falls, whereas Hyndman and colleagues (2009) reported decreased sway during the dual-task condition for all participants, even those with a history of falls. Hyndman et al. suggest that reduced sway under the dual-task conditions was a strategy to preserve balance; participants prioritized the balance task over the secondary task (what others have termed "posture-first strategy"). However, the authors did not report changes in the secondary task under any of the conditions; thus, it is difficult to determine whether preserving balance (the posture-first hypothesis) was done at the expense of performance on the secondary task.

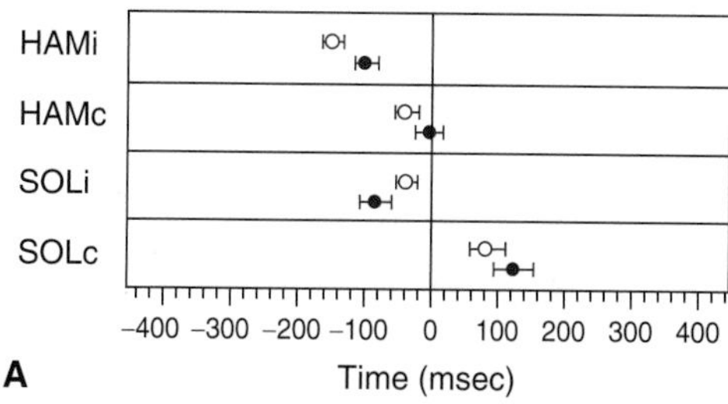

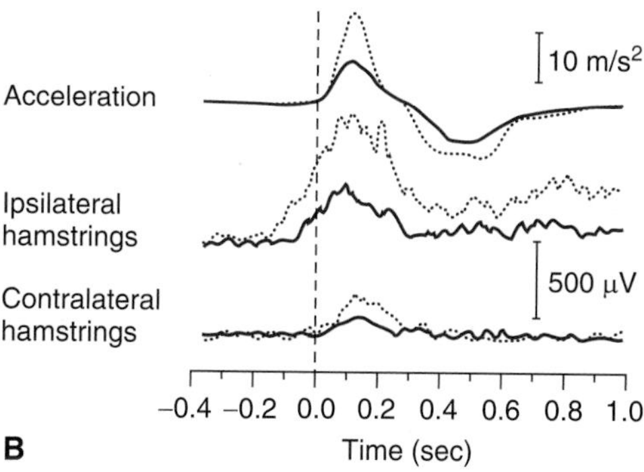

FIGURE 10.20 Changes in anticipatory postural control associated with an arm movement in the first month of recovery following a stroke. A, Just after stroke, the onset latency of the nonparetic hamstrings (HAM_i) preceded arm movement (indicated by time "0"); however, the paretic hamstrings (HAM_c) muscle was activated at the same time as arm movement. B, Rectified and integrated EMG recordings comparing activation of the ipsilateral (nonparetic) and contralateral (paretic) hamstrings activity in association with arm acceleration. Note that prior to training ipsilateral activity proceeds arm acceleration, while contralateral hamstrings activity is coincident with arm acceleration. After a month of rehabilitation, arm acceleration significantly increased; in addition, there was a significant decrease in the onset latency of both the paretic and nonparetic hamstrings muscles. This can be seen in Figure 10.20A (open circles and with filled circles, respectively) and B (dotted lines and solid lines, respectively). (Reprinted with permission from Garland SJ, Willems DA, Ivanova TD, Miller KJ. Recovery of standing balance and functional mobility after stroke. Arch Phys Med Rehabil 2003;84:1753–1759.)

Impaired dual-task performance has also been reported in children with neurologic pathology. Children (mean age, 5 years) with developmental coordination disorder (DCD) demonstrated increased sway under dual-task conditions (naming objects) as compared with typically developing (TD) children. Cognitive performance was affected by the dual tasks in the TD children but not in those with DCD. Thus, under the dual-task conditions, children with DCD had increased sway but no change in cognitive task performance, suggesting that they were prioritizing the cognitive task (Laufer et al., 2008). Finally, Reilly et al. (2008) examined balance under dual-task conditions in children (ages 10 to 14 years) with cerebral palsy (CP) (either spastic diplegia or ataxia) and two control groups of TD children. Under dual-task conditions (narrow stance, visual memory task), children with CP, similar to the younger group of TD children (4 to 6 years), swayed significantly more and faster as compared with single-task performance. Performance (accuracy) in the secondary task was significantly worse in a narrow- as compared with a wide-stance condition, with the children with ataxia showing the greatest effect.

It is clear from this review that dual-task interference is a significant contribution to instability in many types of neurologic pathology. Instability under dual-task conditions may arise for a number of reasons. Neurologic pathology may affect attentional capacity; under dual-task conditions, limited attentional capacity is exceeded and stability is compromised. Neurologic pathology may produce deficits in executive attention, which influences the allocation of attention under dual-task conditions, also impairing balance. Finally, researchers have shown that maintaining stability requires more attentional resources in persons with neurologic pathology as compared with nondisabled individuals, and this may contribute to instability under dual-task conditions. Regardless of the underlying cause, examining the effect of performing a second task on balance control is critical to understanding stability problems in persons with neurologic pathology.

Postural Control in Persons with Dementia

The relationship between impairments in cognitive function and postural control are being studied by many researchers, in part because of the high rates of falls reported in persons with various types of dementia, including Alzheimer's disease (Ballard et al., 1999; Camicioli & Licis, 2004; Kallin et al., 2005). Cognitive impairment is a known predictor of falls in older adults (Buchner et al., 1987; Morris et al., 1987; Tinetti et al., 1995). The incidence of mortality and morbidity following falls is much higher among persons with cognitive impairments as compared with those with no cognitive impairments (Buchner & Larson, 1987; Lord et al., 2001). Risk factors for falls in persons with dementia include impairments of motor function, balance, and gait (Alexander et al., 1995; Camicioli & Licis, 2004; Kallin et al., 2005; Visser, 1983). Poor performance under dual-task conditions has been reported as a risk factor for falls in some studies (Hauer et al., 2003; Pettersson et al., 2005) but not in others (Camicioli & Licis, 2004; Camicioli et al., 1997).

Researchers have begun to study the effects of impaired cognition on different components of postural control in order to better understand the neural mechanisms underlying the increased risk of falls in persons with dementia.

Motor Coordination

Moving-platform methods have been used to study postural motor activity in individuals with Alzheimer's disease. Problems in central set underlying the ability to change postural motor strategies with changing task conditions were examined in individuals with Alzheimer's disease (Chong et al., 1999). Leg-muscle activity during backward platform translations was examined in people with and without Alzheimer's disease when they stood freely, held on to a supporting frame, or sat. Surprisingly, individuals with Alzheimer's disease were able to quickly suppress leg-muscle activity when in the supported condition, suggesting that central set was not impaired.

Anticipatory postural activity preceding a voluntary movement of the arms also appears to be intact in individuals with Alzheimer's disease (Elble & Leffler, 2000). Individuals with Alzheimer's disease were asked to push or pull on a rigid horizontal bar in order to quickly move a cursor into a target window on a computer screen placed in front of them while they were standing unsupported. Although individuals with Alzheimer's disease had slower reaction times and were significantly less accurate in the task than controls, anticipatory postural activity in the legs was the same in the two groups.

In summary, results from studies involving individuals with Alzheimer's-type dementia have shown relatively few deficits in the motor component of postural control, although research is just beginning in this area, and the number of studies available is relatively limited.

Sensory Organization

The ability to organize sensory information for postural control was examined in individuals with mild versus moderate Alzheimer's dementia using the moving-platform and visual-surround methods described earlier (Chong et al., 1999; Dicken & Rose, 2004). Individuals with Alzheimer's disease had difficulty maintaining stability when only vestibular information was available for postural control (conditions 5 and 6 on the SOT test). In addition, individuals with mild Alzheimer's disease had more difficulty than those with moderate disease when visual information was disrupted. The authors interpret these findings to suggest that with increasing severity of dementia, there is a reduced dependence on visual information for postural control. As a result, disrupting visual information has less effect in individuals with moderate-to-severe Alzheimer's disease as compared with those with mild dementia. Research exploring deficits in postural control in persons with dementia is improving our ability to reduce fall rates in this vulnerable population.

IMPAIRED SEATED POSTURAL CONTROL

Postural control underlying the ability to sit independently is a critical part of functional independence in activities of daily living. Impaired sitting balance is a frequent occurrence in both children and adults with neurologic pathology. Acquisition of sitting balance in both children with developmental delays and adults with acquired neurologic pathology has been shown to be a good predictor of functional outcomes. Studies have confirmed the importance of age of sitting onset as a predictor of walking, reporting that sitting by 18 to 24 months predicts walking outcomes in children with spastic diplegia forms of cerebral palsy (Badell-Ribera, 1985; Wu et al., 2004b).

Sitting balance has been shown to be a good prognostic indicator of outcome for persons who have had a stroke (Feigin et al., 1996; Kwakkel et al., 1996; Loewen & Anderson, 1990; Morgan, 1994; Sandin & Smith, 1990) and traumatic brain injury. Impaired sitting balance on admission to rehabilitation was associated with dependence in locomotion and transfers at discharge and at 1 year after traumatic brain injury (Duong et al., 2004). Black et al. (2000) followed 237 patients with traumatic brain injury who were admitted to a rehab unit, and found that, next to age, the ability to sit independently at admission was the best predictor of discharge Functional Independence Measure (FIM) scores.

Because of the importance of independent sitting to functional independence in activities of daily living, and its predictive value in recovery of motor function, understanding postural control impairments that contribute to loss of independent sitting is very important.

Adults with Neurologic Pathology

Many of the studies related to impaired sitting balance following neurologic pathology have focused on persons with stroke. In a prospective study involving 93 patients, 48% were unable to sit independently at the onset of rehabilitation, while 27% were still unable to sit at the end of rehabilitation (Mayo et al., 1991).

During unsupported sitting tasks, patients with acute stroke were more unsteady (greater sway) as compared with healthy controls (Genthon et al., 2008; Harley et al., 2006). In addition, instability during unsupported sitting was increased under dual-task conditions (Harley et al., 2009). Many factors may contribute to an inability to sit independently, including perceptual impairments (Mayo et al., 1991), motor loss (Franchignoni et al., 1997; Hsieh et al., 2002), and impaired postural control (Genthon et al., 2007).

Problems in the activation of trunk muscles may contribute to instability in unsupported sitting in persons with stroke. Messier et al. (2004) examined voluntary trunk flexion in 15 persons who had had a stroke and 13 controls. Individuals were seated on a chair placed on a force plate, with their feet on two additional force plates, and asked to lean forward to touch a target with the forehead. Persons with stroke showed similar amplitude of trunk flexion to controls who had not had a stroke, but there was decreased COP displacement and lower weight bearing under the feet, suggesting smaller anterior displacement of the body mass. The authors suggest that after stroke most of the trunk motion was done with the upper trunk, with little anterior tilt of the pelvis.

Dickstein and colleagues examined muscle activity in 50 persons with stroke and 30 controls during voluntary trunk flexion and extension and while performing voluntary arm and leg movements (2004). Bilateral surface EMGs were used to examine timing, magnitude, and synchronization of trunk muscles during trunk extension. They found that trunk velocity during flexion and extension was lower in persons with stroke as compared with controls, and muscle activity on the paretic side was both reduced in magnitude and delayed relative to the unaffected side. Muscle activity in the trunk was also delayed and reduced during anticipatory postural adjustments associated with voluntary arm or leg movements performed in sitting.

Fujiwara et al. (2001) used transcranial magnetic stimulation to study the relationship between stimulation of affected and nonaffected hemispheres and motor evoked potentials in paretic and nonparetic trunk muscles in 20 persons with hemiplegia and 11 controls. In the stroke group, stimulation of the affected hemisphere resulted in motor evoked potentials in trunk muscles on the paretic side in only 1 person. However, stimulation of the unaffected hemisphere evoked motor potentials in bilateral trunk muscles in 10 of the 11 persons with stroke. In fact, stimulation of the unaffected hemisphere produced larger motor evoked potentials in ipsilateral muscles in the group with stroke than in the control group. The authors suggest that recovery of trunk function following stroke is associated with increased activation of the paretic trunk muscles by the unaffected hemisphere, suggesting a role for compensatory activation of uncrossed pathways in recovery of trunk function.

In addition to trunk muscle activity, activity in the legs is used for support and balance during reaching in the seated position. Peak vertical ground reaction forces occur at the end of a reach; at this time forces through the feet act to brake forward momentum of the body mass and prevent a fall forward. Additional force enables the return of the body to an upright posture. Several factors will increase the level of lower-extremity participation during seated reaching activities, including increasing the distance to be reached, decreasing thigh support, and varying the direction of reaches (Chari & Kibry, 1986; Son et al., 1988). Following stroke, the ability to reach further is linked to the ability to use the affected leg for support and balance. Dean and Shepherd (1997) reported that following stroke there was a decreased ability to recruit leg muscles and generate forces through the floor to control balance while reaching.

In summary, this research suggests that following stroke there appears to be a reduced ability to recruit muscles in the paretic trunk and limbs for seated postural control. This appears to be associated with reduced displacement and velocity of trunk motion during voluntary trunk movements and during reaching movements of the upper extremity. We do not know whether this reduced ability to recruit trunk muscles is also present during recovery of seated balance following an external perturbation. Interestingly, despite these impairments in trunk control, a number of researchers have reported that following stroke, persons commonly begin using trunk movements during reaching to compensate for limitations in reach and grasp (Levin et al., 2002; Michaelsen et al., 2004). Thus, the trunk motion improvement appears to be an important component of recovery of upper-extremity reach and grasp following a stroke.

Pediatric Populations

In contrast to studies in adult neurologic populations, which have focused primarily on trunk activity during voluntary movements, studies in children have examined seated postural control primarily during recovery from external perturbations.

Several studies have examined seated postural control in children with cerebral palsy and other types of developmental motor disorders. These studies used surface EMGs to study muscle activation patterns underlying the recovery of stability in sitting in children with various types of cerebral palsy (Brogren et al., 1996, 1998; van der Heide et al., 2004). They have consistently reported the presence of directionally specific postural responses (muscles opposed to the direction of body sway are activated); however, the recruitment order was not that used in typical children. Rather than a bottom-up recruitment pattern seen in typically developing children over 8 to 10 months, children with cerebral palsy showed a top-down recruitment order and had difficulty modulating muscle activity in response to changing task context. In addition, there was a high level of coactivation in the antagonist muscles.

Similar findings were reported by Washington et al. (2004), who compared muscle activation patterns in response to seated perturbations in typically developing infants at 8 months of age and in high-risk infants with developmental delays. In general, muscle activity in high-risk infants was characterized by increased tonic rather than phasic muscle activity. In addition, when high-risk infants did recruit muscles phasically, the patterns were direction-specific, but recruited in a top-down rather than a bottom-up order, and there was considerable coactivation.

Is impaired postural control in children with cerebral palsy due to biomechanical reasons (children seated in a crouched posture) or to a neural deficit? To answer this question Brogren et al. (2001) examined reactive postural adjustments during sitting in an erect and a crouched position in 20 children 3 to 7 years of age with mild to severe forms of spastic diplegia and 10 age- and sex-matched typically developing children. Children with severe spastic diplegia had significantly impaired muscle activation patterns during recovery from platform translations. This included loss of direction-specific activation of muscles during recovery from backward sway, which was more pronounced in the erect sitting posture as compared with the crouched position. The authors suggest that the crouched sitting pattern adopted by many children with cerebral palsy may in part be a compensatory solution to the problem of impaired postural control leading to instability in the seated position.

A CASE STUDY APPROACH TO UNDERSTANDING POSTURAL DYSCONTROL

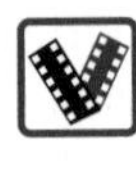

Until now, our discussion of postural dyscontrol following neurologic impairment has focused on presenting a wide variety of sensory, motor, and cognitive problems leading to instability. You can see that the range of problems is great, and this reflects the complexity of problems that affect the CNS. In the last section of this chapter we use our case studies to summarize postural control problems by diagnosis. Several warnings must be stated prior to beginning this section. Remember that even persons with the same diagnosis can be very different. Differences in postural control problems can result from variability in type, location, and extent of neural lesions. Other factors, such as age, premorbid status, and degree of compensation, also have a profound impact on the behavior seen. Before reading the case studies, complete Lab Activity 10.1. The answers to this lab activity may be found in the case studies.

Jean J: Postural Problems following Cerebral Vascular Accident

Jean J, our 82-year-old woman who has a right hemiparesis following a stroke, has significant postural control problems affecting her ability to function independently. Her postural responses are delayed in the paretic right limb.

The synergistic organization of muscles in the paretic limb are also disrupted. During recovery from challenges to balance, proximal muscles in

LAB ACTIVITY 10-1

Objective: To translate research on the physiological basis for abnormal postural control into hypotheses about the potential underlying cause(s) of instability in a patient with a specific neurologic diagnosis.

Assignment

1. For each patient case study listed at the end of this chapter, generate a list of hypotheses regarding the potential sensory, motor, and cognitive factors contributing to instability in each patient. How would you expect these impairments to impact steady state and reactive and proactive balance in sitting and standing?
2. Based on the information presented in this chapter, what research supports your hypotheses?

the hemiparetic limb contract in advance of distal muscles, but in some persons with stroke, these muscles may contract quite late in relationship to distal muscles.

Loss of anticipatory activation of postural muscles during voluntary movements is also present. This makes her unsteady when she carries out functional activities such as lifting, reaching, or carrying physical loads. She has difficulty modifying and adapting postural movements to changing task demands. This makes it difficult for her to maintain stability in response to a change in the base of support, or in appropriately responding to challenges to balance that vary in speed and amplitude.

Neuromuscular problems resulting from her stroke have also produced secondary musculoskeletal problems that affect postural control. Weakness has developed in both the hemiparetic and the nonparetic limb. Limitations in range of motion in the arm and leg have developed, associated with reduced motion. Jean's static alignment is asymmetric and characterized by displacement of the center of body mass away from the paretic limb.

In addition to her motor changes, Jean has a number of sensory problems that are contributing to her impaired postural control. Though Jean does not, many persons with stroke have reduced sensory information from the visual system (hemianopsia), as well as reduced somatosensation in the hemiparetic limbs. Jean does have difficulty in adapting sensory information to changing environmental demands. This affects her ability to maintain stability in certain environments, such as under low light levels or when the surface is soft or unsteady. Inability to maintain balance in conditions in which there is a loss of sensory redundancy is a critical factor in understanding Jean's balance problems.

In addition, Jean has difficulty maintaining balance while performing other tasks. Finally, because of her sensory/motor impairments, Jean has had numerous falls, and is at increased risk for falls in the future.

Mike M: Postural Problems in Parkinson's Disease

Mike is our 67-year-old man with Parkinson's disease. He is having increasing difficulty with mobility skills, including bed mobility, transfers, and gait. Postural problems affecting orientation and stability are a significant factor in his declining independence. Interestingly, despite the fact that he has significant bradykinesia, or slowed voluntary movement, which is common in Parkinson's disease, the onset latencies of his automatic postural responses are likely to be normal. If we were to do an EMG study of his postural muscle responses, we would likely find that he uses a complex pattern of muscle activity involving muscles on both sides of the body when responding to instability. This coactivation of muscles on both sides of his body results in a rigid body and an inability to recover stability adequately.

In addition, he is unable to modify movement patterns quickly in response to changing task demands. This problem with central set causes him to use the same pattern of muscle activity when responding to perturbations to balance while sitting or standing. Because of impaired anticipatory postural control he is unsteady when carrying out functional tasks that are potentially destabilizing, such as lifting or reaching for objects. In addition to primary neuromuscular impairments such as rigidity and bradykinesia, secondary musculoskeletal problems have developed, further limiting movements for postural control.

Mike, like many others with Parkinson's disease has sensory organization problems. He has difficulty organizing and selecting sensory information for postural control. In addition, he is likely to have difficulty maintaining balance under dual task conditions.

John C: Postural Problems in Cerebellar Disorders

John C is our 33-year-old man with spinocerebellar degeneration, type 2, resulting in severe ataxia. Much of the research on postural control in persons with cerebellar disorders has been with persons who have anterior-lobe cerebellar degeneration. Thus, findings from these studies may not necessarily completely apply to John, who has more generalized damage to the cerebellum, or to other persons with specific lateral hemisphere lesions or vestibulocerebellar lesions. Certainly, however, impaired postural control is a hallmark of cerebellar disorders.

Onset of contraction of postural muscles in John are likely to be normal, although in children with ataxic forms of cerebral palsy, contraction onsets are often delayed. John has difficulty scaling postural activity, resulting in hypermetric postural responses. This means that in response to a small backward perturbation to balance John overcorrects and this results in significant oscillation of his body. Research suggests that this overcorrection results from hypermetric muscle responses, that is, responses that are too large compared to the size of the challenge. Thus, he overshoots when trying to return to a stable position.

John also has problems with adapting how sensory information is used for postural control in response to changing environmental demands. He has difficulty when trying to maintain balance in conditions in which he must adapt sensory information for postural control.

Thomas L: Postural Problems in Cerebral Palsy 

Thomas is a 7-year-old boy with the spastic diplegia form of cerebral palsy. He has both neuromuscular and musculoskeletal problems affecting postural control. In response to balance threats, the onset of contraction of his postural muscles is quite delayed, despite the presence of hyperactive stretch reflexes in spastic muscles. If we were to do an EMG analysis of responses in stretched spastic muscles it would likely show that muscle activity is slow and reduced in amplitude. In addition to delayed onset of spastic muscles, he is likely to show a disruption of the normal sequencing of muscle activation patterns. Other factors contributing to muscle sequencing problems are changes in postural alignment (specifically, his crouched stance posture) and the use of AFOs. He has anticipatory postural control problems that also affect his stability during performance of voluntary motor acts. Musculoskeletal problems, including weakness, reduced range of motion and changes to the structure and function of skeletal muscles will also contribute to balance problems.

Problems in sensory adaptation do not appear to be present consistently in all children with spastic hemiplegia forms of cerebral palsy; however, they do appear to be a problem in spastic diplegia and ataxic forms of CP. This can be seen in John's reduced ability to maintain stance stability when standing under altered sensory conditions.

SUMMARY

1. An enormous range of problems can contribute to postural dyscontrol in individuals with a neurologic deficit. In the therapeutic environment, the ability to retrain postural control requires a conceptual framework that incorporates information on the physiological basis for normal postural control, as well as knowledge regarding the basis for instability.
2. Neurologic pathology can affect many aspects of balance control, including the ability to maintain and recover stability during quiet and perturbed stance. Sway during quiet stance (as indicated by COP excursion) is often, but not always increased. Many factors contribute to atypical sway patterns, including problems in alignment, changes in muscle tone, impairments in the sensory/perceptual system, and secondary musculoskeletal problems.
3. Neuromuscular problems that disrupt the coordination of postural movement strategies affect the ability to recover from an external perturbation. Coordination problems include: (a) sequencing problems, (b) problems with the timely activation of muscle response synergies, (c) disorders related to the scaling of postural muscle activity, and (d) problems adapting motor responses to changing task conditions.
4. Sensory problems can disrupt postural control by: (1) affecting a person's ability to adapt sensory inputs to changes in task and environmental demands, and (2) preventing the development of accurate internal models of the body for postural control.
5. Differences in postural control problems can result from variability in type, location, and extent of the neural lesion. Other factors, such as age, premorbid status, and degree of compensation, also have a profound impact on postural behavior.

CHAPTER 11

CLINICAL MANAGEMENT OF THE PATIENT WITH A POSTURAL CONTROL DISORDER

LEARNING OBJECTIVES

Following completion of this chapter, the reader will be able to:

1. Understand the relationship between research on normal and abnormal postural control and clinical methods for assessing and treating impaired postural control in patients with movement disorders.
2. Discuss the clinical implications of both the ICF and Systems framework on the assessment and treatment of balance disorders.
3. Discuss clinical tests and measures for assessing balance and consider the evidence regarding the reliability, validity, sensitivity, and specificity of these tests in pediatric, geriatric, and neurologic populations.
3. Describe a task-oriented approach to improving postural control in sitting and standing; providing a rationale for intervention practices based on a systems theory of normal and abnormal postural control.
4. Discuss the evidence for best practices related to balance retraining in geriatric and neurologic populations.

INTRODUCTION

This chapter focuses on clinical methods for assessing and treating patients with postural control disorders. We will examine research evidence that supports the effectiveness of specific therapeutic methods used to assess and treat postural disorders, including those related to orientation and balance. Although there is a growing body of research related to the effectiveness of balance training, it is often difficult to apply this research to the clinical treatment of patients with balance problems. In many cases, researchers have demonstrated the efficacy of training on a variety of balance outcomes but have provided limited information on what specific strategies were used to improve balance. In addition, while there is growing evidence examining the effect of improved balance on functional activities, there is limited evidence on the effects of improved balance on participation in social roles and complex daily life activities. This makes it difficult for clinicians to identify best practices related to balance rehabilitation.

Conceptual Framework for Balance Rehabilitation

How then shall we assess and treat postural control in our patients? In this book we use a task-oriented approach to balance rehabilitation. Our task-oriented approach incorporates both the International Classification of Functioning, Disability and Health (ICF) and the Systems framework. The ICF framework examines the effects of impaired balance on activities and participation, as well as the underlying impairments of body structure and function that contribute to impaired balance. A systems framework examines the sensory, motor, and cognitive contributions to steady-state, reactive, and proactive balance control in a wide variety of tasks and under varying environmental conditions. The clinical examination of postural control requires the use of multiple tests and measures, since no single test examines all aspects of postural control. Thus, clinicians must make decisions about which constellation of tests and measures are most appropriate for a given patient in the specific context in which the clinician is providing service. Unfortunately, there is rarely enough time to assess all aspects of balance. Therefore, it is essential that clinicians pick tests that are not redundant, and instead choose tests that evaluate different aspects of balance control and examine the effect of impaired balance on functional activities.

EXAMINATION

Safety—The First Concern

During the course of examining postural control, patients will be asked to perform a number of tasks that will likely cause instability. Safety is of paramount importance. All patients should wear an ambulation belt during testing and be closely guarded at all times. In determining which tasks and activities cause loss of balance, the patient must be allowed to experience instability. However, the therapist should protect the patient at all times to prevent a fall.

Examining the Effect of Balance on Participation

An important part of balance assessment is gathering self-report information on the effect of balance on participation in social roles and activities considered by the patient (or the patient's family) to be essential to daily life. This includes asking about the number of recent falls and the circumstances leading to the fall(s) or loss of balance. Self-report information on conditions of instability can help the clinician to generate hypotheses about which aspects of postural control are impaired and to determine the next steps in the examination process. For example, if a patient reports instability when leaning over to pick something up, the clinician may hypothesize impaired anticipatory aspects of postural control. In contrast, a patient reporting loss of balance when washing her hair in the shower suggests a hypothesis related to sensory components of balance control, specifically, difficulty in maintaining balance when visual cues are removed. These hypotheses can then be tested specifically, for example, by observing whether the patient increases sway or requires assistance to prevent a fall when standing with eyes closed versus eyes open.

Additional insight can be gained from understanding a patient's perceptions regarding balance abilities, and the impact of balance on participation in daily life. Assessing the patient's perceptions related to balance can be aided by the use of self-report scales such as the Activities-specific Balance Confidence (ABC) scale (Powell & Myers, 1995) or the Falls Efficacy Scale (Tinetti et al., 1990). The Falls Efficacy Scale is a 10-item scale in which subjects rate their fear of falling on a scale of 1 to 10 during the performance of 10 activities of daily living. The ABC scale (Assessment Tool 11.1) is a 16-item test that asks subjects to rate their confidence (0% = no confidence to 100% = complete confidence) when performing a range of activities of daily living. Older adults with a history of recent falls had lower mean scores on the ABC as compared with those who had not fallen.

Patients can be questioned regarding the impact of balance on daily life activities. Researchers have shown that reduced confidence in the ability to maintain balance (poor balance self-efficacy) as well as fear of falling are associated with activity restrictions and avoidance behavior in order to reduce the risk for additional falls (Delbaere et al., 2004; Deshpande et al., 2008). Reduced self-efficacy and associated activity restrictions appear to be important factors in predicting declines in physical function and increased risk for disability (Delbaere et al., 2004; Deshpande et al., 2008).

Examining the Effect of Balance on Functional Activities

Examination of balance from a functional perspective uses tests and measures that indicate how well a patient can perform a variety of functional tasks that require postural control. Tasks may reflect the need for improvements in: (a) steady-state postural control (e.g., maintaining a safe independent sitting or standing position), (b) anticipatory postural control (e.g., ability to maintain stability while performing tasks that are potentially destabilizing, such as reaching, leaning, or lifting), and (c) reactive postural control (e.g., recovering a stable position following an unexpected perturbation). However, when using performance of functional skills to infer balance abilities, clinicians need to remember that balance is only one of many factors that have an impact on functional performance. Thus, reduced ability to perform functional skills may be the result of impaired balance alone or of impaired balance in conjunction with other underlying sensory, motor, and cognitive impairments.

Standardized measures of functional balance skills provide the clinician with information on the patient's ability relative to established norms. Results can

Assessment Tool 11-1

Two Examples of Self-Report Measures of Balance Confidence

ACTIVITIES-SPECIFIC BALANCE CONFIDENCE (ABC) SCALE[a]

Rate confidence in ability to carry out the following activities (0 = no confidence, 100 = complete confidence). Total score is average of 16 individual scores.

1. Walk around house
2. Up and down stairs
3. Pick up slipper from floor
4. Reach at eye level
5. Reach up on tiptoes
6. Stand on chair to reach
7. Sweep floor
8. Walk outside to nearby car
9. Get in/out of car
10. Walk across parking lot
11. Walk up and down ramp
12. Walk in crowded mall
13. Walk in crowd/bumped
14. Ride escalator holding on
15. Ride escalator not holding rail
16. Walk on icy sidewalk

FALLS EFFICACY SCALE[b]

Rate level of confidence in doing each of the activities without falling (0 = not at all, 10 = completely confident). Total score is sum of 10 individual scores (range: 0 [low self-efficacy] to 100 [high self-efficacy]).

1. Cleaning house
2. Getting dressed and undressed
3. Preparing simple meals
4. Taking a bath or shower
5. Simple shopping
6. Getting in and out of car
7. Going up and down stairs
8. Walking around neighborhood
9. Reaching into cabinets and closets
10. Hurrying to answer the phone

[a]Reprinted with permission from Powell LE, Myers AM. The Activities-specific Balance Confidence (ABC) scale. J Gerontol A Biol Sci Med Sci 1995;50A(1):M28–M34.

[b]Reprinted with permission from Tinetti ME, Richman D, Powell L, Falls efficacy as a measure of fear of falling. J Gerontol Psychol Sci 1990;45:P239–P243.

indicate the need for therapy, serve as a baseline level of performance, and when repeated at regular intervals, can provide both the therapist and the patient with objective documentation about a change in functional status. There are a number of tests available to measure functional skills related to postural control. Many of these tests have been used to determine the risk for falls as well.

Timed Up and Go Test (TUG)

The Get Up and Go test (Mathias et al., 1986) was developed as a quick screening tool for detecting balance problems affecting daily mobility skills in elderly patients. The test requires that subjects stand up from a chair, walk 3 ms, turn around, and return. Performance is scored according to the following scale: 1 = normal; 2 = very slightly abnormal; 3 = mildly abnormal; 4 = moderately abnormal; and 5 = severely abnormal. An increased risk for falls was found among older adults who scored 3 or higher on this test.

The Timed Up and Go test (TUG) modifies the original test by adding a timing component to performance (Podsiadlo & Richardson, 1991). Neurologically intact adults who are independent in balance and mobility skills are able to perform the test in less than 10 seconds. This test correlates well to functional capacity as measured by the Barthel index. Adults with neurologic pathology who took longer than 30 seconds to complete the test were dependent in most activities of daily living and mobility skills. Isles et al. (2004) published normal values for a variety of balance tests, including the TUG in 456 community-dwelling, independently ambulatory women, 20 to 80 years of age with no known neurologic or musculoskeletal diagnoses. Age-related changes in time(s) taken to complete the TUG are summarized in Table 11.1. Also shown in this table is a comparison of data from

TABLE 11.1 Comparison of Timed Up and Go Values

	Age					
	20–29 (n = 40)	30–39 (n = 47)	40–49 (n = 95)	50–59 (n = 93)	60–69 (n = 90)	70–7 (n = 91)
Mean ± SE	5.31 ± 0.25	5.39 ± 0.23	6.24 ± 0.67	6.44 ± 0.17	7.24 ± 0.17	8.54 ± 0.17
Published normative value	NA	NA	NA	NA	8 (60–88) Steffen 8.42 (65–85) Shumway-Cook 13.05 (65–86) Hughes	8.5 (70–84) Podsiadlo 8 (60–88) Steffen 8.42 (65–85) Shumway-Cook

Adapted with permission from Isles RC, Chow NL, Stur M, Witz JC. Normed values of balance tests in women 20–80. J Am Geriatr Soc 2004;53:1370 (Table 1).

the two oldest age groups, with other data from other published studies. There are also age- (65 years and older) and gender-based norms for an 8 foot version of the TUG (an individual walks 8 feet rather than 10 feet as is used in the original test), developed as part of the Functional Fitness Test for neurologically intact older adults (Rikli & Jones, 2001).

The TUG examines primarily proactive or anticipatory aspects of postural control associated with rising from a chair, turning, and sitting down. Sensory conditions are not manipulated during the test, so sensory components of postural control are not tested. By adding a secondary task to the TUG, clinicians can examine the effect of cognitive demand on anticipatory aspects of postural control. The dual-task TUG (TUG_{DT}) was originally created to see whether adding a secondary task would increase the sensitivity and specificity of the TUG as a measure of fall risk in community-living older adults (Shumway-Cook et al., 2000).

Older adults with and without a history of falls were asked to complete the TUG under three different conditions. In the first condition, the TUG alone was performed. In the $TUG_{DT\ cognitive}$ subjects were asked to complete the TUG while counting backward by 3s. Finally in the $TUG_{DT\ manual}$ subjects were asked to complete the TUG while carrying a cup of water. Because so many older adults have difficulty maintaining stability while performing multiple tasks, it was hypothesized that performing the TUG under dual-task conditions would be a more sensitive way to identify fall-prone elders. Table 11.2 compares the sensitivity and specificity of the TUG for identifying fall-prone elders in the three conditions. While the time taken to complete the TUG was significantly longer in the dual-task conditions, the study found that the TUG alone was a sensitive and specific indicator of fall status in community-dwelling older adults. Thus, this relatively simple screening test, which takes only minutes to complete, appears to be a valid method for screening for both level of functional mobility and risk for falls in community-dwelling elders. The addition of a secondary task to the TUG provides insight into how well a patient is able to maintain balance under multitask conditions.

The TUG has also been shown to be a reliable and valid test for examining mobility following stroke (Faria et al., 2009; Ng & Hui-Chan, 2005) and Parkinson's disease (Campbell et al., 2003; Dibble & Lange, 2006; Morris et al., 2001). Faria et al. (2009) reported that following a stroke, the time taken to complete the TUG was significantly slower as compared with controls who had not had a stroke; however, TUG times did not vary with the direction of turn (toward the paretic vs. the nonparetic side). Following stroke, the time to complete the TUG was significantly associated with strength in the hemiparetic plantar flexors (but not spasticity), gait parameters (e.g., gait velocity and step length) and walking endurance (distance covered on the 6-minute walk test) (Ng & Hui-Chan, 2005).

TUG time was significantly slower among persons with Parkinson's disease as compared with age-matched controls (Campbell et al., 2003; Dibble & Lange, 2006; Morris et al., 2001), and associated with increased risk for falls (Dibble & Lange, 2006). Several authors have suggested modifications to the TUG, including adding a secondary task (Campbell et al., 2003) or instrumented technology, such as

TABLE 11.2 Comparison of the Sensitivity and Specificity for Identifying Fall Status in Older Adults

	Sensitivity (% fallers)	Specificity (% nonfallers)	Overall Prediction
TUG	13/15 (87%)	13/15 (87%)	26/30 (87%)
TUG_{manual}	12/15 (80%)	14/15 (93%)	26/30 (87%)
$TUG_{cognitive}$	12/15 (80%)	14/15 (93%)	26/30 (87%)

accelerometers or inertial sensors (Zampieri et al., 2009) to increase the sensitivity of the TUG.

The TUG has also been shown to be a valid and reliable test of mobility function in children with and without physical disabilities (Gan et al., 2008; Williams et al., 2005). Minor modifications to testing procedures (e.g., beginning to time when the child starts to move rather than with the instruction to go), has allowed the test to be used in children as young as 3 years of age (Williams et al., 2005). In typically developing children 3 to 5 years of age, the mean (±SD) time to complete the TUG was 6.7 ± 1.2 sec, but decreased to 5.1 ± 0.08 sec in children 5 to 9 years of age. Among children with disabilities, performance on the TUG was significantly slower as compared with typically developing children and was inversely related to scores on the Standing and Walking dimensions of the Gross Motor Function Measure (Williams et al., 2005).

Reach Tests

Functional Reach Test. The Functional Reach Test is a single-item test developed as a quick screen for balance problems and falls risk in older adults (Duncan et al., 1990). As shown in Figure 11.1A, subjects stand with feet shoulder distance apart and with one arm (hand in a fist) raised to 90 degrees of flexion. Without moving their feet, subjects reach as far forward as they can while still maintaining their balance (Fig. 11.1B). The distance reached is measured and compared with that of age-related norms, shown in Table 11.3. The Functional Reach Test has good interrater reliability and has been shown to be predictive of falls among neurologically intact older adults (Duncan et al., 1990).

A modified version of the Functional Reach test (modified Functional Reach Test [MFRT]) has been developed and tested in the acute (14 to 21 days) post–stroke phase. The test involves measuring unsupported reaching in the forward and lateral direction in the seated position and has high reliability and is responsive to improved motor performance on the paretic side (effect size, 0.80) (Katz-Leurer et al., 2009).

The Pediatric Reach Test (PRT) measures forward and lateral reach in both the seated and standing positions and has been shown to have good interrater and intrarater reliability in both typically developing children and those with cerebral palsy. Construct validity was established through a high correlation with the Gross Motor Function Classification System (Bartlett & Birmingham, 2003).

Multi-Directional Reach Test. The Multi-Directional Reach Test (MDRT) was proposed to examine the limits of stability in not only the forward and backward direction, but also in the medial and lateral directions. As shown in Figure 11.2, a yardstick is fixed to a telescoping tripod, allowing the vertical height of the yardstick to be adjusted so that it is at the level of the subject's acromion process. Instructions are "without moving your feet or taking a step, reach as far [direction given] as you can and try to keep your hand along the yardstick" (Newton, 2001, p. M249). Subjects are allowed to use their arm of choice for the forward and backward reaches, but both the right and the left arms are tested. Newton examined the MDRT in 254 community-dwelling older persons; the mean distance reached (in inches) for this group is shown in Table 11.4. The MDRT was correlated with the Berg Balance Scale (r = 0.476 to 0.356) and inversely related to scores on the TUG (r = −0.26 to −0.442), with the strongest correlations shown for the forward direction.

Performance-Oriented Mobility Assessment (POMA)

Mary Tinetti, a physician-researcher at Yale University, has published a test to screen for balance and mobility skills in older adults and to determine the likelihood for falls (Tinetti, 1986; Tinetti & Ginter, 1988). Assessment Tool 11.2 presents Tinetti's balance

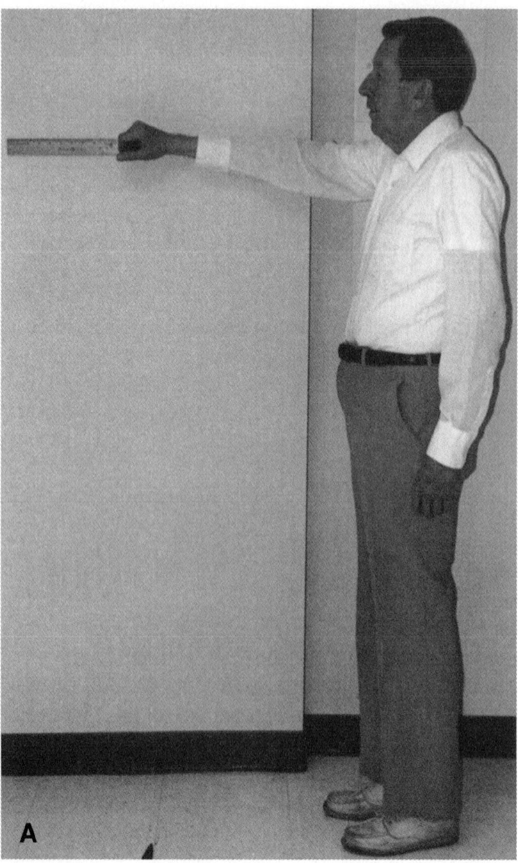

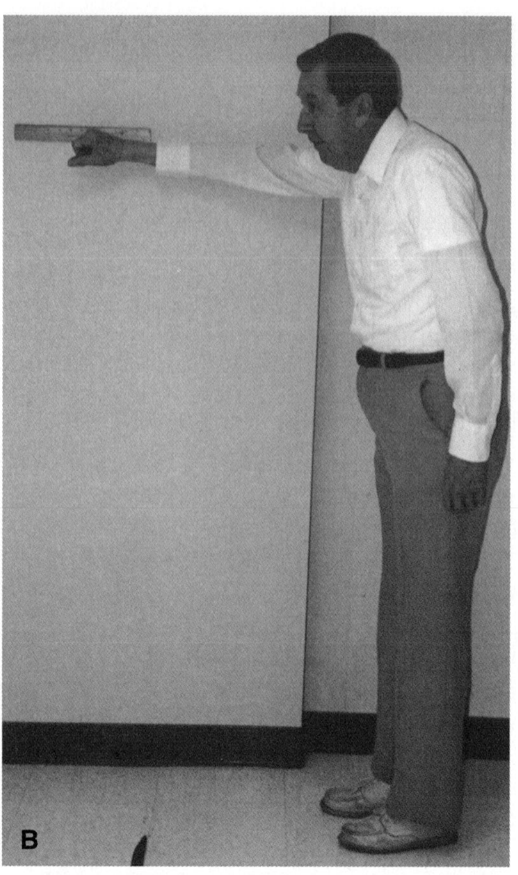

FIGURE 11.1 Functional Reach Test. A, Subjects begin by standing with feet shoulder distance apart, arm raised to 90 degrees of flexion. B, Subjects reach as far forward as they can while still maintaining their balance.

TABLE 11.3 Functional Reach Norms

	Men (means & SD in inches)	Women (means & SD in inches)
20–40 yr	16.7±1.9	14.6±2.2
41–69	14.9±2.2	13.8±2.2
70–87	13.2±1.6	10.5±3.5

Reprinted with permission from Duncan PW, Weiner DK, Chandler J, Studenski S. Functional reach: a new clinical measure of balance. J Gerontol 1990;45:M195.

and mobility scale, which rates performance on a three-point scale. The maximum score is 28 points. An examination of the individual items in the balance portion of the POMA suggests that it evaluates steady-state balance in sitting and standing (items 1 and 5), proactive balance (items 2, 3, 6, and 9), reactive balance (item 6), and includes a sensory component (item 7).

The POMA has been shown to be a good measure of fall risk in neurologically intact older adults living in the community. A score of less than 19 indicates a high risk for falls. Scores in the range of 19 to 24 indicate a moderate risk for falls. The test takes about 10 to 15 minutes to administer, and the interrater reliability of this test is good (Tinetti & Ginter, 1988). In a comparison of four tests of balance (TUG, One-Leg Stand, Functional Reach, and POMA) the POMA was found to have the best test–retest reliability and discriminant and predictive validities for fall risk in 1,200 people 65 years of age or older and was the most responsive to change in status with regard to activities of daily living (Lin et al., 2004).

Berg Balance Scale

The Berg Balance Scale (BBS) was developed by Kathy Berg, a Canadian physical therapist (Berg, 1993). This test, shown in Assessment Tool 11.3, uses 14 different

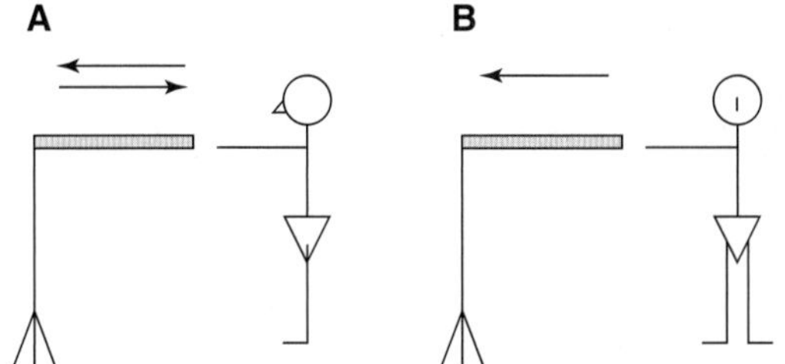

FIGURE 11.2 Positions for the Multi-Directional Reach Test. A, Position for the forward and backward reach. B, Position for the right lateral lean (yardstick would be repositioned for left lateral lean). (Reprinted with permission from Newton R. Validity of the Multi-Directional Reach Test: a practical measure for limits of stability in older adults. J Gerontol Med Sci 2001;56A:M249.)

items, which are rated 0 to 4. The test is reported to have good test–retest and interrater reliability (intraclass correlation coefficient = 0.98) and good internal consistency (Cronbach's alpha = 0.96) (Berg et al., 1989). It has been shown to be correlated with other tests of balance and mobility, including the Tinetti mobility index (r = 0.91) and the TUG (r = 0.76) (Berg et al., 1992).

Shumway-Cook and colleagues (1997a) reported that the BBS was the best single predictor of fall status in community-dwelling older adults without neurologic pathology. Declining BBS scores were associated with increased fall risk, but as can be seen in Figure 11.3, this relationship was nonlinear. In the range of 56 to 54, each 1-point drop in the Berg score was associated with a 3 to 4% increase in fall risk. However, in the range of 54 to 46, a 1-point change in the Berg score was associated with a 6 to 8% increase in fall risk. Below the score of 36, fall risk was close to 100%. Thus, a 1-point change in the Berg score can lead to a very different predicted probability for a fall, depending on where the baseline score is on the scale.

A study by Berg and colleagues (Muir et al., 2008) examined the predictive validity of the BBS in identifying single versus recurrent falls among 187 older adults followed prospectively for 1 year. Like Shumway-Cook et al. (1997a) they reported a nonlinear relationship between fall risk and BBS scores, showing an increasing gradient of risk associated with decreasing Berg scores, shown in Table 11.5. They reported that while 58% of those scoring lower than 45 (the commonly used cutoff point for fall risk) fell, 39% of older adults who scored greater than 45 also fell. The authors conclude that the BBS had good discriminative ability to predict multiple falls; however, the use of the BBS as a dichotomous scale, with a threshold of 45, was inadequate for the identification of the majority of people at risk for falling in the future. They therefore recommend discontinuing the use of 45 as a cutoff point for identifying fall-prone elders.

The BBS may not necessarily be a good predictor of fall risk in individuals with neurologic impairment. Harris et al. (2005) examined the relationship between BBS and falls in 99 community-dwelling people with chronic stroke and found that performance on the Berg Balance Test (BBT) was not different between those with a high risk of falling and those with a low risk, and therefore suggested that clinicians use caution when using the BBT to predict fall risk in a patient with chronic stroke.

The BBS has been shown to be a reliable and valid measure of balance in children with cerebral palsy (Gan et al., 2008; Kembhavi et al., 2002). The BBS was correlated to GMFM total scores, but did

TABLE 11.4 Multi-Directional Reach Test Scores in a Sample of 254 Community-Dwelling Older Adults (mean [±SD] age, 74.1 ± 7.9 yr)

Test	Mean	SD	Min	Max
FR (in.)	8.89	3.4	0.5	16.8
BR (in.)	4.64	3.1	0.4	14.0
RR (in.)	6.86	3.0	0.7	18.2
LR (in.)	6.61	2.9	0.0	14.4

FR = arm stretched forward; BR = leaning backward; RR = arm stretched to the right; LR = arm stretched to the left.
Adapted with permission from Newton R. Validity of the Multi-Directional Reach Test: a practical measure for limits of stability in older adults. J Gerontol Med Sci 2001;56A:M250.

Assessment Tool 11-2

Performance-Oriented Mobility Assessment[a]

I. BALANCE TESTS

Initial instructions: Subject is seated in a hard, armless chair. The following maneuvers are tested.

1. Sitting balance _____
   Leans or slides in chair = 0
   Steady, safe = 1
2. Arises _____
   Unable without help = 0
   Able, uses arms to help = 1
   Able without using arms = 2
3. Attempts to arise _____
   Unable without help = 0
   Able, requires >1 attempt = 1
   Able to rise, 1 attempt = 2
4. Immediate standing balance (first 5 seconds) _____
   Unsteady (staggers, moves feet, trunk sways) = 0
   Steady, but uses walker or other support = 1
   Steady without walker or other support = 2
5. Standing balance _____
   Unsteady = 0
   Steady but wide stance (medial heels >4 inches apart) and uses cane or other support = 1
   Narrow stance without support = 2
6. Nudged (subject at maximum position with feet as close together as possible, examiner pushes lightly on subject's sternum with palm of hand three times) _____
   Begins to fall = 0
   Staggers, grabs, catches self = 1
   Steady = 2
7. Eyes closed (at maximum position no. 6) _____
   Unsteady = 0
   Steady = 1
8. Turning 360 degrees _____
   Continuous steps = 0
   Discontinuous steps = 1
   Unsteady steps (grabs, staggers) = 2
9. Sitting down _____
   Unsafe (misjudged distance, falls into chair) = 0
   Uses arms, or not a smooth motion = 1
   Safe, smooth motion = 2

Balance score:_____ /16

II. GAIT TESTS

Initial instructions: Subject stands with the examiner, walks down hallway or across room, first at usual pace, then back at rapid, but safe pace (usual walking aids)

10. Initiation of gait (immediately after told to "go") _____
    Any hesitancy, or multiple attempts to start = 0
    No hesitancy = 1
11. Step length and height _____
    a. Right swing foot
       Does not pass left stance foot with step = 0
       Passes left stance foot = 1
       Right foot does not clear floor completely with step = 0
       Right foot completely clears floor = 1
    b. Left swing foot
       Does not pass right stance foot with step = 0
       Passes right stance foot = 1
       Left foot does not clear floor completely with step = 0
       Left foot completely clears floor = 1
12. Step symmetry _____
    Right and left step length not equal (estimate) = 0
    Right and left step appear equal = 1
13. Step continuity _____
    Stopping or discontinuity between steps = 0
    Steps appear continuous = 1

(continued)

Assessment Tool 11-2

Performance-Oriented Mobility Assessment[a]

14. Path (estimated in relation to floor tiles, 12-inch diameter; observe excursion of 1 foot over about 10 ft of the course) ______

    Marked deviation = 0

    Mild/moderate deviation or uses walking aid = 1

    Straight without walking aid = 2

15. Trunk ______

    Marked sway or uses walking aid = 0

    No sway, but flexion of knees or back pain or spreads arms out while walking = 1

    No sway, no flexion, no use of arms, and no use of walking aid = 2

16. Step width ______

    Heel apart = 0

    Heels almost touching while walking = 1

Gait score: ______ /12

Balance and gait score:______/28

[a] Reprinted with permission From Tinetti, M. Performance-oriented assessment of mobility problems in elderly patients. J Am Geriatr Soc 1986;34:119–126.

Assessment Tool 11-3

Berg Balance Test[a]

1. SITTING TO STANDING

Instruction: Use a chair with arms. Ask the patient to stand up. If the patient stands up using the arms of the chair, ask him or her to stand up without using his or her hands, if possible.

Grading: Mark the lowest category that applies. ______
______ (4) able to stand, no hands, and stabilize independently
______ (3) able to stand independently using hands
______ (2) able to stand using hands after several tries
______ (1) needs minimal assistance to stand or to stabilize
______ (0) needs moderate or maximal assistance to stand

2. STANDING UNSUPPORTED

Instruction: Stand for 2 minutes without holding on to any external support.

Grading: Mark the lowest category that applies. ______
______ (4) able to stand safely for 2 minutes
______ (3) able to stand for 2 minutes with supervision
______ (2) able to stand for 30 seconds unsupported
______ (1) needs several tries to stand for 30 seconds unsupported
______ (0) unable to stand for 30 seconds unassisted
If subject is able to stand 2 minutes safely, score full marks for sitting unsupported. Proceed to position change from standing to sitting.

3. SITTING UNSUPPORTED FEET ON FLOOR

Instruction: Sit with arms folded for 2 minutes.

Grading: Mark the lowest category that applies. ______
______ (4) able to sit safely and securely for 2 minutes
______ (3) able to sit for 2 minutes under supervision
______ (2) able to sit for 30 seconds
______ (1) able to sit for 10 seconds
______ (0) unable to sit without support for 10 seconds

4. STANDING TO SITTING

Instruction: Sit down.

Grading: Mark the lowest category that applies. ______
______ (4) sits safely with minimal use of hands
______ (3) controls descent by using hands
______ (2) uses backs of legs against chair to control descent
______ (1) sits independently but has uncontrolled descent
______ (0) needs assistance to sit

5. TRANSFERS

Instruction: Move from this chair (chair with arm rests) to this chair (chair without arm rests) and back again.

Grading: Mark the lowest category that applies. ______
______ (4) able to transfer safely with only minor use of hands
______ (3) able to transfer safely with definite need for hands

(continued)

Assessment Tool 11-3

Berg Balance Test

_____ (2) able to transfer with verbal cueing and/or supervision
_____ (1) needs one person to assist
_____ (0) needs two people to assist or supervise to be safe

6. STANDING UNSUPPORTED WITH EYES CLOSED

Instruction: Close your eyes and stand still for 10 seconds.

Grading: Mark the lowest category that applies. _______
_____ (4) able to stand for 10 seconds safely
_____ (3) able to stand for 10 seconds with supervision
_____ (2) able to stand for 3 seconds
_____ (1) unable to keep eyes closed for 3 seconds but stays steady
_____ (0) needs help to keep from falling

7. STANDING UNSUPPORTED WITH FEET TOGETHER

Instruction: Place your feet together and stand without holding on to any external support.

Grading: Mark the lowest category that applies. _______
_____ (4) able to place feet together independently and stand for 1 minute safely
_____ (3) able to place feet together independently and stand for 1 minute with supervision
_____ (2) able to place feet together independently but unable to hold for 30 seconds
_____ (1) needs help to attain position but able to stand for 15 seconds feet together
_____ (0) needs help to attain position and unable to hold for 15 seconds

The following items are to be performed while standing unsupported.

8. REACHING FORWARD WITH OUTSTRETCHED ARM

Instruction: Lift arm to 90 degrees. Stretch out your fingers and reach forward as far as you can. Examiner places a ruler at end of fingertips when arm is at 90 degrees. Fingers should not touch the ruler while reaching forward. The recorded measure is the distance forward that the fingers reach while the subject is in the most forward-leaning position.

Grading: Mark the lowest category that applies. _______
_____ (4) can reach forward confidently > 10 inches
_____ (3) can reach forward >5 inches safely
_____ (2) can reach forward > 2 inches safely
_____ (1) reaches forward but needs supervision
_____ (0) needs help to keep from falling

9. PICK UP OBJECT FROM THE FLOOR

Instruction: Pick up the shoe/slipper that is placed in front of your feet.

Grading: Mark the lowest category that applies. _______
_____ (4) able to pick up slipper safely and easily
_____ (3) able to pick up slipper, but need supervision
_____ (2) unable to pick up but reaches 1 to 2 inches from slipper and keeps balance independently
_____ (1) unable to pick up, and needs supervision while trying
_____ (0) unable to try, and needs assistance to keep from falling

10. TURNING TO LOOK BEHIND OVER LEFT AND RIGHT SHOULDERS

Instruction: Turn to look behind you over your left shoulder. Repeat to the right.

Grading: Mark the lowest category which applies. _______
_____ (4) looks behind from both sides and shifts weight well
_____ (3) looks behind one side only, other side shows less weight shift
_____ (2) turns sideways only, but maintains balance
_____ (1) needs supervision when turning
_____ (0) needs assist to keep from falling

11. TURN 360 DEGREES

Instruction: Turn completely around in a full circle. Pause. Then turn a full circle in the other direction.

Grading: Mark the lowest category that applies. _______
_____ (4) able to turn 360 degrees safely in < 4 seconds each side
_____ (3) able to turn 360 degrees safely one side only in > 4 seconds
_____ (2) able to turn 360 degrees safely but slowly
_____ (1) needs close supervision or verbal cueing
_____ (0) needs assistance while turning

(continued)

Assessment Tool 11-3

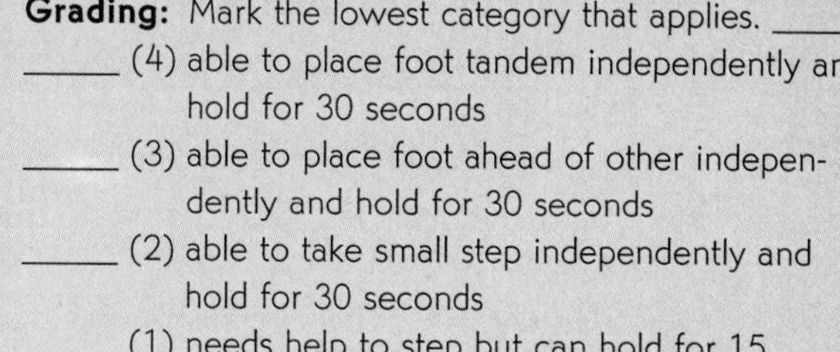

Berg Balance Test

12. COUNT NUMBER OF TIMES STEP STOOL IS TOUCHED

Instruction: Place each foot alternately on the stool. Continue until each foot has touched the stool four times for a total of eight steps.

Grading: Mark the lowest category that applies. _______

_____ (4) able to stand independently and safely and complete eight steps in 20 seconds

_____ (3) able to stand independently and complete eight steps in >20 seconds

_____ (2) able to complete four steps without aid with supervision

_____ (1) able to complete less than 4 steps, needs minimal assistance

_____ (0) needs assistance to keep from falling/ unable to try

13. STANDING UNSUPPORTED, ONE FOOT IN FRONT

Instruction: (Demonstrate to subject) Place one foot directly in front of the other. If you feel that you cannot place your foot directly in front, try to step far enough ahead that the heel of your forward foot is ahead of the toes of the other foot.

Grading: Mark the lowest category that applies. _______

_____ (4) able to place foot tandem independently and hold for 30 seconds

_____ (3) able to place foot ahead of other independently and hold for 30 seconds

_____ (2) able to take small step independently and hold for 30 seconds

_____ (1) needs help to step but can hold for 15 seconds

_____ (0) loses balance while stepping or standing

14. STANDING ON ONE LEG

Instruction: Stand on one leg as long as you can without holding on to an external support.

Grading: Mark the lowest category that applies. _______

_____ (4) able to lift leg independently and hold for >10 seconds

_____ (3) able to lift leg independently and hold for 5–10 seconds

_____ (2) able to lift leg independently and hold for 3 seconds or more

_____ (1) tries to lift leg, unable to hold for 3 seconds, but remains standing independently

_____ (0) unable to try or needs assistance to prevent fall

[a] Reprinted with permission from Berg K. Measuring balance in the elderly: validation of an instrument. Dissertation. Montreal: McGill University, 1993.

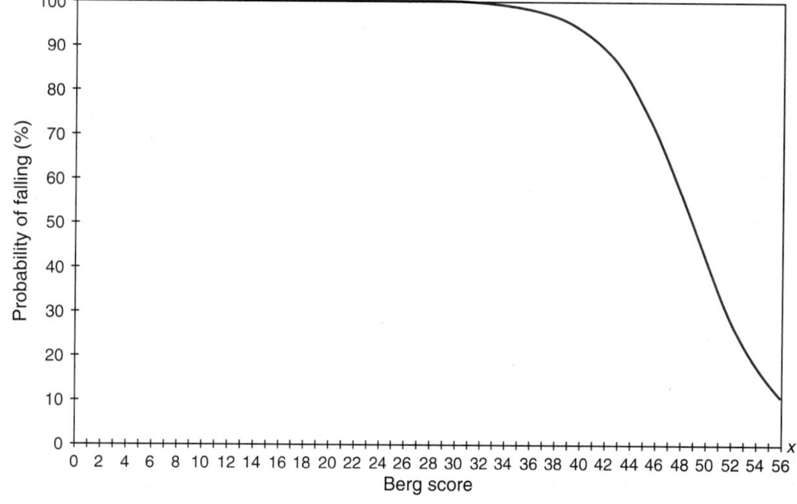

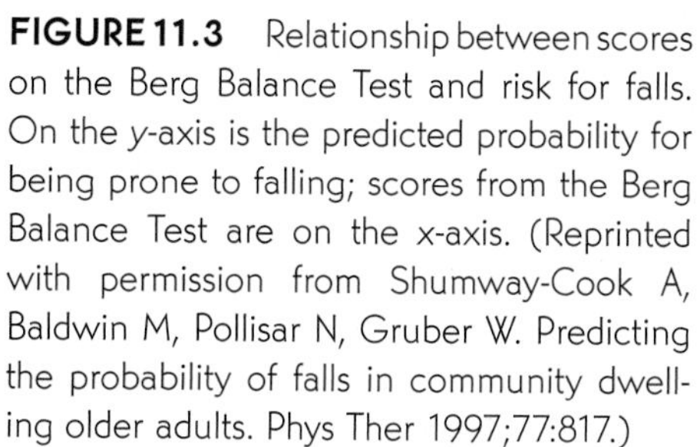

FIGURE 11.3 Relationship between scores on the Berg Balance Test and risk for falls. On the *y*-axis is the predicted probability for being prone to falling; scores from the Berg Balance Test are on the x-axis. (Reprinted with permission from Shumway-Cook A, Baldwin M, Pollisar N, Gruber W. Predicting the probability of falls in community dwelling older adults. Phys Ther 1997;77:817.)

TABLE 11.5 Gradient of Fall Risk and Berg Balance Scale Scores in Community-Living Older Adults[a]

BBS Score	Likelihood for multiple falls
≥55	10%
50–54	11%
45–49	16%
40–44	31% (2.07 × more likely to fall)
<40	54% (5.19 × more likely to fall)

[a]Adapted from Muir SW, Berg K, Chesworth B, Speechley M. Use of the Berg Balance Scale for predicting multiple falls in community-dwelling elderly people: a prospective study. Phys Ther 2008;88:449–459.

not distinguish between children with cerebral palsy with GMFCS levels I and II (Gan et al., 2008). The Pediatric Balance Scale is based on the BBT; it includes the original 14 items, but with a changed order and a slight modification to the scoring procedures (Franjoine et al., 2003).

Donoghue and Stokes (2009) reported that the minimal detectable difference in the Berg Balance test varies as a function of the baseline score. The minimal detectable difference is 4 points when the baseline Berg score is between 45 and 56; 5 points if the score is between 35–44; 7 points if the score is between 25–34 and 5 points if the score is within 0 to 24.

What aspects of postural control does the BBS assess? Take a moment and complete Lab Activity 11.1. Review each item in the BBS. Does it measure steady-state, reactive, or proactive balance? Is the BBS a complete measure of balance control? If a clinician chooses to use the BBS, what additional tests and measures will have to be selected to give a complete view of the patient's balance control?

Short Physical Performance Battery

The Short Physical Performance Battery (SPPB) is an increasingly common test used to measure lower-extremity performance in older adults. It includes a strength, balance, and mobility component, and is shown in Assessment Tool 11.4 (Guralnik et al., 1994). The SPPB involves timing performance on the following items: five chair stands (no arms), 8-ft walk test, and three hierarchical balance tests (side-by-side stance, modified tandem stance, or tandem stance). Time measurements for each of the three tests (strength, balance, and gait) are then converted to ordinal-scale values (0 to 4). Scores from the three areas are summed, for a total score range from 0 (lowest performance) to 12 (highest performance). Test–retest reliability of data

LAB ACTIVITY 11-1

Objective: To examine the relationship between a clinical test of balance, and specific aspects of the systems framework of postural control, specifically the range of tasks and environments examined.

Procedures: Examine Assessment Tool 11.3, which outlines the Berg Balance Test. By each test item, indicate whether the task requires steady-state, reactive, or proactive postural control. Examine the environmental condition for each item.

Assignment:

1. How many items test steady-state balance control?
2. How many items test anticipatory balance control?
3. How many items test reactive postural control?
4. Do any of the items examine the same task under different conditions?

Assessment Tool 11-4

Short Physical Performance Battery[a]

1. REPEATED CHAIR STANDS

Instructions: Do you think it is safe for you to try and stand up from a chair five times without using your arms? Please stand up straight as quickly as you can five times, without stopping in between. After standing up each time, sit down and then stand up again. Keep your arms folded across your chest. Please watch while I demonstrate. I'll be timing you with a stopwatch. Are you ready? Begin.

Grading: Begin stopwatch when subject begins to stand up. Count aloud each time subject arises. Stop the stopwatch when subject has straightened up completely for the fifth time. Also stop if the subject uses arms, or after 1 minute, if subject has not completed rises, and if concerned about the subject's safety. Record the number of seconds and the presence of imbalance. Then complete ordinal scoring.

Time: _____sec (if five stands are completed)

Number of Stands Completed: 1 2 3 4 5

Chair Stand Ordinal Score: ______

0 = unable

1 = ≥16.7 sec

2 = 16.6–13.7 sec

3 = 13.6–11.2 sec

4 = ≤11.1 sec

2. BALANCE TESTING

Begin with a semitandem stand (heel of one foot placed by the big toe of the other foot). Individuals unable to hold this position should try the side-by-side position. Those able to stand in the semitandem position should be tested in the full tandem position. Once you have completed time measures, complete ordinal scoring.

A. Semitandem Stand

Instructions: Now I want you to try to stand with the side of the heel of one foot touching the big toe of the other foot for about 10 seconds. You may put either foot in front, whichever is more comfortable for you. Please watch while I demonstrate.

Grading: Stand next to the participant to help him or her into semitandem position. Allow participant to hold onto your arms to get balance. Begin timing when participant has the feet in position and lets go.

Circle one number

2. held for 10 sec

1. held for less than 10 sec; number of seconds held

____

0. not attempted

B. Side-by-Side Stand

Instructions: I want you to try to stand with your feet together, side by side, for about 10 sec. Please watch while I demonstrate. You may use your arms, bend your knees, or move your body to maintain your balance, but try not to move your feet. Try to hold this position until I tell you to stop.

Grading: Stand next to the participant to help him or her into the side-by-side position. Allow participant to hold onto your arms to get balance. Begin timing when participant has feet together and lets go.

Grading

2. Held for 10 sec

1. Held for less than 10 sec; number of seconds held

____

0. Not attempted

C. Tandem Stand

Instructions: Now I want you to try to stand with the heel of one foot in front of and touching the toes of the other foot for 10 sec. You may put either foot in front, whichever is more comfortable for you. Please watch while I demonstrate.

Grading: Stand next to the participant to help him or her into the side-by-side position. Allow participant to hold onto your arms to get balance. Begin timing when participant has feet together and lets go.

Grading

2. held for 10 sec

1. held for less than 10 sec number of seconds held

____

0. not attempted

Balance Ordinal Score: _______

0 = side by side 0–9 sec or unable

1 = side by side 10 sec, <10 sec semitandem

2 = semitandem 10 sec, tandem 0–2 sec

3 = semitandem 10 sec, tandem 3–9 sec

4 = tandem 10 sec

3. 8-Foot Walk (2.44 meters)

Instructions: This is our walking course. If you use a cane or other walking aid when walking outside your home,

(continued)

Assessment Tool 11-4

Short Physical Performance Battery[a]

please use it for this test. I want you to walk at your usual pace to the other end of this course (a distance of 8 feet. Walk all the way past the other end of the tape before you stop. I will walk with you. Are you ready?

Grading: Press the start button to start the stopwatch as the participant begins walking. Measure the time taken to walk 8 feet Then complete ordinal scoring.

Time: _____ **sec**

Gait Ordinal Score: _______

0 = could not do

1 = >5.7 sec (<0.43 m/sec)

2 = 4.1–5.6 sec (0.44–0.60 m/sec)

3 = 3.2–4.0 sec (0.61–0.77 m/sec)

4 = <3.1 sec (>0.78 m/sec)

Summary Ordinal Score:_____

Range: 0 (worst performance) to 12 (best performance). Shown to have predictive validity showing a gradient of risk for mortality, nursing home admission, and disability.

[a] Reprinted with permission from Guralnik JM, Simonsick EM, Ferrucci L, Glynn RJ, Berkman LF, Blazer DG, Scherr PA, Wallace RB. A short physical performance battery assessing lower extremity function: association with self-reported disability and prediction of mortality and nursing home admission. J Gerontol Med Sci 1994;49(2):M85–M94.

obtained with the SPPB is good, with intraclass correlation coefficients for measurements taken 1 week apart ranging from 0.88 to 0.92 (Ostir et al., 2002). The SPPB has been shown to be a strong predictor of decline in physical function in older adults (Guralnik et al., 2000; Simonsick et al., 2001).

Fullerton Advanced Balance Scale

The Fullerton Advanced Balance Scale (FAB) was developed for higher-functioning older adults to avoid the ceiling effect sometimes found when using the BBT (Rose, 2003). The FAB includes 10 items (shown in Assessment Tool 11.5) scored from 0 to 4, with a score range of 0 (poor balance) to 40 (good balance).

Balance Evaluation Systems Test

The Balance Evaluation Systems Test (BESTest) was developed by Horak and colleagues (2009) to examine multiple aspects of postural control. The BESTest consists of 36 items, grouped into six systems: Biomechanical Constraints, Stability Limits/Verticality, Anticipatory Postural Adjustments, Postural Responses, Sensory Orientation, and Stability in Gait. It has good reliability and is correlated with scores on the Activities Balance Confidence test (Horak et al., 2009). By systematically examining different components of balance, this test allows a clinician to determine the specific factors contributing to instability, increasing the specificity of treatment aimed to improve balance. Rasch analysis was used to develop a shorter version of the BEST test, called the mini-BESTest (Franchignoni et al., 2009). The mini-BESTest contains 14 items that group into four of the original six sections: Anticipatory Postural Adjustments (sit to stand, rise to toes, stand on one leg); Postural Responses (stepping in four different directions); Sensory Orientation (stance—eyes open;

Assessment Tool 11-5

Ten Test Items from the Fullerton Advanced Balance Scale (FAB)[a]

1. Stand with feet together, eyes closed
2. Reach forward to retrieve object
3. Turn in a full circle to the right and left
4. Step up and over bench
5. Tandem walk
6. Stand on one leg, eyes open
7. Stand on foam, eyes closed
8. Two-footed jump for distance
9. Walk with head turns
10. Unexpected backward release

[a] Reprinted with permission from Rose D. Fall proof: a comprehensive balance and mobility program. Champaign, IL: Human Kinetics, 2003.

foam surface—eyes closed; incline—eyes closed); and Balance during Gait (gait during speed change, head turns, pivot turns, obstacles; timed Get Up and Go with dual tasks). In addition, the mini-BESTest uses a three-level ordinal scoring system instead of the original four levels. Table 11.6 summarizes the categories and items for both the original and mini-BESTest. For a complete copy of the BESTest, including instructions see http://www.bestest.us.

New measures for examining posture and balance developed for specific patient populations are emerging constantly (e.g., the Postural Control and Balance for Stroke Test [Pyoria et al., 2005], the Maximal Step Length and Rapid Step Test [Cho et al., 2004]). A complete review of all measures is not feasible. It remains to be seen which of these new tools will emerge as useful and efficient ways to measure balance, and thus become widely adopted for clinical use.

Limitations of Functional Tests and Measures

How well do functional tasks capture postural control from a systems perspective? Most functional measures have limitations. First a patient's performance is examined under a limited set of environmental conditions; thus, it may not always predict actual performance in more complex environments. In addition, few tests examine all three aspects of postural control, including steady-state, reactive, and anticipatory postural control. Finally, most functional tests provide little insight into the quality of movement used to accomplish the task and provide no way to identify specific neuronal or musculoskeletal subsystems within the body responsible for a decline in performance. To gain insight into the quality of movement used to accomplish balance and the underlying system impairments contributing to imbalance, additional tests are needed.

TABLE 11.6 Summary of BESTest Items and Subsystem Categories

The 14 items forming the mini-BESTest for dynamic balance are in bold. Only the worst performance in items 11 (Stand on one leg) and 18 (Lateral stepping) have to be taken into account for the score. Moreover, the performance in item 27 (Cognitive Get up and Go) must be compared with that in the baseline item 26.

I	II	III
Biomechanical Constraints	**Stability Limits**	**Anticipatory—Transitions**
1. Base of support	6 a. Lateral lean L	**9. Sit to stand**
2. Alignment	b. Lateral lean R	**10. Rise to toes**
3. Ankle strength	c. Sitting verticality L	**11. Stand on one leg**
4. Hip strength	d. Sitting verticality R	**(both right and left)**
5. Sit on floor and stand up	7. Reach forward	12. Alternate stair touch
	8 a. Reach L	13. Standing arm raise
	b. Reach R	
IV	**V**	**VI**
Postural Responses	**Sensory Orientation**	**Dynamic Gait**
14. In-place forward	**19 a. Stance EO**	21. Gait natural
15. In-place backward	**(firm surface)**	**22. Change speed**
16. Stepping forward	b. Stance EC	**23. Head turns**
17. Stepping backward	(firm surface)	**24. Pivot turns**
18. Lateral stepping	c. Foam EO	**25. Obstacles**
(both right and left)	**d. Foam EC**	26. Get up and Go
	20. Incline EC	**27. Cognitive Get up and Go**

EC = eyes closed; EO = eyes open; L = left; R = right.

Reprinted with permission from Franchignoni F, Horak F, Godi M, et al. Using psychometric techniques to improve the Balance Evaluation System's Test: the mini-BESTest. J Rehabil Med 2010;42:323–331.

Assessing Strategies for Balance

Understanding balance impairments requires insight into the sensory and motor strategies used to maintain or regain stability.

Motor Strategies

Examination of motor strategies for postural control determines both the alignment of body segments during unperturbed sitting and standing and the patient's ability to generate multijoint movements, or strategies that effectively control motion of the center of mass (COM) and/or the base of support (Shumway-Cook & Horak, 1990; Shumway-Cook & McCollum, 1990; Woollacott & Shumway-Cook, 1990).

Alignment. Examination of postural control includes observation of the patient's alignment in sitting and standing. Is the patient vertical? Is weight symmetrically distributed right to left and forward and backward? A plumb line in conjunction with a grid can be used to quantify changes in alignment at the head, shoulders, trunk, pelvis, hips, knees, and ankles. In addition, the width of the patient's base of support upon standing can be measured and recorded using a tape to measure the distance between the medial malleoli (or alternatively, the metatarsal heads).

Alternative ways to quantify placement of the COM in the standing position include the use of static force plates to measure placement of the center of pressure (COP) or the use of two standard scales to determine whether there is weight discrepancy between the two sides (Fig. 11.4).

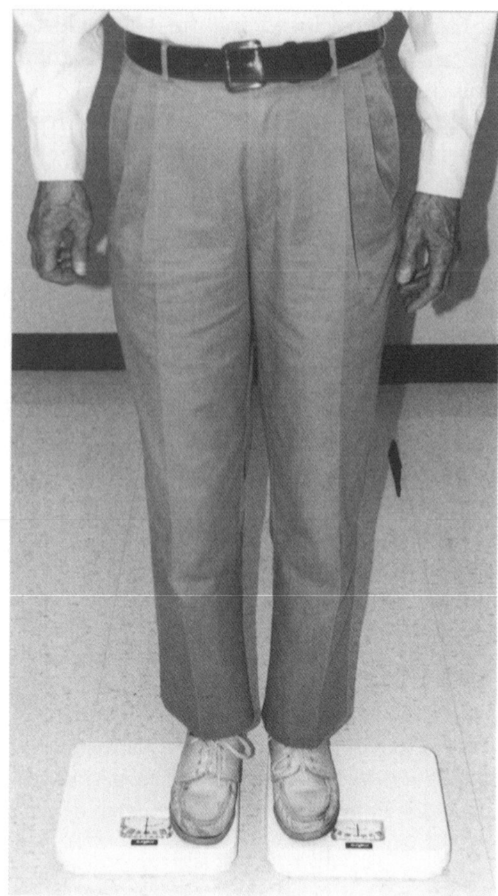

FIGURE 11.4 Two standard scales can be used to quantify static asymmetric standing alignment.

Movement Strategies. Both in-place and change-of-support strategies are necessary for postural stability. In addition, because instability is not confined to one plane, we must be able to control movements of the COM in all planes of movement in a variety of contexts. Movement strategies used to control the body in space are often examined during self-initiated sway, in response to externally induced sway, and anticipatory to a potentially destabilizing upper-extremity movement.

Movements used to control self-initiated body sway are observed while the patient voluntarily shifts the weight forward, then backward, then side to side. The patient is tested in both the sitting and standing positions. Figure 11.5 illustrates the range-of-movement patterns seen in a seated neurologically intact individual as she shifts the trunk further and further laterally while seated. As weight is transferred to one side of the body, the trunk begins to curve toward the unweighted side, resulting in elongation of the weight-bearing side and shortening of the trunk on the unweighted side (Fig. 11.5A). As weight continues to be shifted laterally, maintaining stability requires the subject to abduct the arm and leg in order to keep the trunk mass within the base of support (Fig. 11.5B). Finally, the arm is extended, changing the base of support and preventing a fall (Fig. 11.5C).

Figure 11.6 illustrates two types of movement strategies being used to control voluntary sway in standing. Two patients have been asked to sway forward as far as they can without taking a step. Patient A (Fig. 11.6A) is swaying forward primarily about the ankles, using what has been referred to as an ankle strategy to control COM motion. In contrast, Patient B (Fig. 11.6B) is moving primarily the trunk and hips (a hip strategy), which minimizes forward motion of the COM.

The presence of coordinated movement strategies can also be examined during recovery from an external perturbation. Figure 11.7 illustrates one approach to assessing movement patterns used to recover stability in response to an external displacement at the hips (Carr & Shephard, 1998; Shumway-Cook & Horak,

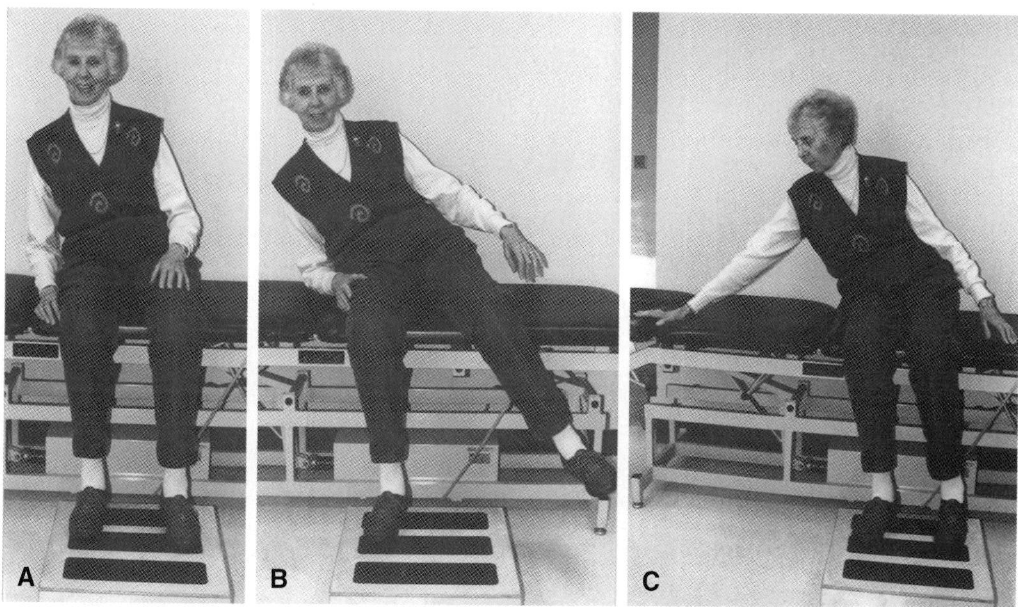

FIGURE 11.5 Maintaining stability during self-initiated weight shifts with trunk movements in sitting. A, Small movements produce adjustments at the head and trunk. B, Larger movements require counterbalancing with the arms and legs. C, When movements of the head and trunk can no longer control stability with the current base of support, the arm reaches out to change the base of support and prevent a fall.

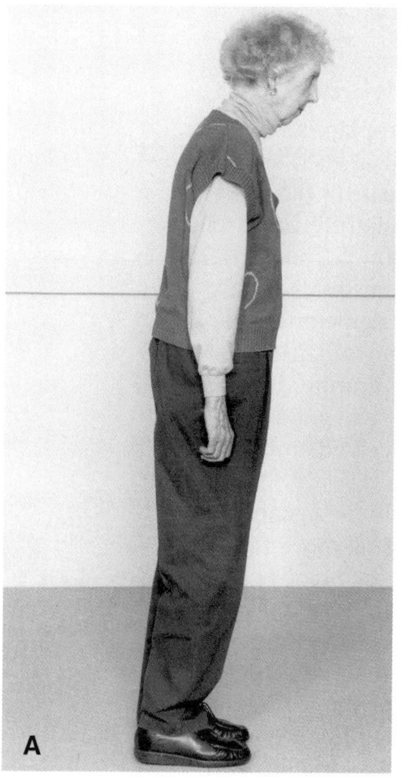

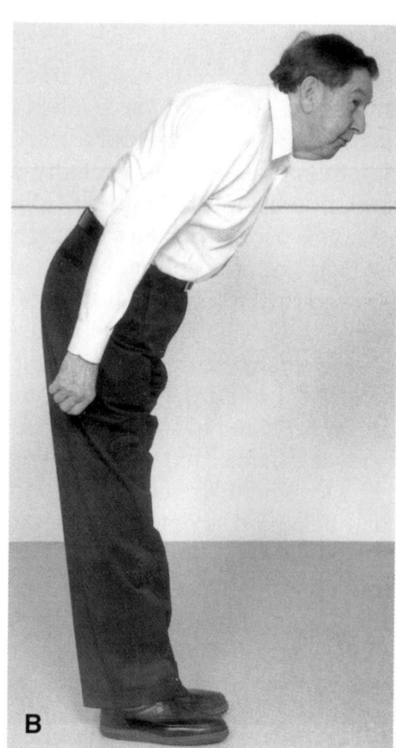

FIGURE 11.6 Controlling stability during voluntary sway in stance. Shown are two types of movement strategies being used to control self-initiated voluntary sway in standing: the ankle strategy (A) and the hip strategy (B).

1992). Holding the patient about the hips, the therapist displaces the hips in multiple directions (forward, backward, side to side, and on diagonals). Strategies to recover stability in response to sagittal-plane perturbations are shown in Figure 11.7, A and B; in-place strategies (ankle or hip) are used to recover from small displacements, while a step (Fig. 11.7 C) may be used to recover stability when in-place strategies will not suffice. An alternative approach to examining reactive balance is described in the BESTest and shown

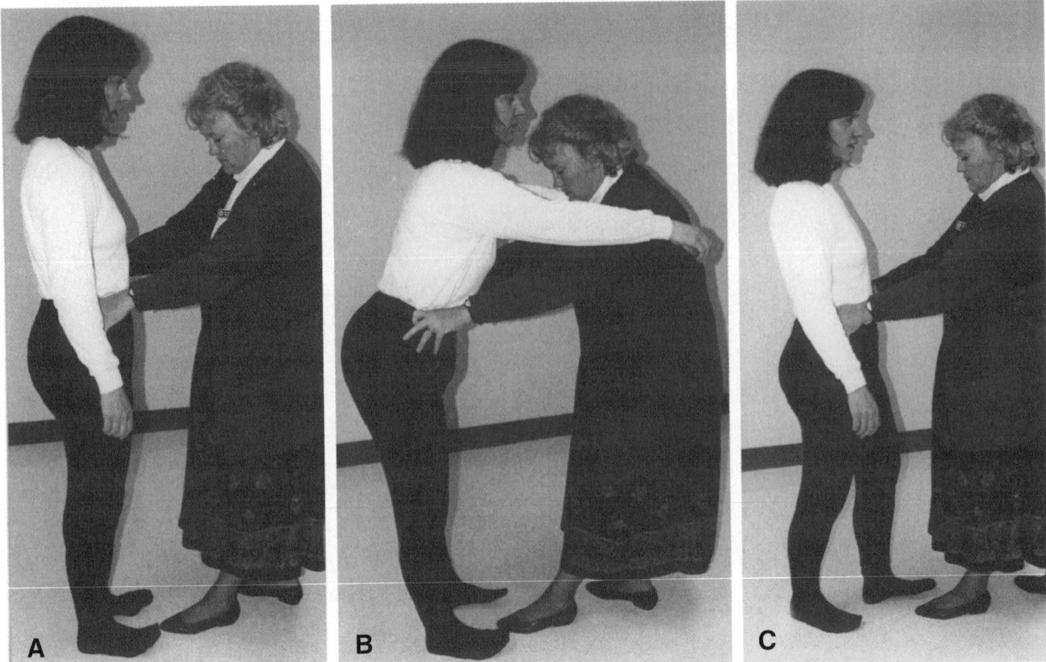

FIGURE 11.7 Movement strategies used to recover from an external perturbation to balance. A, An ankle strategy is used to recover from a small displacement at the hips. B, A larger displacement produces a hip strategy. C, When in-place strategies can no longer control the COM with respect to the existing base of support, a step is used to change the base of support and thus prevent a fall.

in the case-study videos. To elicit an in-place strategy, a small amount of pressure is applied at each shoulder, then released unexpectedly. Increasing the pressure, and asking the patient to lean slightly prior to release is used to elicit a stepping response. The BESTest examines the ability to recover from small versus large perturbations in all directions. Remember that many factors will determine how and when motor strategies are changed, including the amplitude and velocity of the destabilizing stimulus, as well as perceptions related to stability limits, perceived ability to recover balance, and fear of falling.

Movement strategies used to minimize instability in anticipation of potentially destabilizing movements can be assessed by asking a patient to lift a heavy object as rapidly as possible (Fig. 11.8), or by placing one foot on top of a stool. Both of these tasks require subtle shifts of the COM prior to the voluntary movement (of the arms in the lifting task or the leg in the stepping task) in order to maintain stability. Delayed or absent anticipatory adjustments are associated with reduced stability during performance of the task, and in some cases the task may be performed more slowly. Finally, observing movements made to maintain stability in response to changing task demands can provide insight into the range of coordinated movement strategies available for postural control. Commonly used

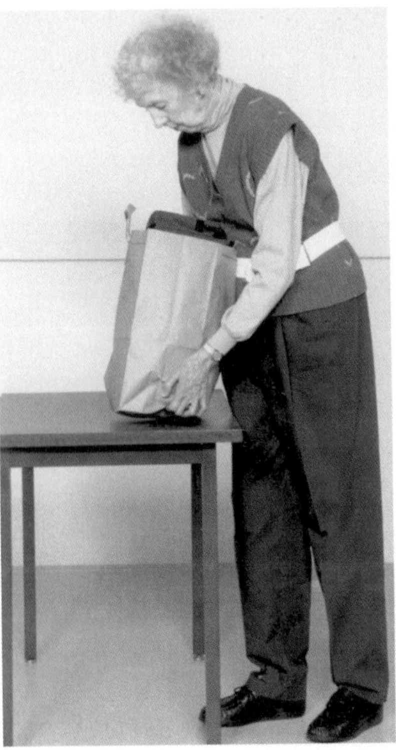

FIGURE 11.8 Anticipatory postural control can be examined by having patients perform tasks that are potentially destabilizing, such as lifting a heavy bag of groceries.

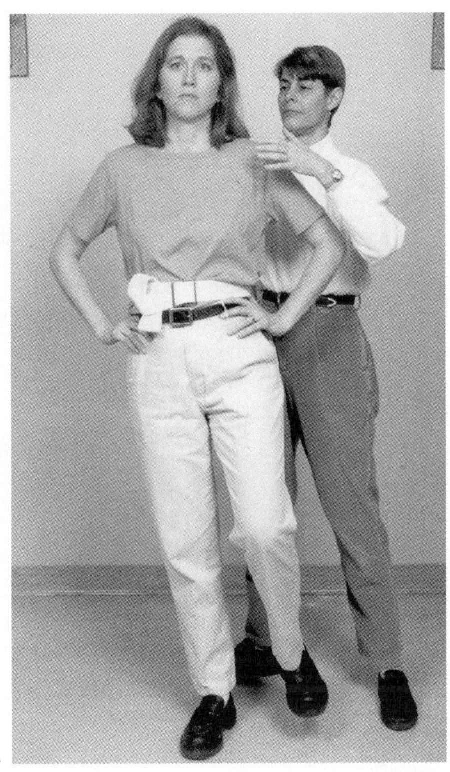
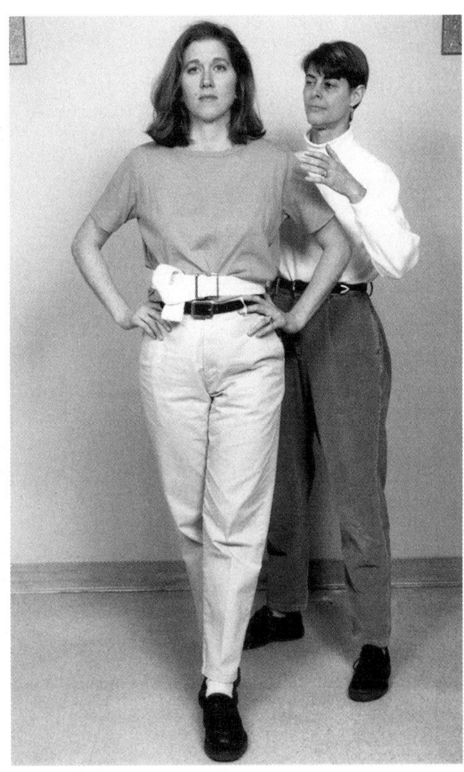

A B

FIGURE 11.9 Adapting movement strategies to changes in the base of support either through the one-foot stand (A) or tandem Romberg (B) position.

balance tasks such as standing on one foot (Fig. 11.9A) or in a tandem Romberg (heel/toe) position (Fig. 11.9B) reduce the base of support and increase the demands for frontal plane stability. They often result in the use of a hip or a stepping strategy to maintain stability and prevent a fall.

Research has shown that muscles in the leg and trunk are activated synergistically during recovery of stability, and this multijoint coordination is a hallmark of normal postural control. The most common clinical approach to evaluating multijoint dyscoordination within movement strategies used for postural control is through observation and description during tests such as the nudge test (Tinetti, 1986) or the reactive balance items from the BESTest (Horak et al., 2009). Following a small perturbation in the backward direction (Fig. 11.10A), the clinician may note that during recovery of stance balance the patient demonstrates excessive flexion of the knees or excessive flexion or rotation of the trunk. Differences in onset of muscle responses in the two sides can often be noted by testing for symmetry when the toes come up in response to a backward perturbation (Fig. 11.10, B and C). However, determining the underlying nature of the dyscoordination, that is, specific timing and or amplitude errors in synergistic muscles responding to instability, most often requires the use of technical tests such as electromyography (Shumway-Cook & McCollum, 1990).

Sensory Strategies

Stability must be maintained in a wide variety of environments (in well-lit environments, in the dark, in the presence of moving visual cues, and on surfaces with different geographic and physical features), necessitating a change in the way sensory information is used for postural control. An important part of assessing postural control is examining a person's ability to organize and select sensory information in response to changing sensory conditions. Instability when certain sensory cues are unavailable can provide insight into environmental conditions likely to produce instability.

Clinical Test For Sensory Interaction In Balance. Shumway-Cook and Horak suggested a method for assessing sensory organization components of stance postural control (Horak, 1987; Shumway-Cook & Horak, 1986). The Clinical Test for Sensory Interaction in Balance (CTSIB) uses a 24-by-24-inch piece of medium-density Temper foam in conjunction with a modified Japanese lantern. A large Japanese lantern is cut down the back and attached to a headband. Vertical stripes are placed inside the

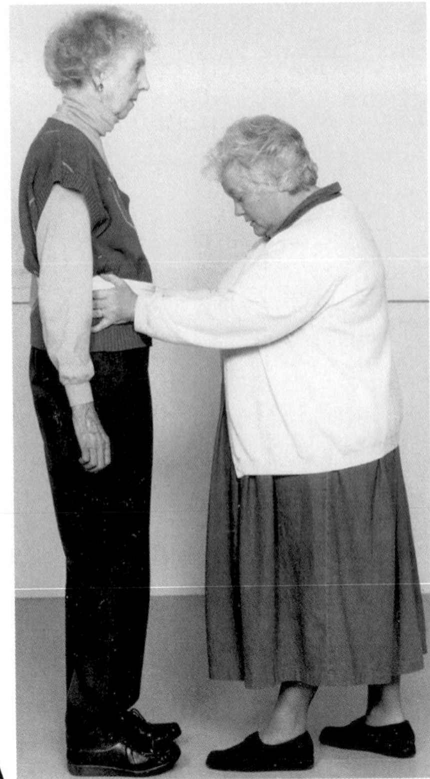

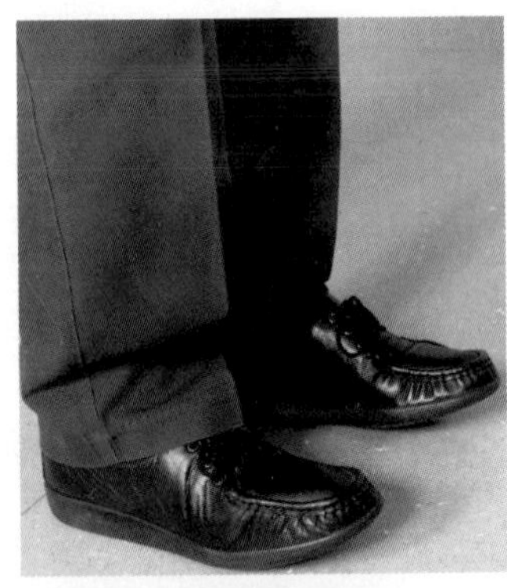

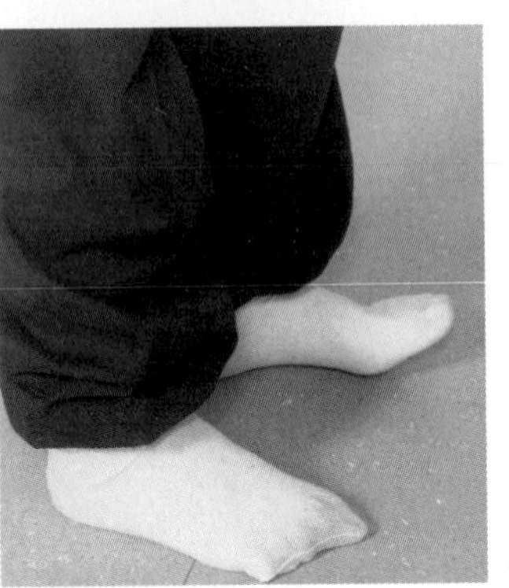

FIGURE 11.10 Symmetry of muscle responses at the ankle can be observed in response to displacement in the backward direction. A, The patient is given a small displacement in the backward direction. B, Normal response is dorsiflexion of both feet. C, An abnormal response in a patient with hemiparesis is loss of the dorsiflexion response in the hemiparetic leg.

lantern, and the top and bottom of the lantern are covered with white paper (Fig. 11.11).

The method is based on concepts developed by Nashner (1982), and it requires the subject to maintain standing balance for 30 seconds under six different sensory conditions that either eliminate input or produce inaccurate visual and surface orientation inputs. These six conditions are shown in Figure 11.12. Patients are tested in the feet-together position, with hands placed on the hips. Using condition 1 as a baseline reference, the therapist observes the patient for changes in the amount and direction of sway over the subsequent five conditions. If the patient is unable to stand for 30 seconds, a second trial is undertaken (Horak et al., 1992).

Neurologically intact young adults are able to maintain balance for 30 seconds on all six conditions with minimal amounts of body sway. As was true for the computerized sensory organization testing, normal adults sway on the average 40% more in conditions 5 and 6, than in condition 1 (Horak et al., 1992). A modified version of the CTSIB has been proposed, eliminating the dome conditions, and retaining four conditions—firm surface eyes open and closed and foam surface eyes open and closed—eliminating the two dome conditions (Allison, 1995; Whitney & Wrisley, 2004).

Results from a number of research studies that have used either a moving platform or the CTSIB (Cohen et al., 1993; DeFabio & Badke, 1990; Horak et al., 1992; Peterka & Black, 1990) suggest the following scoring criteria. A single fall, regardless of the condition, is not considered abnormal. However, two or more falls are indicative of difficulties adapting sensory information for postural control.

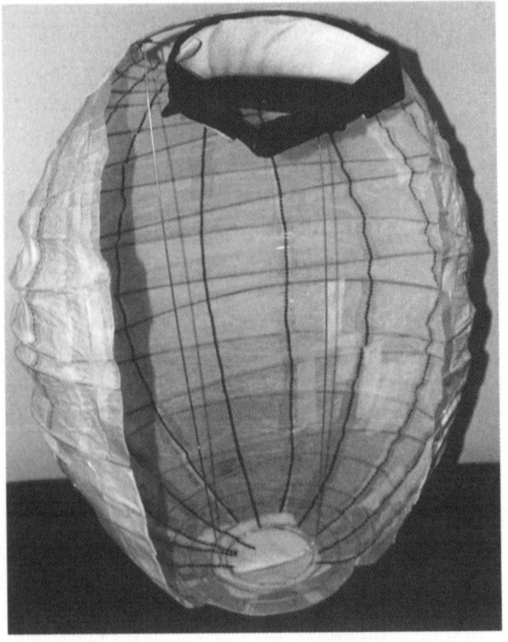

FIGURE 11.11 A modified Japanese lantern is used to change the accuracy of visual input for postural orientation.

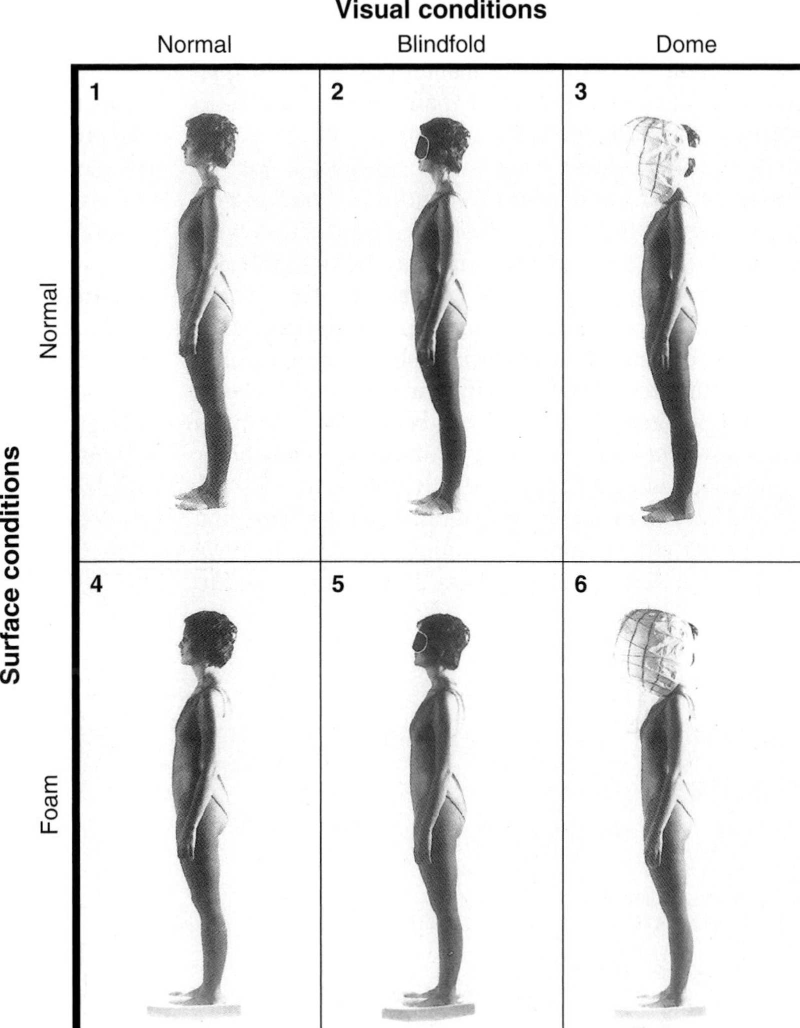

FIGURE 11.12 Six sensory conditions used to examine postural orientation under altered sensory contexts. The approach tests the ability to adapt how senses are used to maintain orientation. (Reprinted from Shumway-Cook A, Horak F. Assessing the influence of sensory interaction on balance. Phys Ther 1986;66:1549, with permission of the American Physical Therapy Association. This material is copyrighted, and any further reproduction or distribution requires written permission from APTA.)

A proposed model for interpreting results is summarized in Figure 11.13. Patients who show increased amounts of sway or lose balance on conditions 2, 3, and 6 are thought to be visually dependent, that is, highly dependent on vision for postural control. Patients who have problems on conditions 4, 5, and 6 are thought to be surface-dependent, that is, dependent primarily on somatosensory information from the feet in contact with the surface, for postural control (Shumway-Cook & Horak, 1990). Patients who sway more, or fall, on conditions 5 and 6, demonstrate a vestibular-loss pattern, suggesting an inability to select vestibular inputs for postural control in the absence of useful visual and somatosensory cues. Finally, patients who lose balance on conditions 3, 4, 5, and 6 are said to have a sensory selection problem. This is defined as an inability to effectively adapt sensory information for postural control (Shumway-Cook & Horak, 1992).

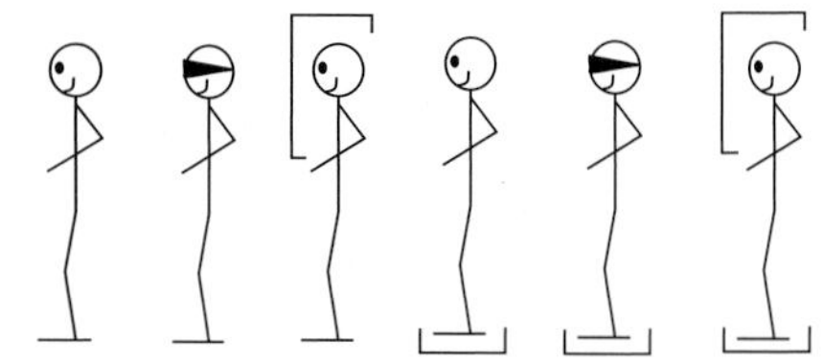

Patterns	1	2	3	4	5	6
		A				
Visually dependent	N	N/A	A	N	N/A	A
Surface dependent	N	N	N	A	A	A
Vestibular loss	N	N	N	N	A	A
Sensory selection	N	N	A	A		A

N = Body sway within normal limits
A = Body sway abnormal

FIGURE 11.13 Proposed model for interpreting the CTSIB test based on information gained through dynamic posturography testing.

It is important to remember the following caution when interpreting results showing increased sway on a compliant surface. While we suppose that the primary effect of standing on a foam surface relates to altering the availability of incoming sensory information for postural orientation, additional factors can affect performance in this condition. Standing on foam changes the dynamics of force production with respect to the surface, and this may be a significant factor affecting performance in this condition. There has been no research examining the dynamics of standing on foam; thus, clinicians should be careful in interpreting results when using the foam condition.

The six-item CTSIB test has been shown to have good test–retest reliability in community-dwelling older adults and young adults (r = 0.99) (Cohen et al., 1993), is a valid way to evaluate and monitor change over time in patients with vestibular dysfunction (Allison, 1995; Cohen et al., 1993; Weber & Cass, 1993), and is used to determine fall risk in older adults (Anacker & DeFabio, 1992) and following stroke (DeFabio & Badke, 1990).

A pediatric version of both the CTSIB (Crowe et al., 1990; Gagnon et al., 2006; Richardson et al., 1992) and the modified CTSIB (Geldhof et al., 2006) has been used to examine sensory-organization components of postural control in typically developing children and those with traumatic brain injury (Gagnon et al., 2004).

Incline Test. Horak and colleagues (2009) in their Balance Evaluation Systems Test (BESTest) have proposed another approach to examining the ability to maintain balance in the absence of useful vision and somatosensory inputs for postural control. In this test, orientation and sway are measured with eyes closed while standing on a firm surface as compared with on a 10–degree-angle incline board (Fig. 11.14, A and B). This test is based on research by Kluzik et al. (2005, 2007), who demonstrated that healthy subjects stood

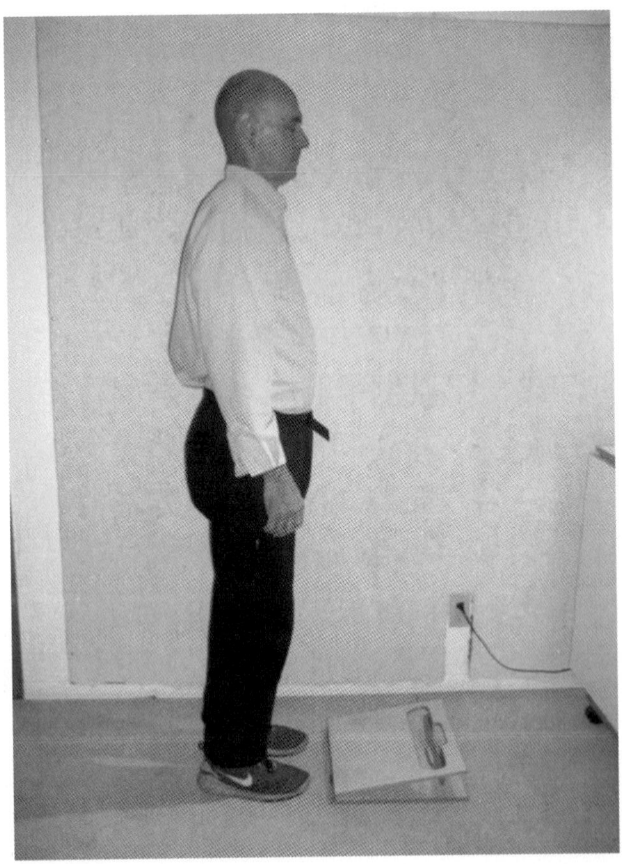

A

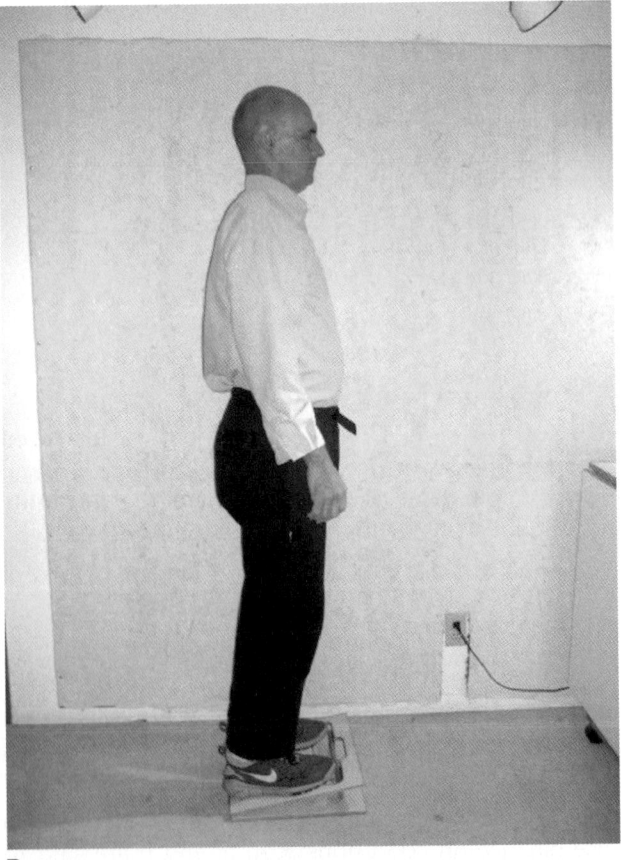

B

FIGURE 11.14 Incline Test. The Incline Test is part of the Balance Evaluation Systems Test (BESTest) and examines the individual's ability to maintain balance using vestibular inputs to orient to vertical in the absence of useful visual cues (eyes closed) and surface inputs (standing on an incline). Patients are tested with eyes closed standing on a firm flat surface (A), then while standing with eyes closed on a 10-degree-angle incline board (B).

with trunk and legs aligned near to gravity-vertical in both conditions. Patients with vestibular loss, however, have difficulty maintaining balance and orienting to vertical while standing on the inclined surface with eyes closed (Horak et al., 2009).

Examination of Underlying Impairments

The final step in a task-oriented approach is examining the sensory, motor (neural and musculoskeletal), and cognitive subsystems that contribute to postural control. During this portion of the examination, the emphasis is on examining impairments that will have the most direct impact on postural control. Thus, examination of strength may focus on examining lower-extremity muscle strength, with particular attention to ankle muscles such as the anterior tibialis and gastrocnemius/soleus, because of the role of these muscles in control of upright stance. For that same reason, examining range of motion at the ankle is also considered critical. Understanding the integrity of sensory inputs critical to postural control, such as vision and somatosensation in the feet and ankles, is also an important part of examination at the impairment level. For a discussion of methods for examining impairments, refer to Chapter 5. Before moving on to treatment, the reader is encouraged to complete Lab Activity 11.2, applying a task-oriented approach to examination.

EVALUATION: INTERPRETING THE RESULTS OF THE EXAMINATION

After completing the examination, the clinician must interpret results, identify the problems, and establish short- and long-term goals and a plan of care for achieving those goals. An important part of establishing an appropriate plan of care is considering the evidence to support different therapeutic approaches to improving balance, restoring function, and maximizing participation.

TASK-ORIENTED BALANCE REHABILITATION

The goals of a task-oriented approach to treating the patient with postural control problems include therapeutic strategies to: (a) resolve, reduce, or prevent impairments in systems that are important to balance; (b) develop effective task-specific sensory, motor, and cognitive strategies, and (c) retrain functional tasks with varying postural control demands (e.g., steady-state, reactive, and anticipatory control) under changing environmental contexts. The ultimate goal of task-oriented balance rehabilitation is to improve participation outcomes, reflected in an improved ability to participate in the social roles, tasks, and activities that are important in the daily life of the patient. Improved participation can be demonstrated by increased frequency of participation or increased independence and safety (reduced falls) when performing daily tasks and activities. Improved participation may also be reflected in increased confidence, reduced fear, and increased satisfaction with one's level of participation. The following sections review our task-oriented approach to improving balance, and includes a review of the research evidence to support specific types of interventions to improve balance and reduce falls.

LAB ACTIVITY 11-2

Objective: To apply a task-oriented approach to examining postural control to a patient with hemiplegia and to establish goals and a plan of care for improving posture and balance based on assessment information.

Procedure: Read the case study of Jean J in Assessment Tool 11.6. (or use a real case study if you have access to a patient with a neurologic diagnosis).

Assignment: Based on the information you have, answer the following questions:

1. What are her functional limitations?
2. Based on her Berg Balance Test score, what is her current fall risk (see Fig. 11.3)?
3. Does she have steady-state balance problems? Anticipatory control problems? Reactive control problems?
4. What movement strategies does she use for control of balance? What impairments are contributing to her choice of movement strategy?
5. How well is she able to organize sensory information for postural control? Based on the results from her CTSIB test, in what environments would you expect her to have difficulty maintaining balance?

Assessment Tool 11-6

Assessment Case Study

Jean J, is a 82-year-old woman with right-sided hemiplegia, referred for evaluation of balance 4 weeks after her stroke.

Medical history: Positive for hypertension. Following her 5-day acute hospital stay for a middle cerebral artery infarct, she spent 2 weeks in rehabilitation and was discharged to her home.

Social history: She lives alone in an assisted living complex. She had been a full-time legal assistant.

Reason for referral: Continued problems with balance.

ON EXAMINATION:

Self-report fall/balance history: She reports two falls since her return home; one occurred while walking to the bathroom at night, and one occurred while lifting a suitcase onto her bed that was heavier than she expected. She indicates she loses her balance several times a day, often when arising, turning to look at something, when lifting heavy objects, and when walking.

TESTS AND MEASURES:

A. Function Balance Test (performed without her single-point cane)

Test Item		*Test Item*	
1. Sit to stand	3	8. Functional Reach	2
2. Stand to sit	3	9. Look over shoulder	3
3. Transfers	3	10. Slipper reach	2
4. Standing 2 minutes	4	11. 360-degree turn	2
5. Sitting	4	12. Stool touch	0
6. Standing feet together	2	13. One-foot stand	0
7. Standing eyes closed	3	14. Tandem stand	0

B. Strategy Assessment

1. Motor

- Alignment in sitting and standing—shifted to the left
- Voluntary sway—tends to bend at the hips when leaning forward or backward; has difficulty shifting weight laterally to the right.
- Nudge test: small perturbations—tends to bend at the hips, does not show a toes-up response to backward displacement in the right foot. Large perturbations—can step with the right foot (but slowly), cannot step with the left

2. Sensory

Modified CTSIB (feet shoulder distance apart, no cane)

Surface, Visual Condition	*Trial 1*	*Trial 2*	*Surface, Visual Condition*	*Trial 1*	*Trial 2*
Firm, Open	30		Foam, Open	0	5
Firm, Closed	30		Foam, Closed	0	0

C. Underlying impairments

1. Decreased cognitive status; specific problems with judgment, and safety issues;
2. Musculoskeletal impairments, including: 5 degrees of ankle dorsiflexion in the right leg;
3. Neuromuscular impairments, including reduced ability to generate force voluntarily (2/5 manual muscle testing in right-lower-extremity muscles), decreased ability to recruit ankle muscles in the right leg for postural control, and moderate increase in muscle tone in the right elbow flexor and ankle extensors;
4. Sensory/perceptual problems, including decreased sensory discrimination (somatosensation) in the right arm and leg and right hemianopsia.

Intervention at the Impairment Level

The goal of intervention aimed at the impairment level is to correct impairments that can be corrected and to prevent the development of secondary impairments. Alleviating underlying impairments enables the patient to resume using previously developed strategies for postural control. When permanent impairments make resumption of previously used strategies impossible, new strategies that are effective in meeting task requirements in the face of persisting impairments will have to be developed.

The focus of intervention at the impairment level is to have an impact on the impairments that have the greatest effect on postural control. For example, in our case study of Jean J, improving underlying impairments related to range of motion and strength are a critical part of balance rehabilitation. What is the evidence to suggest that improving underlying impairments such as strength or flexibility will result in improved balance?

Effect of Strength Training on Balance

A number of studies have found that muscle-strength deficits are at least partially reversible in pediatric, geriatric, and neurologic populations. The evidence demonstrating the relationship between increased muscle strength and improved balance remains mixed, however.

Among older adults, many studies have shown that resistance strength training is effective in increasing strength; however, while in some studies this was associated with improved balance (Chandler & Hadley, 1996; Fiatarone et al., 1994; Fiatarone et al., 1990; Hess et al., 2006; Hess & Woollacott, 2005; Wolfson et al., 1996), in others it was not (Judge et al., 1994). Orr et al. (2008) conducted a systematic review of randomized, controlled trials to examine the effect of progressive resistive strength training on balance in older adults. A total of 29 studies met their inclusion criteria; 14 reported improvements in balance following strength training. Orr and colleagues suggest that inconsistent effects of resistance training on balance in older adults may in part be explained by methodological differences in the studies included in their review; however, they also suggest that resistance training alone may not be a robust enough intervention to improve balance control in older adults.

Similar to the research with older adults, the results of strength training on balance control in neurologic populations is mixed. Among persons with multiple sclerosis (MS), DeBolt and McCubbin (2004) reported that resistance exercise resulted in a significant increase in lower-extremity power; however, there was no significant effect on postural-sway measures (anteroposterior and mediolateral sway and sway velocity) or on TUG performance. The authors conclude that resistance strength training is possible in persons with MS, with no adverse effects on the disease, but while this form of exercise improves power, it does not result in improved balance and mobility (as determined by their measures). Ada et al. (2006) reviewed data from 15 trials to determine whether strength training in participants who have had a stroke improves strength without increasing spasticity and whether increased strength resulted in improved function, though balance was not specifically identified. The meta-analysis found that strengthening interventions had a small positive effect on both strength and functional activities, with very little effect on spasticity. They concluded that strengthening programs should be a part of stroke rehabilitation. These studies suggest that while there is considerable evidence demonstrating the effect of training on improved strength, the degree to which strength training alone will result in improved balance remains unclear.

Activities to Improve Strategies for Postural Control

The goal of interventions aimed at the strategy level is to facilitate the development of sensory, motor, and cognitive strategies that are effective in meeting postural control demands associated with a variety of functional tasks that require steady-state, anticipatory, and reactive aspects of balance control. Movement strategies must successfully control the COM relative to the base of support. This includes the development of strategies for maintaining alignment of the body, strategies for moving the COM relative to a stationary base of support (in-place strategies), and strategies that change the base of support to regain stability of the COM (e.g., taking a step to recover stability in standing, or reaching for support).

Development of sensory strategies includes learning to organize and select the most appropriate sensory input(s) for postural control. Cognitive strategies include learning to allocate attentional resources for postural control during the performance of multiple tasks.

At the heart of balance training is practicing progressively challenging tasks and activities that facilitate the development of postural behaviors needed for the (re)acquisition of skilled functional movement. The selection and sequencing of tasks, activities, and contexts, integrated into a schedule of practice consistent with motor learning principles, is a powerful tool in retraining balance. For example, in initial stages of balance retraining, when the patient has minimal ability to control the COM, he or she may practice tasks with minimal demands for postural control in "closed" environments (e.g., constant and predictable conditions), such as seated upright on a firm flat surface in a supported or semisupported position. As postural control improves, sitting tasks with increasing postural demands are introduced, such as sitting unsupported on the edge of the mat or bed (steady-state postural control), sitting unsupported while turning the head or reaching for an object (anticipatory postural control), or recovery of stable seated position following displacements (reactive balance). As balance improves, seated tasks can be practiced in "open" environments (e.g., changing and less predictable), such as seated on an unstable or foam surface while catching objects thrown from different directions, or while holding a cup of water. Retraining balance within mobility tasks will be discussed in Chapter 15.

Alignment

The goal when retraining alignment is to help the patient develop an initial position that: (a) is appropriate for the task, (b) is efficient with respect to gravity, that is, with minimal muscle activity requirements for maintaining the position, and (c) maximizes stability, that is, places the vertical line of gravity well within the patient's stability limits; this allows the greatest range of movements for postural control. Many tasks use a symmetrical vertical position, but this may not be a realistic goal for all patients (Shumway-Cook & McCollum, 1990).

A number of approaches can be used to help patients develop a symmetrically vertical posture. Commonly, verbal and manual cues are used by the clinician to assist a patient in finding and maintaining an appropriate vertical posture. Patients practice with eyes open and closed, learning to maintain a vertical position in the absence of visual cues. Mirrors can also be used to provide patients with visual feedback about their position in space. The effect of a mirror can be enhanced by having the patient wear a white T-shirt with a vertical stripe down the center and asking him or her to try to match the stripe on the T-shirt to a vertical stripe on the mirror (Fig. 11.15). The patient can use the mirror and T-shirt approach while performing a variety of tasks, such as reaching for an object, which require that the body be moved away from the vertical line and then reestablish a vertical position. Given the results from motor learning research on the frequency of knowledge of results (KR) summarized in Chapter 2, learning might be better if visual feedback regarding midline alignment is given intermittently, rather than during every trial. For example, the therapist could turn or cover the mirror and ask the patient to repeat the task in the absence of visual feedback.

Another approach to retraining vertical alignment, shown in Figure 11.16, uses flashlights attached to the patient's body in conjunction with targets on the wall (Shumway-Cook & Horak, 1992). In this task, the patient is asked to bring the light (or lights) in line with the target(s). Again, lights can be turned on and off during the task so that visual feedback is intermittent.

Another approach to retraining vertical posture involves having patients stand (or sit) with their backs against the wall, which provides enhanced somatosensory feedback about their position in space. This feedback can be further increased by placing a yardstick or small roll vertically on the wall (Fig. 11.17) and having the patient lean against it. Somatosensory feedback can be made intermittent by having the patient lean away from the wall, only occasionally leaning back to get KR.

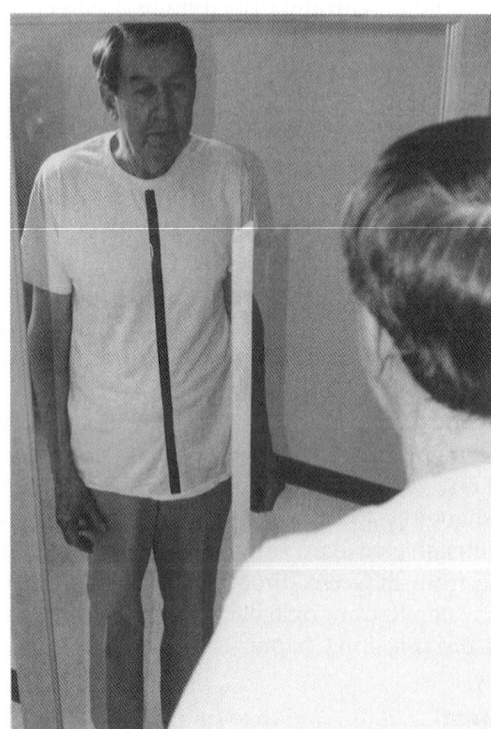

FIGURE 11.15 Using a mirror when retraining alignment. The patient is asked to line up the vertical stripe on his T-shirt with a vertical stripe on the mirror.

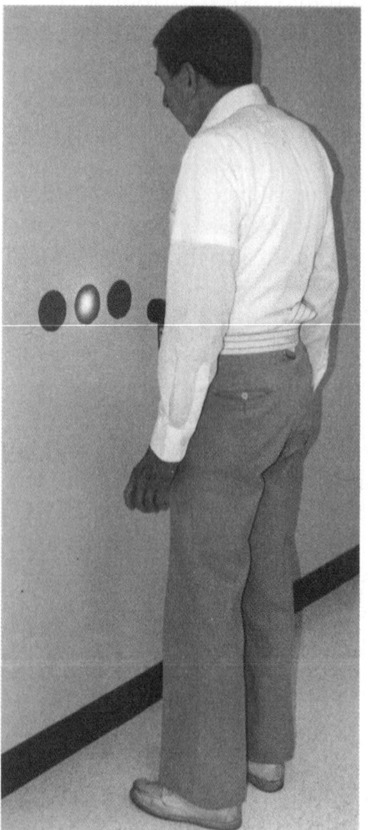

FIGURE 11.16 Using a flashlight in conjunction with targets on a wall to help a patient learn to control COM movements.

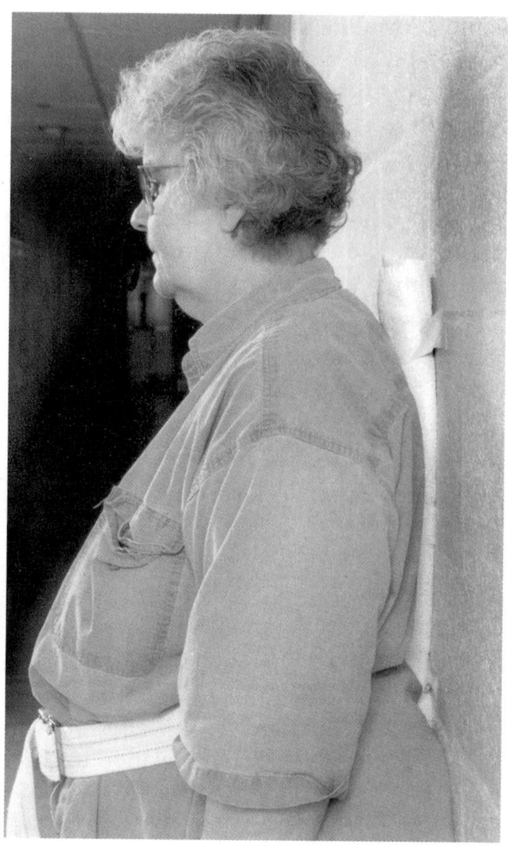

FIGURE 11.17 Enhancing somatosensation regarding verticality when retraining vertical posture by having the patient lean against a small roll placed vertically on the wall.

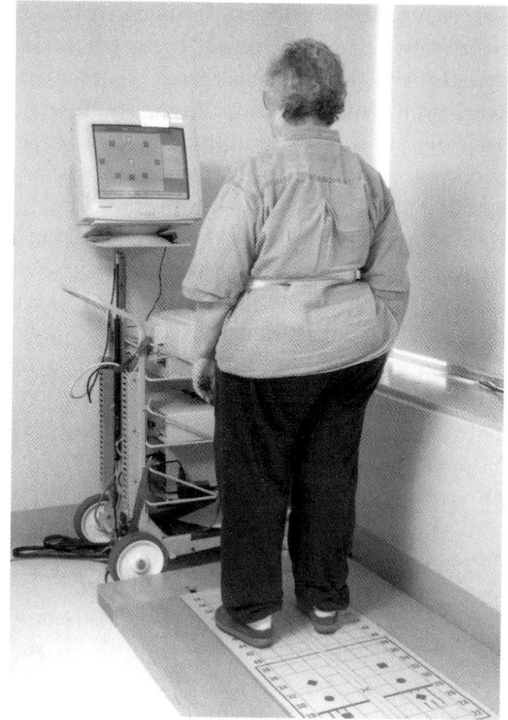

FIGURE 11.18 Use of a force-plate biofeedback system to provide visual feedback regarding alignment and weight-bearing status.

Kinetic- or force-feedback devices are often used to provide patients with information about postural alignment and weight-bearing status (Herman, 1973; Shumway-Cook et al., 1988). Kinetic feedback can be provided with devices as simple as bathroom scales. Alternatively, kinetic feedback can be given through either load-limb monitors (Herman, 1973), feedback canes (Baker et al., 1979), or force-plate biofeedback systems such as the one shown in Figure 11.18.

Research Evidence. What evidence do we have that the use of force-plate biofeedback methods helps patients reestablish symmetrical postural alignment? In one of the earliest studies, Shumway-Cook and colleagues (1988) compared the effect of postural sway biofeedback to usual-care physical therapy in reestablishing symmetrical weight bearing in standing in patients with hemiparesis. Six months after a cerebrovascular accident (CVA), 16 patients were randomly assigned to feedback or usual-care groups. Prior to treatment, all patients carried about 70% of their total body weight on the noninvolved leg. The feedback group received 15 minutes of stance force-plate visual biofeedback twice a day for 2 weeks. The usual-care group received 15 minutes of balance retraining for the same amount of time. Following 2 weeks of training, the experimental group had significantly less lateral displacement than did the patients in the control group (six of whom were more asymmetric at the end of 2 weeks of therapy).

Winstein and colleagues (1989) also examined the effects of providing visual feedback about relative weight distribution over paretic and nonparetic limbs on standing balance and locomotor performance in patients with hemiplegia. They provided visual feedback through a standing feedback trainer to 21 patients randomly assigned to the experimental treatment; 21 patients served as controls and received conventional therapy. Consistent with the previous study, results showed that stance symmetry significantly improved with the visual-feedback therapy; however, there was no change in the asymmetrical locomotor pattern. These authors remind us that while control mechanisms for balance and locomotion may be highly interrelated, a reduction in standing asymmetry will not necessarily lead to a reduction in asymmetric locomotion patterns.

There have been two systematic reviews examining the effectiveness of force-plate biofeedback methods to improve standing balance after stroke. In their review, Barclay-Goddard et al. (2004) concluded that providing feedback from a force platform resulted in patients standing more symmetrically; however, this did not result in improved balance during functional activities, nor did it improve overall independence. The review by van Peppen et al. (2006) found a nonsignificant effect in favor of visual-feedback therapy on weight distribution, postural sway, balance, and gait speed in persons with stroke. They concluded that visual-feedback therapy did not show an advantage over conventional therapy for improving weight-bearing asymmetry after stroke. Similar to Winstein et al.'s (1989) caution, they suggest that many questions remain regarding the relationship between asymmetrical alignment and balance during stance and gait following stroke.

Clinicians routinely provide unsteady patients with assistive devices such as canes or walkers. What effect does providing external support such as a cane have on postural alignment and stability? An assistive device such as a cane increases the base of support. Since stability requires keeping the center of gravity within the base of support, increasing the base of support makes the task of stability easier. Milczarek and colleagues (1993) studied the effects of a cane on standing balance in patients with hemiparesis, using a force plate to record changes in COP under various conditions of support. As illustrated in Figure 11.19, they found that using a cane resulted in a significant shift in the position of the COP toward the cane side, and a decrease in both anteroposterior and mediolateral postural sway. Thus, although using a cane reduced postural sway, it increased the asymmetric alignment of patients toward the side holding the cane (Milczarek et al., 1993). More recently, Bateni et al., (2004a) demonstrated that in healthy subjects the use of a cane or walker interfered with compensatory stepping responses. Use of an assistive device resulted in collisions between the swing foot and the assistive device and a significant reduction in lateral step length, pointing out the inherent limitations in assistive devices during recovery of postural stability in response to external perturbations.

Movement Strategies

The goal when retraining movement strategies is to help the patient develop coordinated multijoint movements that are effective in meeting the demands for postural control in sitting and in standing. This includes movements that move the COM relative to a stationary base of support (in-place strategies), as well as movements that change the base of support relative to the COM (changing-base-of-support strategies). Movement strategies can be practiced within the context of retraining reactive and proactive balance control.

Retraining Reactive Balance Control. Training reactive balance control involves exposing the patient

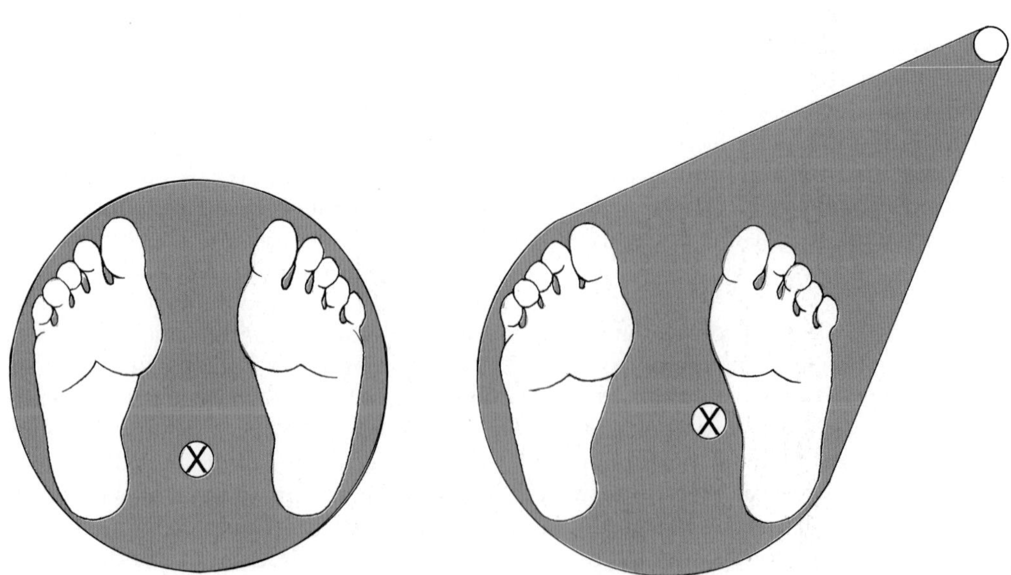

FIGURE 11.19 The effects of holding a cane while standing include widening the base of support and shifting the mean position of the COP laterally toward the cane side. (Adapted from Milczarek JJ, Kirby LM, Harrison ER, MacLeod DA. Standard and four-footed canes: their effect on the standing balance of patients with hemiparesis. Arch Phys Med Rehabil 1993;74:283.)

to external perturbations that vary in direction, speed, and amplitude. External perturbations can include manual pulls and pushes applied to the hips or shoulders, or the use of moving surfaces. Small perturbations can facilitate the use of in-place strategies for balance control, while larger and faster perturbations encourage the use of a step. The amplitude, speed, and direction of perturbations can be systematically varied by the therapist so that both in-place and stepping strategies are practiced.

Stepping can be facilitated manually by clinician's shifting the patient's weight to one side and quickly bringing the COM toward the unweighted leg (Fig. 11.20). The clinician can further assist the patient with a step by manually lifting the foot and placing it during the maneuver. To ensure a patient's safety, stepping can be done within the parallel bars or near a wall. When helping a patient develop the ability to step for postural control, it is important to tell the patient that the goal of the exercise is to take a step to prevent a fall.

Responses to external perturbations should be practiced in multiple directions and under varying sensory (e.g., with and without vision and on firm, foam, and inclined surfaces) and cognitive conditions (alone and while practicing other tasks).

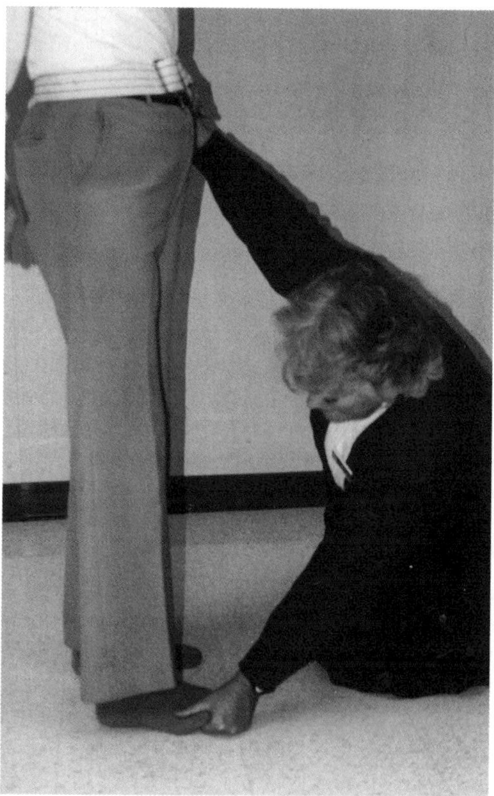

FIGURE 11.20 Facilitating a stepping strategy by manually shifting the patient's COM laterally and manually moving the patient's foot into a step.

Research Evidence. There is mounting evidence that training of reactive balance control does improve the organization and timing of postural responses in patients with neurologic deficits. Marigold et al. (2005) found improvements in the onset latency of paretic lower-extremity muscles in response to platform perturbations in people with chronic stroke after 10 weeks of balance training. Improvements in the onset latency and organization of lower-extremity muscle responses to platform perturbations were also reported in children with spastic hemiplegic and diplegic forms of cerebral palsy following 5 days of intensive reactive balance training on a movable platform (Shumway-Cook et al., 2003; Woollacott et al., 2005).

Other forms of training have also been shown to improve the organization and timing of muscle responses used to recover balance following an unexpected perturbation. Gatts and Woollacott (2006, 2007) examined the effect of three weeks of intense (1½ hour, 5 days per week) of Tai Chi training on the ability to recovery from an unexpected perturbation while walking in balance-impaired older adults. The authors found that Tai Chi training significantly enhanced balance responses by improving the organization and timing of stepping strategies of the swing leg. Participants in the Tai Chi training significantly reduced tibialis anterior (TA) response time from 148.92±45.11 msec to 98.67±417.22 msec ($p \leq 0.004$). In addition, there was a significant reduction in co-contraction of antagonist muscles ($p \leq 0.003$) of the perturbed leg. These studies provide evidence that training can improve the organization and timing of muscle responses used to recover stability following an unexpected perturbation to stance or gait. More research is needed to determine the types of interventions that are effective in improving reactive postural control in both neurologic and geriatric populations.

Retraining Anticipatory Balance Control. Movement strategies can also be practiced during voluntary sway in all directions, as patients learn to control COM movements over increasingly larger areas while varying speed. Knowledge of results regarding how far the COM is moving during self-initiated sway can be facilitated using static force-plate retraining systems. Flashlights attached to the patient in conjunction with targets on the wall can also be used to encourage patients to move from side to side.

Patients who are very unsteady or extremely fearful of falling can practice movement while in the parallel bars or when standing close to a wall or in a corner with a chair or table in front of them

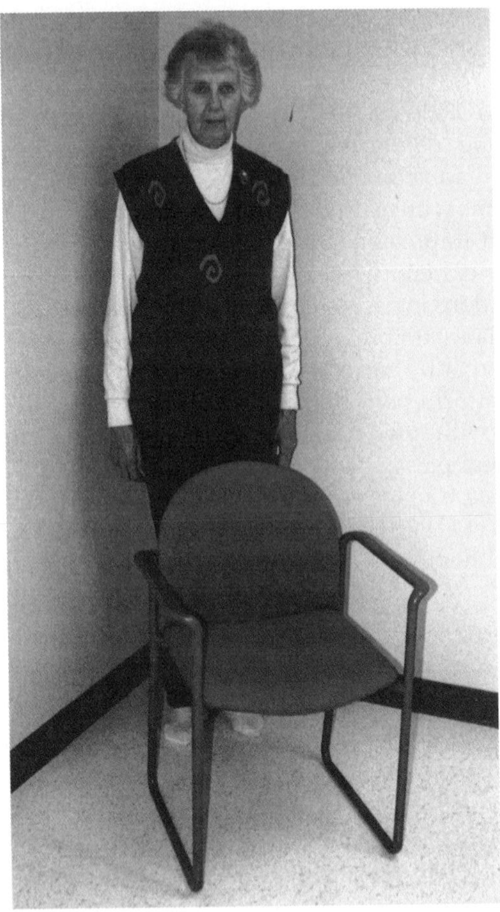

FIGURE 11.21 Placing a patient near a wall with a chair in front of her increases safety when retraining standing balance in a fearful or unstable patient.

(Fig. 11.21). Modifying the environment (either home or clinic) in this manner allows a patient to continue practicing movement strategies for balance control safely and without the continual supervision of a therapist.

When training anticipatory postural control, patients can be asked to carry out a variety of manipulation tasks, such as reaching, lifting, and throwing, thus helping patients to develop strategies for anticipatory postural control. A hierarchy of tasks reflecting increasing anticipatory postural demands can be helpful when retraining patients in this important area. The magnitude of anticipatory postural activity is directly related to the potential for instability inherent in a task. Potential instability relates to speed, effort, degree of external support, and task complexity. Thus, asking a patient who is externally supported by the therapist to lift a light load slowly requires minimal anticipatory postural activity. Conversely, an unsupported patient who must lift a heavy load quickly must use a substantial amount of anticipatory postural activity to remain stable.

Research Evidence. While many studies have documented that repetitive practice of functional tasks (so-called task-oriented treatment) significantly improves performance on functional balance measures such as the Berg Balance Scale, the Functional Reach, and the Timed Up and Go, few studies have examined the underlying muscle activity to determine whether improved task performance is associated with improved anticipatory aspects of postural control. Garland et al. (2003) used surface electromyography to examine the timing of muscle activity in the lower extremities (hamstrings and soleus) relative to the initiation of arm movement in an arm-raising task in persons with poststroke hemiparesis. Prior to rehabilitation, muscles in the paretic lower extremity were activated after the initiation of arm movement, rather than before, as was true in the nonparetic limb. Following 1 month of rehabilitation, arm movement was faster and recruitment of hamstring and soleus muscles was significantly faster in both limbs. While 10 of 27 patients showed activation of anticipatory muscle activity in the hemiparetic limb prior to arm movement (what the authors refer to as "true recovery"), 12 showed no change in the timing of muscle activity in the hemiparetic side, though it improved timing in the nonhemiparetic limb (a compensatory strategy). This research provides some evidence that anticipatory aspects of postural control can be improved with training in some patients. More research is needed to verify and expand these findings to other patient populations.

Sensory Organization Strategies

The goal when retraining sensory organization strategies is to help the patient learn to effectively coordinate and select appropriate sensory information for postural control. Treatment strategies generally require the patient to maintain balance during progressively more difficult static and dynamic movement tasks while the clinician systematically varies the availability and accuracy of one or more senses for orientation (Shumway-Cook & Horak, 1989, 1990).

Patients who show increased reliance on vision for orientation are asked to perform a variety of balance tasks when visual cues are absent (eyes closed or blindfolded) or reduced (blinders or diminished lighting). Alternatively, visual cues can be made inaccurate for orientation through the use of glasses smeared with petroleum jelly (Fig. 11.22) or Frenzel glasses. Decreasing a patient's sensitivity to visual motion cues in their environment can be done by asking the patient to maintain balance during exposure to optokinetic stimuli, such as moving curtains with stripes, moving large cardboard posters with vertical lines, or even moving rooms.

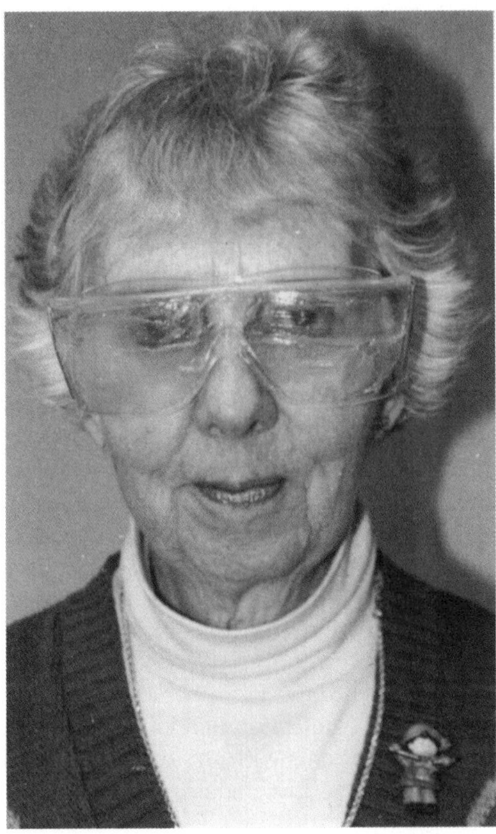

FIGURE 11.22 Training sensory adaptation for postural control. Petroleum jelly–covered glasses are used to obscure but not completely remove visual cues for postural control.

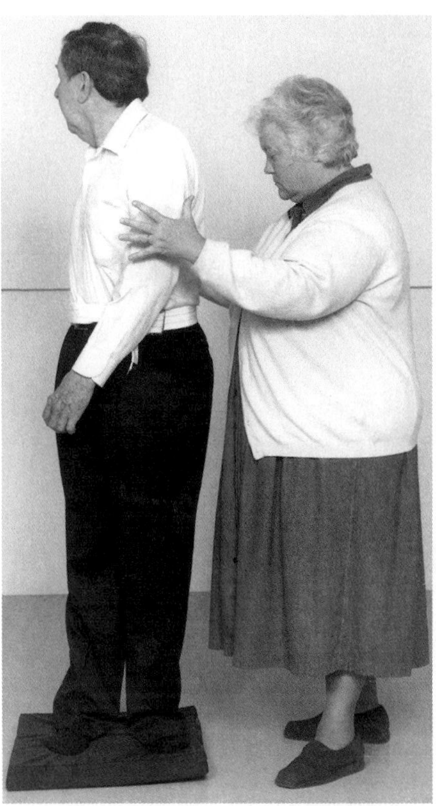

FIGURE 11.23 Training sensory adaptation for postural control. The patient is asked to turn the trunk while standing on foam, which is purported to reduce the availability of somatosensory inputs for postural control and thus increases the weighting of vision/vestibular inputs for postural control.

Patients who show increased reliance on the surface for orientation are asked to perform tasks while sitting or standing on surfaces providing decreased somatosensory cues for orientation, such as carpet or compliant foam surfaces, or on moving surfaces, such as a tilt board. Finally, to enhance the patient's ability to use remaining vestibular information for postural stability, exercises are given that ask the patient to balance while both visual and somatosensory inputs for orientation are simultaneously reduced, such as standing on compliant foam, thick carpet, or an inclined surface with eyes closed. In Figure 11.23 the patient is asked to turn his or her trunk while standing on foam, which is purported to reduce the availability of somatosensory inputs for postural control, and thus increase the weighting of vision/vestibular inputs for postural control. In Figure 11.24, the subject wears petroleum jelly–covered glasses and stands on foam while reaching for a cup. The rationale for this exercise is to increase reliance on vestibular inputs for postural control by reducing the availability of both somatosensory and visual inputs.

Research Evidence. Is there research evidence to suggest that practicing tasks under altered sensory contexts can improve the way people organize and select sensory information for balance control? The answer appears to be yes in both geriatric and neurologic populations. A number of studies have demonstrated improvements in the organization of sensory information for postural control through training in older adults (Hu & Woollacott; 1994a, 1994b), adults with vestibular dysfunction (Cass et al., 1996) or stroke (Bayouk et al., 2006; Bonan et al., 2004; Smania et al., 2008), and children with sensorineural hearing loss and vestibular impairment (Rine et al., 2004).

A study by Hu and Woollacott (1994a, 1994b) used a balance-training protocol that focused on the use of different sensory inputs and the integration of these inputs under conditions in which sensory inputs were reduced or altered. Subjects (65 to 87 years of age) participated in five 1-hr training sessions per week for 2 weeks. The training conditions consisted of standing on a force plate under the following sensory conditions: normal support surface,

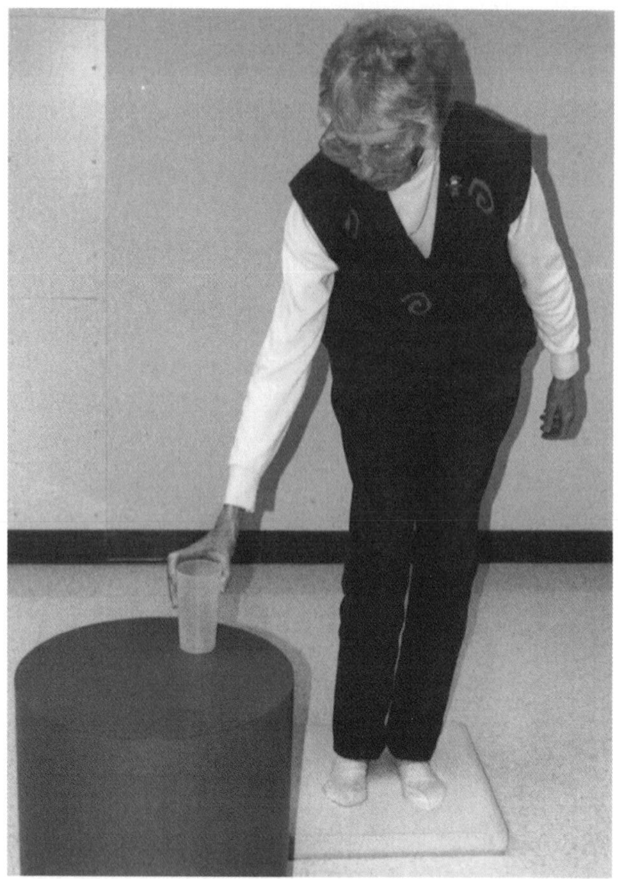

FIGURE 11.24 Training sensory adaptation for postural control. The patient wears petroleum jelly–covered glasses and stands on foam while reaching for a cup. The rationale for this exercise is to increase reliance on vestibular inputs for postural control by reducing the availability of both somatosensory and visual inputs.

eyes open, head neutral; normal surface, eyes closed, head neutral; normal support surface, eyes open, head extended; and normal surface, eyes closed, head extended; then all trials were repeated on the foam surface. They found significant improvements in the sway of the training group between the first and the last day of training in five of the eight training conditions (foam surface and eyes closed, head extended on the normal surface).

Bayouk et al. (2006) examined the effects of a task-oriented exercise program with and without altered sensory input on postural stability in subjects with stroke. Sixteen patients participated in an 8-week training program; half performed task-oriented training with sensory manipulation, while half performed the same set of exercises without sensory manipulation. Both groups significantly improved on the 10-m walk test; however, only the group that practiced under altered sensory conditions showed an improved ability to stand under altered sensory conditions. The authors suggest that "balance senses have to be specifically targeted when designing balance-retraining programs for hemiparetic subjects" (Bayouk et al., 2006, p. 57). Other researchers have also reported that sensory manipulation, including changing vision (Bonan et al., 2004), or a combination of both vision and somatosensory inputs (Smania et al., 2008) was more effective in improving balance than similar training without sensory manipulation in patients with impaired balance following stroke.

Researchers are also developing and testing approaches to enhance sensory feedback related to postural control. Paradoxically, this research has introduced noise-enhanced signals using vibratory shoe inserts to improve the utilization of somatosensory inputs from the lower extremity for postural control (Priplata et al., 2002). It is based on studies in a variety of systems showing that certain levels of noise can enhance the detection and transmission of weak signals (a process referred to as "stochastic resonance"). Introducing noise to the vibrotactile system has been shown to improve detection of a vibrotactile stimulus in older adults, patients with stroke, and patients with diabetic neuropathy (Liu et al., 2002).

Cognitive Strategies

The growing evidence that instability and falls increase during the performance of multiple tasks in both neurologic and geriatric populations suggests the need for training balance under both single- and dual-task conditions. Training balance under dual-task conditions involves practicing tasks requiring steady-state, anticipatory, and reactive balance control while simultaneously varying the cognitive demands through the use of secondary tasks. This aspect of balance rehabilitation is relatively new; thus, we have limited evidence to guide and support the use of dual-task training in balance rehabilitation.

Research Evidence. Silsupadol et al. (2006, 2009a, 2009b) described the outcomes of three approaches to training balance—single-task, dual-task with fixed-priority instructions, and dual-task with variable-task instructions—in older adults with balance impairment. Outcome measures for this series of studies included the BBT, the Dynamic Gait Index (DGI), the single- and dual-task TUG, and the ABC scale. In addition, laboratory measures of walking under single- and dual-task conditions (novel tasks not specifically trained) were also analyzed. Participants were older adults who volunteered for balance training because of a self-reported history of falls in the previous year or concern about impaired balance in the absence of neurologic or musculoskeletal diagnoses. Participants were randomly assigned to one of the three balance-training approaches. Balance training was done three times a week for 4 weeks. For all participants, balance training was based on a systems theory of postural control and used a progression of activities designed to improve steady-state, anticipatory, and reactive balance control. In addition, training targeted sensory and motor components of postural control. Examples of the balance-training strategies used are summarized in Table 11.7. Dual-task training was done under either a fixed (maintain attention on both tasks all the time) or variable (attentional focus was on balance activities for half of each session and on secondary tasks for the other half) instructional set. A summary of the types of secondary tasks used in this study is also found in Table 11.7. All three forms of balance training improved balance on the BBT ($p < 0.001$, effect size = 0.72) and gait speed on the 10-m walk ($p = 0.02$, effect size = 0.27). However only participants who received dual-task training improved gait speed under dual-task conditions (Silsupadol et al., 2009a). In addition, using a variable-priority instructional set during dual-task balance training was more effective at improving balance under dual-task training conditions than either single-task or fixed-priority training strategies. The use of a variable-priority strategy during dual-task training appears to improve both single-task automatization and the ability to coordinate multiple tasks (Silsupadol et al., 2009b). The authors conclude that training balance under single-task conditions may not generalize to balance control under dual-task conditions. In addition, explicit instructions regarding attentional focus may significantly impact the results of dual-task balance training.

The only other study related to dual-task training focused on gait training in stroke. Yang et al. (2007a) used a randomized, controlled trial to examine the effect of 4 weeks of dual-task gait training in persons with chronic stroke. Patients in the control group received no training. Patients in the experimental group showed significant improvements in

TABLE 11.7 List of Activities Used during Balance Retraining under Single- and Dual-Task Conditions

Balance Activities	Secondary Tasks
Stance Activities	**Secondary Task Activities**
1. Semitandem, eyes open, arm alternation	Spell words forward
2. Semitandem, eyes closed, arm alternation	Spell words backward
3. Draw letters with right foot	Name any words starting with letters A to K
4. Draw letters with left foot	Name any words starting with letters L to Z
5. Perturbed forward standing while holding a ball	Remember prices (e.g., bill payment)
6. Perturbed backward standing while holding a ball	Remember prices (e.g., groceries)
Gait Activities	Count backward by 3s
7. Walk forward/backward, normal base of support	Remember words
8. Walk forward/backward, narrow base of support	Tell the opposite direction of a ball toss
9. Walk narrow base of support, step, forward avoiding the obstacles (holding a basket)	Visual imaginary task (tell the road directions from home to the lab)
10. Walk narrow base of support, step, sideways, backward avoiding the obstacles (holding a basket)	Recount daily activities
11. Walk and kick a ball to hit the cans	
12. Walk and reach and trunk twisting	

Adapted from Silsupadol P, Shumway-Cook A, Woollacott M. Training of balance under single and dual task conditions in older adults with balance impairment: three case reports. Phys Ther 2006;86:269–281, with permission of the American Physical Therapy Association.

gait tested under single- and dual-task conditions, suggesting that dual-task exercise programs are both feasible and beneficial for improving walking ability following stroke. Their impact on balance after stroke is unknown.

Intervention at the Functional-Task Level

The ability to perform skilled functional movements in a natural (home or community) environment requires the ability to adapt postural strategies to changing task and environmental demands. Patients who have a neurologic disorder may have difficulty in perceiving relevant factors within a specific task or environment that serve to regulate postural control. Hence, they may have difficulty in adapting sensory and movement strategies appropriately. Thus, optimal recovery requires practicing the maintenance of postural control in a wide variety of tasks and environments, requiring the adaptation of postural strategies to changing conditions.

Research Evidence. What evidence do we have that task-oriented training improves balance and the performance of functional activities in both geriatric and neurologic populations? Despite the growing research in this area, it can be difficult to draw conclusions because of differences in how task-oriented intervention is defined. In some cases, task-oriented therapy is defined by the repetitive practice of functional tasks, with no interventions targeting underlying impairments such as strength. In other cases, a task-oriented approach to therapy uses multidimensional exercises, including strength, flexibility, balance, functional-task practice and endurance training. Because of these varying definitions, meta-analyses comparing task-oriented therapy to other forms of intervention can be difficult.

Several studies have demonstrated the positive effects of a multidimensional exercise program on balance and mobility function in community-living older adults. Shumway-Cook and colleagues (1997b) used a multidimensional exercise program including combinations of lower-extremity strength and flexibility exercises, static and dynamic balance exercises, repetitive functional-task practice, and participation in an aerobic activity (usually a progressive walking program) to improve balance and mobility function in balance-impaired older adults. Activities targeted improving steady-state balance in sitting, standing, and walking; anticipatory balance activities, including reaching, lifting, turning, changing the base of support (narrow base of support, single-limb stance, tandem stance), stepping over and around obstacles, walking forward and backward at different speeds, and walking on different surface types and configurations with and without packages; reactive balance (perturbations of varying sizes, speeds, and directions performed while sitting and standing); and sensory training (varying availability of visual and somatosensory cues). Exercises became progressively more challenging over the 8-week program. Compared to the nonexercising control group, the group that exercised had significant improvement on all balance measures, including the BBS, DGI, and POMA.

Similar results have been reported in other studies. Wolf et al. (2001) undertook a randomized, controlled trial to investigate the effects of a multidimensional exercise program based on a systems theory of postural control to improve balance in older adults (≥75 years of age). They found that 12 sessions of individualized balance training (over 4 to 6 weeks) significantly improved performance on the BBS and the DGI, which was maintained at 1 month, but was not maintained at 1 year. Judge et al. (1993) studied community-dwelling older adults (62 to 75 yr) in a training program that combined lower-extremity resistance training, brisk walking, and Tai Chi training versus flexibility training alone (three times per week for 6 months). They found that balance performance did improve in the Tai Chi/resistance training group, but not in the flexibility group. Single-leg-stance center of force displacement decreased by 18% in the Tai Chi/resistance training group ($p = 0.02$).

A number of studies have examined the effectiveness of exercise on improving balance and functional performance in persons with different types of neurologic pathology. Vearrier and colleagues (2005) used a task-oriented approach, delivered as intensive massed practice (6 hr/day for 2 consecutive weeks) to retrain balance in 10 patients with chronic stroke disability. In addition to significant improvements in the steady-state and anticipatory aspects of balance control, patients also showed significant improvements in their ability to recover from unexpected perturbations to stance. Weight-bearing symmetry improved, and patients significantly reduced the number of falls following training.

Duncan and colleagues (1998) compared the effects of a 12-week multidimensional home-based exercise program (resistance strength training, balance exercises, functional training of upper extremities, and an aerobic component of progressive walking or progressive bicycling) to usual care in patients with poststroke hemiparesis. Both groups showed equivalent improvements on other measures, including the Berg Balance Test, 6-Minute Walk Test, Barthel Activities of Daily Living, and other tests; however, the home-based exercise group performed significantly better than the usual-care group on the Fugl-Meyer Test (lower-extremity function portion) and in gait velocity.

Marigold et al. (2005) compared two types of community-based group exercise on functional balance, mobility, postural reflexes, and falls in 61 older adults with chronic stroke (> 6 months after stroke). Thirty patients were randomly assigned to an agility program involving a series of progressively more difficult balance tasks, including standing in various postures, walking with various challenges, and standing perturbations (instructor pushing participant). Tasks were performed with eyes open and eyes closed and when standing on both firm and foam surfaces. Thirty-one patients were randomly assigned to a stretching/weight-shifting program focused on slow, low-impact movements that incorporated Tai Chi–like movements stressing increased weight bearing of the paretic lower limb. Both exercise interventions were effective in improving performance on all outcome measures, including the BBT, TUG, and ABC, and these improvements were maintained at 1 month after testing. On the platform recovery measures, only the agility group improved onset latencies of postural muscles in the paretic limb, and this was associated with a concomitant decrease in falls.

Hammer et al. (2008) completed a systematic review of 14 randomized, controlled studies related to balance training after stroke. This review concluded that balance following stroke could be improved at all stages of recovery. In addition, a variety of interventions were effective in improving balance after stroke.

Impaired balance and walking is a significant problem among patients with cerebellar pathology. Gill-Body and colleagues (1997) examined the effect of a 6-week staged, home-based intervention approach that provided progressive challenges to body stability in standing and walking in two patients with cerebellar dysfunction (a 36-year-old woman with a 7-month history of unsteadiness and dizziness following surgical resection of a recurrent astrocytoma in the cerebellar vermis, and a 48-year-old man with a 10-year history of progressive balance problems due to cerebrotendinous xanthomatosis and diffuse cerebellar atrophy). Table 11.8 shows the rehabilitation treatment program and its rationale, used with the female patient who had a resected cerebellar tumor. Both patients reported improved steadiness during stance and gait (significant improvements on the Dizziness Handicap Index). In addition, there was a concomitant improvement on both clinical and laboratory tests of balance. Kinematic analysis showed a decrease in sway in the standing position. Posturography tests showed that the ability to stand under altered sensory conditions improved, as did the ability to respond to external perturbations to balance. Patients were able to more quickly take a step as needed, and in addition, were better able to scale the magnitude of postural responses to perturbations of differing sizes. The authors conclude that patients with cerebellar lesions (whether acute or chronic) can significantly improve postural stability following a structured exercise program (Gill-Body et al., 1997).

Results from research in both geriatric and neurologic populations are remarkably similar. It appears that exercise is an effective way to improve balance and that these improvements are associated with enhanced performance on functional tasks and a reduction in falls. Multidimensional exercises appear to be more effective in improving balance than exercises targeting a single system (e.g., strength, flexibility, or aerobic conditioning). Finally, effective interventions for improving balance include activities that target specific components of postural control; in addition, activities should be systematically progressed to increase the challenge to balance over the duration of intervention.

Improving Participation — Evidence-Based Fall Prevention

As discussed earlier, the overall goal of task-oriented balance rehabilitation is to improve participation outcomes, reflected in an improved ability to participate in the social roles, tasks, and activities that are important in the daily life of the patient. Improved participation can be demonstrated by increased frequency and independence when performing daily tasks and activities. Improved participation may also be reflected in a reduced frequency of falls, as well as increased confidence. Because of the social and economic impact of falls, considerable research has focused on strategies to reduce the risk for falls among older adults. Less research is available on the impact of therapeutic interventions to reduce falls among patients with neurologic pathology.

Research Evidence. There have been several systematic reviews examining the effects of various therapeutic interventions, including exercise and balance training, on reducing falls in older adults (Campbell & Robertson, 2007; Gillespie et al., 2009; Howe et al., 2007; Rubenstein & Josephson, 2001; Sherrington et al., 2008). The Cochrane review by Gillespie et al. (2009) included 111 randomized, clinical trials and examined the effect of different types of interventions

TABLE 11.8 Rehabilitation Treatment Program for a Patient with Imbalance Caused by a Resected Cerebellar Tumor

Rationale	Treatment Activity
Phase 1	
Promote use of VOR and COR for gaze stability	Visual fixation, EO, stationary target, slow head movements
Promote use of saccadic eye movements for gaze stability	Active eye and head movements between two stationary targets
Promote VOR cancellation	EO, moving target with head movement, self-selected speed
Improve ability to use somatosensory and vestibular inputs for postural control	Static stance, EO and EC, feet together, arms close to body, head movements
Improve ability to use vestibular and visual inputs for postural control	Static stance on foam surface, EC intermittently, feet 2.54–5.08 cm (1–2 in.) apart
Improve postural control using all sensory inputs	Gait with narrowed base of support, EO, wide turns to right and left
Improve postural control using visual and vestibular inputs	March in place, EO, on firm and foam surfaces, prolonged pauses in unilateral stance
Phase 2	
Promote use of VOR and COR for gaze stability	Visual fixation, EO, stationary and moving targets, slow and fast speeds, simple static background; imaginary visual fixation, EC
Promote use of saccadic eye movements for gaze stability	Active eye and head movements between two targets, slow and fast speeds
Promote VOR cancellation	EO, moving target with head movement, fast and slow speeds
Improve ability to use somatosensory and vestibular inputs for postural control	Semitandem stance, EO and EC, arms crossed
Improve ability to use vestibular inputs for postural control	Stance on foam, EC intermittently, feet 2.54–5.08 cm apart
Improve postural control using visual and vestibular inputs	Gait with EO with sharp 180-degree turns to the right and left, firm and padded surfaces
Improve postural control using vestibular and somatosensory inputs	March in place, EC, prolonged pauses in unilateral stance
Improve postural control using all sensory inputs	Walking sideways and backward; standing EO and EC, heel touches forward, toe touches backward
Improve postural control with head moving using all sensory inputs	Gait with EO, normal base of support, slow head movements
Phase 3	
Promote use of VOR and COR for gaze stability	Visual fixation, EO, stationary and moving targets, various speeds, complex static and dynamic backgrounds; imaginary visual fixation, EC
Promote use of saccadic eye movements for gaze stability	Active eye and head movements between two targets, various speeds
Promote VOR cancellation	EO, moving target with head movement, various speeds, complex static and dynamic backgrounds

(continued)

TABLE 11.8 Rehabilitation Treatment Program for a Patient with Imbalance Caused by a Resected Cerebellar Tumor

Improve ability to use somatosensory and vestibular inputs for postural control	Semitandem stance with EC continuously, and with EO on firm and padded surfaces
Improve postural control using vestibular and somatosensory inputs	Gait with EC with base of support progressively narrowed, firm and padded surfaces; march in place slowly, EO and EC on firm and foam surfaces
Improve postural control using visual and vestibular inputs	Gait with EO, rapid sharp turns to right and left, firm and padded surfaces
Improve postural control when head is moving using all sensory inputs	Gait with normal base of support, EO, fast head movements
Improve postural control using all sensory inputs	Braiding; active practice of ankle sway movements; bending and reaching activities

COR = cervico-ocular reflex; EO = eyes open; EC = eyes closed; VOR = vestibulo-ocular reflex.

Reprinted with permission from Gill-Body KM, Popat RA, Parker SW, Krebs DE. Rehabilitation of balance in two patients with cerebellar dysfunction. Phys Ther 1997;77:534–552.

on both the rate of falls (falls per person-year shown as the rate ratio) and the number of participants sustaining at least one fall during follow-up (risk ratio). This review included 43 clinical trials related to exercise. The main findings from the review included: (1) assessment and multifactorial intervention reduced the rate of monthly falls (rate ratio, 0.75; 95% confidence interval [CI], 0.65 to 0.86), but not the number of people who fell; (2) home safety interventions did not reduce either the rate of falls or the number of people who fell, but were effective in people with severe visual impairment, and in others at higher risk of falling; and (3) medication management, including withdrawal of psychotropic medications reduced the rate of falls (rate ratio, 0.34; 95% CI, 0.16 to 0.73), but not the risk of falling. The review also reported the effects of different types of exercise programs on fall rate and risk for falls. Multiple-component group exercise reduced both the rate of falls (rate ratio, 0.78; 95% CI, 0.71 to 0.86) and the number of people at risk for falls (risk ratio, 0.83; 95% CI, 0.72 to 0.97), as did Tai Chi (rate ratio, 0.63; 95% CI, 0.52 to 0.78; risk ratio, 0.65; 95% CI, 0.51 to 0.82). In addition, individually prescribed multiple-component home-based exercise significantly reduced both the rate of falls (rate ratio, 0.66; 95% CI, 0.53 to 0.82) and the number of persons falling (risk ratio, 0.77; 95% CI, 0.61 to 0.97). While the review found evidence to support the role of exercise in fall prevention among older adults, it also cautioned that it may not be possible to prevent falls completely, but among people who fall frequently, it may be possible to reduce the number of falls. In addition, the report concluded that there was no evidence to support the efficacy of any intervention on falls among persons with stroke or Parkinson's disease or after a hip fracture.

Several studies have found that a single intervention such as exercise can be as effective in reducing falls as complex multifactorial interventions (Campbell & Robertson, 2007; Gardner et al., 2000; Sherrington et al., 2008). However, these reviews are consistent in suggesting that exercise by itself is effective in reducing the rate of falls only if: (1) it targets people whose primary risk factors are improved by exercise (e.g., impaired balance, gait, and lower-extremity strength), and (2) it is of sufficient intensity to modify these risk factors (Gardner et al., 2000; Sherrington et al., 2008). How much exercise, and what type, is needed to reduce falls? Critical attributes of successful fall-prevention exercise trials included a total dose (a combination of frequency of exercise on a weekly basis with total duration) of >50 hours of training, and the presence of highly challenging balance training.

These systematic reviews suggest that exercise (including combinations of balance, strength, and endurance training) can improve balance and reduce falls in community-living older adults. In order to be effective, exercise has to be of sufficient duration and intensity (although optimal range and intensity has yet to be completely defined) and targeted to people whose primary risk factors for falls can be reduced by exercise.

Putting It All Together

In our task-oriented approach to retraining the patient with postural control problems, therapeutic strategies are used to: (a) improve impairments in underlying systems critical to postural control (e.g., exercises to improve strength and range of motion); (b) develop and refine task-specific sensory, motor and cognitive strategies used for postural control; and (c) learn to maintain postural control during changing task and environmental conditions, thus maximizing the person's ability to participate in the social roles, tasks, and activities that are essential to the quality of their lives.

It is important to realize that one does not work on these goals sequentially, but rather in parallel. Thus, therapeutic strategies for achieving these goals are intertwined; this reciprocal interweaving of exercises, tasks, and activities supports the goal of recovery of postural control, enabling the reestablishment of functional independence and participation.

In addition, rehabilitation of the patient with postural-control problems needs to be organized around learning theory. This will help to ensure that improvements in performance gained through therapy are converted to permanent changes in behavior and retained in varied and novel environments. Patients need to practice the desired behavior (in the case of balance, effective control of the COM within the context of a goal-directed functional task) with sufficient duration and intensity to induce plasticity within the central nervous system.

How much practice is enough to induce neural change? Views on this issue are changing. Traditionally, practice was restricted to the hours a patient spent in therapy sessions. With increasing awareness that more practice is needed to induce permanent change, patients were given "homework," that is, exercises, tasks and activities to be practiced for varying amounts of time (usually 30 to 60 minutes) daily.

New views are emerging suggesting that even this amount of practice may be insufficient to induce permanent change in functional-movement behavior in patients following a neurologic injury. Edward Taub, a psychologist at the University of Alabama, developed Constraint-Induced (CI) Movement Therapy, an approach to retraining upper-limb function based on the concept of learned nonuse (Taub, 1980, 1993). Working with other colleagues, he found that significant changes in both the frequency and the quality of functional movement of the paretic arm occurred after 10 days of intensive therapy, involving 6 hours of forced use of the paretic limb (the noninvolved limb was constrained in a sling) (Liepert et al., 1998; Miltner et al., 1999; Taub et al., 1998). These authors go on to suggest that the same improvement in function can be found with conventional therapy delivered over the same period, suggesting that the critical variable in recovery may not be the nature of the therapy, but rather the frequency and intensity with which it is delivered (Liepert et al., 1998).

Motor learning theory also tells us that in order to optimize motor schemas, practice needs to be under varied conditions. Retraining under varied conditions helps a patient learn the "rules" for postural control, rather than a single way for controlling the COM. This ensures that the individual will be able to maintain stability in the face of new and changing task and environmental conditions.

Evidence-based balance rehabilitation means integrating the best available research evidence, with clinical expertise and a patient's preferences regarding treatment. Research related to treatment of instability can help guide a clinician to make choices regarding how to treat impaired balance. Research can provide a rationale for treatment selection, and help determine probable outcomes in a patient. Lab Activity 11.3 provides a framework for developing a treatment program for the patient from Lab Activity 11.2, Jean J, our patient with impaired balance following a stroke. Complete the table proposed in Lab Activity 11.3, identifying the specific individual system to be targeted (column 1), the task or activity to be practiced (column 2), the environmental conditions under which practice will occur (column 3), and the research evidence that supports this aspect of treatment.

SUMMARY

1. A task-oriented approach to examining postural control uses a variety of tests, measurements, and observations to: (a) document functional abilities related to posture and balance control, (b) examine sensory, motor, and cognitive strategies used to maintain or regain stability, and (c) determine the underlying impairments contributing to abnormal postural control. In addition, an important part of examination is understanding the impact of impaired balance on the person's ability to participate in the social roles, activities, and tasks important to their lives.
2. Following completion of the examination, the clinician must interpret results, identifying functional limitations and underlying impairments, and establish the goals and plan of care.

LAB ACTIVITY 11-3

Objective: Apply a task-oriented approach to retraining posture and balance to a patient with post stroke hemiparesis. To identify the research evidence to support clinical decisions regarding specific treatment interventions.

Procedure: Reread the case study presented in Assessment Tool 11.6 and your assignment from Lab Activity 11.2. Review the list of functional problems, strategies, and impairments you outlined.

Assignment: Create a table identifying the various treatments you will use to improve balance in Jean. List the specific individual system to be targeted (column 1), the task or activity to be practiced (column 2), the environmental conditions under which practice will occur (column 3), and the research evidence that supports this aspect of treatment. For example, you may select to do progressive resistance strength training with Jean because weakness is an underlying impairment contributing to her impaired balance and function. The individual component listed in the table is Motor: Strength, the task is strength training, the specific environmental conditions you choose may be free weights at 60% 1 repetition maximum (RM). Several research studies support your decision to incorporate progressive resistive strength training with Jean, including the meta-analysis by Ada et al. (2006). Is strength training alone enough to ensure recovery of balance? What other aspects of balance will you train? What research supports your decision?

Individual Component of Balance	Task or Activity	Environmental Conditions	Research Evidence
Motor: Strength	Progressive resistance strength training	Free weights, 60% of 1 RM	Ada et al. (2006)

3. The plan of care for retraining postural control in the patient with a neurologic deficit will vary widely, depending on the constellation of underlying impairments and the degree to which the patient has developed compensatory strategies that are successful in achieving postural demands in functional tasks.
4. The goals of a task-oriented approach to retraining postural control include: (a) resolve or prevent impairments, (b) develop effective task-specific strategies, and (c) adapt task-specific strategies so that functional tasks can be performed in changing environmental contexts, thereby maximizing the recovery of participation and minimizing disability.
5. The goals of interventions aimed at the impairment level are to correct the impairments that can be changed and prevent the development of secondary impairments.
6. The goal of intervention at the strategy level involves helping patients recover or develop sensory, motor, and cognitive strategies that are effective in meeting the postural demands of functional tasks. This requires that the clinician understand the inherent requirements of the task being performed so that patients can be guided in developing effective strategies for meeting task demands.
7. The goal of intervention at the functional level focuses on having patients practice successfully the performance of a wide collection of functional tasks in a variety of contexts. Since the ability to perform postural tasks in a natural environment requires the ability to modify strategies to changing task and environmental demands, the patient's developing adaptive capacities is a critical part of retraining at the task level, thus enabling participation and reducing disability.
8. The development of clinical methods based on a systems theory of motor control is just beginning. As systems-based research provides us with an increased understanding of normal and abnormal postural control, new methods for assessing and treating postural disorders will emerge.

ANSWERS TO THE LAB ACTIVITIES

Lab Activity 11-1

1. The Berg Balance Test is heavily weighted toward tasks requiring steady-state and anticipatory postural control. Steady-state balance in sitting and standing is tested in items 2 and 3.
2. Anticipatory postural control could be inferred from items 1, 4, 5, 7, 8, 9, 10, 11, 12, 13, and 14. One item (6) manipulates vision, testing a sensory component of postural control. Items 7, 13, and 14 examine balance with a reduced base of support, which increases the demands for mediolateral stability, and is often associated with a shift in movement strategy.
3. There is no task (such as the nudge test in Tinetti's POMA test) that requires reactive postural control. In addition, most items are performed while standing; hence, stability during walking tasks is not tested. This does not mean that the Berg Balance Test is a poor test; it just indicates the limitations of the test with respect to the systems conceptual framework.

Lab Activity 11-2

1. A review of her examination findings suggest that Jean's functional limitations are primarily found in stance and gait (although her mobility problems will be discussed in the next section of the book), while seated activities can be performed without loss of balance.
2. Based on a Berg Balance Scale score of 32, her estimated fall risk would be 99%, however, it is important to remember that the relationship between the Berg score and fall risk was developed with community-dwelling older adults with no history of stroke. We therefore have to be careful applying this information to someone who has had a stroke.
3. Problems in stance include a reduced ability to lift heavy objects, lean over to retrieve things from the floor, step up onto surfaces without support, stand with a reduced base of support, or maintain stance stability when she turns her head and trunk. In addition, she has difficulty recovering a stable stance position following a perturbation, particularly one that requires a change in base of support (step). This suggests problems primarily in anticipatory and reactive (but not in steady-state) postural control in stance.
4. She appears to move primarily at the hips when recovering balance (hip strategy) and has difficulty stepping with the paretic limb.
5. She is able to stand on a firm surface with eyes open and closed, but is unable to maintain stability on a foam surface with eyes open (or closed), suggesting she may rely on somatosensory inputs for postural control. This suggests that she might have problems maintaining stability when on uneven surfaces, inclines, or moving surfaces.

With a better understanding of the functional limitations she is experiencing and the components of balance control that may be contributing to her balance problems, we can turn to establishing a plan of care that incorporates a balance-retraining program to improve her balance, enhance function, and reduce her risk for falls.

Lab Activity 11-3

It is important to remember that there is no single correct way to train balance in Jean. It is essential that all aspects of postural control be included in her rehabilitation program (e.g., steady-state, anticipatory, and reactive) and that a range of tasks and conditions be used to help her develop a variety of postural control strategies so that she is able to maintain balance in a wide diversity of tasks and conditions. The specific order, duration, and timing of each activity may vary from therapist to therapist.

We begin by determining Jean's main concern and goals related to her balance. She expresses concern that she be able to perform the activities done during standing and while walking (dressing, grooming, transferring, etc.) safely (with confidence that she will not fall) and without assistance. She is confident in her ability to maintain balance while performing sitting activities, and this is consistent with her performance on the tests and measures used to evaluate balance.

So our approach to training balance will focus both on improving underlying impairments (her weakness and reduced range of motion) and on practicing functional tasks in standing and walking, since she appears to have fairly good balance in the seated position (the specifics of training mobility will be discussed in later chapters).

Activities will progress from more "static" balance activities, such as practice maintaining a steady position in sitting and standing (steady-state balance) without support in a simple, fairly predictable environment (flat surface/well lit), to more dynamic activities performed in less predictable environments (on unstable surfaces) and under varying visual conditions (low light, and in the presence of external visual motion cues). She will practice a variety of skilled functional activities that are goal-directed and that involve varying requirements for anticipatory (reaching, lifting, turning, weight shift, stepping, sit to stand, stand to sit, etc.) and reactive (responding to unexpected perturbations in different directions, speeds, and amplitudes) postural control.

We will systematically vary the conditions under which she practices functional tasks, including varying the sensory and cognitive demands. This will allow her to solve stability problems under varying conditions, developing flexibility and adaptability critical to her ability to maintain stability when she performs functional tasks in her own environment.

We will try to incorporate motor learning principles into her training. Initially, we will have her practice functional tasks in a blocked manner (practicing each task for a time, before switching to a different task). As she improves we

TABLE 11.9 Evidence-Based Treatment of Balance

Individual Component of Balance	Task or Activity	Environmental Conditions	Research Evidence
Motor: Strength	Progressive Resistance Strength Training	Free weights, 60% of 1RM	Ada et al., 2006
Motor: Alignment and symmetrical weight bearing	Sitting Sit to stand Standing	Scales, visual feedback on force plate	Barclay-Goddard et al., 2004; Shumway-Cook et al., 1988; van Peppen et al., 2006; Winstein et al., 1989
Motor: Organization of muscle responses used for reactive balance	Manual perturbations in unsupported sitting and standing.	Vary the direction, speed and amplitude of perturbations to stimulate inplace and stepping responses.	Marigold et al., 2005; Vearrier et al., 2005
Sensory: Organization of sensory inputs for balance	Steady-state, reactive and proactive balance tasks	Eyes open, closed, while wearing opaque glasses, Firm, foam surface, Carpeted surfaces	Bayouk et al., 2006; Bonan et al., 2004; Smania et al., 2008
Cognitive: Dual-task balance training	Steady state, reactive and proactive balance tasks.	Practice balance tasks under dual-task conditions, adding secondary cognitive tasks	Silsupadol et al., 2009a,b Yang et al., 2007a

will shift to a more random practice pattern (alternating the types of tasks she practices), modifying the conditions under which she practices as well (variable practice). As she is reacquiring balance ability, we will vary the timing and extent of the external feedback she is given. Initially we may provide continuous feedback using verbal and manual cues, perhaps providing her a mirror to augment visual cues related to postural stability in sitting and standing as well. As she progresses, we will fade the external cues given, allowing her to develop intrinsic feedback mechanisms for postural control.

There is considerable research to support our clinical decision making regarding this approach to treatment. Table 11.9 presents some examples. What other research can you find to support your evidence-based balance rehabilitation program?

PART III

MOBILITY FUNCTIONS

A key feature of our independence as human beings is mobility.

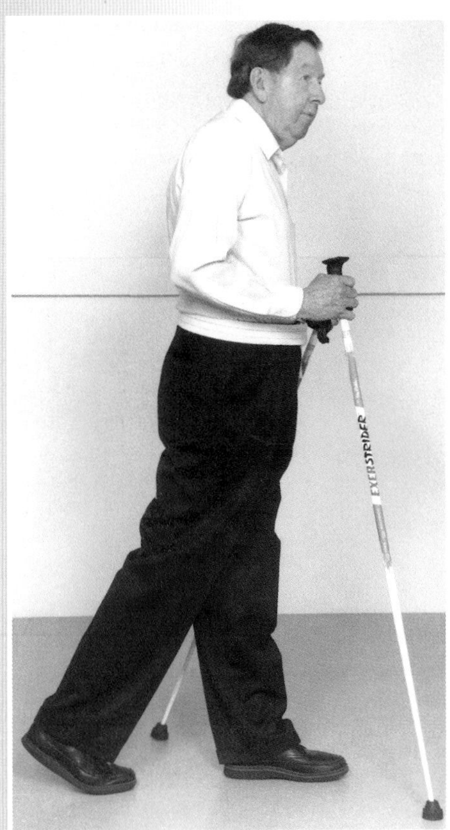

CHAPTER 12

CONTROL OF NORMAL MOBILITY

LEARNING OBJECTIVES

Following completion of this chapter, the reader will be able to:

1. Define the major requirements of locomotion, as well as the goals of each phase of locomotion.
2. Describe the major kinematic, kinetic, and electromyographic parameters that contribute to normal gait.
3. Describe the contributions of neural (sensory, motor, and higher cognitive) and nonneural subsystems to the control of gait.
4. Define the requirements of other forms of mobility, including stair-climbing and transfers

INTRODUCTION

A key feature of our independence as human beings is mobility. We define *mobility* as the ability to independently and safely move oneself from one place to another. Mobility incorporates many types of tasks, including the ability to stand up from a bed or chair, to walk or run, and to navigate through often quite complex environments. During rehabilitation, a primary goal of treatment is to help patients regain as much independent mobility as possible. Often, regaining mobility is the primary goal of a patient. This is reflected in the constantly asked question, "Will I walk again?"

In this chapter we discuss many aspects of mobility, including gait, transfers, bed mobility, and stair walking, examining the contributions of the individual, task, and environment to each of these abilities. We begin with a discussion of locomotion, defining the requirements for successful locomotion and discussing the contributions of the different neural and musculoskeletal systems to locomotor control. In addition, we discuss mechanisms essential for the adaptation of gait to a wide variety of task and environmental conditions. Finally, we consider transitions in mobility, including the initiation of gait and transfers.

Gait is an extraordinarily complex behavior. It involves the entire body and therefore requires the coordination of many muscles and joints. Navigating through complex and often cluttered environments requires the use of sensory inputs to assist in the control and adaptation of gait. Finally, locomotor behavior includes the ability to initiate and terminate locomotion, to adapt gait to avoid obstacles, and to change speed and direction as needed (Patla, 1991). Because of these complexities, understanding both the control of normal gait and the mobility problems of patients with neurologic impairments can seem like an overwhelming task.

To simplify the process of understanding the control of gait, we describe a framework for examining gait that we have found useful. The framework is built around understanding the essential requirements of locomotion and how these requirements are translated into goals accomplished during the different phases of gait. When examining both normal and abnormal gait, it is important to keep in mind both the essential requirements of gait and the conditions that must be met during the stance and swing phases of gait to accomplish these requirements.

ESSENTIAL REQUIREMENTS FOR SUCCESSFUL LOCOMOTION

Locomotion is characterized by three essential requirements: progression, postural control, and adaptation (Das & McCollum, 1988; Patla, 1991). **Progression** is ensured through a basic locomotor pattern that produces and coordinates rhythmic patterns of muscle activation in the legs and trunk that successfully move the body in the desired direction. Progression also requires the ability to initiate and terminate locomotion, as well as to guide locomotion toward end points that are not always visible (Patla, 1997).

The requirement for **postural control** reflects the need to establish and maintain an appropriate posture for locomotion and the demand for dynamic stability of the moving body. Dynamic stability involves counteracting not only the force of gravity, but also other expected and unexpected forces (Patla, 1997).

The third essential requirement of locomotion is the ability to **adapt** gait to meet the goals of the individual and the demands of the environment. Successful locomotion in challenging environments requires that gait patterns be adapted in order to avoid obstacles, negotiate uneven terrain, and change speed and direction as needed.

Finally, these requirements must be accomplished with strategies that are both energy-efficient and effective in minimizing stress to the locomotor apparatus, thus ensuring the long-term structural integrity of the system over the lifespan of the person (Patla, 1997).

Human gait can be subdivided into stance (or support) and swing phases. Certain goals need to be met during each of these phases of gait in order to achieve the three task invariants of successful locomotion (progression, postural control, and adaptability). During the support phase of gait, we need to generate both horizontal forces against the support surface (to move the body in the desired direction [progression]), and vertical forces (to support the body mass against gravity [postural control]). In addition, strategies used to accomplish progression and postural control must be flexible to accommodate changes in speed and direction or alterations in the support surface (adaptation).

The goals to be achieved during the swing phase of gait include advancement of the swing leg (progression) and repositioning the limb in preparation for weight acceptance (postural control). Both the progression and postural control goals require sufficient foot clearance so that the toe does not drag on the supporting surface during swing. In addition, strategies used during the swing phase of gait must be sufficiently flexible to allow the swing foot to avoid any obstacles in its path (adaptation).

The movement strategies used by normal subjects to meet the task requirements of locomotion have been well defined. Kinematic studies describing body motions suggest a similarity in movement strategies across subjects. This is consistent with intuitive observations that we all walk somewhat similarly. In contrast, studies that have described the muscles and forces associated with gait suggest that there is a tremendous variability in the way these gait movements are achieved. Thus, there appears to be a wide range of muscle activation patterns used by normal subjects to accomplish the task requirements of gait.

DESCRIPTION OF THE HUMAN GAIT CYCLE

Let's think about the human body and the control of gait for a moment. We have discussed the essential requirements for normal gait, that is, progression, postural control, and adaptability. The normal human perception–action system has developed elegant control strategies for solving these task requirements.

Although other gait patterns are possible (i.e., we can skip, hop, or gallop), humans normally use a symmetrical alternating gait pattern, probably because it provides the greatest dynamic stability for bipedal gait with minimal control demands (Raibert, 1986). Thus, normal locomotion is a bipedal gait in which the limbs move in a symmetrical alternating motion, which can be described by a phase lag of 0.5 (Grillner, 1981).

A phase lag of 0.5 means that one limb initiates its step cycle as the opposite limb reaches the midpoint of its own cycle (Fig. 12.1). Thus, if one complete stride cycle is defined as the time between two ipsilateral foot strikes (right heel contact to right heel contact (Fig. 12.1), then the contralateral limb begins its cycle midway through the ipsilateral stride cycle.

Traditionally, all descriptions of gait, whether kinematic, electromyographic (EMG), or kinetic are described with reference to different aspects of the gait cycle. Thus, an understanding of the various phases of gait is necessary for understanding descriptions of normal locomotion.

Phases of the Step Cycle

As we mentioned above, the single limb cycle consists of two main phases: stance, which starts when the foot strikes the ground, and swing, which begins when the foot leaves the ground (Fig. 12.1). At freely chosen walking speeds, adults typically spend approximately 60% of the cycle duration in stance, and 40% in swing. As shown in Figure 12.1, approximately the first and the last 10% of the stance phase are spent in double support—the period of time when both feet are in contact with the ground. Single-support phase is the period when only one foot is in contact with the ground, and in walking, this consists of the time when the opposite limb is in swing phase (Murray et al., 1984; Rosenrot et al., 1980).

The stance phase is often further divided into five subphases: (a) initial contact, (b) the loading response (together taking up about 10% of the step cycle, during double-support phase), (c) midstance, (d) terminal stance (about 40% of the stance phase, which is in single support), and (e) preswing (the last 10% of stance, in double support). The swing phase is often divided into three subphases: initial swing, midswing, and terminal swing (all of which are in single-support phase and in total make up 40% of the step cycle) (Enoka, 2002; Perry & Burnfield, 2010).

Typically, researchers and clinicians use electromyography and kinematic and kinetic analysis to analyze gait. For a review of the technology used to analyze gait from these various perspectives, refer to the technology boxes found in Chapter 7.

Temporal and Distance Factors

Gait is often described with respect to temporal and distance parameters such as velocity, step length, step frequency (called "cadence"), and stride length (Fig. 12.1). Velocity of gait is defined as the average horizontal speed of the body measured over one or

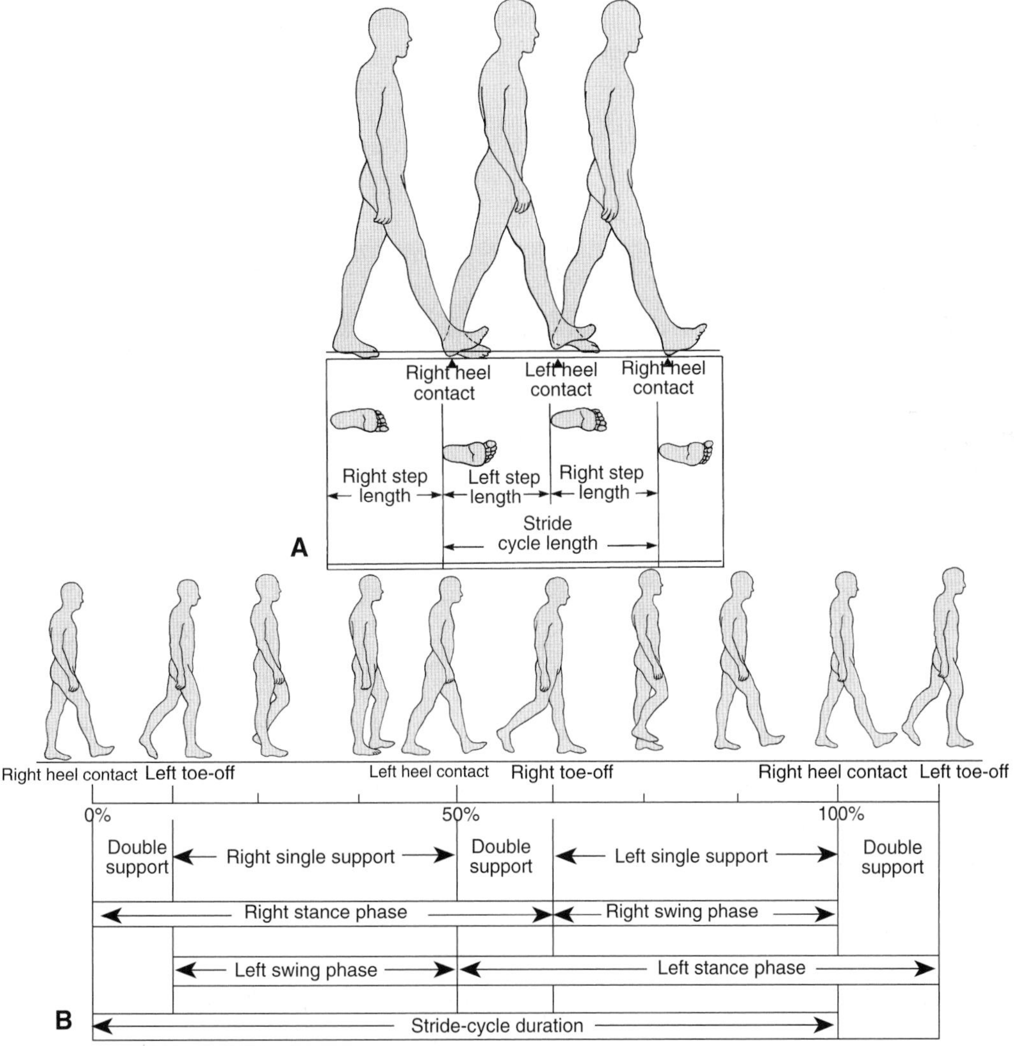

FIGURE 12.1 Temporal and distance dimensions of the gait cycle. A, Step length and stride length characteristics. B, Swing and stance phase characteristics (Adapted with permission from Inman VT, Ralston H, Todd F. Human walking. Baltimore: Williams & Wilkins, 1981.)

more strides. In the research literature, it is usually reported in the metric system (e.g., meters per second) (Perry & Burnfield, 2010). In contrast, in the clinic, gait is usually described in nonmetric terms (feet), and in either distance or time parameters. For example, one might report that the patient is able to walk 50 ft, or that the patient is able to walk continuously for 5 minutes. Because of this difference in convention between the clinic and the lab, we offer information in both metric and nonmetric terms.

Cadence is the number of steps per unit of time, usually reported as steps per minute. **Step length** is the distance from one foot strike to the foot strike of the other foot. For example, the right step length is the distance from the left heel to the right heel when both feet are in contact with the ground. **Stride length** is the distance covered from one heel strike to the next heel strike by the same foot. Thus, right stride length is defined by the distance between one right heel strike and the next right heel strike.

Normal and abnormal gait are often described with reference to these variables. When performing a clinical assessment, there is an advantage to measuring step length, rather than stride length. This is because you will not be able to note any asymmetry in step length if you evaluate only stride length.

How fast do people normally walk? Normal young adults tend to walk about 1.46 m/sec (3.26 mi/hr), have a mean cadence (step rate) of 1.9 steps/sec (112.5 steps/min) and a mean step length of 76.3 cm (30.05 in.) (Craik, 1989).

How do variables such as step length and cadence vary as a function of gait velocity? Complete Lab Activity 12.1 to find out. Walking velocity is a function of step length and step frequency or cadence. When people increase their walking speed, they typically lengthen their step and increase their pace. Although normal adults have a wide range of walking speeds, self-selected speeds tend to center around a small range of step rates, with averages of about 110 steps/min for men and about 115 steps/min for women (Finley & Cody, 1970; Murray et al., 1984). Preferred step rates appear to be related to minimizing energy requirements (Ralston, 1976; Zarrugh et al., 1974). In fact, it has been found that in locomotion we exploit the pendular properties of the leg and the elastic properties of the muscles. Thus, swing phase requires little energy expenditure. A person's comfortable or

LAB ACTIVITY 12-1

Objective: To learn how to calculate temporal and distance parameters of gait.

Procedure: Materials needed for this lab: roll of white paper (1/2-m wide), moleskin cut into 1inch triangle and square shapes, one bottle each of water-soluble red and blue ink, masking tape, cotton swabs, and a stopwatch. Tape a strip of paper 6 m long to the floor at the beginning of each trial. Seat the subject on a chair at one end of the paper. Place one triangle and one square of moleskin approximately at the midline of the sole of each shoe, on the toe and heel, respectively. Saturate the moleskin on the right shoe with red ink and the moleskin on the left shoe with blue ink. Have your subject walk down the paper pathway at a comfortable pace. Use the stopwatch to record the time needed to walk the entire length of the paper. Repeat these procedures, asking subject to walk at his or her fastest pace. You may wish to repeat the lab activity, asking the subject to walk with a variety of assistive devices, such as a cane or walker.

Assignment

From the ink prints on the paper calculate the following for each leg:

1. Step length: vertical distance between heel marker of one foot and the next heel marker of the opposite foot.
2. Stride length: vertical distance between heel marker of one foot and heel marker of the same foot on the next successive step.
3. Step width: horizontal distance between center of heel markers of one foot and the next foot.
4. Cadence: number of steps taken per unit of time (the amount of time taken to walk across the paper divided by the total number of steps).
5. Establish norms (means and standard deviations) for each of these parameters for the subjects tested. Compare your norms with those presented in this chapter. How do spatial and temporal factors change as a function of gait speed? How do they change if an assistive device is used for gait?

(Adapted with permission from Boenig DD. Evaluation of a clinical method of gait analysis. Phys Ther 1977;7:795–798.)

preferred walking speed is at his or her point of minimal energy expenditure per unit distance. At slower or higher speeds, passive pendular models of gait break down, and much more energy expenditure is required (Mochon & McMahon, 1980).

As we increase walking speed, the proportion of time spent in swing and stance changes, with stance phase becoming progressively shorter in relation to swing (Herman et al., 1976; Murray, 1967). Finally, the stance/swing proportions shift from the 60/40 distribution of walking to the 40/60 distribution as running velocities are reached. Double-support time also disappears during running.

As walking speed slows, stance time increases, while swing times remain relatively constant. The double-support phase of stance increases most. For example, double support takes up 25% of the cycle time with step durations of about 1.1 sec, and 50% of the cycle time when cycle duration increases to about 2.5 sec (Herman et al., 1976). In addition, variability increases at lower speeds, probably because of decreased postural stability during the single-support period, which also lengthens with slower speeds.

Within an individual, joint angle patterns and EMG patterns of lower-extremity muscles are quite stable across a range of speeds, but the amplitude of muscle responses increases with faster speeds (Murray et al., 1966; Winter, 1983b; Zarrugh et al., 1974). In contrast, joint torque patterns appear more variable, though they also show gain increases as walking velocity increases.

Kinematic Description of Gait

Another way of describing normal versus abnormal gait is through the kinematics of the gait cycle, that is, the movement of the joints and segments of the body through space. Figure 12.2 shows the normal movements of the pelvis, hip, knee, and ankle in the sagittal, frontal, and transverse planes (Perry, 1992).

The elegant coordination of motion at all the joints ensures the first requirement of gait: the smooth forward progression of the center of body mass. While motion at each individual joint is quite large, the coordinated action of motion across all the joints results in the smooth forward progression of the body.

In the 1950s, Saunders and colleagues (1953) wrote a paper that has significantly affected our ideas regarding the determinants of normal and pathological gait. In that paper, they identified "determinants" of normal walking that they proposed were responsible for saving body energy by minimizing the displacement of the body's center of gravity during gait. This theory is based on simple kinematic arguments. For example, it was noted that if one were to measure hip motion in the sagittal plane during gait, one would see a large amount of flexion and extension (Fig. 12.2). It was proposed that if gait were accomplished solely through these hip movements, the center of mass (COM) would follow these large motions of the hip, and you would see large vertical displacements of the COM. This has been called a "compass gait," and it is seen in people who walk with a stiff knee (Perry & Burnfield, 2010).

According to the theory, the addition of pelvic rotation about the vertical axis to motion at the hip would change the gait pattern, allowing stride length to increase and the amplitude of the sinusoidal oscillations of the COM to decrease. It was suggested that this should result in a smoother path of the COM and a less abrupt transition from step to step.

It was also proposed that the addition of pelvic tilt (rotation of the pelvis about an anteroposterior axis) would flatten the path of the COM even further. Pelvic tilt occurs during swing, when the swing hip lowers in preparation for toe-off. In normal gait, there is a lateral shift in the pelvis that occurs as stance is alternately changed from one limb to the other. The width of the step contributes to the magnitude of the lateral shift of the COM.

It was next proposed that the addition of knee flexion would significantly improve the coordinated efficiency of gait, with knee flexion during stance further flattening the vertical movements of the COM and knee flexion during swing shortening the vertical length of the swing limb and allowing the foot to clear the ground.

Further it was proposed that ankle motion also makes an important contribution to smooth gait (Fig. 12.2). In particular, plantar flexion of the stance ankle would allow a smooth transition from step to step and contribute to the initial velocity of the swing limb (Perry, 1992).

It was also proposed that motion at the three major articulations within the foot is also important in the control of progression and postural control during gait. For example, the subtalar joint, the junction between the talus and calcaneus, allows the foot to tilt medially (inversion) and laterally (eversion). Eversion of the foot begins as part of the loading response, immediately after heel strike, and reaches its peak by early midstance. Following this, the motion slowly reverses, reaching the peak of inversion at the onset of preswing. During swing, the foot drifts back to neutral and then into inversion just before heel strike. Subtalar motion is an essential component of shock absorption during limb loading. In addition, rigidity in this area contributes to foot stability, as weight is transferred to the forefoot in terminal stance.

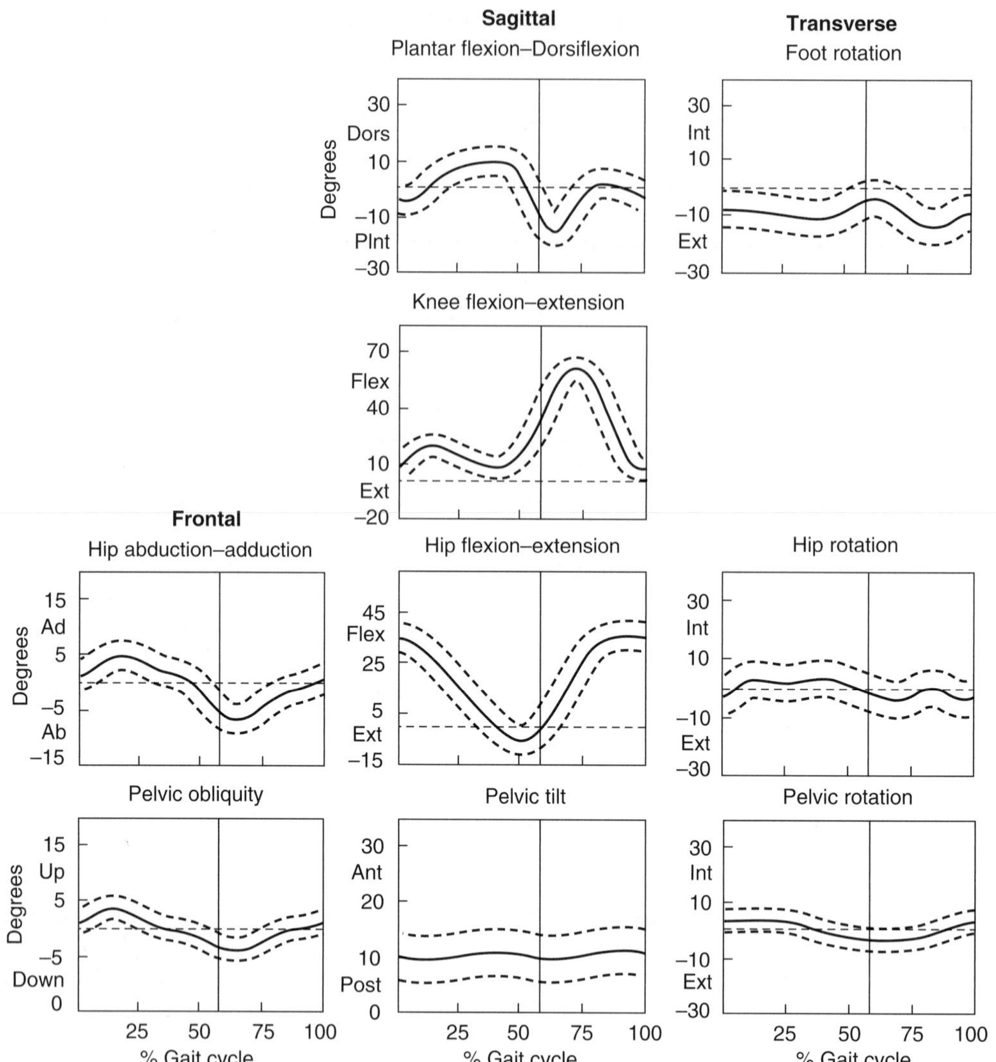

FIGURE 12.2 Normal movements of the pelvis, hip, knee, and ankle in sagittal, frontal, and transverse planes during the gait cycle. (Adapted from DeLuca PA, Perry JP, Ounpuu S. The fundamentals of normal walking and pathological gait. AACP and DM Inst. Course 2, London: Mac Keith Press, 1992.)

The midtarsal joint is the junction of the hindfoot and the forefoot. During loading, the arch flattens quickly; this should allow forefoot contact, and thus contribute to shock absorption. Finally, motion at the metatarsophalangeal joints would allow the foot to roll over the metatarsal heads rather than the tips of the toes during terminal stance (Perry & Burnfield, 2010).

Researchers have noted that this theory of the determinants of gait has a logical appeal, but for many years little research had tested the theory rigorously (Vaughan & Sussman, 1993). Thus, researchers have begun to examine whether gait determinants do reduce the vertical movement of the body during walking, thus decreasing the energy cost. Gard and Childress (1997, 1999) investigated one of the determinants of gait, pelvic obliquity, to determine its effect on the trunk's vertical displacement during walking. Contrary to the predictions of Saunders et al. (1953), they found that pelvic obliquity did not significantly decrease the peak-to-peak vertical movement of the trunk, but simply reduced the mean elevation of the trunk by 2 to 4 mm and shifted the phase of the vertical displacement of the trunk by about 10 to 15 degrees (Gard & Childress, 1997).

They also examined a second determinant of gait, stance-phase knee flexion, and also found that it did not significantly decrease the amplitude of the trunk's vertical displacement. Their data and previous work by others support the concept that stance-phase knee flexion serves a different function, that of shock absorption (Gard & Childress, 1999; Lafortune et al., 1996).

Walking is energy-efficient, but what is responsible for this efficiency? Saunders et al. (1953) suggested that minimization of vertical COM motion is responsible. However, Farley and Ferris (1998) suggest that it is not minimizing vertical COM motion that reduces the metabolic cost of walking, but the smooth mechanical transfer of kinetic and gravitational energies. In fact, the COM must fluctuate in a sinusoidal fashion to achieve efficient transfer of mechanical energy. Research has shown that during walking the body vaults over a relatively stiff stance limb and that the COM reaches its highest point at the middle of the stance phase. Thus, the gravitational potential energy of the COM is at its highest during the midstance phase. In contrast, the kinetic energy of the COM reaches its minimum value at midstance, since the horizontal ground reaction force decelerates the body during the first half of the stance phase and accelerates it during the second half (Farley & Ferris, 1998).

In summary, the step cycle is made up of a complex series of joint rotations, which when coordinated into a whole, provide for a smooth forward progression of the COM. Although Saunders and colleagues (1953) originally predicted that this reduced the energy cost of walking, it is now clear that it is other factors, such as the transfer of mechanical energy (which requires sinusoidal fluctuation of the COM), that reduce the metabolic cost of walking.

Clinical gait assessment relies in part on the observation and description of body motion and joint kinematics. To practice your ability to observe and describe the movements associated with normal and atypical gait patterns, practice Lab Activity 12.2.

Muscle Activation Patterns

Next, we examine the muscle responses during locomotion in terms of their function at each point in the step cycle (Basmajian & De Luca, 1985; Perry & Burnfield, 2010). Despite the variability between subjects and conditions in the EMG patterns that underlie a typical step cycle, certain basic characteristics have been identified.

In general, muscles in the stance limb act to support the body (postural control) and propel it forward (progression). Muscle activity in the swing limb is largely confined to the beginning and end of the swing phase, since the leg swings much like a jointed pendulum under the influence of gravity (McMahon, 1984). Typical EMG patterns during the different phases of the step cycle are shown in Figure 12.3.

LAB ACTIVITY 12-2

Objective: To begin learning how to observe the kinematics of gait.

Procedure: You will need to do this lab in a large room, where your partner can walk for 20 to 30 ft, and you can observe him or her from the side (sagittal plane). Your partner will need to wear shorts. Have your partner walk back and forth. Choose a reference leg, and observe the following from the sagittal plane:

- Observe the stance versus the swing phase of gait.
- Within the stance phase, identify the following events: heel strike, midstance, and push-off.
- Within the swing phase, identify the following events: early swing and late swing.
- Observe the hip at these five points in the gait cycle, and determine whether the hip is flexed, extended, or in a neutral position (i.e., thigh segment is vertical).
- Observe the knee at these five points in the gait cycle, and determine whether the knee is flexed or extended.
- Observe the ankle at these five points in the gait cycle, and determine whether the ankle is dorsiflexed, plantar-flexed, or neutral (90 degrees).

Assignment

You are going to create a graph that plots angular change at each of the three joints as a function of the events observed in the gait cycle. Create a graph for each joint similar to the ones shown in Figure 12.2. On the x-axis, mark the five events you were observing across the step cycle. On the *y*-axis is the angular displacement of the joint. Neutral joint position is represented by a line. Flexion of the joint is above the line, while extension is below the line. Roughly graph the motions you observed at each of the three joints on the graphs. Now compare your results with those found in Figure 12.2. How closely do your graphs approximate those shown in Figure 12.2? If your graphs differ significantly from those shown in the figure, again observe your partner walking, and determine why there is a discrepancy between the two. Is your partner walking with an atypical gait pattern? Or, alternatively, were there errors in your observations?

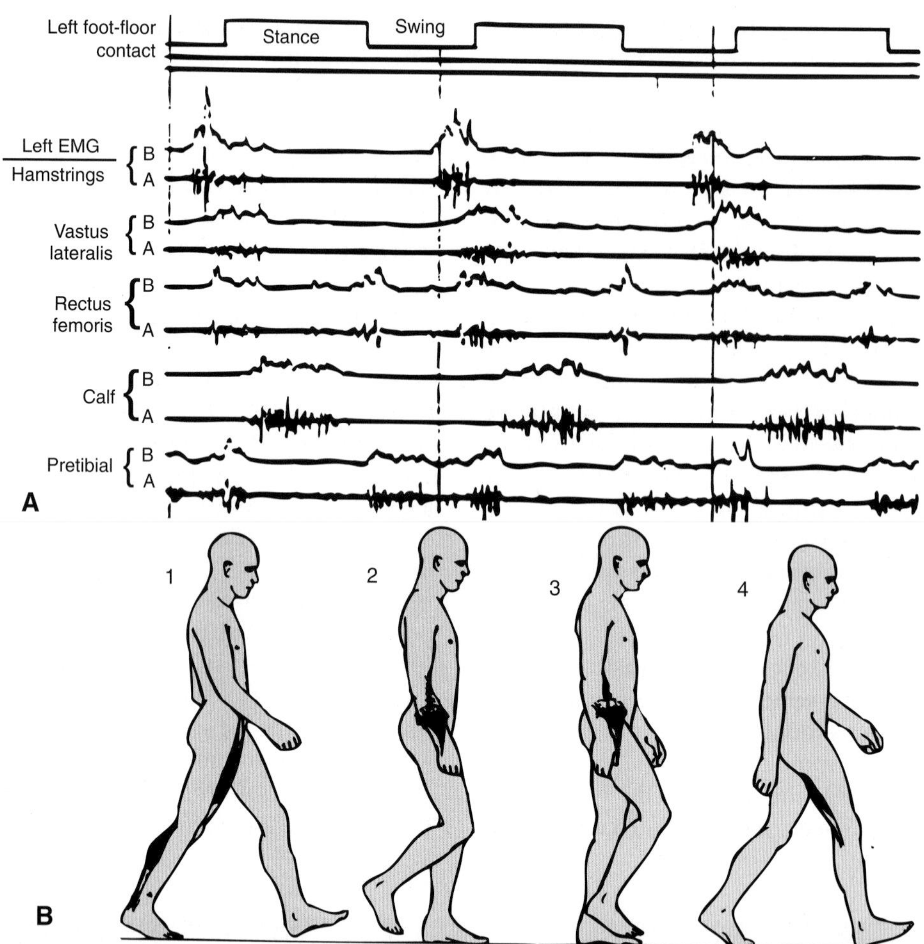

FIGURE 12.3 A, EMG patterns associated with the adult step cycle. Repeatability of muscle activity across three gait cycles. AA, Raw EMG; AB, Rectified and integrated EMG. All muscles are recorded from the left leg. The vertical lines are left foot–floor contact B, Diagram of muscle activity from toe-off until heel strike: 1, Plantar flexors rotate the foot around the ankle and quadriceps straighten the knee, generating a ground reaction force that propels the body forward. 2 and 3, Contraction of the iliopsoas tugs the right leg forward while the knee flexes passively. 4, Hamstrings contract near the end of swing to brake the movement, and heel strike occurs. (Panel A: Adapted with permission from Murray MP, Mollinger LA, Gardner GM, Sepic SB. Kinematic and EMG patterns during slow, free, and fast walking. J Orthop Res 1984;2:272–280; Panel B: Adapted from Lovejoy CO. Evolution of human walking. Sci Am 1988;5:121.)

Remember, there are two goals to be accomplished during the stance phase: (a) postural control: securing the stance limb against the impact force of foot strike and supporting the body against the force of gravity, and (b) progression: subsequent force generation, to propel the body forward into the next step.

To accomplish the first goal, that is, impact absorption for postural stability, knee flexion occurs at the initiation of stance, and there is a distribution of the foot-strike impact from heel contact to the foot-flat stance. At the initiation of stance, eccentric activation of the knee extensors (quadriceps) controls the small knee flexion wave that is used to absorb the impact of foot strike. Eccentric activation of the ankle dorsiflexors (anterior tibialis) decelerates the foot on touchdown, opposing and slowing the plantar flexion that results from heel strike. Thus, both muscle groups initially act to oppose the direction of motion. In addition, postural stability during the stance phase involves activating extensor muscles at the hip, knee, and ankle, which keeps the body from collapsing into gravity. Activation of the hip extensor muscles controls forward motion of the head, arm, and trunk segments as well. By midstance, the quadriceps is predominantly inactive, as are the pretibial muscles.

The second goal in the stance phase is generating a propulsive force to keep the body in motion. There is debate among researchers as to the primary strategy used to propel the body forward during locomotion (Chen & Patten, 2008; Kepple et al., 1997; Neptune et al.,

2001; Perry, 1992; Perry & Burnfield, 2010; Sadeghi et al., 2000; Winter, 1990). Several authors have suggested that generating propulsive forces for progression involves primarily the concentric contraction of the plantar flexors (gastrocnemius and soleus) at the end of stance phase of gait with the assistance of the hip flexors, which provide pull-off (Chen & Patten, 2008; Eng & Winter, 1995; Kepple et al., 1997; Winter, 1990). The "active push-off" theory hypothesizes that the energy generated by the plantar flexor group is transferred to the trunk to provide support and forward progression (Chen & Patten, 2008; Kepple et al., 1997; Neptune et al, 2001; Winter, 1990). The hip extensors are also recognized as a source of both balance and propulsion. During stance, the hip extensors give the body a "push from behind" and also contribute to controlling the movement of the head, arms, and trunk and preventing stance collapse (Eng & Winter, 1995; Sadeghi et al., 2000; Winter, 1990).

In contrast to the active push-off theory, some researchers suggest that forward velocity during walking is generated by a roll-off rather than a push-off (Neptune et al., 2001; Perry, 1992; Perry & Burnfield, 2010). The "controlled roll-off" theory describes forward progression during single-leg stance as a controlled fall. In this theory, the primary action of the ankle plantar flexors during the controlled roll-off is to decelerate tibia rotation and prevent knee flexion as the body rotates over the stance leg. Forward progression is accomplished passively, not actively, because the body moves forward as a result of momentum and inertia (Neptune et al., 2001; Perry, 1992; Perry & Burnfield, 2010).

To clarify the role of the ankle-joint muscles in forward progression, Winter examined the power output at the ankles and knees during walking and found that the generation of forward velocity was associated with a plantar flexor push-off rather than a passive roll-off (Kepple et al., 1997; Winter, 1983a). This was supported by research by Gottschall and Kram (2003), who showed that the generation of propulsive forces by the gastrocnemius makes up about half of the metabolic cost of walking.

The ability of the body to move freely over the foot, in conjunction with the concentric contraction of the gastrocnemius, also means that the COM of the body will be anterior to the supporting foot by the end of stance; this creates the forward fall, noted by Perry (1992), that is also critical to progression. The hip and knee extensors (hamstrings and quadriceps, respectively) may exhibit a burst of activity late in stance as a contribution to propulsion. This activity, however, typically is less important than the activity observed during the impact-absorption phase (Gottschall & Kram, 2003; Kepple et al., 1997; Winter, 1990).

The primary goal to be accomplished in the swing phase of gait is to reposition the limb for continued forward progression. This requires both accelerating the limb forward and making sure the toe clears the ground.

Much of the energy for swing initiation occurs during the preswing phase of gait (Chen & Patten, 2008; Fox & Delp, 2010; Neptune et al., 2001). Preswing has been identified as a key portion of the gait cycle because the muscle forces produced during preswing determine knee flexion velocity at toe-off, and this is correlated to swing-phase peak knee flexion (Fox & Delp, 2010; Reinbolt et al., 2008). Preparation for swing begins in double support, with most of flexion acceleration occurring before the toe leaves the ground; this results in a peak knee-flexion velocity around toe-off (Fox & Delp, 2010). During preswing, hip flexors (iliacus and psoas), with the assistance of the biceps femoris, accelerate the knee into flexion (Fox & Delp, 2010). Forward acceleration of the thigh in the early swing phase is also associated with a concentric contraction of the quadriceps (Fig. 12.3B1). By midswing, however, the quadriceps is virtually inactive as the leg swings through, much like a pendulum driven by an impulse force at the beginning of swing phase. However, the iliopsoas contracts to aid in this forward motion, as shown in Figure 12.3B, 2 and 3. The hamstrings become active at the end of swing to slow the forward rotation of the thigh, in preparation for foot strike (Fig. 12.3B4). Knee extension at the end of swing in preparation for loading the limb for stance phase occurs, not as the result of muscle activity, but as the result of passive nonmuscular forces (Winter, 1984).

Foot clearance is accomplished through flexion at the hip, knee, and ankle, which results in an overall shortening of the swing limb as compared with the stance limb. Again, flexion of the hip is accomplished through activation of the quadriceps muscle. Flexion at the knee is accomplished passively, since rapid acceleration of the thigh will also produce flexion at the knee. Activation of the pretibial muscles produces ankle dorsiflexion late in the swing to ensure toe clearance and to prepare for the next foot fall.

Joint Kinetics

Thus far, we have examined the kinematics or movements of the body during the step cycle and looked at the patterns of muscle activity in each of the phases of gait. What are the typical forces that these movements and muscle responses create during locomotion? The dominant forces at a joint do not necessarily mirror the movements of the joint, as you will see in the discussion that follows.

Determination of the forces generated during the step cycle is considered a kinetic analysis. The kinetic or force parameters associated with the normal gait pattern are less stereotyped than the kinematic or movement parameters. The active and passive muscle forces (called "joint moments") that generate locomotion are themselves quite variable.

Stance Phase

Remember, the goals during stance phase include stabilizing the limb for weight acceptance, shock absorption, and generating propulsive forces for continued motion. Figure 12.4 shows the averaged joint-angle and joint-moment changes observed during one stride cycle. Note that the support moment (top trace of joint-moment graph) during the stance phase of the step cycle (0 to 60% of stride) is the algebraic sum of the joint moments at the hip, knee, and ankle (lower traces) (Winter, 1990). This net extensor moment keeps the limb from collapsing while bearing weight, allowing stabilization of the body and thus accomplishing the stability requirements of locomotion.

However, researchers have shown that people use a wide variety of force-generating strategies to accomplish this net extensor moment. For example, one strategy for achieving a net extensor moment involves combining a dominant hip extensor moment, to counter a knee flexor moment. Alternatively, a knee and ankle extensor moment can be combined to counterbalance a hip flexor moment and still maintain the net extensor support moment (Winter, 1980, 1984, 1990; Winter et al., 1990).

Why is it important to have this flexibility in the individual contributions of joint torques to the net extensor moment? Apparently, this flexibility in how torques are generated is important to controlling balance during gait.

Winter and his colleagues have researched gait extensively and suggest that balance during unperturbed gait is very different from the task of balance during stance (Winter et al., 1991). In walking, the center of gravity does not stay within the support base of the feet, and thus the body is in a continuous state of imbalance. The only way to prevent falling is to place the swinging foot ahead of and lateral to the center of gravity as it moves forward.

In addition, the mass of the head, arms, and trunk (the HAT segment) must be regulated with respect to the hips, as the HAT segment represents a large inertial load to keep upright. Winter and colleagues propose that the dynamic balance of the HAT segment is the responsibility of the hip muscles, with almost no involvement of the ankle muscles. They suggest that this is because the hip has a much smaller inertial load to control, that of the HAT segment, as compared with the ankles, which would have to control the entire body. Thus, they propose that balance during ongoing gait is different from stance balance control, which relies primarily on ankle muscles (Winter et al., 1991).

They note that the hip muscles are also involved in a separate task, that of contributing to the extensor

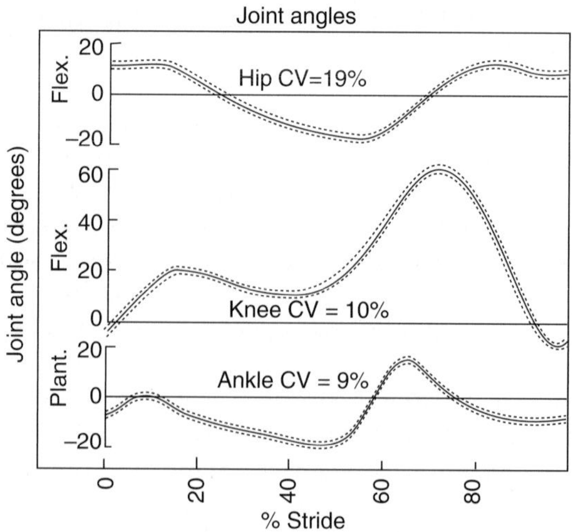

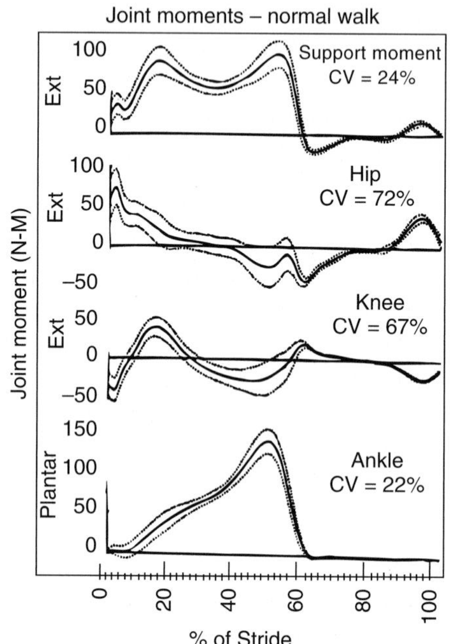

FIGURE 12.4 Top, Joint-angle changes occurring in the hip, knee, and ankle associated with the adult step cycle. Bottom, Individual joint moments (ankle, knee, hip) and the net support moment associated with the adult step cycle during normal walking (normal walk). CV = coefficient of variation; N-M = Newton-meters. Stance phase is approximately the first 60% of the cycle (Adapted with permission from Winter DA. Kinematic and kinetic patterns of human gait: variability and compensating effects. Hum Mov Sci 1984;3:51–76.)

support moment necessary during stance, and view the muscles controlling the HAT segment and those controlling the extensor support moment as two separate synergies. We mentioned above that the net extensor moment of the ankle, knee, and hip joints during stance was always the same, but that the individual moments were highly variable from stride to stride and individual to individual. One reason for this variability is to allow the balance control system to continuously alter the anteroposterior motor patterns on a step-to-step basis. However, the hip balance adjustments must be compensated for by appropriate knee moments in order to preserve the net extensor moment essential for the stance phase of gait (Winter, 1990; Winter et al., 1991).

Does walking speed affect COM displacement? This is an important issue to explore, as many patient populations use a reduced walking speed, which may actually increase COM displacements and make them more unstable. In order to answer this question Orendurff and colleagues (2004) examined COM excursion in normal adults during several walking speeds. They found that the mean (±SD) mediolateral COM displacement was 6.99 ± 1.34 cm at the slowest walking speed (0.7 m/sec) and was reduced significantly, to 3.85 ± 1.41 cm, at the fastest speed (1.6 m/sec). Thus, even normal individuals show substantial mediolateral COM displacement at slow speeds.

Swing Phase

The major goal during swing is to reposition the limb, making sure that the toe clears the ground. Researchers have found that the joint moment patterns during the swing phase are less variable than during the stance phase, indicating that adults use fairly similar force-generating patterns to accomplish this task. This is illustrated by the large standard deviations around the mean joint torques during stance (0 to 60% of stride) as compared with the small standard deviations in swing (60 to 100% of stride), shown in Figure 12.4, bottom graph.

At normal walking speeds, early in swing, there is a flexor moment at the hip that contributes to flexion of the thigh. Early hip flexion is assisted by gravity, reducing the need for a large flexor hip joint moment.

Once swing phase has been initiated, it is often sustained by momentum. Then, as swing phase ends, an extensor joint moment may be required to slow the thigh rotation and prepare for heel strike (Woollacott & Jensen, 1996). Thus, even though the thigh is still flexing, there is an extensor moment on the thigh at this point.

What controls knee motions during swing? Interestingly, during swing, joint torque at the knee is basically used to constrain knee motion rather than to generate motion. In early swing, an extensor moment slows knee-joint flexion and contributes to reversal of the knee joint from flexion to extension. Later in swing, a flexor knee-joint moment slows knee extension to prepare for foot placement (Cavanagh & Gregor, 1975; Winter, 1990, 1993).

At the end of swing phase and during the initial part of stance phase, a small dorsiflexing moment occurs at the ankle, which helps control plantar flexion at heel strike. So even though the ankle motion is one of plantar flexion, the ankle-joint force is a dorsiflexion moment.

Moving through the stance phase, ankle plantar flexion moment increases to a maximum point just after knee flexion, when the ankle begins to plantar flex. The ankle-joint torque is the largest of all the moments of the lower limb and is the main contributor to the acceleration of the limb into swing phase.

So, in many of the previous examples, we see that the joint torque is opposite to that of the limb movement itself. In other words, the joint torque shows us that the combined forces may be acting to brake the movement or control foot fall, rather than simply accelerate the limb.

CONTROL MECHANISMS FOR GAIT

How is locomotor coordination achieved? What are the control mechanisms that ensure that the task requirements for successful locomotion are met? Much of the research examining the neural and nonneural control mechanisms essential for locomotion has been done with animals. It is through this research on locomotion in animals that scientists have learned about pattern formation in locomotion, the integration of postural control to the locomotor pattern, the contribution of peripheral and central mechanisms to adaptation and modulation of gait, and the role of the various senses in controlling locomotion.

The following section reviews some of the research on locomotor control in animals, relating it to experiments examining the neural control of locomotion in humans.

Pattern Generators for Gait

Research in the past 30 years has greatly increased our understanding of the nervous system control of the basic rhythmic movements underlying locomotion. Results of these studies have indicated that central pattern generators within the spinal cord play an important role in the production of these movements (Grillner, 1973; Smith, 1980; Wallen,

1995). A rich history of research has enhanced our understanding of the neural basis of locomotion.

In the late 1800s, Sherrington and Mott (Mott & Sherrington, 1895; Sherrington, 1898) performed some of the first experiments to determine the neural control of locomotion. They severed the spinal cord of animals to eliminate the influence of higher brain centers and found that the hindlimbs continued to exhibit alternating movements.

In a second set of experiments, in monkeys, they cut the sensory nerve roots on one side of the spinal cord, eliminating sensory inputs contributing to stepping on one side of the body. They found that the monkeys did not use the limbs that had undergone de-afferentation during walking. This led them to the conclusion that locomotion required sensory input. A model of locomotor control was created that attributed the control of locomotion to a set of reflex chains, with the output from one phase of the step cycle acting as a sensory stimulus to reflexly activate the next phase.

Graham Brown (1911) performed an experiment only a few years later showing the opposite result. He found that by making bilateral dorsal (sensory)-root lesions in animals whose spinal cord had been transected (called "spinalized animals"), he could see rhythmic walking movements.

Why did the two labs get different results? It appears that it is because Sherrington cut sensory roots on only one side of the spinal cord, not both.

In later experiments, Taub and Berman (1968) found that animals did not use a limb when the dorsal roots were cut on one side of the body, but they would begin to use the limb again when dorsal roots on the remaining side were sectioned. Why? Since the animal has appropriate input coming in from one limb and no sensation from the other, the animal prefers not to use the limb which has no sensation. Interestingly, researchers have found that they can make animals use a single limb that has undergone deafferentation by restraining the intact limb. These results are the rationale behind a therapy approach called the "constraint-induced (or forced-use) paradigm." In this approach, patients with hemiplegia are forced to use their hemiplegic arm, since the intact side is restrained (Taub et al., 1993, 2004; Wolf et al., 1989b).

Other studies have confirmed and extended the results of Graham Brown. These studies have found that muscle activity in spinalized cats is similar to that seen in normal cats walking on a treadmill (Forssberg et al., 1977), with the extensor muscles of the knee and ankle activated prior to paw contact in stance phase. This demonstrates that extension is not simply a reflex in response to contact, but is part of a central program. In addition, the spinalized cat is capable of fully recruiting motor units within the spinal cord when increasing gait from a walk to a gallop (Smith et al., 1979).

Can a spinalized cat adapt the step cycle to clear obstacles? Yes. If a glass rod touches the top of the cat's paw during swing phase, it activates a flexion response in the stimulated leg, with simultaneous extension of the contralateral leg. This lifts the swing leg up and over the obstacle and gives postural support in the opposite leg. Interestingly, the same stimulation of the dorsal surface of the paw during stance causes increased extension, probably to get the paw quickly out of the way of the obstacle. Thus, the identical stimulus to the skin activates functionally separate sets of muscles during different phases of the step cycle, to compensate appropriately for different obstacles perturbing the movement of the paw (Forssberg et al., 1977).

Graham Brown proposed that there was a central pattern generator (CPG) creating the rhythmic alternating flexor and extensor activity in spinal locomotion, which was later called the "half-center" model for gait control. The organization of the half-center CPG involves the following principles. First, each of the limbs is separately controlled by its own CPG. Second, CPGs have two groups of excitatory interneurons—the half-centers—that control the activity of flexor and extensor motoneurons. Third, inhibitory connections between the half-centers allow only one center to be active at a time. Fourth, a fatigue process gradually reduces excitation in the active half-center, allowing phase switching to happen when the reduction in the excitability of one half-center falls below a critical value and the opposing center is released from inhibition. Finally, inhibition of antagonist and agonist motoneurons is tightly coupled (McCrae & Rybak, 2008).

More recently a two-level CPG model has been proposed to address a number of limitations of Graham Brown's model. This model includes both a rhythm generator (RG) and a pattern formation (PF) network. An important characteristic of the model is its ability to independently regulate gait speed (step-cycle periods and phase durations) at the RG level and level of motor neuron activity at the PF level (as this has its own independent mesencephalic locomotor region input). This creates a flexible network for both sensory and descending control of gait that the one-level CPG was not able to accommodate (McCrae & Rybak, 2008).

The pattern-generating circuits in the brainstem reticular formation and spinal cord of a simple vertebrate, the lamprey, have been characterized in great detail in order to understand how network units are precisely coordinated to achieve a proper timing of the different muscle groups in locomotion. Studies have shown that different modulatory systems act on the spinal networks to change the rate of burst activity. For example, brainstem systems activate two types of glutamate receptors (*N*-methyl-D-aspartate [NMDA] and non-NMDA) within the spinal network to activate locomotion. The relative amount of activation of these two types of receptors determines the rate of burst activity. In addition, serotonin systems reduce the burst rate (Grillner et al., 1995; Pearson & Gordon, 2000).

As you can see from this research, although the spinal pattern generators are able to produce stereotyped locomotor patterns and perform certain adaptive functions, descending pathways from higher centers and sensory feedback from the periphery allow the rich variation in locomotor patterns and adaptability to task and environmental conditions.

Descending Influences

Descending influences from higher brain centers are also important in the control of locomotor activity. Much research has focused on identifying the roles of higher centers in controlling locomotion, through transecting the brain of animals along the neuraxis and observing the subsequent locomotor behavior (Pearson & Gordon, 2000). The three preparations that are most often studied are the spinal, the decerebrate, and the decorticate preparations, as shown in Figure 12.5.

In the spinal preparation (which can be made at a level to allow the observation of only the hindlimbs or of all four limbs as part of the preparation), one needs an external stimulus to produce locomotor behavior. This can be either electrical or pharmacological.

The decerebrate preparation leaves the spinal cord, brainstem, and cerebellum intact. An area in the brainstem called the "mesencephalic locomotor region" (MLR in Fig. 12.5) is important in the descending control of locomotion (see Chapter 3 for more information on its control of posture and locomotion). Decerebrate cats will not normally walk on a treadmill, but will begin to walk normally when tonic electrical stimulation is applied to the mesencephalic locomotor region (Shik et al., 1966). Neurons from the MLR activate the medial reticular formation (MRF in Fig. 12.5), which then activates the spinal locomotor system. Weight support and active propulsion are locomotor characteristics seen in this preparation.

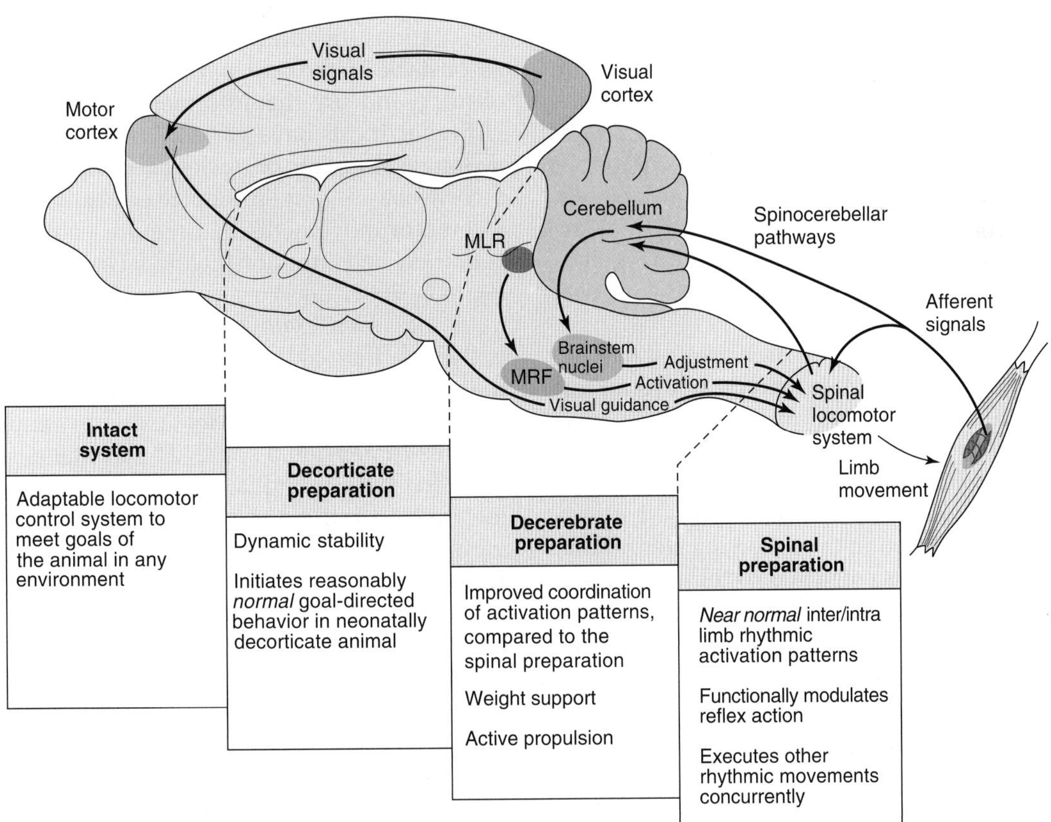

FIGURE 12.5 Diagram of the brain and spinal cord, showing the different sites of lesions used in the study of the contributions of different neural subsystems to gait. (Adapted with permission from Patla AE. Understanding the control of human locomotion: a prologue. In: Patla AE, ed. Adaptability of human gait. Amsterdam: North-Holland, 1991:7.)

When spinal pattern-generating circuits are stimulated by tonic activation, they produce, at best, a bad caricature of walking due to the lack of important modulating influences from the brainstem and cerebellum. This is because normally, within each step cycle, the cerebellum receives afferent feedback from sensory receptors related to locomotion (via spinocerebellar pathways) and sends modulating signals to the brainstem that are relayed to the spinal cord (see Fig. 12.5) via brainstem nuclei (vestibulospinal, rubrospinal, and reticulospinal pathways), which act directly on motor neurons, to fine-tune the movements according to the needs of the task (Grillner & Zangger, 1979).

The cerebellum also may have a very important role in modulation of the step cycle. Experiments suggest that two tracts are involved in this modulation. First, the dorsal spinocerebellar tract is hypothesized to send information from muscle afferents to the cerebellum and is phasically active during locomotion. Second, the ventral spinocerebellar tract is hypothesized to receive information from spinal neurons concerning the CPG output and to send this information also to the cerebellum (Arshavsky et al., 1972a, 1972b).

It is also possible that the cerebellum has an additional role in the modulation of the step cycle. It has been shown that automatic aspects of gait control are regulated by the medial zone of the cerebellum, which receives input from somatosensory, visual, and vestibular systems and sends outputs to the reticular formation of the brainstem. The intermediate zones largely regulate gait through somatosensory input from the limbs, while the lateral cerebellum may adjust gait in novel contexts and when visual guidance is critical (Takakusaki et al., 2008).

Results of this and other research suggest that the cerebellum may also modulate activity, not to correct error but to alter stepping patterns. For example, as an animal crosses uneven terrain, the legs must be lifted higher or lower depending on visual cues about the obstacles encountered. The muscle response patterns may be modulated through the following steps. First, the locomotor rhythm is conveyed to the cerebellum. The cerebellum extrapolates forward in time to specify when the next flexion (or extension) is to occur. The cerebellum would then facilitate descending commands that originate from visual inputs to alter the flexion (or extension) phase at precisely the correct time (Keele & Ivry, 1990).

The decorticate preparation also leaves the basal ganglia intact, with only the cerebral cortex removed. As mentioned in Chapter 3, basal ganglia–brainstem–spinal cord pathways contribute to automatic control of movements such as locomotion and postural tone mainly via pathways originating in the substantia nigra. The substantia nigra–tegmental pathways appear to maintain appropriate postural muscle tone as well as to modulate rhythmic stepping movements and to initiate locomotion. In this preparation, an external stimulus is not required to produce locomotor behavior, and the behavior is reasonably normal goal-directed behavior.

However, the cortex is important in skills such as walking over uneven terrain. In this preparation, vision may have a major role in modulating locomotor outputs (see Fig. 12.5). As reviewed in Chapter 3, the two major pathways involved in visual processing from the primary visual cortex go to the posterior parietal cortex and inferotemporal cortex, often called the "where and what" pathways, or more recently, the "perception and action" pathways (Milner & Goodale, 1993). These pathways help us to visually recognize objects and events from different viewpoints and to process this information from an egocentric perspective, so that we can move efficiently in space. In addition, visual input to the superior colliculus is involved in orienting to novel stimuli in the visual field. It is of interest that walking subjects are aware of the objects around them and alter their steps even when no visual information is currently available about obstacle locations. In addition, cats that have stepped over an obstacle in the past remember the location of that obstacle and use this information to guide stepping. However, if cats have parietal cortex lesions, they can no longer negotiate obstacles successfully. In addition, a corticobasal ganglia loop may also be involved in locomotor movements that require volitional control, cognition, and attention (Lajoie & Drew, 2007; McVea & Pearson, 2009; Takakusaki et al., 2008).

It has been hypothesized that the hippocampus is the site that codes topological information, while the parietal cortex (receiving visual and somatosensory information) provides a metric representation of three-dimensional space. The frontal cortex, along with the basal ganglia, would then transform this information into appropriate spatially directed locomotor movements in an egocentric frame (Paillard, 1987; Patla, 1997).

Do spinal CPGs also contribute to the control of gait in humans? A large amount of evidence from spinal cord–injured individuals during partial-weight-support treadmill walking suggests that CPGs contribute to pattern generation during gait (Dietz, 1997; Zehr & Duysens, 2004). Zehr and Duysens (2004) note that modulation of motor activity correlated with changes in peripheral feedback during gait can also infer CPG activity in humans, and thus activity in a feedback pathway can be used as a probe of CPG activity. As a result of this logic, the modulation of cutaneous reflexes during locomotion in humans has been used to infer the presence of activity of a CPG in humans.

As might be expected, in humans the most convincing evidence for CPGs comes from neonates, as descending pathways from the brain are not developed. For example, stepping is observed in newborns, though they do not have mature pyramidal tracts; in addition, newborns have reflexes to perturbations during walking (Pang & Yang, 2000, 2001, 2002; Pang et al., 2003). In addition, research evidence indicates that limb loading (activating Golgi tendon organs [GTOs]) and hip position (activating muscle spindles) regulate stepping patterns in newborns as they also do in spinalized cats (Pang & Yang, 2000; Yang et al., 1998; Zehr & Duysens, 2004).

Research suggests that, of the two bursts of activity that occur in the tibialis anterior (TA) muscle during unperturbed gait in humans (one at the end of stance and one at the end of swing), the first is primarily activated through the CPG, while the second is primarily cortical in origin. This is supported by clinical evidence that in patients with stroke most problems occur with the second burst (Zehr & Duysens, 2004).

Additional evidence regarding cortical control of locomotion in primates shows that injections of muscimol into the hindlimb region of the motor cortex (M1) cause local paresis of the contralateral hindlimb when walking. This same injection into trunk and hindlimb areas of the supplementary motor area (SMA), which has connections to the reticular formation, disturbed postural control rather than paralyzing the limb. It is also likely that premotor cortex and SMA contribute to planning and programming of locomotion, in addition to postural control, as patients with lesions in these areas show problems with gait initiation and with freezing of gait. This may be because corticoreticular pathways are important for postural preparation before gait initiation (Takakusaki et al., 2008). (See Chapter 3 for more detailed information on locomotor pathways.)

Functional Neural Imaging during Human Gait

It is now possible to record cerebral activity during the gait cycle through neuroimaging techniques like single-photon-emission tomography (SPECT), measuring regional cerebral blood flow, and near-infrared spectroscopy (NIRS), measuring oxygenated versus deoxygenated hemoglobin levels. SPECT studies during gait have shown increased activity in the supplementary motor area, medial primary sensorimotor area, striatum, cerebellar vermis, visual cortex, and dorsal brainstem (Fukuyama et al., 1997; Hanakawa et al., 1999). NIRS techniques have also shown that activity increases in the prefrontal and premotor cortex as locomotor speed increases, while sensorimotor cortex activity was not influenced by speed (Bakker et al., 2007; Suzuki et al., 2004). This research is in its infancy, but it reminds us of the many brain regions that contribute to the control of gait.

Sensory Feedback and Adaptation of Gait

One of the requirements of normal locomotion is the ability to adapt gait to a wide range of environments. Sensory information from all the senses is critical to our ability to modify how we walk. In animals, when all sensory information is taken away, stepping patterns tend to be very slow and stereotyped. The animal can neither maintain balance nor modify its stepping patterns to make gait truly functional. Gait ataxia is a common consequence among patients with sensory loss, particularly loss of proprioceptive information from the lower extremities (Sudarsky & Ronthal, 1992).

There are two ways that equilibrium is controlled during locomotion—reactively and proactively. One uses the reactive mode when, for example, there is an unexpected disturbance, such as a slip or a trip. One uses the proactive mode to anticipate potential disruptions to gait and to modify the way to sense and move in order to minimize the disruption. As in stance, the somatosensory, visual, and vestibular systems all play roles in reactive and proactive postural control of locomotion. The next section describes how sensory information is used to modify ongoing gait.

Reactive Strategies for Modifying Gait

All three sensory systems—somatosensory, visual, and vestibular—contribute to reactive or feedback control of gait. Research on animals and humans has contributed to our understanding of the somatosensory contributions to gait.

Somatosensory Systems. As noted earlier in the chapter, researchers have shown that animals that have both been spinalized and undergone deafferentation can continuously generate rhythmic alternating contractions in muscles of all the joints of the leg, with a pattern similar to that seen in the normal step cycle (Grillner & Zangger, 1979). Does this mean that sensory information plays no role in the control of locomotion? No. Although these experiments have shown that animals can still walk in the absence of sensory feedback from the limbs, the movements show characteristic differences from those in the normal animal. These differences help us to understand the role that sensory input plays in the control of locomotion (Smith, 1980).

First, sensory information from the limbs contributes to appropriate stepping frequency. For example, the duration of the step cycle is significantly longer in cats that have undergone deafferentation than in a chronic spinalized cat (i.e., spinalized previously and allowed to recover) without deafferentation.

Second, joint receptors and muscle-spindle afferents (from the stretched hip flexors) appear to play a critical role in normal locomotion, with the position of the ipsilateral hip joint contributing to the onset of swing phase (Grillner & Rossignol, 1978; Pearson, 1995; Smith, 1980). Studies of decerebrate cats have shown that input from muscle spindles can reset the locomotor rhythm. Activation of both ankle extensor Ia afferents and group II flexor afferents reset the rhythm to extension in fictive locomotion. In addition, small movements about the hip joint produce entrainment of the locomotor rhythm. This continues after anesthetizing the joint capsule, and it gradually is reduced in strength when more hip muscles are denervated. This and other research suggests that muscle spindle afferents from hip flexors influence the rhythm-generating neurons by exciting hip flexor activity. Figure 12.6 shows how hip extension controls the transition from stance to swing. The hip flexor muscle spindle afferents (shown in the diagram of a cat whose hip is oscillating in flexion and extension) are stretched sufficiently at the end of stance phase to excite their own muscle (hip flexor) and inhibit the hip extensors, thus aiding in the stance to swing phase transition (Kriellaars et al., 1994; Pearson & Gordon, 2000).

This information has been used to aid individuals in relearning gait after a stroke. Gait has been retrained using partial body weight support during treadmill walking, and the hip extension as the leg is drawn backward during stance phase on the treadmill aids in the activation of hip flexors to initiate swing phase.

The GTO afferents (the Ib afferents) from the leg extensor muscles can also strongly influence the timing of the locomotor rhythm, by inhibiting flexor burst activity and promoting extensor activity. A decline in their activity at the end of the stance phase may be involved in regulating the transition from stance to

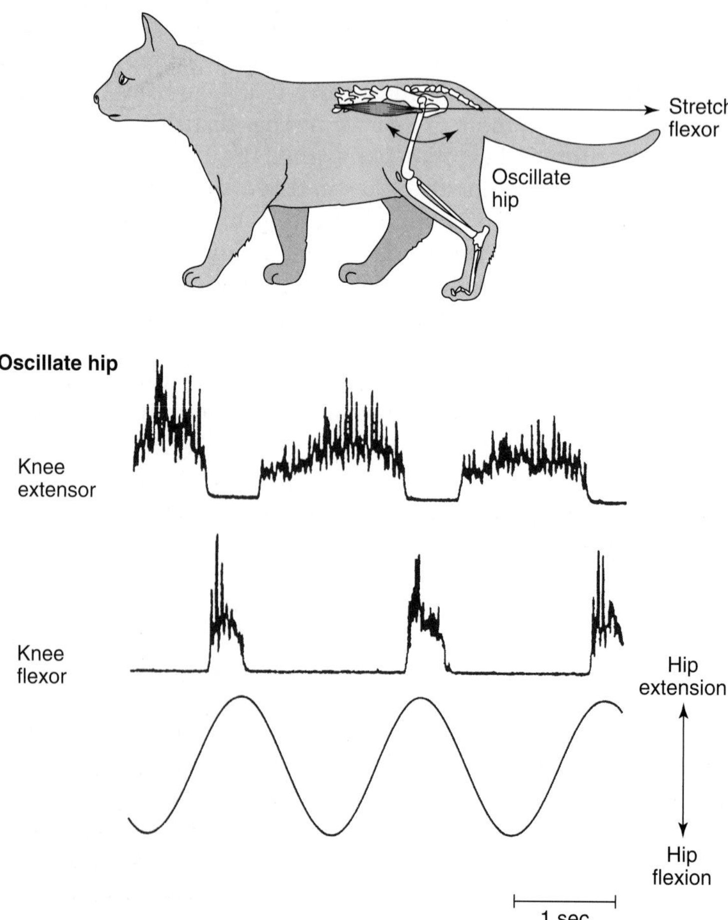

FIGURE 12.6 Cat whose hip is being oscillated in flexion and extension. The flexor muscle is stretched during extension (e.g., in the stance phase of locomotion), and flexor muscle spindle afferents then excite the flexors and inhibit the extensors. (Reprinted with permission from Pearson K, Gordon J. Locomotion. In: Kandel E, Schwartz JH, Jessell TM, eds. Principles of neural science, 4th ed. New York: McGraw-Hill, 2000:748, Fig. 37-8.)

swing. In addition, they may provide a mechanism for automatically compensating for changes in loads carried by extensor muscles. For example, when one walks up an incline, the load increase on the extensor muscles would increase the feedback from the GTOs and automatically increase the activity in the extensor motor neurons. Note that this activity of the GTOs is exactly the opposite of their activity when they are activated passively, when the animal is at rest. At rest, the GTOs inhibit their own muscle, and excite the antagonist muscles, while during locomotion they excite their own muscle and inhibit antagonists (Pearson & Gordon, 2000; Pearson et al., 1992).

Third, cutaneous information from the paw of the chronic spinalized cat has a powerful influence on the spinal pattern generator in helping the animal navigate over obstacles, as discussed above (Forssberg et al., 1977).

It is of interest that in human research on normal adults it is difficult to produce a strong effect on gait transition when performing loading and unloading experiments on the extensor muscles, unlike what was noted above in the cat (Stephens & Yang, 1999). Why do we see this difference? It is probably the case that these cues do not operate in isolation in humans, and other influences may override the unloading effect (Zehr & Duysens, 2004). However, it appears that cutaneous input and stretch reflexes are more tightly controlled during human gait than are loading reflexes. For example, human research, similar to animal research, has shown that these reflexes are enhanced during gait as compared with quiet stance and are highly modulated in locomotion during each phase of the step cycle; this allows them to adapt functionally to the requirements of each phase (Stein, 1991; Zehr et al., 1997).

As was shown in research on cats, cutaneous reflexes actually showed a complete reversal from excitation to inhibition during the different phases of the step cycle. For example, in the first part of swing phase, when the TA is active, the foot is in the air and little cutaneous input would be expected, unless the foot strikes an object. If this happens, a rapid flexion would be needed to lift the foot over the object to prevent tripping. This is when the reflex is excitatory to the TA. However, in the second TA burst, the foot is about to contact the ground, which is a time when a lot of cutaneous input would occur. Limb flexion would not be appropriate at this time, since the limb is needed to support the body. In addition, at this time, the reflex shows inhibition of the TA (Stein, 1991; Zehr & Duysens, 2004). It is interesting that humans have both P1 (short latency) and P2 (middle latency, 75–80 msec) responses to cutaneous stimulation, unlike cats, who show most evidence for P1 responses. It is the P2 responses in humans that show the phase-dependent modulation.

Stretch reflexes in the ankle extensor muscles are small in the early part of the stance phase of locomotion, since this is the time that the body is rotating over the foot and stretching the ankle extensors. A large reflex at this phase of the step cycle would slow or even reverse forward momentum.

On the other hand, the stretch reflex is large when the COM is in front of the foot during the last part of stance phase, since this is the time when the reflex can help in propelling the body forward. This phase-appropriate modulation of the stretch reflex is well suited to the requirements of the task of locomotion as compared with stance. Stretch reflex gains are reduced in running, probably because a high gain reflex response would destabilize the gait in running. Stretch reflex gain changes alter quickly (within 150 msec) as a person moves from stance to walking to running (Stein, 1991).

It is important to note that modulation of stretch reflex amplitudes is sometimes different from that seen in cutaneous reflexes. For example, biceps femoris stretch reflexes are facilitated at the end of swing, supporting the hypothesis that part of this muscle's activation at this time is due to stretch reflex input. This is at a time when cutaneous reflexes to this muscle are suppressed (Zehr & Duysens, 2004).

These studies have shown that spinal reflexes can be appropriately integrated into different phases of the step cycle to remain functionally adaptive. The same outcome occurs in the integration of compensatory automatic postural adjustments into the step cycle. Studies were performed in which subjects walked across a platform that could be perturbed at different points in the step cycle to simulate a slip during walking. Results showed that automatic postural responses were incorporated appropriately into the different phases of the step cycle (Nashner, 1980). For example, postural muscle responses were activated at about 100-msec latencies in the gastrocnemius when this muscle was stretched faster than normal in response to backward surface displacements pitching the body forward. This helped slow the body's rate of forward progression to realign the COM with the backward-displaced support foot. Similarly, responses occurred in the TA muscle when it was shortened more slowly than normal because of forward surface displacements that displaced the body backward. This helped increase the rate of forward progress to realign the body with the forward-displaced foot.

Previous research on the control of steady-state walking has shown that one of the main control issues is keeping the HAT segment well balanced and that the trunk and hip muscles play an active role in this control (Winter et al., 1990). The previous work discussed above on reactive control of balance during gait has shown that the distal perturbed leg muscles are important in this type of control (Gollhofer et al., 1986; Nashner, 1980). However, when a slip occurs, there is not only stretch of the ankle musculature but a challenge to upper-body balance as well. Thus, it is possible that proximal hip and trunk muscle activity may be a primary contributor to both steady-state gait and to the recovery of balance during slips.

Studies recording from bilateral leg, thigh, hip, and trunk muscles have shown that proximal muscles are not the primary muscles contributing to recovery from balance threats during slips in healthy, young adults. Although proximal muscle activity was often present during the first slip trial in young adults, adaptation tended to eliminate it during subsequent trials. However, activity in anterior bilateral leg muscles as well as anterior and posterior thigh muscles showed early (90 to 140 msec), high-magnitude (four to nine times the activity in normal walking), and relatively long duration bursts (Tang et al., 1998). As shown previously for recovery of balance during quiet stance, muscle response patterns to balance threats during walking were activated in a distal-to-proximal sequence. As shown in Figure 12.7 for a forward slip at heel strike, first the tibialis anterior on the ipsilateral side was activated (TAi), followed by the rectus femoris (RFi) and biceps femoris (BFi), and then the gluteus medius (GMEi) and abdominal muscles (ABi) (in initial trials).

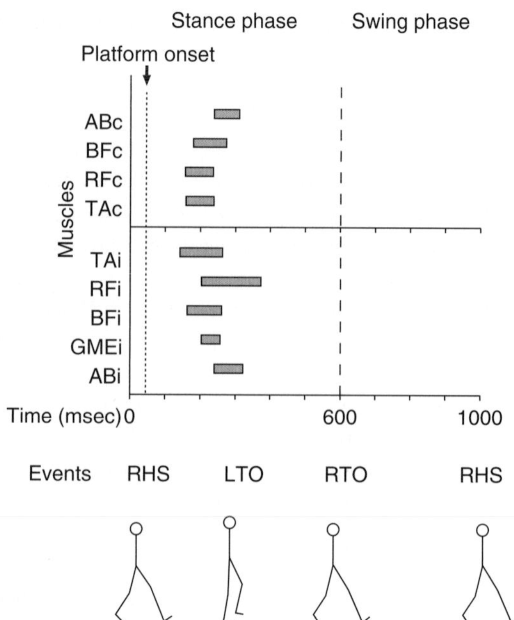

FIGURE 12.7 The organization of the postural responses of the anterior muscles and the biceps femoris in response to a forward slip at heel strike. The horizontal bars indicate the duration of postural activity in these muscles. The stick figures indicate the events during normal walking. AB = rectus abdominis; BF = biceps femoris; c = contralateral side; GME = gluteus medius; i = ipsilateral to the perturbed side; LTO = left toe-off; RF = rectus femoris; RHS = right heel strike; RTO = right toe-off; TA = tibialis anterior. (Adapted with permission from Tang PF, Woollacott MH, Chong RKY. Control of reactive balance adjustments in perturbed human walking: roles of proximal and distal postural muscle activity. Exp Brain Res 1998;119:141–152.)

Research has shown that arm movements are typically used during balance recovery, as well. Forward arm elevation evoked in response to a slip during locomotion aids to counteract the backward fall of the COM. Arm movements also may be used in a protective role, with hands either being directed to nearby handrails, or if a fall occurs, with arms absorbing force at the point of impact. These are often called "whole-body responses." In fact, both cutaneous and stretch reflexes in arm muscles are modulated according to the phase of the arm swing during the step cycle (Maki & McIlroy, 2006; Marigold & Misiaszek, 2009; Zehr & Duysens, 2004).

When given multiple slip perturbations, young adults adapt their strategy of recovery (Bhatt et al., 2006; Marigold & Patla, 2002). On the first slip (subjects unexpectedly stepped on rollers as they walked) individuals used a rapidly activated flexor synergy, with the TA and biceps femoris being activated, along with a large arm elevation and modified swing trajectory, as noted above. With repeated slips, individuals modified the strategy, using a more flat-footed landing, a shift of the mediolateral COM closer to the support limb at foot contact with the rollers, thus allowing them to attenuate the responses and use a "surfing strategy" as they went across the rollers. This suggests that they incorporated proactive adjustments in subsequent trials as they crossed the slippery surface.

In a study to determine how strategies for dealing with slippery floors are altered when subjects know in advance of a possible hazard, Cham and Redfern (2002) asked individuals to walk across either dry (baseline conditions) or water-, soap-, or oil-covered floors, for which they did not know the identity of the possible contaminant in advance. They found that when individuals anticipated a slippery surface they produced peak required coefficient of friction values that were 16 to 33% less than during baseline conditions, in order to reduce the potential for a slip. This was accomplished by reductions in stance duration and loading speed on the supported foot, taking shorter stride lengths, and using a slower angular velocity at heel strike. Interestingly, during a recovery condition in which subjects knew the floor was again dry, gait characteristics did not return to normal, but showed 5 to 12% reductions in coefficient of friction values.

Many falls in older adults occur as the result of trips. How is balance recovery accomplished during trips? Research analyzing responses to a tripping perturbation have found that the type of strategy used to maintain stability depends on when in the swing phase the trip occurs. As shown in Figure 12.8, if the trip occurs early in the swing phase of walking, the most common movement outcome is an elevating strategy of the swing limb with muscle responses occurring at 60 to 140 msec. Figure 12.8 shows the increased flexion at the hip, knee, and ankle (dashed lines) after obstacle contact (shown by the arrow) in the trial in which the subject was tripped, compared with the control trial (solid lines). The elevating strategy consisted of a flexor torque component of the swing limb, with the temporal sequencing of the swing limb biceps femoris occurring prior to the swing limb rectus femoris to remove the limb from the obstacle before accelerating the limb over it. An extensor torque component in the stance limb generated an early heel-off to increase the height of the body.

Use of the elevating strategy would be dangerous if a trip occurred late in the swing phase, since flexion of the swing limb as it is approaching the ground would increase, not decrease, instability; thus, a lowering strategy was used by subjects, as shown in Figure 12.9. Note the early plantar flexion of the ankle. The lowering strategy was accomplished by inhibitory responses in the swing limb vastus lateralis and an excitatory response of the swing limb biceps femoris, resulting in a shortened step length (Eng et al., 1994).

In a study examining recovery from trips in more detail (Schillings et al., 2000), researchers asked individuals to walk on a treadmill, and at different times in the swing phase a rigid obstacle unexpectedly blocked the forward movement of the foot. As noted above, all subjects showed an elevation strategy for early-swing and a lowering strategy for late-swing perturbations. The muscle responses responsible for the elevation strategy were due to the ipsilateral biceps femoris, causing extra knee flexion, and the TA, causing ankle dorsiflexion. Later rectus femoris responses were associated with knee extension as the foot was placed back on the treadmill. In the lowering strategy, the foot was placed quickly on the treadmill and was lifted over the obstacle in the subsequent swing phase. Foot placement was controlled by the ipsilateral rectus femoris and biceps femoris, associated with knee extension and deceleration of forward sway. Activation of the ipsilateral TA preceded the main ipsilateral soleus response.

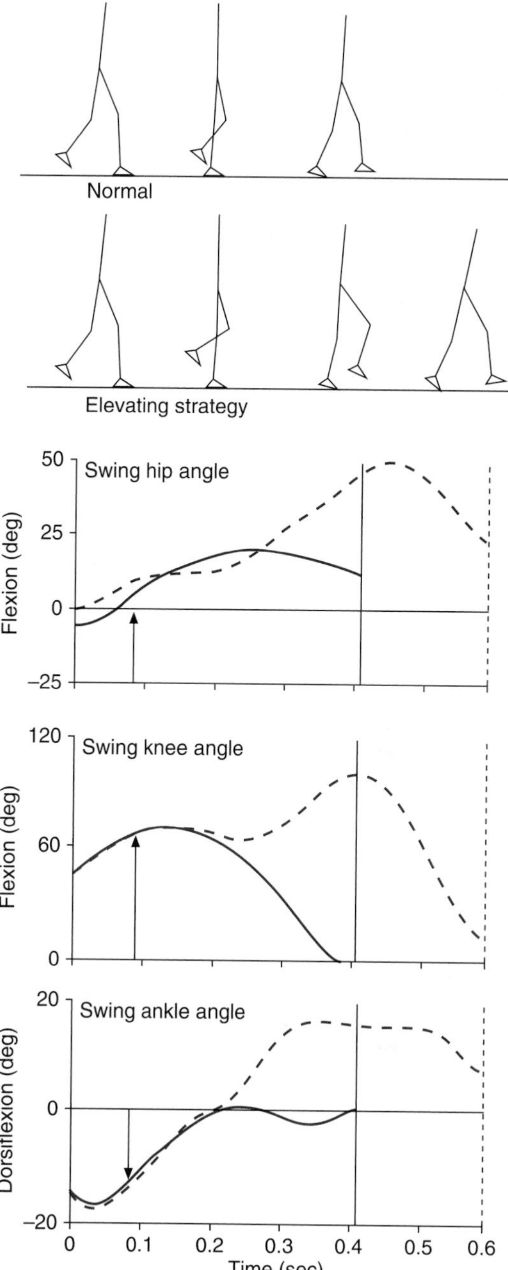

FIGURE 12.8 Hip, knee, and ankle trajectories of the swing limb observed in response to a trip during early swing phase of walking, showing the elevation strategy. Solid line = normal trial; dashed line = perturbed trial. Time 0 = toe-off; arrow = contact of foot with obstacle; vertical solid line = normal heel contact; vertical dashed line = perturbed heel contact. (Adapted with permission from Eng JJ, Winter DA, Patla AE. Strategies for recovery from a trip in early and late swing during human walking. Exp Brain Res 1994;102:344.)

Midswing perturbations could activate either elevation or lowering strategies. The first response was typically a short-latency stretch reflex, caused by the impact of the collision with the foot. This was not functionally related to the subsequent behavioral

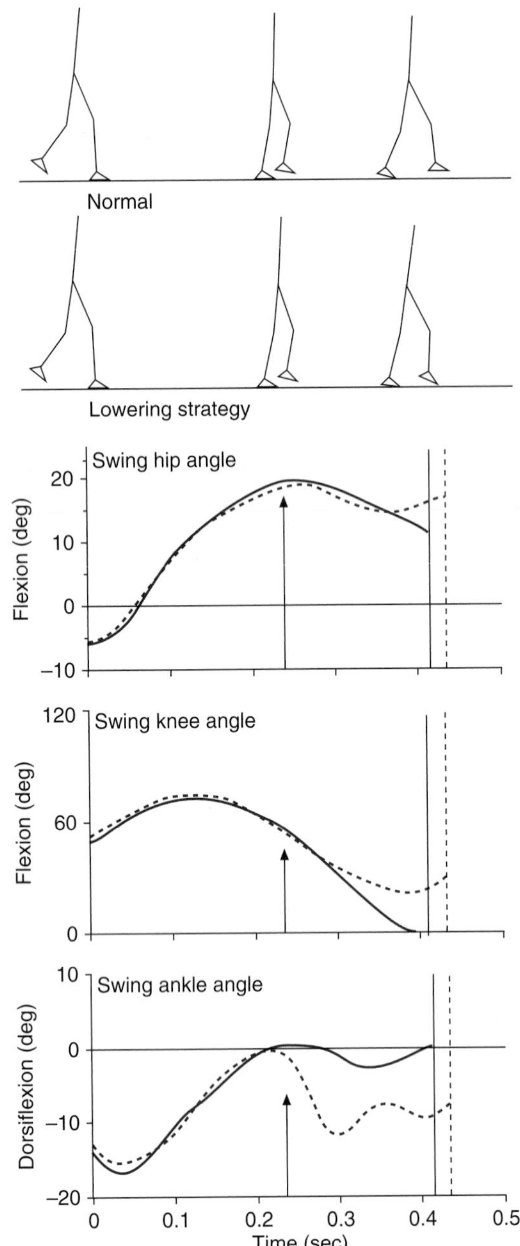

FIGURE 12.9 Hip, knee, and ankle trajectories of the swing limb observed in response to a trip during the late swing phase of walking, showing the lowering strategy. Solid line = normal trial; dashed line = perturbed trial. Time 0 = toe-off; arrow = contact of foot with obstacle; vertical solid line = normal heel contact; vertical dashed line = perturbed heel contact. (Adapted with permission from Eng JJ, Winter DA, Patla AE. Strategies for recovery from a trip in early and late swing during human walking. Exp Brain Res 1994;102:345.)

strategy. The first responses associated with elevation or lowering strategies occurred at about 110 msec.

More recent work has shown that the nervous system also takes advantage of passive dynamics to control the recovery from a trip during the swing phase of gait. Kinematic data were analyzed using inverse dynamics techniques (see Technology Tool 12.1) to determine the joint moment and mechanical power (kinetic) profiles and to partition the joint moments into active and passive components. Results showed that the nervous system used the passive dynamics of the musculoskeletal system to aid in balance recovery. Active control of one joint, the knee joint, passively contributed to the flexion at the hip and the ankle joints following a trip in early swing (Eng et al., 1997). Thus, it is important to consider both the passive and the active joint moments produced during balance recovery, in addition to the muscle response patterns of involved muscles, in order to understand the interactions between passive and active components of the control systems.

How do humans modify gait when walking or running on surfaces with different compliance or compressibility? If humans used the same muscle stiffness for all surfaces, the dynamics of walking and running would be strongly affected by surface stiffness or compliance. Although no studies have examined *walking* on compliant surfaces, work by Ferris et al. (1998) on *running* has shown that humans adjust muscle stiffness according to the surface they are running across. They found that the central nervous system modulates joint displacements and joint moments according to surface stiffness, probably in order to keep COM movement and ground contact time the same. Research on animals has shown that this is done within one step of moving on to the new surface. The above-mentioned research on human stretch reflex and GTO contributions to the step cycle suggests that proprioceptive feedback may be a factor in this stiffness modulation (Pearson et al., 1992; Stein, 1991). However, research has also shown that when lower-limb reflexes are temporarily blocked by ischemia, adults run with a normal ground contact time, suggesting that leg stiffness is unchanged (Dietz et al., 1979). Thus, there may be multiple contributions to stiffness regulation.

Vision. Work with humans suggests that there are a variety of ways in which vision modulates locomotion in a feedback manner. First, visual flow cues help us determine our speed of locomotion (Lackner & DeZio, 1988). Studies have shown that if one doubles the rate of optic flow past subjects as they walk, 100% of them will increase their stride length. In addition, about half will perceive that the force exerted during each step is less than normal. However, other subjects will perceive that they have nearly doubled their stepping frequency (Lackner & DeZio, 1992).

Visual flow cues also influence the alignment of the body with reference to gravity and the environment

TECHNOLOGY TOOL 12-1 Kinetic Analysis—Inverse Dynamics

Inverse dynamics is a process that allows researchers to calculate the joint moments of force (torque) responsible for movement—in this case, locomotion. Researchers begin by developing a reliable model of the body using anthropometric measures such as segment masses, center of mass, joint centers, and moments of inertia. Because these variables are difficult to measure directly, they are usually obtained from statistical tables based on the person's height, weight, and sex (Winter, 1990).

Using extremely accurate kinematic information on the limb trajectory during the step cycle, in combination with a reliable model, researchers can calculate the torque acting on each segment of the body. They can then partition the net torque into components due to gravity, the mechanical interaction among segments (motion-dependent torques), and a generalized muscle torque. This type of analysis allows researchers to assess the roles of muscular and nonmuscular forces in the generation of the movement (Winter et al., 1990).

during walking. For example, when researchers tilted the room surrounding a treadmill on which a person was running, it caused the person to incline the trunk in the direction of the tilted room to compensate for the visual illusion of body tilt in the opposite direction (Lee & Young, 1986).

Vestibular System. An important part of controlling locomotion is stabilizing the head, since it contains two of the most important sensors for controlling motion: the vestibular and visual systems (Berthoz & Pozzo, 1994). The otolith organs, the saccule and the utricle, detect the angle of the head with respect to gravity, and the visual system also provides us with the so-called visual vertical.

Adults appear to stabilize the head, and thus gaze, by covarying both pitch (forward) rotation and vertical displacement of the head to give stability to the head in the sagittal plane (Pozzo et al., 1990, 1992). The head is stabilized with a precision (within a few degrees) that is compatible with the efficiency of the vestibulo-ocular reflex, an important mechanism for stabilizing gaze during head movement.

It has been hypothesized that during complex movements, like walking, postural control is not organized from the support surface upward, in what is called a "bottom-up mode," but is organized in relation to the control of gaze, in what is called a "top-down mode." Thus, in this mode, head movements are independent from the movements of the trunk. It has been shown that the process for stabilizing the head is disrupted in patients with bilateral labyrinthine lesions (Berthoz & Pozzo, 1994).

Proactive Strategies

Proactive strategies for adapting gait focus on the use of sensory inputs to modify gait patterns. These strategies are used to modify and adapt gait in two different ways. First, vision is used proactively to identify potential obstacles in the environment and to navigate around them. Second, prediction is used to estimate the potential destabilizing effects of simultaneously performing tasks like carrying an object while walking, and anticipatory modifications to the step cycle are made accordingly. In the section on reactive control of slips during gait, discussed above, we mentioned how reactive control of gait shows both adaptation and anticipatory modifications with repeated exposure.

Proactive visual control of locomotion does not require repeated exposure to a situation, but it can be used in any environmental setting. It has been classified into both avoidance and accommodation strategies. Avoidance strategies include: (a) changing the placement of the foot, (b) increasing ground clearance to avoid an obstacle, (c) changing the direction of gait, when it is perceived that objects cannot be cleared, and (d) stopping. Accommodation strategies involve longer-term modifications, such as reducing step length when walking on an icy surface, or shifting the propulsive power from the ankle to hip and knee muscles when climbing stairs (Patla, 1997).

Most avoidance strategies can be successfully carried out within a step cycle. An exception occurs when changing directions, and this requires planning one step cycle in advance. It has been suggested that there are various rules associated with changing the placement of the foot. For example, when possible, step length is increased, rather than shortened, and the foot is placed inside rather than outside an obstacle, as long as the foot does not need to cross the midline of the body. Adapting strategies for foot placement does not involve simply changing the amplitude of the normal locomotor patterns, but is complex and task-specific (Patla, 1997).

The decision to step over an obstacle rather than move around it is related to the object size as compared with the body size. For example, when the ratio of obstacle size to leg length is 1:1, subjects prefer to go around it (Warren, 1988). It is probable that this choice relates to stability issues, as the risk of tripping increases as we step over obstacles of increased height.

Our experience with an object also determines our avoidance strategy. For example, perceived fragility of an obstacle influences the amount of toe clearance, with clearance being larger for the more fragile objects (Patla, 1997).

How do we sample the environment for proactive visual control? Visual processing time is shared with other tasks, and thus the terrain is typically sampled for less than 10% of our travel time when walking over even surfaces. However, when uneven surfaces are simulated by requiring subjects to step on specific locations, visual monitoring goes up to about 30% (Patla, 1997; Patla et al., 1996). In an experiment in which individuals were asked to wear opaque liquid crystal glasses and press a handheld switch to make the glasses transparent when they wanted to sample the environment, results showed that even in a novel environment individuals could walk safely while sampling less than 50% of the time. Visual sampling was increased when specific foot placement was required or if there was a hazard in the path (Patla et al., 1996).

To what extent do we use central versus peripheral vision in proactive control of gait? To answer this question researchers asked participants to wear goggles that could occlude the upper, lower, or circumferential peripheral visual field, while they were walking over obstacles. The researchers found that even without cues from the lower or peripheral visual field, the participants could complete the task safely, suggesting that subjects used central visual information in a feedforward manner to help them negotiate the obstacles. However, participants were much more variable in their performance under the peripheral occlusion conditions, increased minimum foot clearance, and decreased walking speed and step length, suggesting that peripheral visual information is used for online control of the legs during obstacle crossing (Graci et al., 2009, 2010).

How do we navigate in a large-scale spatial environment? Humans use what is called a "piloting strategy," which requires a mental representation of the spatial environment. These cognitive maps include both topological information (relationships of landmarks in the environment) and metric information (specific distances and directions). Topological information is needed when obstacles constrain our travel path. The fact that most animals can also accurately take shortcuts to reach a goal supports the concept that metric information is also used in navigation (Patla, 1997).

Stepping Over Obstacles. Controlling balance when walking over obstacles requires increased control as compared with normal locomotion, as imbalance of the body may occur and cause a fall. In order to determine the motion of the COM when stepping over obstacles of different heights, Chou and colleagues (2001) asked young adults to step over obstacles of 2.5 to 15% of their body height, while walking at their own comfortable walking speed. They found that stepping over higher obstacles caused significantly greater ranges of COM motion in both the anteroposterior (AP) and vertical directions (but not the mediolateral [ML] direction), along with a greater AP distance between the COM and center of pressure (COP). These small shifts in ML COM may reflect control strategies used by healthy individuals to keep the COM well within safe limits for balance control. Balance-impaired older adults and patient populations appear to have more difficulty with this control (see Chapters 13 and 14).

Cognitive Systems in Locomotion

As mentioned in Chapter 7, although posture and locomotion are often considered to be automatic, they require attentional processing resources, and the amount of resources required varies depending on the difficulty of the postural or locomotor task. Experiments using a dual-task design have led researchers to propose a hierarchy of postural and gait tasks based on attentional processing requirements of the tasks. The least resources are required for nondemanding postural tasks such as sitting or standing with feet shoulder width apart; attentional demands increase when standing in tandem Romberg position, walking (Lajoie et al., 1993), during obstacle avoidance while walking (Chen et al., 1996), and during recovery from external perturbations (Brown et al., 1999; Rankin et al., 2000).

Normal Gait

In a study by Lajoie et al. (1993), young adults were asked to perform an auditory reaction-time task while sitting, while standing with a normal versus a reduced base of support, and during walking (single- vs. double-support phase). Reaction times were fastest for sitting and slowed for the standing and walking tasks. Reaction times were slower in the single-support phase as compared with the double-support phase of the step cycle.

Lajoie et al.'s study focused on examining the attentional demands associated with gait (i.e., its effect on the performance of a secondary task) and reported no change in gait parameters associated with the performance of a simple reaction-time task in young adults. In contrast, Ebersbach et al. (1995) specifically studied the effect of concurrent tasks on the control of gait. They measured gait parameters (stride time, double-support time) under a single-task condition (walking without a concurrent task) and four dual-task conditions presented in random order: (1) memory-retention task (digit-span recall), (2) fine-motor task (opening and closing a coat button continuously while walking), (3) a combination task (digit-recall and buttoning task), and (4) finger tapping at 5 Hz or faster. The only dual-task condition that produced a significant decrease in stride time (increased stride frequency) was finger tapping. The other gait parameter measured, double-support time, was significantly affected when the fine-motor and memory tasks were performed synchronously with the walking; no other dual-task condition affected this parameter. Interestingly, the authors noted that performance of the gait task did affect the digit-recall task. The mean digit-span recall was 6.7 (range, 6 to 8) during quiet stance, but reduced to 5.8 (range, 4 to 8) during walking. In this study, even the significant changes in gait parameters are fairly small, again suggesting that performance of multiple tasks during a relatively simple task such as unperturbed gait does not present a significant threat to stability in healthy, young adults.

Obstacle Crossing

Chen and colleagues (1996) examined the effect of dividing attention on the ability to step over obstacles efficiently. In this study individuals were asked to walk down a walkway and to step over a virtual object (a band of light) when a red light turned on at the end of the walkway. On some trials they were asked to perform a secondary task involving giving a vocal response. The authors measured obstacle contact in single- versus dual-task conditions. Results indicated that obstacle contact was increased when attention was divided.

One interesting question regarding the attentional requirements of obstacle crossing is the time course of attentional demands, and when they are the highest. To answer this question, Brown and colleagues (2005) compared the attentional demands associated with steady-state walking and the precrossing and crossing phases of an obstacle task. They found that young adults directed more attention to gait during precrossing than during obstacle crossing.

Walk–Run Transition

It has also been shown that cognitive–perceptual processes contribute to the walk–run transition. Young adults were asked to walk on a treadmill while performing a mathematical task; the treadmill speed was gradually increased, and the point of walk–run transition was noted. The transition speed increased when performing the mathematical task, suggesting that the cognitive load distracts an individual's focus from physiological cues that typically contribute to the walk–run transition (Daniels & Newell, 2003).

Nonneural Contributions to Locomotion

So far, we have looked at neural contributions to the control of locomotion, but there are also important musculoskeletal and environmental contributions. Biomechanical analyses of locomotion in cats have determined the contributions of both muscular and nonmuscular forces to the generation of gait dynamics (Hoy & Zernicke, 1985, 1986; Hoy et al., 1985; Smith & Zernicke, 1987). This involves a type of kinetic analysis called "inverse dynamics." To understand more about inverse dynamics, refer to the Technology Tool 12.1.

As discussed in earlier chapters, nonmuscular forces, such as gravity, play a role in the construction of all movement. When an inverse dynamics analysis of limb dynamics is used, it is possible to determine the relative importance of the muscular and nonmuscular contributions. For example, during locomotion, each segment of the cat hindlimb is subjected to a complex set of muscular and nonmuscular forces. Changes in speed lead to changes in the interactive patterns among the torque components (Hoy & Zernicke, 1985; Wisleder et al., 1990).

Very often during locomotion in the cat, there are high passive extensor torques at a joint, which must be counteracted by active flexor torques generated by the muscles, when the animal is moving at one speed, or in one part of the step cycle. When the speed is increased, or the animal moves to a different part of the cycle, the passive torques that must be counteracted change completely. How does the dialogue between the passive properties of the system and the neural pattern-generating circuits occur? This is still unclear, although the discharge from somatosensory receptors plays a role (Hoy et al., 1985; Smith & Zernicke, 1987; Wisleder et al., 1990). What is revealed in the dynamic analysis of limb movements is the intricacies of the interaction among active and passive forces.

The results from these studies suggest that in normal locomotion there is a continuous interaction between the CPGs and descending signals. Higher centers contribute to locomotion through feedforward modulation of patterns in response to the goals of the individual and to environmental demands. As noted briefly above, sensory inputs are also critical for feedback and feedforward modulation of locomotor activity in order to adapt it to changing environmental conditions.

INITIATING GAIT AND CHANGING SPEEDS

How do we initiate walking? Before we describe the initiation of gait, complete Lab Activity 12.3.

Research studies confirm what you no doubt noticed from your own experiment: the initiation of gait from quiet stance begins with the relaxation of specific postural muscles, the gastrocnemius and the soleus (Carlsoo, 1966; Herman et al., 1973). In fact, the initiation of gait has the appearance of a simple forward fall and regaining of one's balance by taking a step. This reduction in the activation of the gastrocnemius and soleus is followed by activation of the TA, which assists dorsiflexion and moves the COM forward in preparation for toe-off. But, as you noticed, and as research on gait confirms, the initiation of gait is more than a simple fall.

In tracing the COP during the initiation of gait in normal adults, the following sequence of events is evident. Prior to movement onset, the COP is positioned just posterior to the ankle and midway between both feet, as shown in Figure 12.10. As the person begins to move, the COP first moves posteriorly and laterally toward the swing limb and then shifts toward the stance limb and forward.

Movement of the COP toward the stance limb occurs simultaneously with hip and knee flexion and ankle dorsiflexion as the swing limb prepares for toe-off. Then the COP moves quickly toward the stance limb. Toe-off of the swing limb occurs with the COP shifting from lateral to forward movement over the stance foot (Mann et al., 1979).

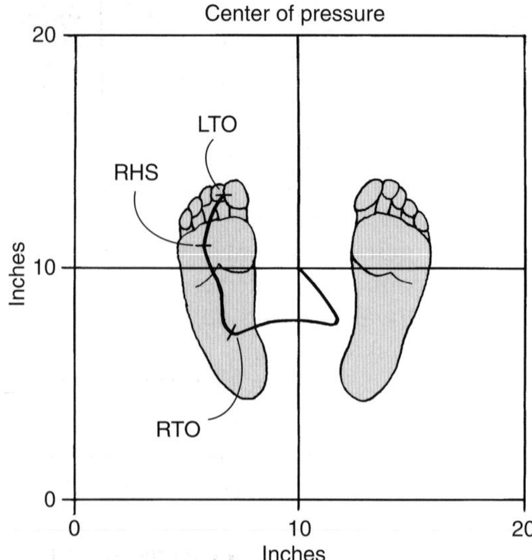

FIGURE 12.10 Trajectory of the COP during the initiation of gait from a balanced, symmetric stance. Prior to movement, the center of pressure is located midway between the feet. LTO = left toe-off; RHS = right heel strike; RTO = right toe-off. (Adapted with permission from Mann RA, Hagy JL, White V, Liddell D. The initiation of gait. J Bone Joint Surg Am 1979;61:232–239.)

What neural patterns are correlated with these shifts in COP? As the COP moves posteriorly and toward the swing limb, both limbs are stabilized against backward sway by activation of anterior leg and thigh muscles, the TA and the quadriceps. Subsequent activation of the TA then causes dorsiflexion in the stance ankle, pulling the lower leg over the foot,

LAB ACTIVITY 12-3

Objective: To understand the movements essential to the initiation of gait.

Procedure: Get up and stand next to a wall, with your shoulder touching the wall. First try to start walking with the foot that is next to the wall. Then try to start walking with the foot that is away from the wall.

Assignment

In each condition (e.g., gait initiation with the leg nearer versus farther from the wall) note the following:

1 What muscles contract and relax?
2. Which way does the body move in the process of preparing to take a step?
3. Under which condition is it easiest to initiate gait?
4. When you tried to initiate gait with the leg farther away from the wall, did you notice that you had more problems?
5. Why?

as the body moves forward in preparation for toe-off. Anterior thigh muscles are activated to keep the knee from flexing so that the leg rotates forward as a unit. Activation of hip abductors counters lateral tilt of the pelvis toward the swing limb side as this limb is unloaded. Also, activation of the peroneals stabilizes the stance ankle. After toe-off, the gastrocnemius and hamstrings muscles in the stance leg are used for propelling the body forward (Herman et al., 1973; Mann et al., 1979). How long after initiation does it take to reach a steady velocity in gait? Steady state is reached within one to three steps, depending on the magnitude of the velocity one is trying to achieve (Breniere & Do, 1986; Cook & Cozzens, 1976).

Turning Strategies

One of the times when many patients and older adults fall is when making a sudden turn while walking. In order to determine the turning strategies used by healthy, young individuals while turning, Hase and Stein (1999) asked subjects to walk at a comfortable speed and to turn in a specific direction when they felt an electrical stimulus. Results showed that two different turning strategies were used, depending on which foot the subject had in front, for braking before the turn. To turn to the right with the right foot in front, individuals typically spun the body around the right foot (termed a "spin-turn"). In turning left with the right foot in front, they shifted weight to the right leg, then externally rotated the left hip and stepped onto the left leg, continuing to turn until the right leg stepped in the new direction (termed a "step-turn").

They noted that the step-turn was easy and stable because the base of support during the turn is wider, so some subjects preferred this method. The deceleration of walking before the turn involved activation of muscles in a sequence similar to the "ankle strategy" for balance control, starting at the distal soleus muscle and moving proximally to the hamstrings and erector spinae, showing that balance synergies may be used in a variety of tasks. Most subjects completed the turn without the need to reset the walking rhythm (Hase & Stein, 1999).

Walk–Run Transition

As we increase our speed during walking or decrease our speed during running, there comes a point at which a gait transition occurs. The selection of this transition point occurs over a relatively narrow range of speeds across adults. Since humans are capable of walking and running at both higher and lower speeds than the transition speed, a number of researchers have tried to determine the factors that may influence this transition (Hreljac 1993b, 1995a,b; Kram et al., 1997).

It has traditionally been assumed by many researchers that both humans and other animals change gait at a speed that minimizes their metabolic energy consumption, since many animals select a transition speed within a particular gait that minimizes metabolic energy cost (Alexander, 1989; Cavagna & Franzetti, 1986; Grillner et al., 1979; Hoyt & Taylor, 1981). If this were the case, the preferred transition speed for humans between a walk and a run would be about 2.24 to 2.36 m/sec (Margaria, 1976). However, it has been noted that the preferred transition speed is more typically 1.88 to 2.07 m/sec (Hreljac, 1993b; Thorstensson & Roberthson, 1987). Thus, more recent research has attempted to determine the primary factors contributing to this transition.

A set of studies has shown that subjects changing from a walk to a run at these lower speeds perceived that their sense of exertion decreased by 26%, even though the energy cost increased by 16% (Hreljac, 1993b). Thus, it is unlikely that the energy cost of locomotion is the primary factor contributing to the speed of gait transition. In horses it has been shown that the trot-to-gallop transition occurs when the ground reaction forces reach a critical level, with peak forces decreasing by about 14% when the horses shifted from a trot to a gallop (Farley & Taylor, 1991). Since ground reaction forces are related to musculoskeletal forces, this might be a way to prevent injuries caused by high musculoskeletal forces. However, it has been shown that in humans there is an increase in ground reaction forces during the transition from a walk to a run and thus this does not appear to be a critical factor for the walk-to-run transition (Hreljac, 1993a).

Instead, it has been proposed that peak ankle angular velocity and acceleration are critical components in triggering this transition (Hreljac, 1995a). Why would this be the case? It has been hypothesized that high levels of activity in ankle dorsiflexors close to the time of toe-off at the walk–run transition point are necessary to rotate the foot quickly to prevent toe drag and to position the heel for the next stance phase. At this time, there is also cocontraction of the ankle plantar flexors, requiring increased output from the dorsiflexors to rotate the foot. Thus, one outcome of the gait transition would be a reduction in muscular stress or fatigue in the dorsiflexors (Hreljac, 1995a). By shifting to a run, the stress would be removed from the dorsiflexors and shifted to the larger muscles of the upper leg.

It has also been shown that body size is moderately correlated ($r = 0.54$ to 0.60) with the preferred transition speed. This follows from the assumption that people of different heights would reach the same ankle angular accelerations at different walking speeds (Hreljac, 1995b).

STAIR-WALKING

Understanding the sensory and motor requirements associated with stair-walking is critical to retraining this skill. Stairs represent a significant hazard even among the nondisabled population. Stair-walking accounts for the largest percentage of falls occurring in public places, with four out of five falls occurring during stair descent. Stair-walking is similar to level walking in that it involves stereotypical reciprocal alternating movements of the lower limbs (Craik et al., 1982; Simoneau et al., 1991). Like locomotion, successful negotiation of stairs has three requirements: the generation of primarily concentric forces to propel the body upstairs or eccentric forces to control the body's descent downstairs (progression); while controlling the COM within a constantly changing base of support (stability); and the capacity to adapt strategies used for progression and stability to accommodate changes in stair environment, such as height, width, and the presence or absence of railings (adaptation) (McFadyen & Winter, 1988).

Sensory information is important for controlling the body's position in space (stability) and to identify critical aspects of the stair environment so that appropriate movement strategies can be programmed (adaptation). Researchers have shown that normal subjects change movement strategies used for negotiating stairs when sensory cues about stair characteristics are altered (Craik et al., 1982; Simoneau et al., 1991).

Similar to gait, stair-climbing has been divided into two phases, a stance phase lasting approximately 64% of the full cycle and a swing phase lasting 36% of the cycle. In addition, each phase of stair-walking has been further subdivided to reflect the objectives that need to be achieved during each phase.

Ascent

During ascent, the stance phase is subdivided into weight acceptance, pull-up, and forward continuance, while swing is divided into foot clearance and foot placement stages.

During stance, weight acceptance is initiated with the middle to front portion of the foot. Pull-up occurs because of extensor activity at the knee and ankle, primarily concentric contractions of the vastus lateralis and soleus muscles. Stair ascent differs from level walking in two ways: (a) forces needed to accomplish ascent are two times greater than those needed to control level gait, and (b) the knee extensors generate most of the energy to move the body forward during stair ascent. Finally, during the forward-continuance phase of stance, the ankle generates forward and lift forces; however, ankle force is not the main source of power behind forward progression in stair-walking. In controlling balance during stair ascent, the greatest instability comes with contralateral toe-off, when the ipsilateral leg takes the total body weight, and the hip, knee, and ankle joints are flexed (McFadyen & Winter, 1988).

The objectives of the swing phase of stair-climbing are similar to level gait and include foot clearance and placing the foot appropriately so weight can be accepted for the next stance phase. Foot clearance is achieved through activation of the TA, dorsiflexing the foot, and activation of the hamstrings, which flex the knee. The rectus femoris contracts eccentrically to reverse this motion by midswing. The swing leg is brought up and forward through activation of the hip flexors of the swing leg and motion of the contralateral stance leg. Final foot placement is controlled by the hip extensors and ankle foot dorsiflexors (McFadyen & Winter, 1988).

Descent

Walking upstairs is accomplished through concentric contractions of the rectus femoris, vastus lateralis, soleus, and medial gastrocnemius. In contrast, walking downstairs is achieved through eccentric contractions of these same muscles, which work to control the body with respect to the force of gravity. The stance phase of stair descent is subdivided into weight acceptance, forward continuance, and controlled lowering, while swing has two phases: leg pull-through and preparation for foot placement (Craik et al., 1982; McFadyen & Winter, 1988).

The weight-acceptance phase is characterized by absorption of energy at the ankle and knee through the eccentric contraction of the triceps surae, rectus femoris, and vastus lateralis. Energy absorption during this phase is critical, since ground reaction forces as much as two times body weight have been recorded when the swing limb first contacts the stair. Activation of the gastrocnemius prior to stair contact is responsible for cushioning the landing (Craik et al., 1982).

The forward-continuance phase reflects the forward motion of the body, and precedes the controlled-lowering phase of stance. Lowering of the body is controlled primarily by the eccentric contraction of the quadriceps muscles and, to a lesser degree, the eccentric contraction of the soleus muscle.

During swing, the leg is pulled through, because of activation of the hip flexor muscles. However, by midswing, flexion of the hip and knee is reversed, and all three joints extend in preparation for foot placement. Contact is made with the lateral border of the foot, and is associated with TA and gastrocnemius activity prior to foot contact.

Adapting Stair-Walking Patterns to Changes in Sensory Cues

Researchers have shown that neurologically intact people adapt the movement strategies they use for going up and down stairs in response to changes in sensory information about the task. Thus, when normal subjects wear large collars that obstruct their view of the stairs, anticipatory activation of the gastrocnemius prior to foot contact is reduced. This anticipatory activity is further reduced when the subject is blindfolded. In this study, subjects still managed a soft landing by changing the control strategy used to descend stairs. Subjects moved more slowly, protracting swing time and using the stance limb to control the landing (Craik et al., 1982).

Foot clearance and placement are critical aspects of movement strategies used to safely descend stairs. Good visual information about stair height is critical. When normal subjects wear blurred-vision lenses and are unable to clearly define the edge of the step, they slow down and modify movement strategies so that foot clearance is increased and the foot is placed further back on the step to ensure a larger margin of safety (Simoneau et al., 1991). Thus, information from the visual system about the step height appears to be necessary for optimal programming of movement strategies used to negotiate stairs.

MOBILITY OTHER THAN GAIT

Although mobility is often thought of solely in relationship to gait or locomotion, there are many other aspects of mobility that are essential to independence in activities of daily living. The ability to change positions, whether moving from sitting to standing, rolling, rising from a bed, or moving from one chair to another, is a fundamental part of mobility. These various types of mobility activities are often grouped together and referred to as "transfer tasks."

Retraining motor function in the patient with a neurologic impairment includes the recovery of these diverse mobility skills. This requires an understanding of: (a) the essential characteristics of the task, (b) the sensory motor strategies that normal individuals typically use to accomplish the task, and (c) the adaptations required for changing environmental characteristics.

All mobility tasks share three essential task requirements: motion in a desired direction (progression), postural control (stability), and ability to adapt to changing task and environmental conditions (adaptation). The following sections briefly review some of the research on these other aspects of mobility function. As you will see, compared to the tremendous number of studies on normal gait, there have been relatively few studies examining these other aspects of mobility function.

Transfers

Transfers represent an important aspect of mobility function. One cannot walk if one cannot get out of a chair or rise from a bed. Inability to safely and independently change positions represents a great hindrance to the recovery of normal mobility. Several researchers have studied transfer skills from a biomechanical perspective. As a result, we know quite a bit about typical movement strategies used by neurologically intact adults when performing these tasks. However, use of a biomechanical approach has provided us with little information about the perceptual strategies associated with these various tasks. In addition, because most often research subjects are constrained to carry out the task in a unified way, we have little insight into ways in which sensory and movement strategies are modified in response to changing task and environmental demands.

Sitting to Standing

Sitting-to-standing (STS) behaviors emerge from an interaction among characteristics of the task, the individual, and the constraints imposed by the environment. While the biomechanics of STS have been described, there are many important questions that have not yet been studied by motor control researchers. For example, how do the movements involved in STS vary as a function of the speed of the task, the characteristics of the support, including height of the chair, the compliance of the seat, or the presence or absence of hand rests? In addition, do the requirements of the task vary depending on the nature of the task immediately following? That is, do we stand up differently if we are intending to walk instead of stand still? What perceptual information is essential to establishing efficient movement strategies when performing STS?

The essential characteristics of the STS task include: (a) generating sufficient joint torque needed to rise (progression), (b) ensuring stability by moving the center of mass from one base of support (the chair) to a base of support defined solely by the feet (stability), and (c) the ability to modify movement strategies used to achieve these goals depending on environmental constraints such as chair height, the presence of armrests, and the softness of the chair (adaptation).

The STS task has been divided into different phases, either two, three, or four, depending on the researcher. Each phase has its own unique movement and stability requirements. A four-phase model of the STS task is shown in Figure 12.11 (Millington et al., 1992; Schenkman et al., 1990). This figure also shows the movements of the joints and the muscle activity used by a normal subject when completing this task.

The first phase, called the "weight shift" or "flexion momentum" stage, begins with the generation of forward momentum of the upper body through flexion of the trunk. The body is quite stable during this phase, since the COM, although moving forward, is still within the base of support of the chair seat and the feet. Muscle activity includes activation of the erector spinae, which contract eccentrically to control forward motion of the trunk (Millington et al., 1992; Schenkman et al., 1990).

Phase 2 begins as the buttocks leave the seat, and involves the transfer of momentum from the upper body to the total body, allowing lift of the body. Phase 2 involves both horizontal and vertical motion of the body and is considered a critical transition phase.

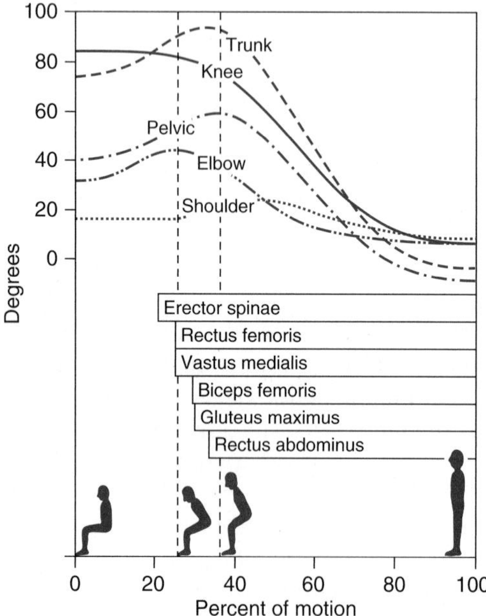

FIGURE 12.11 Four phases of the STS movement, showing the kinematic and EMG patterns associated with each phase. (Adapted from Millington PJ, Myklebust BM, Shambes GM. Biomechanical analysis of the sit-to-stand motion in elderly persons. Arch Phys Med Rehabil 1992;73:609–617.)

Stability requirements are precise, since it is during this phase that the COM of the body moves from within the base of support of the chair to that of the feet. The body is inherently unstable during this phase because the COM is located far from the center of force. Because the body has developed momentum prior to liftoff, vertical rise of the body can be achieved with little lower-extremity muscle force. Muscle activity in this phase is characterized by coactivation of hip and knee extensors, as shown in Figure 12.11 (Schenkman et al., 1990).

Phase 3 of the STS task is referred to as the "lift" or "extension" phase, and is characterized by extension at the hips and knees. The goal in this phase is primarily to move the body vertically; stability requirements are less than in phase 2 since the COM is well within the base of support of the feet. The final phase of STS is the stabilization phase; it is the period following complete extension when task-dependent motion is complete and body stability in the vertical position is achieved (Schenkman et al., 1990).

STS requires the generation of propulsive impulse forces in both the horizontal and vertical directions. However, the horizontal propulsive force responsible for moving the COM anteriorly over the base of support of the foot must change into a braking impulse to bring the body to a stop. Braking the horizontal impulse begins even before liftoff from the seat. Thus, there appears to be a preprogrammed relationship between the generation and braking of forces for the STS task. Without this coordination between propulsive and braking forces, the person could easily fall forward upon achieving the vertical position.

Horizontal displacement of the COM appears to be constant, despite changes in the speed of STS. Controlling the horizontal trajectory of the COM is probably the invariant feature controlled in STS to ensure that stability is maintained during vertical rise of the body (Millington et al., 1992).

This strategy could be referred to as a "momentum-transfer strategy," and its use requires: (a) adequate strength and coordination to generate upper-body movement prior to liftoff, (b) the ability to eccentrically contract trunk and hip muscles in order to apply braking forces to slow the horizontal trajectory of the COM, and (c) concentric contraction of hip and knee muscles to generate vertical propulsive forces that lift the body (Schenkman et al., 1990).

Accomplishing STS using a momentum-transfer strategy requires a trade-off between stability and force requirements. The generation and transfer of momentum between the upper body and the total body reduces the requirement for lower-extremity force because the body is already in motion as it begins to lift. On the other hand, the body is in a precarious state of balance during the transition stage, when momentum is transferred.

An alternative strategy that ensures greater stability but requires greater amounts of force to achieve liftoff includes flexing the trunk sufficiently to bring the COM well within the base of support of the feet prior to liftoff. However, the body has zero momentum at liftoff. This strategy has been referred to as a "zero-momentum strategy," and it requires the generation of larger lower-extremity forces in order to lift the body to vertical (Schenkman et al., 1990).

Another common strategy used by many older adults and people with neurologic impairments involves the use of armrests to assist in STS. Use of the arms assists in both the stability and force generation requirements of the STS task.

Understanding the different strategies that can be used to accomplish STS, including the trade-offs between force and stability, will help the therapist when retraining STS in the patient with a neurologic deficit. For example, the zero-momentum strategy may be more appropriate to use with a patient with cerebellar pathology who has no difficulty with force generation, but who has a major problem with controlling stability. On the other hand, the patient with hemiparesis, who is very weak, may need to rely more on a momentum strategy to achieve the vertical position. The frail elderly person who is both weak and unstable may need to rely on armrests to accomplish STS.

Supine to Standing

The ability to assume a standing position from a supine position is an important milestone in mobility skills. This skill is taught to a wide range of patients with neurologic impairments, from young children with developmental disabilities first learning to stand and walk, to frail older people prone to falling. The movement strategies used by normal individuals moving from a supine to a standing position have been studied by a number of researchers. An important theoretical question addressed by these researchers relates to whether rising to standing from supine follows a developmental progression, and whether by the age of 4 or 5 years the mature, or adult-like, form emerges and remains throughout life (VanSant, 1988a). By performing Lab Activity 12-4, you can come to your own conclusions about some of these questions.

Researchers have studied supine-to-standing movement strategies in children, ages 4 to 7 years, and young adults, ages 20 to 35 years (VanSant, 1988b). These researchers found that while there was a slight tendency toward age-specific strategies for moving from supine to standing, there was also great variability among subjects of the same age. Their findings do not appear to support the traditional assumption of a single mature supine-to-standing pattern, which emerges after the age of 5 years.

The three most common movement strategies for moving from supine to standing are shown in Figure 12.12. When analyzing strategies used for moving from supine to standing, the body is divided into three components—upper extremities, lower extremities, and axial—which includes the trunk and the head. Movement strategies are then described in relationship to the various combinations of movement patterns within each of these segments. The research on young adults suggests that the most common pattern used involves symmetrical movement patterns of the trunk and extremities, and the use of a symmetrical squat to achieve the vertical position (Fig. 12.12A). However, only one-fourth of the subjects studied used this strategy.

LAB ACTIVITY 12-4

Objective: To observe the strategies used to move from a supine to a standing position in healthy adults.

Procedures: For this lab you will need a stopwatch, four or five partners, and room to observe each individual moving from a supine (flat on the floor) to a standing position. Time each person as they move from a supine to a full standing position. Observe the movement patterns used by each individual to arise. Pay specific attention to the use of arms, symmetry of foot placement, and trunk rotation.

Assignment

Were all subjects able to arise independently without physical assistance of another? How did times vary across subjects? How many different strategies were observed among the subjects? Did any two subjects move in the same way? How do your results compare with VanSant's (1988b) results shown in Figure 12.12? What are the primary muscles that are active in each of the strategies? How would weakness or loss of joint range of motion affect each of these strategies?

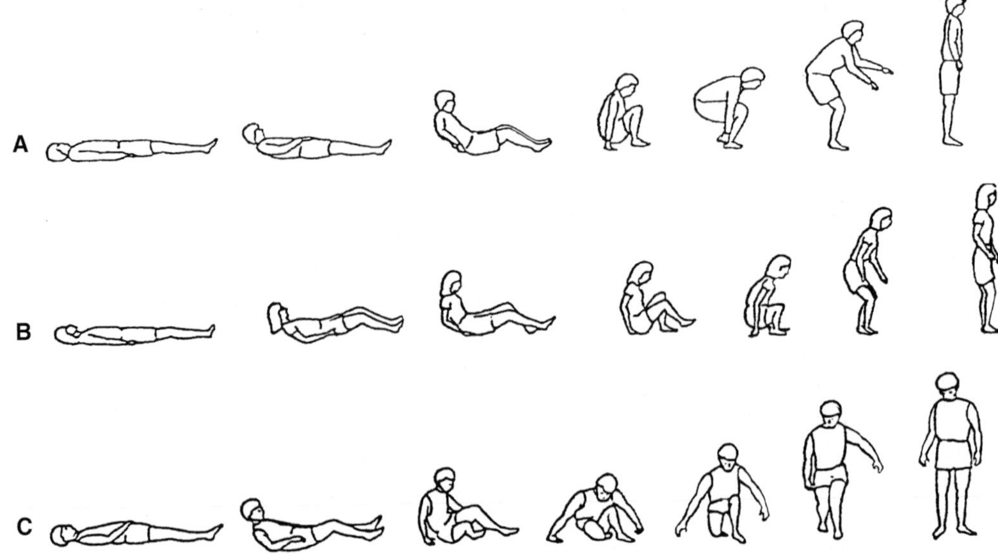

FIGURE 12.12 The three most common movement strategies identified among young adults for moving from a supine to a standing position. A, Strategy involving symmetrical trunk and symmetrical squat. B, Strategy involving symmetrical trunk and asymmetrical squat. C, Strategy involving asymmetrical trunk movement. (Adapted from VanSant AF. Rising from a supine position to erect stance: description of adult movement and a developmental hypothesis. Phys Ther 1988;68:185–192, with permission of the American Physical Therapy Association. This material is copyrighted, and any further reproduction or distribution requires written permission from APTA.)

The second most common movement pattern involved an asymmetric squat on arising (Fig. 12.12B), while the third most common strategy involved asymmetric use of the upper extremities, a partial rotation of the trunk, and assumption of stance using a half-kneel position (Fig. 12.12C).

Additional studies have characterized movement patterns used to rise from supine in middle-aged adults, ages 30 to 39 years, and found some differences in movement strategies as compared with younger adults (Green & Williams, 1992). In addition, this study looked at the effect of physical activity levels on strategies used to stand up. Results from the study found that strategies used to stand up are influenced by lifestyle factors, including level of physical activity.

Many factors probably contribute to determining the type of movement strategy used to move from supine to standing. Traditionally, nervous system maturation, specifically, the maturation of the neck-on-body righting reactions and body-on-body righting reactions, were considered the most significant factors affecting the emergence of a developmentally mature supine-to-standing strategy. However, a switch from an asymmetric rotation to a symmetric sit-up strategy may be constrained by the ability to generate sufficient abdominal and hip flexor strength.

Developmental changes in moving from supine to standing are considered further in Chapter 13, on age-related aspects of mobility.

Rising from Bed

Clinicians are often called on to help patients relearn the task of getting out of bed. In therapeutic textbooks on retraining motor control in patients with neurologic impairments, therapists are instructed to teach patients to move from supine to side-lying, then to push up to a sitting position and from there, to stand up. These instructions are based on the assumption that this pattern represents that typically used to rise from a bed (Bobath, 1990; Carr & Shepherd, 1992).

To test these assumptions, researchers examined movement patterns used by young adults to rise from a bed (McCoy & VanSant, 1993; Sarnacki, 1986). These studies report that movement patterns used by nondisabled people to rise from a bed are extremely variable. Eighty-nine patterns were found among 60 subjects. In fact, no subject used the same strategy consistently in 10 trials of getting out of bed.

Figure 12.13 shows one of the most common strategies used by young adults to rise from a bed. Essential components of the strategy include pushing with the arms (or grasping the side of the bed and

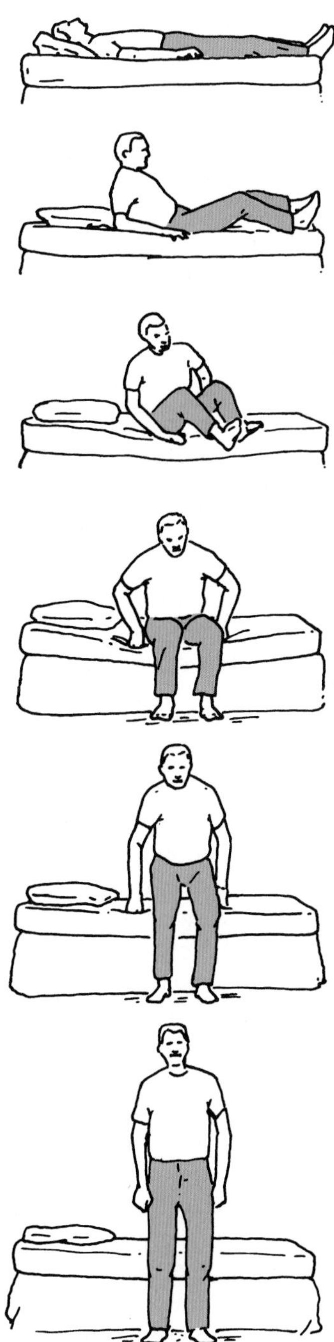

FIGURE 12.13 Most common movement strategy used by young adults for getting out of bed. (Adapted from Ford-Smith CD, VanSant AF. Age differences in movement patterns used to rise from a bed in subjects in the third through fifth decades of age. Phys Ther 1992;73:305, with permission of the American Physical Therapy Association. This material is copyrighted, and any further reproduction or distribution requires written permission from APTA.)

then pushing with the arms), flexing the head and trunk, pushing into a partial sit position, and rolling up to standing. Another common strategy found was a push-off pattern with the arms, rolling to the side and coming to a symmetrical sitting position prior to standing up.

While the authors of this study have not specifically stated the essential features of this task, its similarity to the STS task suggests that they share the same invariant characteristics. These include: (a) the need to generate momentum to move the body to vertical, (b) stability requirements for controlling the COM as it changes from within the support base defined by the horizontal body to that defined by the buttocks and feet, and finally to a base of support defined solely by the feet, and (c) the ability to adapt how one moves to the characteristics of the environment.

In trying to better understand why people move as they do, and in preparation for understanding why patients move as they do, it might be helpful to reexamine descriptions of movement strategies used to rise from a bed in light of these essential task characteristics. In doing so, it might be possible to determine common features across diverse strategies that are successful in accomplishing invariant requirements of the task. It would also be possible to examine some trade-offs between movement and stability requirements in the different strategies. For example, in the roll-off strategy, is motion achieved with greater efficiency at the expense of stability? Alternatively, the come-to-sit pattern may require more force to keep the body in motion, but stability may be inherently greater.

This research demonstrates the tremendous variability of movement strategies used by neurologically intact subjects when getting out of bed. It suggests the importance of helping patients with neurologic impairments to learn a variety of approaches to getting out of bed.

Rolling

Rolling is an important part of bed mobility skills and an essential part of many other tasks, such as rising from bed. Movement strategies used by nonimpaired adults to roll from supine to prone are very variable. Figure 12.14 shows one of the most common movement patterns used by adults to roll from a supine to a prone position (Richter et al., 1989). Essential features of this strategy include a lift-and-reach-arms pattern, with the shoulder girdle initiating motion of the head and trunk, and a unilateral lift of the leg.

A common assumption in the therapeutic literature is that rotation between the shoulders and pelvis is an invariant characteristic in rolling patterns used by normal adults (Bobath, 1965); however, in this study on rolling, many of the adults tested did not show this pattern. Similar to the findings from studies on rising from a bed, the great variability used by normal subjects to move from a supine to a prone position

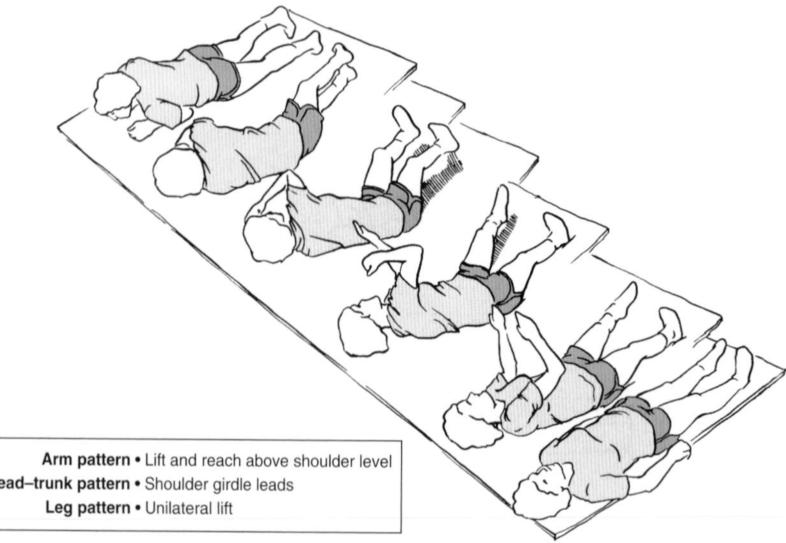

FIGURE 12.14 Most common movement strategy used by young adults when rolling from a supine to a prone position. (Adapted from Richter RR, VanSant AF, Newton RA. Description of adult rolling movements and hypothesis of developmental sequences. Phys Ther 1989;69:63–71, with permission of the American Physical Therapy Association. This material is copyrighted, and any further reproduction or distribution requires written permission from APTA.)

suggests that therapists may use greater freedom in retraining movement strategies used by patients with neurologic impairments. Clearly, there is no one correct way to accomplish this movement.

SUMMARY

1. There are three major requirements for successful locomotion: (a) progression, defined as the ability to generate a basic locomotor pattern that can move the body in the desired direction; (b) stability, defined as the ability to support and control the body against gravity; and (c) adaptability, defined as the ability to adapt gait to meet the individual's goals and the demands of the environment.
2. Normal locomotion is a bipedal gait in which the limbs move in a symmetrical alternating relationship. Gait is divided into a stance and swing phase, each of which has its own intrinsic requirements.
3. During the support phase of gait, horizontal forces are generated against the support surface to move the body in the desired direction (progression), while vertical forces support the body mass against gravity (stability). In addition, strategies used to accomplish both progression and stability must be flexible in order to accommodate changes in speed, direction, or alterations in the support surface (adaptation).
4. The goals to be achieved during the swing phase of gait include advancement of the swing leg (progression) and repositioning the limb in preparation for weight acceptance (stability). Both the progression and stability goals require sufficient foot clearance, so the toe does not drag on the supporting surface during swing. In addition, strategies used during the swing phase of gait must be sufficiently flexible in order to allow the swing foot to avoid any obstacles in its path (adaptation).
5. Gait is often described with respect to temporal distance parameters such as velocity, step length, step frequency (cadence), and stride length. In addition, gait is described with reference to changes in joint angles (kinematics), muscle activation patterns (electromyographic), and the forces used to control gait (kinetics).
6. Many neural and nonneural elements work together in the control of gait. Although spinal pattern generators are able to produce stereotyped locomotor patterns and to perform certain adaptive functions, descending pathways from higher centers and sensory feedback from the periphery allow the rich variation in locomotor patterns and adaptability to task and environmental conditions.
7. One of the requirements of normal locomotion is the ability to adapt gait to a wide-ranging set of environments, and this involves using sensory information from all the senses, both reactively and proactively.
8. An important part of controlling locomotion is stabilizing the head, since it contains two of the most important sensors for controlling motion: the vestibular system and visual system. In neurologically intact adults, the head is stabilized with great precision, allowing gaze to be stabilized through the vestibulo-ocular reflex.

9. Stair-walking is similar to level walking in that it involves stereotypical reciprocal alternating movements of the lower limbs and has three requirements: the generation of primarily concentric forces to propel the body upstairs, or eccentric forces to control the body's descent downstairs (progression); controlling the center of mass within a constantly changing base of support (stability); and the capacity to adapt strategies used for progression and stability to accommodate changes in stair environment, such as height, width, and the presence or absence of railings (adaptation).
10. Although mobility is often thought of in relation to gait, many other aspects of mobility are essential to independence. These include the ability to move from a sitting to a standing position, rolling, rising from a bed, or moving from one chair to another. These skills are referred to as "transfer tasks."
11. Transfer tasks are similar to locomotion in that they share common task requirements: motion in a desired direction (progression), postural control (stability), and the ability to adapt to changing task and environmental conditions (adaptation). Researchers have found great variability in the types of movement strategies used by neurologically intact young adults when performing transfer tasks.
12. Understanding the stability and strength requirements for different types of strategies used to accomplish transfer tasks has important implications for retraining these skills in neurologically impaired patients with different types of motor constraints.

ANSWERS TO LAB ACTIVITY ASSIGNMENTS

Lab Activity 12-1

1. Step length: mean step length of about 76.3 cm (30.05 in.).
2. Stride length: approximately twice the step length, unless the participant has an asymmetric gait.
3. Step width: about 8–9 cm.
   Cadence: mean cadence (step rate) of about 1.9 steps/sec (about 112.5 steps/min).
4. There is a linear relationship between step length and step frequency over a wide range of walking speeds. However, once an upper limit to step length is reached, continued elevation in speed comes from step rate. Stance phase shortens as walking speed increases. Also, the addition of an assistive device most often decreases gait velocity even among nonimpaired individuals.

Lab Activity 12-2

For answers, see Figure 12.2. Determine whether your numbers are similar to those in the individual graphs.

Lab Activity 12-3

1. Gastrocnemius and soleus relax and tibialis anterior contracts.
2. COP first moves posteriorly and laterally toward the swing limb and then shifts toward the stance limb and forward.
3. With the leg closer to the wall.
4. Yes.
5. You could not easily shift your weight in preparation for stepping.

Lab Activity 12-4

Answers will vary.

CHAPTER 13

A LIFE SPAN PERSPECTIVE OF MOBILITY

LEARNING OBJECTIVES

Following completion of this chapter, the reader will be able to:

1. Describe the time course of emergence during development of the three major requirements of locomotion—progression (pattern generation), stability (balance during gait), and adaptation (proactive control, including obstacle avoidance and reactive control to slips and trips)—and the changes in these requirements with aging.
2. Describe the major kinematic, kinetic, and electromyographic changes that occur during the development and maturation of independent gait in children and the changes in these parameters that occur with aging.
3. Describe the contributions of neural (sensory, motor, and higher cognitive) and nonneural subsystems to the development of gait in children and changes with aging.
4. Discuss the changes across the life span associated with other forms of mobility, including stair-climbing and transfers.

INTRODUCTION

It is wonderful to see children develop their first mobility skills as they begin to crawl, creep, walk, and run—finally, navigating expertly through complex environments. How do these skills develop? When do they first begin to emerge? What key features of normal locomotor development should we incorporate into our measurement tools so that we can better understand the delayed or disordered development of the child with central nervous system pathology?

Falls, and the injuries that often accompany them, are a serious problem in the older adult. Many of these falls occur during walking. Problems with balance and gait are considered major contributors to falls in the older adult. Nevertheless, not all older adults have difficulties with mobility skills. Much like the study of balance control, it is important to distinguish between age-related changes in mobility affecting all older adults and pathology-related changes, which affect only a few.

This chapter discusses mobility skills from a lifespan perspective. We first review the development of mobility skills in neurologically intact children and summarize research from different theoretical perspectives that explore the factors contributing to the emergence of this complex ability. In the latter half of the chapter, we discuss how mobility skills change in older adults.

DEVELOPMENT OF LOCOMOTION

Independent locomotion may at first seem to be a fairly simple and automatic skill, but it is really a very intricate motor task. A child learning to walk needs to activate a complex pattern of muscle contractions in many body segments to produce a coordinated stepping movement, meeting the goal of progression. To accomplish the goal of stability, the child must be strong enough to support body weight and stable enough to compensate for shifts in balance while walking. Finally, the child must develop the ability to adapt gait to changing environmental circumstances, allowing navigation around and over obstacles, and across uneven surfaces (Thelen & Ulrich, 1991).

In the following section, we summarize research evidence suggesting that in the development of locomotion, these three requirements emerge sequentially, during the first years of life. How does this complex behavior develop? What are the origins of this behavior during prenatal development?

Prenatal Development

Researchers have actually traced the origins of locomotor rhythms back to embryonic movements that begin to occur in the first stages of development. Ultrasound techniques have been used to document the movements of human infants prenatally. This research has shown that all movements except those observed in the earliest stages of embryonic development (7 to 8 weeks) are also seen in neonates and young infants. Isolated leg and arm movements develop in the embryo by 9 weeks of age, while alternating leg movements, similar to walking movements seen after birth, develop by about 16 weeks of embryonic age (De Vries et al., 1982; Prechtl, 1984).

Animal research has also explored the prenatal development of locomotor circuitry. Detectable limb movements appear to emerge in a cephalocaudal sequence, with movements in the forelimbs preceding those in the hindlimbs (Bradley & Smith, 1988). Intralimb coordination develops prior to interlimb coordination, with the first detectable movements occurring at proximal joints, and moves distally with development. Finally, interlimb coordination develops, first with alternating patterns, then with synchronous patterns (Stehouwer & Farel, 1984).

Many newborn animals, such as rats, do not normally show coordinated locomotor movements until about 1 week after birth (Bradley & Bekoff, 1989). If, however, rats are placed in water at birth, they swim, demonstrating the maturity of their locomotor system. In addition, adult forms of locomotion can be elicited in 3-day-old kittens by placing them on a treadmill (Bradley & Smith, 1988). However, gait in kittens is uncoordinated, because of their poor postural abilities.

These results suggest that a primary constraint on emerging locomotor behavior is the immaturity of the postural system and thus the inability to achieve upright stability. In addition, these findings remind us to be careful about assuming that because a behavior is not evident there is no neural circuitry for it.

Early Stepping Behavior

Because locomotor patterns have been developing for some months prenatally, it is not surprising to find that stepping behavior can be elicited in newborns under the right conditions (Forssberg, 1985; Prechtl, 1984; Thelen et al., 1989). For example, when newborn infants are held under the arms in an upright position, tilted slightly forward, with the soles of the feet touching a surface, they often perform coordinated movements that look much like erect locomotion. Surprisingly, stepping becomes progressively more difficult to elicit during the first month of life, tending to disappear in most infants by about 2 months of age and reappear with the onset of self-generated locomotion many months later.

This pattern of appearance and disappearance of newborn stepping was found in a study that examined 156 children longitudinally (Forssberg, 1985). It was found that 94 infants stepped at 1 month, 18 stepped at 3 months, and only 2 stepped at 4 and 5 months. Then, at 10 months, after a 4- to 8-month period of no stepping, all 156 infants stepped with support and 18 stepped without support. Thus, the stepping pattern appeared to be temporarily lost in 98 to 99% of the infants.

What causes these changes? Different theoretical approaches explain changes in infant behavior in very different ways. From a reflex hierarchy perspective, newborn stepping is thought to result from a stepping reflex. Its disappearance is assumed to be mainly the result of inhibition by maturing higher neural centers. Figure 13.1 illustrates seven phases in the development of infant locomotion, beginning with the observation of this reflex (phase 1) and its disappearance (phase 2), continuing with its reappearance (phase 3) and the emergence of assisted locomotion (phase 4), and concluding with three phases of erect independent walking, in which the hands gradually move from a high guard position (phase 5) down to the side (phase 6) and the trunk and head become more erect (phase 7) (McGraw, 1945).

In contrast to a reflex hierarchical model, researchers using a dynamic systems approach have examined the emergence of stepping in relation to the contributions of multiple neural and nonneural systems. In particular, these studies have explored the conditions leading to the emergence of newborn stepping and the changes that cause its disappearance. Esther Thelen, a psychologist, and her colleagues have applied a dynamic systems approach to the study of locomotor development (Thelen et al., 1989). This approach views locomotion as an emergent property of many interacting complex processes, including sensory, motor, perceptual, integrative, respiratory, cardiac,

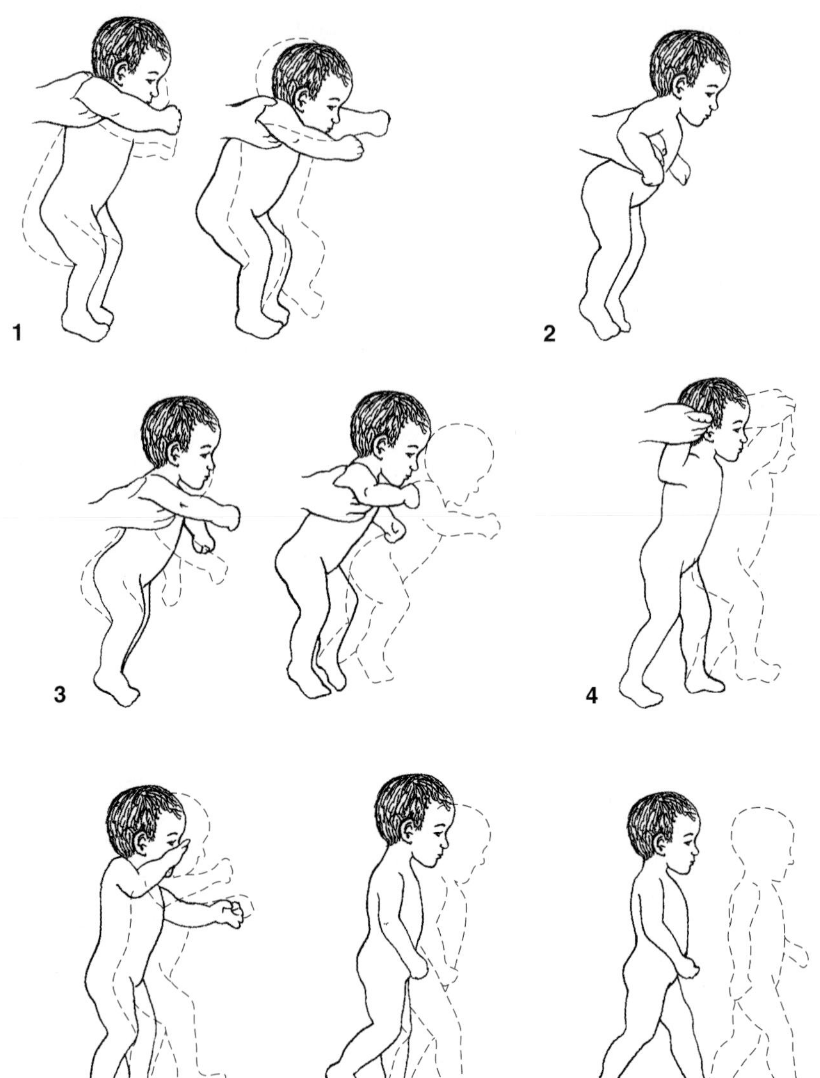

FIGURE 13.1 The seven phases of erect locomotion according to McGraw. 1, Stepping reflex; 2, its disappearance; 3, its reappearance; 4, assisted locomotion; 5–7, three phases of erect independent walking in which the hands gradually move from a high guard position (5) down to the side (6) and the trunk and head become more erect (7). (Adapted from McGraw MB. The neuromuscular maturation of the human infant. New York: Hafner Press, 1945.)

and anatomical systems. According to a dynamic systems approach, moving and developing systems have certain self-organizing properties, that is, they can spontaneously form patterns that arise simply from the interaction of the different parts of the system.

A dynamic systems model stresses that actions always occur within specific contexts. As a result, a given neural code will produce very different behavioral outcomes, depending on the contributions of the other elements of the system, as in the position of the child with relation to gravity. Thus, dynamic systems researchers suggest that the specific leg trajectory seen in newborn stepping is not coded precisely anywhere in the nervous system. Instead, the pattern emerges through the contributions of many elements. These include the neural substrate, anatomical linkages, body composition, activation or arousal level, and the gravitational conditions in which the infant is kicking (Thelen et al., 1989).

From a dynamic systems perspective, the disappearance of the neonatal stepping pattern at about 2 months of age results from changes in a number of components of the system that reduce the likelihood of seeing this behavior. For example, body build changes greatly in the first 18 months of life. Infants add a lot of body fat in the first 2 months of life and then slim down toward the end of the first year. It has been suggested that the stepping pattern goes away at 2 months because infants have insufficient strength to lift the heavier leg during the step cycle (Thelen et al., 1989).

When 4-week-old infants are submerged up to their trunk in water, thus making them more buoyant and counteracting the effects of gravity, stepping increases in frequency (Thelen et al., 1984). This suggests that the infant's weight is a factor that affects the step cycle. Further support for the weight hypothesis related to the disappearance of newborn stepping comes from research examining newborn kicking patterns. Supine kicking has the same spatial and temporal patterning as newborn stepping. For example, the swing phase of locomotion is similar to the flexion and extension phases of the kick, while the stance phase is similar to the pause between kicks. As stepping speeds up, the stance phase is reduced, and as kicking speeds up, the pause phase is reduced (Thelen et al., 1989).

This suggests that the same pattern generator may be responsible for both supine kicking and newborn stepping. Yet supine kicking continues during the period when newborn stepping disappears. One explanation for the persistence of supine kicking is that it does not require the same strength as stepping, since the infants are not working against gravity (Thelen et al., 1984).

Other researchers (Forssberg, 1985; Okamoto et al., 2001) have examined in more detail the contribution of the nervous system to the emergence of locomotion. Forssberg (1985) postulated that human locomotion is characterized by the interaction of many systems with certain hierarchical components. His research suggests that an innate pattern generator creates the basic rhythm of the step cycle, which can be seen in newborn stepping. In the first year, the gradual development of descending systems from higher neural centers gives the child the ability to control this locomotor activity. Adaptive systems for equilibrium control, organized at a higher level than those controlling the pattern generator, develop over a longer period.

According to this research, the emergence of walking with support is not the result of critical changes in the stepping pattern per se, but appears to be due to maturation of the equilibrium system. In addition, the gradual emergence of mature gait over the next year is hypothesized to result from a new higher-level control system influencing the original lower level network and modifying it (Forssberg, 1985).

Forssberg's research, using electromyography (EMG) and motion analysis, has examined how the locomotor pattern changes over the first 2 years of development. Studies using motion-analysis techniques have shown a gradual transformation of the locomotor movement from a synchronous pattern of joint movements in newborn stepping to a more adult-like dissociated pattern of joint motion by the end of the first year of development. The transformation to adult-like gait patterns happens during the latter part of the second year. At this point, heel strike begins to occur in front of the body. Figure 13.2 shows the kinematics of neonatal versus adult stepping movements. Note that the infant shows high levels of hip flexion as compared with the adult.

The EMG analysis supported the findings of the motion analysis. For example, in the neonate, the motor pattern was characterized by a high degree of synchronized activity. In other words, the extensor muscles of different joints were active simultaneously, and there was much coactivation of agonist and antagonist muscles at each joint. As with the movement patterns, the EMG patterns also began to look more mature during the latter part of the second year, with asynchronous patterns emerging at the different joints (Forssberg, 1985).

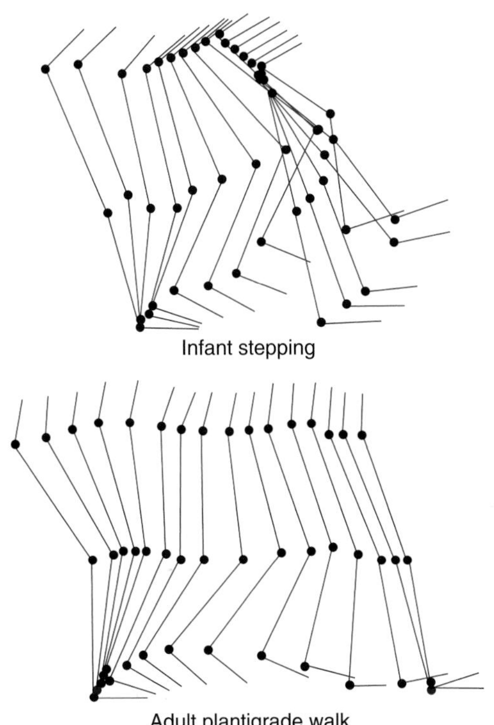

FIGURE 13.2 Stick figures taken from motion analysis of one step cycle of walking in an infant versus an adult. Note the high amounts of hip flexion in the infant. (Source: Forssberg H. Ontogeny of human locomotor control: 1. Infant stepping, supported locomotion and transition to independent locomotion. Exp Brain Res 1985;67:481.)

Another set of longitudinal studies explored the developmental changes in control of the leg muscles from newborn stepping through the first 4 months of life, and from the onset of independent walking through 3 years of age (Okamoto & Okamoto, 2001; Okamoto et al., 2001) and supported and extended the results of Forssberg. The researchers found that neonatal stepping showed cocontraction patterns of agonists and antagonists, especially during the stance phase. They found that EMG patterns began to change to reciprocal patterns in infant stepping after the first month, but excessive muscular contraction accompanying their slightly squatted posture and forward lean were still present. Results showed that strong leg extensor activation before floor contact, not seen in the neonatal period, began to appear in the young infant period from 1 month to 3 months of age.

Okamoto and colleagues (Okamoto et al., 2001; Okamoto & Okamoto, 2001) noted that the EMG characteristics of infant gait up to about 1 month after learning to walk were clearly distinct from those in the adult. For example, in the stance phase from foot contact until push-off, the vastus medialis appeared to be critical for maintaining stability, with a slightly squatted position being used to lower the center of gravity. Subsequently, reciprocal or cocontraction patterns of activity in the rectus femoris and biceps femoris or in the tibialis anterior and gastrocnemius were associated with the return of the body's center of mass (COM) toward its initial position. Finally, toward the end of the swing phase, the vastus medialis and gastrocnemius were strongly activated for active leg extension, possibly used to prevent falling. The authors suggest that this excessive muscle activation in infant walking may be due to weak muscle strength and an immature balancing system. Like Forssberg, Okamoto and colleagues suggest that the gradual changes of leg muscular activity from newborn stepping through more mature walking are due to the development of subsystems underlying postural control and muscle strength, thus modulating the neonatal stepping reflex.

Locomotion in human neonates may be similar to that of quadrupeds who walk on the their toes, like cats, dogs, and horses. For example, newborns show high knee/hip flexion and do not have heel strike. Since extensor muscle activity occurs prior to foot touchdown, it appears to be driven by an innate locomotor pattern generator, as has been found in quadrupeds, rather than being reflexly activated by the foot in contact with the ground. It has also been suggested that the neural network for stepping must be organized at or below the brainstem level, since anencephalic infants (infants born without a cerebral cortex) can perform a similar pattern of infant stepping (Peiper, 1963).

Interestingly, some researchers believe that the abnormal gait patterns found in many patients with neurologic pathology are actually immature locomotor patterns. Thus, children with cerebral palsy, children with mental retardation, and children who habitually toe-walk may persist in using an immature locomotor pattern, while adults with acquired neurologic disease may revert to immature locomotion because of the loss of higher-center modulation over the locomotor pattern generator (Forssberg, 1985).

One kinematic characteristic of mature walking is its pendular movement, associated with the COM of the body vaulting over the stance leg in an arc. This is called the "inverted pendulum mechanism of bipedal walking." Researchers have explored whether the pendulum mechanism is innate or, alternatively, is acquired with walking experience (Ivanenko et al., 2004). The kinematics of locomotion from infants taking their first unsupported steps (at about 1 year of age) were compared with that in older children and adults. Results indicated that the pendulum mechanism was not implemented at the onset of unsupported locomotion.

To determine whether differences were due to the infants walking much more slowly than older children, the researchers normalized the locomotor speed and found that the percentage of recovery of mechanical energy in children older than 2 years was roughly similar to that of the adults, while the percentage of recovery in toddlers was about 50% lower. They found that pendulum-like behavior along with a fixed coupling of the angular motion of the lower limb segments rapidly moved toward mature values within a few months of independent walking, suggesting that independent walking experience could be a functional trigger for these developmental changes. They concluded that the emergence of the pendulum mechanism is not an inevitable mechanical consequence of a system of linked segments, but requires active neural control and an appropriate pattern of intersegmental coordination (Ivanenko et al., 2004).

One of the rate-limiting factors hypothesized to constrain the emergence of independent locomotion is the development of postural control, and it has been hypothesized that one factor contributing to unusual EMG and kinematic characteristics of newly walking toddlers is their postural instability. In order to determine the extent to which instability can explain why toddlers walk with a different gait, Ivanenko et al. (2005) compared kinematics and EMGs in toddlers performing their first independent steps with versus without hand or trunk support. They found that hand support significantly improved postural stability and reduced the percentage of falls, step width, lateral hip deviations, and trunk oscillations. However, in spite of these improvements, many kinematic and EMG patterns were unaffected by increased postural stability. In particular, they found that the covariance of the angular motion of the lower limb segments, the pattern of bilateral coordination of the vertical movement of the two hip joints, the high variability of the foot path, the single peak trajectory of the foot in the swing phase, and characteristic EMG bursts at foot contact remained similar in both supported and unsupported walking. The toddler pattern was, rather, found to show features similar to those of an adult stepping in place. They also found that characteristics of walking kinematics did not basically change until the occurrence of a child's first unsupported steps; then they quickly matured. They thus propose that many of the idiosyncratic features of newly walking toddlers are not due to poor balance control but may represent an innate kinematic template of stepping (Ivanenko et al., 2005).

So what are the elements that contribute to the emergence of locomotion in the infant? Remember that in development, some elements of the nervous and musculoskeletal systems may be functionally ready before others, but the systems must wait for the maturation of the slowest component before the target behavior can appear. A small increase or change in the development of the slowest component can act as the control parameter, becoming the impetus that drives the system to a new behavioral form.

The research we just discussed shows that many of the components that contribute to independent locomotion are functional before the child takes any independent steps. Function of the locomotor pattern generator is present in a limited capacity at birth and is improved during the second half of the first year, as the tight intralimb synergies become dissociated and capable of more complex modulation and control. As we noted in Chapter 8 on the development of postural control, infants are able to use optic flow information at birth to modulate head movements and at least by 5 to 6 months of age for modulation of stance. Motivation to navigate toward a distant object is clearly present by the onset of creeping and crawling, and voluntary control over the limbs is certainly present by this time for many behaviors (Thelen et al., 1989).

So what is the constraint that keeps upright bipedal locomotion from emerging before 9 to 12 months of age? Most researchers believe that it is primarily due to limitations in balance control, and possibly also limitations in strength (Forssberg, 1985; Thelen et al., 1989; Woollacott, 1989). Of course, balance control and the stepping pattern continue to mature after the emergence of independent walking (Ivanenko et al., 2005).

For example, when an infant is creeping, one foot at a time can be picked up, so there is always a tripod stance available and, thus, balance is much less demanding. Normal infants who are about to take their first steps have developed motor coordination within the locomotor pattern generator; they also have functional visual, vestibular, and somatosensory systems and the motivation to move forward. Infants may also have sufficient muscle strength at least to balance, if not for use in propelling the body forward. But they will not be able to use these processes in effective locomotion until the postural control system can effectively control the shift of weight from leg to leg, thus avoiding a fall. When these processes hit a particular threshold for effective function, then the dynamic behavior of independent bipedal locomotion can emerge.

When looking at the three requirements for successful locomotion: a rhythmic stepping pattern (progression), the control of balance (stability), and the ability to modify gait (adaptation), clearly, a rhythmic stepping pattern develops first. It is present in limited form at birth, and is refined during the first year of life. Stance stability develops second, toward the end of the first year and the beginning of the second year of life. As we discuss in the next section, it appears that adaptability is refined in the first years after the onset of independent walking.

Specificity of Perceptual Learning During Locomotor Development

When infants begin to crawl, cruise, and walk, they need to learn to take advantage of the environments and surfaces that afford safe locomotion and to avoid contexts that are not safe (e.g., cliffs or steep stairs). What constitutes a safe environment will also change as the infant gains new locomotor skills and learns to navigate steeper slopes and narrower surfaces with agility. How do infants acquire these perceptual skills? Researchers have studied this by changing surface properties that infants move over, including the friction, surface rigidity, slant, bridge width over a steep drop, cliff edges, height of stairs and pedestals and availability of handrails (Berger & Adolph, 2007). Figure 13.3 shows examples of some of these contexts that have been studied.

Figure 13.4 shows both cross-sectional and longitudinal data that indicate that infants learn to perceive affordances for locomotion through crawling and walking experience. For example, in their first weeks of both crawling and walking infants attempted to navigate slopes that were well beyond their ability (positive numbers on the x-axis of the graph show that the slope is well beyond their ability to navigate). With experience, this behavior decreased, with their perceptual judgments becoming similar to their actual motor ability, such that attempts to navigate a slope matched the infant's probability of success. Interestingly, results show no transfer between crawling and walking postures. For example, infants who were new walkers avoided a 36-degree descent in crawling but would plunge down the same slope when walking (Adolph & Berger, 2006).

Maturation of Independent Locomotion

Bril and Breniere, two French researchers, studied the emergence of locomotion and hypothesized that learning to walk is a two-stage process (Bril & Breniere, 1993; Breniere & Bril, 1998). In the initial phase (3 to 6 months after the onset of walking), infants learn to

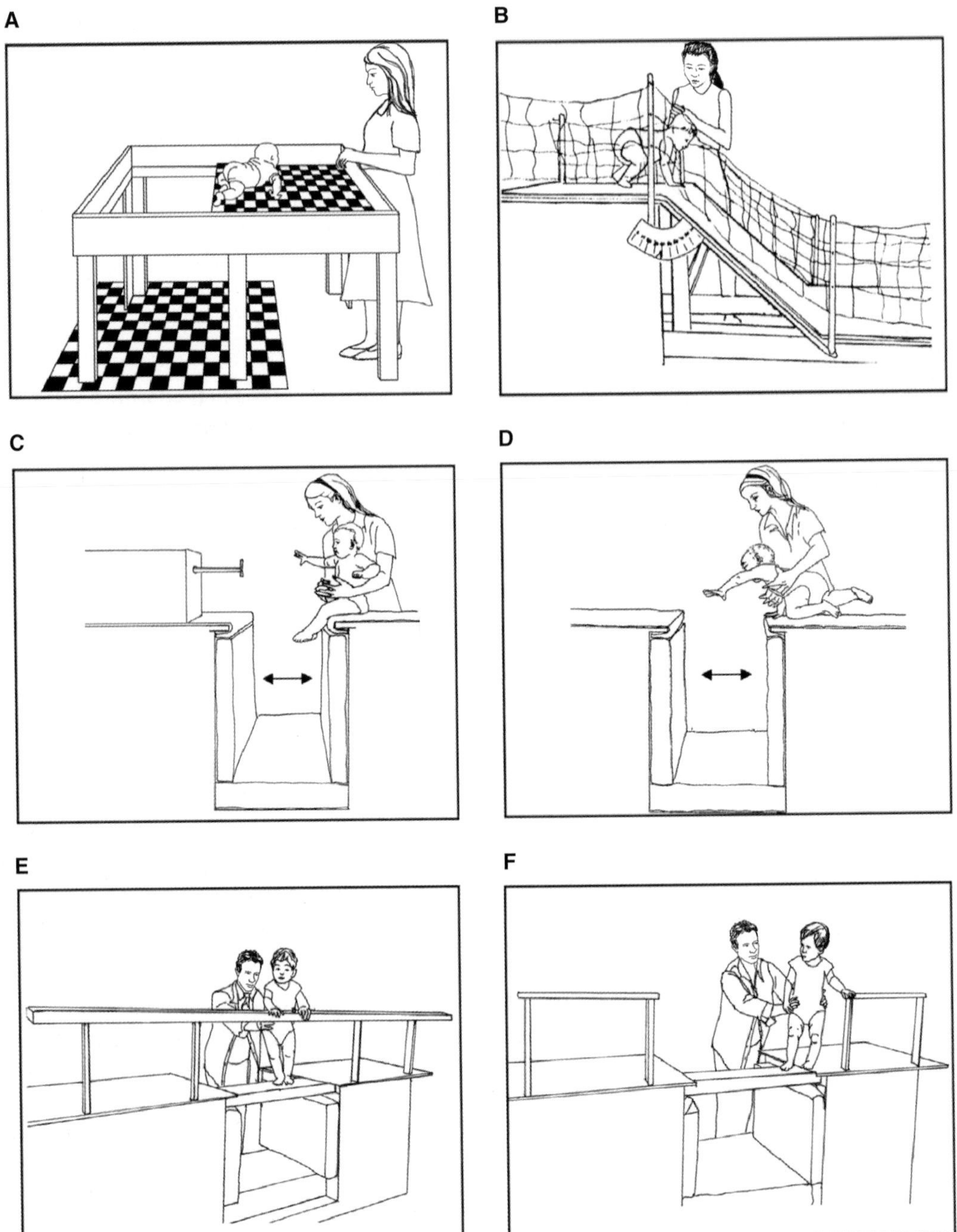

FIGURE 13.3 Examples of paradigms that have been used to test infants' perception of affordances for locomotion: A, A crawling infant approaching a "visual cliff" with an apparent drop off. B, A crawling infant at the top of a changeable slope. C, A sitting infant reaching forward over an adjustable gap in the surface. D, A crawling infant approaching a gap in the support surface. E, A walking infant using a handrail to help balance on a narrow bridge. F, A walking infant exploring a narrow bridge. (Reprinted with permission from Adolph KE, Berger SE. Motor development. In: Damon W, Lerner R, series eds.; Kuhn D, Siegler RS, vol. eds. Handbook of child psychology, vol. 2. Cognition, perception, and language, 6th ed. New York: Wiley, 2006:192. Copyright © 2006 John Wiley & Sons, Inc. Reproduced with permission of John Wiley & Sons, Inc.).

control balance, while in the second phase (lasting through 5 years of independent walking), the locomotor pattern is progressively refined.

They studied children longitudinally during the first 6 years of life to see how gait patterns change as independent locomotion develops. Significant changes in emerging gait patterns are summarized in Figure 13.5. Figure 13.5A illustrates the decrease in the duration of the double-support phase of gait that shows a dramatic drop in the first 4 months of

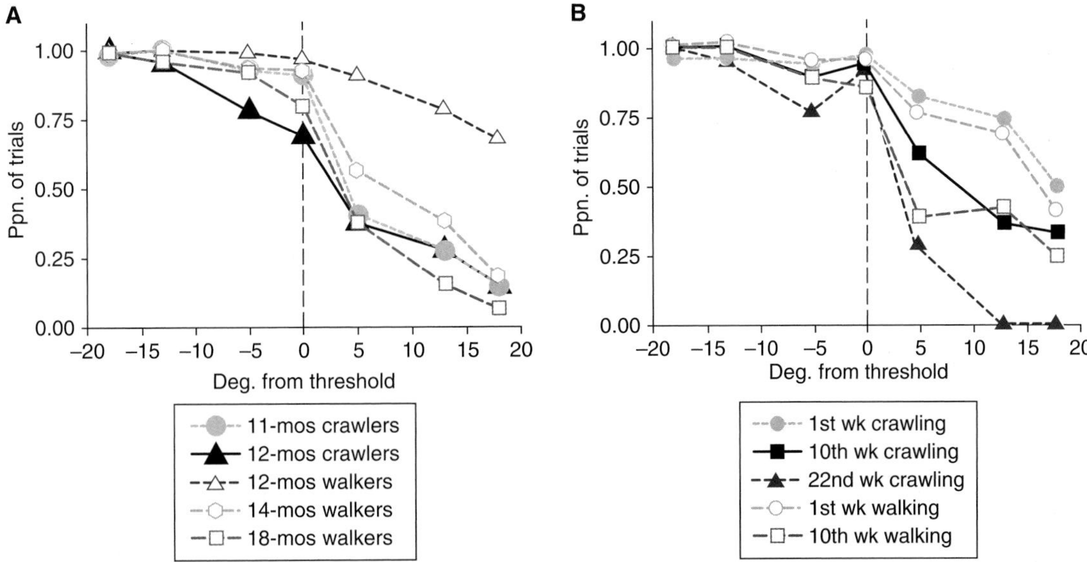

FIGURE 13.4 Perceptual judgments of infants (indicated by attempts to crawl and walk down slopes. A, Cross-sectional data. B, Longitudinal data. Data are normalized to each infant's motor threshold (indicated by 0 on the x-axis). Negative numbers on the x-axis indicate safe slopes that were shallower than the infants' motor thresholds. Positive numbers indicate risky slopes steeper than the infants' motor thresholds. Graphs show that perceptual errors (attempts to locomote on risky slopes) depend on the motor experience of the infant within a posture, not on their age or the specific locomotor posture. (Reprinted with permission from Adolph KE, Berger SE. Motor development. In: Damon W, Lerner R, series eds.; Kuhn D, Siegler Rs, vol. eds. Handbook of child psychology, vol. 2. Cognition, perception, and language, 6th ed. New York: Wiley, 2006:194. Copyright © 2006 John Wiley & Sons, Inc. Reproduced with permission of John Wiley & Sons, Inc.).

walking, and then continues to drop until about 35 months of independent walking. Figure 13.3B shows the dramatic increase in step length that occurs in the first 4 months of walking, along with a decrease in step width that continues through about 10 months of walking experience. They noted that in newly walking children, walking velocity was very low, with the duration of the swing phase being very short and that of the double-support phase being long, probably because the children needed a long double-support phase to regain balance.

The authors asked what factors might constrain the development of these postural abilities during walking (Breniere & Bril, 1998). They proposed that high levels of strength are required to control gravitational forces that tend to destabilize the upper body. In fact, it has been predicted that requirements of musculotendinous forces at the hip may reach six to eight times body weight at certain points in the stance phase of gait (McKinnon & Winter, 1993). Thus, Breniere and Bril (like Okamoto & Okamoto, 2001) hypothesized that newly walking children may lack the muscular strength to control balance. In order to test this hypothesis, the authors measured vertical center of gravity acceleration under the assumption that vertical ground reaction forces reflect the ability of the musculoskeletal system to compensate for body weight.

In adults, the vertical acceleration of the COM at heel strike is positive, indicating that they have both the muscular capacity and the control to counter destabilizing forces associated with initial contact. In contrast, Breniere and Bril (1998) found (as shown in Fig. 13.5C) that at the onset of independent walking in infants, the vertical acceleration of the COM at heel strike was always negative, indicating an initial deficit in muscular capacity. In the first 5 months of independent walking, the infants increased walking velocity substantially, due in large part to increases in step length. This increases the vertical instability, and interestingly, the vertical acceleration of the COM becomes even more negative. Thus, during this period, muscle strength appears to remain low compared with balance requirements. As shown in Figure 13.5C, by about 6 months of independent walking the vertical acceleration of the COM at heel strike finally showed a change in direction toward positive values, indicating a change in postural control. Now the infants stopped "walking by falling" and began controlling this forward "fall" during walking. The vertical acceleration of the COM at heel strike finally reached 0 value at about 3 to 4 years of walking experience (4 to 5 years of age), showing that they could control the inertial and gravity forces induced by walking (Fig. 13.5C). By 5 years of walking experience, three

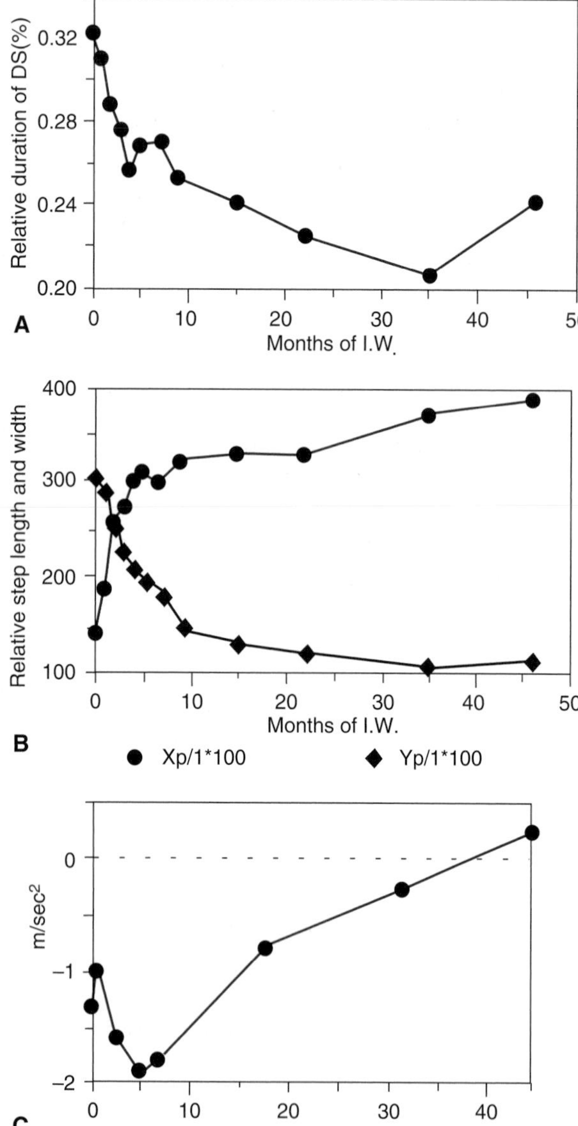

FIGURE 13.5 Changes in different walking parameters during the first 4 years of walking. A, Relative duration of the double-support (DS) phase. B, Changes in relative step length and width. C, Changes in vertical acceleration of the center of gravity. IW = independent walking; Xp = step length; Yp = step width. (Reprinted with permission from Bril B, Breniere Y. Posture and independent locomotion in childhood: learning to walk or learning dynamic postural control? In: Savelsbergh GJP, ed. The development of coordination in infancy. Amsterdam: North-Holland, 1993:337–358.)

of the five children showed positive values similar to those of adults (Breniere & Bril, 1998). Since the changes in step width, step length, and double-support phase relate to the mastery of balance control, their findings support the idea that it is during the first phase of walking that a child learns to integrate posture into locomotor movements.

Studies of changes in EMG characteristics and kinematics from the onset of walking through the mastery of mature forms of gait have been performed by other laboratories as well (Dierick et al., 2004; Okamoto & Kumamoto, 1972; Okamoto & Okamoto, 2001; Sutherland et al., 1980).

As noted above, in the first days of independent walking, stepping patterns are immature. For example, the push-off motion in the stance phase is absent, the step width is very wide, and the arms are held high. The infant appears to generate force to propel the body forward by leaning forward at the trunk. The swing phase is short because the infant is unable to balance on one leg.

By 10 to 15 days of independent walking, the infant begins to reduce cocontraction, and at 50 to 85 days after the onset of walking, the muscle patterns begin to show a reciprocal relationship. Okamoto and Kumamoto (1972) state that if infants are supported during walking, the reciprocal relationship between muscles emerges, but with the additional requirement of stabilizing the body while walking independently, the coactivation returns. This is in contrast to the results of Ivanenko et al. (2005), noted above, that indicated that most EMG and kinematic patterns were unaffected by giving additional postural support to new walkers.

Other common gait characteristics in the first year of walking include a high step frequency, absence of the reciprocal swinging movements between the upper and lower limbs, a flexed knee during stance phase, and an increased hip flexion, pelvic tilt, and hip abduction during swing phase. There is also ankle plantar flexion at foot strike and decreased ankle flexion during swing, giving a relative foot drop (Sutherland et al., 1980). By 2 years of age, the pelvic tilt and abduction and external rotation of the hip are diminished. At foot strike, a knee-flexion wave appears, and reciprocal swing in the upper limb is present in about 75% of the children. The relative foot drop disappears as the ankle dorsiflexes during swing. By the end of 2 years, the infant begins to show a push-off in stance. During the years from 1 until 7, the muscle amplitudes and durations gradually reduce toward adult levels. By the age of 7, most muscle and movement patterns during walking look very similar to those of adults (Sutherland et al., 1980).

Sutherland et al. (1980) list five important characteristics that determine mature gait, including: (a) duration of single limb stance, (b) walking velocity, (c) cadence, (d) step length, and (e) the ratio of pelvic span to step width.

Duration of single-limb stance increases steadily from 32% in 1-year-olds to 38% in 7-year-olds (39% is a typical adult value). Walking velocity and cadence decrease steadily, while step length increases. Step length is short in the newly walking child, due to lack of stability of the supporting limb, and lengthens with increasing balance abilities. Finally, the ratio of pelvic span, which is defined as body width at the level of the pelvis, to step width increases until age 2½, after which it stabilizes. By 3 years of age, the gait pattern is essentially mature, although small improvements continue through age 7 (Sutherland et al., 1980).

Because control of the COM during walking has been found to be a good indicator of stability, one study further examined changes in the displacement of COM in walking during development in children from 1 to 9 years. Results showed that vertical and lateral amplitudes of the COM (when controlled for leg length) were greater for children before 4 years of age and that the forward amplitude was greater for children before 7 years of age. The authors concluded that the development of COM displacement during gait is a gradual process, evolving through 7 years of age (Dierick et al., 2004).

Table 13.1 summarizes some of the characteristic changes in the step cycle from the initiation of independent walking through the development of mature patterns at about the age of 3 (Gallahue, 1989). These changes can be seen more graphically in Figure 13.6. To better understand changes in gait associated with development, complete Lab Activity 13.1.

Run, Skip, Hop, and Gallop

Running is often described as an exaggerated form of walking. It differs from walking as the result of a brief flight phase in each step. The flight phase that distinguishes a run from a walk is seen at about the second year of age. Until this time, the infant's run is more like a fast walk, with one foot always in contact with the ground. By 4 years of age, most children can hop (33%) and gallop (43%). The development of the gallop precedes the hop slightly. In one study, by 6.5 years, children were skillful at hopping and galloping. However, only 14% of 4-year-olds could skip (step-hop) (Clark & Whitall, 1989).

If central pattern generators (CPGs) control walking, are there separate CPGs for hopping, galloping, and skipping? Probably not. Then why do they emerge in a fixed order of appearance? It is possible to explain their emergence from the dynamic systems perspective. Remember that walking and running are patterns of interlimb coordination in which the limbs are 50% out of phase with one another. This is the easiest stepping pattern to produce, and thus it appears earliest. Running appears later than walking, probably because of its increased strength and balance requirements as compared with walking. Galloping requires that the child produce an asymmetrical gait with unusual timing and a differentiation in force production in each

TABLE 13.1 Developmental Sequence for Walking

I. Walking
- A. Initial stage
  1. Difficulty maintaining upright posture
  2. Unpredictable loss of balance
  3. Rigid, halting leg action
  4. Short steps
  5. Flat-footed contact
  6. Toes turn outward
  7. Wide base of support
  8. Flexed knee at contact followed by quick leg extension
- B. Elementary stage
  1. Gradual smoothing of pattern
  2. Step length increased
  3. Heel–toe contact
  4. Arms down to sides with limited swing
  5. Base of support within the lateral dimensions of trunk
  6. Out-toeing reduced or eliminated
  7. Increased pelvic tilt
  8. Apparent vertical lift
- C. Mature stage
  1. Reflexive arm swing
  2. Narrow base of support
  3. Relaxed, elongated gait
  4. Minimal vertical lift
  5. Definite heel–toe contact

II. Common problems
- A. Inhibited or exaggerated arm swing
- B. Arms crossing midline of body
- C. Improper foot placement
- D. Exaggerated forward trunk lean
- E. Arms flopping at sides or held out for balance
- F. Twisting of trunk
- G. Poor rhythmic action
- H. Landing flat-footed
- I. Flipping foot or lower leg in or out

Reprinted with permission from Gallahue DL. Understanding motor development: infants, children, adolescents. Indianapolis: Benchmark, 1989:236.

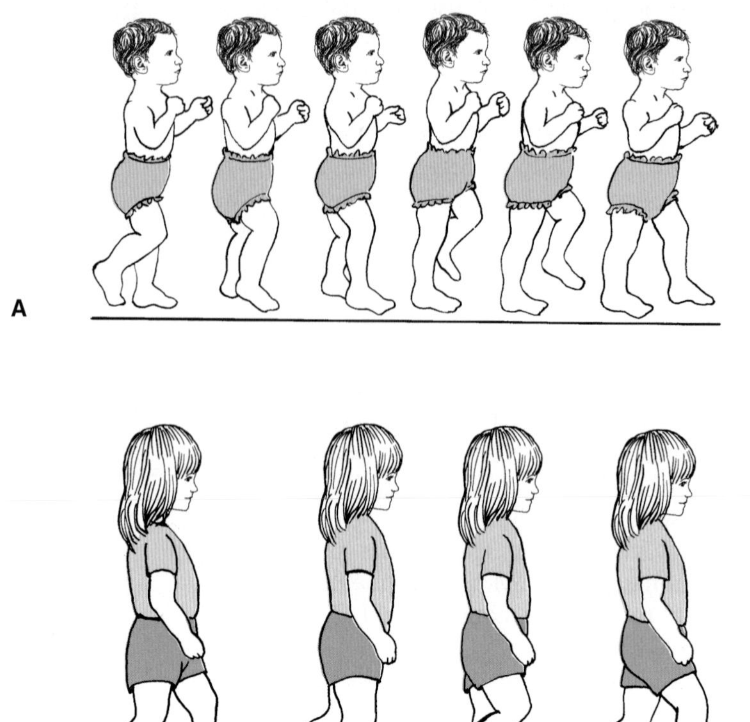

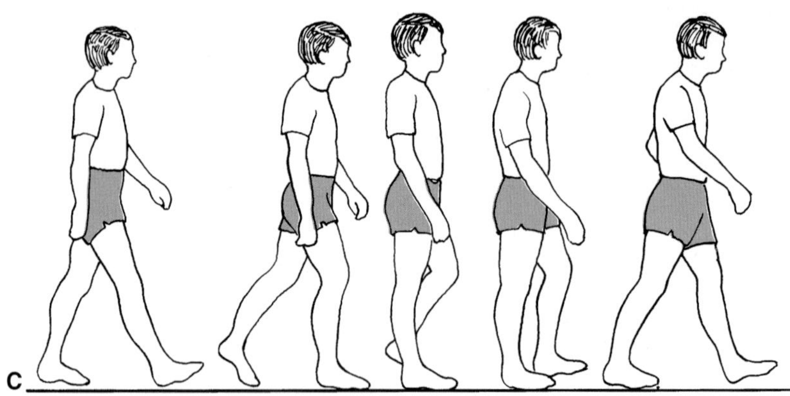

FIGURE 13.6 Body motions associated with developing gait. A, Initial forms of gait. B, Elementary forms of gait. C, Mature forms of gait. (Adapted from Gallahue DL. Understanding motor development: infants, children, adolescents. Indianapolis: Benchmark, 1989:237.)

limb, and it may have additional balance requirements. Hopping emerges next, possibly because it requires the ability to balance the body's weight on one limb and it requires additional force to lift the body off the ground after landing. Skipping (a step-hop) emerges last, possibly because one locomotor coordination pattern is imbedded into another, and thus it requires additional coordination abilities (Clark & Whitall, 1989).

It has been proposed that developmental milestones such as walk, run, gallop, hop, and skip are better indicators of balance development than chronological age. For example, in a study that compared EMG (timing and amplitude) and kinetic (center of pressure [COP] and torque production) characteristics of reactive postural responses in children, the highest level of significance between groups across development was found when children were grouped by the above developmental milestones rather than by chronological age (Sundermier et al., 2001).

Development of Adaptation

How do children learn to adapt their walking patterns so they can navigate over and around obstacles, on

LAB ACTIVITY 13-1

Objective: To examine the kinematics of developing gait.

Procedures: Observe gait patterns in one or two infants of the following ages: 8–10 mo (prewalkers), 12–18 mo (new walkers), and 18–24 mo (experienced walkers). Document age-related changes in spatial and temporal aspects of gait across these age groups. Also observe and describe the following gait characteristics in each child: (1) Ability to maintain an upright posture, (2) ability to control stability (How often does the child fall within a fixed time period?), (3) initial contact at foot strike, and (4) position of arms.

Assignment:

1. Compare your descriptions among the children observed. How do each of the parameters change with age and experience walking?
2. Compare your descriptions of the development of gait to those described in Table 13.1. When do gait parameters begin to approximate those of adults?

different surfaces, and while performing other tasks? As we mentioned in Chapter 12, both reactive and proactive strategies are used to modify gait to changes in the environment. There has been very little research examining the development of adaptation in normal children.

Reactive Strategies

Reactive strategies for adapting gait relate to the integration of compensatory postural responses into the gait cycle. Researchers have looked at compensatory postural muscle responses to perturbations during locomotion and have compared them with those during perturbed quiet stance.

In response to fast-velocity stance perturbations, children respond with both an automatic postural response and a monosynaptic reflex response. As children mature, the stretch reflex response gets smaller in amplitude, while the postural response gets faster. In very young children, there is considerable coactivation of antagonist muscles (Berger et al., 1985).

Perturbations during gait produce a monosynaptic reflex response in children from 1 to 2.5 years but not in older children, as shown in Figure 13.7. This figure shows large monosynaptic reflexes before the automatic postural response in the 1-year-old, which is reduced in the 2.5-year-old, and has disappeared in the 4-year-old and adult. Similar to stance perturbations, automatic postural responses to gait perturbations become faster with age, with mature responses occurring by about 4 years. Coactivation of antagonist muscles also is reduced with age.

Changes in the characteristics of compensatory postural activity are associated with increased stability during gait and increased ability to compensate for perturbations to gait (Berger et al., 1985). This study suggests that children as young as a year old who are capable of independent locomotion can integrate

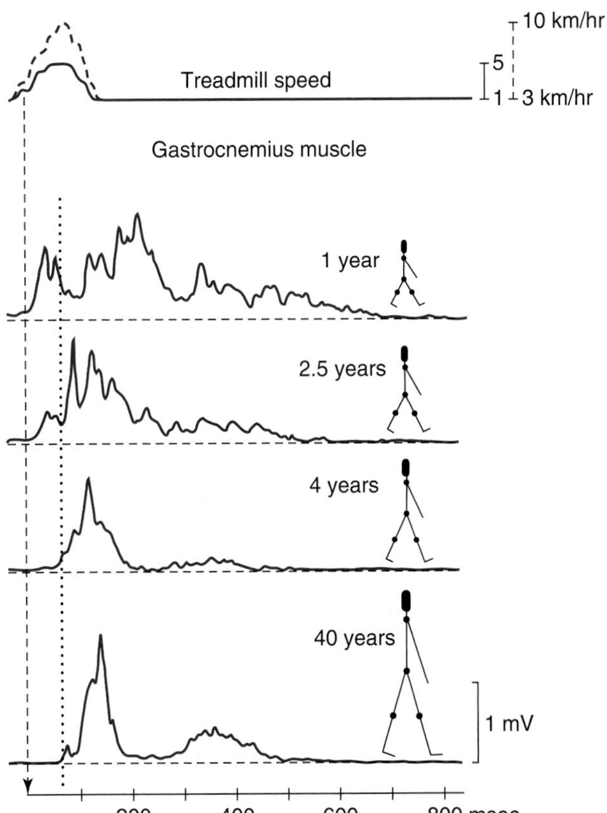

FIGURE 13.7 Examples of the gastrocnemius EMG responses of individual children of 1, 2.5, and 4 years of age and of an adult when their balance is perturbed during walking on a treadmill by briefly increasing treadmill speed. The leftmost vertical line is the onset of the treadmill acceleration and the dotted line to its right is the onset of the EMG response. Note that there is a large monosynaptic reflex in the youngest children, before the automatic postural response. This disappears by 4 years of age. (Reprinted with permission from Berger W, Quintern J, Dietz V. Stance and gait perturbations in children: developmental aspects of compensatory mechanisms. Electroencephalogr Clin Neurophysiol 1985;61:388.)

compensatory postural activity into slow walking when gait is disturbed, although their responses are immature.

Compensatory Stepping Skills During Balance Recovery. The ability to step independently is a fundamental skill required both for locomotion and for balance recovery when threats to balance are large, requiring a step. Interestingly, it appears that the ability to take independent steps in walking does not automatically translate into the ability to use a step for balance recovery. In a study examining the emergence of the ability to step in response to increasing velocities of balance threats, "standers" (children who could stand but not walk), new walkers (children capable of three steps but with less than 2 weeks of walking experience), intermediate walkers (children with 1 to 3 months of walking experience), and advanced walkers (children with 3 to 6 months of walking experience) were given backward support-surface translations. Results showed that the ability to adapt balance responses to increasing balance threats is not present in new standers and new walkers, since almost no children in these two categories were able to take a step to recover balance. Stepping to recover balance begins to develop in infants with 1 to 3 months of walking experience and is relatively refined by 6 months of walking experience (Roncesvalles et al., 2000).

Proactive Strategies

Proactive strategies for adapting gait use sensory information to modify gait patterns in advance of encountering obstacles to gait. When do children begin integrating these strategies into the step cycle? It has been suggested that children first learning to walk acquire feedback control of balance before feedforward control (Hass & Diener, 1988). The results of experiments by Bril and Breniere (1993) support this idea, since children seem to spend the first 4 to 5 months of walking learning to integrate balance into the step cycle.

There is little research on the development of proactive strategies during gait. However, Grasso et al. (1998) examined the ability of children from 3.5 to 8 years to use anticipatory head movements when turning a 90-degree corner while walking. The results showed that predictive head orientation movements occurred in all the 3.5-year-old children in at least one trial, beginning at about 1 second before the turn, as it did in the older children and adults. However, the peak of the head rotation coincided with turning the 90-degree corner for the children, while it occurred about 250 msec earlier in adults. The results suggest that proactive strategies for goal-directed walking are in use early in the development of gait, although they do not mature until later in childhood.

Studies by McFadyen and others (McFadyen et al., 2001; Vallis & McFadyen, 2005) have examined the ability of midchildhood-aged children (7 to 12 years) to use proactive locomotor control to avoid obstacles. These studies showed that these children use adult-like limb displacements and general dynamic strategies for obstacle clearance. However, when data were normalized to body mass, the amplitudes of muscle power bursts related to anticipatory locomotor adjustments were reduced as compared with those of adults.

They also found that when adults and children altered their mediolateral (ML) COM trajectory, adults reoriented the head and trunk segments at the same time as the COM, while children reoriented the head and trunk before changing COM direction. Finally, adults changed their gait patterns well before obstacle crossing, while children initiated ML adjustments to gait patterns just prior to obstacle crossing. The authors conclude that children partition obstacle avoidance into two tasks, initially steering with proactive movement of the head and trunk segments and then making adjustments to their gait trajectory, through stride and step width changes, to obtain the necessary obstacle clearance just before obstacle crossing. The different head and trunk anticipatory coordination patterns imply that the way children obtain visual information is different from that in adults when avoiding obstacles, and they depend more on visual input to guide their locomotor strategy (Vallis & McFadyen, 2005).

Head and Trunk Stabilization during Gait

An important part of controlling locomotion is learning to stabilize the head. Adults stabilize the head with great precision, allowing a steady gaze. Thus, control of the head, arm, and trunk (HAT) segments is a critical part of controlling mobility. How do children control the trunk, arms, and head during locomotion to ensure stabilization of the head and gaze?

Assaiante and Amblard (1995; Assaiante et al., 2005) performed experiments in children from early walkers through children 10 years of age to explore changes in control of these body segments. They suggest that balance and locomotion can be organized according to one of two stable reference frames, either the support surface on which the subject stands and moves or the gravitational reference of vertical.

They noted that when using the support surface as reference, the subject organized balance responses from the feet upward toward the head, using mainly proprioceptive and cutaneous cues. In contrast, when the subject stabilized the head using vision and vestibular information, balance was organized from the head down toward the feet. These researchers explored the changing use of these two strategies in balance control during locomotor development in children.

They also noted that the head can be stabilized on the trunk in one of two modes, in an en bloc mode, in which it moves with the trunk, or in an articulated mode, in which it moves freely, minimizing movements away from vertical. This study explored locomotor strategies through kinematic analysis of walking in infants and children up to 8 years of age.

The authors found that from the acquisition of stance until about 6 years of age, children organize locomotion in a bottom-up manner, using the support surface as a reference and controlling head movements in an en bloc mode, which serves to reduce the degrees of freedom to be controlled. During this period, the children gradually learn to stabilize the hips, then the shoulders, and finally the head. At about 7 years of age, with mastery of control of the head, there is a transition, and the head control is changed to an articulated mode, and top-down organization of balance during locomotion becomes dominant. The authors hypothesized that at 7 to 8 years of age, information specifying head position in relation to gravity becomes more available to the equilibrium-control centers and thus allows the child to use an articulated mode of head control. They suggest that there may be a transient dominance of vestibular processing in locomotor balance at this age (Assaiante & Amblard, 1995; Assaiante et al., 2005).

Research by Ledebt et al. (1995) has shown that hip stabilization in space is present at the onset of walking while head and trunk stabilization improve considerably during the following 3 to 4 months, after which they do not change for about a year.

Studies of the development of canal and otolith vestibulo-ocular reflexes (VORs) have shown that their developmental time courses are very different. The canal VOR is relatively stable in young walkers. However, the onset of walking is a transition point in otolith VOR development, with clear changes in the slow-phase velocity of the VOR. It has thus been proposed that otolith VOR development may play a critical role in the development of postural control during the first months of walking. The authors noted that although the canal VOR does not change during this period, it is very different from that of older children, thus suggesting that it is still immature. They propose that this may be related to the fact that new walkers adopt a stiff neck posture during walking, which is also used by adults with bilateral vestibular deficits. This strategy reduces the amplitude of head rotations in the pitch and roll planes in order to limit instability in the movement of the visual field due to problems with gaze stabilization (Wiener-Vacher et al., 1996).

Initiation of Gait

Chapter 12 on locomotion in adults showed that gait initiation involves anticipatory shifts in the COP backward and toward the stepping foot, which cause a forward and lateral shift of the center of gravity toward the stance leg. Some research has shown that an anticipatory backward shift in the center of pressure is present in children as young as 2½ years of age, and becomes habitual by 6 years of age (Ledebt et al., 1998).

In adults, the anticipatory changes in the COP are accompanied by inhibition of the soleus muscle and activation of the tibialis muscles prior to heel-off (Breniere et al., 1981; Herman et al., 1973). In a study using motion analysis and muscle-response patterns to characterize step initiation in both prewalkers and in children with 1 month to 4 years of walking experience (Assaiante et al., 2000), anticipatory postural adjustments before step initiation were not found in prewalkers, but were present in children with as little as 1 to 4 months of walking experience. These adjustments included a clear anticipatory lateral tilt of the pelvis and of the stance leg, in order to unload the opposite leg shortly before its swing phase. In addition, there was an anticipatory activation of the hip abductor muscle of the leg in stance phase prior to heel off, suggesting the control of pelvis stabilization. These anticipatory postural adjustments did not occur consistently until 4 to 5 years of age. Between 1 and 4 years of age there was a shift from the use of both upper and lower parts of the body (an en bloc strategy) in the lateral shift of the body toward the stance leg, to the inclusion of only the pelvis and leg (articulated operation) in the older children, similar to results from adults. Accompanying these kinematic changes were lower use of hip and knee muscles and greater use of ankle muscles in the older children during the gait initiation process (Assaiante et al., 2000).

Development of Other Mobility Skills

The first part of this chapter describes the emergence of independent locomotion. We now turn briefly to a review of some of the information on the emergence of other mobility behaviors during development, including rolling, prone progression, and movement from lying in a supine position to standing.

There are two approaches to describing motor development in infants and children. One approach relies on normative studies that describe the age at which various motor behaviors emerge. Normative studies have given rise to norm-referenced scales that compare an infant's motor behavior with the performance of a group of infants of the same age. Normative studies can provide clinicians with rough guidelines about the relative ages associated with specific motor milestones. However, they have universally reported that there is incredible variability in the time at which normal children achieve motor milestones (Palisano, 1993).

Another approach to describing motor development is with reference to the stages associated with the emergence of a single behavior, such as rolling or coming to standing. Stages within the emergence of a skill are often used by clinicians as the basis for a treatment progression, with the assumption that a mature and stable adult-like pattern is the last stage in the progression. However, some research has raised doubts about the concept that there is a consistent stable sequential pattern during the emergence of a particular motor behavior (Fishkind & Haley, 1986; Horowitz & Sharby, 1988).

Given these cautions about timing, variability, and the sequential nature of the emergence of motor skills, we review some of the studies that have examined the stages in the emergence of rolling, prone progression, and the assumption of the vertical position from supine. As we mentioned in Chapter 8 on development of postural control, much of the information we have on the emergence of motor behavior in children is largely the result of efforts in the 1920s and 1930s by two developmental researchers, Arnold Gesell and Myrtle McGraw, who observed and recorded the stages of development in normal children (McGraw, 1945).

Development of Rolling

Rolling is an important part of mobility skills because rotation or partial rotation is a part of movement patterns used to achieve supine-to-sitting or supine-to-standing behavior. Babies first roll from the side-lying to the supine position at 1 to 2 months of age and from the supine to the side-lying position at 4 to 5 months. Infants roll from prone to supine at 4 months of age and then from supine to prone at 6 to 8 months. Infants change their rolling pattern as they mature, from a log-rolling pattern, in which the entire body rolls as a unit, to a segmental pattern. By 9 months of age, most infants use a segmental rotation of the body on the pelvis (McGraw, 1945; Towen, 1976).

Development of Prone Progression

According to McGraw (1945), the prone progression includes nine phases that take the infant from the prone position to creeping and crawling and span the months from birth to 10 to 13 months. Figure 13.8 illustrates the nine phases reported by McGraw and the relative time in which the behavior was seen. The age at which the behavior was seen and the percentage of children in which the behavior was observed are graphed. The first phase is characterized by lower-extremity flexion and extension in a primarily flexed posture. In phase 2, spinal extension begins, as does the development of head control. In the third phase, spinal extension continues cephalocaudally, reaching the thoracic area. The arms can extend and support the chest off the surface. Propulsion movements begin in the arms and legs during phases 4 and 5. In phase 6, the creeping position is assumed. Phase 7 is characterized by fairly disorganized attempts at progression; however, by phases 8 and 9, organized propulsion in the creeping position has emerged.

Keep in mind that McGraw placed great emphasis on the neural antecedents of maturing motor behavior. Her emphasis was on describing stages of motor development that could be related to the structural growth and maturation of the central nervous system (CNS). Current research has shown that many factors contribute to the emergence of motor skill during development, including but not limited to maturation of the CNS (Thelen & Ulrich, 1991).

Development of Moving from Supine to Standing

Just as the pattern used to roll changes as infants develop, so does the movement pattern used to achieve standing from a supine position. The pattern initially seen in infants moving from supine to standing includes rolling to prone, then moving into an all-fours pattern, and using a pull-to-stand method to achieve the erect position. With development, the child learns to move from the all-fours position to a plantigrade position and from there to erect stance. By the age of 2 to 3 years, the supine-to-prone portion is modified to a partial roll and sit-up pattern, and by ages 4 to 5, a symmetrical sit-up pattern emerges (Fig. 13.9). This is considered a mature or adult-like movement pattern used for this task (McGraw, 1945). But as you remember from Chapter 12 on normal mobility skills, researchers have found tremendous variability in how adults move from supine to standing. Just as was true for adults, most likely, strength in the abdominals and hip flexors plays a major role in the type of pattern used by infants when moving from supine to standing (VanSant, 1988a).

Development of Sit to Stand

Studies have also examined variations in sit–to-stand behavior in children as compared with adults (Cahill et al., 1999; Guarrera-Bowlby & Gentile, 2004). When comparing children of 12 to18 months, 4 to 5 years, and 9 to 10 years, researchers found that even the youngest children had mastered the basic intersegmental

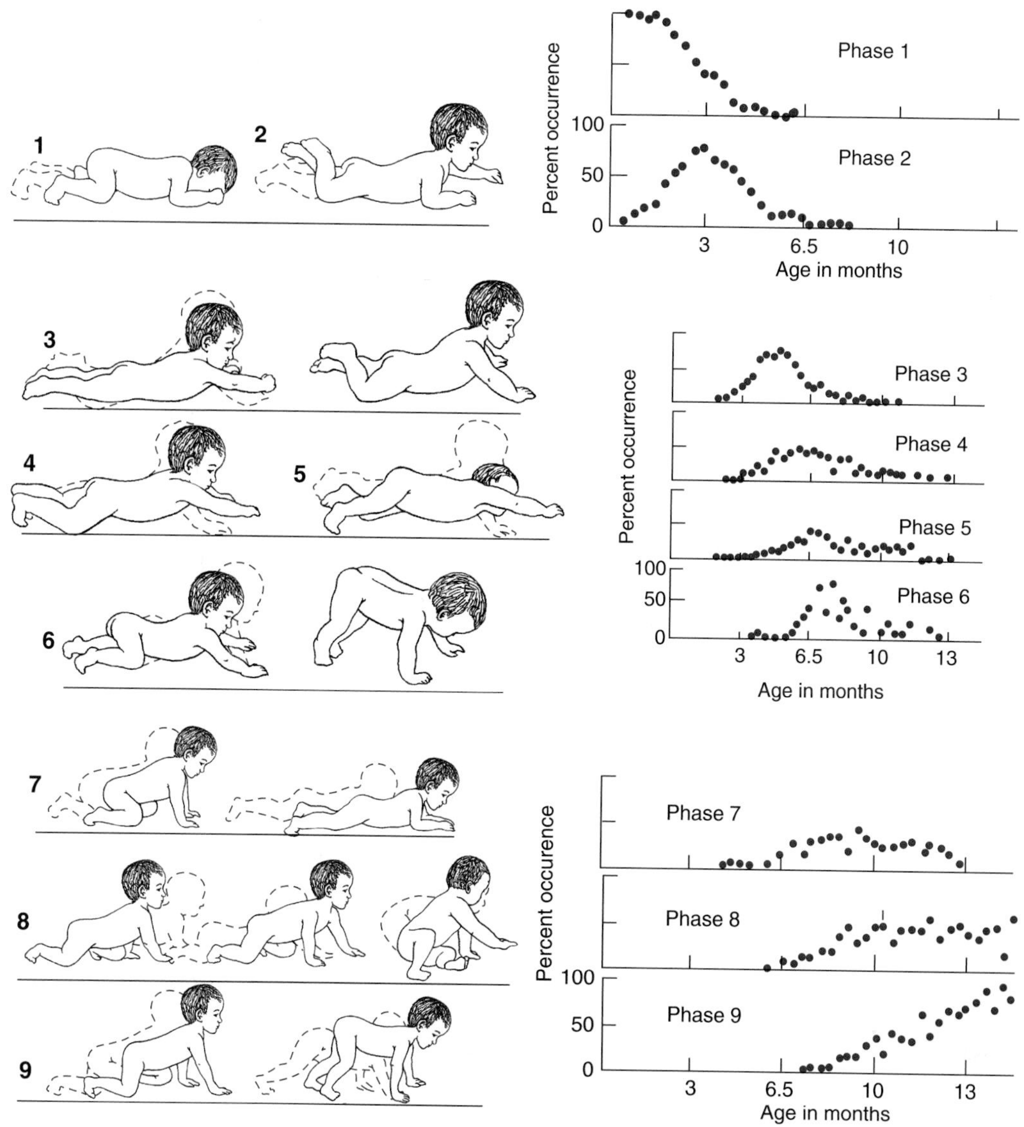

FIGURE 13.8 Left, Illustration of the nine phases of prone progression as reported by McGraw. Right, Graphs for each phase, showing the ages at which the behavior was seen (x-axis) and the percentage of children in which the behavior was observed (y-axis). See the text for details of each stage. (Adapted from McGraw M. The neuromuscular maturation of the human infant. New York: Hafner Press, 1945.)

pattern seen in adults. However, the youngest children were not able to perform the movement as efficiently because they ended the movement by either rising up on toes or taking a step forward. In addition, movement time, amplitude and peak angular velocity of trunk flexion increased with development. Children in the older age groups showed ground reaction force patterns that were similar to those of adults, while younger children reached peak force gradually, with fluctuations. Other studies have shown that children who are 6 to 7 years old have twice the intraindividual variability across trials as adults (Guarrera-Bowlby & Gentile, 2004). It is possible that these changes are related to the development of children's ability to control horizontal momentum and balance (Cahill et al., 1999).

LOCOMOTION IN OLDER ADULTS

Falls and the injuries that often accompany them are a serious problem in older adults. In fact, falls are the seventh leading cause of death in people over 75 years of age (Ochs et al., 1985). Forty-eight percent of adults over 75 years who have had an injurious fall acquire a fear of falling, and 26% of these people begin avoiding

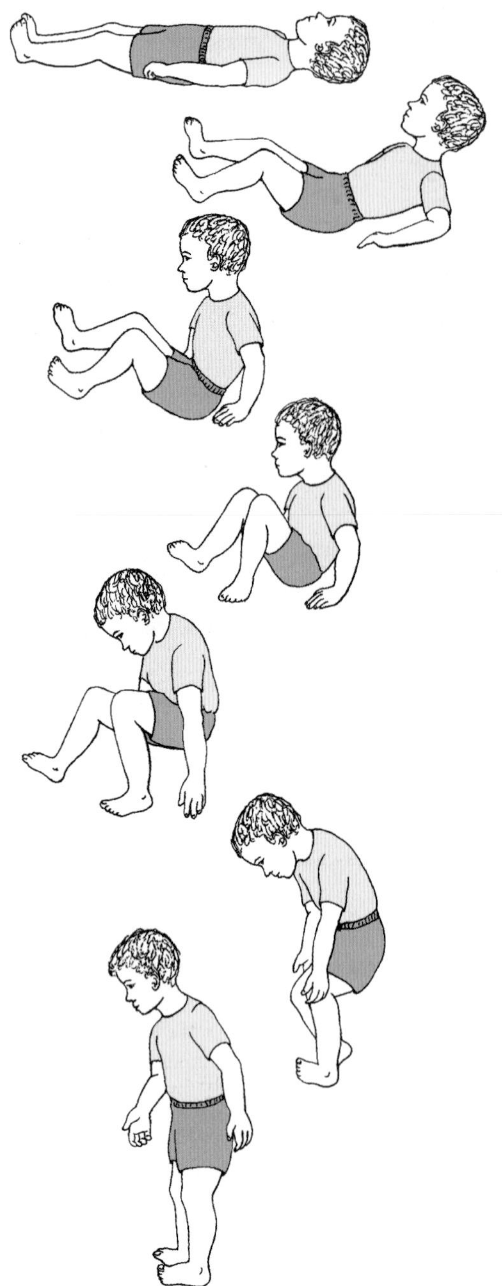

FIGURE 13.9 Common pattern used to move from supine to standing in children ages 4 to 5. Note that the child uses a symmetrical pattern. (Adapted from Van-Sant AF. Age differences in movement patterns used by children to rise from a supine position to erect stance. Phys Ther 1988;68:1130–1138, with permission of the American Physical Therapy Association. This material is copyrighted, and any further reproduction or distribution requires written permission from APTA.)

situations that require refined balance skills, thus leading to further declines in walking and balance skills.

Many of the falls experienced by the elderly occur during walking. It is thus important to understand the changes in the systems contributing to normal gait in the elderly to fully understand the cause of increased falls in this population. As we stated in the first section of this chapter, many researchers now believe that balance control is a primary contributor to stable walking. In addition, decreased balance control is a major factor affecting loss of independent mobility in many elderly persons. The following sections describe locomotor changes commonly seen in older adults and the systems contributing to these changes.

Gait Dysfunction: Aging or Pathology?

Again, age-related changes in locomotion may be due to primary or secondary aging phenomena. Primary factors affecting aging include changes in gene expression that result in changes in hormonal function, aging, and death. Also, individuals may have a genetic predisposition to specific diseases, which results in an inevitable decline of neuronal function within a particular system. Secondary factors are experiential, and include nutrition, exercise, stress level, and acquired pathologies, among others. The extent to which gait disorders in the elderly are due to primary or secondary factors is a very important point to consider as we begin to look at the literature on changes in gait characteristics in older adults (Karasik et al., 2005).

The older clinical literature referred to many different walking patterns as age-related gait disorders. These diverse gait disorders included gait apraxia (slow, halting, short-stepped, shuffling, or sliding gait), hypokinetic–hypertonic syndrome (slow, deliberate gait, but without the shuffling or sliding components described above), and marche à petits pas (small, quick shuffling steps, followed by a slow cautious, unsteady gait), vestibular dysfunction gait (difficulties in turning), and proprioceptive dysfunction gait (cautious, with a tendency to watch the feet and make missteps) (Craik, 1989).

As was true in the postural-control literature, care must be taken when reviewing studies discussing age-related changes in gait. When interpreting the results of a study, one should examine carefully the population studied, and ask questions such as: What criteria were used in selecting older subjects? Did researchers exclude anyone with pathology under the assumption that pathology is not a part of primary aging? Results will vary tremendously depending on the composition of the group of older adults under study. For example, one study noted that in an unselected group of subjects 60 to 99 years of age, walking velocities were much slower than those for young adults and also slower than those shown in other published studies on older adults (Imms & Edholm, 1981). It is quite possible that the subjects in the study were less fit, and many subjects reported symptoms likely to impair gait. In contrast, a study that screened 1184 older adults and chose 32 who had no pathology, found no changes in the gait parameters tested (Gabell & Nayak, 1984).

Thus, more recent research has begun to indicate that many gait disorders considered to be age-related, such as gait apraxia, hypokinetic–hypertonic syndrome, and marche à petits pas, are really manifestations of pathology rather than characteristics of a generalized aging process. However, as we note in the following sections, there are distinctive changes in gait that occur in many, even healthy, older adults.

Temporal and Distance Factors

Studies examining changes in walking patterns with age have used a number of different experimental approaches. In one approach, which we might call a "naturalistic approach," adults were observed walking spontaneously in a natural setting. This paradigm was used to try to minimize the constraints on walking style that are often necessary when quantifying gait parameters in a laboratory setting.

In these studies, researchers observed people of different ages walking along the streets of New York City (Drillis, 1961) or Amsterdam (Molen, 1973). In the first study, of 752 pedestrians in New York City, as age increased from 20 to 70 years, there was a decrease in walking velocity, step length, and step rate (no statistical analysis was reported). In the second study on 533 pedestrians in Amsterdam, similar results were found. Gender differences were also found; both younger and older women walked with slower velocity, shorter step length, and higher cadence than men. While there are advantages in allowing subjects to walk in a natural environment, the disadvantages include being unable to control for variables such as different walking goals, such as taking a stroll versus hurrying to work, and relative health of the subjects (Craik, 1989).

Kinematic Analysis

Later studies of age-related changes in gait focused on a kinematic analysis of stepping patterns in older adults. In one study, subjects were healthy men, with normal strength and range of motion, ranging in age from 20 to 87 years of age (Murray et al., 1969). Each was tested at his preferred and at a fast walking speed. Men over 67 years of age showed significantly ($p < 0.01$) slower walking speeds (118 to 123 cm/sec) than the young adults (150 cm/sec). Stride length was also significantly shorter, especially during fast walking. Vertical movement of the head during the gait cycle was smaller, while lateral movement was larger. Stride width tended to be wider for men over 74. Toeing out was also greater for men over 80. Over age 65, the stance phase was longer, with a commensurate shortening of time in the swing phase.

Finally hip, knee, and ankle flexion were less than in young adults, and the whole shoulder rotation pattern was shifted to a more extended position, with less elbow rotation as well. Figure 13.10 is adapted from the study of Murray et al. (1969), showing the differences in the limb positions of a younger versus an older man at heel strike. In a second study (Murray et al., 1970), age-related changes in gait patterns were investigated in women, and similar changes were noted, including reduced walking speeds and shorter steps. These changes occurred in the 60- to 70-year-old age group.

Interestingly, the researchers concluded that the older adults studied did not have a pathologic gait pattern. Instead, their walking was reported as guarded, possibly with the aim to increase stability. Gait patterns were similar to those used by someone walking on a slippery surface or someone walking in darkness. This sounds like a postural-control problem. From reading this description, one might hypothesize that gait changes in the elderly person relate more to the loss of balance control than to changes in the step cycle itself (Murray et al., 1969).

How do these slower walking speeds affect function in daily life? Many of the previous studies report that older adults are unable to walk faster than 1.4 m/sec. This is the minimal speed required to cross a street safely. Lundgren-Lindquist et al. (1983) have shown

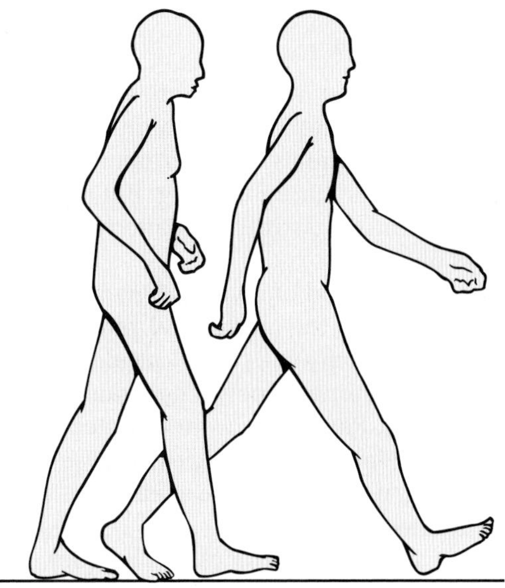

FIGURE 13.10 Example of the walking pattern of a young adult (right) versus a healthy older man (left). (Adapted from Murray MP, Kory RC, Clarkson BH. Walking patterns in healthy older men. J Gerontol 1969; 24:169–178.)

that none of the 205 subjects studied who were 79 years old could cross a street before the traffic light changed when walking at their preferred speed. Thus, many of the older adults studied would not be considered independent community ambulators.

Muscle Activation Patterns

The studies discussed above show clear changes in certain kinematic characteristics of the gait cycle in the average older adult. How do these changes relate to changes in muscle response patterns? In a study comparing patterns of muscle activity in younger (19 to 38 years of age) and older (64 to 86) women, average EMG activity levels in gastrocnemius, tibialis anterior, biceps femoris, rectus femoris, and peroneus longus were higher in the older than in the younger age group (Finley et al., 1969).

In addition, there were changes in the activity of individual muscles at specific points in the step cycle. For example, at heel strike, the peroneus longus and gastrocnemius muscles were moderately to highly active in the older women, but showed little or no activity in the younger group. The authors suggested that this increased activity resulted from an effort to improve stability during the stance phase of gait. For example, increased coactivation of agonist and antagonist muscles at a joint may be used to improve balance control, by increasing joint stiffness. This strategy is often seen in subjects who are unskilled in a task, or who are performing in a situation that requires increased control (Woollacott, 1989).

Kinetic Analysis

We have just noted several studies indicating that older adults show higher levels of muscle responses and different activation sequences among leg muscles than young adults during walking. But how do these changes in muscle activation patterns change the dynamics of gait?

Using the method of inverse dynamics, moments of force, as well as the mechanical power generated and absorbed at each joint, can be calculated. This process allows the amount of power generated by muscles to be estimated. Remember from Chapter 12 on locomotion that an increase in muscle energy is needed to initiate swing, while a decrease in energy is needed to prepare for heel strike.

Using inverse dynamics techniques, Winter and colleagues (1990) compared the gait patterns of 15 healthy older adults (62 to 78 years of age) to 12 young adults (21 to 28). They found that older adults had significantly shorter stride length and longer double-support time than did young adults. In addition, in elderly subjects, plantar flexors generated significantly less power at push-off, while the quadriceps muscle absorbed significantly less energy during late stance and early swing.

These researchers concluded that the reduction of plantar flexor power during push-off could explain the shorter step length, flat-footed heel strike, and increased double-support duration. Two alternative explanations were proposed for a weaker push-off in the older adult. One explanation suggested that a reduction in muscle strength in the ankle plantar flexors in the older adults could be responsible for the weaker push-off. An alternative explanation argued that reduced push-off could be an adaptive change used to ensure a safer gait, since high push-off power acts upward and forward and is thus destabilizing (Winter et al., 1990).

In the study by Winters et al., an index of dynamic balance was computed to determine the ability to coordinate the anterior/posterior balance of the HAT segment while simultaneously maintaining an appropriate extensor moment in the ankle, knee, and hip during the stance phase. It was found that the older adults showed a reduced ability to covary movements at the hip and knee. This means that older adults had trouble controlling the HAT segment while simultaneously maintaining an extensor moment in the lower stance limb. In evaluating the older group individually, it was noted that two-thirds were within the normal young adult range, while one-third had very low covariances of moments at the hip and knee. It was concluded that some older adults may have had problems with dynamic balance during locomotion, indicative of balance impairments not detected in their medical history or simple clinical tests.

In order to determine whether the decreased joint torques and powers that are found in older adults during gait are due to slower self-selected walking speeds or are true gait-limiting factors, researchers examined these parameters in young and older adults when they were walking at the same speed (DeVita & Hortobagyi, 2000). They found that support angular impulse was the same in both groups, but older adults used 58% more angular impulse and 279% more work at the hip, 50% less angular impulse and 39% less work at the knee, and 23% less angular impulse and 29% less work at the ankle. Thus, the older adults showed a redistribution of joint torques and powers compared with young adults, using hip extensors more and knee extensors and ankle plantar flexors less than young adults when walking at the same speed.

Numerous research studies have described changes in gait patterns found among many older adults. These changes are summarized in Table 13.2. To better understand age-related changes to gait, complete

TABLE 13.2 Summary of Gait Changes in the Older Adult

Temporal/distance factors
- Decreased velocity
- Decreased step length
- Decreased step rate
- Decreased stride length
- Increased stride width
- Increased stance phase
- Increased time in double support
- Decreased swing phase

Kinematic changes
- Decreased vertical movement of the center of gravity
- Decreased arm swing
- Decreased hip, knee, and ankle flexion
- Flatter foot on heel strike
- Decreased ability to covary hip/knee movements
- Decreased dynamic stability during stance

Muscle activation patterns
- Increased coactivation (increased stiffness)

Kinetic changes
- Decreased power generation at push-off
- Decreased power absorption at heel strike

LAB ACTIVITY 13-2

Objective: To examine age-related changes in the spatial, temporal, and kinematic parameters of gait.

Procedures: Find two older adults from your community, one who is very active and well-balanced, and the other who has reported gait and balance problems. Document changes in spatial and temporal aspects of gait in these two adults. Also observe and describe the following gait characteristics in each adult: (1) ability to maintain an upright posture, (2) ability to control stability (how often does the older adult fall within a fixed time period), (3) initial contact at foot strike, and (4) position of arms.

Assignment:

1. Compare the data you have gathered from healthy young adults with that gathered from your two older subjects. What parameters of gait are similar between the young and the elderly?
2. What parameters differ?
3. How similar or dissimilar are gait parameters between the two older adults?
4. How do your data compare with those described in Table 13.2?

Lab Activity 13.2. Compare your findings to the research summarized in Table 13.2.

Changes in Adaptive Control

Many falls by older adults occur while walking and may be due to slipping and tripping. Several research groups have examined proactive adaptive strategies during gait in the elderly. In addition, studies on age-related changes in reactive balance control have been published (Chambers & Cham, 2007; Lockhart et al., 2003; Tang & Woollacott, 1998, 1999).

Proactive Adaptation

Proactive adaptation depends in large part on the ability to use visual information to alter gait patterns in anticipation of upcoming obstacles (Patla, 1993). Patla et al. (1992) studied whether a possible cause of poor locomotor abilities in older adults might be a reduced ability to sample the visual environment during walking. They wanted to know whether visual sampling of the environment changed with age.

In their experiment, subjects wore opaque liquid crystal eyeglasses and pressed a switch to make them transparent whenever they wanted to sample the environment. Subjects walked across a floor that was either unmarked, or that had footprints marked at regular intervals, on which the subjects were supposed to walk. When subjects were constrained to land on the footprints, the young subjects sampled frequently, though for shorter intervals than older subjects, who tended to sample less often, but for longer time periods. Thus, older adults seem to monitor the terrain much more than the young adults (Patla, 1993).

What is the minimum time required to implement an avoidance strategy in a younger versus an older adult? In a second study, healthy young and older adults were asked to walk along a walkway, and when cued by a light at specific points along the walkway, to either lengthen or shorten their stride to match the position of the light (Patla et al., 1992).

Compared with young adults, older adults had more difficulty in modulating their step length when the cue was given only one step duration ahead. Young adults succeeded 80% of the time, while older adults succeeded 60% of the time when lengthening the step and only 38% of the time when shortening the step. Both groups were equally successful when the cue was given two step durations in advance (Patla et al., 1992).

The authors suggest that older adults have more difficulty in shortening a step because of balance constraints. Shortening the step requires regulating the forward pitch of the HAT segment, which if not controlled, could result in a fall. Remember in the review of Winter's study presented earlier, older adults had more trouble than young adults in controlling dynamic balance during gait.

These results suggest that the older adult may need to begin making modifications to gait patterns in the step prior to a step requiring obstacle avoidance. This may be one cause of increased visual monitoring.

What strategies do older adults use to avoid obstacles during walking? To answer this question, researchers analyzed the gait of 24 young and 24 older (mean age, 71 years) healthy adults while they stepped over obstacles of varying heights. Obstacles were made the height of a 1-in. or 2-in. door threshold or a 6-in. curb, and performance was compared with a 0-mm condition (tape marked on the walkway). No age-related changes in foot clearance over the obstacles were found, but older adults used a significantly more conservative strategy when crossing obstacles. Older adults used a somewhat slower approach speed, a significantly slower crossing speed, and a shorter step length. Also, 4 of the 24 older adults inadvertently stepped on an obstacle, while none of the young adults did (Chen et al., 1991).

Other research on changes in obstacle-avoidance ability has focused on the control of the COM during obstacle crossing (Hahn & Chou, 2004). During obstacle crossing, older adults showed anterior-direction COM velocities that were significantly slower than those of young adults. They also showed reduced anteroposterior distances between the COM and the COP, which indicates a conservative strategy, reducing the mechanical load on the supporting limb. The authors note that this strategy may be the result of reduced muscle strength in the older adults.

Reactive Adaptation

Trips. Research on falls (Gabell et al., 1985; Overstall et al., 1977) has indicated that 35 to 47% of falls in older adults result from tripping over an object. In order to study the determinants of balance recovery from a trip, Chen (1993) used a biomechanical model simulation. He showed that the critical muscles for recovery from a trip are the hip flexors of the swing leg and the ankle plantar flexors of the stance leg. In addition, he found that the rate of torque development, rather than available strength, was critical to balance recovery. Thus, the factor critical to recovery of balance following a trip appears to be how quickly restorative forces can be generated. Figure 13.11 shows the effects of different joint torques and torque development rates on balance recovery after tripping. Figure 13.11A shows a stick figure of the response to tripping if a subject had maximum joint torques and torque development rates, while B and C show a response if a subject had 75 and 50%, respectively, of reference torques and rates available. For subject C, the swing foot recontacts the ground, tripping again, with his upper body COM in front of his base of support, causing an additional perturbation to balance (Schultz, 1995).

A second study (Pijnappels et al., 2005), both supporting and extending these results, was designed to determine whether: (a) timing and sequencing of muscle activation and (b) the magnitude and rate of development of muscle activation during recovery after a trip differs between young and older subjects.

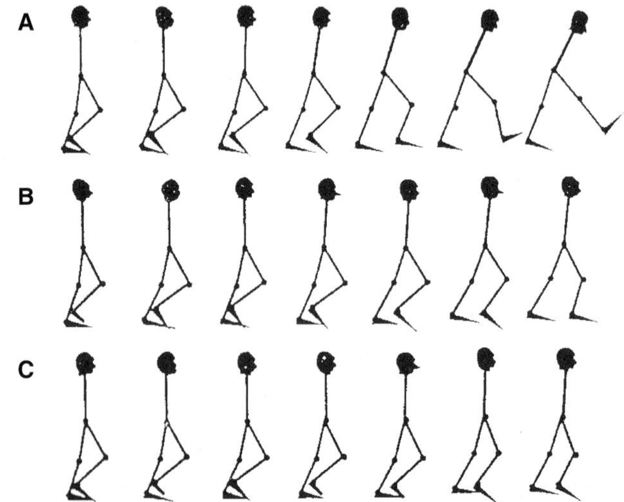

FIGURE 13.11 A, Stick figure of the response to tripping if a subject had maximum joint torques and torque development rates. B and C, Response that would be seen if a subject had 75% and 50%, respectively, of reference torques and rates available. For the hypothetical subject in C, the swing foot recontacts the ground, tripping again, with his upper body COM in front of his base of support, causing an additional perturbation to balance (Reprinted with permission from Schultz AB. Muscle function and mobility biomechanics in the elderly: an overview of some recent research. J Gerontol 1995;50A(special issue):60–63.)

In this study, young (mean age, 25 years) and older (mean age, 68 years) adults walked over a platform and were tripped several times at different points in the gait cycle. The results showed that after tripping, rapid EMG responses (60 to 80 msec) were activated in both the hamstrings and gastrocnemius/soleus muscles of the stance leg in both young and older subjects, with the older subjects showing a delay (11 msec) in activation of the soleus muscle. The sequencing of the muscle activity patterns was similar in the two groups; however, the magnitude and rate of development of muscle activity were significantly lower in the older adults. These results and those from previous studies suggest that a lower rate of development of muscle activation in the support limb of older subjects may contribute to inadequate recovery from slips, leading to falls (Pijnappels et al., 2005; Schultz, 1995; Thelen et al., 1996).

In a study designed to determine the risk of falling following a trip, Pavol and colleagues (1999) gave older adults (mean [±SD] age, 72 ± 5 years) a single unexpected trip while walking, by activating without warning the elevation of a concealed mechanical obstacle in their footpath; 22% of the trips resulted in a fall into a harness, while 61% resulted in a full recovery, and 17% resulted in a rope-assisted recovery. Results showed that women fell more than four times more often than men.

Slips. Slips also account for a high percentage (27 to 32%) of falls and subsequent injuries in community-dwelling older adults (Gabell et al., 1985). This phenomenon suggests that although active and healthy older adults preserve a mobility level comparable with that of young adults, these older adults may have difficulty generating efficient reactive postural responses when they slip. A study by Tang and Woollacott (1998) tested the hypothesis that active and healthy older adults use a less effective reactive balance strategy than young adults when experiencing an unexpected forward slip occurring at heel strike during walking. They predicted that less effective balance strategies would be manifested by slower and smaller postural responses, altered temporal and spatial organization of the postural responses, and greater upper-trunk instability after the slip in older adults.

In the study, young adults (n = 33; mean age, 25 ± 4 years) and community-dwelling older adults (n = 32; mean age, 4 ± 14 years) walked down a ramp and across a force plate that moved forward at heel strike, creating a forward slip. Both muscle-response characteristics and body-segment movements used in the recovery of balance were analyzed.

Tang and Woollacott noted that, behaviorally, older adults were less stable after the slips than young adults. For example, when recovering from a slip, older adults tended to trip more, as the advancing swing limb caught on the surface. Trips occurred 66% of the time in older adults, as compared with 15% in the younger adults. Older adults also showed greater trunk hyperextension and higher arm elevation in response to the slip than the young adults, as shown in Figure 13.12A. The figure shows a stick figure drawn from the motion analysis of the movements of a young and an older adult responding to a forward slip at heel strike. Note the backward extension of the trunk and the raising of the arm in the older adult at the onset of the slip. In addition, older adults had an earlier contralateral foot strike and shortened stride length, suggesting a more conservative balance strategy and an attempt to quickly reestablish the base of support after the slip.

What changes in neuromuscular response characteristics could be the cause of these difficulties in regaining balance in the older adults? A summary of the analysis is shown in Figure 13.12C. Older adults (darker bars) showed longer onset latencies and smaller magnitudes in the postural muscles activated in balance recovery (e.g., tibialis anterior, rectus femoris, and abdominal muscles of the perturbed leg) as compared with the younger adults (lighter bars). These delayed and weaker muscle responses thus contributed to the trunk hyperextension and trips seen in the older adults during recovery. In order to compensate for these deficiencies in responses, the older adults showed longer muscle-response burst duration (Fig. 13.12B) and the use of the arms to aid in recovery. They also showed a longer coactivation time for the agonist/antagonist muscle pairs at the ankle, knee, and trunk of the perturbed leg, possibly to stiffen the joints as an additional aid in balance control (Tang & Woollacott, 1998).

How do older adults adapt their responses to balance threats at different phases in the gait cycle? When young adults experience a balance threat at midstance rather than at heel strike, the threat to stability is less, and they reduce the amplitude of responses appropriately. However, when older adults experience a midstance slip, their responses are actually the same size as at heel strike, showing little to no adaptation. Why is this the case? It is possible that their reduced response capacity (i.e., smaller burst magnitudes) at heel strike (see Fig. 13.12B) is the key constraint. They may be showing a normal response at midstance, but simply do not have the response capacity to increase the response to appropriate levels for the increased balance threat at heel strike (Tang & Woollacott, 1999).

In another study examining the gait changes in older adults and the effects of these changes on slips and the frequency of falls, Lockhart et al. (2003) asked young and older adults to walk around a circular track and placed a slippery (oily) surface over

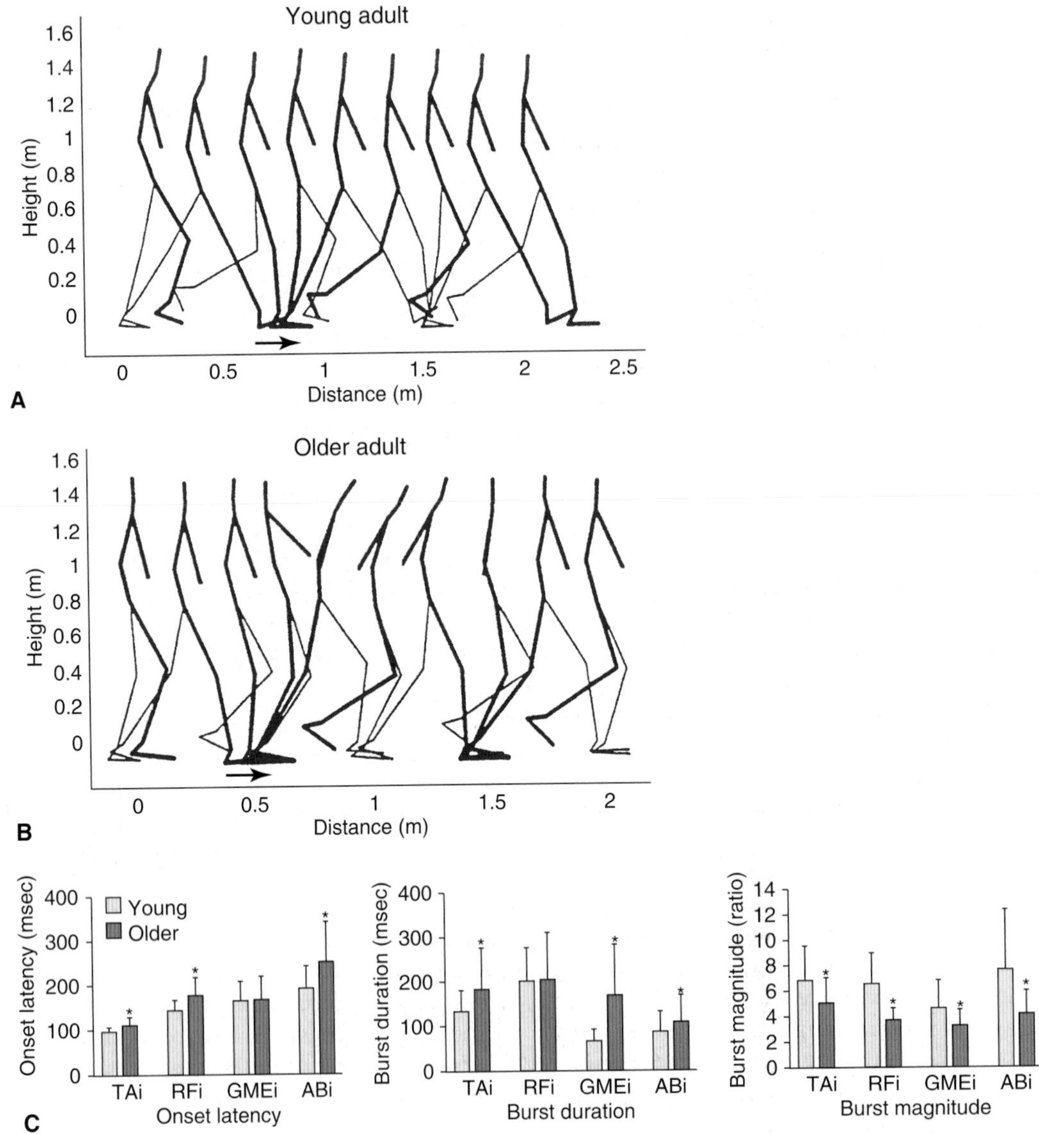

FIGURE 13.12 A, Stick figures drawn from the motion analysis of the movements of a young and an older adult responding to a forward slip at heel strike. Note the backward extension of the trunk and the raising of the arm in the older adult at the onset of the slip, indicated by the arrow. B, Means and standard deviations of onset latencies, burst durations, and burst magnitudes of postural responses in young (lighter bars) and older (darker bars) adults, for the anterior muscles of the perturbed leg. ABi = ipsilateral abdominal; GMEi = ipsilateral gluteus medius; RFi = ipsilateral rectus femoris; TAi = ipsilateral tibialis anterior. (Reprinted with permission from Tang PF, Woollacott MH. Inefficient postural responses to unexpected slips during walking in older adults. J Gerontol 1998; 53:M471–M480.)

the force plate at random times without the participant's awareness. The experimental setup is shown in Figure 13.13. Results showed that the older adults' horizontal heel-contact velocity was significantly faster and the step length was shorter. Older adults also slipped longer and faster and fell more often than younger participants. The researchers noted that participants who fell had a faster horizontal heel contact velocity than those who did not fall, suggesting that gait changes associated with aging affect the initiation of and recovery from slips. Examination of muscle responses underlying slips on oily surfaces has shown that older adults did not increase the power and duration of their muscle responses when responding to a highly hazardous as compared with a less hazardous slip, unlike young adults. This may be related to reduced lower-extremity strength in older adults (Chambers & Cham, 2007).

When young and older adults were alerted to expect a slippery surface, they added a proactive

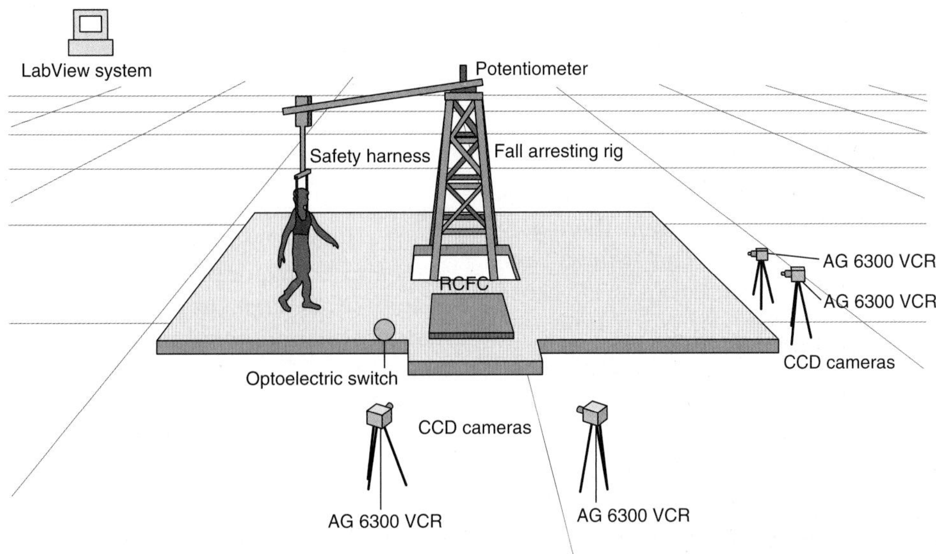

FIGURE 13.13 Layout of experiment examining age-related gait changes associated with slips and falls. The participant was in a safety harness and walked a 20-m circular track into which was incorporated a force plate. The force plate was covered with outdoor carpet for control trials and oily vinyl tile for the unexpected slip trials. Charge-coupled device (CCD) cameras recorded the kinematic data for each trial. A remote-controlled floor changer (RCFC) was used to change the test floor surfaces unexpectedly. (Reprinted with permission from Lockhart TE, Woldstad JC, Smith JL. Effects of age-related gait changes on the biomechanics of slips and falls. Ergonomics 2003;46:1140.)

component to their balance response, coactivating the muscles at the ankle and knee and increasing the power of their muscle responses; however, older adults showed less proactive increase in muscle power than young adults. Subjects also took shorter steps, reducing the foot-floor angle and the vertical heel velocity at heel strike, as well as increasing knee flexion and hip moment, which resulted in a decrease in the potential of a slip and fall (Chambers & Cham, 2007).

Gait Changes in Balance-Impaired Older Adults

How do the walking characteristics of older adults who fall compare with those with no history of falls? While the previous studies have shown that the gait characteristics of healthy older adults show few differences when compared with those of younger adults, older individuals with a history of falls show significant differences in walking patterns (Hausdorff et al., 1997; Heitmann et al., 1989; Wolfson et al., 1995). Wolfson et al. (1995) have shown that both stride length (no history of falls, 0.82 ± 0.22 m; history of falls, 0.53 ± 0.21 m) and walking speed (no history, 0.64 ± 0.21 m/sec; history, 0.37 ± 0.17 m/sec) are significantly reduced in older adults who fall. Hausdorff et al. (1997, 2001) found that all measures (stride time, stance time, and swing time) of gait variability were significantly greater in those with a history of falls as compared with elderly subjects with no history of falls and young adults. They also noted that increased gait (stride time) variability predicted falls in these community-dwelling adults. Stride-time variability was also significantly correlated with strength, balance, gait speed, functional status, and mental health, but these other performance measures did not discriminate those who would fall in the future from those who would not.

Heitmann et al. (1989) have found that older female subjects with poor balance performance have increased step width during gait. Other studies have reported that step width measured at the heel was significantly larger in older persons with a history of falls when they walked at a fast speed (6 km/hr) when compared with subjects without a history of falls. It was also noted that older subjects with a history of falls had balance problems unrelated to gait because they were unable to stand with their feet in tandem position and their eyes open as long as those with no history of falls. Of course, it is likely that older adults with a history of falls have an undiagnosed pathological condition. Therefore, it is important to examine these subjects carefully, to determine underlying pathology that may contribute to gait disturbances, when performing studies on older adults who fall (Gehlsen & Whaley, 1990; Heitmann et al., 1989).

Adaptive Gait Control in Older Adults with Imbalance

One of the causes of falls in older adults is trips during obstacle crossing. A review of studies examining obstacle-crossing performance in older adults showed that older adults had more frequent obstacle contacts during crossing than young adults when there was limited time to avoid the obstacle. The authors note that it is likely that increased obstacle contact is a cause of trips and falls in these contexts. When time was not constrained, older adults adopted a slower more conservative strategy when stepping over obstacles, allowing them to adjust foot placement and reduce the risk of tripping (Galna et al., 2009).

Chou and colleagues (2003) have studied COM motion during obstacle crossing in older adults with imbalance to determine whether excessive lateral COM motion may be a cause of their instability in these situations and thus to identify persons at great risk of imbalance and falls. Although elders with imbalance did not have differences in temporal-distance gait parameters such as walking velocity and stride length, they did show greater and faster lateral motion of the COM when crossing over obstacles that were 15% of body height. Figure 13.14 shows the mediolateral COM position and velocity trajectories for a healthy (solid line) and balance-impaired (dashed line) older adult. Note the large deviation of COM position and velocity as the individual with imbalance crosses the obstacle.

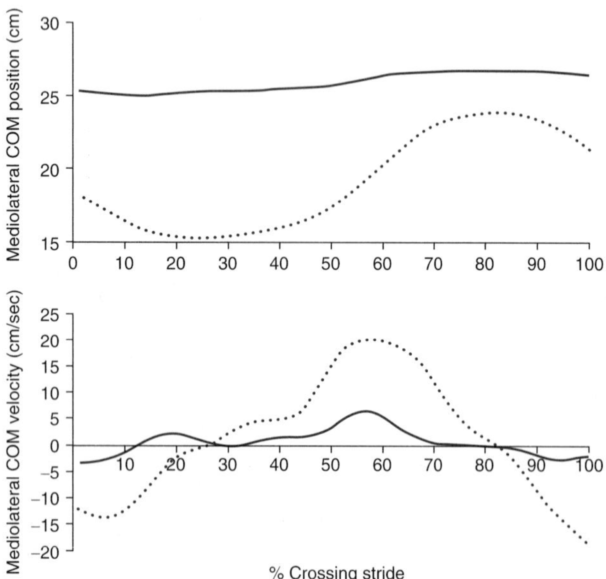

FIGURE 13.14 Mediolateral COM position and velocity data from a single trial of a representative healthy older adult (solid line) and an older individual with imbalance (dashed line) while crossing an obstacle of 15% body height. (Reprinted with permission from Chou L-S, Kaufman KR, Hahn ME, Brey RH. Medio-lateral motion of the center of mass during obstacle crossing distinguishes elderly individuals with imbalance. Gait Posture 2003;18:129.)

In fact, the authors found that COM motion distinguished patients with balance disorders from healthy older adults better than the motion of markers at the hip, trunk, or pelvis, because of large variations in individual segment motion. These results suggest that information about an elderly person's ability to control the COM trajectory during obstacle crossing could help identify persons at risk for falls and allow for interventions before falls occur (Chou et al., 2003; Hahn & Chou 2003).

Variability in Gait Patterns within the Individual: Does This Contribute to Imbalance?

Most studies on age-related deterioration in balance and gait have focused on overall performance differences in older versus young adults. Although these studies have shown substantial and significant differences in performance in older as compared with younger adults, a second performance variable that may also contribute to balance constraints in the elderly is the extent to which the individual varies in their performance from trial to trial in a repeated task, that is, intraindividual variability. Intraindividual variability may reflect processing fluctuations or lack of processing robustness, indicating "noise" within the physiological system underlying behavioral control (Li et al., 2004). This is an important factor in balance control, as increased variability of COM motion, for example, when an individual is already near his or her stability limits during gait could result in the COM moving outside the stability limits and thus result in loss of balance and a subsequent fall.

A number of research labs have begun to explore stride-to-stride variability in older adults who fall. For example Hausdorff and colleagues (Hausdorff, 2007; Hausdorff et al., 1997) evaluated the variability of gait in community-dwelling older fallers, nonfallers, and young adults. They found that stride-time and swing-time variability were significantly larger in the fallers as compared with both young adult and elderly nonfallers. In contrast, gait speed was similar in the fallers and nonfallers. Although both elderly groups had similar walking speed and muscle strength, the elderly fallers had significant increases in stride variance.

In addition, Studenski and colleagues (Brach et al., 2005) have shown that either too much or too little step-width variability is associated with older adults who fall. They sampled a population of 503 older adults (mean age, 79 years) who were independent walkers. They found that individuals with extreme step-width variability (either low or high variability) were more likely to report a fall in the past year than individuals with moderate variability. The association between step-width variability and fall history was not significant in individuals who walked less than 1 m/sec.

It has also been shown that walking variability, and specifically, stride-time variability, increases when older adults are asked to perform a simultaneous arithmetic task (Beauchet et al., 2005). This increase in variability in dual-task settings is assumed to be due to insufficient attentional processing resources for performing the two tasks simultaneously, causing increased processing noise.

To be useful as a clinical tool for the assessment of falls, it is helpful to be able to use measures of gait for early identification of persons at risk of falls. Hausdorff et al. (2001) tested the hypothesis that in community-dwelling elders, altered gait variability would predict future fallers. Older adults were assessed at baseline and then followed for 12 months, monitoring fall status weekly. During the 12-month follow-up period, 39% of the participants reported at least one fall. At baseline, gait instability measures were significantly increased in those who subsequently fell as compared with those who did not. In addition, baseline measures of gait instability were also *predictive* of future falls. These results suggest that measures of gait instability may provide a useful assessment tool for fall risk in older adults.

Role of Pathology in Gait Changes in the Elderly

What is the role of secondary aging factors, particularly the role of pathology, in gait abnormalities observed in older adults? In many studies examining apparently healthy older adults, participants are considered pathology-free if they do not have a known neurologic, cardiovascular, or musculoskeletal disorder. Yet, when this population is examined carefully, many show subtle pathologies. For example, in a study on idiopathic gait disorders among older adults Sudarsky and Ronthal (1983) found that, on closer medical evaluation, this type of gait pattern could actually be attributed to a number of specific disease processes. This suggests that in many instances pathological conditions may be an underlying contributing factor to changes in gait pattern seen in older adults. Pathology within a number of systems can potentially affect locomotor skills in the older adult.

In a study examining the effects of multiple impairments on severe walking disability, researchers analyzed data from 1002 women 65 years of age or older who performed tests of both muscle strength (hand-held dynamometer test of knee extension strength) and balance (feet together, semitandem and tandem Romberg) in their homes. The results showed that the risk of being severely walking-disabled was 10 times greater for persons having both strength and balance impairments as compared with those with only one impairment. Thus, an effective method for reducing walking disabilities could be the prevention or remediation of multiple impairments, with improvement in just one impairment having a substantial impact on the probability of having a walking disability (Rantanen et al., 1999).

Cognitive Factors

The ability to divide attention between two or more tasks is an important aspect of locomotion during many activities of daily life. For example, an older adult may be required to walk across a street while talking to a friend while simultaneously looking both ways to avoid oncoming traffic. A number of studies have been performed to study the ability of older adults to simultaneously perform locomotor and other cognitively demanding tasks, in order to determine whether attentional problems could be a factor contributing to falls. In Chapters 7, 9 and 12 we defined attention and discussed the research on the attentional requirements of balance and locomotion and the changes in the attentional requirements of balance in the elderly. In this chapter we will focus on changes in the attentional requirements of locomotion in healthy and balance-impaired older adults.

It has been suggested that as the functional capacity of older adults is stressed while walking and performing a secondary motor or cognitive task, problems in gait or in the performance of a secondary task will be revealed, due to either: (1) a limited capacity to perform either task, requiring more attentional resources or (2) limitations in the information-processing capacity of the older adults, causing problems in allocating attention efficiently between the two tasks.

In order to determine whether older adults show problems with attention when performing a secondary task while walking, Eichhorn et al. (1998) asked older (mean age, 73 years) and young (mean age, 24 years) adults to respond vocally to a tone cue (say "soft" to a low and "loud" to a high tone) as quickly as possible while walking. They found that the reaction time of the older adults on the auditory task was significantly reduced when walking, while that of the younger adults was not. Thus, older adults showed problems performing both tasks efficiently when they were performed simultaneously. Other studies have shown that the type of cognitive task is important to the dual-task interference with walking. For example, a simple push-button reaction-time task did not affect gait performance in older recurrent fallers, while a visual-spatial reaction time task significantly slowed gait in a dual-task setting (Faulkner et al., 2007).

In a slightly more complex walking task, Chen et al. (1996) asked healthy older (mean age, 72 years) and young (mean age, 24 years) adults to walk down a walkway and step over a virtual object (a band of light) while responding vocally when a red light was turned on at the end of the walkway. Figure 13.15 shows the experimental setup. They found that both young and older adults showed increased obstacle contact when performing the secondary task, but this was greater in the older adults. Thus, decrements in obstacle avoidance occur in both younger and older adults when performing a secondary cognitive task, but older adults show higher decrements. This decreased ability to avoid obstacles when performing a secondary cognitive task could contribute to many falls in older adults.

Not only do older adults have more obstacle contact as compared with young adults when performing obstacle crossing in a dual-task situation, the above research has shown that the secondary task is affected as well. Older adults also show higher error rates than young adults on the secondary task, suggesting that the attentional demands of obstacle avoidance increase with age as well. Brown et al. (2005) have also shown that the attention directed toward obstacle avoidance in the precrossing phase was more than in the crossing phase in young adults. However, for older adults, both precrossing and crossing phases of obstacle negotiation required equal attention, suggesting decreased balance control during the crossing phase in older adults.

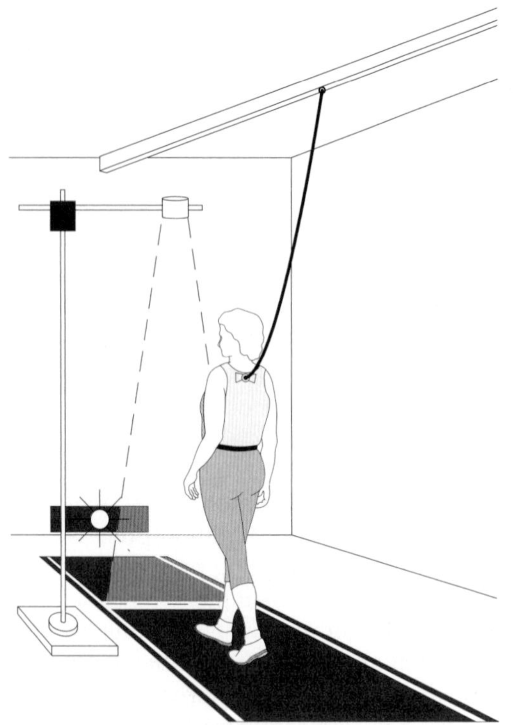

FIGURE 13.15 Experimental setup for study of attentional demands associated with performing a secondary task while avoiding an obstacle. Young and older adults walked down a walkway and stepped over a virtual object (a band of light) while responding vocally when a red light was turned on at the end of the walkway. (Adapted with permission from Chen HC, Schultz AB, Ashton-Miller JA, et al. Stepping over obstacles: dividing attention impairs performance of old more than young adults. J Gerontol 1996;51A:M116–M122.)

In another study young, middle-aged, and older adults were asked to memorize word lists while either sitting, standing, or walking on two narrow tracks with different path complexities. The authors predicted that dual-task costs would increase from early adulthood through old age. Results showed that there was greater reduction in memory accuracy when walking as compared with sitting or standing. In addition, individuals showed greater reductions in walking speed and accuracy when they were performing the dual tasks as compared with walking alone. The decrements were already present in 40- to 50-year-olds with respect to memorizing and walking speed. With respect to walking accuracy, they were apparent only in the 60- to 70-year-olds. The authors propose that the consistency in findings across so many studies of this type suggests a more general phenomenon of aging, which they call the "age-associated permeation of behavior and cognition." This view holds that sensory/motor aspects of performance require more cognitive control and supervision as individuals age, because of frailty, sensory deficits, and problems in sensory integration (Lindenberger et al., 2000).

Studies have shown that after repeated falls, older persons develop a fear of falling, and this fear may contribute to changes in gait characteristics as well. For example, it has been shown that preferred walking pace, anxiety level, and depression are good predictors of the extent of fear of falling in community-dwelling older adults (Tinetti et al., 1990). Older adults who avoid activities because of a fear of falling tend to walk at a slower pace and to have higher levels of anxiety and depression as compared with adults who have little fear of falling. This has led several investigators to propose that slowed gait velocity among older adults reflects a conscious strategy to ensure safe gait, rather than the consequence of specific constraints on walking speed (Craik, 1989; Murray et al., 1969; Winter et al., 1990).

In other studies examining balance control in older adults with a fear of falling, researchers were not sure whether these adults had real problems with balance control or whether the fear of falling itself was affecting stability in an artifactual way (Maki et al., 1991). Thus, it is possible that cognitive factors, such as fear of falling, may contribute to changes in gait patterns in older adults.

Research has shown that executive attentional function is essential for successful dual-task performance. For example, the InCHIANTI study showed that poor performance on the Trail Making Test, a test of executive function, was related to reduced gait speed over an obstacle course and to a variety of dual-task physical tests (Coppin et al., 2006). Liu-Ambrose and colleagues (2009) examined the extent to which different aspects of executive function contribute to reduced dual-task walking abilities in older adults. They found that deterioration in set shifting abilities were significantly associated with poor dual-task gait performance. However, executive function played a role in dual-task performance only when cognitive load was high. They also found that balance confidence was independently associated with dual-task gait performance in community-dwelling older women.

Sensory Impairments

As noted in Chapter 9 on changes in postural control in the older adult, pathologies within visual, proprioceptive, and vestibular systems are common among many older adults, reducing the availability of information from these senses for posture and gait. If reduction in sensory function is part of normal aging, it will be important to determine ways to optimize environmental factors and use training to improve stability during walking in older adults.

Muscle Weakness

Decreased muscle strength has been indicated as a contributor to locomotor changes in older adults. In the section on kinetics of the gait cycle, we noted that Winter and colleagues (1990) reported a significant decrease in push-off power during gait in healthy older adults, which was possibly related to decreased muscle strength. Chapter 9 discusses in detail issues related to age-related reductions in muscle strength.

Effects of Exercise Programs on Gait Function

A number of studies have examined the effect of a variety of exercise programs on gait function in older adults. For example, Meier (1992) gave intensive daily physical therapy to six nursing home residents over a 5-week period and found a high degree of improvement in gait in this group as compared with six controls. Sauvage et al. (1992) used a 12-week moderate- to high-intensity strengthening and aerobic exercise program on a nursing home resident population and found significant improvements in clinical mobility scores, strength, muscular endurance, and some gait parameters, including velocity.

High-intensity resistance training has also been shown to increase knee extensor muscle strength and muscle size and to enhance functional mobility in frail adults in their 90s. Mean tandem gait speed was increased by 48% in this group after an 8-week training program. In addition, two of these frail subjects no longer used canes as an aid in walking at the end of the training period (Fiatarone et al., 1990).

Lord et al. (1996) used a 22-week randomized, controlled trial of exercise to determine whether a program of regular exercise could improve gait patterns in older women (mean age, 71 years) and whether improvements were mediated by increased lower-limb strength. They found improvements in muscle strength; increased walking speed, cadence, and stride length; and shorter stride times due to reduced swing and stance durations, while no changes were found in an age-matched control group. They noted that increased cadence was associated with improved ankle dorsiflexion strength and that increased stride length was associated with increased hip extension strength.

As might be expected, subjects with slower initial walking speeds showed the greatest improvements, while those with higher velocities showed little change. Older women with gait speeds of less than about 1 m/sec (these people have difficulties with functional activities such as crossing roads in urban environments) benefited most from the intervention (Lloyd, 1990; Lord et al., 1996). These studies suggest that both exercise and strength-training programs have positive effects on gait parameters in older adults, especially in those with slower gait velocities prior to training.

Gait Initiation and Backward Gait

Gait initiation requires dynamic balance control, since it is a transitional phase between static standing balance and dynamic balance requirements associated with walking. One way of examining the ability to control gait initiation is to measure both center of gravity (COG) changes, reflecting body position, and COP changes, reflecting both weight shifts and muscular control during dynamic postural changes. Gait initiation requires the separation of the COG and the COP in order to push off and begin gait. This separation between the COG and COP, known biomechanically as the "COG–COP moment arm," helps predict an individual's ability to tolerate dynamic unsteadiness.

Thus, a small moment arm would indicate that the COP and COG are being kept closely aligned during gait initiation, minimizing dynamic unsteadiness. Chang and Krebs (1999) have shown that the length of COG–COP moment arm during gait initiation clearly differentiates healthy older adults, who show a COG–COP moment arm of 21 ± 8 cm, from disabled older adults who show a moment arm of 15 ± 3 cm. This shortened moment arm could be due to either the result of muscle weakness (a primary impairment) or a compensatory strategy used to minimize dynamic unsteadiness.

Since backward walking is used in rehabilitation programs to improve balance, strength, and coordination, a study by Laufer (2005) compared the ability of older adults to perform backward walking with that of young adults. It was found that older adults showed significantly decreased stride length for backward walking as compared with young adults. In addition, they could increase velocity only by increasing cadence, while young adults used both cadence and stride length increases to increase velocity.

Stair-Walking

Research has documented that walking on stairs is associated with the highest proportion of falls in public places and that most of these falls occur as subjects walk down the stairs. To understand the physical requirements of stair-walking in older adults, characteristics of stair descent were studied in a group of 36 healthy women between the ages of 55 and 70 (Simoneau et al., 1991). Participants were asked to walk down a set of stairs under conditions of poor or distorted visual inputs; for example: (a) stairs were painted black, (b) vision of the stair was blurred (stairs were painted black and the subject wore a headband with a light-scattering plastic shield), or (c) stairs were painted black with a white stripe at the edge of each tread. A striped corridor surrounded the stairs.

The results of high-speed film analysis showed significantly slower cadence, larger foot clearance, and more posterior foot placement while subjects walked under the blurred condition as compared with the other two conditions. The authors further observed that foot clearance was larger than that obtained during pilot work from their laboratory on young adults. They concluded that older subjects walked with larger foot clearance during stair descent as compared with young adults and that gait patterns during stair descent were affected by visual conditions. It has also been shown that when going down stairs, older adults show a greater medial inclination angle during the stair-to-floor transition phase as compared with young adults. This inability to regulate body sway during the stair-to-floor transition, could increase the risk of falling in older adults (Lee & Chou, 2007).

Age-Related Changes in Other Mobility Skills

Sitting to Standing

The task of rising from a seated position is often associated with falling in older adults (Tinetti et al., 1986). Research indicates that 8% of community-dwelling older adults over 65 years of age show some problems in rising from a chair or bed. As a result, several studies have examined the sit-to-standing task in older adults (Alexander et al., 1991; Millington et al., 1992; Pai et al., 1994).

One study compared movement strategies, forces used, and the time taken to rise from sitting among young adults, older adults able to rise without armrests (old able), and older adults unable to rise without armrests (old unable). Average rise times from a chair were similar in the young and old able groups (1.56 vs. 1.83 seconds), but significantly longer in the old unable group (3.16 seconds). In addition, the hand forces used by the old able group were significantly less than those used by the old unable group.

The old able were different from the young mainly in the amount of time they spent in the initial phase of rising from the chair, which included the time from start to lifting off from the seat. They flexed their legs and trunks more during trials in which they used no hands to help themselves rise. Other studies (Mourey et al., 2000; Pai et al., 1994) showed that the peak vertical momentum of the center of mass, the maximal COM velocity in the horizontal axis and the COM velocity at the instant of lifting off were lower in elderly compared with young subjects. This was probably due to lower levels of muscle strength in the older adults.

In a study by Papa and Cappozzo (2000), different sit-to-stand motor strategies were identified for young versus community-dwelling older adults. The strategies were associated with both a different initial posture (ankle dorsiflexion angle) and speed of execution of the motor task. Prior to lifting off from the seat, the elder group tended to flex the trunk more than the younger group, bringing the COM closer to the base of support. They also used a higher movement velocity, thus gaining higher momentum. After lifting off from the seat, the older adults rotated the body forward and, only after having brought their COM over the base of support, effectively started elevation. Results showed that both global muscular effort and coordination effort associated with the achievement of balance and raising the COM were lower. However, maximal speed was also lower. The authors suggested that this may indicate that the elders had a lower functional reserve than the young individuals, thus choosing an optimal strategy for their limited reserve capacity.

Dubost et al. (2005) examined stand-to-sit characteristics in older versus young adults. The results showed that older adults tended to minimize the forward body displacement during sitting down. The authors suggested that this strategy was an adaptive mechanism to decrease the risk of anterior disequilibrium during sitting.

Rising from a Bed

Are there age-related differences in the movement patterns used in rising from a bed? To answer this question, adults ranging from 30 to 59 years of age were videotaped while rising from a bed (Ford-Smith & VanSant, 1993). As had been reported for young adults, there was considerable variability in patterns for rising from a bed among the slightly older group, aged 50 to 59. As was mentioned in Chapter 12, the most common patterns of bed-rising in the 30-to-39-year-old group involved a grasp-and-push pattern with the upper extremities, a roll-off or come-to-sit pattern, and a synchronous lifting of the lower limbs off the bed, with one limb extending to the floor in front of the other. The slightly older group, consisting of 50-to-59-year-olds, tended to use a more synchronous lifting pattern, with both legs moved to the floor simultaneously, as shown in Figure 13.16. No studies have been published to date on patterns used by the elderly when rising from the bed. Since many elderly people report falls at night associated with getting out of bed, such a study is essential.

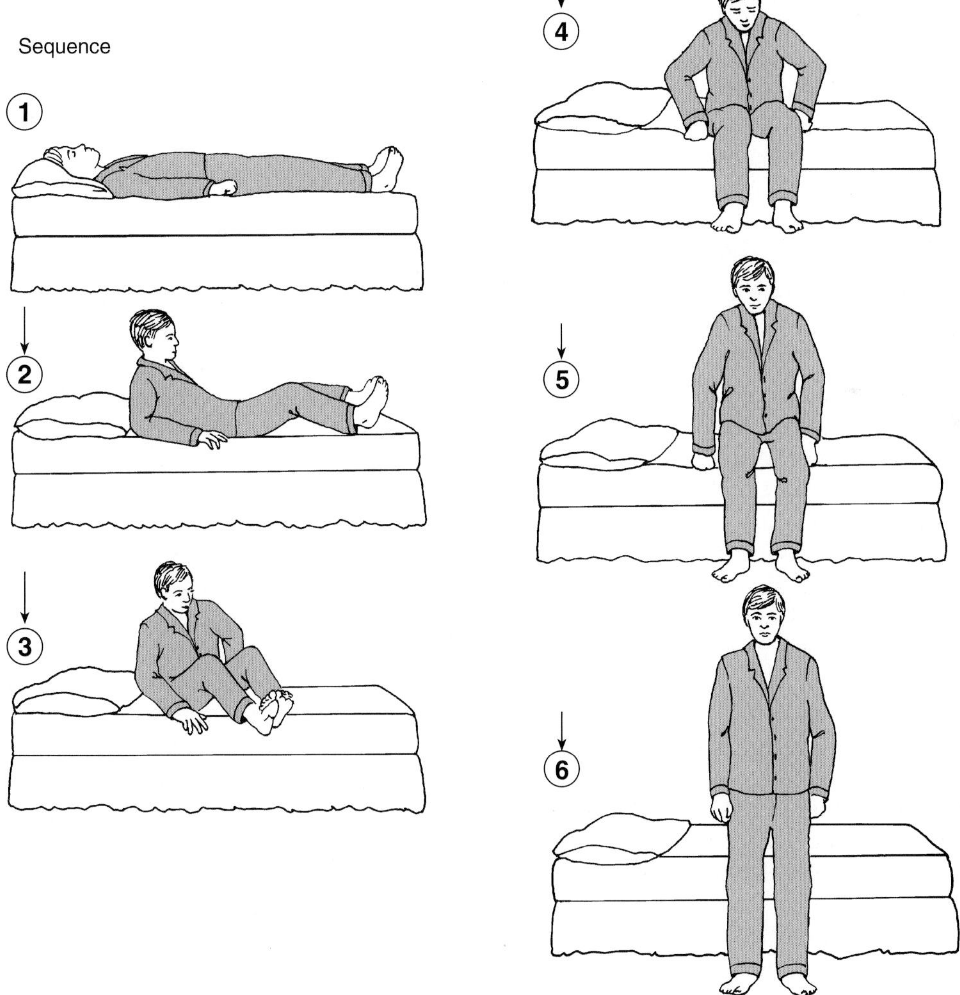

FIGURE 13.16 Frequent pattern of rising from a bed seen in 50- to-59-year-old subjects. (Adapted from Ford-Smith CD, VanSant AF. Age differences in movement patterns used to rise from a bed in subjects in the third through fifth decades of age. Phys Ther 1993;73:305, with permission of the American Physical Therapy Association. This material is copyrighted, and any further reproduction or distribution requires written permission from APTA.)

Supine to Standing

Moving from a supine to a standing position is an important task, even in older adults. The ability to stand up after a fall is a key element for functional independence. A number of studies have examined patterns of supine-to-standing movements across the lifespan and have shown that there is a progression across childhood to adulthood from asymmetrical to symmetrical movement patterns, with older adults more likely to show asymmetrical patterns like those seen in children (VanSant, 1990). One study investigated the relationship of age, activity level, lower-extremity strength, and range of motion to the movement patterns and time required to rise to a standing position from the floor (Thomas et al., 1998). They confirmed previous results regarding movement patterns and found that symmetrical movement patterns were associated with younger age, greater plantar flexion and hip extension strength, and greater dorsiflexion range of motion. This suggests that symmetrical patterns like those seen in young adults require higher levels of extensor muscle strength; however, alternative asymmetrical standing strategies are available to older adults with extensor weakness.

COMPARING GAIT CHARACTERISTICS OF INFANTS AND ELDERLY: TESTING THE REGRESSION HYPOTHESIS

It has been suggested that changes in the gait pattern among the elderly are related to the reemergence of immature walking patterns seen in young infants. Thus, it has been hypothesized that, as aging occurs, there is a regression to immature reflex patterns that characterized movement in young infants. This regression is thought to result from loss of higher-center control over the primitive reflexes that reemerge in the very old (Shaltenbrand, 1928). What are the similarities and differences between the gait characteristics of the very young and the very old?

Both groups show a shorter duration of single-limb stance and a greater relative duration of double support. This has been interpreted in both groups as an indication of decreased balance abilities (Bril & Breniere, 1993; Gabell & Nayak, 1984; Murray et al., 1969; Sutherland et al., 1980).

The gait of young walkers has also been described as having a wide base of support along with toeing-out, a characteristic observed in the elderly as well (Bril & Breniere, 1993; Murray et al., 1969). It has been suggested in both groups that an increased base of support is used to ensure better balance control.

Finally, both young children (Forssberg, 1985) and older adults (Finley et al., 1969) show coactivation of agonist and antagonist muscles during gait. This again has been described as a way of increasing joint stiffness, which helps in balance control (Woollacott, 1986).

Clearly, there are many similarities in the gait characteristics of young children and older adults. These similarities appear to relate to difficulties with balance control common to both groups. Thus, it is not necessarily true that similarities between the very old and the very young are due to a reappearance of primitive reflexes. In this case, the reason is a functional one: the two groups, often for very different reasons, have difficulties with the balance system, but use similar strategies to compensate for those difficulties.

A CASE STUDY APPROACH TO UNDERSTANDING AGE-RELATED CHANGES IN MOBILITY

Bonnie B is our 90-year-old woman with impaired balance and gait resulting in multiple falls, two of which required hospitalization. She lives alone in an apartment and has a home health aide who assists her with shopping, cooking, cleaning, and laundry. Bonnie's main concerns relate to her declining balance and frequent falls, many of which occur while she is walking. She is very fearful of falling again and restricts her mobility because of this.

Bonnie, like many older adults with a history of falls, shows significant differences in her walking pattern as compared with young and healthy older adults (Hausdorff et al., 1997; Heitmann et al., 1989; Wolfson et al., 1985). She shows a decrease in walking velocity, shorter step and stride length, and longer double support time. Bonnie is unable to walk without the use of her four-wheeled walker. With a gait velocity of 0.4 m/sec, she is unable to walk fast enough to cross a street safely. In the community, she uses her walker when ambulating for short distances, but most often relies on a wheelchair for mobility. Her gait pattern, including stride time, stance time, and swing time, are likely more variable, an indication of her high risk for falls (Hausdorff et al., 1997, 2001).

A kinematic analysis of her walking would find that joint-angle excursions at the hip, knee, and ankle flexion are less than in young adults (Winter et al., 1990). She walks with a flexed posture, in part because of her use of a walker.

An EMG analysis of muscle activity during walking would probably find increased coactivation of agonist and antagonist muscles, a strategy to increase joint stiffness and improve balance control. A kinetic analysis would probably find that plantar flexors generated significantly less power at push-off, while the quadriceps muscles absorbed significantly less energy during late stance and early swing (Winter et al., 1990).

Reduced plantar-flexor torque could be due to either muscle weakness or, alternatively, could be a strategy to improve stability during gait (Winter et al., 1990).

Bonnie has difficulty maintaining balance during complex walking tasks. She has considerable difficulty with obstacle avoidance. She is unable to lift her walker over an obstacle, and this has contributed to several falls in the community. Research has shown that during obstacle crossing, older adults with a history of falls frequently make contact with the obstacle, which increases their risk for falls (Chen et al., 1991).

A reduced ability to recover from slips and trips while walking is a major factor contributing to Bonnie's increased fall risk. Several factors contribute to her reduced ability to recover from a trip. Muscle responses used to recover stability following a slip or trip are likely delayed and weak (Tang & Woollacott, 1998). In addition, she likely has a reduced ability to generate torque quickly in the hip flexors of the swing leg, and the ankle plantar flexors of the stance leg, critical muscles for regaining stability following a trip (Chen et al., 1996).

Finally Bonnie has a reduced independence in other mobility tasks, including transfers and stairs. She must use her hands when moving from sitting to standing and often requires several tries in order to stand. She has difficulty on the Timed Up and Go test (TUG), a test of mobility requiring her to stand up from a chair, walk 10 ft, turn around and walk back to her chair and sit. She completes the test in 24 seconds, considerably slower than the 8 to 10 seconds taken by healthy older adults. When she performs the TUG with the addition of a secondary task, her time slows to 33 seconds and she is unsteady on her turns.

Many factors contribute to Bonnie's mobility impairments, including age-related changes in the systems critical to the control of balance and gait. In addition, because of her fear of falls, Bonnie has significantly reduced her activity level. This sedentary lifestyle also contributes to her impaired gait and mobility skills, and increases her risk for falls.

SUMMARY

1. There are three requirements for successful locomotion: (a) the ability to generate a rhythmic stepping pattern to move the body forward (progression), (b) postural control, ensuring orientation and stability, and (c) the ability to adapt gait to changing task and environmental requirements (adaptation). In the development of locomotion, these three factors emerge sequentially, with the stepping pattern appearing first, equilibrium control next, followed by adaptive capabilities.
2. The emergence of independent gait is characterized by the development of many interacting systems with certain hierarchical components. An innate pattern generator creates the basic rhythm of the step cycle, which can be seen in newborn stepping. In the first year, the gradual development of descending systems from higher neural centers gives the child increasing control over this locomotor behavior. The control of equilibrium, organized at a higher level than that of the pattern generator, develops over a longer period, as do adaptive systems essential to the integration of reactive and proactive strategies into gait.
3. The development of locomotor behavior begins prenatally and continues until the emergence of mature gait at about 7 years of age. Stepping behavior is present at birth and can be elicited in most infants if they are supported and inclined slightly forward. This early behavior resembles quadrupedal stepping, with flexion of the hip and knee, synchronous joint motion, and considerable coactivation of agonist and antagonist muscles.
4. In many infants, early stepping disappears at about 2 months of age, possibly because of biomechanical changes in the infant's system, such as an increase in relative body weight. Early stepping gradually transforms into a more mature pattern over the first 2 years of life.
5. There seems to be agreement among researchers that the ability to integrate postural control into the locomotor pattern is the most important rate-limiting factor on the emergence of independent walking.
6. The most significant modifications to the gait pattern occur during the first 4 to 5 months of independent walking. Most of these changes reflect the child's growing ability to integrate balance control with locomotion in these first months.
7. Studies characterizing gait patterns in older adults have consistently shown that healthy older adults have reduced walking speed, shorter stride length, and shorter step length than young adults.
8. Proactive locomotor abilities also change with age, with older adults taking more time to monitor the visual environment, taking more time to alter an upcoming step to avoid an obstacle, and using strategies such as slowing of approach and crossover time when stepping over obstacles.
9. Changes in the characteristics of gait patterns in older adults are influenced by balance

ability, leg muscle strength, and changes in the availability of sensory information. Cognitive factors such as fear of falling and attentional problems may also be important contributors.

10. When evaluating gait patterns of older people, consideration must be given to the underlying mechanisms contributing to these changes. In this way, one can differentiate between contributions related to pathology versus aging per se. Only after the systems contributing to walking-pattern dysfunction are identified can a clinician design effective and appropriate interventions to improve gait and thus help older adults achieve a safe and independent lifestyle.

ANSWERS TO LAB ACTIVITY ASSIGNMENTS

Lab Activity 13-1

See Table 13.1.

Lab Activity 13-2

See Table 13.2 for changes expected for older adults.

CHAPTER 14

ABNORMAL MOBILITY

LEARNING OBJECTIVES

Following completion of this chapter, the reader will be able to:

1. Discuss current approaches to classifying gait impairments in individuals with neurologic pathology.
2. Discuss the effects of neuromuscular impairments on gait, including the effects of spasticity, paresis, and dyscoordination.
3. Discuss the effects of other central nervous system (CNS) impairments, including those in the sensory, perceptual, and cognitive systems, on gait.
4. Discuss the recovery of walking following neurologic pathology, including the factors restricting participation in the mobility domain.
5. Discuss the prevalence and cause of other types of mobility problems, including those related to stair climbing, bed mobility, and transfers in people with CNS pathology.
6. Compare and contrast gait abnormalities in individuals with stroke, Parkinson's disease, cerebellar disorders, and cerebral palsy.

INTRODUCTION

Impaired mobility function, specifically disorders of gait, is one of the earliest and most characteristic symptoms of a wide variety of neurologic disorders. Mobility is a critical part of maintaining independence and an essential attribute of quality of life (Patla & Shumway-Cook, 1999). Mobility is one of the nine domains of activities and participation in the International Classification of Functioning, Disability, and Health (ICF) framework, and encompasses a spectrum of activities, including the ability to move oneself from one location to another by walking, running, climbing, or using other forms of transportation (World Health Organization, 2001). Walking in the ICF includes walking forward, backward, or sideways as well as walking both short and long distances, around obstacles, and over variable terrain (WHO, 2001).

Walking limitations resulting in restricted participation in the mobility domain (often referred to as "mobility disability" or "locomotor disability") have been identified as one of the most debilitating consequences of neurologic pathology, including stroke (Keenan et al., 1984; Lord et al., 2004; Perry et al., 1995; Pound et al., 1998), Parkinson's disease (Schenkman et al., 2002), and multiple sclerosis (Johansson et al., 2007). Mobility disability is reflected in reduced performance on functional walking activities such as walking on different terrains, up and down stairs or curbs, while carrying loads, or while talking to others. These limitations play a significant role in limiting participation in social roles as well as tasks and activities critical to daily life (Guralnik et al., 1993; Shumway-Cook et al., 2007).

This chapter describes impaired mobility function, including abnormalities of gait, stair walking, and transfers, in people with neurologic pathology. We begin by discussing the effect of motor, sensory and cognitive impairments on gait, and examine factors influencing the recovery of walking, including those that restrict participation in the mobility domain.

ABNORMAL GAIT

While abnormal gait is a common characteristic of many neurologic disorders, the constellation of underlying problems that produces disordered gait varies from patient to patient, even among patients with the same pathology. The type of gait abnormality observed depends on the type and extent of central nervous system (CNS) pathology, the constellation of resulting impairments, and the extent to which the patient is able to compensate for those impairments. Understanding the contribution of these elements to gait abnormalities can be very difficult. As a result, technology such as electromyography (EMG) and kinematic and/or kinetic analysis is often necessary to distinguish impairment from compensation. Technology is thus used extensively in studies examining gait problems in people with a neurologic disorder.

Classification Systems

While a number of classification schemes have been proposed, there is little consensus on the best framework for classifying gait disorders. Gait classification uses a set of defined variables to group individuals into categories based on distinct gait patterns (Dobson et al., 2007). Gait classification is designed to arrange individuals into homogeneous groups that can be used to assist clinicians with communication and clinical decision-making regarding therapeutic interventions to improve gait. Gait-classification systems are different from gait indexes and other methods for assessing gait, which provide a method for quantifying deviations from normal gait without assigning an individual patient to a specific subgroup (Dobson et al., 2007).

The most common framework for classifying disorders of gait is based on the neurologic diagnosis itself—for example, Parkinsonian gait, cerebellar ataxic gait, or spastic hemiparesis gait. A limitation of this approach is the assumption that a specific diagnosis results in a homogeneous gait pattern. However, this assumption is not supported by current research. For example, O'Byrne and colleagues (1998) classified gait patterns in 312 children with cerebral palsy (hemiplegia or diplegia) into eight categories, one of which was "crouch gait." However Rozumalski and Schwartz (2009) found that children with cerebral palsy who walked with a crouch gait (defined as excessive knee flexion at initial contact) were not a homogeneous sample, but instead could be further subdivided into five unique clusters, each of which was related to underlying clinical pathology, specifically, variations in strength, selective motor control, and spasticity. Similarly, Kinsella and Moran (2008) analyzed gait in 23 individuals with chronic stroke who walked with an equinus gait pattern and found three distinct subgroups. Thus, there appears to be significant heterogeneity among persons walking with an apparently homogeneous gait pattern.

Dobson et al. (2007) described two approaches, qualitative and quantitative, to subclassifying gait patterns in children with cerebral palsy. Qualitative methods classify gait patterns based primarily on gait speed and sagittal-plane gait kinematics. An example of this approach was the system proposed by Winters et al. (1987), which classified children with cerebral palsy hemiplegia into one of four categories based on kinematic gait deviations at the ankle or proximal joints (Kerr et al., 2009; McDowell et al., 2008).

Quantitative methods such as cluster analysis have also been used to classify gait patterns (Dobson et al., 2007). Cluster analysis is a generic term for a wide range of statistical techniques that are used to examine multivariate data in order to establish clusters of homogeneous subgroups (Dobson et al., 2007). For example, Mulroy et al. (2003) used cluster analysis to identify poststroke gait patterns using gait velocity and two kinematic parameters: knee extension in midstance and ankle dorsiflexion in midswing. Their analysis identified four homogeneous subgroups of walking patterns in poststroke hemiplegia. Strength, not spasticity, was the only clinical parameter that distinguished among the groups.

Researchers have also classified gait according to the primary pathophysiologic mechanism producing disordered gait. Crenna and Inverno (1994) have suggested a conceptual framework based on four main impairments contributing to disordered gait in individuals with supraspinal lesions: (1) defective muscle activation (paretic component); (2) abnormal velocity-dependent EMG recruitment during muscle lengthening (spastic component), (3) loss of selectivity in motor output (cocontraction component), and (4) changes in mechanical properties of the muscle tendon system (nonneural component). This conceptual framework has found support from research by Knutsson and Richards (1979) that has identified similar components in the gait of adults who have had a stroke. A limitation of this approach is that to date, the classification system is based solely on problems within the motor systems and does not include gait disorders due to sensory or perceptual problems.

As you can see, a wide variety of classification systems has been proposed to help researchers and clinicians understand abnormal gait. However, while groups of individuals may appear homogeneous based on one parameter of gait, they may vary widely on other parameters. For example, following stroke, gait classification based on velocity alone was associated with widely variable kinematic and EMG patterns (Olney et al., 1998). Classification based on velocity in conjunction with gait kinematics was associated with variable EMG activity and clinical parameters (de Quervain et al., 1996). Finally, classification based on similar EMG patterns was associated with widely varying kinematics and gait velocities (Knutsson & Richards, 1979; Shiavi et al., 1987). Thus, no single classification system appears to describe the full range of gait deviations in any neurologic population. In addition, there is relatively little information on how classification subgroups relate to specific underlying motor impairments (Dobson et al., 2007).

In this chapter we use both a pathophysiologic and a diagnostic framework to discuss disorders of gait. We begin with a pathophysiologic framework to examine how impairments in motor, sensory, perceptual, and cognitive systems contribute to disorders of gait, and we consider some common compensatory strategies used to maintain function in light of these impairments. Finally, we use our case studies to summarize gait problems from a diagnostic perspective. Regardless of the type of classification system used, understanding the effects of sensory, motor, and cognitive impairments on mobility function, as well as the types of patients likely to have these problems, is essential knowledge for examining and treating the patient with mobility problems.

Effect of Motor Impairments on Gait

Motor problems affecting gait include disruptions to both neuromuscular and musculoskeletal systems. In individuals with neurologic pathology, musculoskeletal problems develop secondary to primary neuromuscular problems that limit movement.

Neuromuscular Impairments

The neuromuscular control of gait includes the generation of the basic locomotor patterns for progression, the control of posture for maintaining orientation and stability, and the adaptation of gait patterns to changing task and environmental demands. The nervous system must be able to generate and adapt locomotor patterns while maintaining an appropriate posture for locomotion. In addition, since the mass of the head, arms, and trunk is large, and a significant amount of time is spent in single-leg support, balance is inherently unstable and the control of dynamic equilibrium is essential (Patla, 2003).

WEAKNESS/PARESIS An analysis of abnormal gait in various neurologic pathologies has shown that reduced ability to generate force, the so-called paretic component, is a primary contributor to disordered gait (Chen & Patten, 2008; Jonkers et al., 2009; Perry & Burnfield, 2010). Paresis, or weakness, is a primary neuromuscular impairment affecting the number, type, and discharge frequency of motor neurons essential for force production during gait (Duncan & Badke, 1987).

Paresis affects both the neural and nonneural components of force production. The neural component of weakness/paresis results from insufficient supraspinal recruitment of motor neurons in specific leg muscles either during certain parts of the gait cycle or throughout the gait cycle. Nonneural contributions to weakness reflect secondary changes in the muscle fibers themselves that affect the patient's ability to generate tension.

Muscles in gait act both concentrically to generate motion and eccentrically to control motion. Thus, weakness can result in both the inability to generate forces to move the body forward (e.g., the effect of weak plantar flexors in terminal stance) as well as unrestrained motions resulting from lack of control (e.g., foot slap following heel strike due to loss of eccentric control by the tibialis anterior [TA] and uncontrolled plantar flexion).

How much does weakness affect the ability to walk independently? This depends on which muscles are weak, the extent of the weakness, and the capacity of other muscles to substitute for weak muscles in achieving the requirements of gait. Walking normally does not tax the various lower-extremity muscle groups to their full capacity (Buchner & DeLateur, 1991; Patla, 2003). The only muscles that come close to their maximum output during gait are the ankle plantar flexors, which normally provide a major source of propulsive power. The following section briefly reviews the effect of weakness in select groups of lower-extremity muscles on gait.

Plantar-Flexor Weakness. In their classic study, Knutsson and Richards (1979) examined gait in 26 hemiparetic subjects, 9 (about one-third) showed a paretic pattern of gait. The paretic component resulted from a lack of muscle activation in gait. As shown in Figure 14.1A, EMG activity indicated a complete lack of phasic activation of the paretic calf muscles in stroke patients (dotted line) as compared with the normal controls (solid line). As shown in Figure 14.1B, there was relatively low activity of the TA in the subjects with hemiparesis (dotted line) as compared with normal controls (solid line). Behaviorally, strong hyperextension of the knee in the stance phase and lack of knee flexion characterized this gait pattern in the swing phase. This can be seen in Figure 14.1C, an angle diagram showing changes in knee motion in normal subjects (solid line) and in patients (dotted line). Interestingly, for several of the patients examined, poor muscle recruitment in gait was associated with preserved recruitment when the muscle was activated voluntarily, suggesting that injury disturbs the central generation of preprogrammed gait activation but leaves the capacity to activate muscles voluntarily relatively intact (Knutsson & Richard, 1979). Similar results were reported by Shiavi et al. (1987), who reported that reduced muscle activity was the most common EMG pattern found during gait analysis in the acute phase of stroke.

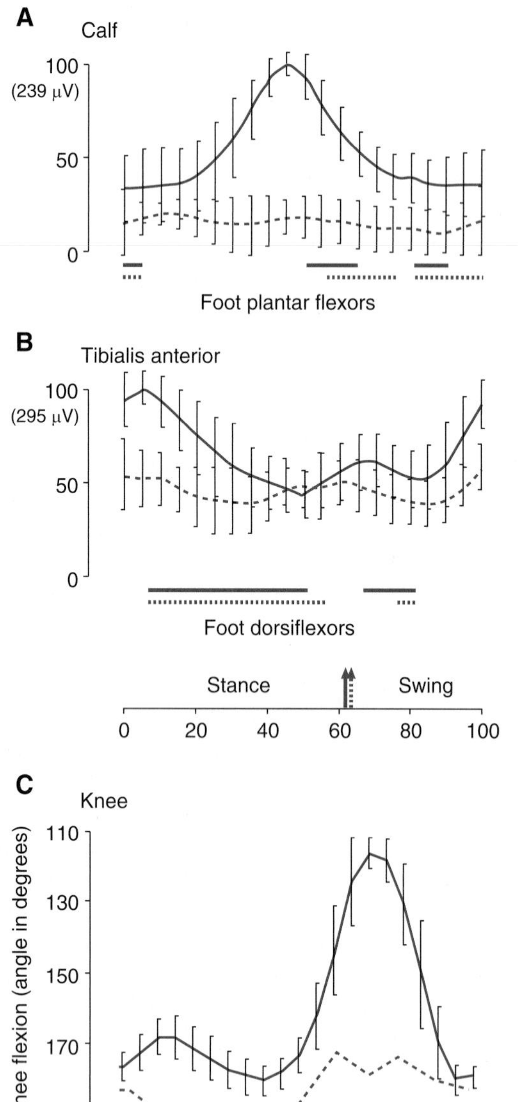

FIGURE 14.1 Effects of paresis on gait. A and B, Rectified, integrated EMG activity from ankle plantar flexors and dorsiflexors across the gait cycle in normal healthy controls (solid lines) and a group of subjects with hemiparesis (dotted line). EMG in the patient group shows a lack of phasic activation of the calf muscles and relatively low activity of the tibialis anterior. C, Changes in knee motion in normal subjects (solid line) and in patients (dotted line). (Adapted with permission from Knutsson E, Richards C. Different types of disturbed motor control in gait of hemiparetic patients. Brain 1979;102:420.)

More recently, a number of research studies have documented the contribution of weakness, specifically in the plantar flexors, to impaired gait following stroke (Chen & Patten 2008; Jonkers et al., 2009; Lamontagne et al., 2002; Mulroy et al., 2003) and Parkinson's disease (Svehlík et al., 2009). Chen and colleagues compared the mechanical work produced by the hip, knee, and ankle moments during preswing in the paretic limb of 23 individuals with poststroke hemiparesis with that of nondisabled controls walking at comparable speeds (Chen & Patten, 2008; Chen et al., 2005). In comparison with control subjects, leg kinetic energy at toe-off and peak knee flexion during swing were significantly reduced in the poststroke group. Reduced leg kinetic energy during preswing was largely the result of reduced ankle plantar flexor work.

This can be seen in Figure 14.2, which compares mean ankle moment (Fig. 14.2A) and ankle work (Fig. 14.2B) during preswing as a function of gait velocity in controls (shown as stars) and subjects with stroke (filled circles represent subjects who used an ankle–foot orthosis [AFO]; open circles are hemiparetic subjects without an AFO). Among the participants with poststroke hemiparesis, plantar-flexor work in the paretic limb was very low as compared with the nondisabled subjects walking at similar slow speeds. Increased knee and hip moments partially offset the reduction in plantar-flexor work during preswing. Chen and Patten's (2008) work is consistent with that of other researchers (Nadeau et al., 1997; Olney et al., 1998), who reported that strong hip flexor activity during pull-off can partially compensate for reduced plantar flexor strength and power in the paretic limb.

Mulroy et al. (2003) used cluster analysis to identify four gait patterns in patients with poststroke hemiparesis. Group 1, labeled "fast," had the fastest velocity (44% of normal), slightly decreased knee extension in midstance (7 degrees of flexion) and adequate (1 degree) ankle dorsiflexion in swing. Group 2, labeled "moderate/slight flexion," had intermediate velocity (21% of normal) and slightly greater knee flexion in midstance (14 degrees). Group 3, labeled "flexed," had a very slow gait velocity (10% of normal), excessive knee flexion in midstance (23 degrees) and inadequate dorsiflexion in swing (–8 degrees).

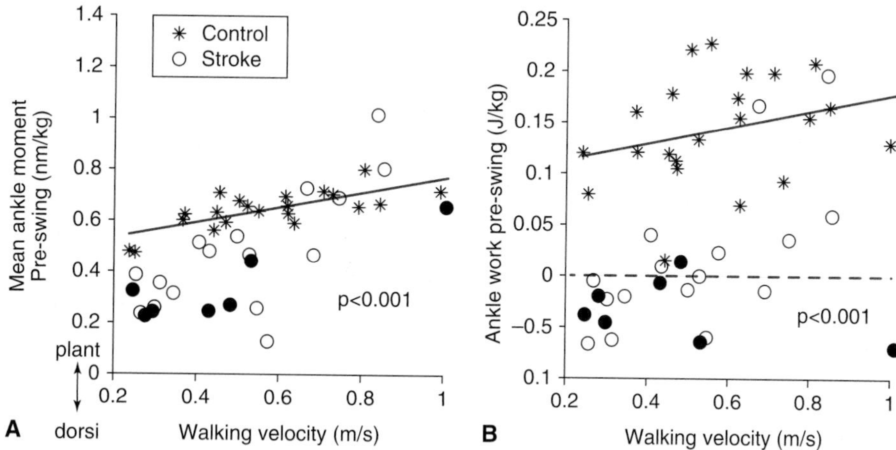

FIGURE 14.2 Effects of weakness on stance-to-swing transition following stroke. Mean ankle moment (A) and ankle work (B) during preswing as a function of gait speed in nondisabled controls (asterisks) and individuals with hemiparesis with (filled circles) and without (open circles) an ankle-foot orthosis. dorsi = dorsiflexors; plant = plantarflexors. (Adapted with permission from Chen G, Patten C. Joint moment work during the stance to swing transition in hemiparetic subjects. J Biomechanics 2008;41:880).

Group 4, labeled "extended," also had very slow velocity (11% of normal), knee hyperextension in midstance (–6 degrees), and inadequate dorsiflexion in swing (–11 degrees).

In this study, strength was the only clinical parameter that distinguished among the four groups. Isometric torques for the ankle plantar flexors, knee extensors, and hip extensors were significantly reduced in the three slower groups (17 to 36% of normal) compared to the fastest group (53 to 70% of normal). For patients with significant plantar-flexor weakness, velocity was decreased and the compensatory pattern of gait adopted depended on the relative strength of the knee and hip extensors. Patients in Group 3 walked with excessive knee flexion in midstance and had greater strength in the quadriceps as compared with the hip extensors and thus used prolonged activity in the quadriceps to support the flexed-knee posture. In contrast, participants in Group 4 demonstrated knee hyperextension in midstance and had greater strength in the hip extensors as compared with the quadriceps; they thus used hip-extensor strength and passive knee extension to ensure stability.

Finally, a reduced ability to increase ankle and hip power limits the potential to increase walking speed among persons with lower gait function following stroke (Jonkers et al., 2009).

Quadriceps Weakness A weak quadriceps (grades 3+ to 4) will lead to difficulty controlling knee flexion during loading. A very weak quadriceps (grades 0 to 3) will lead to trouble stabilizing the knee during midstance. The primary compensation for this is hyperextension of the knee during midstance, since the forward movement of the body weight will serve as the knee extensor force (Mulroy et al., 2003; Perry & Burnfield, 2010). When hyperextension is continued into preswing, it prevents the knee from moving freely during the swing phase. This can slow progression and result in toe drag.

Compensation for a weak quadriceps may involve a forward trunk lean, which brings the body vector anterior to the knee, resulting in knee hyperextension. While this is an effective compensatory strategy for stabilizing the knee, there are disadvantages to the use of a knee-hyperextension strategy as a compensation for a weak quadriceps. First, it limits knee flexion during loading and increases the impact of body weight on the structures of the stance limb. It traumatizes the internal structure of the knee and can damage these structures in the long term. It also requires good hip extensor strength to control the forward trunk lean (Mulroy et al., 2003). The advantage of the knee-hyperextension strategy is that it allows a more stable posture, and therefore may be a reasonable and appropriate strategy for people with a weak quadriceps (Mulroy et al., 2003; Perry & Burnfield, 2010).

Hip Flexor Weakness. Normal gait requires only a grade 2+ (poor plus) muscle strength in the hip flexors (Perry & Burnfield, 2010). Hip-flexor weakness, producing inadequate hip flexion, primarily affects the swing phase of gait. Hip flexion is used during swing to assist progression by producing a hip-flexor moment at the initiation of swing (Chen & Patten; 2008; Neptune et al., 2001; Winter, 1984). Knee flexion is lost in swing when there is inadequate hip flexion; thus, the patient is unable to develop sufficient momentum at the hip to indirectly flex the knee. As a result, toe clearance is reduced or lost. A shortened step is also associated with inadequate hip flexion, and it can affect the position of the foot at heel strike. When the hip cannot be flexed at the initiation of swing, limb advancement and thus progression are hampered. At the same time, placement of the foot in preparation for weight acceptance is affected, challenging stability. Impaired hip-flexor strength affecting pull-off has been shown in a number of neurologic populations including stroke (Chen & Patten, 2008) and Parkinson's disease (Svehlík et al., 2009). This may be particularly problematic, since use of the hip flexors to increase pull-off has been shown to be an effective compensatory strategy for persons with significantly reduced plantar-flexor force (Nadeau et al., 1999; Olney & Richards, 1996).

There are several compensatory strategies people use to achieve foot clearance during swing despite inadequate hip flexion; these are shown in Figure 14.3. The first uses a posterior tilt of the pelvis and activation of the abdominal muscles to advance the swing limb (Fig. 14.3A). The second uses circumduction, defined as hip-hike, forward rotation of the pelvis, and abduction of the hip, to advance the limb (Fig. 14.3B). The other strategies used to advance the limb despite hip flexor weakness include contralateral vaulting (Fig. 14.3C), involving coming up onto the forefoot of the stance limb, or leaning the trunk laterally toward the opposite limb (Fig. 14.3D).

Hip-Extensor Weakness. Activation of the hip extensors is critical to control of the head, arms, and trunk (HAT) segment (Winter, 1984). In addition, hip-extensor strength relative to quadriceps strength is a significant determinant in how persons compensate for weak plantar-flexors following stroke (Mulroy et al., 2003). Hip-extensor weakness can produce a forward trunk lean that threatens stability. Backward lean in stance compensates for hip-extensor weakness by bringing the center of mass (COM) behind the hips; it is used for stability. However, TA activity is needed to prevent falls in the backward direction. Following stroke, hip-extensor weakness has been shown to be positively correlated with gait velocity and is a major determinant of compensatory frontal-plane pelvic motions (Cruz & Dhaher, 2009).

Hip-Abductor Weakness. Weak hip abductors (gluteus medius) can result in drop of the pelvis on the side contralateral to the weakness, called a "Trendelenburg gait." A common compensation for hip-abductor weakness is a lateral shift of the COM over the stance leg in conjunction with lateral lean of the trunk toward the stance leg. This shift of the upper body over the stance side moves the ground reaction force (GRF) in the same direction. When the GRF passes directly through the center of the femoral head, the internal moment generated by the hip abductors (that normally produces a stabilizing force) is no longer needed (Gage, 1993; Perry & Burnfield, 2010). This same compensatory mechanism is used when the problem is a painful hip, in order to reduce the proportion of force passing through the hip joint (Gage, 1991). Hip-abductor weakness is a contributing factor to hip deformities, including subluxation, in children with cerebral palsy. Metaxiotis et al. (2000) examined compensatory gait strategies in 23 children with cerebral palsy (19 diplegic and 4 hemiplegic) and found that 21 compensated for hip subluxation with an ipsilateral trunk lean and contralateral pelvic drop. They reported hip-abductor weakness as the main cause of the hip deformity.

Hip abductors also make an important contribution to achieving an appropriate step width, an essential part of ensuring mediolateral stability of the center of body mass. Thus, weakness of these muscles can result in instability in the frontal plane, a factor in increased risk for falls in older adults (Krebs et al., 1998) and patients with neurologic pathology (Basford et al., 2003; Chou et al., 2003).

Effect of Paresis / Weakness on Gait Speed. The effect of paresis on gait speed following stroke has been examined by a number of researchers (Chen & Patten, 2008; Kim & Eng, 2003; Lamontagne et al., 2002; Nadeau et al., 1997; Olney et al., 1986, 1991). Olney et al.'s studies compared joint power profiles at the ankle, knee, and hip in patients with hemiparesis due to stroke. Subjects were sorted into three groups based on self-selected gait speed (fast = 0.63 m/sec, medium = 0.41 msec, and slow = 0.25 m/sec). Power profiles in the patients with hemiparesis were very similar in shape to those of controls who had not had a stroke, with major positive work done by ankle plantar flexors at push-off (A2) and at the hip during the pull-off phase (H3). While peak profiles were similar, there was a significant difference in amplitude between affected and unaffected limbs. Peak power at the ankle and hip were correlated with gait speed, underscoring the effect of weakness on gait performance following stroke.

These findings were consistent with the finding of Nadeau et al. (1997) that gait speed was somewhat correlated with isokinetic plantar-flexor torque ($r = 0.41$); however, hip flexor torque was highly correlated with both self-selected gait speed ($r = 0.83$) and maximum pace ($r = 0.88$). Kim and Eng (2003) also examined the relationship between lower-extremity muscle torque

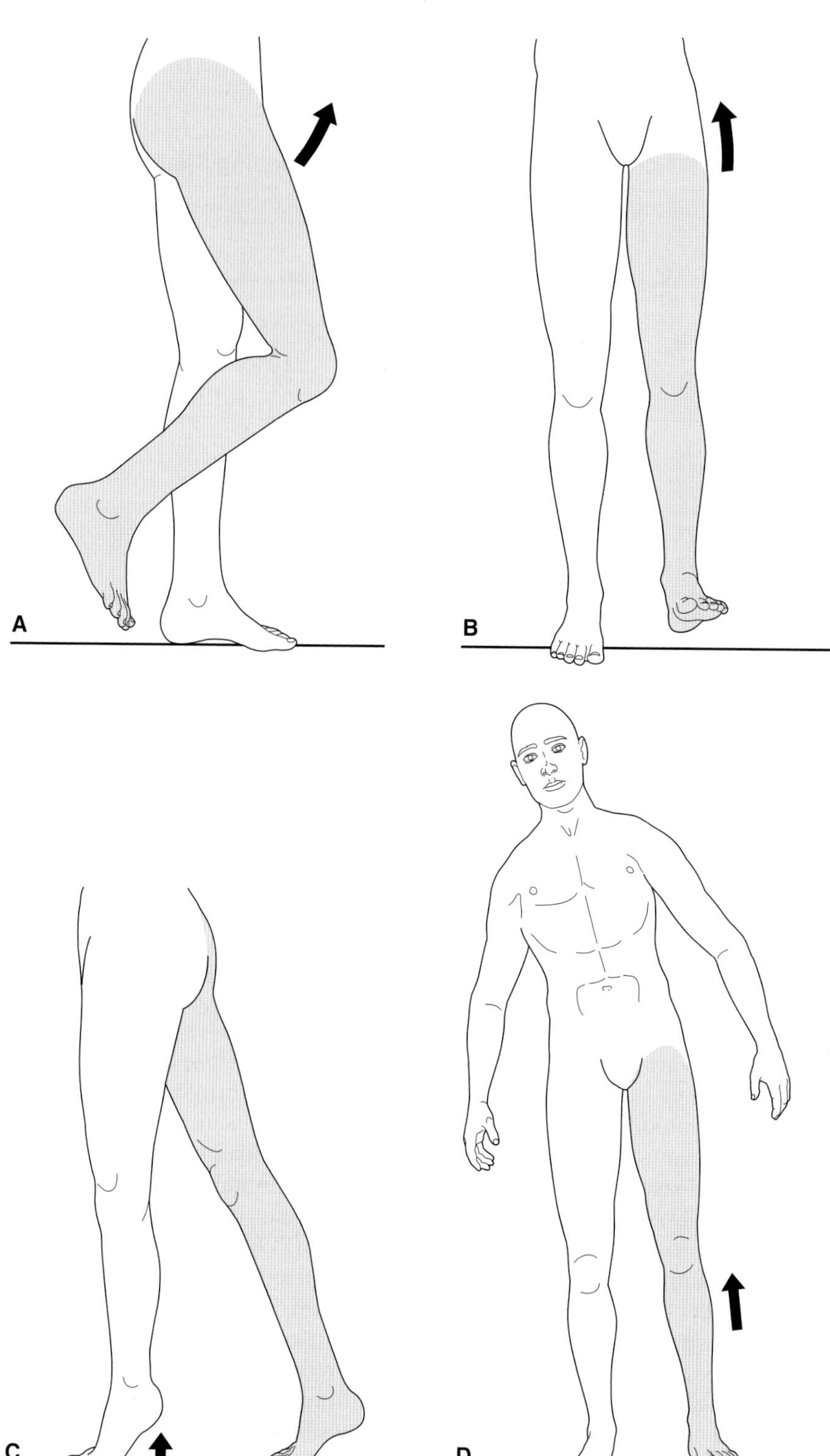

FIGURE 14.3 Compensatory strategies used to advance the swing leg despite inadequate hip flexion include: A, activation of the abdominal muscles in conjunction with a posterior tip of the pelvis; B, circumduction; C, contralateral vaulting; and D, leaning the trunk laterally toward the opposite limb.

and locomotor performance in people with stroke. They examined the relationship between gait speed and concentric isokinetic torques of the flexor and extensor muscles at the ankle, knee, and hip bilaterally in 20 independently ambulatory participants with stroke. They reported moderate to high correlations (r = 0.5 to 0.8) between gait and stair-climbing speeds and torques of the paretic ankle plantar flexors, hip flexors, and knee flexors. The relationship between muscle torques in the paretic and nonparetic sides and gait speed is shown in Table 14.1. As you can see, paretic ankle plantar flexor torque has the highest correlation

TABLE 14.1 Correlation between Average Torque Values versus Self-Selected Gait Speed and Stair-Climbing Speed in 20 Persons with Stroke

Side	Test	Gait Speed (m/sec)	Stair-Climbing Speed (m/sec)
Paretic	Hip extension	0.351	0.273
	Hip flexion	0.574[a]	0.544[b]
	Knee extension	0.408	0.337
	Knee flexion	0.555[b]	0.482[b]
	Ankle plantar flexion	0.845[a]	0.709[a]
	Ankle dorsiflexion	0.329	0.328
Nonparetic	Hip extension	0.346	0.324
	Hip flexion	0.380	0.289
	Knee extension	0.331	0.443
	Knee flexion	0.615[a]	0.477[b]
	Ankle plantar flexion	0.486	0.450[b]
	Ankle dorsiflexion	0.294	0.367

[a] $p < 0.01$.
[b] $p < 0.05$.
Reprinted from Kim CM, Eng JJ. The relationship of lower extremity muscle torque to locomotor performance in people with stroke. Phys Ther 2003;83:54, Table 4, with permission of the American Physical Therapy Association. This material is copyrighted, and any further reproduction or distribution requires written permission from APTA.

(r = 0.845) to gait speed. Stepwise multiple-regression analyses identified paretic ankle plantar-flexor torque as the single most important variable in predicting gait speed, and alone explained 67 to 72% of the variance in gait speed on level surfaces.

A study by Lamontagne et al. (2002) investigated the role of paresis, antagonist coactivation, passive stiffness, and spasticity on the reduced-stance-phase plantar-flexor moment and swing-phase dorsiflexor moment during gait in 30 people with hemiparesis due to a recent (<6 months) stroke. The study found reduced plantar-flexor (PF) moment in both the paretic and nonparetic side in subjects with stroke compared with controls. On the paretic side, reduced ankle moments were associated with low medial gastrocnemius (MG) activation levels (paresis) but excessive coactivation levels on the nonparetic side. Half of the patients had reduced dorsiflexion (DF) during the swing phase of gait compared with controls. However, reduced DF on the paretic side was not in general associated with decreased TA activation, excessive ankle coactivation, or excessive PF spasticity. Instead in some but not all patients, increased PF passive stiffness resisted swing-phase dorsiflexion. Similar to the findings of Kim and Eng (2003), more than 50% of the variance in gait speed could be explained by peak PF activation on the paretic side during the stance phase of gait.

This relationship between gait speed and lower-extremity power has also been shown in older adults with mobility disability in the absence of a neurologic diagnosis (Cuoco et al., 2004; Bean et al., 2002). However, this relationship between gait speed and lower-extremity power may or may not apply to persons with Parkinson's disease (PD). While Sofuwa et al. (2005) found a significant reduction in ankle (push-off) and hip-flexor (pull-off) power generation in the PD group, there was no correlation between ankle power and gait speed. In contrast, Svehlík et al. (2009) found a positive relationship between gait velocity and ankle and hip power in 20 persons with PD tested off medication.

In summary, a reduced ability to generate force is a major factor contributing to disordered gait in both older adults and in those with neurologic pathology. Paresis and weakness affect both control of movement through loss of eccentric contractions and generation of movement through loss of concentric contractions, and this seems to be a significant factor in reduced gait velocity in many patients.

Spasticity. Because spasticity is a frequent accompaniment of neurologic disorders, many researchers have looked at its effect on gait. Spasticity can have an impact on gait in two ways. First, spasticity results in the inappropriate activation of a muscle at points during the gait cycle when it is being rapidly lengthened. In addition, spasticity alters the mechanical properties of a muscle, producing increased stiffness (a musculoskeletal problem) (Dietz et al., 1981). Increased stiffness affects the freedom of body segments to move rapidly with regard to one another; this limits the transfer of momentum during gait, affecting the progression requirements of locomotion.

In order to determine the contribution of spasticity to disordered gait, a number of researchers have examined activation levels of muscles in response to stretch during perturbed and nonperturbed gait. Some studies have examined activation of spastic muscles during lengthening contractions in unperturbed gait (Crenna, 1998; Knutsson & Richards, 1979; Lamontagne et al., 2001; Sinkjaer et al., 1996). Others have used perturbations to gait to study spasticity in gait, either by rapidly stretching the calf muscles using mechanical devices fixed to the subject's leg (Anderson & Sinkjaer, 1996) or by abruptly changing belt speed during treadmill walking (Berger et al., 1984b).

Regardless of the methods used, a key to understanding the contribution of spasticity to disordered gait requires knowing when muscles undergo lengthening during the gait cycle. This allows the researcher to examine the activity of spastic muscles during critical lengthening periods. For example, Figure 14.4A summarizes data from 10 healthy children showing the lengthening phases in representative lower limb muscles, including the quadriceps (Quad), medial hamstrings, soleus, and TA. As can be seen in this graph, the Quad is lengthened twice over the gait cycle, in early stance phase, during knee yielding associated with loading, and when the knee flexes during toe-off. One would expect, therefore, that the effect of a spastic quadriceps muscle would be greatest during these two points in the gait cycle. In contrast, the hamstring has one lengthening period in late swing, associated with knee extension in preparation for initial contact. Therefore, one would expect the effect of spasticity in the hamstring to be heightened activation of this muscle during late swing.

In patients for whom spasticity is the primary impairment contributing to disordered gait, one does in fact see heightened activity in spastic muscles undergoing lengthening. However, often spasticity is not the sole contributor to disordered gait. This is best illustrated in Figure 14.4B, which shows the activation of four representative muscles in a child with spastic diplegia. In this figure, the filled boxes represent muscle activity that is comparable to normal. The open boxes represent an absence of muscle activity that is normally seen (see, for example, Quad L1), and the gray boxes represent muscle activity that is found in children with cerebral palsy, but never in the normal control children. Thus, one can see from looking at this figure that spasticity is not the only component contributing to disordered gait (Crenna, 1998).

The following section briefly reviews the effects of spasticity in certain key muscles.

Plantar Flexor Spasticity. Spasticity in the ankle plantar-flexors (triceps surae) is a common problem following neurologic injury, and it has been reported in patients with stroke and cerebral palsy and following

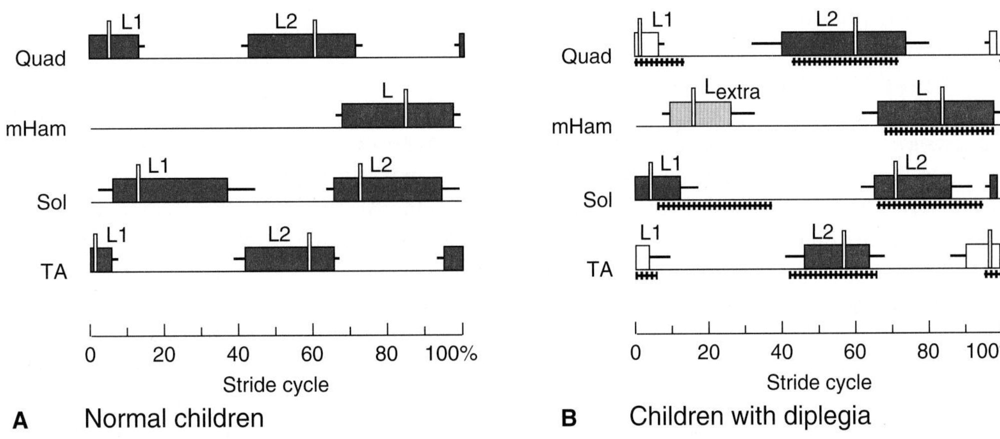

FIGURE 14.4 Lengthening phases in representative lower limb muscles, including the quadriceps (Quad), medial hamstrings (mHam), soleus (Sol), and tibialis anterior (TA) in normal healthy children (A) and children with spastic cerebral palsy (B). See text for explanation. (Adapted with permission from Crenna P. Spasticity and "spastic" gait in children with cerebral palsy. Neurosci Biobehav Rev 1998;22:573.)

traumatic brain injury (Crenna & Inverno, 1994; Knutsson & Richards, 1979; Perry, 1992).

Knutsson and Richards (1979) studied 26 adults with spastic hemiplegia secondary to stroke and found that 9 (about one-third) showed a "spastic" pattern of gait, characterized primarily by abnormal activation of the triceps surae (TS) muscles during the early part of the stance phase of walking. Figure 14.5A compares averaged EMG activity (normalized to 239 mV) of the TS during the gait cycle in 10 control subjects and 9 individuals with spastic hemiparesis. As compared with controls, in individuals with spastic hemiparesis, the TS activation began early in the stance phase and had relatively lower peak amplitude. Following initial contact, stretching of the TS resulted in the early activation of the muscles. The resultant shortening of the muscle before the body had passed ahead of the foot, pulled the lower leg backward and produced knee hyperextension. This is seen in the graph of knee angle during the gait cycle, in the lower part of the figure. Figure 14.5B is a stick figure of lower-limb motion in a control participant (left) versus a person with hemiparesis (right). It illustrates the effect of premature contraction of the TS in the hemiparetic limb, which impedes muscle lengthening and forward rotation of the tibia, resulting in knee hyperextension as the body moves forward. This reduces the ability of the TS to build tension for push-off.

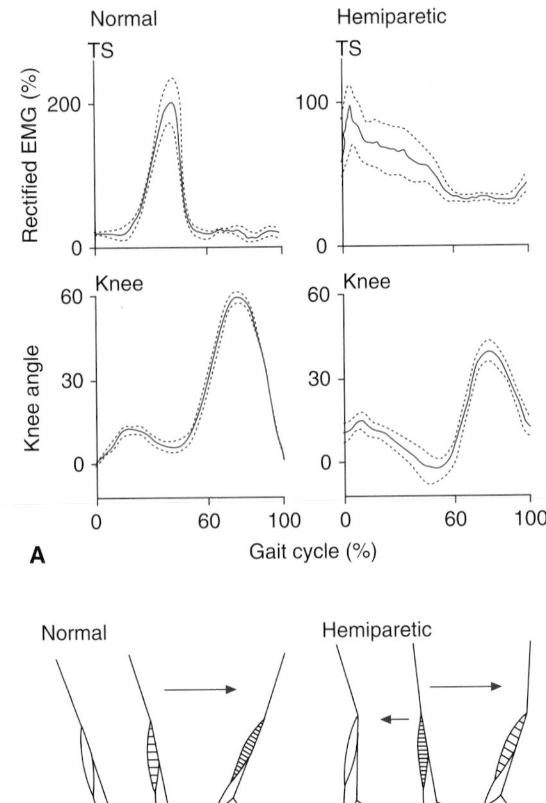

FIGURE 14.5 Effect of spastic triceps surae (TS) on gait in patients with hemiplegia. A, Averaged EMG activity (normalized to 239 mV) of the TS during the gait cycle in 10 normal control subjects and 9 patients with spastic hemiparesis, along with the corresponding knee angular changes. Note the high activation of TS during the entire stance phase in the patients with hemiparesis. B, Effect of early TS activation on knee position in normal and hemiparetic gait. (Adapted with permission from Knutsson E. Can gait analysis improve gait training in stroke patients? Scand J Rehab Med Suppl 1994;30:78.)

Lamontagne et al. (2001) studied the effect of spasticity in the medial gastrocnemius (MG) during walking in 30 persons with hemiparesis following stroke (time since stroke, <6 mo) and 15 control subjects. EMG activity in the MG was recorded using surface EMGs; kinematics of lower-extremity motion were recorded with a two-dimensional motion-analysis system. Gait analysis measures were correlated with clinical measures of spasticity (modified Ashworth scale [MAS]), ankle clonus, and ankle plantar-flexor strength (using a handheld dynamometer).

A locomotor-specific measure of spasticity was developed that related plantar-flexor activity (EMG activity) and the velocity of muscle lengthening. The slope of this relationship was used as a measure of the velocity-sensitive response of the MG during walking. Consistent with Knuttson and Richards' (1979) findings, this study also showed premature activation (one or more bursts of low amplitude) of the plantar-flexor muscles (MG) in the spastic hemiparetic limb, which occurred during peak lengthening velocity in the stance phase of gait in two-thirds of the individuals with hemiparesis.

Figure 14.6 compares lengthening velocity in the MG and EMG activity in a control subject (A), and in the paretic (B) and nonparetic (C) limbs of a person with stroke. The top panel in A shows two critical lengthening periods identified for the MG—one in stance and one in swing. The middle panel plots EMG activity in the MG. The bottom panel plots the normalized EMG value (to its maximal value) as a function of lengthening velocity. The slope of this relationship is a measure of locomotor spasticity. Note that in the paretic limb (Fig. 14.6B), EMG activity in the MG is early and is characterized by multiple small bursts of activity. The relationship between MG activity and lengthening velocity is positively related, and the slope is 261 (as compared with an inverse slope of −93.0 in the control subject and −51.6 in the nonparetic limb). Interestingly, the authors did not find excessive activation of the MG when it was lengthened during the swing phase of gait, suggesting that locomotor

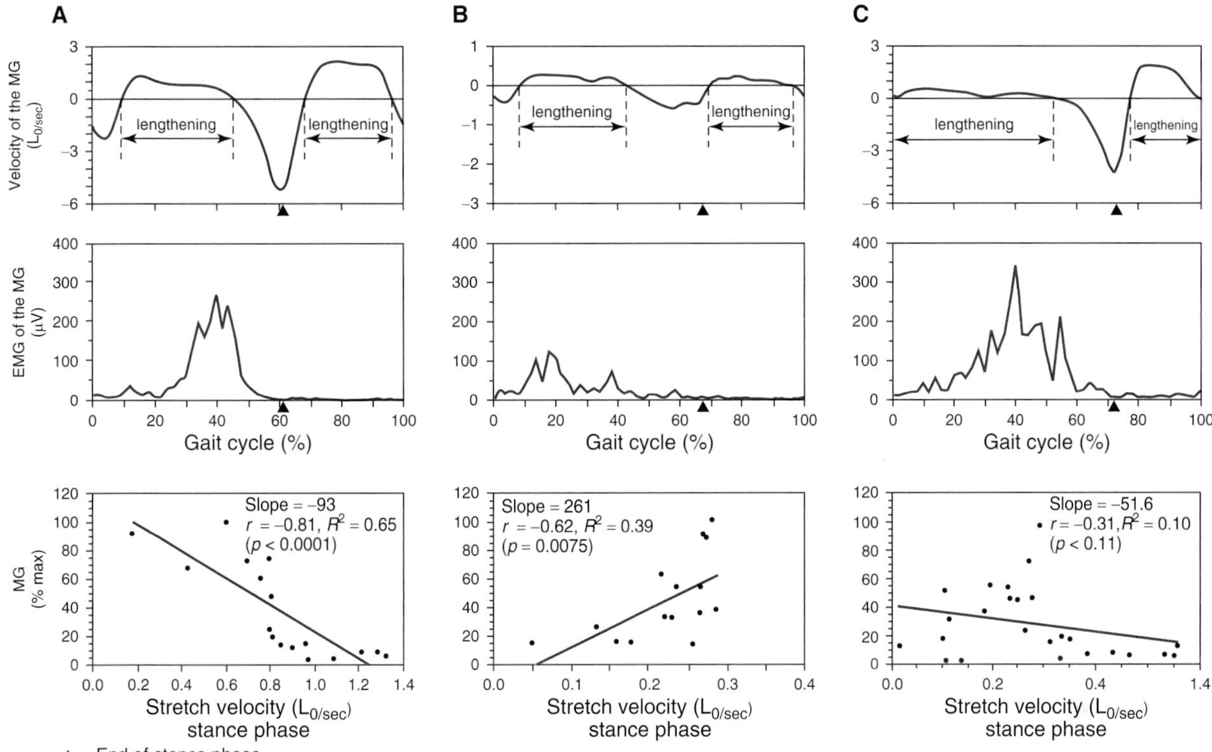

FIGURE 14.6 Effect of spasticity in the MG in gait. A comparison of lengthening velocity in the MG and EMG activity in a normal control subject (A) and in paretic (B) and nonparetic (C) limbs of a patient with stroke. The top panels show the two critical lengthening periods identified for the MG—one in stance and one in swing. The middle panel plots EMG activity in the MG. The lowest box plots the normalized EMG value (to its maximal value) as a function of lengthening velocity. The slope of this relationship is a measure of locomotor spasticity. Note that in the paretic limb (panel B), EMG activity in the MG is early and is characterized by multiple small bursts of activity. The relationship between MG activity and lengthening velocity is positively related, and the slope is 261 (as compared with an inverse slope of −93.0 in the control subject and −51.6 in the nonparetic limb). Adapted from Lamontagne A, Malouin F, Richards CL, Dumas F. Mechanisms of disturbed motor control in ankle weakness during gait after stroke. Gait Posture 2002;15:244–255.

spasticity is phase-dependent. Locomotor spasticity was inversely related to gait speed, suggesting that early premature activation of the MG in response to lengthening velocity impairs ankle push-off in late stance. Finally, locomotor spasticity was correlated with clinical measures of spasticity (using the MAS) and clonus, but only weakly associated with static muscle strength.

Crenna and Inverno (1994) identified spasticity as one of four factors contributing to disordered gait in children with spastic forms of cerebral palsy (diplegia and hemiplegia). The effect of a spastic muscle on gait parameters in stance versus swing is shown in Figure 14.7. It compares activity of the soleus muscle when it is being lengthened in early stance (A) and in swing (B) in a normal control child and in a child with spastic diplegia. The child with diplegia shows excessive activation of the soleus (increased EMG amplitude) in the early stance-lengthening phase. Interestingly, there was no excessive activation of the soleus muscle in the child with spastic diplegia when the soleus muscle underwent a second lengthening during the swing phase of gait (Fig. 14.7B). The effects of spasticity on an equinus gait pattern in children with cerebral palsy are increased at faster walking speeds; thus, children may walk at a slower gait velocity in an attempt to decrease the effect of spasticity on gait kinematics (van der Krogt et al. 2009).

Sinkjaer et al. (1996) found that impaired gait in individuals with multiple sclerosis (MS) was in part due to impaired stretch-reflex modulation of the soleus muscle and concomitant increased ankle-joint stiffness. Normally, the soleus stretch reflex is modulated in a phase-dependent way during walking (Figure 14.8A), with stance phase showing a large-magnitude stretch response, the transition from stance to swing phase showing a minimal response, and the swing phase showing a response that is 50% of the stance-phase magnitude. In five of the seven persons with MS studied, the soleus muscle's response

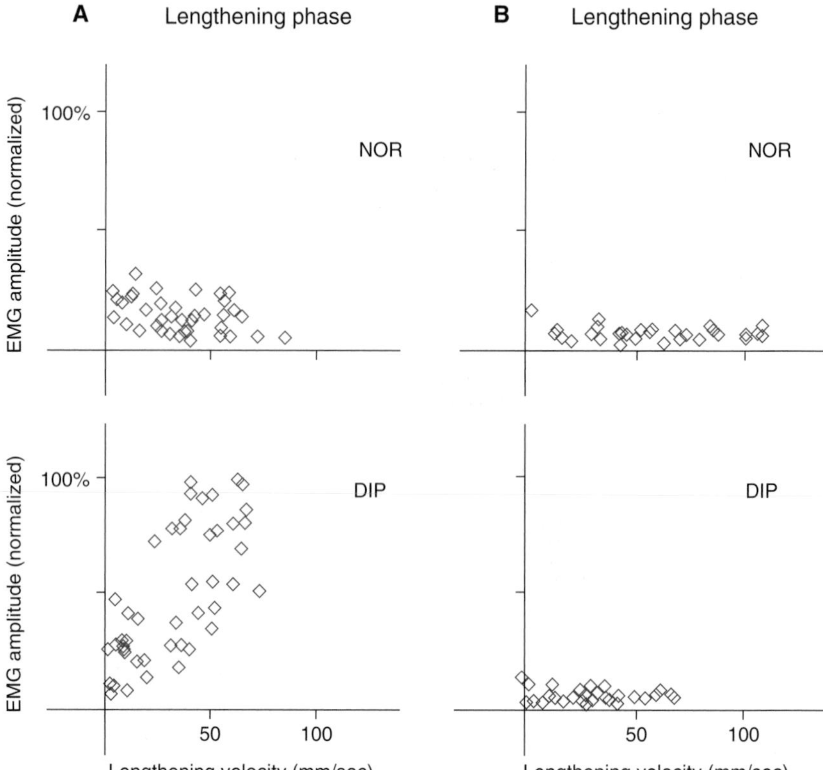

FIGURE 14.7 Comparison of activity of the soleus muscle when it is being lengthened in early stance (A) and in swing (B) in a normal control child (NOR) and a child with spastic diplegia (DIP). (Adapted with permission from Crenna P, Inverno M. Objective detection of pathophysiological factors contributing to gait disturbance in supraspinal lesions. In: Fedrizzi E, Avanzini G, Crenna P, eds. Motor development in children. New York: John Libbey, 1994:110.)

to stretch during walking was faster (shorter-onset latency) and increased in amplitude by 241%, and there was virtually no phase-dependent modulation of the stretch reflex during the different phases of gait (as shown in Fig. 14.8B). Interestingly, the two individuals who showed some stretch-reflex modulation were also those who walked the fastest of all the persons with MS; thus, the authors suggest that locomotor impairments are strongly linked to stretch-reflex modulation in persons with this diagnosis.

In summary, spasticity in the plantar-flexors can contribute to pathologic gait patterns in both the stance and swing phases of gait. Research has shown that in stance phase, plantar-flexor spasticity will affect foot position at initial contact, thus having an impact on the stability component of gait. Spastic plantar-flexors limit dorsiflexion and thus prevent heel strike at initial contact. When initial contact is made with a flat foot, the ground reaction force vector is anterior to the knee, producing knee extension. This is shown in

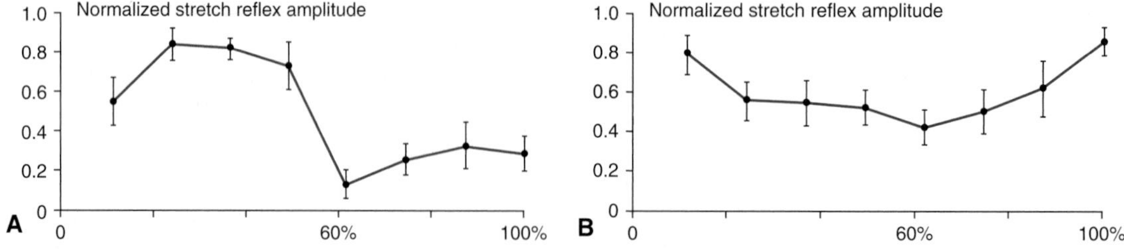

FIGURE 14.8 Normal modulation of the soleus stretch reflex during the different phases of gait (A) in comparison with minimal modulation in patients with MS (B), who have a spastic soleus muscle. In normal subjects (A), note the large-magnitude stretch response in stance phase, minimal response to stretch in the transition from stance to swing (60% of gait cycle), while in the swing phase the stretch reflex is 50% of that in stance phase. In contrast, patients with multiple sclerosis (B) show very little modulation of stretch reflex amplitude throughout the gait cycle. (Adapted from Sinkjaer T, Andersen JB, Nielsen JF. Impaired stretch reflex and joint torque modulation during spastic gait in multiple sclerosis patients. J Neurol 1996;243:570.)

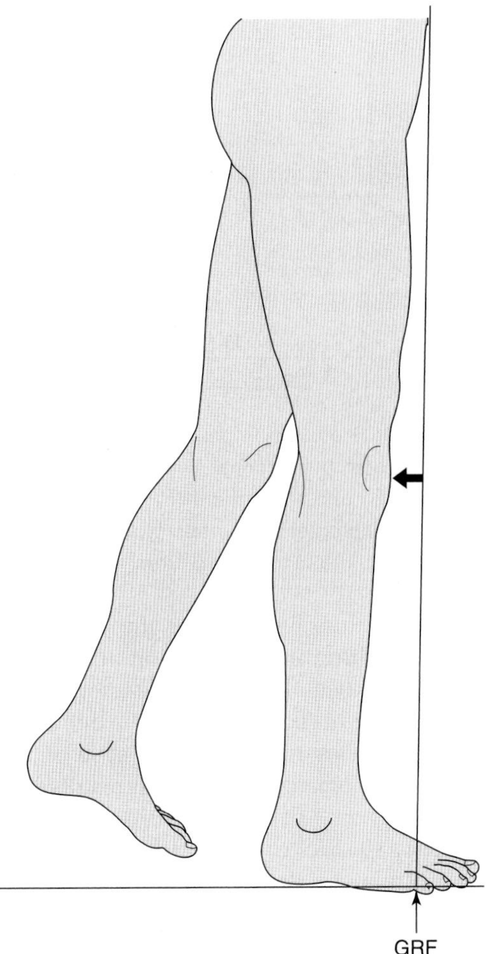

FIGURE 14.9 When initial contact is made with a flat foot, the ground reaction force (GRF) vector is anterior to the knee, producing knee extension.

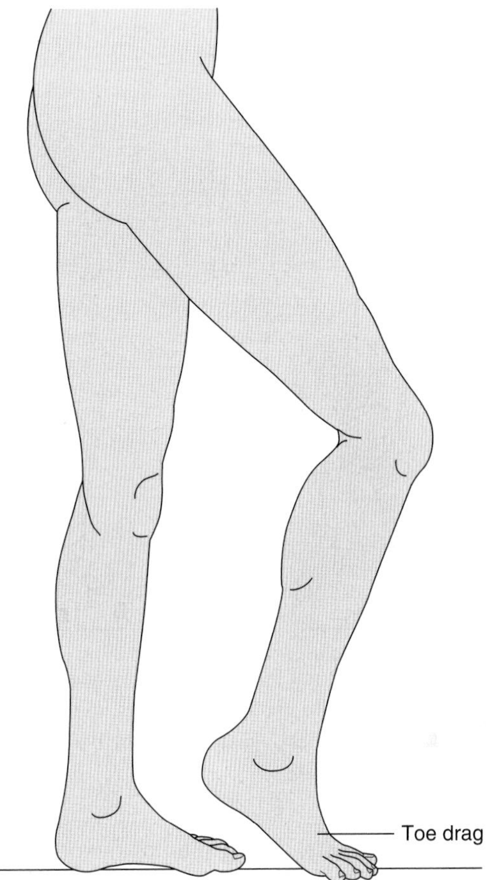

FIGURE 14.10 Spastic plantar-flexors affect forward foot clearance during swing; the subsequent consequence is toe drag.

Figure 14.9. Major compensations for excessive plantar flexion include hyperextension of the knee and forward trunk lean. Another compensation involves shortening the step length of the other limb. Which compensatory strategy is used will depend on a number of factors. Knee mobility is critical to the hyperextension strategy. In contrast, strong hip and trunk extensors are necessary for the trunk-flexion strategy (Mulroy et al., 2003; Perry & Burnfield, 2010).

In the swing phase of gait, spasticity in the plantar-flexors results in inadequate toe-off due to an extended knee position at terminal stance. Inability to adequately flex the knee makes toe-off more difficult and requires the hip and knee flexors to work harder to lift the limb and clear the foot during swing. Spastic plantar-flexors affect forward foot clearance during swing; the subsequent consequence is toe drag (Fig. 14.10). In terminal swing, spastic plantar-flexors resist extension at the knee and dorsiflexion of the foot, critical to positioning the leg for heel strike at initial contact. Compensatory strategies include a shortened stride length and reduced gait velocity.

Spasticity in the plantar-flexors in conjunction with other ankle-joint muscles produces coronal plane problems at the foot. A combination of excessive activity of the TS and posterior tibialis muscles produces inversion and an equinovarus foot position. An equinovarus foot position in the sagittal plane is shown in Figure 14.11A and in the frontal plane in Figure 14.11B. This is seen clinically as the elevation of the first metatarsal head from the floor, with the subsequent foot contact made on the lateral border of the foot only.

In contrast, in equinovalgus gait, foot contact is made with the medial border of the foot. Equinovalgus gait can result from excessive activation of the TS in conjunction with the peroneus brevis muscle. An alternative cause of valgus gait is weakness or inaction by the ankle invertors, for example, a weak or inactive soleus. Thus, a flaccid paralysis can also lead to a valgus foot posture.

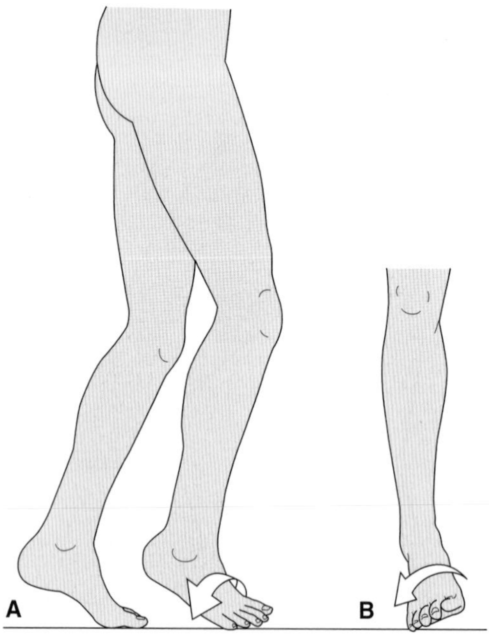

FIGURE 14.11 A combination of excessive activity of the TS and posterior tibialis muscle produces inversion and an equinovarus foot position, illustrated from both the sagittal (A) and frontal (B) planes.

Quadriceps Spasticity. Like plantar-flexor spasticity, quadriceps spasticity can also result in excessive knee extension in the stance phase of gait. Remember that during weight acceptance, there is a brief flexion of the knee that assists in absorbing the shock of loading. Quadriceps spasticity results in an excessive response to knee flexion and subsequent lengthening of the quadriceps, triggering a stretch-reflex response that can limit flexion and result in hyperextension of the knee (Montgomery, 1987; Perry & Burnfield, 2010). An early study by Norton et al. (1975) found no relationship between spasticity at the knee (quadriceps or hamstrings) and gait velocity in patients with stroke. Similarly, a study by Bohannon and Andrews (1990) also found no relationship between knee-extensor spasticity (measured on a Cybex II dynamometer) and gait speed after stroke. However, a study by Lewek et al. (2007) examined the underlying mechanisms for stiff knee gait following stroke and reported that hyperexcitable heteronymous reflex connections from hip flexors to knee extensors resulted in prolonged quadriceps activity that contributed to reduced knee flexion at toe-off.

Hamstring Spasticity. Hamstring spasticity producing excessive knee flexion is a frequent problem in certain types of cerebral palsy; it manifests as a crouched gait pattern, as shown in Figure 14.12. In the terminal swing phase of gait, excessive activation of the hamstrings muscles prevents the knee from fully extending, resulting in knee flexion at initial contact (A). Excessive knee flexion persists throughout the stance phase of gait (B), increasing the demand on the quadriceps muscles to prevent collapse of the limb into flexion. A shortened step length results.

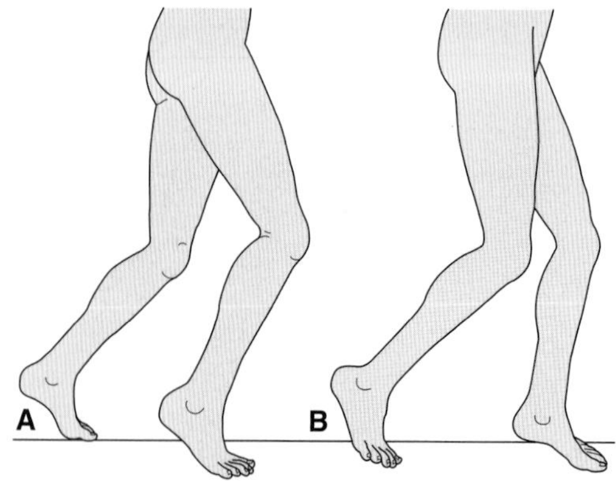

FIGURE 14.12 Hamstring spasticity producing excessive knee flexion in both the terminal swing phase and the initiation of stance (A) and throughout the stance phase of gait (B), is a frequent problem in certain types of cerebral palsy and manifests as a crouched gait pattern.

Hip-Adductor Spasticity. Hip adductor spasticity produces a contralateral drop in the pelvis during stance, as the femur is drawn in medially. Adductor spasticity can result in scissors gait, which is characterized by excessive adduction. During the swing phase of gait, as the hip flexes, excessive adduction produces a severe medial displacement of the entire limb. This results in a reduced base of support affecting stability. In severe cases, the adducted swing leg catches on the stance limb and impedes progression (Montgomery, 1987; Perry & Burnfield, 2010).

In summary, spasticity contributes to disordered gait through the inappropriate activation of a muscle during the portions of the gait cycle during which it is lengthened and through changes in stiffness resulting from alterations in the mechanical properties of the muscle itself.

Coordination Problems. Coordination problems, or difficulties coordinating multijoint movements, are a hallmark of neurologic pathology. However, multijoint coordination problems are not immediately apparent by looking at one joint at a time; rather we must look at multiple joints. As will be seen in the following discussion, multijoint coordination problems can manifest in many different ways.

Abnormal Synergies. Abnormal synergies are defined as the simultaneous recruitment of muscles at multiple

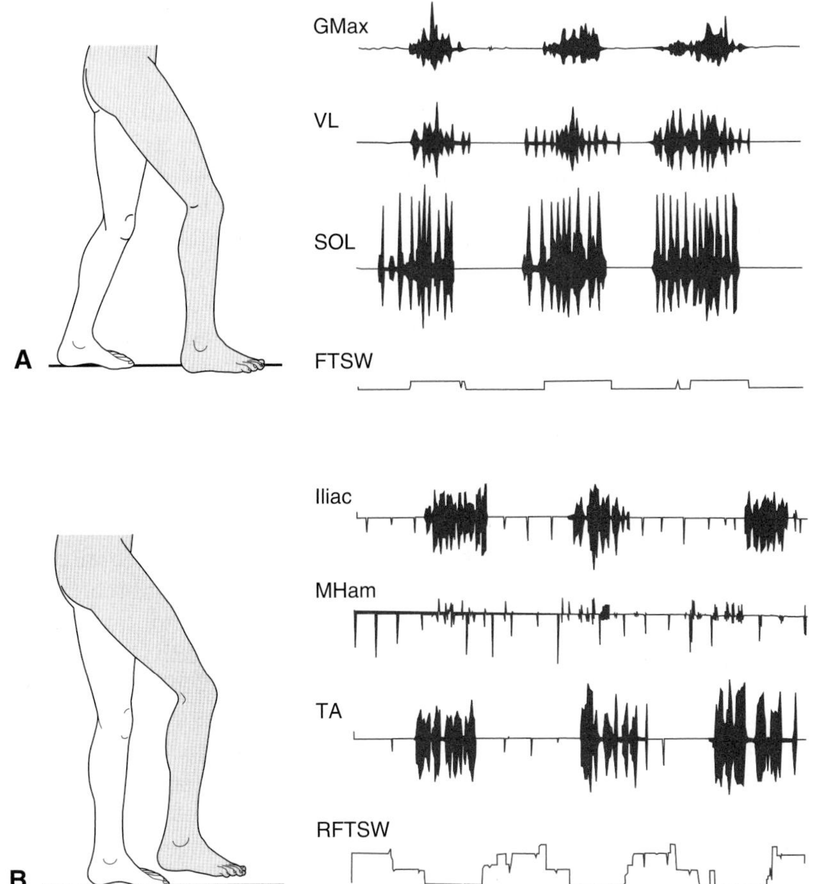

FIGURE 14.13 Synergies manifest in gait as either total extension (A) or total flexion (B) patterns. The right panels are EMG traces of extensor muscles (A) and flexor muscles (B), while the left panels illustrate the behavior observed: excessive extension in stance (A) and flexion in swing (B). FTSW = footswitch; GMax = gluteus maximus; Iliac = iliacus; MHam = medial hamstring; RFTSW = right footswitch; SOL = soleus; TA = tibialis anterior; VL = vastus lateralis. (Adapted with permission from Perry J. Gait analysis: normal and pathological function. Thorofare, NJ: Slack, 1992:313.)

joints and body segments resulting in stereotypical and relatively fixed patterns of movement. The presence of abnormal synergies reflects loss of fractionation of movement (muscle recruitment) and is due to corticospinal lesions.

Abnormal synergies manifest in gait as either total extension (Fig. 14.13A) or total flexion (Fig. 14.13B) patterns. This can be seen in the EMG traces as simultaneous activation of either extensors (A) during the stance phase of gait or flexors (B) during the swing phase. Thus, persistent flexion of the knee throughout the swing cycle is often associated with the use of a flexor synergy or total flexor pattern at all three joints. Use of the flexor synergy results in an inability to extend the knee while flexing the hip during terminal swing. Knutsson and Richards (1979) reported that mass patterns of flexion and extension were one of four characteristic gait patterns found in persons with hemiparesis following stroke.

Chen et al. (2003) reported a higher prevalence of synergistic mass patterns and reduced stability in patients with poor locomotor recovery following stroke as compared with those with good recovery. Similarly, DeQuervain et al. (1996) found that patients with the slowest gait velocity (0.08 to 0.24 m/sec, or 4.8 to 14.4 m/min) had significant muscle weakness and the presence of a primitive mass synergy pattern, while patients with intermediate gait velocity (0.4 to 0.7 m/sec, or 24 to 42 m/min) had mild weakness and were able to isolate joint movements. The one patient who walked at a nearly normal gait velocity (1.04 m/sec, or 62.4 m/min) had no weakness or evidence of abnormal muscle synergy.

Disordered Patterns of Activation (Control Problems). Central lesions of the CNS result in impaired programming affecting leg-muscle activation. Impaired programming can manifest in gait as: (1) an inability to recruit a muscle appropriately, (2) increased activation of a muscle that is unrelated to spasticity-mediated stretch, (3) inability to modulate a muscle's activity throughout the gait cycle, or (4) abnormal phasing of multijoint movement, leading to poor intersegmental coordination.

Reduced Muscle Recruitment. Loss of the ability to selectively recruit the TA muscle during gait following stroke is a common example of impaired programming. Inability to activate the TA results in a flat foot at foot strike, or alternatively, the heel may strike, but the foot drops quickly (foot slap) because of inadequate eccentric contraction of the TA. The presence of a rapid foot drop following heel strike suggests that the underlying impairment is an inactive TA rather than a spastic or contracted gastrocnemius or soleus (Knutsson & Richards, 1979; Montgomery, 1989; Perry & Burnfield, 2010).

Non–Stretch-Related Muscle Overactivity. Overactivity of the hamstring muscle unrelated to stretch has been reported in both adult patients following stroke (Knutsson & Richards, 1979) and children with cerebral palsy (Crenna, 1998; Perry & Burnfield, 2010). Hamstring hyperactivity can manifest as either premature or prolonged activation of the hamstring (Crenna, 1998; Perry, 1992). It was originally thought that hamstring over activity was the result of spasticity (e.g., velocity-dependent hyperactivity of the stretch reflex). But researchers have subsequently found that performing a dorsal rhizotomy, which involves selectively cutting the sensory-nerve roots, does not decrease hamstring over activity in children with cerebral palsy. This suggests that the basis for hamstring over activity is abnormal coordination, not a simple hyperactive stretch reflex (Crenna, 1998; Perry & Burnfield, 2010).

Impaired Intersegmental Coordination. Impaired intersegmental coordination is a hallmark characteristic of "ataxic gait," a common characteristic in many people with cerebellar pathology. Ataxic gait is characterized by staggering, veering, irregular stepping, and high steppage. In patients with cerebellar pathology, ataxic gait is associated with delays in the relative movement of the knee and ankle throughout the gait cycle (Palliyath et al., 1998). Intersegmental coordination problems also result in delays in the timing of peak knee flexion during the swing phase of gait (Palliyath et al., 1998).

Coactivation of Agonist and Antagonist Muscles. Normal gait is characterized by a remarkable degree of selectivity of muscle activity. There is a reciprocal recruitment pattern during gait such that coactivation of agonist and antagonist muscles is minimized. Cocontraction is defined as the loss of selective recruitment of physiologically antagonistic muscles. Coactivity among antagonist muscles during gait has been reported in many individuals with supraspinal lesions, including stroke and cerebral palsy. Researchers have hypothesized several possible reasons for the presence of coactivation, including: (a) pathologically disorganized central programs, (b) additional postural support activity, (c) immature gait programs, and (d) compensatory programming—that is, the use of coactivation to increase stiffness (Crenna, 1998; Knutsson, 1994).

Knutsson and Richards (1979) found a coactivation pattern of activity in 4 of 26 individuals with hemiparesis following stroke. Increased coactivation in the leg-muscle groups began at the end of the swing phase and continued throughout the stance phase of gait. While this pattern is not commonly seen in adult-onset spastic hemiparesis, it is a common finding in cerebral palsy (Knutsson, 1994). More recently, Lamontagne et al. (2002) reported excessive antagonist coactivation as a factor contributing to reduced swing-phase dorsiflexion in the nonparetic side in subjects with hemiparetic gait due to stroke. Crenna and colleagues reported that the presence of coactivation of lower-extremity muscles was a common finding among children with spastic-type cerebral palsy (Crenna, 1998). A comparison of coactivation between the hamstring (medial hamstring) and quadriceps (vastus medialis) muscles in a typically developing child versus a child with spastic diplegia is shown in Figure 14.14. Note that the filled areas (activity in both muscles greater than 20% of maximum locomotor output) cover a much greater part of the step cycle in the child with spastic diplegia as compared with the typically developing child. Coactivation between the TA and MG has been reported as a factor contributing to equinus ankle during the swing phase of gait in children with cerebral palsy (Wakeling et al., 2007).

Musculoskeletal Impairments

Problems in the musculoskeletal system include weakness, loss of range of motion and contractures, and changes in alignment. Passive properties of the muscle–tendon system contribute to development of torque during walking. Thus, abnormal joint stiffness and limited range of motion not only reduce joint motion but also affect the ability of muscles to generate power at various speeds (Patla, 2003).

In both children with cerebral palsy and adults with hemiplegia, changes in the passive properties of the musculoskeletal system have been found to be relevant factors in disordered locomotion. Among these neurologic populations, both soft-tissue contractures and bony constrictions limit joint range of motion, constrain movement, and increase the workload on the muscles, thus affecting a patient's ability to meet the requirements of gait. In general, decreased joint mobility during stance restricts forward motion of the body over the supporting foot, thus affecting progression. In swing, decreased joint mobility reduces foot clearance, affecting progression, and appropriate

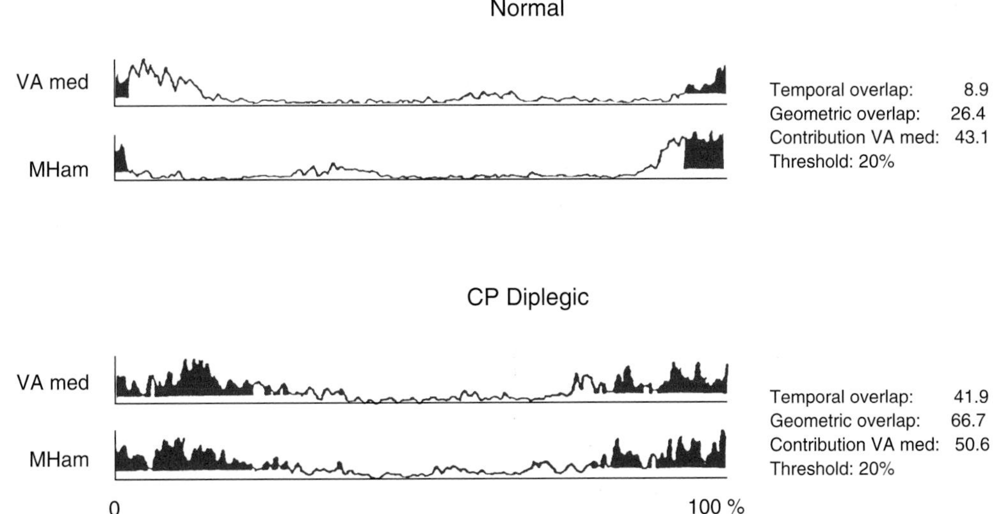

FIGURE 14.14 Quantitative assessment of cocontraction between quadriceps (VA med) and hamstrings (MHam) in a child with spastic diplegia and an age-matched typically developing child walking at comparable speed. Filled areas represent coactivation of agonist and antagonist muscles. (Reprinted with permission from Crenna P, Inverno M. Objective detection of pathophysiological factors contributing to gait disturbance in supraspinal lesions. In: Fedrizzi E, Avanzini G, Crenna P, eds. Motor development in children. New York: John Libbey, 1994:112.)

foot placement for weight acceptance, affecting stability. Limited range of motion also limits a patient's ability to modify movement strategies, thus affecting adaptation. For example, a person with limited ankle and knee flexion will be unable to increase limb flexion during the swing phase of gait to step over an obstacle.

As we mentioned in Chapter 10 on abnormal postural control, musculoskeletal limitations found in persons with neurologic dysfunction most often develop secondary to a CNS lesion. Musculoskeletal impairments that particularly affect gait include ankle-extensor contractures, knee- and hip-flexor contractures, and reduced pelvic and spinal mobility.

A wide range of musculoskeletal problems occurring at the ankle, knee, and hip joints can reduce a person's ability to use a heel-strike strategy during the initiation of stance, and result in low heel contact, foot-flat contact, forefoot contact, contact made with the medial (or lateral) border of the foot, and/or foot slap during loading. During stance, a smooth progression over the supporting foot requires a minimum of 5 degrees of ankle dorsiflexion; thus, ankle plantarflexor contractures can impair a person's ability to move the limb over the foot. The effect of a plantarflexion contracture on foot strike will vary, depending on its severity. Fifteen degrees of plantar-flexion contracture is common in adults with acquired disability, and it usually results in a low heel contact and early flat foot during loading. A 30-degree contracture is not uncommon in children with spastic cerebral palsy, and produces a forefoot contact at foot strike (Perry & Burnfield, 2010).

Plantar-flexor contractures limit tibial advancement over the stationary foot during stance. If the contracture is elastic (i.e., able to lengthen in response to body weight), the only result may be an inappropriate foot position at foot contact, since body weight will lengthen the plantar-flexors, allowing the tibia to advance (Perry & Burnfield, 2010). However, if the contracture is not elastic, recurvatum results. Recurvatum occurs when the knee has sufficient mobility to move posteriorly past neutral. Knee hyperextension can occur quickly or slowly, and it usually begins in midstance or terminal stance and continues into preswing. Excessive knee extension means the tibia cannot advance over the stationary foot in the stance phase (Perry & Burnfield, 2010). Plantar-flexor contractures also affect foot clearance during swing by preventing ankle flexion sufficient to allow toe clearance.

Hip-flexion contractures result in inadequate hip extension, which can affect both stability and progression. During midstance, if the hip cannot extend to neutral, the trunk will flex forward, bringing the COM anterior to the hip joint. Gravity will pull the trunk forward into more flexion, and this places an additional demand on the hip extensors to prevent collapse of the forward trunk and causes loss of stability (Perry, 1992). Hip-flexion contractures that limit hip extension have a great effect on terminal stance, as it is during this phase that the hip is normally hyperextended. Lack of hip extension produces an anterior pelvic tilt and an inability to move the thigh posterior to the hip. This results in a shortened step length and reduces forward progression of the body.

One way to compensate for a hip-flexion contracture is to flex the knees. This allows the pelvis to be normally aligned despite the hip-flexion contracture. Flexion of the hip and knees is called a "crouched gait," and it is often seen in spastic cerebral palsy as a compensatory gait pattern for inadequate hip extension (Montgomery, 1987; Perry & Burnfield, 2010; Rozumalski & Schwartz, 2009). However, this compensatory strategy has its own limitations, since it increases the demands on the quadriceps muscle to control the knee (Mulroy et al., 2003). Increased knee flexion also requires either excessive ankle dorsiflexion or heel rise onto the forefoot during stance, and thus constrains progression. Knee-flexion contractures prevent the knee from fully extending at the end of swing. This affects the patient's ability to place the foot appropriately for weight transfer, reducing stability and increasing the need for muscular action to control the knee.

In summary, a wide variety of motor impairments contribute to disorders of gait in persons with neurologic dysfunction. These impairments can occur alone or in combination, which can make sorting out their relative contributions difficult. We now turn our attention to sensory impairments that also contribute to disordered gait.

Effect of Sensory Impairments on Gait

The control of gait is based on the integration of both peripheral sensory inputs and descending supraspinal inputs. Sensation is a critical determinant for maintaining gait in natural environments, in which we are required to constantly modify how we move in response to changes in our surroundings. Sensory inputs play several important roles in the control of locomotion. Sensory inputs serve as a trigger for the initiation of swing. Thus, loss of proprioceptive cues that normally signal hyperextension in the hip and the termination of stance can result in delayed initiation of the swing phase (Smith, 1980). In addition, sensory inputs are necessary in adapting locomotor patterns to changes in environmental demands. This includes signaling unanticipated disruptions to gait, as well as the ability to predict and anticipate upcoming obstacles. Thus, the effects of sensory impairments on gait are varied, depending on which sense is affected and the age at which the sensory loss occurs.

Somatosensory Deficits

Abnormal somatosensory inputs result in gait ataxia. Gait problems in persons with sensory ataxia can be due to interruption of either peripheral or central proprioceptive pathways. When this occurs, the individual is usually no longer aware of the position of the legs in space, or even of the position of the body itself. With mild sensory dysfunction, walking may not appear to be abnormal, if the person can use vision. However, ataxia is worse when visual cues are reduced or inappropriate. Staggering and unsteadiness increase, and some people lose the ability to walk.

Normally, proprioceptively mediated stretch reflexes are modulated throughout the gait cycle. They are facilitated in the gastrocnemius and soleus at the end of stance phase, allowing for compensation for ground irregularities and assisting in push-off, but they are inhibited during the swing phase, to prevent stretch-reflex–mediated plantar-flexion during ankle dorsiflexion (Sinkjaer et al., 1996). Loss of proprioceptive inputs results in reduced modulation throughout the gait cycle.

Visual Deficits

Vision is critical to the feedforward control of equilibrium during gait. Visual inputs are used to regulate gait on a local level (step-by-step basis) and on a more global level (route-finding) (Patla, 2003). Loss of vision affects the stability and adaptation aspects of gait. Visually impaired and blind patients tend to walk more slowly. In addition, they appear able to use auditory cues to assist in locating obstacles in space (Ashmead et al., 1989).

Vision is critical for obstacle avoidance during gait, since visual inputs regarding upcoming obstacles are used to alter gait patterns in an anticipatory manner. For example, loss of the visual field on one side (hemianopsia) can have an impact on the person's ability to perceive potential threats to stability on the impaired side. This is shown in Figure 14.15, which illustrates a bus coming from the left that would be invisible to a person with left hemianopsia (Tobis & Lowenthal, 1960). Thus, loss of visual inputs will affect both route-finding and obstacle-avoidance.

Vestibular Deficits

The functional consequence of the loss of vestibular inputs appears to depend on the age of the individual at the time of the sensory loss. For example, individuals who lost vestibular function as infants had near-normal posture and gait control (Horak et al., 1994). However, loss of vestibular function in adulthood can

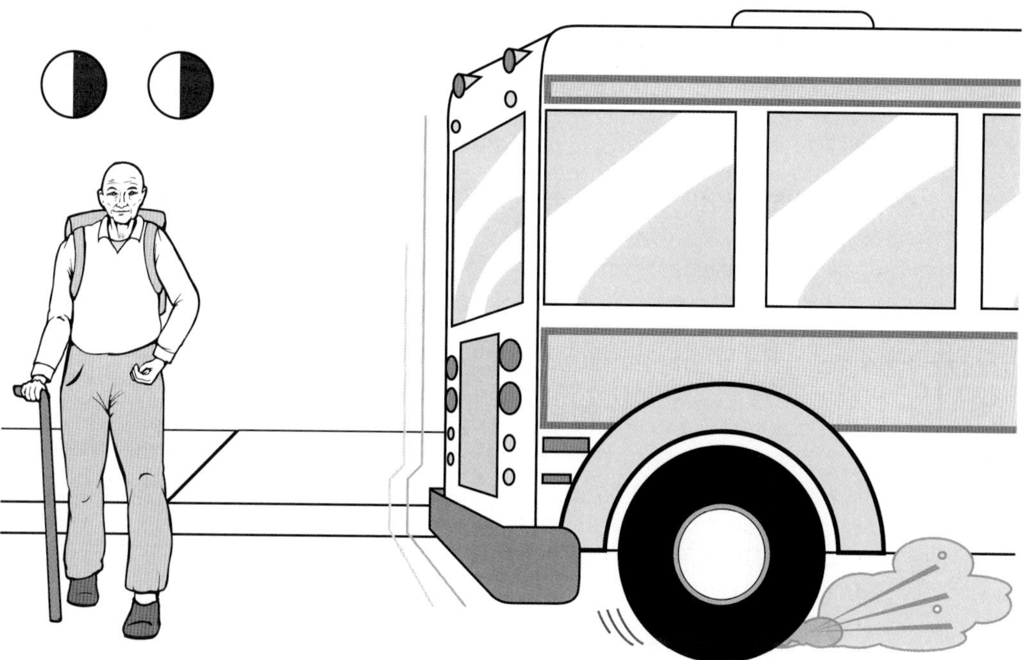

FIGURE 14.15 Functional effects of visual hemianopsia. A patient with a left hemianopsia would not perceive a bus coming from the left. (Adapted with permission from Tobis JS, Lowenthal M. Evaluation and management of the brain damaged patient. Springfield IL: Charles C Thomas, 1960:78.)

produce gait ataxia and difficulty in stabilizing the head in space.

Adult patients with vestibular deficits may walk more slowly than nonimpaired individuals. Other changes include a prolonged double-support phase, and a 6.5% longer cycle time than in normal subjects (Takahashi et al., 1988). Interestingly, when individuals with vestibular deficits were asked to walk at a normal velocity, using a metronome to establish the pace, the duration of their double-support phase became more normal. It is not clear why individuals with vestibular deficits seem to prefer a slower gait speed and whether practicing at faster speeds would improve the kinematics of their gait cycle.

It has been reported that persons with vestibular deficits may also show impairments in head stabilization during gait, especially when walking in the dark (Pozzo et al., 1991; Takahashi et al., 1988). Gaze is equally stable for individuals with vestibular deficits and normal subjects during sitting and standing. However, when walking, the ability to stabilize gaze is impaired; thus, persons with vestibular deficits report impaired vision and oscillopsia. In addition, eye movements compensate for head movements more effectively during active head rotations than during similar movements made while walking. It has been suggested that this may be due to the predictable nature of active voluntary head movements versus the passive head movements that happen during locomotion (Grossman & Leigh, 1990).

When normal subjects walk or run in the dark, the amplitude and velocity of head rotations are decreased as compared with head movements during normal walking. However, these parameters increase for subjects with bilateral vestibular deficits when they walk in the dark (Pozzo et al., 1991).

Effect of Cognitive and Perceptual Impairments on Gait

As mentioned in Chapter 5, perceptual and cognitive problems can have a devastating effect on functional movement capability, including mobility function.

Body Image/Scheme Disorders

Body image deficits can result in a number of gait deviations, including ipsilateral trunk lean toward the stance leg, resulting in loss of stability. Impaired body image can also result in inappropriate foot placement and difficulty in controlling the center of body mass relative to the changing base of support of the feet (Perry, 1992). Individuals with unilateral spatial neglect (USN; defined as the inability to perceive and

TABLE 14.2 Scores on the Video Face Test in Patients With Unilateral Spatial Neglect: Number of Correct Identifications of Faces Presented on the Right or Left Side in Sitting, Standing, and Walking

		Sitting		Standing		Stepping	
Subject No.	Hemisphere Lesion Side	RT	LT	RT	LT	RT	LT
1	Right	15	15	15	15	14	0
2	Right	15	15	15	15	15	7
3	Right	14	15	15	15	13	7
4	Right	14	13	15	15	15	0
5	Right	15	15	15	15	15	0
6	Right	15	15	15	15	15	0
7	Right	15	15	15	15	15	9
8	Right	15	0	15	0	15	0
9	Right	15	15	15	15	15	15
10	Right	14	15	15	15	15	15
11	Left	14	15	15	15	10	15
12	Left	0	15	0	15	0	15

Total possible, 15. RT = right; LT = left.
Reprinted with permission from Suzuki E, Chen W, Kondo T. Measuring unilateral spatial neglect during stepping. Arch Phys Med Rehabil 1997;78:176.

integrate stimuli on one side of the body), affecting the left side, tend to veer to the right when walking, or bump into objects on the left side when walking or propelling a wheelchair.

Suzuki et al. (1997) used a dual-task method to examine the relationship between USN and gait in 31 individuals who had had a stroke, 15 with left hemiplegia (right hemisphere damage), and 19 with right hemiplegia (left hemisphere damage). They created a video face test involving use of a video monitor, placed in front of the patient, which showed a video of scenery associated with walking along a corridor. Faces appeared on the video periodically, positioned to the right or left of midline. The ability to perceive faces presented on the right versus the left side was examined while individuals were sitting, standing, or stepping continuously. Results from this study are summarized in Table 14.2. They found that many of the individuals with USN (see, e.g., subjects 1, 5, and 6) were able to observe all 15 faces presented on the side contralateral to the lesion when sitting or standing; however, they were unable to perceive faces (score of 0) while stepping. In contrast, subjects 8 and 12 show USN (as indicated by 0 scores) in sitting, standing, and stepping. These findings indicate that in some individuals USN is context-specific.

Interestingly, two of the individuals with USN (subjects 9 and 10) who performed normally on the video face test in stepping (score of 15), required more assistance to step during the test, suggesting that they allocated attention to the video task rather than to the stepping task. Other subjects were able to keep stepping with minimal or no assistance (Suzuki et al., 1997).

Spatial Relation Disorders

Purposeful locomotion toward a goal that is not visible from the start requires navigational strategies that depend on stored spatial knowledge (Patla, 2003). The impact of deficits in spatial cognition on mobility is considerable, and particularly affects the ability to navigate safely through the environment, avoiding collisions with obstacles that are not readily perceived. Inability to remember the relationship of one place to another, called "topographic disorientation," can significantly affect route-finding aspects of locomotion (Patla, 2003).

Pain

Pain can also cause an alteration of movement patterns used for gait. An antalgic gait is defined as a gait pattern that results from pain. Compensatory strategies used in the presence of pain are movements that: (1) reduce-weight bearing time on the painful limb (e.g., shortening stance phase of gait), (2) avoid impact loads, (3) reduce joint excursion (e.g., limiting knee flexion during the stance phase of gait), and (4) decrease joint compressive forces by minimizing activity in muscles that cross the joint (e.g., side bending over a painful hip to bring the COM closer to the joint's center of rotation, reducing the need for hip-abductor activity and concomitant joint compressive forces) (Eyring & Murray 1964). Antalgic gait is often characterized by decreased gait velocity, shortened stance phase on the painful limb, a tendency to stiffen the limb in order to minimize joint motion, and a reduction in forceful foot contact or push-off.

Cognitive Impairments

Cognitive impairments also have an impact on mobility function, specifically, the ability to initiate gait, to adapt gait patterns to changing environmental demands, and to navigate in both familiar and unfamiliar locations. Cognitive impairments, as discussed in Chapter 5, include deficits affecting memory, attention, and executive functions. A more complete discussion of higher-order gait disorders resulting from impaired cognitive function can be found elsewhere (Nutt et al., 1993, 1997).

Many studies have found that dementia is a major risk factor for falls (Alexander et al., 1995; Tinetti et al., 1988). Alexander and colleagues (1995) studied 17 subjects with Alzheimer's disease (AD). They found that the individuals with AD walk at half the speed of healthy older adults, have a higher obstacle-contact rate, and tend to land more closely to the obstacle. These factors could contribute to falls, particularly trips, in persons with AD. In addition, falls during gait may be the result of impaired judgment, resulting in attempts to perform tasks that are beyond a person's physical capabilities (Nutt & Horak, 1997).

Effect of Attentional Demands on Gait. Researchers have shown that posture, balance, and gait, although considered "automatic," require attentional resources (Lajoie et al., 1993; Teasdale et al., 1993; Woollacott & Shumway-Cook, 2002). Attentional demands associated with postural control appear to be greater in individuals with impaired balance as compared with nonimpaired individuals. Balance appears to be more attentionally demanding after stroke. Brown et al. (2002) examined attentional demands associated with three postural tasks (sitting, standing, and standing with feet together) in six people with stroke (<1 year since onset) and six age- and gender-matched controls. Reaction times (RTs) on the secondary verbal-reaction-time task in the stroke group were significantly slower (mean [±SD], 410 ± 72 msec) in all conditions than RTs in the controls (320 ± 54 msec). In addition, in subjects with stroke (but not in controls), RT scores on the secondary task performed in standing (feet together) were significantly slower than those in sitting. Figure 14.16 compares the difference in average RT in sitting, standing feet apart, and standing feet together in subjects with stroke as compared with age- and gender-matched controls. Results suggest that individuals who have suffered a stroke showed increased attentional demands for tasks of static postural control compared with healthy, age-matched participants. Regnaux et al. (2005) also used a dual-task paradigm and found that attentional demands associated with sitting, standing, and walking were greater in persons with stroke as compared with nonimpaired controls; in addition, walking required more attentional resources than either sitting or standing.

Changes in RT on secondary tasks performed simultaneously with postural-control tasks have been

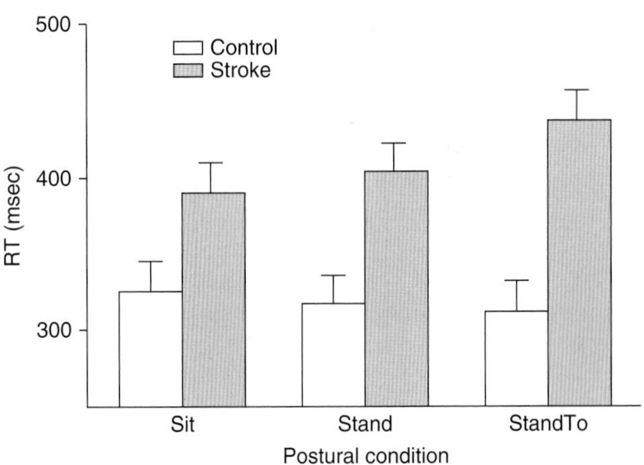

FIGURE 14.16 Attentional demands associated with three different postural tasks (sitting, standing, and standing with feet together [StandTo]) in persons with stroke and age- and gender-matched controls. Reaction times (RTs) to a secondary verbal RT task are slower in subjects with stroke as compared with controls in all three conditions. In addition, RT is significantly faster in sitting as compared with standing tasks in stroke patients but not in controls, suggesting that postural control is more demanding after stroke. (Reprinted from Brown LA, Sleik RJ, Winder TR. Attentional demands for static postural control after stroke. *Arch Phys Med Rehabil* 2002;83:1732–1735, Figure 1.)

used to infer increasing automaticity of postural control during recovery of balance control (Harley et al., 2006; Geurts et al., 1991). Geurts and colleagues (1991) used a dual-task design to study changes in attentional resources associated with recovery of stance balance in patients undergoing rehabilitation services following amputation of a lower extremity. Initially, RT in the group of individuals with amputations was significantly different from that in the control group; however, RT improved significantly through the recovery process. The authors suggest that dual tasks give information about the restoration of automaticity of postural control as an essential characteristic of the central reorganization process associated with recovery of postural stability.

Performance of a secondary task while walking can impair stability in patients with various types of neurologic pathology, including stroke, PD, and traumatic brain injury. Bowen and colleagues (2001) compared the effects of a secondary task on gait speed in 12 persons with hemiparesis following a stroke (average time since stroke, 4 mo) with those in nonimpaired controls. Their results, shown in Figure 14.17, found that performance of a secondary task decreased gait velocity in some but not all persons with stroke. We have added the Berg Balance Scale scores listed for each patient to this figure to illustrate that performance on the Berg test (a nongait balance measure) did not predict who would have difficulty in the dual-task gait conditions. Other researchers have confirmed the presence of dual-task interference on gait following stroke (Plummer-D'Amato et al., 2008; Yang et al., 2007a). Following stroke, impaired dual-task gait performance was present even among individuals who were considered full community ambulators (Yang et al., 2007a).

A number of researchers have reported on the effects of attentional demands on walking in individuals with PD (Bloem et al., 2006; Campbell et al., 2003; Galletly & Brauer, 2005; O'Shea et al., 2002; Plotnik et al., 2009; Rochester et al., 2004; Yogev et al., 2007). Campbell and colleagues (2003) tested the effect of two types of cognitive tasks (a low-attention task, and a high-attention task) on gait using the timed up and go (TUG) test. Their results are shown in Figure 14.18, which compares times on the TUG test in the 10 healthy older adults and 9 individual subjects with PD in the three conditions (no task and the two secondary tasks). While the low-attention task did not interfere with TUG performance, the high-attention task did, with the greatest effect found in persons with the most disease progression.

Rochester et al. (2004) examined the effects of various types of secondary tasks: motor (carrying a tray), cognitive (answering questions), and multiple (both tasks together) on gait (speed, step length) in 20 subjects with idiopathic PD and 10 controls. Performance of both the cognitive task and the multiple tasks (but not motor alone) decreased both gait speed and step length in both groups (results shown in Figure 14.19); however, the greatest effect was in the group with PD. A secondary task influences many aspects of gait in persons with PD, including velocity, gait variability, bilateral coordination and rhythmicity (Hausdorff et al., 1998; O'Shea et al., 2002; Plotnik et al., 2009; Yogev et al., 2005).

Finally, a number of researchers have reported that performance of a secondary task can impair stance and gait in persons with traumatic brain injury, even those with a relatively mild concussion (Brauer et al., 2004; Catena et al., 2007; Fait et al., 2009; Kern & Mateer, 1996; McCulloch, 2007; Pare et al., 2009; Parker et al., 2005; Rasmussen et al., 2008). Parker et al. (2005) studied the effects of a secondary task on gait 48 hours after a concussion injury. For subjects who had had a concussion, walking while performing a concurrent

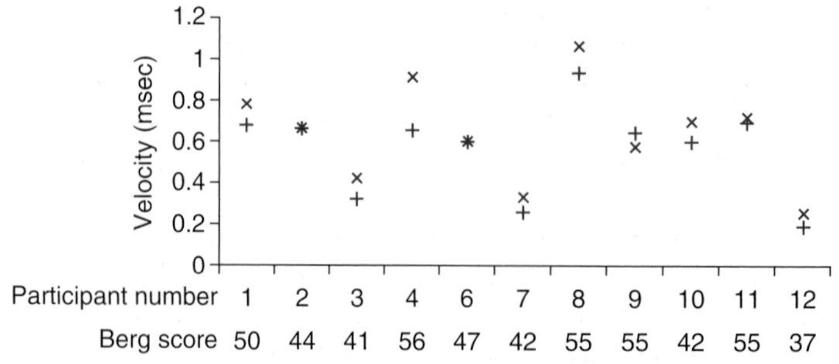

FIGURE 14.17 Effect of a secondary task on gait speed after stroke. Gait speed (m/sec) in 12 persons with stroke under single- and dual-task conditions. Also shown are the score on the Berg Balance Scale for each individual subject, illustrating the relationship between the Berg test and gait performance in single- and dual-task conditions. (Adapted with permission from Bowen A, Wenman R, Mickelborough J, Foster J, Hill E, Tallis R. Dual-task effects of talking while walking on velocity and balance following a stroke. *Age Ageing* 2001;30:319–323.)

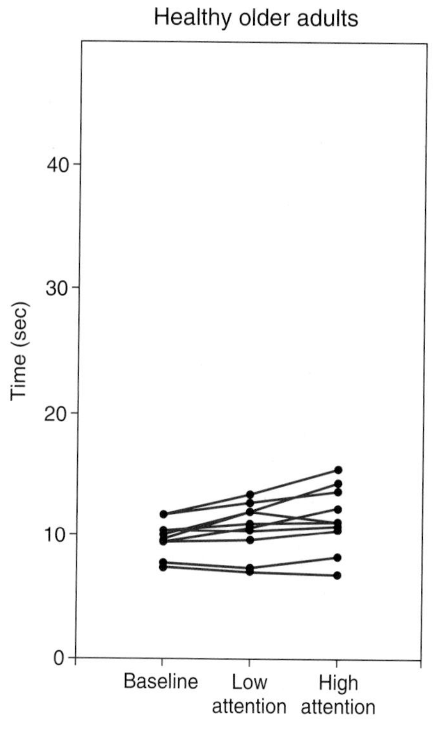

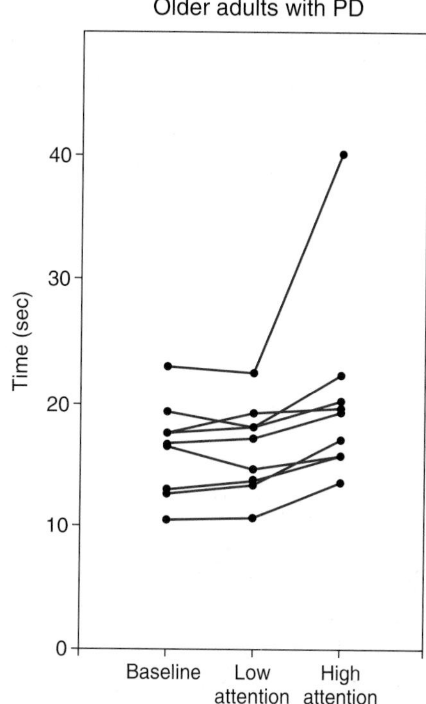

FIGURE 14.18 Effect of two types of secondary tasks on performance of the TUG test. Change in time on the TUG in three conditions, single task (baseline), low-attention task, and high-attention task is compared in healthy older adults and subjects with PD. While the low-attention task did not interfere with TUG performance, the high-attention task did. (Reprinted with permission from Campbell C, Rowse J, Ciol MA, Shumway-Cook A., The effect of attentional demands on the Timed Up and Go test in older adults with and without Parkinson's disease. Neurol Rep 2003;3:2–7, Figure 1.)

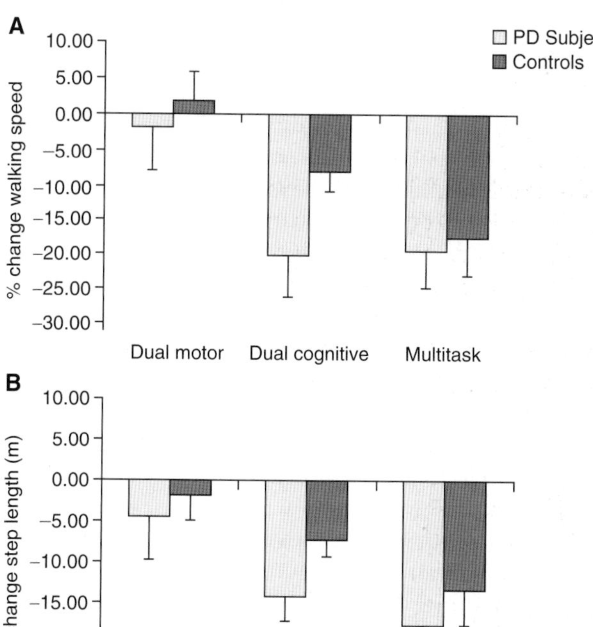

FIGURE 14.19 Effect of a motor, cognitive, and combined task on gait speed (A) and step length (B) in persons with PD and age-matched controls. (Modified with permission from Rochester L, Hetherington V, Jones B, et al. Attending to the task: interference effects of functional tasks on walking in Parkinson's disease and the roles of cognition, depression, fatigue and balance. *Arch Phys Med Rehabil* 2004;85:1581, Figure 2.)

cognitive task resulted in significant changes in gait variables (decreased gait speed and step length, increased stride time) and an increase in mediolateral displacement and velocity of the COM as compared with age-matched controls. Thus, following concussive injury, there is a decrease in stability in gait that can be observed during dual-task conditions. Dual-task gait assessment was more sensitive in detecting instability following concussion than single-task level walking (Catena et al., 2007). Following traumatic brain injury, measures of cognitive function, specifically executive function, can predict locomotor behavior, particularly in complex environments (Cantin et al., 2007). These studies suggest the potential importance of evaluating walking function under more complex conditions in persons with neurologic pathology.

Impairments on Complex Walking Tasks

Inability to adapt gait to walking under more complex conditions may be a significant factor in the recovery of mobility function in persons with neurologic pathology. Complex walking tasks involving adaptation to changing task and environmental demands, require physiological resources beyond those needed for walking under less difficult conditions, and thus reflect the demands associated with walking in home and community environments (Shumway-Cook et al., 2007). Performance on complex walking tasks is a good predictor of adverse health outcomes in both geriatric and neurologic populations, including falls, fractures, and incident mobility limitations (Cho et al., 2004; Dargent-Molina et al., 1996; Shumway-Cook et al., 2000). Many researchers have examined the effect of neurologic pathology on the ability to manage complex walking tasks. For example, impaired obstacle crossing has been reported following stroke (Lu et al., 2010; Said et al., 2005, 2008, 2009); traumatic brain injury (Catena et al., 2009; Cantin et al., 2007; Chou et al., 2004; Fait et al., 2009; Vallee et al., 2006), in patients with PD (Galna et al., 2009; Snijders et al.. 2010; Vitorio et al., 2010), and in children with cerebral palsy (Law & Webb, 2005). Gait impairments during obstacle crossing in these populations include slower gait velocity when approaching and crossing an obstacle, reduced (or alternatively excessive) toe clearance in both the leading and trailing limbs, increased step variability, increased mediolateral instability during crossing, and a reduced ability to modify gait parameters appropriately to changing obstacle height. All of these impairments result in an increased likelihood for striking an obstacle during crossing, increasing the individual's risk for a trip-related fall.

Impairments on complex walking tasks are not limited to obstacle crossing, but have been reported in a wide variety of tasks, including changing gait speed and direction, while carrying objects, walking on uneven or inclined surfaces (Robinson, 2010), during turns or movements of the head (Hong & Earhart, 2010; Huxham et al., 2008; Mak et al., 2008), and, as discussed earlier, during the performance of a wide variety of secondary cognitive and motor tasks. Impaired ability to adapt gait in response to complex task and environmental demands affects the ability to walk safely in home and community environments and is a major factor in the development of mobility disability (Robinson et al., 2009; Shumway-Cook et al., 2007).

RECOVERY OF WALKING: WHAT FACTORS LIMIT PARTICIPATION IN THE MOBILITY DOMAIN?

Limited participation in the mobility domain (referred to as mobility disability and defined by a limited ability to walk in a home and community environment) has been identified as one of the most debilitating aspects of neurologic pathology, including stroke (Lord et al., 2004; Robinson et al., 2007), and PD (Schenkman et al., 2002). The prevalence of mobility disability is high. For example, only 50% of survivors of stroke regain the ability to walk in the community, and 30% of individuals are unable to walk without the assistance of another person (Lord et al., 2004). Walking in the community, with its complex task demands, is particularly difficult. In one study on community walking following stroke, 4% of survivors of stroke reported moderate difficulty walking at home; however, 72% reported moderate difficulty when walking outdoors on a slope or on uneven ground (Robinson et al., 2010). In addition, as difficulty with walking increased, satisfaction with community walking skills decreased (Robinson et al., 2010). The ability to manage complex environmental challenges is necessary to achieving successful participation in community walking (Lord et al., 2006), and an inability to manage specific environmental challenges is a critical determinant of impaired mobility function (Hirvensalo et al., 2000; Jette et al., 1998). Understanding the factors that limit participation in the mobility domain and contribute to mobility disability is critical to developing effective strategies for the rehabilitation of gait disorders.

Research suggests that good outcomes on clinical measures of mobility such as gait speed and distance (referred to as "capacity" in the ICF framework), do not reliably predict the ability to walk in the community ("performance" in the ICF framework) (Lord et al., 2004). For example, balance, paretic-leg strength (Kollen et al., 2005: Patterson et al., 2007), cardiovascular fitness (Michael et al., 2005; Patterson et al., 2007), and gait speed (Kollen et al., 2006; Lord et al., 2004; Michael et al., 2005; Perry et al., 1995) have been associated with clinical measures of functional ambulation skills, but not with participation in community walking. Robinson et al. (2007, 2010) examined the factors associated with participation in community ambulation among participants with chronic (>6 months) stroke. Following stroke, participation in community ambulation was reduced, as indicated by both a decrease in the number of trips made into the community and the number of walking-related activities on each trip (on average, 1) as compared with controls, who performed, on average, 2 or more walking-related activities per trip in the community.

The following factors were significantly correlated with participation in community ambulation: balance, usual gait velocity as well as velocity on complex walking tasks, and strength in the hemiparetic limb. However, regression modeling found that these factors, while significant, explained only a small portion of the variance in participation in community walking (Robinson et al., 2007). In a follow-up study, Robinson et al. (2010) found that personal factors, specifically balance and falls self-efficacy, depression, and fatigue were also significantly associated with participation in community walking following stroke and that they explained a much larger portion of the variance in participation in the mobility domain. Poor balance self-efficacy and fear of falling resulting in avoidance of physical activity including walking in the community have been reported in a number of studies (Basler et al., 2008; Bertera & Bertera, 2008; Deshpande et al., 2008; Hellstrom et al., 2003; Pound et al., 1998; Salbach et al., 2006). In addition, depression has also been associated with reduced walking participation and function in activities of daily living in patients with neurologic dysfunction (Chemerinski et al., 2001; Goodwin & Devanand, 2008).

This research confirms that among persons with neurologic impairments, the ability to participate in community walking is perceived as very important. In addition, the prevalence of reduced participation (mobility disability) is very high among persons with neurologic pathology. It also suggests that poor participation results from a combination of factors including physical, psychological, and environmental factors. Impaired gait, while important, is only one of many factors influencing the recovery of mobility. Other factors, such as self-efficacy, fear, depression, and fatigue may have a greater influence on long-term recovery of mobility in the home and community. Understanding the constellation of factors influencing participation is important to the development of treatment strategies effective in ensuring recovery of participation in persons with neurologic pathology.

DISORDERS OF MOBILITY OTHER THAN GAIT

Stair Walking

Like level walking, stair walking involves reciprocal movements of the legs through alternating stance and swing phases. Climbing stairs requires the generation of concentric forces at the knee and ankle (mostly the knee) for forward and vertical progression. Stability demands are greatest during the single-limb stance phase, when the swing leg is advancing to the next step (McFadyen & Winter, 1988).

In contrast to stair ascent, descent is achieved largely through eccentric contractions of the hip, knee, and ankle extensors, which control body position in response to the accelerating force of gravity. Energy absorption and a controlled landing are ensured through anticipatory activation of the gastrocnemius prior to foot contact with the step (McFadyen & Winter, 1988).

This means that in a person with a neurologic deficit, decreased concentric control will primarily affect stair ascent, while decreased eccentric control will primarily affect stair descent. Persons with a CNS lesion tend to walk stairs slowly, require the use of rails for support and progression, and in severe cases of dyscontrol, are unable to use a reciprocal pattern for stair walking. Instead, they bring both feet to the same step prior to progressing to the next step.

Impaired visual sensation affects anticipatory aspects of this task. For example, gastrocnemius activity, which precedes foot contact, is less when visual cues are reduced (Simoneau et al., 1991).

Transfers and Bed Mobility

During the performance of transfer activities such as sitting to standing (STS), rolling, and rising from a bed, healthy young adults tend to use momentum to move the body smoothly and efficiently from one position to another. An alternative strategy that can be used when performing transfer tasks is the zero-momentum or force-control strategy (refer to Chapter 2 to review this material).

There are many reasons why persons with neurologic impairments might use a force-control strategy during transfers. Postural-control problems limiting stability, cardiovascular problems such as orthostatic hypotension, and episodes of dizziness may require a person to move slowly and make interim stops during the task. For example, when rising from a bed, a person with orthostatic hypotension would need to sit for a moment on the side of the bed before standing up or risk a sudden drop in blood pressure and loss of balance. The over reliance on a force-control strategy and upper-extremity control during transfer tasks, however, can limit a person's ability to adapt to changing environmental conditions. For example, they may find it difficult to stand up independently from a chair without arms (Carr & Shepherd, 1998; Schenkman et al., 1990).

There have been many studies examining pathologic gait in neurologic populations. In contrast, few studies have systematically explored problems constraining other mobility skills in this population.

Sitting to Standing

Many persons with neurologic pathology report difficulty rising from a chair. In a survey of 379 older adults with varying neurologic diagnoses, 42% reported difficulty with rising from a chair at home (Munton et al., 1981). In a survey of persons with PD, 81% reported difficulty standing up (Brod et al., 1998). There are many impairments that potentially constrain the ability to move from sitting to standing effectively and efficiently. However, the majority of research has focused on the impact of neuromuscular impairments on STS in stroke, PD, and cerebral palsy.

A number of studies have identified reduced force production as a major factor in difficulty with rising to stand. Lomaglio and Eng (2005) studied the relationship of lower-extremity joint torques and weight-bearing symmetry to STS performance in individuals with chronic stroke. A motion analysis system (kinematics) and two force plates (ground reaction forces) were used to quantify characteristics of STS under self-paced and fast-paced conditions. An isokinetic dynamometer measured maximum concentric joint torques of the paretic and nonparetic ankle, knee, and hip (normalized to body mass).

The study found that paretic-ankle dorsiflexion and knee-extension torques were significantly correlated to the time taken to complete the self-paced STS condition, while paretic-ankle dorsiflexion, plantar flexion, and knee-extension torques related to the time taken to complete fast-paced STS condition. Faster performance on STS was associated with greater weight-bearing symmetry.

Cameron et al. (2003) compared kinetic energy and duration of the task during STS and curb climbing in 15 individuals with hemiparetic stroke and age-matched controls. In addition, they compared performance on STS to standing balance, maximum weight-bearing ability of the paretic extremity, and knee-extension strength. They reported that as compared with controls, STS in subjects with stroke was characterized by reduced kinetic energy and prolonged duration, with a significant correlation between STS kinetic energy and knee-extension strength, standing balance, and maximum weight bearing.

Cheng et al. (2004) examined leg-muscle activation patterns (tibialis anterior [TA] and soleus) and ground reaction forces (GRFs) during self-paced STS from an armless chair in an individual with hemiparesis due to stroke (with and without a history of falls). They found that in 70% of the individuals with stroke who had a history of falls, TA activity was either absent or slow with low amplitude. In addition, for half the subjects with poststroke hemiparesis and a history of falls, the soleus muscle exhibited early or excessive activity. This pattern of activity in the affected limb during STS was associated with compensatory excessive TA and quadriceps muscle activation in the unaffected limbs.

In an earlier study, Cheng et al. (1998) reported that the rate of rise in force production was significantly lower in persons who had a stroke and a positive history of falls than in those with no history of falls and healthy subjects. In addition, the center of pressure movement in the mediolateral direction during rising and sitting down was much greater in persons with a history of falls than in those with no history of falls or healthy subjects. Patients with stroke exhibited an asymmetric body-weight distribution, with significantly more body weight on their sound side (Cheng et al., 1998).

Impaired rate of force production has also been reported in persons with PD. Bishop and colleagues (2005) examined lower-extremity muscle activation patterns in 41 people with PD (grouped according to time taken to complete the task) asked to stand up from a bench. Dual force plates were used to quantify GRFs, including peak acceleration and vertical GRF, the slopes of peaks, and the timing of events, while surface EMG was used to measure activity of the soleus and TA.

Results showed that in subjects with PD, increased duration of STS was due to a longer time for the seat-off phase. In addition, slower subjects demonstrated a slower rate of force production, took longer to complete the flexion-momentum phase (64%, vs. 56% in faster subjects) and used more cocontraction. The authors noted that deficits recruiting the TA may contribute to the decreased rate of production of the acceleration forces and the longer time required for the seat-off phase and suggest that treatment strategies designed to facilitate TA activation may improve the functional performance of this task.

Inkster and colleagues (2003) reported lower hip- and knee-extensor torques in subjects with PD, with greater deficits found at the hip. Greater hip strength was related to better STS ability in subjects with PD; in contrast, greater knee strength was related to better STS ability in controls. The authors conclude that reduced strength, particularly at the hip, may be one factor that contributes to difficulty rising from a chair in persons with PD. These findings are supported by Mak et al. (2003), who reported smaller hip-flexion torque and a slower torque build-up rate in seven subjects with PD, as compared with age-matched controls. The PD group demonstrated joint kinematic patterns similar to those of controls, but slower angular displacement. The authors conclude that slowness of STS in people with PD could be due to reduced hip-flexion joint torque and a prolonged rate of torque production. In addition to smaller hip-flexion and ankle-dorsiflexion joint torques, and prolonged time to peak torque, subjects with PD appear to have difficulty switching from flexion to extension during sitting to standing (Mak & Hui-Chan, 2002).

Force production has also been implicated in impaired STS in children with cerebral palsy. Park et al. (2003) compared the kinetic and kinematic characteristics of sitting to standing in 27 children with spastic cerebral palsy (CP; 15 with spastic diplegia, 12 with spastic hemiplegia) and 21 typically developing children. All children with CP performed the task more slowly than typically developing children. In addition, STS in the children with CP was characterized by increased anterior pelvic tilt and hip flexion, an early abrupt knee extension (in diplegia only) decreased maximal knee-extensor moment, and decreased extensor power generation of the hip and knee joints.

Finally, while impaired anticipatory postural control has been hypothesized to contribute to impaired STS in persons with PD, a study by Inkster and Eng (2004) did not support this hypothesis in subjects with mild PD. Their study found that subjects with PD used an exaggerated hip-flexion strategy and moved their COM further forward during the preparation stage than did controls. The authors speculate that an exaggerated hip-flexion strategy used in preparation for rising from a chair may have been compensatory to increased stiffness and reduced flexibility of the trunk. It could also be a strategy to reduce balance demands in the task by increasing the time the COM stays within the base of support. The authors caution that their study included only subjects with mild PD (9 of 10 scored normally on the STS item on the Unified Parkinson Disease Rating Scale [UPDRS]); hence, it may not apply to persons with more advanced disease.

Rise-to-Walking Task

Are similar impairments described in the STS task also found when the task required is to rise and walk? Biomechanical studies have shown that different motor strategies are used when healthy subjects rise to stand versus rise to walk. During STS, forward momentum of the body COM must be stopped on arising, whereas during rise to walking, forward momentum is maintained and stepping is initiated before reaching a full standing position (Dion et al., 2003). Thus, non–neurologically impaired subjects use a fluid motor strategy when performing the rise-to-walk (RTW) task. In contrast, after stroke, RTW is characterized by a nonfluid strategy, with the majority of individuals with stroke arresting forward motion before initiating stepping (Dion et al., 2003).

A scale to measure difficulty in the RTW task has been developed and is shown in Table 14.3 (Malouin et al., 2003). The relationship between scores on the RTW and patterns of forward momentum during the RTW task in subjects with hemiparetic stroke are shown in Figure 14.20. COM horizontal momentum mean curves are shown for controls (heavy line) and patient subgroups in each of the four categories of RTW scores. Note that horizontal momentum of the COM increases, peaking just before the seat-off phase, then rises again as subjects rise to walk. Lowest scores on the RTW scale (0 category subgroup) are associated

TABLE 14.3 Fluidity Scale for the Rise-to-Walk Task

Score	Descriptors
3	The foot (heel and toes)* is lifted off the ground while the subject's body is still moving forward; the trunk remains slightly flexed forward even when the subject stands up.†
2	The forward movement of the body stops and as soon as the subject stands up with his body fully vertical, he lifts his foot.
1	The forward movement of the body stops, the subject stands up with his body fully vertical and then stops momentarily before he lifts his foot.
0	The forward movement of the body stops, the subject stands up with his body fully vertical, then stops momentarily before reaching for his cane, stops and then lifts his foot.

**The stepping limb is the affected limb.*

†Stands up: is the maximal vertical position of the shoulder.

Description of the rise to walk task

Starting position

Subjects are seated on a chair without backrest and armrest, with the feet on the floor and two-thirds of the thighs in contact with the seat; they are asked to keep their arms folded in front of them during the task.

Instructions

Subjects are instructed to look ahead, to distribute their weight evenly and, upon an auditory signal to stand up, without using their hands, and walk, at a natural pace, toward the target (a table placed about 2 m in front of the subject), but are not required to cover the full distance.

Conditions

Patients are allowed to use a walking aid (cane) and wear their orthosis, but are not provided external support. The stepping limb is the affected limb.

Reprinted with permission from Malouin F, McFadyen B, Dion L, Richards CL. A fluidity scale for evaluating the motor strategy of the rise to walk task after stroke. Clin Rehabil 2003;17:674–684 (appendix).

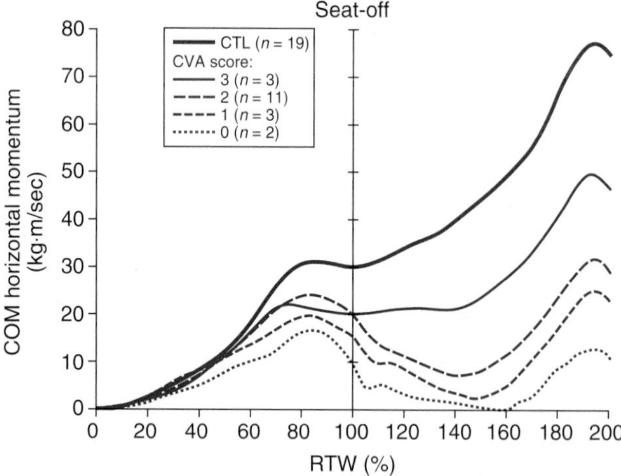

FIGURE 14.20 Relationship between scores on the rise-to-walk (RTW) scale and patterns of forward body momentum in persons with stroke and controls. Shown are COM horizontal momentum mean curves in the control group and in patient subgroups in each category of the RTW scale. In contrast to controls, who maintain forward momentum on arising (seat-off), subjects with the lowest score (0) arrest forward momentum on arising, then initiate gait. CTL = control subject; CVA = cerebral vascular accident. (Reprinted with permission from Malouin F, McFadyen B, Dion L, Richards CL. A fluidity scale for evaluating the motor strategy of the rise to walk task after stroke. *Clin Rehabil* 2003;17:679, Figure 2.)

with a stop on arising (arresting forward momentum) (Malouin et al., 2003).

Bed Mobility Skills

Bed mobility skills include changing position while in bed (rolling supine to side-lying or prone) and getting out of bed, either to a chair or standing up. Researchers have found that normal young adults use a variety of momentum-related strategies when performing bed mobility skills. There is incredible variety in how people move; in fact, none of the young adults tested used exactly the same strategy twice.

In contrast, force-control movement strategies are frequently used by neurologically impaired patients, and are characterized by frequent starts and stops. As mentioned previously, there are many reasons why a force-control strategy may be more appropriate than a momentum strategy in a patient with neurologic impairments (Richter et al., 1989).

The most common approach to rolling shown by normal young adults involves reaching and lifting with the upper extremity, flexing the head and upper trunk, and lifting the leg to roll onto the side, then over to prone. Most healthy young adults did not show rotation between the shoulders and pelvis, assumed by many clinicians to be an invariant feature of rolling (Richter et al., 1989). Because bed mobility skills are primarily initiated by movement of the head, upper trunk, and shoulders, impairments that affect these structures (such as weakness and or range-of-motion limitations) will limit performance of these skills.

A CASE STUDY APPROACH TO UNDERSTANDING MOBILITY DISORDERS

We now turn to summarizing mobility disorders by diagnosis, using our case studies as examples. Again, as in the abnormal postural control chapter it is important to remember that there is a great deal of heterogeneity among patients even with the same diagnosis. Thus, not all patients who have had a stroke will have a gait disorder similar to that in our case example.

Jean J: Poststroke Hemiparesis

Stroke is considered to be a leading cause of disability throughout the world (Dombovy et al., 1987). The ability to walk is often a prime factor in determining residential status and level of productivity following a stroke. Loss of independent ambulation, particularly outdoors, is reported as one of the most debilitating consequences of stroke (Pound et al., 1998). A study of 115 stroke survivors reported that despite good mobility outcomes on standardized measures of balance and gait, nearly one-third of those studied reported that they were unable to go into the community without assistance (Lord et al., 2004).

Jean, our patient with right hemiparesis, has significant balance and gait impairments, and as a result has had numerous falls, particularly during walking-related activities. With her walker, she walks at 0.5 m/sec, which is 50% more slowly than individuals her age who have no neurologic impairment. With her cane, her gait velocity is further slowed, to 0.3 m/sec. Her slow gait velocity is the result of a number of factors, including her extensive muscle weakness, moderate spasticity, and presence of abnormal synergy patterns of movement. Because she is unable to achieve a walking speed of at least 48 m/min and has difficulty managing curbs and stairs, she relies on a wheelchair for community mobility and is not a community ambulator (Perry et al., 1995).

Jean demonstrates abnormal spatial temporal parameters associated with her hemiparetic gait, including increased double-support time, decreased stance time by the involved leg, and a shortened step by the noninvolved leg. This results in a significant step asymmetry (Olney & Richards, 1996). On kinematic analysis of Jean's gait, we observe in the stance phase: (a) equinovarus foot position, leading to a forefoot or flat-foot strike during loading; (b) knee hyperextension in midstance, with a forward lean of the trunk; and (c) limited hip extension during stance phase, resulting in an inability to place the hemiparetic leg in a trailing position during terminal stance. The pelvis is retracted on the stance leg and drops on the swing side, probably due to abductor weakness. In the swing phase of gait we observe: (a) toe drag, impeding progression because of inadequate flexion at the hip, knee, and ankle; (b) delayed hip flexion until after toe-off; (c) reduced knee flexion during preswing and swing; and (d) inappropriate foot placement because of incomplete knee extension and ankle dorsiflexion at the end of the swing phase (Montgomery, 1987; Olney et al., 1998).

If the technology were available we might do an EMG analysis of Jean's gait in order to determine the muscle patterns used for walking and to try to determine the underlying cause of abnormal gait patterns. By analyzing the activation of muscles during gait we may be able to place Jean into one or more of the following categories of gait disorders: (1) "spastic pattern," characterized by exaggerated stretch response; (2) "paretic pattern," characterized by decreased (or absent) centrally generated patterned muscle activation; or (3) "coactivation pattern," produced by abnormal coactivation of multiple muscle groups (Knutsson, 1981, 1994; Knutsson & Richards, 1979). These patterns were described in more detail in early sections of this chapter.

A kinetic analysis of work and power may well indicate a reduction in Jean's ability to generate a plantar flexion moment for push-off during stance, because of paresis. She may compensate for this by increasing hip-flexor moment at pull-off in swing to help her advance her swing limb (Nadeau et al., 1997; Olney et al., 1991). These limitations in muscle strength will affect her gait speed.

If we analyze her energy expenditure while walking, we may be surprised to find that the oxygen cost for walking is quite low, despite the abnormal appearance of her gait. The inefficiency associated with abnormal gait patterns appears to be offset by slow gait speed. This suggests that ambulation is not physiologically stressful for the typical stroke patient unless there are cardiovascular problems as well (Waters & Mulroy, 1999; Waters et al., 1988). But this study examined energy costs in stroke patients based on time walked. When distance walked is considered, energy expenditure associated with hemiparetic gait is twice as much as that of normal gait, because it takes stroke patients, who walk at half the velocity of normal adults, twice as long to cover the same distance (Montgomery, 1987).

Jean has significant problems with dynamic gait activities, indicating a reduced ability to adapt locomotor patterns to changing task and environmental demands. She has difficulty traversing uneven terrains—modifying her step height and length to step over obstacles. Control of posture and gait is less automatic and requires more attentional resources. Stability while walking is further compromised when she performs other attentionally demanding tasks. Using her cane, she performs the Timed Up and Go (TUG) test under single task conditions in 32 seconds, and this increased to 42 seconds when performing the TUG under dual-task conditions. In addition, she makes multiple errors on the secondary task while walking, which are not present when she is sitting.

Jean demonstrates asymmetry in gait initiation (Hesse et al., 1997). Patients with hemiparesis demonstrate significant differences in timing, step length, mediolateral displacement of the center of pressure (COP), and pattern of velocity of COM movements when starting with the affected versus the nonaffected leg. Figure 14.21A shows the movement of the COP during gait initiation for a control subject with an anticipatory shift of the COP over the stance leg prior to initiating stepping. Figure 14.21B shows the movement of the COP of a subject with hemiparesis initiating gait with the affected side, while Figure 14.21C shows gait initiation with the unaffected side. This figure illustrates that when patients initiate gait with the affected limb, there is nearly normal anticipatory movement of the COP over the nonimpaired leg in preparation for step initiation. In contrast, when stepping is initiated with the nonimpaired leg, there is a reduction in movement of the COP over the affected leg associated with minimizing the amount of time during which the body is supported by the paretic limb alone.

Finally, Jean has difficulty with other mobility tasks, including transfers such as sitting to standing and rise to walk. Reduced ability to develop symmetric torques result in an asymmetric sitting-to-standing pattern, with the majority of work being done by her unaffected leg. She moves slowly and stops on arising prior to initiating steps to walk.

Mike M: Parkinson's Disease

Mike has significant gait problems, which increase his probability for falls. The degree of his gait abnormality depends on both the progression of his disease and his medication state. Blin et al. (1990, 1991) studied 21 patients at various stages in the clinical

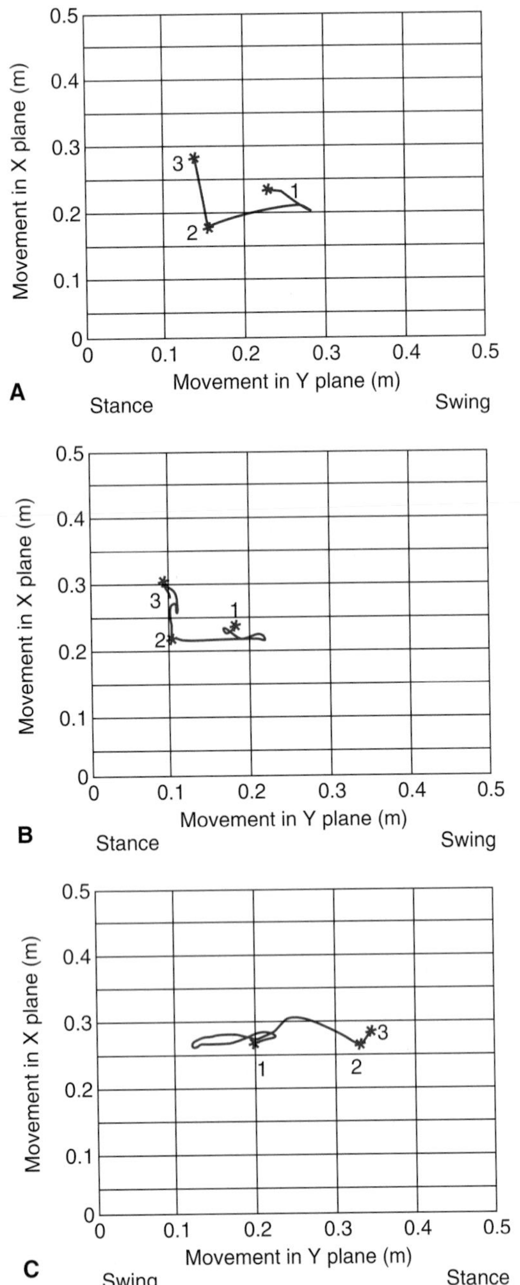

FIGURE 14.21 Movement of the COP during gait initiation for a control subject (A) and a subject with hemiparesis initiating gait with the affected (B) and unaffected (C) side. Note the similarities in gait initiation between the upper and middle traces. (Adapted with permission from Hesse S, Reiter F, Jahnke M, et al. Asymmetry of gait initiation in hemiparetic stroke subjects. *Arch Phys Med Rehabil* 1997;78:722.)

progression of the disease (Hoehn and Yahr stages I through IV [Hoehn & Yahr, 1967]). Compared with normal elderly controls, patients with PD showed a slower walking velocity, a shorter and more variable stride length, and longer stride duration. In addition, patients with PD showed an increased duration of stance and double-support phase and a concomitant decrease in the swing phase. Table 14.4 compares selected gait characteristics in patients with PD with those of healthy age-matched controls. Researchers have found a significant relationship between walking velocity in patients with PD and the stages of disability as described by the Schwab Classification of Progression (Schwab, 1960) or the Hoehn and Yahr Classification (Hoehn & Yahr, 1967).

Kinematic analysis of Mike's gait, especially when walking while in the off-medication state, indicate a reduction in the speed and amplitude of leg movements (resulting in characteristic short, shuffling steps) and arm movements (resulting in diminution of arm swing). Specific alterations in the stance phase of gait include: (a) lack of heel strike; instead, he makes contact with the foot flat or with the forefoot; (b) incomplete knee extension during midstance; (c) inability to extend the knee and plantar-flex the ankle in terminal stance, resulting in decreased forward thrust of the body; (d) forward trunk lean; (e) diminished trunk motion; and (f) reduced or absent arm swing. Decreased motion of the joints is apparent in swing phase as well, with decreased hip and knee flexion resulting in diminished toe clearance. In addition, reduced speed and amplitude of motion of the swing leg affect forward thrust of the body (Knutsson, 1972; Sofuwa et al., 2005; Stern et al., 1983).

An EMG study of Mike's gait may allow us to categorize him into one of three types of muscle activation patterns: (a) continuous EMG activity instead of cyclical activity; (b) reduced amplitude of muscle activation; and (c) abnormal coactivation of muscles (Knutsson, 1972). A kinetic analysis will likely show a reduction in ankle push-off power generation and a reduce hip-flexion pull-off power even in the "on" phase of medication (Sofuwa et al., 2005).

When he is in the off-medication state, Mike demonstrates problems with freezing while walking, particularly when he is turning or trying to step over obstacles or when he is moving through doorways. Gait in patients with PD has been characterized by an inability to control momentum. If a patient is unable to generate sufficient momentum, forward progression is arrested. This is often referred to as "freezing" (or "gait ignition failure"). Freezing episodes are transient, lasting from seconds to minutes. Freezing most often affects gait initiation (start hesitation) during turns, in narrow spaces, or when approaching obstacles (Fahn, 1995; Giladi et al., 1997). We may be able to help Mike reduce his freezing episodes using trick maneuvers such as counting or stepping over real or imagined lines (Stern et al., 1980).

TABLE 14.4 Comparison of Selected Gait Characteristics in Patients with Parkinson's Disease and Healthy Age-Matched Controls

	PD Patients (N = 21)	Controls (N = 58)	PD Patients Versus Controls	
	Mean±SD	Mean±SD	z Value	*p* Value
Velocity (m/sec)	0.44±0.20	0.83±0.23	5.25	<0.01
Stride length (m)	0.57±0.26	0.97±0.22	4.95	<0.01
Stride duration (sec)	1.29±0.16	1.19±0.15	2.17	<0.05
Swing duration (sec)	0.40±0.08	0.46±0.05	2.88	<0.01
Stance duration (sec)	0.88±0.16	0.74±0.12	3.50	<0.01
Swing velocity (m/sec)	1.36±0.44	2.12±0.46	5.03	<0.01
Peak velocity (m/sec)	2.00±0.66	3.28±0.72	5.31	<0.01
Double-support duration (sec)	0.23±0.08	0.13±0.05	5.21	<0.01
Relative double-support duration (sec)	35.8±9.80	21.8±6.80	5.24	<0.01
Stride-duration variability	5.51±5.10	4.75±2.30	0.12	NS
Stride-length variability	6.68±4.27	5.17±3.80	1.92	<0.05

Reprinted with permission from Blin O, Ferrandez AM, Serratrice G. Quantitative analysis of gait in Parkinson patients: increased variability of stride length. J Neurosci 1990;98:95.

In addition to freezing, Mike's gait is characterized by unrestrained momentum that leads to uncontrolled progression, called a "propulsive gait pattern." Propulsive gait disorders may be due to an exaggerated forward inclination of the body, resulting in an anterior displacement of the COM beyond the supporting foot. In some instances, however, propulsive gait is seen in patients who have normal vertical posture but seem unable to oppose forward momentum (Knutsson, 1972).

Mike, like many patients with PD, has problems with gait initiation, leading to akinesia (defined as loss of willed movement). Gait initiation has been cinematically studied in 31 patients with PD (Rosin et al., 1997). Gait initiation was divided into two phases, movement preparation time and movement execution. Patients with PD had significantly longer movement preparation time, but not execution time. In addition, while initiation of ankle, knee, hip, arm, and trunk movements was delayed, the sequencing and timing of submovements was comparable between groups. The authors suggest that gait-initiation problems in PD were not the result of dyscoordinated movements, but rather were due to a deficit within the basal ganglia's internal cueing for movement sequences (Rosin et al., 1997).

Mike is taking medication to help control the symptoms of his PD; however, he shows considerable fluctuations in his motor performance, both throughout the course of the day as well as from one day to the next. Contributions to motor fluctuations include variation in levels of anti-PD medications, time of day, fatigue, stress, diet, and change in responsiveness to the medication (Nutt et al., 1984). A number of studies have examined the effect of medication (L-DOPA) on various gait parameters (Blin et al., 1991; MacKay-Lyons, 1998; Morris et al., 1996). Gait parameters particularly sensitive to changes in drug levels are walking velocity and stride length (Blin et al., 1991; MacKay-Lyons, 1998; Morris et al., 1996). In contrast, other variables, such as cadence, stride time, and swing duration did not vary as a function of medication cycle (Blin et al., 1991; Pedersen et al., 1991). Morris et al. (1996) concluded that characteristics of gait in patients with mild PD are reproducible during the "on" phase of medication (both across 30 minutes of peak dosage or at 24-hour intervals) but are more variable during the "off" phase. In contrast, MacKay-Lyons (1998) found extensive variability throughout the entire L-dopa cycle in patients with moderately severe PD. Not all fluctuations in motor performance are predictable, however. Poewe (1994) found that approximately 15% of patients with PD have random fluctuations in motor performance that were not related to L-dopa doses. This led Poewe to categorize fluctuations in motor performance in patients with PD as either predictable or random.

Mike relies heavily on visual cues during walking. Prokop and Berger (1996) found that when an optical flow pattern was imposed during stepping on a treadmill, patients with PD continuously modulated their speed in response to changing visual flow patterns, while healthy controls did not. It has been hypothesized that increased reliance on visual cues to regulate gait is the result of impaired proprioceptive reflexes (Bronstein & Guerraz, 1999). In contrast to patients with spasticity, patients with PD show a reduced reflex sensitivity (Berardelli et al., 1983; Tatton et al., 1984).

Finally, Mike, like Jean, has difficulty with other mobility tasks, such as transfers, sitting to standing, and bed mobility. He takes longer to stand up, particularly off medication, because of a reduced rate of force production.

John C: Degenerative Cerebellar Injury

John, our 33-year-old with spinocerebellar degeneration has significant gait problems. His walking, particularly without his shoes on, is characterized by staggering, irregular stepping, veering from side to side, and excessively high lifting of the feet above the ground (Gilman, 2000; Palliyath et al., 1998). John walks more slowly than his age-matched peers and has a reduced step and stride length and longer stride durations (Earhart & Bastian, 2001). Palliyath et al. (1998) quantified gait in 10 patients with cerebellar ataxia, 6 with hereditary cerebellar cortical atrophy and 4 with olivopontocerebellar atrophy. Mean quantitative differences in gait characteristics between patients and normal controls are shown in Table 14.5. Patients were, on average, slower than normal controls and showed more variability across all measures. Patients showed reduced step and stride length, and motion at the ankle, knee, and hip. Interestingly, despite current clinical assumptions that cerebellar ataxic gait is characterized by increased step width and high steppage, in this study there was not a significant difference in step width or toe clearance between the two groups. Seidel and Krebs (2002) also found no increase in step width in persons with chronic ataxia.

A kinematic analysis of John's ataxic gait demonstrates poor intersegmental coordination with abnormal rates of motion between ankle and knee. Problems with intersegmental coordination are associated with increased frontal-plane instability, as indicated by increased displacement and velocity of the COM in the mediolateral direction during stepping tasks (Hudson & Krebbs, 2000).

John has problems adapting his gait to changes in external demands (Earhart & Bastian, 2001; Morton & Bastian, 2003; 2007). Researchers have reported that individuals with cerebellar pathology have difficulty adapting locomotor patterns to changing external constraints, including wedges in the walking path (Earhart & Bastian, 2001) and stepping over obstacles (Morton et al., 2004), because of reduced ability to coordinate the relative movement of multiple joints.

Thomas: Spastic Diplegic Cerebral Palsy

Thomas, our 7-year-old with a spastic diplegic form of cerebral palsy, began walking much later than his age-matched peers. He walks much more slowly than his typically developing peers, averaging 0.5 m/sec without his assistive device. He is much faster when walking with his walker. At home and at school, Thomas walks with a walker or no assistive device, but he uses a scooter for community mobility. His gait is characterized by a reduced stride length and step width. He walks with a characteristic crouched gait pattern, with excessive hip and knee flexion, in conjunction with excessive ankle plantar flexion, and anterior pelvic tilt during the stance and swing phases of gait. Foot strike is abnormal, with an equinovarus foot posture and often forefoot contact. This foot position is continued through the stance phase of gait. Excessive plantar-flexion and knee and hip flexion are seen during loading and continue through the stance phase of gait. Excessive flexion persists into the terminal stance, and the preswing phase is minimal or absent because of an inability to extend the hip and knee. The swing phase of gait also shows excessive knee and hip flexion.

If Thomas had spastic hemiplegic, instead of spastic diplegic, cerebral palsy, he would likely present with a genu recurvatum gait pattern instead of a crouched gait pattern. The former gait pattern is characterized by knee hyperextension during stance and excessive ankle plantar flexion. Hip flexion and forward lean of the trunk may occur as the patient leans forward to balance over a plantar-flexed foot. Loading is onto the forefoot because of inadequate knee extension and excessive plantar flexion during swing. During swing, toe drag constrains progression, requiring contralateral trunk lean to free the foot and advance the thigh. The genu recurvatum gait pattern is more common in unilateral motor impairments such as spastic hemiplegia (Crenna et al., 1998; Gage, 1993).

TABLE 14.5 Comparison of Selected Gait Characteristics in Patients with Cerebellar Ataxia and Healthy Age-Matched Controls

Descriptor	Control (Mean ±SD)	Patient (Mean ±SD)	P From *T test*
Cadence (steps/min)	111.00±7.60	102.20±15.90	0.14
Step length (% height)	0.48±0.20	0.29±0.07	0.02*
Stride length (% height)	0.96±0.40	0.59±0.14	0.02*
Step width (% height)	0.16±0.08	0.14±0.03	0.68
Step-length symmetry	1.00±0.06	0.97±0.17	0.64
Stride-length symmetry	1.02±0.02	1.00±0.04	0.35
Step-width symmetry	0.98±0.06	1.02±0.12	0.31
Stance time (sec)	0.66±0.12	0.79±0.17	0.07
Swing time (sec)	0.39±0.05	0.43±0.06	0.18
Step time (sec)	0.54±0.04	0.61±0.11	0.13
Stride time or gait cycle (sec)	1.08±0.08	1.21±0.22	0.11
Gait velocity (mm/sec)	0.90±0.39	0.47±0.17	0.01*
Ankle angle range of motion, degrees	31.50±6.20	23.20±5.10	0.004*
Ankle angle at heel strike	102.50±5.90	103.00±8.50	0.90
Heel-off time (% of gait cycle)	44.00±4.00	50.00±8.00	0.04*
Toe-off time (% of gait cycle)	66.00±1.00	68.00±3.00	0.04*
Knee-angle range of motion	58.50±2.10	53.90±7.70	0.10
Knee-angle range of motion during stance	11.50±4.90	7.50±3.80	0.07
Time of peak flexion of knee during swing (% of gait cycle)	2.70±1.90	75.50±3.20	0.02*
Hip-angle range of motion	34.30±5.90	31.30±4.70	0.23
Foot height (cm)	11.90±1.20	11.50±1.90	0.62

Reprinted with permission from Palliyath S, Hallett M, Thomas SL, Lebiedowska MK. Gait in patients with cerebellar ataxia. Mov Disord 1998;13:962.

An EMG analysis of Thomas's gait might allow us to separate his problems into one of four categories: (a) defective recruitment of motor units, referred to as a "paresis" or "weakness pattern"; (b) abnormal velocity-dependent recruitment during muscle stretch, the so-called spasticity pattern; (c) nonselective activation of antagonist muscles with a loss of a normal reciprocal inhibitory pattern, called the "cocontraction pattern"; and (d) problems associated with musculoskeletal restraint due to changes in mechanical properties of muscles, the nonneural problem pattern (Crenna et al., 1991).

Interestingly, in children with spastic hemiplegic cerebral palsy, a cocontraction pattern of muscle activity was found in both the hemiplegic leg and the noninvolved leg. Thus, researchers are now considering the possibility that cocontraction represents a compensatory strategy aimed at stiffening a joint to compensate for postural instability or paresis (Berger et al., 1984b; Crenna et al., 1991; Leonard et al., 2006). The particular gait profile seen in an individual will reflect a combination of the factors just listed. Thus, each individual with CP will present with a slightly different gait pattern.

When walking, Thomas's heart rate and oxygen rates will be higher than his age-matched peers. Researchers believe that this is because the flexed posture, which is typical of the crouched-gait pattern, requires additional muscle activity for stability. Interestingly, the physiological costs of walking decrease in typically developing children as they get older. In contrast, the physiological costs of walking increase as children with CP get older. Why does this happen? Increased physiological costs of walking are not due to an increase in motor abnormalities in CP, since it is a nonprogressive disease. Instead, researchers believe that oxygen rates associated with walking increase as children with CP get older because changes in body morphology, including increased body weight and size, interact with impaired motor control. This results in an increase in the physiological cost of gait in older children. As a result, the older child with CP may walk less and increasingly rely on a wheelchair (Waters, 1992).

Finally, Thomas has difficulty with other mobility tasks, including standing up, because of neuromuscular impairments affecting his ability to generate and time the forces needed for the sitting-to-standing task.

SUMMARY

1. While abnormal gait is a common characteristic of many neurologic pathologies, the constellation of underlying problems that produce disordered gait will vary from patient to patient depending on: (a) primary impairments, such as inadequate activation of a muscle; (b) secondary impairments, such as contractures; and (c) compensatory strategies developed to meet the requirements of mobility in the face of persisting impairments.
2. Musculoskeletal impairments constrain movement and increase the workload on the muscles, affecting a patient's ability to meet the requirements of gait. Decreased joint mobility during stance restricts forward motion of the body over the supporting foot, affecting progression. In swing, decreased joint mobility reduces foot clearance, affecting progression, and appropriate foot placement for weight acceptance, affecting stability.
3. Neuromuscular impairments affecting gait include weakness, abnormalities of muscle tone, and task-specific control problems. Task-specific control problems consist of: (a) the inability to recruit a muscle during an automatic task such as posture or gait; (b) inappropriate activation of a muscle during gait, which is not related to stretch of the muscle; (c) coactivation of agonist and antagonist muscles around a joint, which increases stiffness and decreases motion; and (d) problems related to scaling the amplitude of muscle activity during gait.
4. Sensory disorders can lead to problems in the following areas of locomotor control: (a) signaling terminal stance and thus triggering the initiation of swing, (b) signaling unanticipated disruptions to gait, and (c) detecting upcoming obstacles important for modifying gait to changes in task and environmental conditions.
5. Impairments can manifest as problems affecting the patient's abilities to meet the progression, stability, and adaptation goals inherent in both the stance and the swing phases of gait. A careful analysis of movement patterns can lead the clinician to generate multiple hypotheses about the potential underlying causes of gait problems.
6. During the performance of transfer activities such as sitting to standing, rolling, and rising from a bed, healthy young adults tend to use a momentum strategy, which requires the generation of concentric and eccentric contractions to control motion, and ensures stability. In contrast, a force-control strategy, characterized by frequent starts and stops, is frequently used by neurologically dysfunctional patients. This is related to impairments affecting both stability and progression aspects of the movement. This is also the strategy most commonly taught by clinicians when retraining transfer tasks.

CHAPTER 15

CLINICAL MANAGEMENT OF THE PATIENT WITH A MOBILITY DISORDER

LEARNING OBJECTIVES

Following completion of this chapter, the reader will be able to:

1. Describe a task-oriented approach to evaluating mobility function in geriatric and neurologic populations.
2. Review functional tests and measures used to quantify functional mobility skills, including limited ability to participate in mobility functions in the context of a home and community environment ("performance" in the ICF framework) as well as clinical measures of functional mobility skills ("capacity" in the ICF framework).
3. Discuss clinical methods for evaluating strategies for gait and other mobility skills, including measures used to assist the process of observational gait analysis.
4. Discuss a task-oriented approach to treating functional mobility limitations, including ambulation, transfers, and bed mobility skills.
5. Review the evidence for mobility training in geriatric and neurologic populations.

INTRODUCTION

Management of mobility problems is often a key to return of functional independence in patients with neurologic pathology. Consider Jean J, our 82-year-old woman with poststroke hemiparesis. Prior to her stroke, she was living independently in her own home. In the hospital, she was dependent in all mobility functions, requiring assistance in moving about her bed, transferring to her wheelchair or commode, and standing up. At that point, she was unable to walk, even with the assistance of another person. Since mobility is essential to many basic activities of daily living (BADLs), such as toileting, transfers, and dressing, as well as many instrumental activities of daily living (IADLs), such as shopping, cleaning, and cooking, regaining mobility function was a critical determinant of Jean's ability to recover functional independence and return to living in her own home. Given the importance of mobility to recovery of functional independence, a critical issue for her therapist was to determine the most effective way to examine and retrain mobility skills.

This chapter presents a task-oriented approach to examining and treating patients with mobility dysfunction, with a main focus on examination and treatment of gait. As is true throughout this book, our task-oriented approach is based on both the International Classification of Functioning, Disability and Health (ICF) and systems framework. We begin with examination, reviewing some of the tests and measurements that can be used to document functional abilities related to mobility including: (1) level of mobility disability, defined as a restriction in participation of mobility-related activities in the person's home and community environment (referred to as "performance" in the ICF framework), and (2) functional mobility skills within a standard setting (referred to as "capacity" in the ICF framework). As part of our task-oriented examination we will explore the process of observational gait analysis, an approach to describing strategies used to accomplish the main tasks of gait. The second half of the chapter addresses issues related to retraining mobility skills in the patient with neurologic pathology, focusing on a task-oriented approach. Included in this section is a review of the research evidence supporting the efficacy of therapeutic strategies designed to improve gait and other mobility functions.

A TASK-ORIENTED APPROACH TO EXAMINATION

In a task-oriented approach, examination of mobility function analyzes performance at three levels: (a) the functional-task level, (b) the essential strategies used to accomplish the requirements of mobility, and (c) the underlying sensory, motor, and cognitive impairments that constrain mobility. The three-level examination attempts to answer the following questions:

1. To what degree can the patient consistently perform functional mobility tasks? What is the effect of impaired mobility function on the ability of the patient to be engaged in daily life activities and social roles (restricted participation)?
2. What strategies does the person use to accomplish mobility tasks, such as walking? Is the person able to adapt strategies to changing task and environmental conditions?
3. What are the cognitive, visual-perceptual, musculoskeletal, somatosensory or other impairments that constrain how they perform mobility tasks? Can these impairments be altered through intervention, thereby enhancing the patient's capabilities?

Examination at the Functional Level

A functional assessment uses tests and measures to determine the person's abilities in his or her actual living environment (performance in the ICF framework), and in a standard (clinical) environment (capacity in the ICF framework). The following section reviews a wide range of tests used to measure mobility function, with a specific focus on gait. Within the ICF, mobility is considered both an activity (e.g., a task performed by an individual) and a domain of participation (e.g., the societal level of functioning). This can make it difficult to classify tests of mobility function. In this chapter, a mobility test performed in a standardized clinical environment is classified as an activity measure considered to capture the ICF's concept of capacity. A test is classified as a measure of participation (performance) when it gathers information about the person's mobility behavior (self-reported or observed) in his or her environment. It is important to remember that outcomes on activities measures (such as gait speed on the 10 Meter Walk clinical test) may or may not predict mobility participation, that is, behavior in the person's own environment (ICF concept of performance). We recognize that not everyone will agree with our approach to classifying tests and measures, and many may disagree with the way a specific test or measure is classified. Though subject to interpretation and error, we feel that it is important to create a consistent framework for the presentation of these materials.

Measuring Participation (Mobility Performance in Home and Community Contexts)

For many people with neurologic pathology, reintegration into community life marks a significant goal in rehabilitation. Ambulation in home and community contexts is an important part of the community reintegration process. As discussed in Chapter 14, mobility in daily life requires the ability to walk in diverse environments, with varying terrains, ambient conditions, and attentional demands. In addition, walking is most often performed in conjunction with other tasks, such as carrying loads, scanning the environment, and engaging in social interactions. A restricted ability to participate in mobility-related activities is referred to as "mobility disability." Mobility measured in a clinical context often does not capture the complexity of walking in natural environments; thus, it may not predict mobility behavior in the person's real-life context. Measures of participation that reflect mobility behavior in the person's daily life are needed.

Most measures of participation rely on self-report (by the individual or his or her proxy) to determine the degree to which the person is mobile during the performance of social roles and daily life activities. Alternatively, technology such as pedometers and activity monitors can be used to measure mobility, specifically walking behavior, directly.

Self-Report Measures of Mobility Participation. A number of self-report instruments designed to examine participation in multiple domains including mobility are available. Examples include the Mobility and Self-Care (MOSES) Questionnaire, which measures perceived difficulty with mobility and self care activities performed in the home and community (Farin et al., 2007), and the Participation Survey/Mobility

(PARTS/M), which measures perceived choice, importance, and satisfaction related to components of participation (Gray et al., 2006). The Craig Handicap Assessment and Reporting Technique (CHART) measures participation (handicap) in multiple dimensions including: physical independence, mobility, occupation, social integration, economic self-sufficiency (Hall et al., 2001; Walker et al., 2003; Whiteneck et al., 1992). The Assessment of Life Habits (LIFE-H) measures level of difficulty, type of assistance, and satisfaction in several domains, including mobility. It also documents the impact of assistive technology on participation (Noreau et al., 2002, 2004).

Another approach to examining mobility participation is through the use of life space, defined as the size of the spatial area a person purposely moves through in his or her daily life, as well as the frequency of travel within a specific time frame. Life space assesses actual mobility performance in the real world, rather than functional capability under hypothetical or experimental conditions (Baker et al., 2003; May et al., 1985). Restriction of life space is a marker for incident frailty, disability, and mortality (Xue et al., 2008). The Life Space Questionnaire (LSQ) is an instrument developed to determine the spatial extent of an older person's mobility; it is used to document a person's mobility within their home and community (Peel et al., 2005; Stalvey et al., 1999).

Activity Monitors. Activity monitoring has been used to gain insight into locomotor activity in a person's own environment. The pedometer is a simple device often used to measure locomotor activity by counting the number of steps taken. However, locomotor activities in daily life consist of walking (and running) on various terrains and at varying speeds or work intensities, while performing other activities, such as carrying loads, and this illustrates one of the limitations of the pedometer. Another limitation is that output from pedometers (and some actigraphs—i.e., accelerometers to measure activity of the body) is confounded by gait speed and pattern (Cyarto et al., 2004).

Orendurff and colleagues (2008) used step activity monitors to examine walking patterns in healthy young adults employed and living in a typical urban environment. They found that walking in daily living for this sample of people was overwhelmingly comprised of short-duration walking bouts. Forty percent of all walking bouts were less than 12 steps in a row; and 60% of all walking lasted 30 sec or less. The authors suggest that walking in daily living is predominantly short duration with lots of initiation, termination, speed modulation, corner negotiation, and maneuvering. This has implications for locomotor training in geriatric and neurologic populations.

Step activity monitors (SAMs) and pedometers have been used to examine walking behavior in various environments following a stroke. Robinson (2010) used pedometers and reported that participants with chronic (>6 mo) stroke walked on an average (±SD) of 2540±2176 steps per day. Studies using a SAM have reported a wide range of steps per day in participations following stroke. In two studies, averages ranged from 2700 to 2800 steps per day (Michael et al., 2005; Shaughnessy et al., 2005). Mudge and Stott (2009) reported an average of 4700 steps; while Manns and Baldwin (2009) reported 6100±2068. Differences may be due to the type of device used, where it was placed on the body, and the environment in which walking was measured (Leicht & Crowther, 2007, 2009; Mudge et al., 2007).

Busse et al. (2004) examined the reliability and validity of an activity monitor in subjects with and without neurologic impairment and reported that the 7-day mean step count was 5951 (range, 2886 to 9955) in healthy subjects, 3818 (1611 to 5391) in patients with Parkinson's disease, 3003 (716 to 5302) in those with muscular disorders, and 2985 (689 to 5340) in those with multiple sclerosis.

Activity monitors, including pedometers, are not routinely used in therapy to either evaluate or treat locomotor function (as a source of feedback to patients). While there are many technical limitations to work out, they may prove to be a useful way to encourage locomotor activity outside the context of a clinical setting, and thus could be useful in facilitating increased participation in mobility. In addition, ambulatory monitoring may prove to be a useful outcome measure for patients involved in mobility-training programs and may provide insight into participation in the mobility domain.

Standardized Measures of Functional Activities (Capacity)

Examination of functional mobility often focuses on determining the distance a patient can walk, the time it takes to traverse this distance, and the level of assistance needed (Katz et al., 1970; Keith et al., 1987; Lawton, 1971). The patient can be asked to walk a specified distance (e.g., 150 ft) and the time taken to walk that distance can be recorded. Alternatively, the patient can be asked to walk for a specified time period, and the distance walked can be recorded.

Gait Velocity. A number of researchers have suggested that velocity alone can be used as a single measure of functional gait since it is simple, quick, and appears to be a composite measure of temporal and distance variables (Brandstater et al., 1983;

LAB ACTIVITY 15-1

Objective: To determine gait velocity under self-paced and fast-paced conditions.

Procedure: Measure a 10-m (33-ft) walking course. You will be calculating a steady-state gait velocity, so you want to be walking at a constant speed, not speeding up or slowing down. Starting at about 3 ft before the first mark, begin walking at a comfortable pace, and keep walking for at least 3 ft after the second mark. Using a stopwatch, calculate the time it takes to walk the middle (marked) 10 m. Repeat this three times, recording the time for each trial. Now, repeat the test walking the 10 m as fast as you can, and record the time. You may also wish to try this test using a distance of 5 m, as recommended by Salbach et al. (2001), to determine differences in gait velocity that occur with distance. In addition, you can repeat the test using various types of assistive devices, such as a single-point cane or a pick-up or front-wheeled walker to determine the effect of an assistive device on gait speed.

Assignment: Average the three trials for each condition and calculate gait velocity (divide the total walking distance of 10 m (or 5 m) by the elapsed time in seconds, multiply by 60 to get meters per minute) for both the self-paced and fast-paced conditions. Convert self-selected gait velocity to a percentage of normal. Compare self-selected gait velocity to fast-paced velocity and calculate the percentage increase in gait speed. How does using an assistive device change your gait velocity?

Murray et al., 1970; Richards et al., 1995). You can gain experience in calculating self-paced and fast-paced gait velocity in Lab Activity 15.1. Converting the patient's self-selected gait velocity to a percentage of normal can be an effective way to communicate locomotor abilities to patients and their families and insurers (Bohannon, 1997; Montgomery, 1987). In order to find the patient's percentage of normal gait velocity, reference values for normal individuals are needed. In some cases a standard reference value of 80 m/min is used. Bohannon (1997) published normative values for comfortable and maximum gait speed based on data from 230 healthy individuals. Reference values are both gender- and age (by decades)-specific and include both actual gait speed (cm/sec) and gait speed normalized to height (actual gait speed [cm/ sec]/height [cm]). Norms from this study (converted to meters per minute) are shown in Table 15.1.

What is the best distance to use when calculating gait velocity? One common method calculates gait speed measured over 10 m (33 ft) indoors (Collen, 1990). Alternatively, patients have been asked to walk 5 m, turn and walk back (so-called 2 × 5 m test) (Collen, 1990). Guralnik and colleagues (1994) reported that the 4-m walk was the distance of choice because it was demonstrated to be feasible in the home as well as the clinical setting, however the longer distance improved measurement accuracy (Guralnik et al., 1994). Dean and colleagues (2001) reported that walking speed over a distance of 10 m overestimated

TABLE 15.1 Reference Values for Gait Speed: Comfortable versus Maximum Velocity by Decade of Age and Gender

	Comfortable (m/min)		Maximum (m/min)	
Decade	Men	Women	Men	Women
20s	83.6	84.4	151.9	148.0
30s	87.5	84.9	147.4	140.5
40s	88.1	83.5	147.7	127.4
50s	83.6	83.7	124.1	120.6
60s	81.5	77.8	115.9	106.4
70s	79.8	76.3	124.7	104.9

Adapted with permission from Bohannon RW. Comfortable and maximum walking speed of adults aged 20 to 79 years: reference values and determinants. Age Ageing 1997;26:15–19.

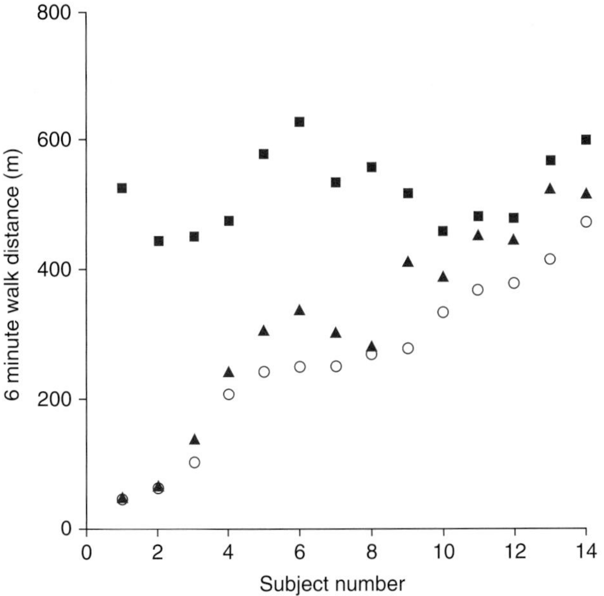

FIGURE 15.1 Relationship between gait speed on the 10-m walk test, estimated distance (triangles) walked in 6 minutes (based on 10-m gait speed) and actual distance (circles) walked in 6 minutes in 14 subjects following stroke. (Adapted from Dean CM, Richards CL, Malouin F. Walking speed over 10 meters overestimates locomotor capacity after stroke. Clin Rehabil 2001;15:419, Figure 2.)

walking capacity in persons with stroke. They measured walking velocity over 10 m in 14 subjects at least 3 months after stroke (mean age, 63±8 years) and 12 controls (mean age, 44±4 years) and used it to estimate distance walked on a 6-minute walk test. Distance was then compared with actual distance walked in 6 minutes. Results from the subjects with stroke are shown in Figure 15.1. Subjects with stroke were unable to maintain their comfortable walking speed (as established on the 10-m walk test) for 6 minutes; in contrast, control subjects walked faster than their comfortable speed for 6 minutes. As a result, on the 6-minute walk, the participants with stroke walked on average half the expected distance predicted by gait velocity measured on the 10-m test. Thus, it may be best to calculate velocity over a short distance for the sake of efficiency, being aware that in many cases, this velocity cannot be sustained over a long period (e.g., 6 minutes).

Does gait velocity measured in the clinic (capacity) correspond to gait velocity used in natural environments (performance)? An important assumption in the measurement of any gait variable, including gait velocity, is that measures taken in the clinic are ecologically valid—that is, reflecting the person's capabilities in the real world. This may not be true. Gait speeds observed in natural environments were slower than those observed in the clinic (Mosely et al., 2004). It is possible that slower gait speed in more complex environments such as in a shopping mall and a busy hospital corridor, were due to additional demands on mobility in these environments.

For any measure to be useful as an outcome measure, the minimal amount of change that is clinically meaningful and associated with an important difference in function needs to be determined. Tilson and colleagues (2010) estimated that the minimally clinical important difference (MCID) for usual gait speed was 0.16 m/sec in persons between 20 and 60 days after stroke.

Schmid et al. (2007) determined that a change in gait speed sufficient to result in a transition within the Perry mobility classification scheme results in better function, participation and quality of life. For example, those who transitioned from household ambulators to limited or full community ambulation had significantly better Stroke Impact Scale (SIS) scores in mobility and participation.

MCID may vary as a function of baseline gait speed and diagnosis. Palombaro et al. (2006) reported that the MCID for gait speed in older adults with hip fracture was 0.10 m/sec. Similarly, Perera et al. (2006) estimated that a substantial change in gait speed was 0.10 m/sec. This estimate was derived from data from a range of participants including older adults with mobility disability, poststroke survivors, and community-dwelling older adults. Among older adults, a change in gait speed of 0.10 m/sec was associated with reduced disability and better survival rates (Hardy et al., 2007).

Being able to calculate a patient's self-selected gait velocity is important, since it represents a cumulative quality score of a patient's ability and confidence in walking (Brandstater et al., 1983; Richards et al., 1995). It can also be used to infer the level of disability related to mobility, since patients who walk at less than 30% of normal do not usually become community ambulators (Perry et al., 1995). However, clinicians need to be careful when assuming that gait speed measured during short distances under relatively ideal clinical conditions reflects walking ability for longer distances and in more natural (and often less than ideal) contexts.

6- or 12-Minute Walk. Independent mobility in the community requires not just sufficient speed, but walking endurance as well (Hesse et al., 1994). Thus, measuring the distance a patient can walk is an important outcome when retraining gait. ADL scales, such as the Functional Independence Measure (FIM), evaluate independence in walking based on distance measures (Keith et al., 1987).

The 12-minute walking test was designed to examine exercise tolerance in patients with chronic respiratory disease (McGavin et al., 1976). However, because the 12-minute test is time-consuming and fatiguing to the patient, several researchers examined the validity of a shortened version of the test, comparing the performance of patients at 2, 6, and 12 minutes (Butland et al., 1982). These researchers concluded that, although the 12-minute test has excellent test–retest reliability, both the 2- and 6-minute tests are equally reliable, although slightly less sensitive in discriminating a patient's level of exercise tolerance. They concluded that the shorter time durations could be used when assessing exercise tolerance (Butland et al., 1982). Age (community-dwelling older adults 65 years of age or older) and gender-specific normative values for the 6-minute walk have been published as part of the Functional Fitness Test (Rikli & Jones, 2001). In addition, in a study examining mobility measures in subjects with chronic stroke, Ng and Hui-Chan (2005) reported that the average distance walked in the 6-minute walk test was 202±88 ft in subjects with stroke, as compared with 416.5±95.7 ft in age-matched controls.

Wise and Brown (2005) estimated that the MCID for the 6-minute walk test is 54 to 80 meters; an individual patient would need to change by about 86 meters to be confident that a statistically significant change had occurred.

Other Temporal and Distance Factors. A number of authors have advocated the inclusion of other temporal and distance factors, such as cadence, step and stride length, including right/left asymmetry in step and stride length in the examination of gait (Holden et al., 1984; Robinson & Schmidt, 1981). These factors are usually documented during ambulation over a short distance (e.g., 20 to 30 ft). Characteristics of constant gait velocity are determined, and thus the first and last 5 ft are not used in the calculations. Patients are usually given one practice trial, followed by two data-collection trials, separated by a rest period.

A number of methods for quantifying temporal and distance factors in the clinic have been suggested, including a footprint analysis using either inked feet and white butcher paper (Holden et al., 1984) or floor grids (Robinson & Schmidt, 1981).

Technological Devices for the Clinic. The use of laboratory methods (e.g., motion analysis, electromyography [EMG], and force plates) for analyzing gait is expensive and time-consuming and requires specialized expertise; as a result, it is not realistic in clinical settings. However, there are a growing number of simple devices being developed that can quantify spatial and temporal aspects of gait and can be used in the clinic. These devices vary in their complexity and cost, but can improve the therapist's ability to measure specific gait parameters within the clinical setting. Examples include portable stride analyzers (insoles that contain four compression-closing foot switches that connect to a lightweight mobile data-collection box worn on a belt) and various types of instrumented walkways.

Measures of Complex Walking Tasks. Measurement of spatial and temporal aspects of gait, while important, is limited to examining gait under rather static conditions (walking at a comfortable speed over level ground, in ideal ambient conditions). A number of mobility scales have been developed to examine a broader range of walking skills that are more characteristic of mobility in community environments, including starts and stops, changes in direction and speed, stepping over and around obstacles, and the integration of multiple tasks such as talking, turning to look at something, or carrying objects during gait. Thus, these tests include not only the examination of unimpeded gait, defined as a closed-skill task, but also the ability to modify and adapt gait to both expected and unexpected disturbances to locomotion. Several mobility tests, including the Timed Up and Go test (TUG) and the Performance-Oriented Mobility Assessment (POMA), were discussed in Chapter 11, because they are tests that are commonly used as measures of balance and fall risk. When selecting a test, clinicians should keep in mind the severity of mobility impairment in the patient being tested and choose a scale that is appropriate, in order to avoid either a ceiling (a test that is too easy) or floor (a test that is too difficult) effect.

Dynamic Gait Index. The Dynamic Gait Index (DGI) was developed by Shumway-Cook et al. (1997a) to evaluate and document a patient's ability to modify gait in response to changing task demands. The test is shown in Assessment Tool 15.1. The test has been used as a measure of mobility in older adults, with a score below 19 (of 24) indicative of increased fall risk. A number of researchers have demonstrated good reliability and validity of the DGI in a variety of patient populations (Hall & Herdman, 2006; Herman et al., 2009; Jonsdottier & Cattaneo, 2007; Marchetti et al., 2008; McConvey & Bennett, 2005; Whitney et al., 2000, 2003; Wrisley et al., 2003). Finally, the MCID for the DGI appears to be 4 points (Wrisley et al., 2002).

Assessment Tool 15-1

Dynamic Gait Index

1. Gait level surface_____

Instructions: Walk at your normal speed from here to the next mark (20 ft)

Grading: Mark the lowest category that applies.

(3) Normal: Walks 20 ft, no assistive devices, good speed, no evidence of imbalance, normal gait pattern.

(2) Mild impairment: Walks 20 ft, uses assistive devices, slower speed, mild gait deviations.

(1) Moderate impairment: Walks 20 ft, slow speed, abnormal gait pattern, evidence of imbalance.

(0) Severe impairment: Cannot walk 20 ft without assistance, severe gait deviations, or imbalance.

2. Change in gait speed_____

Instructions: Begin walking at your normal pace (for 5 ft), when I tell you to "go," walk as fast as you can (for 5 ft). When I tell you "slow," walk as slowly as you can (for 5 ft).

Grading: Mark the lowest category that applies.

(3) Normal: Able to smoothly change walking speed without loss of balance or gait deviation. Shows a significant difference in walking speeds between normal, fast, and slow speeds.

(2) Mild impairment: Is able to change speed but demonstrates mild gait deviations, or no gait deviations but unable to achieve a significant change in velocity, or uses an assistive device.

(1) Moderate impairment: Makes only minor adjustments to walking speed, or accomplishes a change in speed with significant gait deviations, or changes speed but loses significant gait deviations, or changes speed but loses balance but is able to recover and continue walking.

(0) Severe impairment: Cannot change speeds, or loses balance and has to reach for wall or be caught.

3. Gait with horizontal head turns_____

Instructions: Begin walking at your normal pace. When I tell you look right, keep walking straight but turn your head to the right. Keep looking to the right until I tell you, "look left," then keep walking straight and turn your head to the left. Keep your head to the left until I tell you, "look straight," then keep walking straight but return your head to the center.

Grading: Mark the lowest category that applies.

(3) Normal: Performs head turns smoothly with no change in gait.

(2) Mild impairment: Performs head turns smoothly with slight change in gait velocity, i.e., minor disruption to smooth gait path or uses walking aid.

(1) Moderate impairment: Performs head turns with moderate change in gait velocity, slows down, staggers but recovers, can continue to walk.

(0) Severe impairment: Performs task with severe disruption of gait, i.e., staggers outside 15-inch path, loses balance, stops, reaches for wall.

4. Gait with vertical head turns_____

Instructions: Begin walking at your normal pace. When I tell you, "look up," keep walking straight, but tip your head and look up. Keep looking up until I tell you, "look down." Then keep walking straight and turn your head down. Keep looking down until I tell you, "look straight," then keep walking straight, but return your head to the center.

Grading: Mark the lowest category that applies.

(3) Normal: Performs head turns with no change in gait.

(2) Mild impairment: Performs task with slight change in gait velocity, i.e., minor disruption to smooth gait path or uses walking aid.

(1) Moderate impairment: Performs task with moderate change in gait velocity, slows down, staggers but recovers, can continue to walk.

(0) Severe impairment: Performs task with severe disruption of gait, i.e., staggers outside 15-inch path, loses balance, stops, reaches for wall.

5. Gait and pivot turn_____

Instructions: Begin walking at your normal pace. When I tell you, "turn and stop," turn as quickly as you can to face the opposite direction and stop.

Grading: Mark the lowest category that applies.

(3) Normal: Pivot-turns safely within 3 sec and stops quickly with no loss of balance.

(2) Mild impairment: Pivot-turns safely in more than 3 sec and stops with no loss of balance.

(1) Moderate impairment: Turns slowly, requires verbal cueing, requires several small steps to catch balance following turn and stop.

(0) Severe impairment: Cannot turn safely; requires assistance to turn and stop.

(continued)

Assessment Tool 15-1

Dynamic Gait Index

6. Step over obstacle_____

Instructions: Begin walking at your normal speed; when you come to the obstacles, step over them, not around them, and keep walking.

Grading: Mark the lowest category that applies.

(3) Normal: Is able to step over obstacles without changing gait speed; no evidence of imbalance.

(2) Mild impairment: Is able to step over obstacles but must slow down and adjust steps to clear obstacles safely.

(1) Moderate impairment: Is able to step over obstacles but must stop, then step over. Instability may be present. May require verbal cueing.

(0) Severe impairment: Cannot perform without assistance.

7. Step around obstacles_____

Instructions: Begin walking at your normal speed. When you come to the first cone (about 6 ft away), walk around it to the right. When you come to the second cone (6 ft past first cone), walk around it to the left.

Grading: Mark the lowest category that applies.

(3) Normal: Is able to walk around cones safely without changing gait speed; no evidence of imbalance.

(2) Mild impairment: Is able to step around both cones but must slow down and adjust steps to clear cones.

(1) Moderate impairment: Is able to clear cones but must significantly slow speed to accomplish task or requires verbal cueing.

(0) Severe impairment: Unable to clear cones, walks into one or both cones, or requires physical assistance.

8. Steps_____

Instructions: Walk up these stairs as you would at home (i.e., using the rail if necessary). At the top, turn around and walk down.

Grading: Mark the lowest category that applies.

(3) Normal: Alternating feet, no rail.

(2) Mild impairment: Alternating feet, must use rail.

(1) Moderate impairment: Two feet to a stair; must use rail.

(0) Severe impairment: Cannot do safely.

Functional Gait Assessment. The Functional Gait Assessment (FGA) tool is a 10-item gait assessment based on the DGI (Wrisley et al., 2004); it is shown in Assessment Tool 15.2. Wrisley and colleagues examined the psychometric properties of the FGA within a population of patients with vestibular disorders. Interrater reliability was good (ICC = 0.86), as was intrarater reliability (ICC = 0.74). Concurrent validity with other balance measures, including the TUG (r = ~0.50), DGI (r = 0.80), number of falls (r = ~0.66), Activities-specific Balance Confidence Scale (ABC scale) (r = 0.64), and Dizziness Handicap Index (r = ~0.64). A cutoff score of 22/30 was effective in classifying fall risk in older adults and predicting unexplained falls in community-dwelling older adults (Wrisley & Kumar, 2010).

Stops Walking When Talking. The Stops Walking When Talking (SWWT) test examines the effect of a secondary task, talking, on walking. In this test, the examiner begins a conversation with a walking patient; the patient who stops walking in order to talk defines a positive response. The SWWT test has been found to be a good predictor of falls among frail, institutionalized, older adults (Lundin-Olsson et al., 1997), with 95% specificity but only 48% sensitivity. The SWWT test did not predict falls in persons with Parkinson's disease (Bloem et al., 2000). Hyndman and Ashburn (2004) examined the predictive ability of the SWWT test following stroke. Of the 63 subjects tested, 26 stopped walking when talking, and 16 of them fell during the 6-month follow-up period. Thus, in persons with stroke, the SWWT test had a specificity of 70% (23 of 33) and a sensitivity of 53% (16 of 30).

The SWWT test is limited because a positive outcome is defined relative to whether a patient stops walking when talking. Thus, a patient who slows but does not stop walking during the performance of a secondary task will not be identified by the SWWT test. In an effort to capture patients who slow but do not stop walking when talking, clinicians have examined the effect of a secondary task on usual gait speed measured during a 4-, 8-, or 10-m walk test. A reduction in gait speed during performance of a secondary task has been shown in a variety of patients, including those with stroke (Bowen et al., 2001), Parkinson's disease (Rochester et al., 2004), and older adults at risk for falls (Shumway-Cook et al., 2000).

Assessment Tool 15-2

Functional Gait Assessment (FGA)

Requirements: A marked 6-m (20-ft) walkway that is marked with a 30.48-cm (12-in.) width.

1. Gait level surface_____

Instructions: Walk at your normal speed from here to the next mark (6 m [20 ft]).

Grading: Mark the highest category that applies.

(3) Normal—Walks 6 m (20 ft) in less than 5.5 sec, no assistive devices, good speed, no evidence for imbalance, normal gait pattern, deviates no more than 15.24 cm (6 in.) outside the 30.48-cm (12-in.) walkway width.

(2) Mild impairment—Walks 6 m (20 ft) in less than 7 sec but more than 5.5 sec, uses assistive device, slower speed, mild gait deviations, or deviates 15.24 to 25.4 cm (6 to 10 in.) outside the 30.48-cm (12-in.) walkway width.

(1) Moderate impairment—Walks 6 m (20 ft), slow speed, abnormal gait pattern, evidence for imbalance, or deviates 25.4 to 38.1 cm (10 to 15 in.) outside the 30.48-cm (12-in.) walkway width. Requires more than 7 sec to ambulate 6 m (20 ft).

(0) Severe impairment—Cannot walk 6 m (20 ft) without assistance, severe gait deviations or imbalance, deviates more than 38.1 cm (15 in.) outside the 30.48-cm (12-in.) walkway width or reaches and touches the wall.

2. Change in gait speed_____

Instructions: Begin walking at your normal pace (for 1.5 m [5 ft]). When I tell you "go," walk as fast as you can (for 1.5 m [5 ft]). When I tell you "slow," walk as slowly as you can (for 1.5 m [5 ft]).

Grading: Mark the highest category that applies.

(3) Normal—Able to smoothly change walking speed without loss of balance or gait deviation. Shows a significant difference in walking speeds between normal, fast, and slow speeds. Deviates no more than 15.24 cm (6 in.) outside the 30.48-cm (12-in.) walkway width.

(2) Mild impairment—Is able to change speed but demonstrates mild gait deviations, deviates 15.24 to 25.4 cm (6 to 10 in.) outside the 30.48-cm (12-in.) walkway width, or no gait deviations but unable to achieve a significant change in velocity, or uses an assistive device.

(1) Moderate impairment—Makes only minor adjustments to walking speed, or accomplishes a change in speed with significant gait deviations, deviates 25.4 to 38.1 cm (10 to 15 in.) outside the 30.48-cm (12-in.) walkway width, or changes speed but loses balance but is able to recover and continue walking.

(0) Severe impairment—Cannot change speeds, deviates more than 38.1 cm (15 in.) outside 30.48-cm (12-in.) walkway width, or loses balance and has to reach for wall or be caught.

3. Gait with horizontal head turns_____

Instructions: Walk from here to the next mark 6 m (20 ft) away. Begin walking at your normal pace. Keep walking straight; after three steps, turn your head to the right and keep walking straight while looking to the right. After three more steps, turn your head to the left and keep walking straight while looking left. Continue alternating looking right and left every three steps until you have completed two repetitions in each direction.

Grading: Mark the highest category that applies.

(3) Normal—Performs head turns smoothly with no change in gait. Deviates no more than 15.24 cm (6 in.) outside the 30.48-cm (12-in.) walkway width.

(2) Mild impairment—Performs head turns smoothly, with slight change in gait velocity (e.g., minor disruption to smooth gait path), deviates 15.24 to 25.4 cm (6 to 10 in.) outside the 30.48-cm (12-in.) walkway width, or uses an assistive device.

(1) Moderate impairment—Performs head turns with moderate change in gait velocity, slows down, deviates 25.4 to 38.1 cm (10 to 15 in.) outside the 30.48-cm (12-in.) walkway width but recovers, and can continue to walk.

(0) Severe impairment—Performs task with severe disruption of gait (e.g., staggers 38.1 cm [15 in.] outside the 30.48-cm [12-in.] walkway width, loses balance, stops, or reaches for wall).

4. Gait with vertical head turns_____

Instructions: Walk from here to the next mark (6 m [20 ft]). Begin walking at your normal pace. Keep walking straight; after three steps, tip your head up and keep walking straight while looking up. After three more steps,

(continued)

Assessment Tool 15-2

Functional Gait Assessment (FGA)

tip your head down, keep walking straight while looking down. Continue alternating looking up and down every three steps until you have completed two repetitions in each direction.

Grading: Mark the highest category that applies.

(3) Normal—Performs head turns with no change in gait. Deviates no more than 15.24 cm (6 in.) outside the 30.48-cm (12-in.) walkway width.

(2) Mild impairment—Performs task with slight change in gait velocity (e.g., minor disruption to smooth gait path), deviates 15.24 to 25.4 cm (6 to 10 in.) outside the 30.48-cm (12-in.) walkway width, or uses assistive device.

(1) Moderate impairment—Performs task with moderate change in gait velocity, slows down, deviates 25.4 to 38.1 cm (10 to 15 in.) outside the 30.48-cm (12-in.) walkway width but recovers, and can continue to walk.

(0) Severe impairment—Performs task with severe disruption of gait (e.g., staggers 38.1 cm [15 in.] outside the 30.48-cm [12-in.] walkway width, loses balance, stops, reaches for wall).

5. Gait and pivot turn_____

Instructions: Begin walking at your normal pace. When I tell you to turn and stop, turn as quickly as you can to face the opposite direction and stop.

Grading: Mark the highest category that applies.

(3) Normal—Pivot turns safely within 3 sec and stops quickly with no loss of balance.

(2) Mild impairment—Pivot turns safely in <3 sec and stops with no loss of balance, or pivot turns safely within 3 sec and stops with mild imbalance, requires small steps to catch balance.

(1) Moderate impairment—Turns slowly, requires verbal cueing, or requires several small steps to catch balance following turn and stop.

(0) Severe impairment—Cannot turn safely, requires assistance to turn and stop.

6. Step over obstacle_____

Instructions: Begin walking at your normal speed. When you come to the shoe box, step over it, not around it, and keep walking.

Grading: Mark the highest category that applies.

(3) Normal—Is able to step over two stacked shoe boxes taped together (22.86 cm [9 in.] total height) without changing gait speed; no evidence of imbalance.

(2) Mild impairment—Is able to step over one shoe box (11.43 cm [4.5 in.] total height) without changing gait speed; no evidence of imbalance.

(1) Moderate impairment—Is able to step over one shoe box (11.43 cm [4.5 in.] total height), but must slow down and adjust steps to clear box safely. May require verbal cueing.

(0) Severe impairment—Cannot perform without assistance.

7. Gait with narrow base of support_____

Instructions: Walk on the floor with arms folded across the chest, feet aligned heel to toe in tandem for a distance of 3.6 m [12 ft]. The number of steps taken in a straight line are counted, for a maximum of 10 steps.

Grading: Mark the highest category that applies.

(3) Normal—Is able to walk for 10 steps heel to toe with no staggering.

(2) Mild impairment—Walks 7 to 9 steps.

(1) Moderate impairment—Walks 4 to 7 steps.

(0) Severe impairment—Walks less than 4 steps heel to toe or cannot perform without assistance.

8. Gait with eyes closed_____

Instructions: Walk at your normal speed from here to the next mark (6 m [20 ft]) with your eyes closed.

Grading: Mark the highest category that applies.

(3) Normal—Walks 6 m (20 ft), no assistive devices, good speed, no evidence of imbalance, normal gait pattern, deviates no more than 15.24 cm (6 in.) outside the 30.48-cm (12-in.) walkway width. Walks 6 m (20 ft) in less than 7 seconds.

(2) Mild impairment—Walks 6 m (20 ft), uses assistive device, slower speed, mild gait deviations, deviates 15.24 to 25.4 cm (6 to 10 in.) outside the 30.48-cm (12-in.) walkway width. Ambulates 6 m (20 ft) in less than 9 seconds but more than 7 sec.

(1) Moderate impairment—Walks 6 m (20 ft), slow speed, abnormal gait pattern, evidence for imbalance, deviates 25.4 to 38.1 cm (10–15 in.) outside the 30.48-cm (12-in.) walkway width. Requires more than 9 seconds to walk 6 m (20 ft).

(continued)

Assessment Tool 15-2

Functional Gait Assessment (FGA)

(0) Severe impairment—Cannot walk 6 m (20 ft) without assistance, severe gait deviations or imbalance, deviates more than 38.1 cm (15 in.) outside the 30.48-cm (12-in.) walkway width or will not attempt task.

9. Ambulating backward_____

Instructions: Walk backward until I tell you to stop.

Grading: Mark the highest category that applies.

(3) Normal—Walks 6 m (20 ft), no assistive devices, good speed, no evidence for imbalance, normal gait pattern, deviates no more than 15.24 cm (6 in.) outside the 30.48-cm (12-in.) walkway width.

(2) Mild impairment—Walks 6 m (20 ft), uses assistive device, slower speed, mild gait deviations, deviates 15.24 to 25.4 cm (6 to 10 in.) outside the 30.48-cm (12-in.) walkway width.

(1) Moderate impairment—Walks 6 m (20 ft), slow speed, abnormal gait pattern, evidence for imbalance, deviates 25.4 to 38.1 cm (10 to 15 in.) outside the 30.48-cm (12-in) walkway width.

(0) Severe impairment—Cannot walk 6 m (20 ft) without assistance, severe gait deviations or imbalance, deviates more than 38.1 cm (15 in.) outside the 30.48-cm (12-in.) walkway width or will not attempt task.

10. Steps_____

Instructions: Walk up these stairs as you would at home (i.e., using the rail if necessary). At the top turn around and walk down.

Grading: Mark the highest category that applies.

(3) Normal—Alternating feet, no rail.

(2) Mild impairment—Alternating feet, must use rail.

(1) Moderate impairment—Two feet to a stair; must use rail.

(0) Severe impairment—Cannot do safely.

Total score: _____ (Maximum score: 30)

Adapted with permission from Dynamic Gait Index. Modified and reprinted with permission of authors and Lippincott Williams & Wilkins (http://www.lww.com).

(Adapted from Wrisley DM, Marchett GF, Kuharsky DK, Whitney SL. Reliability, internal consistency, and validity of data obtained with the functional gait assessment. Phys Ther 2004;84:906–918, with permission of the American Physical Therapy Association. This material is copyrighted, and any further reproduction or distribution requires written permission from APTA.)

Physical Performance and Mobility Examination. The Physical Performance and Mobility Examination (PPME) was developed to measure performance of physical function and mobility in hospitalized and frail older adults (Winograd et al., 1994). The PPME was designed to assess function without overtaxing frail or acutely ill subjects. Six mobility tasks integral to everyday life were chosen for the test, which does not examine constituent abilities such as strength and range of motion. This test includes both high-level tasks, such as standing up five times from a chair, and lower-level tasks, such as bed mobility and transfer skills. The test is summarized in Table 15.2. Shown are the list of tasks, a description of how the task is to be performed, and the response dimensions.

Rivermead Mobility Index (RMI). The RMI (Collen et al., 1991), shown in Assessment Tool 15.3, quantifies mobility function using 15 activities. Fourteen of these activities are scored via the patient's self-report (1 = yes, 0 = no). Item 5, standing unsupported for 10 seconds, is directly observed. The RMI is simple and quick and can be used in a variety of environments. It has been shown to be both a reliable and valid test of mobility function (Forlander & Bohannon, 1999).

Emory Functional Ambulation Profile. The Emory Functional Ambulation Profile (EFAP) (Baer & Wolf, 2001) is a modification of the Functional Ambulation Profile (FAP) (Wolf, 1979) a timed measure of walking under five environmental challenges shown in Assessment Tool 15.4. The five timed subscores are added to derive a total score. The EFAP has excellent interrater reliability (ICC = 0.999), test–retest reliability (ICC = 0.998) and good correlation with the Berg Balance Test; it thus appears to be a reliable gait assessment measure for patients with stroke.

High-Level Mobility Assessment. To overcome the ceiling effect of many of the current measures of mobility function Williams and colleagues developed the High-Level Mobility Assessment (HiMAT). This test is shown in Assessment Tool 15.5. The test has good interrater and test retest reliability, internal consistency and good concurrent validity (Williams et al., 2006a, b; Williams & Morris, 2009).

Predicting Participation from Functional Activity Measures. An important part of rehabilitation of persons with gait disorders is predicting the ability to participate in mobility-related activities within his

TABLE 15.2 Physical Performance and Mobility Examination

Tasks	Description	Response dimension
1. Bed mobility	Sit up in bed from lying down	Need for assistance, time to complete
2. Transfers	Stand up from bed (from sitting) move to chair, sit down, stand up from chair once	Need for assistance, use of arms
3. Multiple chair stands	Stand up from chair 5 times	Need for assistance, use of arms, time to complete
4. Standing balance	Ability to hold 4 positions for 10 sec, feet apart, feet together, semitandem, tandem	Need for assistance, time
5. Step up	Step up one step with handrail	Need for assistance, use of handrail
6. Ambulation	Walk 5 m, 2 trials	Time at usual pace, number of steps

Reprinted with permission from Winograd CH, Lemsky CM, Nevitt MC, et al. Development of a physical performance and mobility examination. J Am Geriatr Soc 1994;42:743–749.

Assessment Tool 15-3

Rivermead Mobility Index

Ask the patient each question. Score 1 for yes, 0 for no. Observe for question 5.

Topic and Question **Date**

1. Turning over in bed: Do you turn over from your back to your side without help?
2. Lying to sitting: From lying in bed, do you get up to sit on the edge of the bed on your own?
3. Sitting balance: Do you sit on the edge of the bed without holding on for 10 sec?
4. Sitting to standing: Do you stand up from any chair in less than 15 seconds and stand there for 15 sec using hands and/or an aid if necessary?
5. Standing unsupported: Ask to stand. Observe standing for 10 sec without any aid.
6. Transfer: Do you manage to move from bed to chair and back without any help?
7. Walking indoors with an aid if necessary: Do you walk 10 m, with an aid if necessary, but with no standby help?
8. Stairs: Do you manage a flight of stairs without help?
9. Walking outside on even ground: Do you walk around outside on pavements without help?

Topic and Question **Date**

10. Walking inside with no aid: Do you walk 10 m inside with no ankle–foot orthoses, brace, splint, or other aid (including furniture or walls) without help?
11. Picking up off floor: Do you manage to walk 5 meters, pick something up from the floor, and then walk back without help?
12. Walking outside on uneven ground: Do you walk over uneven ground, such as grass, gravel, snow, ice, without help?
13. Bathing: Do you get into and out of a bath or shower by yourself unsupervised and without help?
14. Up and down four steps: Do you manage to go up and down four steps with no rails but using an aid if necessary?
15. Running: Do you run 10 meters without limping in 4 seconds (fast walk, not limping, is acceptable)?

Reprinted with permission from Collen FM, Wade DT, Robb GF, Bradshaw CM. The Rivermead Mobility Index: a further development of the Rivermead Motor Assessment. Int Disabil Studies 1991;13:50–54.

Assessment Tool 15-4

Modified Emory Functional Ambulation Profile Scale (mEFAP)

The mEFAP is composed of five subtasks: (1) floor, (2) carpet, (3) up and go, (4) obstacles, and (5) stairs. Each subject is given a rest period between the performance of each subtask long enough for the examiner to explain and demonstrate the next component. Each subject is instructed to use an assistive device or receive manual assistance as needed and to wear a gait belt during performance of all subtasks. Upon completion of the test the examiner calculates a total mEFAP score.

1. Floor

Setup: A 1-m strip of masking tape is placed on a hard-surfaced floor at the starting point. Five meters ahead of the starting point, a 2-cm piece of masking tape marks the end point. A small piece of tape is used to mark the end point so that subjects do not decelerate in anticipation of the finish line.

Instructions: "When I say 'go,' walk at your normal, comfortable pace until I say 'stop.'" Assist subject as needed in placing toes on starting-line tape.

Scoring: Begin timing when tester says "go"; stop timing when subject crosses the 5-m line. Multiply time recorded by appropriate factor according to level of assistive device used during the task: no assistance, × 1; ankle–foot orthosis (AFO), × 2; single-point cane, × 3; hemiwalker or quad cane, × 4; AFO + single-point cane, × 5; AFO + hemiwalker or AFO + quad cane, × 6.

_____Floor time

_____Multiplying factor (assistive device: ________________________)

_____Total floor score

2. Carpet

Setup: A piece of short-pile carpet, no less than 7 m long and 2 m wide, is taped securely to the floor. Starting point is marked with a 1-m strip of masking tape. End point is marked exactly 5 m from the starting point with a 2-cm piece of masking tape. Both starting point and end point are at least 1 m from the edge of the carpet.

Instructions: "When I say 'go,' walk at your normal, comfortable pace until I say 'stop.'" Provide patient assistance as needed in placing toes on starting-line tape.

Scoring: Begin timing when tester says "go"; stop timing when subject crosses the 5-m line. Multiply time recorded by appropriate factor according to level of assistive device used during the task: no assistance, × 1; AFO, × 2; single-point cane, × 3; hemiwalker or quad cane, × 4; AFO + single-point cane, × 5; AFO + hemiwalker or AFO + quad cane, × 6.

_____Carpet time

_____Multiplying factor (assistive device: ________________________)

_____Total carpet score

3. Up and go

Setup: Standard armchair with a 46-cm seat height is placed on the hard-surfaced floor. Three meters away, a 1-m strip of black tape is placed on the floor.

Instructions: "Next, you will sit in this chair with your back against the back of the chair and your arms resting on the armrests. When I say 'go,' you will stand up from the chair, walk at your normal comfortable pace past this line, turn around, walk back to the chair, and sit down, making sure your back is against the back of the chair."

Scoring: Start timing when examiner says "go"; stop when the subject is fully seated with back against the chair. Multiply time recorded by appropriate factor according to level of assistive device used during the task: no assistance, × 1; AFO, × 2; single-point cane, × 3; hemiwalker or quad cane, × 4; AFO + single-point cane, × 5; AFO + hemiwalker or AFO + quad cane, × 6.

_____Up and go time

_____Multiplying factor (assistive device: ________________________)

_____Total up and go time score

4. Obstacles

Setup: A 1-m piece of masking tape is placed on a hard-surfaced floor to mark the starting point. A brick is placed on the floor at the 1 1/2-m mark and the 3-m mark. A 40-gal rubber trash can is placed at the 5-m mark.

Instructions: "When I say 'go,' walk forward at your normal, comfortable pace and step over each brick. Then, walk around the trash can from either the left or right. Then walk back stepping over the bricks again. Continue walking until I say 'stop.'"

Scoring: Start timing when examiner says "go"; stop when the subject steps crosses the end line. Multiply time recorded by appropriate factor according to level of assistive device used during the task: no assistance, × 1; AFO, × 2; single-point cane, × 3; hemiwalker or quad cane, × 4; AFO + single-point cane, × 5; AFO + hemiwalker or AFO + quad cane, × 6.

_____Obstacle time

_____Multiplying factor (assistive device: ________________________)

_____Total obstacle score

(continued)

Assessment Tool 15-4

Modified Emory Functional Ambulation Profile Scale (mEFAP)

5. Stairs

Setup: Stairs with four steps, hand railings, and the following measurements are used: 26.04-cm stair depth, 75.57-cm stair width, 15.24-cm stair height, 76.20-cm platform depth, and 75.57-cm platform width. A 1-m piece of masking tape is placed 25 cm from the base of the first step.

Instructions: "When I say 'go,' walk up the stairs at your normal, comfortable pace to the top of the stairs, turn around, and come back down. You may use the handrails if needed. I will follow behind you for safety." Assist subject as needed in placing toes on starting-line tape.

Scoring: Start timing when examiner says "go"; stop timing when subject's nonlead foot comes in firm contact with the floor. Multiply time recorded by appropriate factor according to level of assistive device used during the task: no assistance, × 1; AFO, × 2; single-point cane, × 3; hemiwalker or quad cane, × 4; AFO + single-point cane, × 5; AFO + hemiwalker or AFO + quad cane, × 6.

_____Stairs time

_____Multiplying factor (assistive device: _______________________)

_____Total stairs score

Total score_____

Modified with permission from Baer HR, Wolf SL. Modified Emory Functional Ambulation Profile: an outcome measure for the rehabilitation of poststroke gait dysfunction. Stroke 2001;32:973–979.

or her own environment (level of mobility disability). However, there are few guidelines to assist the clinician in the prediction process. The relationships among impairments, limitations in functional abilities (capacity) and level of participation (mobility disability) are not clear. Gait velocity measured in the clinic has been shown to relate to strength (an impairment measure) but neither measure has been shown to correlate well with home versus community independence (a disability measure) (Robinson et al., 2007; 2010; Lord & Rochester, 2005).

Hoffer et al. (1973) suggested a classification of walking disability including the following: nonambulator (a person who cannot meet the requirements of ambulating within the home or community); nonfunctional ambulator (an individual who walks for therapeutic but not functional purposes); household ambulator (an individual who can safely perform the tasks that define mobility within the home environment); and community ambulator (no limitations to the individual's ability to meet the demands of moving within the community). This classification system was expanded and modified by Perry et al. (1995) and is summarized in Table 15.3. Perry and colleagues studied 147 patients who had had a stroke in order to identify the best combination of measures that predicted mobility status. Measures used to predict level of ambulation included a self-report questionnaire regarding walking abilities, calculation of stride characteristics using a footswitch stride analyzer, a test of proprioception, and the upright motor control test. This test is shown and explained in Figure 15.2.

Gait velocity was one of several variables important in predicting walking classification. A velocity of 0.42 m/sec predicted community ambulation. The mean walking velocity of the highest category of community walkers among the stroke subjects was 0.8 m/sec, significantly slower than the normal population value of 1.33 m/sec, and not fast enough to cross a street safely.

In addition to gait velocity, four ambulation tasks were found to be critical to determining the level of mobility disability. These included the ability to manage: (1) changes in surface levels and terrain irregularity, (2) obstacle avoidance, (3) distance, and (4) manual handling of loads. Interestingly, while the ability to manage a change in level such as curbs was found to be critical to leaving home, the ability to manage stairs was not.

Perry's findings were consistent with a study by Lerner-Frankiel and colleagues (1990), who reported that the requirements for being a community ambulator included the ability to: (1) walk at greater than 33% of a normal adult's velocity (0.45 m/sec), or about 1.0 mph; (2) walk 80 m/min for 13 to 27 m in order to cross a street safely in the normal time allotted by stoplights; and (3) negotiate 7- to 8-in. curbs independently (with assistive devices as needed). The study also found that in general clinicians underestimated the distance and speed needed to function independently within a community environment (Lerner-Frankiel et al., 1990). This may be because tests of normal activities of daily living (ADL) skills, for example, the FIM, often define complete independence in locomotor skills as being

Assessment Tool 15-5

HiMAT: High-Level Mobility Assessment Tool

DATE ______________________

DATE OF ACCIDENT ______________

DIAGNOSIS ___________________

AFFECTED SIDE LEFT/RIGHT

PATIENT
ID
LABEL

		SCORE					
ITEM	**PERFORMANCE**	**0**	**1**	**2**	**3**	**4**	**5**
WALK	sec	X	>6.6	5.4-6.6	4.3-5.3	<4.3	X
WALK BACKWARD	sec		>13.3	8.1-13.3	5.8-8.0	<5.8	X
WALK ON TOES	sec		>8.9	7.0-8.9	5.4-6.9	<5.4	X
WALK OVER OBSTACLE	sec		>7.1	5.4-7.1	4.5-5.3	<4.5	X
RUN	sec		>2.7	2.0-2.7	1.7-1.9	<1.7	X
SKIP	sec		>4.0	3.5-4.0	3.0-3.4	<3.0	X
HOP FORWARD (AFFECTED)	sec		>7.0	5.3-7.0	4.1-5.2	<4.1	X
BOUND (AFFECTED)	1) cm 2) 3)		<80	80-103	104-132	>132	X
BOUND (LESS-AFFECTED)	1) cm 2) 3)		<82	82-105	106-129	>129	X
UP STAIRS DEPENDENT (Rail **OR** not reciprocal: if not, score 5 and rate below)	sec		>22.8	14.6-22.8	12.3-14.5	<12.3	
UP STAIRS INDEPENDENT (No rail **AND** reciprocal: if not score 0 and rate above)	sec		>9.1	7.6-9.1	6.8-7.5	<6.8	X
DOWN STAIRS DEPENDENT (Rail **OR** not reciprocal: if not score 5 and rate below)	sec		>24.3	17.6-24.3	12.8-17.5	<12.8	
DOWN STAIRS INDEPENDENT (No rail **AND** reciprocal: if not score 0 and rate above)	sec		>8.4	6.6-8.4	5.8-6.5	<5.8	X
	SUBTOTAL						

TOTAL HIMAT SCORE /54

Please notify Gavin Williams at gavin@neuro-solutions.net or gavin.williams@epworth.org.au so that the use of the HiMAT can be tracked.

(continued)

Assessment Tool 15-5

HiMAT: High-Level Mobility Assessment Tool

INSTRUCTIONS

Subject suitability:	The HiMAT is appropriate for assessing people with high-level balance and mobility problems. The minimal mobility requirement for testing is independent walking over 20 m without gait aids. Orthoses are permitted.
Item testing:	Testing takes 5–10 minutes. Patients are allowed 1 practice trial for each item.
Instructions:	Patients are instructed to perform at their maximum safe speed except for the bounding and stair items.
Walking:	The middle 10 m of a 20 m trial is timed.
Walk backward:	As for walking.
Walk on toes:	As for walking. Any heel contact during the middle 10 m is recorded as a fail.
Walk over obstacle:	As for walking. A house brick is placed across the walkway at the midpoint. Patients must step over the brick without contacting it. A fail is recorded if patients step around the brick or make contact with the brick.
Run:	The middle 10 m of a 20 m trial is timed. A fail is recorded if patients fail to have a consistent flight phase during the trial.
Skipping:	The middle 10 m of a 20 m trial is timed. A fail is recorded if patients fail to have a consistent flight phase during the trial.
Hop forward:	Patients stand on their more affected leg and hop forward. The time to hop 10 m is recorded.
Bound (affected).	A bound is a jump from one leg to the other with a flight phase. Patients stand behind a line on their less affected leg, hands on hips, and jump forward **landing on their more affected** leg. Each bound is measured from the line to the heel of the landing leg. The average of three trials is recorded.
Bound (less-affected).	Patients stand behind a line on their more affected leg, hands on hips, and jump forward **landing on their less affected** leg. The average of three trials is recorded.
Up stairs:	Patients are asked to walk up a flight of 14 stairs as they normally would and at their normal speed. The trial is recorded from when the patient starts until both feet are at the top. Patients who use a rail or a nonreciprocal pattern are scored on **Up Stairs Dependent**. Patients who ascend the stairs reciprocally without a rail are scored on **Up Stairs Independent** and get an additional 5 points in the last column of Up Stairs Dependent.
Down stairs:	As for Up stairs.
Scoring:	All times and distances are recorded in the "performance" column. The corresponding score for each item is then circled and each column is then subtotaled. Subtotals are then added to calculate the HiMAT score.

able to walk 150 ft safely (Keith et al., 1987). However, this standard may underestimate the requirements for being truly independent within the community.

The functional scale proposed by Hoffer and expanded by Perry has been modified by Viosca and colleagues (2005). The Functional Ambulation Classification (FAC) scale includes six functional levels ranging from 0 (absence of walking capacity) to 5 (recovery of normal ambulation). This scale is shown in Table 15.4. This scale was tested on 31 patients with poststroke hemiplegia and a control group of five healthy adults. The test was found to have good inter-rater reliability (k = 0.74) and a strong correlation to walking velocity (Spearman correlation = 0.84).

A functional walking classification scale for children was developed by researchers at Gillette Hospital (Novacheck et al., 2000). The Gillette Functional Walking Scale, shown in Assessment Tool 15.6 is a parent report, 10-level walking scale, encompassing a wide range of walking abilities from nonambulatory

TABLE 15.3 Perry's Proposed Scheme for Classifying Mobility Function

Discriminant Functions	Functional Walking Category					
	Physiological	Limited Household	Unlimited Household	Most-Limited Community	Least-Limited Community	Community
Bathroom	4.32*	11.78*	16.93†	16.96†	16.60†	17.89
Bedroom	3.39*	8.35*	12.68†	11.83†	11.25†	10.83
Enter/exit	1.80‡	3.67‡	5.47*	7.83†	7.24†	7.05
Curb	−0.14‡	1.94‡	4.77*	7.04†	7.94†	8.40
Grocery	−0.06†	−0.37†	−0.01†	−0.03*	1.61†	1.58
Shopping center, uncrowded	0.21†	0.74†	1.54†	1.34*	3.79†	2.98
Shopping center, crowded	0.30‡	0.02‡	0.05‡	−0.22†	−2.10*	1.19
Constant	−6.70	−33.51	−76.24	−88.13	−92.45	−101.47

*Questionnaire item had a strong influence on placement between the two adjacent walking groups.
†Questionnaire item had minimal or no influence on placement between the two adjacent walking groups.
‡Questionnaire item had moderate influence on placement between the two adjacent walking groups.

to community ambulation. In a study with 41 children with neurologic pathology (83% of the children had a diagnosis of cerebral palsy) resulting in a range of ambulation skills, the test was found to have good test–retest reliability among parents and good inter-rater reliability between parents and community caregivers. The test had good content and construct validity, as indicated by a significant correlation with the pediatric version of the Functional Independence Measure (Wee FIM), and a significant inverse correlation to laboratory measures of oxygen consumption.

Patla and Shumway-Cook (1999) suggested that classifying levels of mobility disability first requires an understanding of the external factors that determine the complexity and difficulty of mobility within various environments. They define eight external factors, which they call "dimensions," that operationally define the demands of community mobility. These include both distance and time parameters, as well as ambient conditions (defined by both light levels and weather conditions), terrain characteristics (including both geometric properties such as curbs and stairs, and physical properties such as compliance and friction), external physical loads, attentional demands, postural transitions (e.g., stop, start, head turns, changes in direction), and traffic level (e.g., avoiding collisions with stationary or moving people and objects).

Thus, functional mobility within a community environment requires not only the ability to walk safely in fairly simple and predictable environments, but also the ability to modify and adapt gait to both expected and unexpected disturbances and challenges to locomotion. Mobility disability is defined not by the number of tasks a person can or cannot perform, but rather by the range of environmental contexts under which tasks can be carried out. The more disabled one is, the more restrictive the dimensions under which one can safely move about. For example, the patient can walk only a limited distance, or at a certain speed, the patient cannot carry any physical load because an assistive device is required, or the patient can walk (steady state) but cannot safely perform postural transitions (e.g., start, stop, or turn).

Limitations of Functional Gait Measures

All functional measures, whether of mobility, balance, or general motor control, are indicators of the end product only and do not provide information about the way performance is achieved. Thus, these measures do not provide insight into underlying impairments that require treatment. However, functional measures are good indicators of overall function and, therefore, are important indices of change.

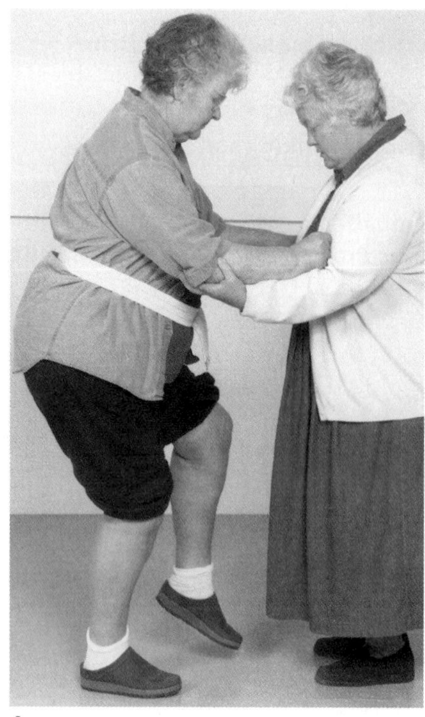

A

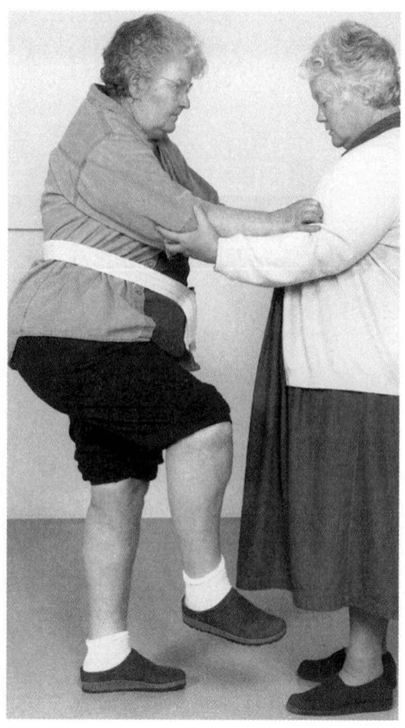

B

FIGURE 15.2 Upright motor control test. A, Knee extension: This test involves extension in control of the body weight during single-limb stance. The patient bends both knees to approximately 30 degrees and then lifts the unaffected leg off the ground. Knee extension grades: strong, straightens the flexed knee to full extension; moderate, supports body weight on the flexed knee; weak, unable to support body weight on the flexed knee. B, Knee flexion: This test involves knee flexion of the unloaded leg during single-limb stance. The patient stands as straight as possible and brings the knee and foot on the affected side up toward the chest as high and as fast as possible, and repeats this three times. Knee flexor grades: strong, joint flexes more than 60 degrees; weak, joint flexes less than 60 degrees or cannot complete three efforts in 10 seconds. (Adapted with permission from Perry J, Garrett M, Gronley JK, Mulroy SJ. Classification of walking handicap in the stroke population. Stroke 1995;26:982.)

Examination at the Strategy Level

Quantitative measures such as gait speed provide an objective measure of function but do not describe the quality of performance (e.g., the ways in which gait patterns deviate from normal). Therefore, examination of gait must include a systematic description of the strategies used by patients to meet the requirements inherent in locomotion.

Observational Gait Analysis

Observational gait analysis (OGA) is the most common method for examining gait in clinical practice (Krebs et al., 1985). OGA is the observation of kinematic patterns of movement used for gait. Observation of atypical kinematic patterns of movement are used to identify major gait deficits; however, nonobservable deficits, such as weakness, coordination, and spasticity, can be inferred only from observation and require confirmation with appropriate testing. OGA is used as both an evaluative tool (e.g., to monitor change over time) and as a diagnostic tool (e.g., to determine the causal factors producing atypical gait) (Lord et al., 1998; Winter, 1993). In OGA, the observer describes characteristics of gait without the aid of electronic devices.

There are many standardized forms available to help clinicians' structure their approach to visual gait analysis. One example was the gait assessment portion of the Performance-Oriented Mobility Assessment described in Chapter 11. Other examples of visual gait analysis forms that are helpful in guiding a clinical examination of gait patterns in the patient with neurologic impairments follow.

Rancho Los Amigos Gait Analysis Form. The Gait Analysis Form, shown in Assessment Tool 15.7, from the physical therapy department at the Rancho Los Amigos Hospital, Downey, CA, is a comprehen-

TABLE 15.4 Functional Ambulation Classification Scale

Score	Description
0	(Nonambulation): Absolute walking incapacity, even with external help.
1	(Nonfunctional ambulation): Dependent walking that requires permanent help of others. The patient must be firmly supported by one or two people and/or walking is possible only within a therapy session at home or at the hospital between parallel bards.
2	(Household ambulation): Walking is only possible indoors, on flat, horizontal surfaces, usually within a known and controlled area, such as in the home.
3	(Neighborhood ambulation): Patients are able to walk indoors and outdoors on uneven surfaces, and they are able to climb an occasional step or stair. Therefore, the patient is able to walk in the street, albeit within a limited and restricted walking distance.
4	(Independent community ambulation): Patients are able to walk on all types of irregular surfaces. They can ascend and descend steps, or stairs, ramps, curbs, etc. They have a considerable, even unrestricted, walking distance so that they are capable of shopping for food and accomplishing other basic chores. However, they are not considered normal walkers because they have aesthetic anomalies, such as an obvious limp.
5	(Normal ambulation): Walking is completely normal in both distance and appearance, both at home and outside and with an unlimited distance. There is no aesthetic anomaly or limp. They can tiptoe, walk on their heels and in tandem.

Reprinted with permission from Viosca E, Martinez JL, Almagro PL, Gracia A, Gonzalez C. Proposal and validation of a new functional ambulation classification scale for clinical use. Arch Phys Med Rehabil 2005;86:1234–1238.

Assessment Tool 15-6

Gillette Functional Walking Scale

Choose one answer below that best describes your child's typical walking ability (with the use of any needed assistive devices).

1. Cannot take any steps at all.
2. Can do some stepping on his/her own with the help of another person. Does not take full weight on feet: does not walk on a routine basis.
3. Walks for exercise in therapy and less than typical household distances. Usually requires assistance from another person.
4. Walks for household distances, but makes slow progress. Does not use walking at home as preferred mobility (primarily walks in therapy).
5. Walks more than 15–50 ft but only inside at home or school (walks for household distances).
6. Walks more than 15–50 ft outside the home, but usually uses a wheelchair or stroller for community distances or in congested areas.
7. Walks outside the home for community distances, but only on level surfaces (cannot perform on curbs, uneven terrain, or stairs without the assistance of another person).
8. Walks outside the home for community distances, is able to perform on curbs and uneven terrain in addition to level surfaces, but usually requires minimal assistance or supervision for safety.
9. Walks outside home for community distances, easily gets around on level ground, curbs, and uneven terrain but has difficulty or requires minimal assistance with running, climbing and/or stairs.
10. Walk, runs, and climbs on level and uneven terrain without difficulty or assistance.

Reprinted with permission from Novacheck TF, Stout JS, Tervo R. Reliability and validity of the Gillette Functional Assessment Questionnaire as an outcome measure in children with walking disabilities. J Pediatr Orthop 2000;20:76 (Table 1).

Assessment Tool 15-7
Rancho Los Amigos Gait Analysis Form

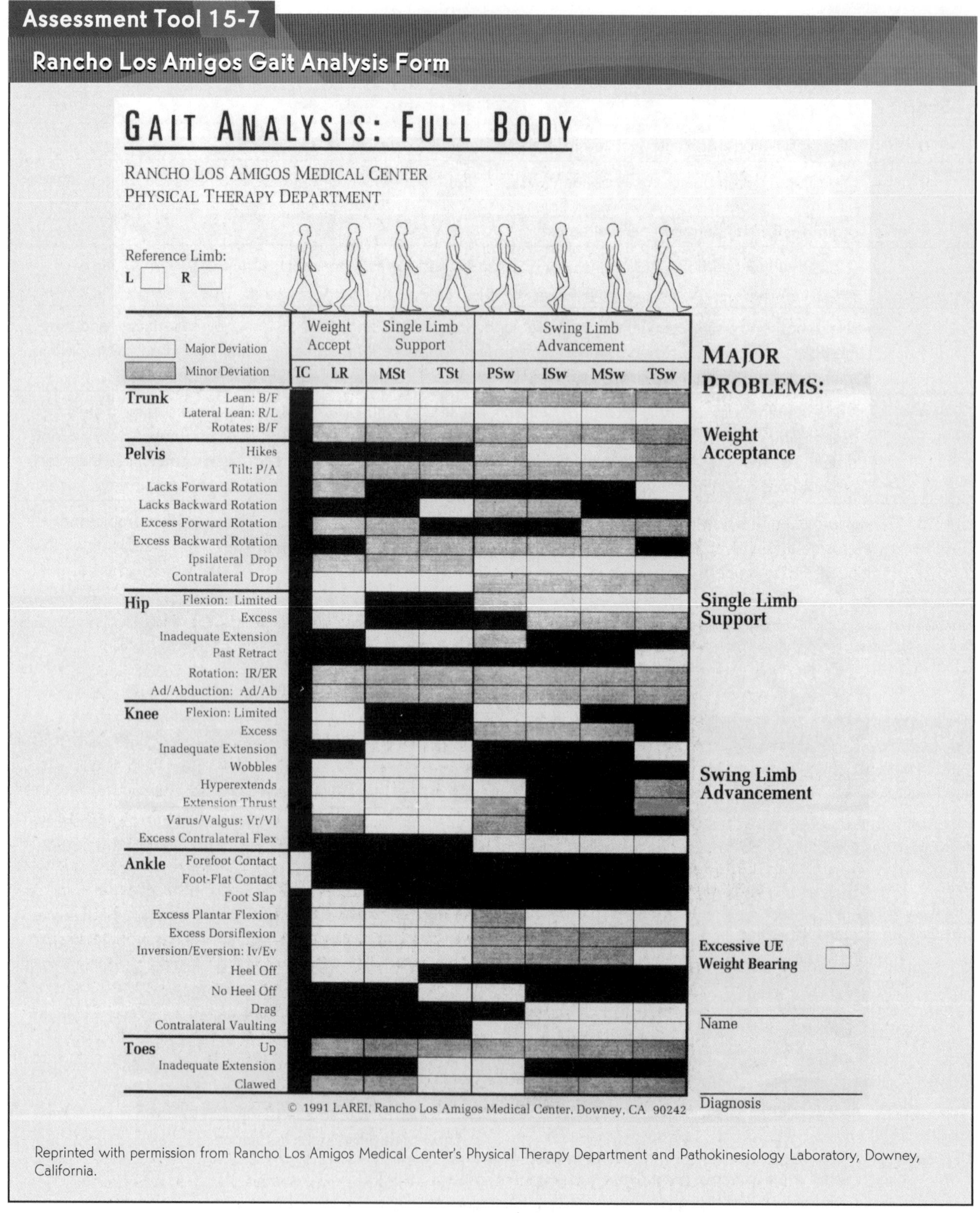

GAIT ANALYSIS: FULL BODY

RANCHO LOS AMIGOS MEDICAL CENTER
PHYSICAL THERAPY DEPARTMENT

Reference Limb:
L ☐ R ☐

☐ Major Deviation
☐ Minor Deviation

	Weight Accept		Single Limb Support		Swing Limb Advancement			
	IC	LR	MSt	TSt	PSw	ISw	MSw	TSw
Trunk Lean: B/F								
Lateral Lean: R/L								
Rotates: B/F								
Pelvis Hikes								
Tilt: P/A								
Lacks Forward Rotation								
Lacks Backward Rotation								
Excess Forward Rotation								
Excess Backward Rotation								
Ipsilateral Drop								
Contralateral Drop								
Hip Flexion: Limited								
Excess								
Inadequate Extension								
Past Retract								
Rotation: IR/ER								
Ad/Abduction: Ad/Ab								
Knee Flexion: Limited								
Excess								
Inadequate Extension								
Wobbles								
Hyperextends								
Extension Thrust								
Varus/Valgus: Vr/Vl								
Excess Contralateral Flex								
Ankle Forefoot Contact								
Foot-Flat Contact								
Foot Slap								
Excess Plantar Flexion								
Excess Dorsiflexion								
Inversion/Eversion: Iv/Ev								
Heel Off								
No Heel Off								
Drag								
Contralateral Vaulting								
Toes Up								
Inadequate Extension								
Clawed								

MAJOR PROBLEMS:

Weight Acceptance

Single Limb Support

Swing Limb Advancement

Excessive UE Weight Bearing ☐

Name

Diagnosis

sive approach to movement analysis during gait. The form is based on the framework for analyzing gait suggested by Perry and colleagues (Perry, 1992; Perry & Burnfield, 2010) and is shown in Figure 15.3. Gait is broken down into component parts. The observer focuses on one period of gait at a time (e.g., stance vs. swing), considers the functional tasks to be performed during those periods

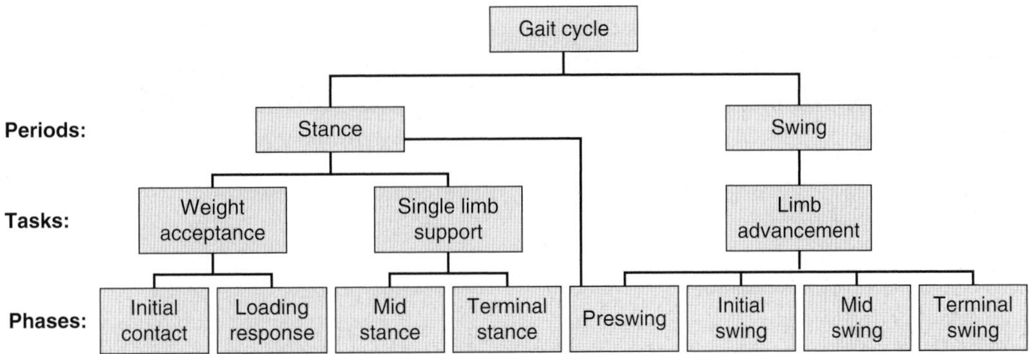

FIGURE 15.3 Conceptual framework for analyzing gait suggested by Perry (1992). See text for explanation.

(e.g., weight acceptance, single-limb support, and limb advancement), and observes motion at each of the major joints (e.g., ankle, knee, hip, pelvis, and trunk) in each of the phases of gait (e.g., initial contact, loading response, midstance, etc.).

Gait Assessment Rating Scale. The Gait Assessment Rating Scale (GARS), developed by Wolfson and colleagues (1990), is shown in Assessment Tool 15.8. The scale also allows the quantification and documentation of three categories of gait abnormalities, a general category, a lower-extremity category, and a trunk, head, and upper-extremity category. The scale has been used to document gait problems in healthy elderly, as well as in older adults with a history of falls. The test has been shown to have high interrater reliability and is a sensitive indicator of changes in gait function among older adults.

Rivermead Visual Gait Assessment. The Rivermead Visual Gait Assessment (RVGA), shown in Assessment Tool 15.9, has also been proposed as a method to structure visual gait assessment. A total of 20 observations are made, and a 4-point scale is used to quantify degree of abnormality, with 0 = normal, 1 = mild, 2 = moderate and 3 = severe abnormality. The test is divided into three parts, observations of the upper-limb position, observations made during stance phase, and observations made during the swing phase of gait. Visual gait analysis includes observation of one side of the body at a time. A global score can be calculated by summing total numbers of deviation scores ranging from 0 (normal) to 59 (severely abnormal gait). This test has been shown to have good reliability and validity (Lord et al., 1998).

OGA Strategies: Expert Versus Novice Clinicians. While many of these scales have been developed for researchers to measure changes in gait patterns with various interventions, few are routinely used in the assessment of gait patterns in the clinic (Patla et al., 1987; Toro et al., 2003). Many of these tests require considerable training, and the reliability of these tests when given by relatively untrained therapists remains a concern.

There is no consensus on the best approach to observing gait and little research to direct clinicians in choosing a strategy to guide them during visual gait analysis. A study by McGough (2005) examined differences in strategies used for OGA in expert versus novice clinicians. Six novice and six expert physical therapists performed OGA on two videotaped patients with central nervous system pathology. Prioritized problem lists and processes used to complete OGA were compared in the two groups. Results indicated that OGA strategies differed between the two groups, with expert clinicians initiating OGA by scanning the whole body and then proceeding to segmental analysis. In contrast, only 6 of 12 novice clinicians reported scanning the whole body first, with the remaining 6 reported performing a segment-by-segment analysis prior to a whole-body or more global gait analysis. In addition, experts tended to observe the trunk first and then the extremities, while the novice clinicians scanned joint by joint, either from head to toe or in the reverse direction. Because of strategy differences, expert clinicians tended to list problems with regard to either multiple segments or the whole body, while novice clinicians tended to list gait problems with reference to single body segments.

McGough suggests that differences in strategies used in OGA may reflect differences in the clinical reasoning framework. Expert clinicians may rely more on forward (inductive) reasoning, with a focus on pattern recognition perhaps derived from whole-body and multiple-segment scanning. In contrast, novice clinicians may rely on backward (hypothetical–deductive) reasoning, performing a segment-by-segment analysis of gait and building a pattern from this component analysis.

Assessment Tool 15-8

Gait Assessment Rating Scale

GENERAL CATEGORIES

1. **Variability**—a measure of inconsistency and arrhythmicity of stepping and of arm movements.
   0 = fluid and predictably paced limb movements
   1 = occasional interruptions (changes in velocity), approximately <25% of time
   2 = unpredictability of rhythm approximately 25–75% of time
   3 = random timing of limb movements
2. **Guardedness**—hesitancy, slowness, diminished propulsion and lack of commitment in stepping and arm swing
   0 = good forward momentum and lack of apprehension in propulsion
   1 = center of gravity of HAT projects only slightly in front of push-off, but still good arm–leg coordination
   2 = HAT held over anterior aspect of foot and some moderate loss of smooth reciprocation
   3 = HAT held over rear aspect of stance phase foot and great tentativeness in stepping
3. **Weaving**—an irregular and wavering line of progression
   0 = straight line of progression on frontal viewing
   1 = a single deviation from straight (line of best fit) line of progression
   2 = two to three deviations from line of progression
   3 = four or more deviations from line of progression
4. **Waddling**—a broad-based gait characterized by excessive truncal crossing of the midline and side bending
   0 = narrow base of support and body held nearly vertically over feet
   1 = slight separation of medial aspects of feet and just perceptible lateral movement of head and trunk
   2 = 3 to 4 in. of separation between feet and obvious bending of trunk to side so that COG of head lies well over ipsilateral stance foot
   3 = extreme pendular deviations of head and trunk (head passes lateral to ipsilateral stance foot) and further widening of base of support
5. **Staggering**—sudden and unexpected lateral partial losses of balance
   0 = no losses of balance to side
   1 = a single lurch to side
   2 = two lurches to side
   3 = three or more lurches to side

LOWER-EXTREMITY CATEGORIES

1. **Percent Time in Swing**—a loss in the percentage of the gait cycle constituted by the swing phase
   0 = approximately 3:2 ratio of duration of stance to swing phase
   1 = a 1:1 or slightly less ratio of stance to swing
   2 = markedly prolonged stance phase but with some obvious swing time remaining
   3 = barely perceptible portion of cycle spent in swing
2. **Foot Contact**—the degree to which heel strikes the ground before the forefoot
   0 = very obvious angle of impact of heel on ground
   1 = barely visible contact of heel before forefoot
   2 = entire foot lands flat on ground
   3 = anterior aspect of foot strikes ground before heel
3. **Hip ROM**—the degree of loss of hip range of motion seen during a gait cycle
   0 = obvious angulation of thigh backward during double support (10 degrees)
   1 = just barely visible angulation backward from vertical
   2 = thigh in line with vertical projection from ground
   3 = thigh angled forward from vertical at maximum posterior excursion
4. **Knee ROM**—the degree of loss of knee range of motion seen during a gait cycle
   0 = knee moves from complete extension at heel strike (and late stance) to almost 90 degrees (70 degrees) during swing phase
   1 = slight bend in knee seen at heel-strike and late-stance and maximal flexion at midswing is closer to 45 degrees than 90 degrees
   2 = knee flexion at late stance more obvious than at heel strike; very little clearance seen for toe during swing
   3 = toe appears to touch ground during swing, knee flexion appears constant during stance, and knee angle during swing appears 45 degrees or less

TRUNK, HEAD, AND UPPER-EXTREMITY CATEGORIES

1. **Elbow Extension**—a measure of the decrease of elbow range of motion
   0 = large peak-to-peak excursion of forearm (approximately 20 degrees), with distinct maximal flexion at end of anterior trajectory

(continued)

Assessment Tool 15-8

Gait Assessment Rating Scale

1 = 25% decrement of extension during maximal posterior excursion of upper extremity
2 = almost no change in elbow angle
3 = no apparent change in elbow angle (held in flexion)

2. **Shoulder Extension**—a measure of the decrease of shoulder range of motion
0 = clearly seen movement of upper arm anterior (15 degrees) and posterior (20 degrees) to vertical axis of trunk
1 = shoulder flexes slightly anterior to vertical axis
2 = shoulder comes only to vertical axis, or slightly posterior to it during flexion
3 = shoulder stays well behind vertical axis during entire excursion

3. **Shoulder Abduction**—a measure of pathological increase in shoulder range of motion laterally
0 = shoulders held almost parallel to trunk
1 = shoulders held 5–10 degrees to side
2 = shoulders held 10–20 degrees to side
3 = shoulders held greater than 20 degrees to side

4. **Arm-Heel Strike Synchrony**—the extent to which the contralateral movements of an arm and leg are out of phase
0 = good temporal conjunction of arm and contralateral leg at apex of shoulder and hip excursions all of the time
1 = arm and leg slightly out of phase 25% of the time
2 = arm and leg moderately out of phase 25–50% of time
3 = little or no temporal coherence of arm and leg

5. **Head Held Forward**—a measure of the pathological forward projection of the head relative to the trunk
0 = earlobe vertically aligned with shoulder tip
1 = earlobe vertical projection falls 1 in. anterior to shoulder tip
2 = earlobe vertical projection falls 2 in. anterior to shoulder tip
3 = earlobe vertical projection falls 3 in. or more anterior to shoulder tip

6. **Shoulders Held Elevated**—the degree to which the scapular girdle is held higher than normal
0 = tip of shoulder (acromion) markedly below level of chin 1 to 2 inches
1 = tip of shoulder slightly below level of chin
2 = tip of shoulder at level of chin
3 = tip of shoulder above level of chin

7. **Upper Trunk Flexed Forward**—a measure of kyphotic involvement of the trunk
0 = very gentle thoracic convexity, cervical spine flat, or almost flat
1 = emerging cervical curve, more distant thoracic convexity
2 = anterior concavity at midchest level apparent
3 = anterior concavity at midchest level very obvious

COG = center of gravity; HAT = head, arms, trunk; ROM = range of motion.

Reprinted with permission from Wolfson L, Whipple R, Amerman P, Tobin JN. Gait assessment in the elderly: a gait abnormality rating scale and its relation to falls. J Gerontol 1990;45:M12–M19.

This research is interesting because it may provide insight into why relatively few clinicians use observational gait analysis forms during routine clinical analysis of gait (Patla et al., 1987; Toro et al., 2003). An OGA form that focuses on a segment-by-segment (or joint-by-joint) analysis will not necessarily be useful to a clinician who relies on pattern recognition derived from full-body and multiple-segment scans. Perhaps the issue facing clinicians and researchers alike is to better comprehend the most useful framework for understanding abnormal gait in patients with varying levels of gait abnormalities.

Interpreting OGA: Framework for Determining Causes of Atypical Gait. Systematically observing and documenting gait abnormalities is the first step in understanding and hypothesizing the possible causes for these deviations. Table 15.5 illustrates a gait diagnostic chart developed by Winter (1993) to serve as a framework for understanding possible causes of gait abnormalities observed during a visual gait analysis. The chart has three columns; the first lists the observed abnormalities, the second column lists the possible causes of the abnormality, and the third column describes the type of biomechanical or neuromuscular evidence that might be gathered to determine which of the possible causes is likely to be producing the observed abnormality. Thus, results from a visual gait analysis are tied to hypotheses regarding possible underlying causes

Assessment Tool 15-9

The Rivermead Visual Gait Assessment

PATIENT:_______________

Scoring: Normal = 0 **Deviations:** 1 = mild, 2 = moderate, 3 = severe (please circle)

UPPER-LIMB POSITION

1	Shoulder Depressed/Retracted/Elevated		0 1 2 3
2	Elbow flexed ≤ 45 degrees (=**0**) 45 to 90 degrees (=**1**) > 90 degrees (=**2**)		0 1 2

Stance Phase *For trunk deviations, 0* = midline

3	Trunk flexed/extended		3 2 1 0 1 2 3 (←→)
		Inclined:	backward / forward
4	Trunk side flexed		3 2 1 0 1 2 3
		Direction:	left / right
5	Trunk and pelvis: lateral displacement		3 2 1 0 1 2 3
		Amount:	excessive / reduced
6	Contralateral drop pelvis		0 1 2 3
7	Hip extension decreased		0 1 2 3
8	*with backward rotation*		0 1 2 3
9A	Knee **flexion** excessive: *at initial contact*		0 1 2 3
10A	*throughout range* **or**		0 1 2 3
9B	Knee **extension** excessive: *at initial contact*		0 1 2 3
10B	*throughout range*		0 1 2 3
11A	Ankle in excessive **plantar** flexion **or**		0 1 2 3
11B	Ankle in excessive **dorsi**flexion		0 1 2 3
12	Inversion excessive		0 1 2 3
13	Plantar flexion decreased at toe-off		0 1 2 3

Swing Phase *For trunk deviations, 0* = *midline*

14	Trunk flexed		3 2 1 0 1 2 3 (←→)
		Direction:	backward / forward
15	Trunk side flexed		3 2 1 0 1 2 3
		Direction:	left / right
16	Hike pelvis (elevation)		0 1 2 3
17	Backward rotation pelvis		0 1 2 3
18	Decreased hip flexion		0 1 2 3
19	Decreased knee flexion		0 1 2 3
20	Ankle in excess plantar flexion		0 1 2 3

Any other deviations noted

.... 0 1 2 3
.... 0 1 2 3

Reference limb _______________
Walking aid _______________
Ankle–Foot–Orthosis
Total score _______________ /59 Date _________

Reprinted with permission from Collen FM, Wade DT, Robb GF, Bradshaw CM. The Rivermead Mobility Index: a further development of the Rivermead Motor Assessment. Int Disabil Stud 1991;13:50–54.

and the types of diagnostic tests needed to confirm the cause. When determining appropriate interventions for retraining gait, a clinician can then use this information.

Limitations to Observational Gait Analysis. Studies have shown that a major limitation of most observational gait analysis is poor reliability even among highly trained and experienced clinicians (Krebs et al., 1985). In addition, a detailed qualitative gait analysis is very time-consuming and often unrealistic in a busy clinical environment. Finally, strong evidence does not exist to indicate that most observational gait analysis forms are sensitive to changes in gait patterns in response to therapy.

An alternative to observational gait analysis is the use of technological systems to quantify movement patterns, muscle activation patterns, and forces used in gait. However, this technology is beyond the reach of the average clinician. In addition to being extremely expensive, this equipment requires considerable time and technical expertise to use.

TABLE 15.5 Winter's Framework for Understanding Atypical Gait Patterns

Observed Abnormality	Possible Causes	Biomechanical and Neuromuscular Diagnostic Evidence
Foot slap at heel contact	Below-normal dorsiflexor activity at heel contact	Below-normal tibialis anterior EMG or dorisflexor moment at heel contact
Forefoot or flat-foot initial contact	(a) Hyperactive plantarflexor activity in late swing (b) Structural limitation in ankle range (c) Short step-length	(a) Above-normal plantarflexor EMG in late swing (b) Decreased dorsiflexion range of motion (c) See (a), (b), (c), and (d) immediately below
Short step length	(a) Weak push-off prior to swing (b) Weak hip flexors at toe-off and early swing (c) Above-normal knee extensor activity during push-off (d) Excessive deceleration of leg in late swing	(a) Below-normal plantarflexor moment or power generation or EMG during push-off (b) Below-normal hip flexor power or power or EMG during late push-off and early swing (c) Above-normal quadriceps EMG or knee extensor moment or power absorption in late stance (d) Above-normal hamstring EMG or knee flexor moment or power absorption late in swing
Stiff-legged weight bearing	(a) Above-normal extensor activity at the ankle, knee, or hip early in stance	(a) Above-normal EMG activity or moments in hip extensors, knee extensors, or plantar flexors early in stance
Stance phase with flexed but rigid knee	(a) Above-normal extensor activity during weight acceptance at the ankle and hip with reduced knee extensor activity (b) Excessive ankle dorsiflexion	(a) Above-normal EMG activity or moments in hip extensors and plantar flexors in early and middle stance (b) Hyperactivity of dorsiflexors or excessive dorsiflexion of ankle orthosis
Weak push-off accompanied by observable pull-off	(a) Weak plantar flexor activity at push-off (b) Normal or above-normal hip flexor EMG activity during late push-off and early swing	(a) Below-normal plantarflexor EMG, moment or power during push-off (b) Normal or above normal hip flexor EMG, moment or power during late push-off and early swing
Hip hiking in swing with or without circumduction of lower limb	(a) Weak hip, knee, or ankle flexor activity during swing (b) Overactive extensor synergy during swing	(a) Below-normal tibialis anterior EMG or hip or knee flexors during swing (b) Above-normal hip or knee extensor EMG or moment during swing
Trendelenburg gait	(a) Weak hip abductors (b) Overactive hip adductors	(a) Below-normal EMG in hip abductors: gluteus medius and minimus, tensor fasciae latae (b) Above-normal EMG in hip adductors, adductor longus, magnus and brevis, and gracilis

Reprinted with permission from Winter DA. Knowledge base for diagnostic gait assessments. Med Prog Technol 1993;19:72.

LAB ACTIVITY 15-2

Objective: To perform a visual gait analysis.

Procedure: Get a partner. Choose one or more of the visual gait analysis forms presented in this chapter. Observe your partner walking at his or her comfortable gait speed, first from the sagittal plane, then from the frontal plane. You may wish to videotape several cycles of gait from both the sagittal plane and frontal plane. If you have access to a patient with an atypical gait pattern you may wish to repeat this assignment with them.

Assignment: Complete the gait analysis form you have chosen. If you use several different forms consider the ease of using each form. How long did it take you to complete a visual gait analysis?

Gait analysis is an integral part of almost every motor control evaluation in the patient with neurologic dysfunction. Gait itself is complex, and understanding the complications of gait is even more difficult. Therefore, it is essential that a clinician have a systematic and consistent approach to observing and analyzing gait. Despite its limitations, an observational gait analysis form provides a framework for systematically observing gait, and is therefore an essential part of the examination of gait.

To practice your skills in observational gait analysis perform Lab Activity 15.2.

Examination at the Impairment Level

A complete examination includes identifying underlying impairments that are potentially constraining mobility function and participation. The physical examination of underlying systems important to gait is often referred to as a "static evaluation," since it evaluates factors such as strength, range of motion (ROM), and tone in passive situations such as while the patient is sitting or lying down. In contrast, a "dynamic evaluation" examines these systems while the patient is performing functional movements such as gait. Examination of underlying impairments was discussed in Chapter 5 and will not be repeated in this chapter.

Do Impairments Predict Gait Performance?

Static examination of factors such as strength, ROM, and spasticity are important; however, they do not always predict gait performance in patients with neurologic lesions. Nadeau et al. (1997) studied the relationship between plantar-flexor strength and gait speed in subjects with hemiplegia. An instrumented dynamometer was used to evaluate muscular parameters (static torque, dynamic torque, power, and maximal rate of tension development) in ankle plantar flexors in the hemiparetic limb of patients who had had a stroke. Muscular parameters were compared with gait speed, performance on the Timed Up and Go test, the Fugl-Myer Assessment, and level of plantar-flexor spasticity.

Results showed that subjects with hemiparesis were significantly weaker than controls. Dynamometric assessment showed that in subjects with hemiparesis, ankle plantar-flexion torque was, on average, 50% of that of normal controls. In addition, torque values for the subjects with hemiparesis declined more rapidly in the initial stages of movement than they did for controls. There was no relationship between dynamometric data and spasticity at the ankle (as measured passively while the patient was sitting), suggesting that plantar-flexor strength was not associated with hyperactivity or spasticity at the ankle joint.

Comfortable gait speed in the hemiplegic subjects was 0.45 m/min, or 76% of that of elderly controls. Maximal plantar-flexor parameters as measured with a dynamometer were not significantly related to gait performance, suggesting that the strength of the plantar flexors was not the most critical determinant of gait velocity in subjects with hemiplegia. Some patients with good plantar-flexor strength walked at relatively slower speeds; in contrast, some patients with decreased plantar-flexor strength could walk at relatively fast velocities (over 60 m/min). These individuals produced the faster gait velocity using alternative movement strategies, such as increased use of hip flexors for "pull-off" during swing as a substitute for decreased push-off in terminal stance (Nadeau et al., 1997).

While ankle strength may not predict gait performance, knee strength might. The upright motor control test, which was described in Figure 15.2, examines hip, knee, and ankle flexion and extension strength in the standing position. Perry and colleagues found that a combination of gait velocity and knee-extension control was highly predictive of mobility function in stroke patients. A combination of a strong grade of knee extension on the upright motor control test (see Figure 15.2: single-limb stance of the affected leg, able to extend the knee from 30 degrees of flexion) and a gait velocity of 16 m/min predicted community ambulation. Moderate and weak knee-extension scores would require at least 24 m/min and 32 m/min, respectively, to achieve community-level ambulation. In these patients, the loss of knee control required the substitution of other mechanisms to achieve the required gait speed.

While strength may not always correlate with gait parameters, sensation appears to. In the study by Nadeau et al. (1997) the patients with the lowest sensory scores tended to be the slowest walkers, supporting the findings of Brandstater et al. (1983) that the quality of gait is poorest in patients with sensory deficit following stroke. This is also consistent with the finding of Perry et al. (1995) that proprioception was a strong predictor of independent mobility function following stroke and that of Lord et al. (1996), who found that sensory impairments predicted gait performance in older adults.

Finally, in the first 6 months following stroke, Mercer et al. (2009) found that performance on the Step Test (an impairment measure of dynamic standing balance) was moderately correlated (R^2 = 0.60 to 0.79) with gait speed, but only weakly associated (R^2 = 0.34 to 0.41) with mobility participation as measured on the Stroke Impact Scale.

Thus, the relationship between impairment and gait parameters is very complex, and depends on many factors, including the type and extent of impairment, the functional level of the patient, and the capacity for compensation by other systems.

Measuring Mobility: Do We Really Need All These Tests and Measures?

As you can see, examination of mobility using a task-oriented approach is very complex. It uses a range of tests and measures to quantify functional status and level of disability, describe gait strategies, and document underlying impairments. In this time of health care reform, when the amount of time available to examine and treat a patient is shrinking rapidly, do we really need all these measures? Is it really necessary to measure functional mobility, perform a visual gait analysis, and examine underlying impairments? We would argue that each provides essential information when establishing a plan of care for the patient.

For example, a static examination of underlying impairments determines the resources and constraints affecting gait and other aspects of mobility function. A dynamic evaluation using visual gait analysis can help a clinician determine the extent to which current strategies meet the requirements of gait in the face of underlying impairments. Functional measures, whether a single measure such as gait velocity or multiple measures available through mobility scales, document level of function and may help to predict disability. These measures are important for justifying the need for therapy and serve as outcome measures, quantifying change over time and in response to intervention. Thus, a clinician can use information from all levels of assessment to develop a comprehensive plan of care designed to maximize functional mobility status.

Before moving on to treatment, the reader is encouraged to review the case study presented in Assessment Tool 15.10, and complete Lab Activity 15.3, applying a task-oriented approach to examination.

TRANSITION TO TREATMENT

Setting Goals

As is true for goal setting related to other physical skills, clinicians need to establish both long- and short-term goals during mobility retraining that are objective, measurable, and meaningful to the patient.

Long-Term Goals (Outcomes)

Long-term goals, or functional outcomes, are often stated in terms of functional performance and level of disability. They usually reflect ambulation outcomes with respect to level of independence and/or the context or conditions under which a patient will be able to walk. Examples of long-term goals might be: the patient will be able to walk independently a minimum of 1000 ft in the community with the use of a cane and orthosis; the patient will be able to walk independently with a quad cane, 50 ft in her home environment; the patient will be able to walk independently using a single-point cane up and down curbs, on inclines and uneven surfaces; and the patient will be able to sustain a walking speed of 32 m/min with the use of a cane and orthosis for a distance of 1/4 mi.

Short-Term Goals

Short-term goals for mobility retraining can be expressed in terms of:

1. Changing underlying impairments. One example would be to decrease flexion contractures at the hip by 20 degrees, at the knee by 15 degrees, and at the ankle by 20 degrees.
2. Improving gait patterns. One example would be to decrease forward trunk flexion by 20 degrees and thereby improve upright posture during the stance and swing phases of gait.

Assessment Tool 15-10

Assessment Case Study

Jean J, is a 82-year-old woman with right-sided hemiplegia, referred for evaluation of walking 4 weeks after her stroke.

Medical history: Positive for hypertension. Following her 5-day acute hospital stay for a middle cerebral artery infarct, she spent 2 weeks in rehabilitation and was discharged to her home.

Social history: She lives alone in a two-story home. She had been a full-time legal assistant.

Reason for referral: Continued problems with balance and walking.

ON EXAMINATION

Self-report participation and fall/balance history: Jean reports walking in her own home with her assistive device. When she goes into the community, she is always accompanied. She walks only short distances, and her companion holds onto her when stepping up and down curbs, or over obstacles. She has had several falls since her return home, often tripping over obstacles while walking.

FUNCTIONAL ACTIVITY MEASURES

1. **10-M Walk:** On the 10-m walk test, her gait velocity is 0.5 m/sec and she walks with a cane.
2. **Dynamic Gait Index:**
   1. Level surface: 2
   2. Change in gait speed: 2
   3. Horizontal head movements: 1
   4. Vertical head movements: 2
   5. Gait with pivot turn: 1
   6. Over obstacles: 1
   7. Around obstacles: 2
   8. Steps: 1
3. **TUG:** Completes the Timed Up and Go test in 22 sec; she must use her left arm when rising, and requires close guarding on the turns. When a secondary task is added, her time increases to 31 sec.

OBSERVATIONAL GAIT ANALYSIS

Jean uses a cane and walks with a stiff-knee gait. She is asymmetric and has a prolonged stance time on her non hemiparetic side, increased swing on her hemiparetic side and unequal step lengths. At initial contact, she has an equinovarus foot position and she strikes with a flat foot. She does not flex her knee during loading, and her knee is hyperextended in midstance. She is unable to achieve a trailing limb position during terminal stance and does not flex her knee during preswing. To advance her swing limb, she circumducts her leg and leans laterally with her trunk. Her foot remains plantar-flexed during swing.

UNDERLYING IMPAIRMENTS

She has reduced ability to selectively activate muscles in her affected arm and leg. She has reduced strength, and mildly limited range of motion at the ankle. She has reduced somatosensation in her hemiparetic arm and leg. She also has visual problems including hemianopsia. To understand her balance problems, review her balance assessment case study found in Chapter 11.

LAB ACTIVITY 15-3

Objective: To apply a task-oriented approach to examining mobility function in a patient with hemiplegia and to establish goals and a plan of care for walking based on assessment information.

Procedures: Read the case study of Jean J in Assessment Tool 15.10. (or use a real case study if you have access to a patient with a neurologic diagnosis).

Assignment: Based on the information you have, answer the following questions:

1. How would you classify Jean using the Perry ambulation classification system?
2. Which aspects of gait are affected in Jean, progression, stability or adaptation?
3. What impairments are contributing to her hemiparetic gait pattern?
4. What factors are contributing to her inability to safely step over obstacles?

3. Accomplishing interim steps toward long-term goals. Examples include: (a) increasing distance walked, with only standby assist, from 10 ft to 25 ft; (b) to increase speed; patient will be able to walk 200 ft, standby assist only, in 45 sec; (c) to become independent in the use of a front-wheeled walker.

Short-term goals usually lead to treatment strategies aimed at resolving underlying impairments and improving the quality of gait strategies. Long-term goals often lead to treatment strategies related to improving the overall performance of ambulation, such as increasing the distance walked or the speed of ambulation. Often, the two are interrelated, as when the goal is to improve a particular aspect of the locomotor pattern to increase the velocity of gait.

Defining Goals Based on the Task Requirements of Gait

Alternatively, goals related to retraining mobility function could be defined in relationship to the three requirements of gait—progression, postural support and stability, and functional adaptation.

Progression. Treatment goals related to progression concern helping the patient develop the capacity to generate momentum to facilitate forward propulsion of the body. Specific examples include:

1. Improve the range and freedom of motion so that momentum can be transferred freely between body segments. This encompasses improving range of motion, decreasing contractures, reducing spasticity, which limits the velocity of motion, and reducing coactivation of muscles, which increases joint stiffness.
2. Increase the speed of walking, because generation of momentum requires a minimum speed of movement. This includes increasing the speed at which segments are moved. For example, increasing the speed and amplitude of hip flexion during the swing phase of gait will advance the thigh segment quickly. This will facilitate passive knee flexion for toe clearance and subsequent knee extension for foot placement. This goal requires facilitation of hip flexion in conjunction with knee extension, thus decreasing reliance on a flexor synergy pattern to accomplish the goals of swing.
3. Improve plantar-flexor strength, since it is the plantar flexors that generate the largest percentage of the forces necessary for forward propulsion.
4. Improve toe clearance during the swing phase of gait so that the swing leg is advanced without contacting the surface, since this decreases, or halts, forward momentum.

Postural Support and Stability. Treatment goals related to postural support and stability reflect the need for: (a) a good foot placement, to facilitate weight bearing during initiation of stance, (b) the presence of sufficient extensor torque to support the body against gravity during single-limb stance, (c) facilitation of hip and trunk extensors to control the hip–arm–trunk (HAT) segment, and (d) hip abductor strength and control, in order to facilitate mediolateral stability. Thus, working toward postural support and stability during gait includes helping the patient to:

1. Achieve a heel-first foot strike, in the absence of coronal-plane deviations. This position will allow the body to move smoothly over the foot, and to take advantage of the full weight-bearing surface of the foot, enhancing stability.
2. Develop coordinated extension at the hip and knee, in order to generate an extensor moment to support body weight during single-limb stance.
3. Develop a vertical posture of the trunk, with good hip and back extension to control the HAT segment, and adequate activation of the abductors to control the pelvis.
4. Facilitate extensor moments at the hip and knee while maintaining the capacity to dorsiflex the ankle, thus avoiding use of a total extensor synergy pattern during stance.

Functional Adaptation. Treatment goals related to functional adaptation require the patient to modify movement and sensory strategies for locomotor control in response to changing task and environmental demands. Examples of functional adaptation goals include:

1. Integration of compensatory aspects of postural control into the ongoing gait cycle.
2. Utilization of visual cues to identify upcoming disturbances to mobility and modify gait strategies in order to minimize their effect.
3. Ability to change the speed and direction of gait safely, without loss of balance.
4. Ability to manage terrain changes, including curbs, ramps, steps, and uneven surfaces, safely and smoothly, with no loss of balance.

With comprehensive and realistic goals established, based on the patient's desires and problems, the clinician can move ahead to planning treatments designed to meet these goals.

"TASK-ORIENTED" APPROACH TO MOBILITY TRAINING

This chapter discusses a task-oriented approach to retraining mobility function, with an emphasis on gait retraining. A task-oriented approach (as defined in this book) stresses therapeutic interventions that are specific to the task being trained. This includes treatments aimed at minimizing impairments, maximizing gait strategies that effectively and efficiently meet the requirements of gait, and developing the ability to adapt functional gait skills to changing task and environmental demands in order to maximize participation and minimize mobility disability. While this approach does not use preambulation skill training, it does use both part and whole practice to retrain functional gait strategies. Finally, there is considerable emphasis on practicing the skill of gait under varied task and environmental conditions.

Interventions at the Impairment Level

The goal of treatment aimed at the impairment level is to maximize the sensory-motor resources available for the performance of functional mobility skills. During retraining the task of walking, special emphasis is given to musculoskeletal impairments that constrain the use of strategies that are effective in meeting the essential requirements of propulsion, postural control, and functional adaptation. For example, impairments that have a specific impact on the goal of propulsion include weakness of the ankle plantar flexors, which limits a forceful push-off in terminal stance, and shortened hip flexors and/or ankle plantar flexors, which limits the ability to advance the body over the stance foot. Impairments that have an impact on the goal of postural control include weakness of the ankle, knee, and hip extensors, limiting the generation of an extensor support moment, and weakness of the hip abductors, which has an impact on mediolateral stability.

Thus, therapeutic exercises that focus on strength and flexibility are used to correct or minimize impairments that can be changed and prevent the development of secondary impairments. Alleviating underlying impairments enables the patient to resume using previously developed strategies for gait. When permanent impairments make resumption of previously used strategies impossible, new strategies will have to be developed. In Chapter 5 we discussed treatment strategies aimed at resolving or preventing underlying musculoskeletal and neuromuscular impairments; this information will not be repeated in this chapter.

Research Evidence: Does Changing Impairments Improve Gait Function?

Although most clinicians use treatment strategies to remediate underlying impairments, the extent to which these types of improvements carry over to functional locomotion is still undetermined. For example, researchers have found that, while therapeutic strategies were effective in significantly increasing hip flexion range of motion and improving trunk strength, improvements in these areas did not significantly improve gait speed (Godges et al., 1993). Judge and colleagues (1993) reported that gait measures did not change significantly in older adults following strengthening exercises. Krebs et al. (1998) examined the effect of moderate-intensity strength training on gait in 132 functionally limited elders. Following 6 months of progressive resistive exercises, strength improved by 17.6%. While gait velocity did not significantly change, mediolateral stability (as measured by mediolateral center-of-mass [COM] excursion and velocity) significantly improved (Krebs et al., 1998). In contrast, Puthoff et al. (2008) reported that among older adults with functional limitations, lower-extremity strength, peak power, and power at both low and high intensity were all related to everyday walking behavior (total steps, distance, and walking speed) measured using an accelerometer activity monitor.

Ouellette and colleagues (2004) used a program of high-intensity resistance training in long-term stroke survivors (average time since stroke, 32 months) and found significant improvements in muscle strength and peak power but no change in performance-based measures of walking distance (6-minute walk) or speed (habitual or maximal gait velocity). Participants in the resistance training group reported improvements on the Late Life Function and Disability Instrument. Flansbjer et al. (2008) also reported improvement in strength and no change in muscle tone after progressive resistance training at 80% of maximum, two times a week for 10 weeks in a group of 15 subjects with chronic stroke. Improvements in lower-extremity strength were not associated with improvements on the TUG or the Stroke Impact Scale (their measure of participation) immediately after the intervention, though there were slight differences between the training and control groups at the 5-month follow-up.

DeBolt and McCubbin (2004) examined the effects of a home-based resistance exercise program on power, balance, and mobility in adults with multiple sclerosis (see Chapter 11 for a more detailed description of the study) and found that resistance strength training resulted in increased lower-extremity power, but no changes in mobility as assessed by the Timed Up and Go test.

Damiano and colleagues (1998; 2010) in a series of studies examined the effect of strength training on physical function in children with cerebral palsy (CP). These studies showed that children with CP had significantly improved strength in the targeted muscles. The effect of improved strength on gait parameters was variable, however. While in some children gait patterns improved, in others gait patterns either did not change or were slightly worse. The authors suggest that given the variability of outcomes in strengthening studies in CP, methods are needed to better identify the individuals who are most likely to benefit from strengthening (Damiano et al., 2010).

Why are there conflicting research results on the effects of strength training on gait velocity? Current research has shown that there is a nonlinear relationship between gait speed and strength in the lower-extremity muscles (Buchner et al., 1996). This is shown in Figure 15.4A, which plots leg strength versus usual gait speed in a group of elderly subjects (Buchner et al., 1996). The regression curve plotting strength to speed is shown for an average age of 76 years and an average body weight of 71 kg. The hypothesized relationship between leg strength and gait speed is shown in Figure 15.4B. Since walking does not require maximum strength, normal walking speed could be maintained in the presence of a range of strength abilities (this is shown as a range of strength marked with an A in Figure 15.4B). Thus, it is proposed that a patient who is already walking at this speed will not show further changes in gait in response to changes in strength. In contrast, the strength range marked by area B corresponds to the range in which decrements in strength will affect walking speed; thus, changes in strength will have an impact on gait speed. Finally, the strength range marked C illustrates the range of strength deficits in which walking is no longer possible.

In summary, current research raises questions about the effect of retraining impairments on functional performance of gait, suggesting that resolution of impairments alone may not be enough to ensure recovery of ambulation skills. In addition to treatments aimed at underlying impairments, interventions aimed at improving gait strategies and functional performance are required.

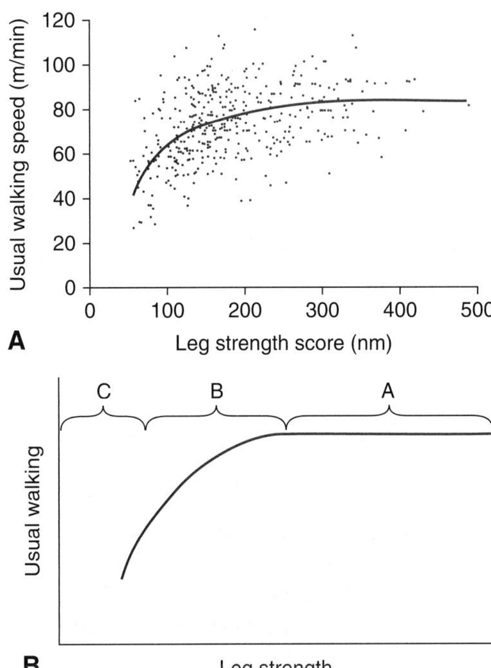

FIGURE 15.4 Relationship between strength and walking speed. A, Plot of leg-strength scores versus usual gait speed in elderly subjects. Shown also is the regression curve plotting strength versus speed for the average age of 76 and average body weight of 71 kg. B, The hypothesized nonlinear relationship between gait speed and strength predicting the effect of changes in strength on gait speed. See text for further explanation. (Redrawn with permission from Buchner DM, Larson EB, Wagner EH, et al. Evidence for a non-linear relationship between leg strength and gait speed. Age Ageing 1996;25:387.)

Intervention at the Strategy Level

The goal of retraining at the strategy level is to assist the patient in developing movement strategies that are effective and efficient in meeting the essential requirements of progression, postural support and stability, and adaptation. While much of gait retraining strives to assist patients in the recovery of previously used "normal" gait patterns, this may not be a realistic goal in the face of permanent sensory and motor impairments. Thus, a better standard for judging the efficacy of a patient's movement strategies is to ask, "Is he or she effective in meeting the demands of the task in the face of current impairments? Are current impairments potentially modifiable, and how will this change the strategies used for gait?"

The framework used below presents therapeutic techniques used to achieve the specific requirements of gait. While techniques are organized around a single requirement, it should be recognized that many of the suggested therapeutic strategies would have an impact on more than one requirement of gait. Therapeutic strategies are based on an understanding of normal and pathologic gait and are drawn from our own efforts related to the application of a systems theory of motor control and motor learning

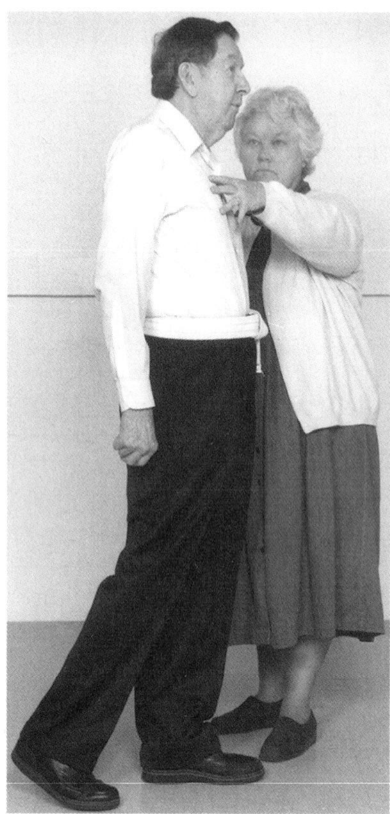

FIGURE 15.5 Assisting a patient learning to maintain a vertical trunk posture during gait with manual cues.

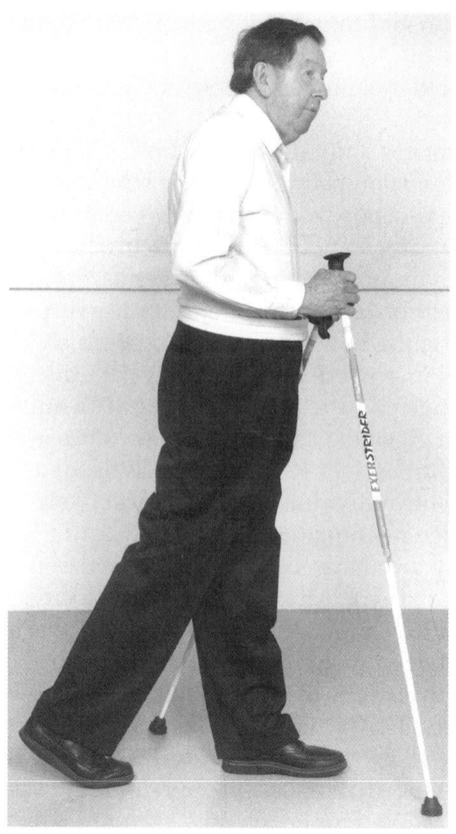

FIGURE 15.6 During gait retraining, long poles can be used to facilitate extension of the HAT segment.

(as well as others) (Carr & Shepherd, 1998), and other sources (including the neurofacilitation approaches) (Bobath & Bobath, 1984; Brunnstrom, 1970; Charness, 1986; Davies, 1985; Voss et al., 1985). It is important to remember that while these techniques are commonly used by clinicians to retrain gait, they have not necessarily been validated through controlled research involving patients with neurologic impairments.

Postural Support and Stability

Treatments aimed at postural control include improving postural alignment of the HAT (head–arms–trunk) segment, effective generation of an extensor support moment in the stance limb, control of mediolateral stability (including placement of the foot at initial contact of stance), improving balance in the single- and double-support phases of gait, and the use of assistive devices that broaden the base of support.

Control of the Hat Segment. Treatment of underlying impairments such as weakness of the hip extensors and shortening of the hip flexors will improve the capacity for vertical alignment of the HAT segment. During gait retraining, manual cues can be given to the patient at the shoulders (shown in Fig. 15.5) or at the hips to facilitate a vertical posture and control of HAT stability over the extended hips. Assistance can progress from light manual guidance to verbal cueing.

Often patients with poor balance look down while walking, bringing the neck and trunk into flexion. To facilitate extension of the neck and trunk, and an upright position of the HAT segment, verbal cues to "look up" in combination with a visual target at eye level can be used. Finally, assistive devices such as long poles (shown in Fig. 15.6) can be used to facilitate extension of the trunk and hips during walking.

Extensor Support Moment. Postural support requires the ability to load the stance limb without collapsing. Treatment varies depending on the underlying cause. When weakness of the hip and knee extensors is the cause, strengthening both concentrically and eccentrically is essential. Stretching of tight hip flexors and ankle plantar flexors, which limit the generation of extensor support, is indicated.

In patients who do not have sufficient knee control to prevent collapse during loading, the knee can be externally supported to prevent collapse, such as with a knee brace (shown in Fig. 15.7). With the knee braced to prevent collapse, the patient can work on

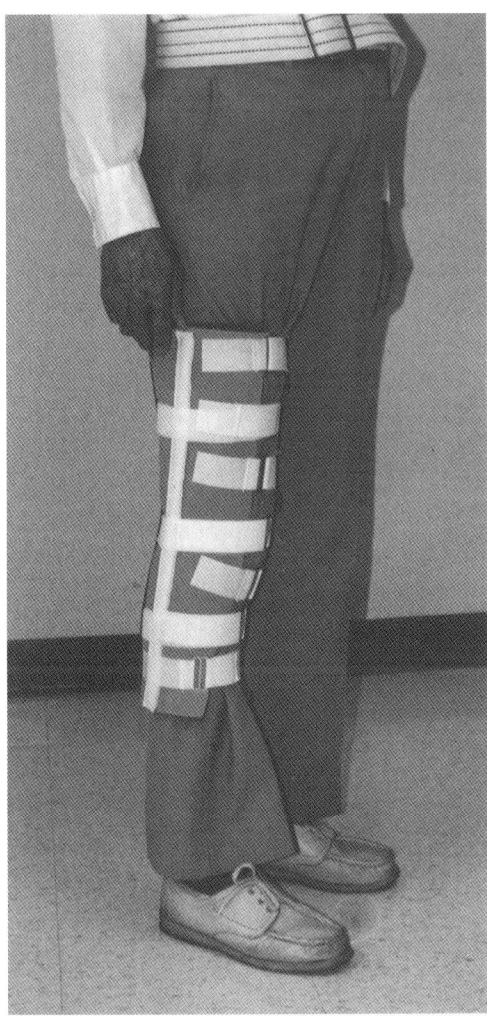

FIGURE 15.7 In patients who do not have sufficient knee control to prevent collapse during loading, the knee can be externally supported with a knee brace to prevent collapse.

weight-bearing activities in stance and gait. For example, the patient can practice stepping with the nonbraced leg, learning to advance the body over the stance foot, keeping the hip extended with the ankle dorsiflexed. Other activities that load the limb include stepping up onto a higher surface, such as a stool or taped newspapers (Fig. 15.8). The advantage of taped newspapers is that they are readily available and cheap and the height can be varied depending on the need of the patient. While the benefit of bracing the knee into extension is to facilitate weight bearing in the stance phase of gait, the benefit is lost during the swing phase, when the patient is required to flex the leg to advance the limb.

A common problem related to postural support involves hyperextension of the knee during loading and midstance. Treatment depends on whether the hyperextension is the primary impairment or compensatory for another problem elsewhere. If hyperextension is due to hyperactivity of the plantar flexors, then an ankle–foot orthosis (AFO) with a plantar-flexion stop can be used (Montgomery, 1987; Mulroy et al., 2003; Perry & Burnfield, 2010; Rosenthal et al., 1975). Alternatively, techniques to decrease muscle tone in the plantar flexors, such as having the patient practice weight bearing with the ankle dorsiflexed, thus lengthening the triceps surae, have been recommended (Carr & Shepherd, 1998; Montgomery, 1987).

When hyperextension of the knee is compensatory for a weak quadriceps, strengthening exercises, electrical stimulation, and electromyographic (EMG) biofeedback have been recommended to facilitate activation of the quadriceps. Orthoses that block knee hyperextension have also been proposed to prevent hyperextension of the knee during gait.

It has also been recommended that patients practice generating an extensor support moment in other tasks, such as moving from a sitting to a standing position, or alternatively, standing against a wall and flexing, then extending, the knees and hips (Bobath & Bobath, 1975; Davies, 1985). Again, it is not known whether practicing the generation of an extensor support moment in a task other than gait will carry over to improvements in stability during the stance phase of gait.

Foot Placement at Initial Contact. Foot placement during initial contact and throughout the stance phase of gait is a major factor in determining stability; thus, improving movement and control of the ankle and foot at initial contact and during loading can significantly improve stability. Heel-strike foot contact with a smooth transition to a stable flat-foot position will facilitate both forward progression and a stable base of support important for stability. The treatment of problems impairing heel strike depends on the underlying cause.

Heel-strike foot contact requires hip flexion in conjunction with knee extension and ankle dorsiflexion at terminal swing. Reducing musculoskeletal impairments that constrain a dorsiflexed position of the foot at initial contact is important. This includes stretching tight plantar flexors and hamstring muscles to allow knee extension and ankle dorsiflexion. The use of myofascial release techniques to reduce tightness in the intrinsic muscles and fascia of the foot can be helpful in preparing the foot to accept weight and allowing motion at the foot as the shank moves forward over the stance foot.

When inadequate knee extension in late swing is the result of knee-flexion contractures, manual stretching, casting, and splinting can be used to alter mechanical constraints. However, contractures will

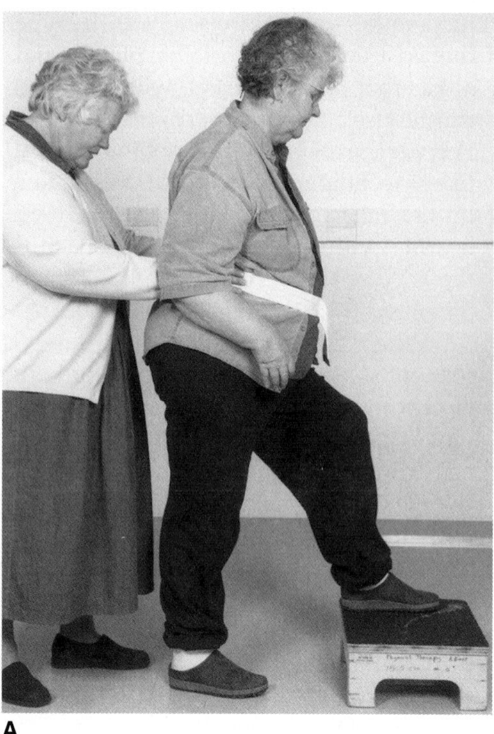

A

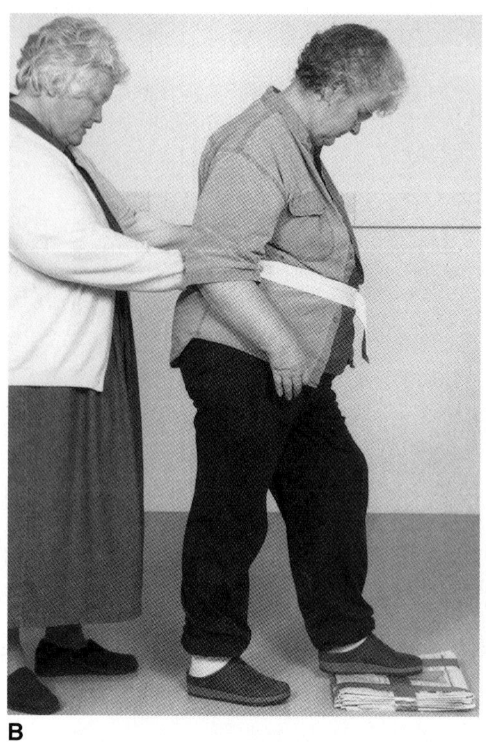

B

FIGURE 15.8 Activities that increase weight bearing in a single-limb stance include stepping up to a low stool (A) or to a taped stack of newspapers (B).

simply recur if the underlying cause is chronic overactivity of the hamstrings muscles during swing. Electrical stimulation of the quadriceps has been used to reciprocally inhibit overactive hamstrings muscles (Bogataj et al., 1989; Montgomery, 1987).

Inability to activate the tibialis anterior (TA) muscle is a common cause of impaired heel strike in the patient with neurologic impairments. Strengthening exercises to increase force production of the TA are important in making sure the TA is capable of generating force in response to descending commands. Unfortunately, the capacity to generate force does not ensure that the muscle will be recruited automatically during gait. Nonetheless, strengthening is necessary to ensure that the capability for force generation is at least present.

Biofeedback and/or electrical stimulation of the TA in conjunction with a foot switch placed inside the patient's shoe has been used effectively to increase activation of the TA at heel strike (Basmajian et al., 1975; Takebe et al., 1975; Waters et al., 1975). Functional electrical stimulation (FES) to multiple muscles may provide even greater improvements to gait. Kesar et al. (2009) examined the effects of FES on gait in 13 participants with poststroke hemiparesis. Compared to FES delivered to only the ankle dorsiflexor muscles during the swing phase, delivering FES to both the paretic-ankle plantar flexors during terminal stance and dorsiflexors during the swing phase resulted in greater swing-phase knee flexion, greater ankle plantar-flexion angle at toe-off, and greater forward propulsion. Thus multimuscle FES timed to the gait cycle corrected gait deficits at multiple joints (Kesar et al., 2009).

Use of an orthotic that has motion at the ankle joint (hinge joint), but a posterior stop is an effective way to control foot drop in an individual who is unable to recruit the TA. The ankle-joint motion of the orthotic allows some dorsiflexion, thus allowing the tibia to advance over the supporting foot. Coronal-plane foot problems affecting foot strike can often be controlled with an AFO. Nolan et al. (2009) examined the effect of wearing an AFO on gait in 18 participations with poststroke (>6 months) hemiparesis. They found that wearing an AFO significantly improved both the distance and the velocity walked, and the effect was greatest among participants with slower gait velocity.

A varus foot position during gait can be controlled with an AFO with a slight buildup of the lateral border of the foot. In addition, electrical stimulation of the toe extensors can reduce varus positioning during stance. A valgus foot position can be controlled with an AFO with a slight buildup of the medial border (Montgomery, 1987). The effect of a wedge insole can vary depending on how it is used. Chen et al. (2010)

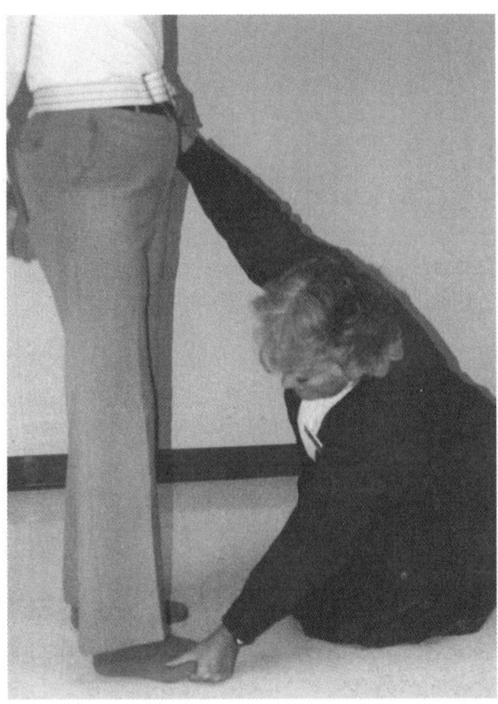

FIGURE 15.9 Helping the patient to accomplish a heel-first foot-strike pattern. This position will allow the body to move smoothly over the foot with good weight-bearing surface, enhancing both postural control and progression.

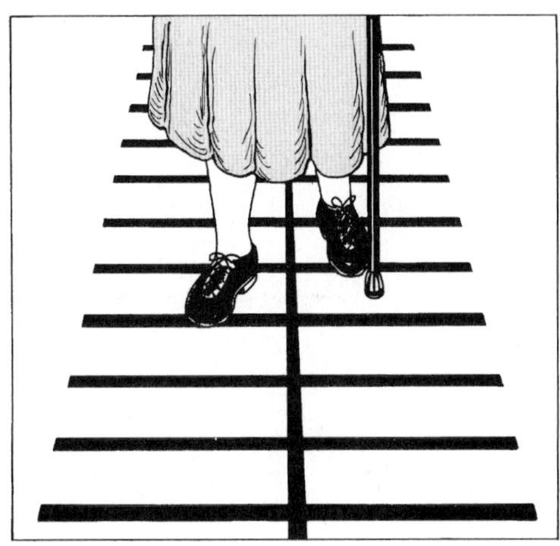

FIGURE 15.10 An example of a floor grid that can be used to visually guide patients toward better foot placement during gait. (Redrawn from Jims C. Foot placement pattern, an aid in gait training: suggestions from the field. Phys Ther 1977;57:286, with permission of the American Physical Therapy Association. This material is copyrighted, and any further reproduction or distribution requires written permission from APTA.)

examined the effect of lateral wedge insoles in the hemiparetic versus the nonhemiparetic limb on stance and gait in 10 individuals with poststroke hemiplegia. Interestingly, applying a 5-degree lateral wedge to the nonparetic limb resulted in improved symmetry in stance but not in gait. There was improved weight bearing at initial contact when the lateral wedge was worn under the varus foot. Finally, a lateral wedge worn on either foot reduced the internal load on the knee abductors, which in turn reduced the adductor external moment. The authors suggest that a reduced adductor load may reduce hip/knee pain in persons with poststroke hemiparesis (Chen et al., 2010).

Manual cues to facilitate hip flexion, knee extension, and ankle dorsiflexion at terminal swing in order to ensure a heel-first foot-strike pattern can be used; this is shown in Figure 15.9.

Improving foot placement by increasing step length can be assisted by making a grid on the floor, which helps to visually guide patients in establishing a better foot-placement pattern. This is shown in Figure 15.10. The distance between horizontal stripes can be individualized to the patient's desired stride length (Jims, 1977).

Balance During Double- and Single-Limb Support. Postural stability (control of the COM in both the frontal and sagittal planes) is critical to functionally independent gait, and emerges through the interaction of many sensorimotor systems. Therapeutic strategies focus on improving balance in both the single- and double-support phases of gait. Stability in the frontal plane is achieved through foot placement (step width) and depends to a large part on strength and coordination of the hip abductors (Patla et al., 1992). A common clinical practice used to help patients learn to improve control and movement of the COM involves having them practice voluntary lateral, anterior/posterior, and diagonal movements of the COM in stance (Fig. 15.11, A and B). However, the degree to which practice of isolated weight shift transfers to improved control of the COM in gait is unknown.

Use of Assistive Devices. Assistive devices contribute to postural stability by widening the base of support and providing additional support against gravity. A variety of assistive devices are available to provide support, including walkers (standard and rolling), canes (quad, tripod, and single-point) and various types of crutches (see Bateni & Maki, 2005, for a review). A number of factors are considered when prescribing an assistive device for a patient with neurologic impairments, including extent of physical disability, cognitive impairment, and the patient's personal motivations and desires (Allet et al., 2009; Schmitz, 1998). Allet et al. (2009) compared the effects of three different walking aids (four-point cane, single-point cane with ergonomic handle, and Nordic walking stick) on characteristics of gait and patient satisfaction in 25 inpatients with poststroke hemiparesis gait. Patients preferred the single-point cane,

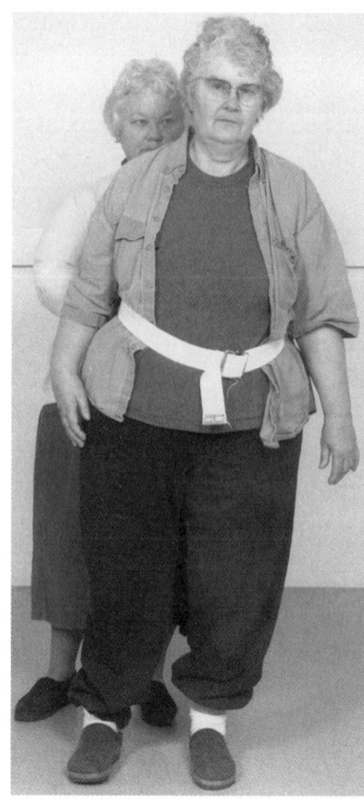

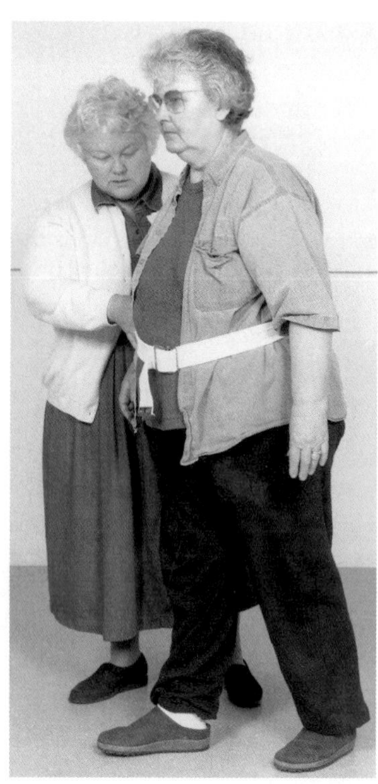

FIGURE 15.11 To improve stability, patients practice controlled movement of the COM in the lateral direction (A), in the anteroposterior direction (B), and in the diagonal direction (not shown).

which was associated with better walking velocity and distance, compared to the other two devices.

Walkers provide the greatest degree of stability during ambulation, further widening the base of support, and improving both lateral and anterior stability. A variety of walkers exist, including straight walkers and rolling walkers with two or four casters. An advantage of rolling walkers is that they allow patients to maintain speed, facilitating the generation of momentum, and thereby facilitating progression. However, the disadvantage of rolling walkers is that they have reduced stability as compared with standard pick-up walkers. New body-weight-support walkers are being developed that allow the extension of body weight support to overground walking training. The Body Weight Supported Walker consists of a light frame with casters, a harness, and a winch system, and enables a single therapist to perform gait training safely even in patients with severe gait impairment (Ochi et al., 2009).

A progression of assistive devices is often prescribed based on the amount of support available (e.g., walker, quad or tripod cane, single-point cane). Some treatment approaches discourage the use of assistive devices (particularly asymmetrical devices such as canes) as it is believed that using a walking aid such as a cane encourages a patient to lean to the sound side in order to apply weight to the assistive device. This then reinforces an asymmetric gait pattern (Davies, 1985). To examine clinical assumptions regarding the amount of weight carried through various assistive devices, one study examined the effect of three types of walking aids (tripod cane, two high sticks, and a single-point cane) on gait in patients following stroke. This study found that the amount of support taken through an assistive device appears to be related to factors associated with severity of hemiplegia (e.g., ability to bear weight through the weak limb during stance), not features of the walking aid per se (Tyson, 1998).

It is important to consider the effects of using various assistive devices on factors other than gait skills, such as attentional resources and their potential interference with balance in certain situations. Wright and Kemp (1992) reported the attentional costs associated with using an assistive device. *Attentional costs* refer to the demand for attentional resources for information processing during the performance of a task. The attentional demands can vary depending on the type of assistive device used and the patient's familiarity with the device. Their study reported that while both a rolling and a standard walker demand attention, a rolling walker is less attention-demanding than a standard pick-up walker (Wright & Kemp, 1992). Since there is some evidence that competing demands for attentional resources by postural and cognitive systems contribute to instability in the elderly (Shumway-Cook et al., 1997b), understanding the attentional requirements of the assistive devices we give patients is an important consideration during gait training.

Bateni and Maki (2005), in their review on the benefits and adverse consequences of assistive devices for balance and mobility, reported that while assistive devices do improve balance and mobility in many patients, some research has shown that the use of assistive devices increases the risk of falling by causing trips or disruption of balance. A number of studies have reported that inappropriate device use, inadequate training, and use of nonprescribed assistive devices contribute to falls (Bateni et al., 2004a, b; Milczarek et al., 1993).

Further information describing types of assistive devices, procedures for measuring, and techniques for training gait with assistive devices on level surface, curbs, and steps may be found in detail in other sources (O'Sullivan & Schmitz, 2001).

Progression

There is an impact on progression by both the generation of energy through concentric contractions and the absorption of energy through eccentric contractions. Thus, weakness will limit the generation of forces necessary for progression, while impairments such as spasticity and muscle shortening may result in inefficient gait through excessive energy absorption.

Energy Generation. As discussed in Chapter 12, there is controversy regarding the mechanisms used to generate energy to advance the body and achieve the goal of propulsion. Many researchers believe that the energy generated for gait comes from the gastrocnemius "pushing off" in terminal stance, and through the hip flexors, which "pull off" during initial swing. Therefore, exercises to improve plantar-flexor strength and reduce limitations in flexibility are critical, as are exercises to improve the strength of the hip flexors.

Patients can practice a forceful push-off (concentric contraction of the plantar flexors) while maintaining an extended leg posture (e.g., hip extension coupled with plantar flexion of the ankle), as shown in Figure 15.12. This includes practicing lifting the heel and moving the body weight anteriorly over the forefoot while the hip is extended and the knee flexes. Manual cues and assistance can be given by the clinician as needed to facilitate this component of gait.

To improve the ability of the hip flexors to participate in generation of power for progression, the patient can also practice pull-off (exaggerating hip flexion) during the initiation of swing. Manual cues and support of the leg can be provided by the therapist as needed. Other activities to facilitate hip flexion during swing have been used, including marching in place and practicing a high-step gait—that is, bringing the knee up into an exaggerated flexed position (Fig. 15.13). Finally, as shown by Olney et al. (1991, 1994), increasing the speed of walking will have a tendency to increase the speed and amplitude of hip flexion during the initiation of the swing phase of gait, and this will facilitate passive knee flexion for toe clearance.

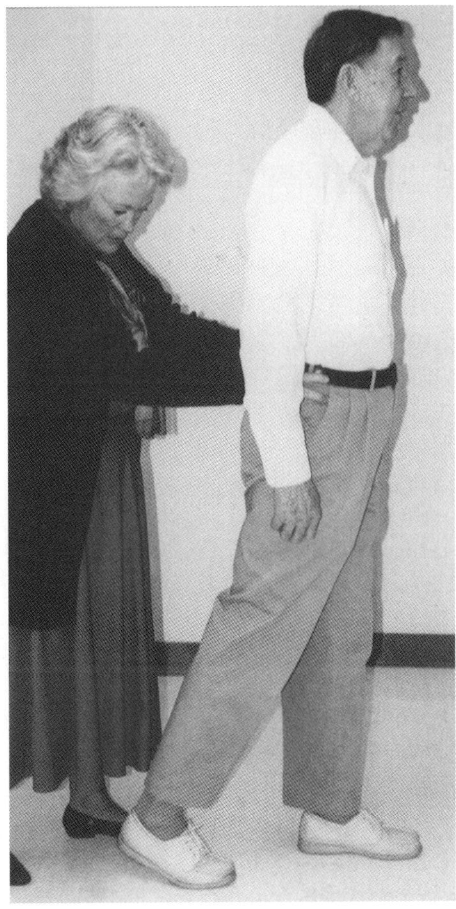

FIGURE 15.12 Patient practices a forceful push-off (concentric contraction) of the gastrocnemius, in an extended leg posture.

Treatments to reduce spasticity in the triceps surae will improve forward movement of the shank over the foot. As discussed in the previous section, treatments to reduce the tone and tightness in intrinsic muscles of the foot will ensure that the foot can roll off, lifting the heel and pushing onto the ball of the foot. Inability to advance the weight to the forefoot due to clawing of the toes can be treated with a shoe insert that spreads and extends the toes (Montgomery, 1987).

Advancement of the Swing Limb. To advance the swing limb, clearing the supporting surface with the foot requires activation of the plantar flexors at

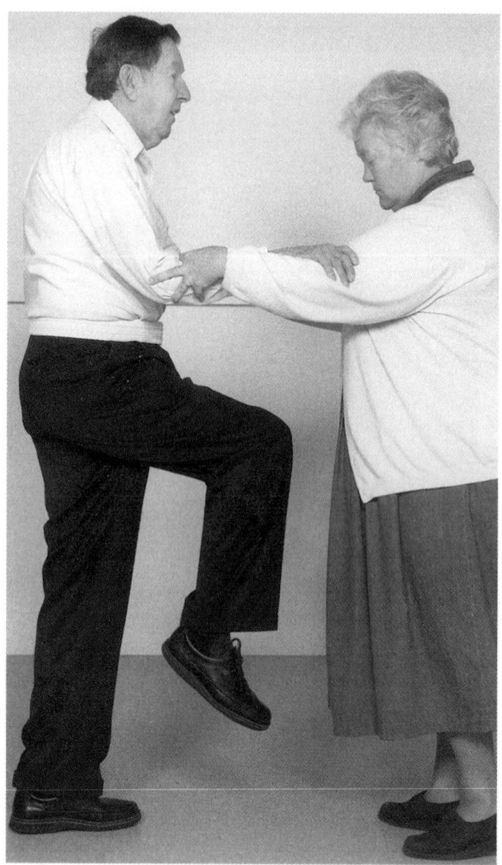

FIGURE 15.13 Improving use of the hip flexors to pull off the swing limb through practice of a high-step gait pattern.

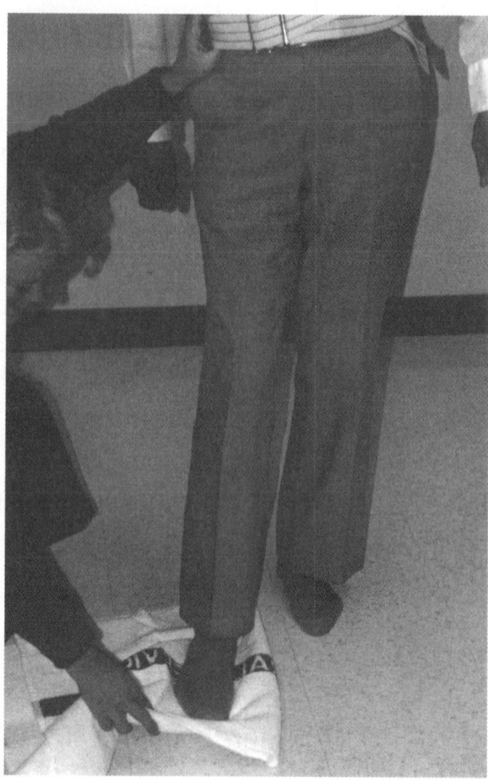

FIGURE 15.14 Placing a towel under the hemiparetic leg to facilitate advancement of the swing limb without lateral trunk lean or hip hike.

push-off in conjunction with hip flexors at the initiation of swing to draw the thigh segment forward with sufficient force to passively flex the knee. In addition, activation of the TA to dorsiflex the ankle is also important to the achievement of foot clearance. Thus, loss of foot clearance can be caused by: (1) weakness of the plantar flexors, hip flexors, and/or TA, (2) spasticity of the ankle plantar flexors and/or hamstrings, or (3) neural control problems affecting the appropriate activation of muscles such as the TA muscle during swing.

Early in gait training, when the patient does not have sufficient control to advance the swing limb using hip and knee flexion, a towel can be placed under the patient's foot to facilitate advancement of the foot (Davies, 1985). This is shown in Figure 15.14. Alternatively, an elastic bandage (Fig. 15.15) can be used to prevent ankle plantar flexion and subsequent toe drag during the swing phase of gait (Davies, 1985).

Additional suggestions to improve flexion of the swing limb were described above, in the section on postural support and stability.

What is the optimal walking speed at which to retrain gait? Several researchers have shown an association between walking speed and characteristics of gait. Olney et al. (1991, 1994) studied changes in gait associated with changes in gait speed in a group of patients with hemiparesis following stroke. Gait changes associated with increased walking velocity included greater hip extension at terminal stance and increased hip flexor moment at the initiation of swing. Wagenaar and Beek (1992) found that patients who had had a stroke, like healthy controls, modified gait characteristics (stride length and frequency) in response to changing gait velocities. Andriacchi et al. (1977) found that following a stroke, the presence of asymmetry in gait is highly dependent on walking speed. Thus, individuals who walk at faster speeds tend to be less asymmetrical than those who walk at slower speeds. This research suggests that one way to have a powerful impact on gait is to increase the speed at which the patient is walking. This may seem counterintuitive to therapists, who often work with patients at relatively slow speeds of walking in order to improve the quality of the movement patterns used to achieve gait.

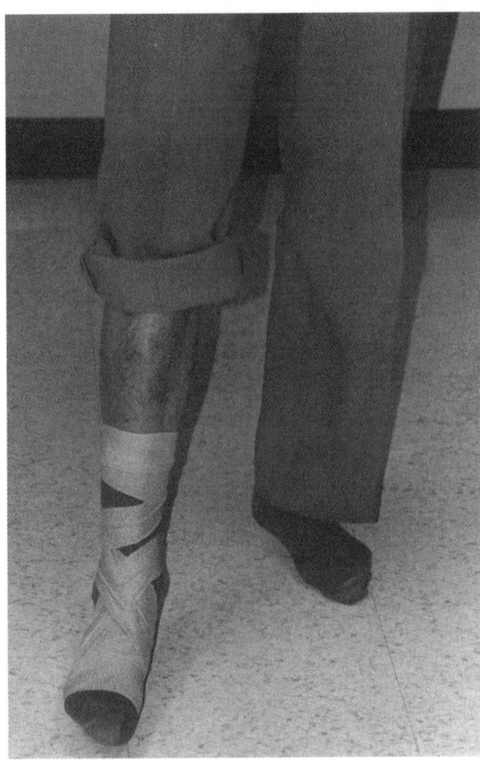

FIGURE 15.15 Using an elastic bandage to maintain the ankle in dorsiflexion and to facilitate toe clearance.

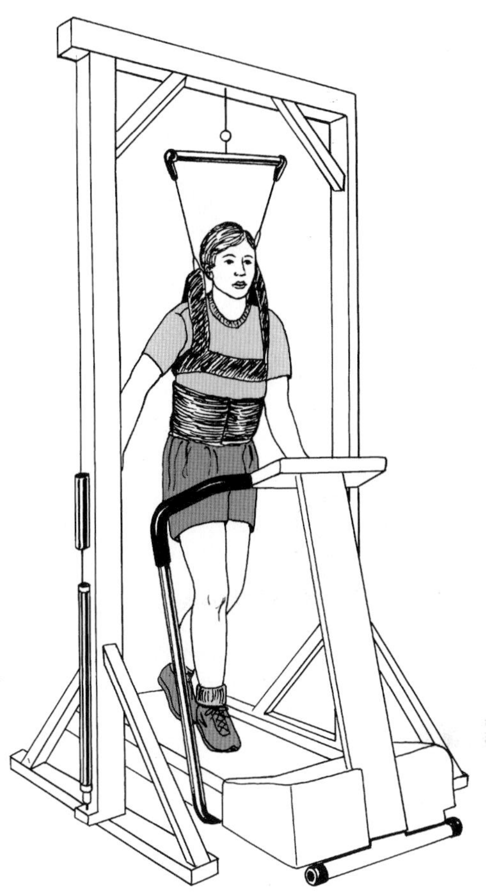

FIGURE 15.16 Gait retraining using a treadmill and harness system for partial support of body weight.

Whole vs. Part Practice in Locomotor Training

The preceding section reviewed strategies for improving components of the gait pattern with a focus on part-task practice. However, as reviewed in Chapter 2, motor learning research suggests that combining part with whole-task practice is necessary to achieve maximal function. Locomotor training using body-weight support on a treadmill (BWST), or robotic devices such as the Lokomat, are examples of whole task training.

Body Weight Support on a Treadmill Training. BWST training uses a harness to provide partial body-weight support in conjunction with a motorized treadmill to facilitate extended practice of the entire gait pattern. As gait improves, support is decreased and the patient is required to control a greater and greater percentage of body weight (Cernack et al., 2008; Finch et al., 1991; Hesse et al., 1994, 1995; Richards et al., 1993; Waagfjord et al., 1990). An example of a partial-weight-support harness system is shown in Figure 15.16.

Researchers examining locomotor training have suggested that training using BWST has several advantages: (1) the body-weight-support harness allows a progressive increase in the demands for postural control, (2) the treadmill allows systematic control and progression of the speed at which walking is performed, and (3) the repetitive training of a complete gait cycle enables a more appropriate pattern of sensory input associated with the different phases of gait to stimulate the locomotor pattern. In addition, locomotor training using BWST allows the therapist to provide manual assistance to help the patient simulate a more normal walking pattern (Barbeau, 2003; Behrman et al., 2005, 2006; Cernack et al., 2008).

A considerable number of research studies have examined the effect of treadmill training alone or in combination with body-weight support on recovery of gait in a variety of patient populations.

Treadmill Training after Stroke. Hesse and colleagues (1994, 1995, 1999) have performed a group of studies comparing the effect of treadmill training with partial weight support (PWS) to other forms of physical therapy. In one study, they compared treadmill training to neurofacilitation treatment in seven patients with hemiparesis following stroke. They used

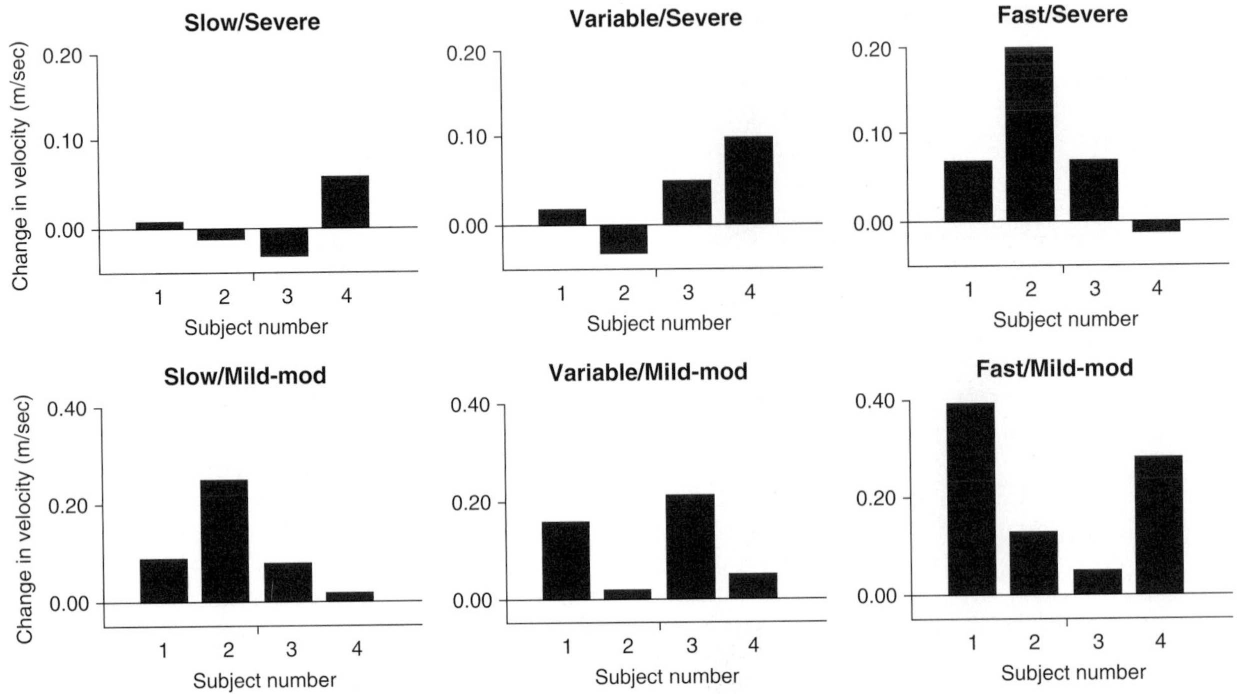

FIGURE 15.17 Individual data from six subjects with stroke, illustrating the interacting effects of speed of treadmill training (slow, fast, or variable) and severity of locomotor impairment (severe versus mild to moderate). Posttraining change in gait velocity (m/sec) is shown in the two groups of subjects under the three training speeds. (Reprinted with permission from Sullivan KJ, Knowlton BJ, Dobkin BH. Step training with body weight support: effect of treadmill speed and practice paradigms on poststroke locomotor recovery. Arch Phys Med Rehabil 2002;83:688.)

an ABA single case study with 3 weeks (15 sessions) of PWS treadmill training (A1), followed by 3 weeks (15 sessions) of neurofacilitation treatment (Bobath approach) (B), and finally 3 more weeks (15 sessions) of PWS treadmill training (A2). Treadmill training sessions lasted 30 minutes, body-weight support was progressively decreased from 70% to 0%, and gait was trained at velocities that ranged from initial speeds of 0.7 to 0.22 m/sec to final speeds of 0.18 to 0.22 m/sec. Gait significantly improved in all patients; with patients able to walk independently at the end of the study. Gait velocity, step and stride length, and cadence all significantly increased during the first treadmill training sessions (A1), but not during the neurofacilitation treatments (B). The authors conclude that practicing components of walking in isolation (the neurofacilitation approach) is not as effective as practicing the entire task of gait in the functional context of walking on a treadmill.

Sullivan and colleagues (2002) used a randomized, repeated-measures design to study the effect of BWST training in 24 individuals with hemiparetic gait with walking speeds that were at least 50% below normal. This study also examined the effect of treadmill speed on outcomes. Participants were stratified by locomotor severity to treadmill training at slow (0.5 mph), fast (2.0 mph), or variable (0.5, 1.0, 1.5, and 2.0 mph) speeds. Training sessions were 20 min, three times a week for 4 weeks. Self-selected walking speed was measured at the onset, middle, and end of training and 1 and 3 months later. For all groups, the percentage of body-weight support progressively decreased from an average of 34% at the beginning of training to an average of 11 to 14% at the end of training. All three training groups improved in self-selected gait speed and continued to make improvements in walking speed across the 1-month follow-up, which were sustained at 3 months. In general, the greatest gains in gait speed were in the group who trained at the fast treadmill speed; however, as can be seen in Figure 15.17, there was considerable variability across participants.

Sullivan and colleagues did not include overground walking training as part of their protocol. A study by Ada et al. (2003) examined a combination of treadmill (without body-weight support) and overground walking training in individuals with hemiparetic gait disorders following a stroke (average time since stroke, 28 months). Participants included 27 subjects randomly assigned to one of two treatment groups; the experimental group performed a 30-minute treadmill and overground walking program three times a week for 4 weeks. Treadmill training was progressed by increasing treadmill speed, reducing hand support, and the performance of a secondary task to increase the automaticity of walking. Overground walking training included practicing walking around an outdoor circuit that included walking forward, backward, sideways, and up and down curbs, slopes, stairs, and rough terrain while conversing with the trainer (dual-task). The control group received a low-intensity home exercise program of strength, flexibility, and balance (low intensity to reduce a training effect, providing a sham program) and regular telephone contact. Results supported the effectiveness of the mobility-training program on improving gait speed and distance (with a significant improvement in step length [but not width]), which were sustained at 3 months. There was no significant difference in mobility disability as measured by the Sickness Impact Profile; however, 58% of the participants in the experimental group reported going out in the community more often as a result of training, as compared with 25% of the control group.

Richards et al. (2004) used a randomized, controlled trial (RCT) to examined two approaches to locomotor training—a technology-based, task-oriented locomotor training program (treadmill training, a Kinetron for muscle strengthening while performing walking movements, and a limb-load monitor to improve loading of the affected limb [n = 32]) to a non–technology-based task-oriented approach (practicing functional mobility skills and dynamic gait activities without technology [n = 31]) in participants approximately 52 days after they experienced a stroke. Training for both groups was 60 minutes, five times a week for 2 months. Their results found that irrespective of training mode, all participants in the subacute phase after stroke who received task-oriented therapy (with or without technology) markedly improved gait speed and maintained that improvement over 3 months.

In a Cochrane database systematic review, Moseley et al. (2003) examined the research evidence for treadmill training and body-weight support for walking after stroke. They performed a systematic review of 11 randomized and quasirandomized or controlled trials (458 participants) using BWST training following stroke. The review concluded that BWSTT was effective in improving gait speed in ambulatory persons; however there was not enough evidence to fully determine the benefits of BWSTT relative to other forms of locomotor training. More research is needed to explore this and to clarify the effects of treadmill training for people who cannot walk independently (Mosely et al., 2003). In a commentary on this review, Helbostad (2003) suggested that despite these results, treadmill training may be of benefit for persons with limited walking ability, since it allows a greater amount of training; in addition, it may be the only alternative for walking training in persons who are not able to walk, even with support from walking aids or other persons.

Does locomotor training alter underlying gait patterns in persons with stroke? The evidence for this is mixed. Mulroy and colleagues (2010) characterized changes in gait parameters in participants with post-stroke hemiparetic gait who had completed 6 weeks of task-specific locomotor training. Gait characteristics were compared among a high-response group (participants who showed an increase in gait speed of greater than 0.08 m/sec) vs. a low-response group (those with less than a 0.08 m/sec improvement). After the intervention, the high-response group had greater improvements in kinematic, kinetic, and muscle activity patterns as compared with the low-response group. These changes—including increased terminal-stance hip extension, hip-flexion power, and intensity of soleus muscle EMG activity—were associated with increases in gait speed. In contrast, Den Otter et al. (2006) found that improvements in gait speed were not associated with a change in the temporal pattern of muscle activity in the lower extremities in persons with stroke participating in 10 weeks of locomotor rehabilitation. Despite improved gait speed and function, duration of muscle coactivity, abnormal muscle timing, and gait asymmetry persisted. The authors conclude that recovery of walking ability following stroke is not dependent on normalization of the temporal coordination of muscle activity. More research is needed to determine the effect of locomotor training on underlying gait mechanisms.

Treadmill Training with Children. Richards and colleagues (1997) have begun exploring the use of treadmill training with partial body-weight support (PBW) in very young children who have cerebral palsy. Their preliminary work suggests that PBW treadmill training is feasible in children as young as 15 months, and can be used in children who are not yet walking independently.

Ulrich et al. (2001) examined whether the use of a treadmill to practice stepping could have an impact on the onset of walking in children with Down syndrome (DS; trisomy 21). Thirty families of infants with DS were randomly assigned to the intervention or control group once the children could sit alone for 30 seconds. All infants received traditional physical therapy at least every other week, and in addition, the intervention infants practiced stepping on a small motorized treadmill, 5 days/week for 8 minutes a day, in their own homes. Their parents, who received training, provided assistance. The results from this study found that infants in the experimental group learned to walk with help and to walk independently significantly more quickly (73.8 days and 101 days, respectively) than the control group. These results provide evidence that treadmill training (with the support of parents trained to assist) can help infants with DS learn to walk earlier than they normally would.

Locomotor training using BWS on a treadmill in conjunction with overground gait training was an effective way to improve ambulatory function in a 13-year-old child with severe cerebellar ataxia; however, the intensity and duration of training required for functionally significant improvements were significantly longer than most traditional rehabilitation programs offer (Cernak et al., 2008). Improvements in functional walking were obtained after 6 months of intensive (5 days/week) locomotor training that included BWST training in conjunction with overground practice (Cernak et al., 2008).

Treadmill Training in Parkinson's Disease. Miyai et al. (2002) used an RCT to investigate whether BWST training was of long-term benefit for patients with Parkinson's disease (PD). Twenty-four patients (Hoehn and Yahr stage 2.5 or 3) were randomized to receive either a 45-minute session of BWST training (up to 20% of body weight supported) or conventional physical therapy (PT), three times a week for 1 month. The BWST training group had significantly greater improvement than the PT group in ambulation speed at 1 month and in the number of steps at 1, 2, 3, and 4 months after training, leading the authors to conclude that BWST training for 1 month had a positive effect on ambulation that lasted for 4 months.

What can we conclude from the research on BWST training? The research in adults suggests that it is as effective as (but not more effective than) task-oriented training (without technology). In addition, it may be particularly beneficial in patients who are unable to walk without assistance, and in children who have not yet learned to walk. A limitation of BWST training in adults is that it is more time- and labor-intensive than overground training, although it gives more intensive training; e.g., it often requires three or more persons to assist the nonambulating patient with walking. The advancement of electromechanical (robotic) gait trainers may enable nonambulatory patients to practice gait-like movements with minimal assistance (Werner et al., 2002).

Robotic Training of Gait. Robotic devices, such as the Lokomat (Hocoma, Inc., Zurich, Switzerland) have been developed to automate locomotor training in neurorehabilitation (Westlake & Patten, 2009). A growing number of studies have examined the effect of robotic gait trainers on walking function in various neurologic populations. Westlake and Patten (2009) compared locomotor training with a robotic device (Lokomat) to body-weight-support treadmill training with manual assistance. Overall, there were no differences between the two approaches to training on self selected walking speed and step-length ratio, though effect size was greater on the Lokomat group on other variables, suggesting a slight advantage to that form of training. Schwartz et al. (2009) also compared the effectiveness of early and prolonged locomotor treatment with the use of a robotically assisted gait-training, to conventional PT alone, on functional ambulation outcomes in 67 patients with subacute stroke. Compared to the control group receiving conventional PT, participants in the robotically assisted group had greater gains on the Functional Ambulatory Capacity Scale, but there were no significant differences on gait velocity or endurance between the two groups. While these and other studies (Husemann et al., 2007; Pohl et al., 2007) suggest that robotic training is as effective as, or in some cases more effective than, conventional training, several studies have reported the opposite. These studies have found that participants with stroke receiving conventional gait training had significantly better gains in walking velocity and distance as compared with those receiving the same amount of training with the Lokomat (Hidler et al., 2009; Hornby et al., 2008). More research is needed to determine the efficacy of locomotor training using robotic devices as compared with other approaches, and the types of patients who will benefit from each. One distinct advantage in robotic training is the reduced number of people needed to carry out the training as compared with BWST training. A disadvantage may be the lack of variability in training parameters associated with robotic training.

Interventions to Improve Functional Locomotor Skills

Intervention at the functional level focuses on having patients practice functional locomotor skills under a variety of task and environment contexts in order to learn to adapt gait to functional demands likely to be encountered in the home and community environment. Task-oriented training of gait and other motor skills focuses on addressing functional activity limitations, not on the isolated remediation of underlying impairments. In their review, Winstein and Wolf (2009) suggest that in order for a training program to be considered task-oriented, it must be:

1. **Challenging** enough to require new learning and to engage attention to solve the motor problem;
2. **Progressive and optimally adapted** such that over practice, the task demand is optimally adapted to the patient's capability and the environmental context; not too simple or repetitive to not challenge, and not too difficult to cause a failure of motor learning or a low sense of competence,
3. Interesting enough to invoke **active participation** to engage a "particular type of repetition" referred to as "problem-solving."

The three criteria (i.e., challenging, progressive and optimally adapted, and active participation) are not necessarily independent, but rather complementary in nature (Winstein & Wolf, 2009).

Thus an important aspect of task-oriented locomotor training is to progressively increase the difficulty of training activities in order to maintain the challenge as patients improve. As patients learn to develop strategies effective in meeting the task requirement of locomotion in relatively non-demanding environments, such as on a level surface, training is broadened to include achieving functional walking skills under more complex and challenging conditions. These types of activities are often referred to as "dynamic gait" or "complex walking activities."

Complex walking activities are designed to improve both anticipatory and reactive components of postural control during ambulation. In Table 15.6 we summarize a framework for organizing dynamic gait activities based on the eight environmental dimensions identified in work by Shumway-Cook and colleagues (Patla & Shumway-Cook, 1999; Shumway-Cook et al., 2002, 2003, 2005). This table lists the eight dimensions, the goal for gait training in each dimension, and examples of some of the activities that could be used to train each dimension of locomotor adaptation. Examples of these activities include the ability to step over obstacles of various heights (Fig. 15.18A) or around obstacles (Fig. 15.18B), to walk a straight path while turning the head (Fig. 15.19), and to walk while interacting with an external physical load, such as carrying an object (Fig. 15.20A) or opening a heavy door (Fig. 15.20B). In this way patients learn to modify gait

TABLE 15.6 Summary of Environmental Dimensions and Associated Activities to Promote Locomotor Adaptation, Based on a Proposed Framework by Patla and Shumway-Cook (1999)

Dimension	Items
Distance	**Goal**: Increase distance walked at comfortable speed, community ambulation goal 1200 ft. **Activities**: • Practice continuous walking while gradually increasing distance walked.
Temporal	**Goal**: Increase comfortable and fast walking speeds, ability to change speeds safely. Community ambulation goal: comfortable walking speed of ≥0.45 m/sec, with ability to walk ≥0.8 m/sec for distances of 40 ft (to cross streets) **Activities**: • Practice continuous walking at comfortable speed, gradually increasing gait velocity. • Practice fast walking, gradually increasing gait velocity. • Practice increasing and decreasing speed safely, with short bursts of fast walking for distances of 40 to 60 ft.
Ambient	**Goal**: Walk safely under different light and weather conditions. **Activities:** • Practice walking under different light-level conditions and during transitions in light (e.g., light to dark, dark to light). • Practice walking outside in different light and weather conditions.
Terrain	**Goal**: Ability to walk safely under changing terrain characteristics. **Activities**: • Practice walking on uneven surfaces, up and down curbs, ramps. • Practice walking up and down stairs

(continued)

TABLE 15.6 Summary of Environmental Dimensions and Associated Activities to Promote Locomotor Adaptation, Based on a Proposed Framework by Patla and Shumway-Cook (1999)

Physical load	**Goal**: Ability to walk safely while interacting with physical loads, including carrying/pushing/pulling loads. **Activities:** • Practice walking while carrying weights, gradually increasing the weight of objects carried. • Practice carrying weight distributed over one or two packages carried in the arms (e.g., grocery bag) or held by hand (e.g., plastic bag with handles). • Practice carrying loads of varying fragility and predictability (e.g., paper cup vs. water glass (filled to various levels), tray with rolling ball or egg). • Practice opening/closing manual doors of varying weights. • Practice walking while pushing/pulling loads of varying weights.
Postural transitions	**Goal**: Ability to walk safely while making postural transitions. **Activities**: • Practice static stance tasks—standing reach above, below, and forward; stepping forward, sideways, backward; stepping up (forward, sideways). • Practice dynamic tasks that require proactive balance control, such as walking with postural transitions, including: walking with head turns; change in direction; pivot turns; walking forward, sideways, and backward; walking with wide/narrow base of support; walking with long/short steps, stops, and starts; sit to stand and walk. • Practice recovery of balance while walking: walking on treadmill with varying speeds, walking against unpredictable and variable resistance from elastic tubing, walking while recovering from small external perturbations given manually.
Attentional demands	**Goal**: Maintain safe ambulation while concurrently performing a secondary manual or cognitive task. Also includes ability to walk in noisy distracting environments and to navigate in novel environments. **Activities**: • Practice walking while simultaneously performing secondary cognitive tasks (see Table 11.11 for examples of tasks used in training). • Practice walking in noisy, crowded, and distracting environments (busy hallways, hospital dining room, therapy rooms with loud distracting music playing, malls). • Practice walking and navigating to familiar and unfamiliar places.
Density and collision Avoidance	**Goal**: Ability to walk safely while avoiding contact with obstacles in the environment. **Activities**: • Practice walking over, around, and under static objects that vary in height/width and fragility. • Practice walking over and around dynamic (moving) obstacles. • Collision avoidance should be practiced with objects presented on the floor as well as overhead, requiring persons to duck under an object.

in anticipation of potentially destabilizing threats to balance during gait.

Strategies to retrain compensatory responses to unexpected perturbations to gait include unexpectedly changing the speed of a treadmill while the patient is walking on it. It is also possible to ask the individual to walk against resistance (using elastic tubing) and to unexpectedly release the resistance to give an unexpected perturbation to forward progression. It is very important to have the patient wear a gait belt (or harness system) and to guard them carefully during dynamic gait tasks in order to prevent a fall.

Research Evidence

Reviewing the research evidence for a task-oriented approach to training walking function can be difficult because there is no consensus on what constitutes

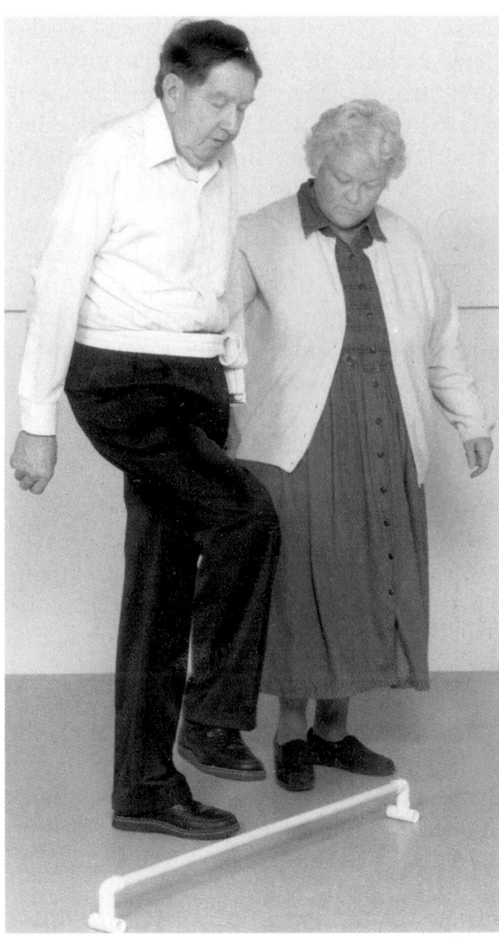
A

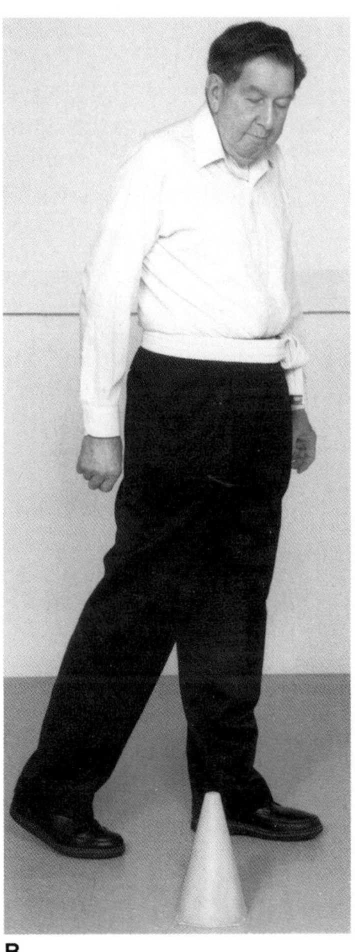
B

FIGURE 15.18 Retraining dynamic gait skills. Practicing collision avoidance by stepping over (A), and around (B) obstacles.

task-oriented training. Some studies use the term *task-oriented* to describe gait training with a body-weight-support system and motorized treadmill. Others use the term to reflect practice of a progression of functional tasks that may or may not include treadmill training. In addition, so-called task-oriented training may or may not also include interventions designed to improve impairments in strength, flexibility, balance, and cardiovascular endurance. Consistent across all task-oriented intervention studies is a primary focus on the practice of functional tasks related to mobility. The following review of research studies is designed to examine the evidence for improving mobility in patients with neurologic pathology and to give the reader a sense of the specific types of therapeutic strategies that were used in these studies to effectively improve mobility.

Mobility Training after Stroke

Much of the research examining the efficacy of mobility training has focused on poststroke training.

Acute and Subacute Stroke. Salbach et al. (2004) used an RCT to examine the efficacy of a task-oriented walking intervention following stroke. Subjects included 91 individuals less than 1 year after they had experienced a stroke, randomly assigned to receive a 6-week intervention (60 minutes, three times a week) that targeted walking or upper-extremity (UE) function. Walking training included a progressive program of 10 functional tasks, including walking on a treadmill, standing up and walking to and sitting down on a chair, kicking a soccer ball against a wall, walking a balance beam, performing step-ups, walking an obstacle course, walking while carrying an object, walking at maximal speed, walking backward, and walking up and down stairs. A control group practiced UE tasks while sitting. Results are shown in Table 15.7 and indicate that as compared with those in the UE training, participants in the walking intervention improved on all measures of gait, with the greatest improvements found in the subjects with moderately severe gait problems.

Duncan and colleagues (2003) examined the effects of an individualized home-based exercise program

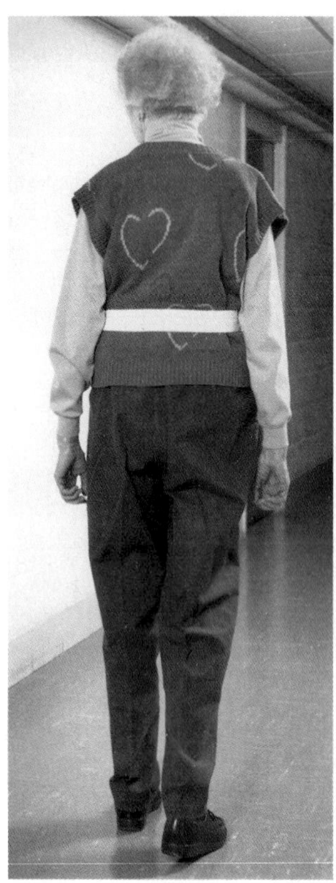

FIGURE 15.19 Retraining dynamic gait skills. Walking a straight path while practicing head turns.

(90-minute sessions, three times a week for 12 weeks) on balance and mobility in subacute stroke (average, 77 days after stroke). Participants were randomly assigned to a usual care versus home exercise program with four components: strengthening, balance (step-ups, chair rise, marching in place, toe rises, wall exercise [standing leaning back to a wall and bouncing upright again]), UE functional use, and endurance (riding a stationary bike, progressing up to 30 minutes with increased resistance). The home-based exercise group made significantly greater improvements in balance (Berg Balance Scale), gait speed (10-m test), and distance (6-minute walk test) compared with the usual care group.

Chronic Stroke. Mudge et al. (2009) used circuit-based rehabilitation to improve walking function in 60 participants at least 6 months after stroke. Participants in the exercise group received 12 sessions of locomotor training at 15 different exercise stations (shown in Table 15.8). The control group participated in 12 sessions of social interaction and education. The exercise group walked a significantly greater distance on the 6-minute walk test compared to the control group immediately after the intervention, but improvements were not retained 3 months later. There was no difference in gait velocity or other measures of usual walking performance between the groups.

Dean and colleagues (2000) examined the effects of 4-week task-related circuit training on patients with chronic stroke randomly assigned to one of two

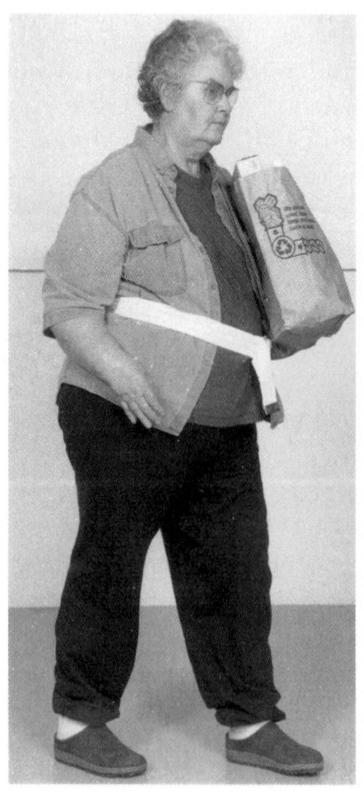

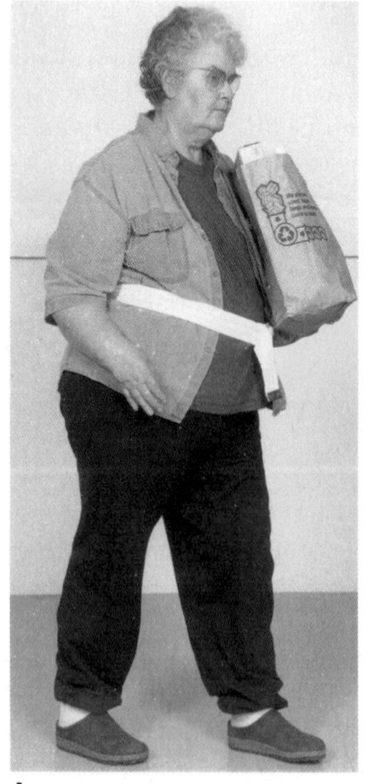

A

B

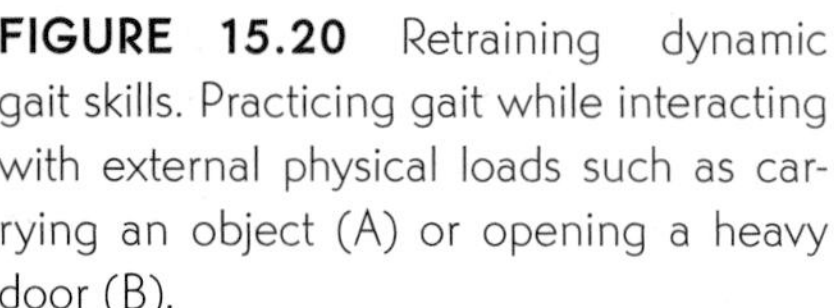

FIGURE 15.20 Retraining dynamic gait skills. Practicing gait while interacting with external physical loads such as carrying an object (A) or opening a heavy door (B).

TABLE 15.7 The Effects of Two Types of Training on Balance and Mobility Following Stroke

Measure	Mobility Training (*n* = 44)		UE Training (*n* = 47)		Group Difference (95% CI)
	Mean ± SD	Range	Mean ± SD	Range	
Six-minute walk test (m)					
Pre	209 ± 126	13–520	204 ± 31	9–594	
Post	249 ± 136	37–530	209 ± 132	4–550	
Change	40 ± 72	−61–381	5 ± 66	−90–379	35 (7–64)
Comfortable walking speed (m/sec)					
Pre	0.64 ± 0.33	0.10–1.41	0.61 ± 0.37	0.08–1.90	
Post	0.78 ± 0.40	0.10–1.58	0.64 ± 0.37	0.01–1.29	
Change	0.14 ± 0.18	−0.31–0.60	0.03 ± 0.20	−0.76–046	0.11 (0.03–0.19)
Maximum walking speed (m/sec)					
Pre	0.79 ± 0.45	0.12–1.84	0.81 ± 0.49	0.08–2.33	
Post	0.99 ± 0.56	0.11–2.33	0.80 ± 0.49	0.01–1.93	
Change	0.20 ± 0.26	−0.24–1.16	−0.01 ± 0.18	−0.68–0.30	0.21 (0.12–0.30)
Timed Up and Go (sec)					
Pre	24.4 ± 18.8	7.9–88.9	25.5 ± 21.7	7.0–100.0	
Post	23.2 ± 20.6	6.3–93.7	27.1 ± 27.1	7.3–154.4	
Change	−1.2 ± 9.7	−22.3–51.7	1.7 ± 13.5	−17.6–58.6	−2.9 (−7.8–2.0)
Berg Balance Scale (/56)					
Pre	42 ± 11	21–56	40 ± 13	5–56	
Post	44 ± 11	11–56	41 ± 13	10–55	
Change	2 ± 6	−12–18	1 ± 6	−12–12	*

UE = upper extremity

* Wilcoxon rank-sum test; p = 0.854

Reprinted with permission from Salbach NM, Mayo NE, Wood-Dauphinee S et al. A task-oriented intervention enhances walking distance and speed in the first year post stroke: a randomized controlled trial. Clin Rehabil 2004;18:514.

exercise classes. The control group (n = 6) practiced UE tasks, while the experimental group (n = 6) practiced functional locomotor tasks in a supervised exercise class set up as a circuit training course (circuit stations are described in Table 15.9). Both groups practiced for 60 minutes, three times a week for 4 weeks (12 sessions). Subjects practiced for approximately 5 minutes at each of the 10 stations, then spent 10 minutes in walking relays and races, providing 1 hour of continuous practice of locomotor-related tasks. Subjects were evaluated prior to, immediately following, and 2 months after training. Results on the clinical measures are shown in Figure 15.21. As compared with the control group, participants in the locomotor training group improved walking speed over 10 m (with and without assistive devices), distance walking on the 6-minute walk, and ability to load the affected limb as indicated by performance on the step test (number of times the person could place their unaffected foot on top of a 7.5-cm-high wooden block in 15 seconds).

TABLE 15.8 Content and Progressions of Circuit Exercise Program

Exercise Station	Progressions
1. Sit to stand	Increase speed until can complete 30, then decrease seat height.
2. Self-sway	Start near wall for support, sway from ankles forward and backward, progress by increasing amplitude, then progress to standing away from wall.
3. Standing balance	Stand in parallel bars with feet close together. Try to balance as long as possible. Progress by adding crossed arms and turns of upper body. Progress further to standing on one leg.
4. Step-ups	Start with low step. Progress by increasing height of step.
5. Balance beam	Step over balance beam, leading with alternate feet. Progress by increasing speed. Progress further to crossovers.
6. Standing hamstring curl	Progress weight and repetitions.
7. Tandem walk	Walk with feet touching line on floor. Progress to heel–toe. Progress further by decreasing speed, looking forward, and crossing arms.
8. Swiss ball squats	Progress depth of squat until thighs are parallel with ground. Add hold, which can be progressed by increasing time. Progress further by adding weights to hands.
9. Tandem stance	Start with hands on wall for balance. Progress base of support until heel–toe. Progress to center of room. Progress to arms crossed.
10. Calf raise	Start with double calf raise. Progress speed. Progress to single calf raise. Progress to jumps.
11. Backward walk	Start near wall for balance. Progress to center of room. Progress to shuttle runs.
12. Lunges	Start holding on for support. Progress depth of lunge. Progress number on each leg. Progress to no support.
13. Side leg lifts	Progress weight and repetitions.
14. Marching in place	Progress to marching with a weight, marching with no hand support, marching on mini-trampoline.
15. Obstacle course	Progress by increasing speed, varying obstacles.

Two minutes at each station, finish with 5 minutes stretching major leg muscle groups.
Reprinted with permission from Mudge S, Barber PA, Stott NS. Circuit-based rehabilitation improves gait endurance but not usual walking activity in chronic stroke: a randomized controlled trial. Arch Phys Med Rehabil 2009;90:1994:Appendix 1.

There were no significant changes in the Timed Up and Go test for either group. In addition, improvements were sustained at the 2-month examination.

Bassile et al. (2003) used a case series of five individuals with chronic stroke to examine the effects of an obstacle-training program on gait. The intervention included twice-weekly, 60-minute sessions for 4 weeks, in which subjects practiced walking on a 10-m walkway over obstacles that varied by both height (6.5, 13, and 27 cm) and width (6.5, 13, and 27 cm). Subjects alternated leading with the affected then the unaffected limb. Ambulation without obstacles was practiced for one-third of the total passes for each session, and task difficulty was increased over the training period. Participants significantly improved gait velocity (mean [±SD] speed before training, 0.97±0.42 m/sec; mean speed after training, 1.15±0.39, which was sustained at 1 month. Distance walked on the 6-minute walk also improved (before, 339 m; after, 407 m) but was not sustained at 1 month.

TABLE 15.9 Exercises Performed in Each of 10 Stations Used to Train Mobility Function after Stroke

1. Sitting at a table and reaching in different directions for objects located beyond arm length to promote loading of the affecting leg and activation of paretic leg muscles.
2. Sit to stand from various chair heights to strengthen affected leg extensor muscles.
3. Stepping forward, backward, and sideways onto blocks of various heights to strengthen affected leg muscles.
4. Heel lifts in standing to strengthen affected plantar-flexor muscles.
5. Standing with base of support constrained, feet in parallel and tandem while reaching for object, including down to the floor, to improve balance.
6. Reciprocal leg flexion and extension using the Kinetron in standing to strengthen leg muscles.
7. Standing up from a chair, walking a short distance, and returning to the chair.
8. Continuous walking on a treadmill.
9. Walking over various surfaces and obstacles.
10. Walking over slopes and stairs.

Reprinted with permission from Dean CM, Richards CL, Malouin F. Task-related circuit training improves performance of locomotor tasks in chronic stroke: a randomized, controlled pilot trial. Arch Phys Med Rehabil 2000;81:409–417.

Parkinson's Disease. Several reviews of RCTs have examined the effect of physical therapy (not specifically task-oriented training) on functional abilities, including gait, in persons with PD. Results were equivocal in part because of numerous methodological issues (Deane et al., 2002; Kwakkel et al., 2007). In their review of evidence-based physical therapy, Morris et al. (2010) suggested that the optimal mix of

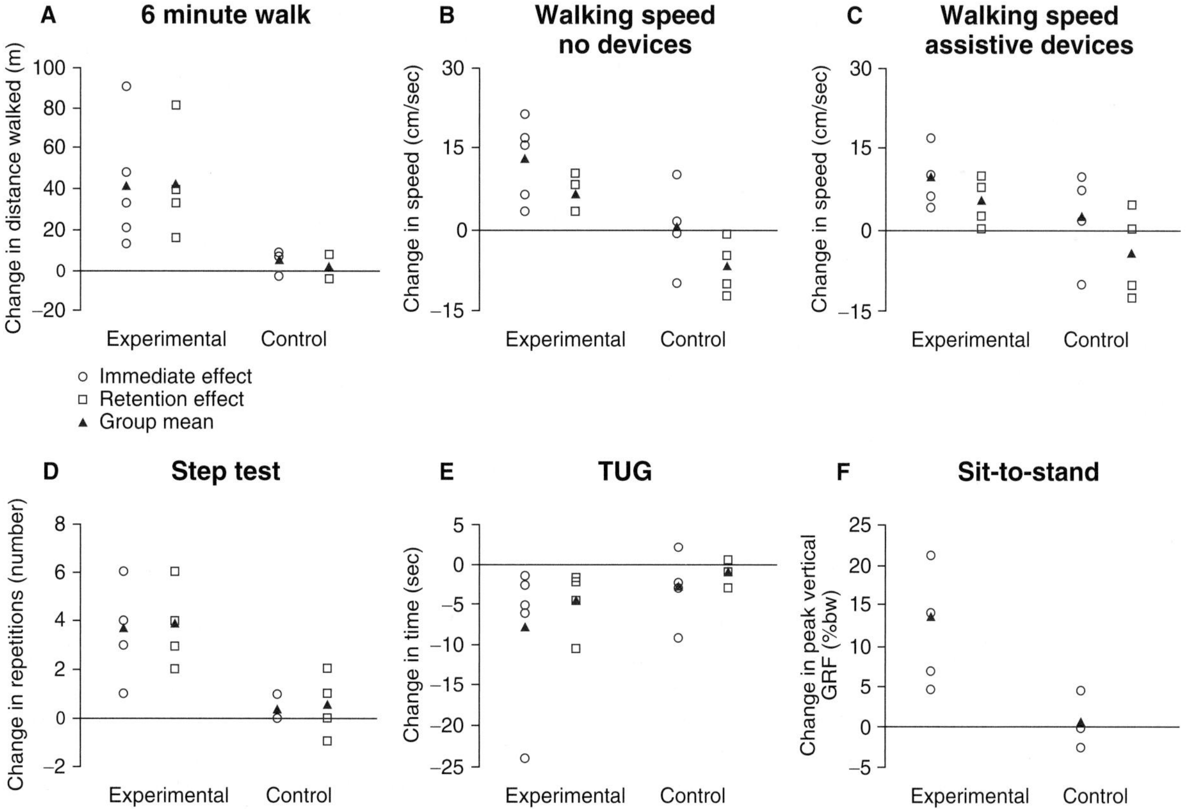

FIGURE 15.21 Effect of task-related circuit training on walking performance in individuals with chronic stroke. (Reprinted with permission from Dean CM, Richards CL, Malouin F. Task-related circuit training improves performance of locomotor tasks in chronic stroke: a randomized, controlled pilot trial. Arch Phys Med Rehabil 2000;81:412, Figure 1.)

interventions varies according to the stage of disease progression, the age and preferences of the patient, as well as their capacity for learning. All reviews agree that more quality research examining the effect of various forms of training is needed.

The studies reviewed offer support for a task-oriented approach to locomotor training in both geriatric and neurologic populations. More research is needed, however, to determine the optimal dosage and the combination of therapies most effective in improving functional mobility.

Is Preambulation Skill Training Necessary to Recovery of Gait?

What is the role of preambulation skill training in recovery of gait? Some clinicians stress the importance of practicing preambulation skills as an essential part of retraining gait. Preambulation skills are activities that are considered precursors to ambulation, and thus preparatory to walking (Bobath, 1978; Davies, 1985; Schmitz, 1998; Voss et al., 1985).

Many of the preambulation gait-training sequences are based on having the patient repeat activities that are part of a normal developmental sequence; thus, extensive mat activities are often used prior to, or in parallel with, retraining gait (Charness, 1986; Schmitz, 1994). The sequence begins by having patients practice mobility and stability skills in prone and supine positions. This includes activities such as rolling, maintaining a prone position on the elbows or hands, supine bridging, and practicing counterrotation trunk motions—that is, movements in which the shoulders rotate in the opposite direction from the hips. As motor control in the supine and prone positions is recovered, patients begin to practice activities on all fours, then sitting, kneeling, half-kneeling, modified plantigrade position, and finally standing (Brunnstrom, 1970; Charness, 1986).

Do developmental skills learned through mat exercise transfer to gait? There are a growing number of researchers and clinicians questioning the requirement that patients regain mobility skills according to a developmental sequence (Carr & Shepherd, 1998; Forssberg, 1980; Mayston, 1992; Shumway-Cook, 1989). However, there has been limited research examining this question. Lord et al. (1998) compared the task-oriented and the neurofacilitation approaches to retraining mobility function in 20 patients with multiple sclerosis (MS). The neurofacilitation approach (as defined by Lord and colleagues) relied heavily on mat exercises and preambulation skill training. The task-oriented approach (as defined by these authors) focused on practicing goal-directed functional tasks, with no treatment aimed at underlying impairments. Results from this study showed that both approaches significantly improved all measures of mobility (10-m timed walk, Rivermead Mobility Index, stride length, Rivermead Visual Gait Assessment, Berg Balance Test). In addition, there was no significant difference found between the two approaches on any measure. In their discussion, the authors state that they were unsure whether the lack of significant difference in outcome measures between the two approaches suggested that the two approaches were equally effective, or alternatively, that despite the purported differences, the two treatment strategies used common interventions.

These authors raise an important point. In order to evaluate the effectiveness of an intervention, or compare the relative effectiveness of two interventions, it is important to be able to clearly identify the essential components of each approach and to be able to determine what elements the two approaches have in common and what elements are unique. Lord et al. explored the effectiveness of a task-oriented approach to retraining mobility. Their definition of a task-oriented approach differs markedly from the definition of a task-oriented approach used in this textbook. Lord's definition of a task-oriented approach stressed the importance of practicing functional tasks while refraining from using interventions aimed at underlying impairments constraining function. In contrast, the task-oriented approach described in this book has at its focus the functional tasks being retrained, but uses interventions aimed at underlying impairments constraining performance of the task, facilitating the development of effective and efficient task-specific strategies and learning to modify task performance to changes in environmental demands. Thus, the same term, *task-oriented,* is being used in very different ways.

Improving Participation in the Mobility Domain

What strategies work to improve mobility in real life contexts? Unfortunately, little is known about the effects of interventions aimed at impairments and functional mobility skills (capacity) on performance of mobility in the person's daily life (participation). This is in part because of the paucity of measures related to participation in the mobility domain. In addition, few studies use measures of participation as outcomes in intervention studies. Often, gait interventions use change in gait velocity measured in the clinic as a primary outcome measure, but this does not necessarily mean improved function in the context of daily life. Mudge et al. (2009) found that among chronic stroke patients, circuit training improved distance walked on the 6 Minute Walk test, but found no change in average steps per day as measured by a step activity monitor.

As discussed in Chapter 14, many factors influence level of participation in the mobility domain. Physical factors such as gait speed, balance, performance on complex walking tasks, and strength contribute to recovery of participation in the mobility domain after stroke; however, they explain relatively little of the variance in participation (Michael et al., 2005; Robinson et al., 2007; Van de Port et al., 2008). Personal factors, particularly balance self-efficacy, may play a more important role in determining level of participation (Robinson, 2010). More research is needed to determine the rehabilitation strategies most effective in improving participation in both geriatric and neurologic populations.

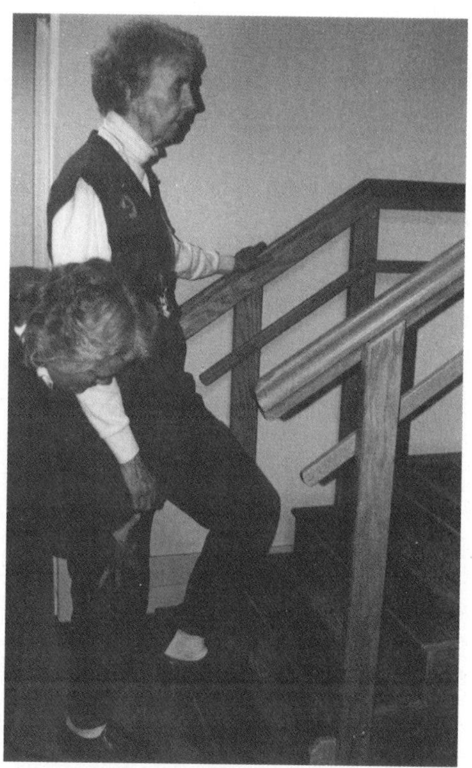

FIGURE 15.22 Assisting stair walking, controlling the involved leg for single-limb stance in stair ascent.

RETRAINING STAIR WALKING AND OTHER MOBILITY SKILLS

Stair Walking

Patients with neurologic impairments with decreased concentric control will have primary problems climbing stairs, while patients with difficulty controlling eccentric forces will have primary problems descending stairs. In addition, sensory impairments will affect a patient's ability to clear the step during swing and to place the foot appropriately for the next step. Published strategies for retraining stair walking have focused primarily on retraining patients who have had a stroke.

During stair ascent, the patient is taught to advance the nonhemiplegic leg first. Manual assistance is given as needed to guide and control the involved leg (Bobath, 1978; Davies, 1985; Voss et al., 1985). This is shown in Figure 15.22. The clinician helps to control the knee to prevent collapse during the single-limb stance phase and assists with knee and ankle flexion to ensure foot clearance in the swing leg (Fig. 15.23).

During stair descent, shown in Figure 15.24, the patient with stroke is taught to advance the hemiplegic leg first. The therapist assists with foot placement as needed and in knee control, to prevent collapse of the leg when the noninvolved leg is advanced during swing.

Research has shown that certain stair features are critical in establishing effective movement strategies for stair walking. Thus, it is possible that accentuating stair features, such as the edge of the step or the height of the step, and drawing the patient's attention to these features, may enhance the ability to develop effective stair-walking strategies.

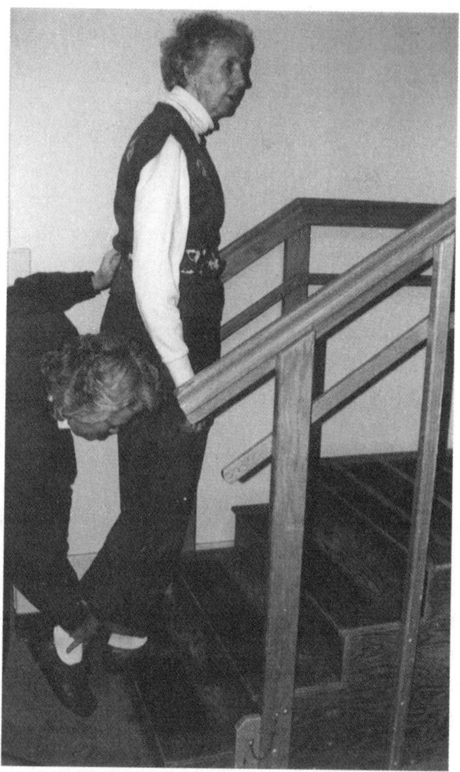

FIGURE 15.23 Manual assistance with knee and ankle flexion to ensure foot clearance in the swing leg during stair ascent.

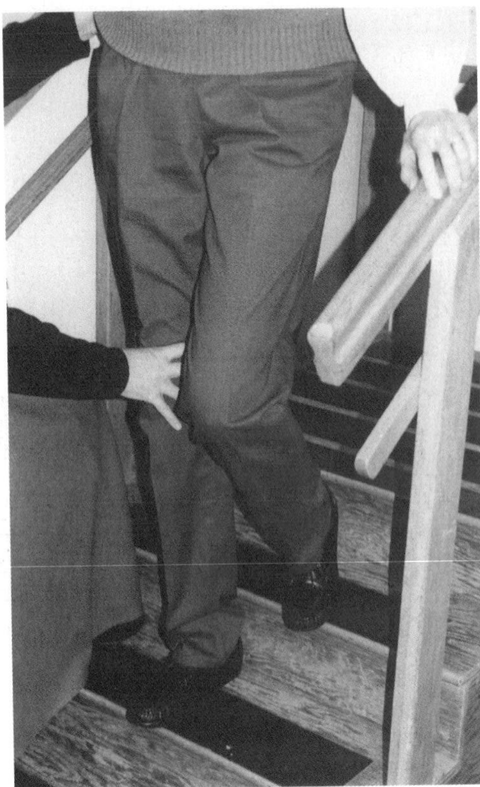

FIGURE 15.24 Manually assisting control of the knee during stair descent.

Transfers and Bed Mobility

When retraining other types of mobility skills, such as transfers and bed mobility, it is important to remember that there is no single correct strategy for patients to learn. Research suggests that healthy young people perform tasks such as rising from a bed, standing up from the floor, or rolling in many different ways. Variability characterizes the movement patterns used by neurologically intact individuals to perform everyday mobility skills. In fact, often the exact same strategy is never repeated. Instead, normal young adults seem to learn the rules for performing a task. This means that they learn what the essential or invariant requirements of a task are and develop a variety of strategies to accomplish these requirements. This suggests that the goal when retraining transfer skills in the patient with neurologic disabilities is to help him or her to develop sensory and motor strategies that are effective in meeting the task requirements, despite persisting impairments.

Patients need to learn new rules for moving and sensing, given their impairments, rather than learning to use a "normal" pattern of movement. Research with neurologically intact subjects suggests that there is no single template for moving that can be used to train patients. Instead, guided by the clinician, patients learn to explore the possibilities for performing a task. Patients learn the boundaries of what is possible, given the demands of the task and the current constellation of impairments.

Sitting to Standing. Standing up is critical to mobility function; thus, learning to transfer from a seated position to standing (and walking) is an important part of mobility training. A task-oriented approach to training transfers, including sit to stand (STS) focuses on having patients practice this functional task in a variety of contexts. Remember from Chapter 12, there are two basic strategies that can be used separately or in combination to stand up: a momentum strategy and a force-control strategy. A patient should be allowed to explore the possibilities for using momentum when performing a transfer task, since this strategy is most efficient and requires the least amount of muscular activity.

Essential elements of teaching a momentum strategy include encouraging the patient to move quickly, but safely, and avoid breaks in the motion. The clinician can verbally instruct the patient to move quickly, with no stops. An appropriate prompt might be, "Now we are going to try standing up again, but this time I want you to move quickly, with no stops." Manual cues can be used at the shoulders to set the pace. Patients who have trouble generating force quickly with the trunk can try swinging their arms freely while standing up, to increase momentum generated in upper body segments.

When teaching a momentum strategy, clinicians should be aware of the stringent stability requirements of this strategy, and adequately safeguard a patient with poor postural control to prevent a fall. The risk for a backward fall will be greatest at the beginning of the movement if the patient tries to transfer momentum from the trunk to the legs for a vertical lift before the COM is sufficiently forward over the feet. This is often characteristic of STS in a patient who is hemiparetic. In contrast, the risk for a forward fall will be greatest at the end of the movement in patients who are unable to control horizontal forces affecting the COM. When this occurs, the COM continues to accelerate forward of the base of support of the feet after the patient reaches a vertical position, resulting in a fall forward. This is often characteristic of STS in patients with cerebellar pathology, who have difficulty scaling forces for movement.

In contrast to the momentum strategy, a force-control strategy is characterized by frequent stops. In using a force-control strategy, patients are taught to bring the buttocks forward toward the edge of

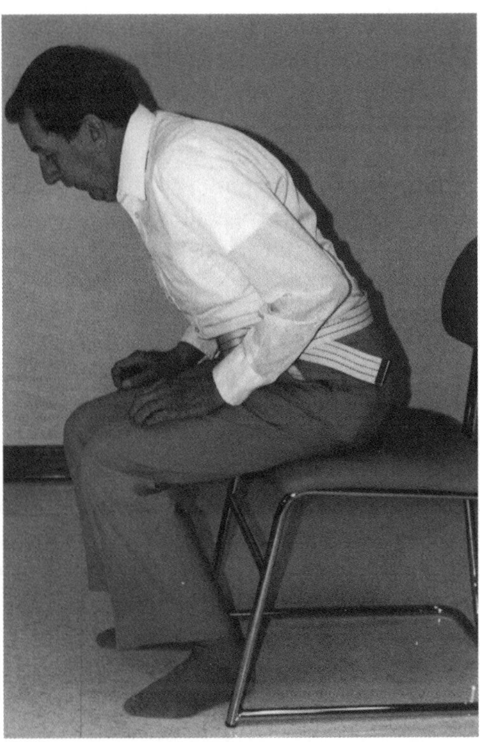

FIGURE 15.25 Teaching a force-control strategy for accomplishing STS involves asking the patient to move forward to the edge of the chair, incline the trunk forward until the "nose is over the toes," and then stand up.

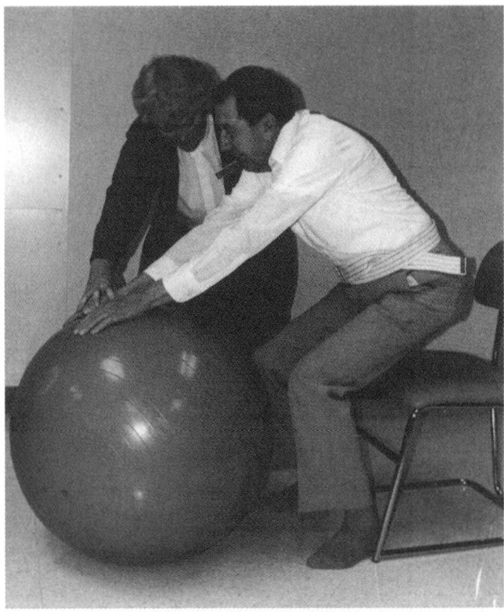

FIGURE 15.26 Encouraging forward inclination of the trunk during STS by bringing the arms forward.

the chair. The trunk is brought forward, bringing the "nose over the toes." This is shown in Figure 15.25. This brings the COM over the base of support of the feet. The patient is then cued to stand up. The patient can be encouraged to bring the arms forward, with or without a support, to assist in bringing the trunk mass forward; this is shown in Figure 15.26. Patients with weakness, making it difficult to achieve a vertical position from a normal-height chair, can begin learning STS from a raised chair, reducing the strength requirement for lifting the body (Fig. 15.27). As the patient improves, the seat height can be lowered.

In patients with asymmetrical force-production problems, facilitating symmetry is important when possible, since symmetrical weight bearing enhances both progression and stability during the task. A symmetrical weight-bearing posture is possible only in patients who can generate sufficient force to control the knee and prevent collapse of the body when the impaired limb is loaded. When this is not the case, the clinician will have to manually control the knee—for example, as illustrated in Figure 15.28. It is important that when manually assisting knee control, forward motion of the knee is not blocked as the patient stands up.

It is often easier for a patient to learn to sit down than to stand up because eccentric force control is often gained prior to concentric force control (Carr & Shepherd, 1998; Duncan & Badke, 1987). When teaching a patient to sit down, the therapist asks the patient to practice flexing the knees in preparation for sitting.

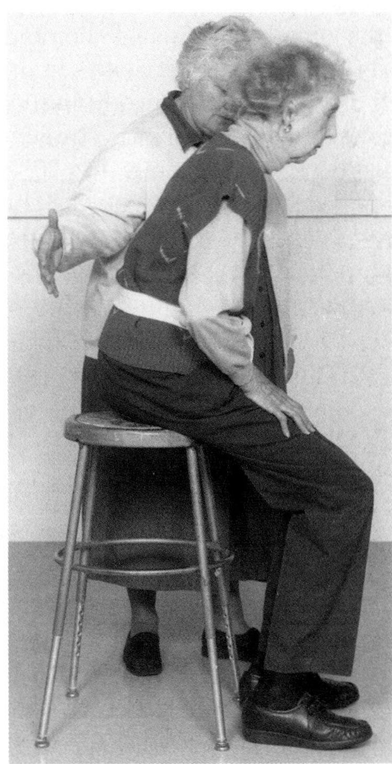

FIGURE 15.27 Teaching STS from a raised chair reduces the strength requirement for lifting the body and allows a weak patient to accomplish the task.

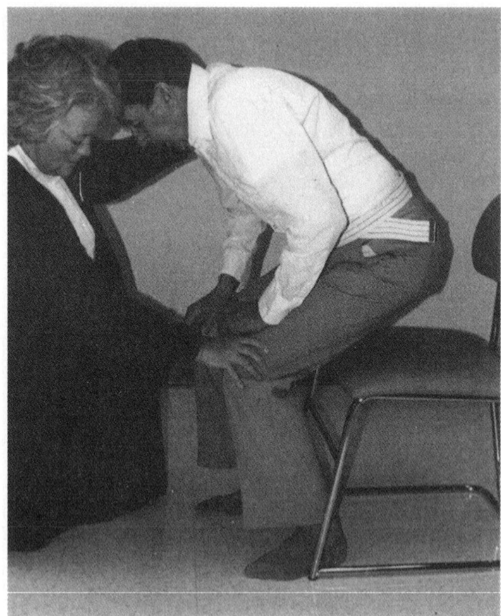

FIGURE 15.28 Manually controlling the knee when assisting a patient who is moving from a sitting to a standing position.

This requires eccentric contraction of the quadriceps to control premature collapse of the knee.

Research Evidence. Monger and colleagues (2002) examined the effect of a 3-week home-based task-oriented exercise program (activities summarized in Table 15.10) on STS performance in individuals with chronic stroke (mean time since stroke, 2.6 years). Exercises were performed daily for 20 minutes; in addition, a researcher worked with each person three times a week in order to progress activities (decreasing seat height, increasing step height, and increasing the number and speed of repetitions). Verbal feedback about weight distribution and encouragement were provided. Five of six subjects improved their score on the standing up item from the Movement Assessment Scale, while all six improved self-selected walking speed (10-m walk test). In addition, laboratory measures found improved timing (but not magnitude) of the peak vertical ground reaction force during sitting to standing. Grip strength, which was not trained, did not change.

Bed Mobility Skills. Retraining bed mobility skills includes tasks such as changing position while in bed (e.g., rolling from the supine position to a side-lying or prone position) and getting out of bed, either to a chair or standing up. As noted earlier, researchers have found that normal young adults use a variety of momentum-related strategies when performing bed mobility skills. In contrast, force-control movement strategies are frequently used by patients with neurologic impairments and are characterized by frequent starts and stops.

Rolling. The most common approach to rolling in normal young adults involves reaching and lifting with the upper extremity, flexing the head and upper trunk, and lifting the leg to roll onto the side, then over to prone. However, there are many variations to this pattern. Most healthy young adults do not show rotation between the shoulders and pelvis, assumed by many clinicians to be an invariant feature of rolling.

There are at least two ways to teach a patient to roll over. The first relies more heavily on the generation of momentum to propel the body from supine to prone. Motion is initiated with flexion of the head and trunk. At the same time, the patient reaches over the body with the upper extremity. In addition, the leg is lifted and rotated over the opposite leg, to assist

TABLE 15.10 Task-Specific Activities for Training Sitting to Standing

Sit–stand–sit	10 times (or maximum number up to 10 that can be performed without a rest). Repeat three times (30 repetitions in total). Move feet backward, look straight ahead, swing trunk forward at the hips and stand up with weight evenly distributed through both feet. Do not use your arms.
Step-ups	Standing, affected foot on 8-cm block, step up and down with other leg: (a) to shift body mass forward on to affected leg and (b) to shift body mass sideways on to affected leg. Exercise near furniture to steady yourself if necessary. Do three sets of 10 repetitions (or a maximum number up to 10 that you can perform without a rest).
Calf stretch	Standing with affected knee straight and extended arm/s resting on wall: keeping body straight, pivot the body forward at the ankles, keeping heel on the floor until you feel that the calf muscle is stretched. Hold for 2 minutes, relax, and repeat 10 times.

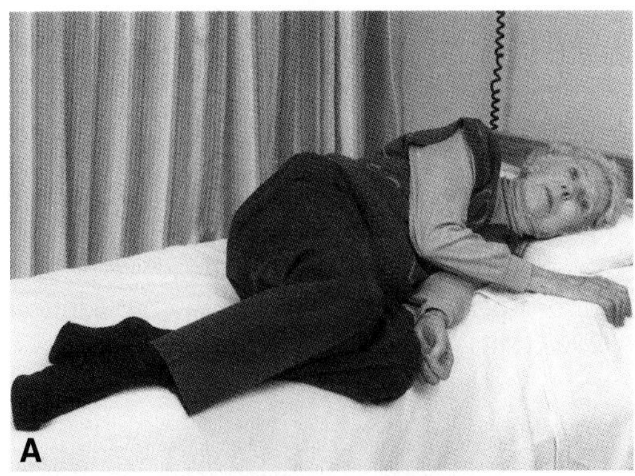

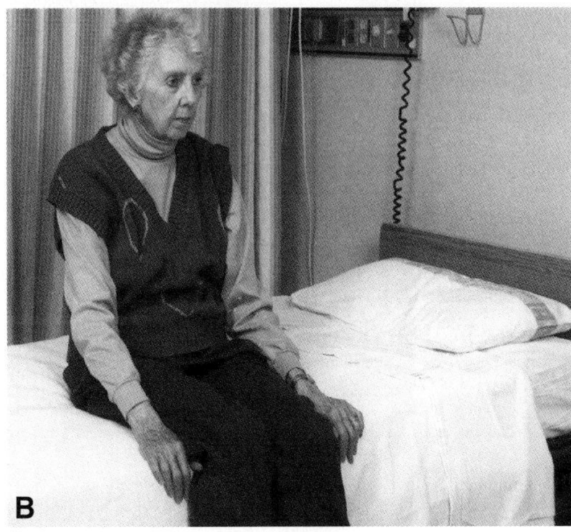

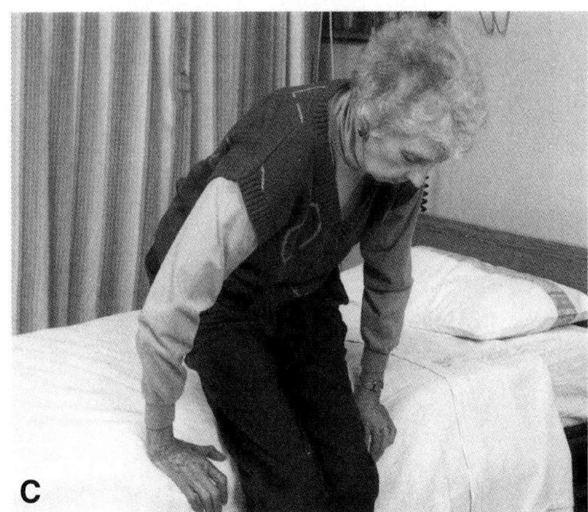

FIGURE 15.29 Learning to rise from a bed using a force-control strategy breaks the movement into three stages, rolling to a side-lying position (A), then to a sitting position (B), and finally from sitting to standing (C).

with the generation of momentum, to roll the body to side-lying and on to prone position. An alternative to a momentum-based strategy is a force-control (or combination) strategy. In this approach, the patient is taught to lift one leg and place the foot flat on the bed. Pressure downward by the leg propels the body to side-lying and on to prone position. Flexion of the head and trunk and reaching movements of the arms can assist in generating force to roll over (Carr & Shepherd, 1998; Davies, 1985; Voss et al., 1985).

Rising from a Bed. Research examining movement patterns used by normal adults to get out of bed again suggests great variability in how this is accomplished. Still, momentum-based strategies are used most often. For example, the movement begins as the person pushes the trunk into flexion with the arms or, alternatively, grasps the side of the bed and pulls and pushes into flexion and immediately into a partial sitting position with the weight on one side of the buttocks. Without stopping, the person continues to roll off the bed into a standing position. This strategy has stringent stability requirements, but because there are no breaks in the movement, uses momentum to move the body efficiently. As noted in Chapter 14, there are many reasons why this strategy is not appropriate for a patient with neurologic dysfunction.

An alternative strategy involves teaching a patient to roll to side-lying (with or without use of a bed rail when available) (Fig. 15.29A), then to push up to a sitting (Fig. 15.29B) position. After the patient is stable in a symmetrical sitting position with the feet flat on the floor, he or she is taught to stand up (Fig. 15.29C) (Davies, 1985; Voss et al., 1985).

Importance of Varying Task and Environmental Demands

Just as in gait, patients must learn to perform functional tasks such as sitting to standing and transfers, under varying task and environmental demands. To assist in the process of exploring movement strategies that are effective in meeting changing task and environmental demands, conditions of training are varied. For example, as shown in Figure 15.30, during the process of learning to move from a sitting to a

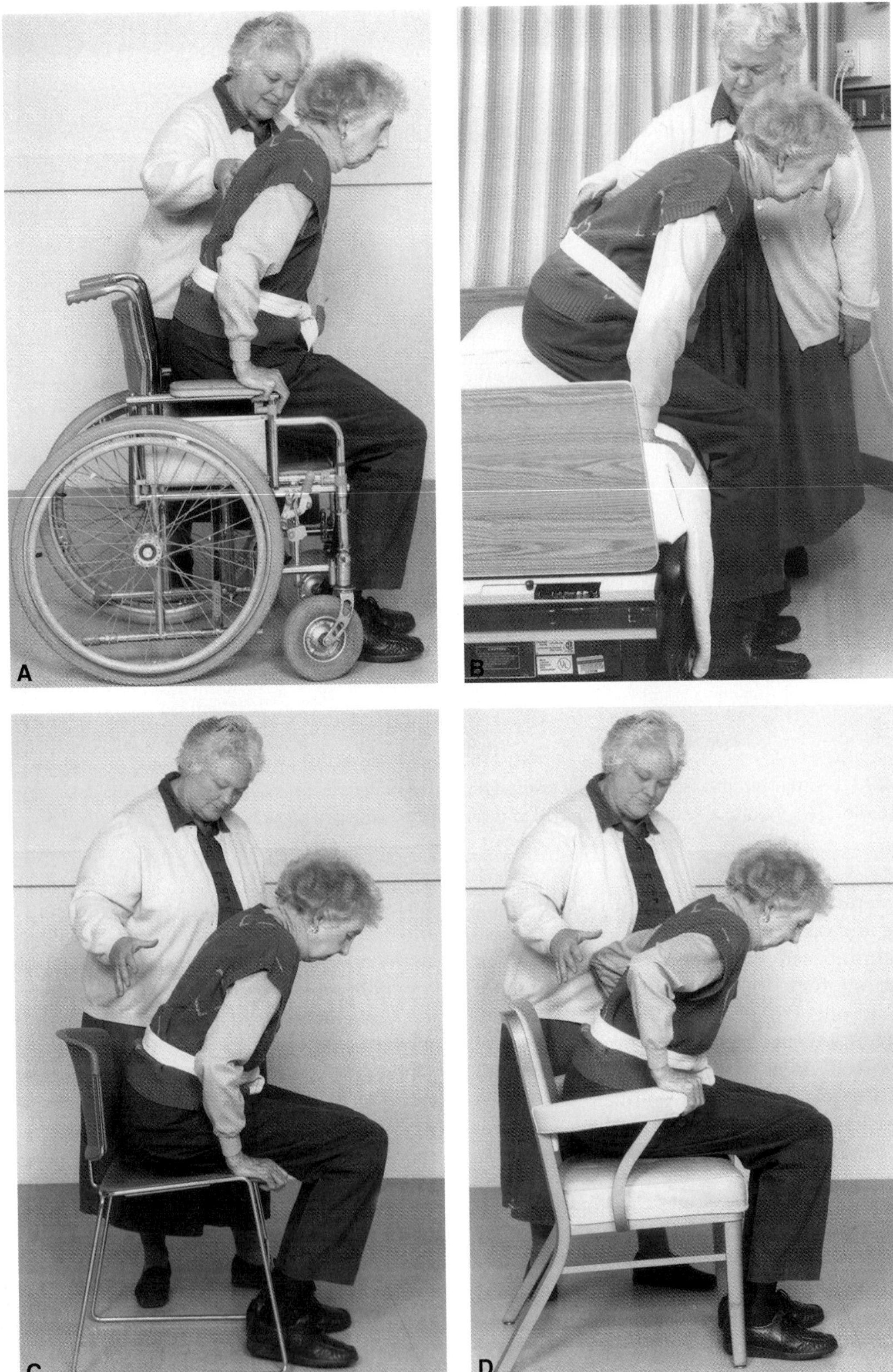

FIGURE 15.30 Varying the environmental conditions while learning the STS task. Practice conditions involve standing up from a wheelchair (A), from the bed (B), from a chair without arms (C), and from a low soft chair (D).

standing position, the patient may practice standing up from a wheelchair (Fig. 15.30A), from the bed (Fig. 15.30B), from a chair without arms (Fig. 15.30C), and from a low soft chair (Fig. 15.30D). In addition, patients may learn to embed STS in a variety of other tasks, such as stand up and stop, stand up and walk, or stand up and lean over. This type of variability encourages the patient to modify strategies used to stand up in response to changes in task and the environment demands.

Often, as therapists, we are quick to guide patients toward the use of strategies that we know will be effective in meeting the demands of the task. Patients rarely have the time to experiment with a variety of solutions that are effective in meeting task demands. This concept of trial-and-error exploration in the learning of strategies that are effective in meeting task goals has a number of important implications for clinicians. Initial performance may be quite poor as patients learn to explore and to find their own solutions. Patients may not progress as quickly as if they were taught a single solution to the task being learned. If we value the importance of multiple solutions to task demands, short- and long-term therapy goals may need to be rewritten to reflect this. For example, the patient will demonstrate the ability to adapt motor responses by performing the STS task in three different ways.

Lab Activity 15.4 provides a framework for developing a treatment program for retraining locomotor function in our patient Jean J. Review our case study in Assessment Tool 15.10, and the information gained through Lab Activity 15.3. Complete the table proposed in Lab Activity 15.4, identifying the specific individual system to be targeted (column 1), the task or activity to be practiced (column 2), the environmental conditions under which practice will occur (column 3), and the research evidence that supports this aspect of treatment (column 4).

LAB ACTIVITY 15-4

Objective: Apply a task-oriented approach to retraining mobility in a patient with poststroke hemiparesis. To identify the research evidence to support clinical decisions regarding specific treatment interventions.

Procedure: Reread the case study presented in Assessment Tool 15.10 and your assignment from Lab Activity 15.3.

Assignment: Create a table identifying the various treatments you will use to improve mobility function in Jean. List the specific individual system to be targeted (column 1), the task or activity to be practiced (column 2), the environmental conditions under which practice will occur (column 3), and the research evidence that supports this aspect of treatment. For example, you may decide to do progressive resistance strength training with Jean because weakness is an underlying impairment contributing to her impaired gait. The individual component listed in the table is motor: strength, the task is strength training, and the specific environmental condition you choose may be free weights at 60% 1 RM. Several research studies support your decision to incorporate progressive resistive strength training with Jean, including the meta analysis by Ada et al. (2006). Is strength training alone enough to insure recovery of gait? What other aspects of mobility will you train? What research supports your decision?

Individual Component of Balance	Task or Activity	Environmental Conditions	Research Evidence
Motor: Strength	Progressive Resistance Strength Training	Free weights, 60% of 1 RM	Ada et al., 2006; Pak & Patten, 2008

RM = Repetition Max.

SUMMARY

1. The key to recovery of mobility skills following neurologic injury is learning to meet the task requirements of progression, postural control, and adaptability, despite persisting sensory, motor, and cognitive impairments. Research examining mobility strategies in neurologically intact subjects suggests that there is no one right strategy that can, or should, be used to meet these requirements.
2. Retraining the patient with impaired mobility skills begins with an examination of: (a) functional mobility skills, (b) strategies used to accomplish stance and swing requirements of gait, and (c) underlying sensory, motor, and cognitive impairments that constrain the performance of functional mobility skills.
3. Visual gait analysis is the clinical tool most commonly used to aid therapists in systematically analyzing a patient's gait strategies.
4. There is considerable evidence to support effectiveness of task-specific mobility training strategies on improving ambulation skills (speed and distance) in patients with neurologic disorders.
5. A task-oriented approach to treatment (as defined in this book) focuses on helping patients to resolve specific impairments constraining the task, to develop strategies effective in meeting essential task requirements, and to learn how to adapt and modify these strategies so performance can be sustained in a wide variety of settings.

ANSWERS TO LAB ACTIVITY ASSIGNMENTS

Lab Activity 15-1

Compare the data from this lab to the norms listed in Table 15.1.

Lab Activity 15-2

If you have analyzed an atypical gait pattern, refer back to Table 15.5, and examine the possible causes of the gait abnormalities you observed.

Lab Activity 15-3

1. Jean walks at 0.4 m/sec and has poor ability to walk safely when on inclines and irregular surfaces, during obstacle avoidance and when trying to when carrying a load. She is unable to walk 500 m, a distance considered critical to community mobility. This information suggests that she is a limited community ambulator.
2. **All three of these aspects of gait are affected in Jean.** She has reduced ability to generate forces for progression; this results in slowed gait speed. She has reduced stability, particularly when initiating gait, turning, walking with head movements and stepping over obstacles, suggesting impaired proactive balance control. In addition she has a reduced ability to recover from a slip or trip while walking, suggesting impaired reactive balance control. She has a reduced ability to adapt her gait to changing task and environmental demands. For example, she cannot modify her gait speed, so she is unable to cross a street safely in the amount of time available. She is unable to modify her step height or length, so has difficulty crossing obstacles. Because she must use a cane for balance, she is unable to carry packages and thus requires assistance on all shopping trips.
3. Refer to Table 15.5 to determine the relationship between her underlying impairments and her gait pattern. For example, her hyperextension in midstance could be the result of one or more of the following: spasticity in her plantar flexors (or quads), reduced range of motion in her ankle, weakness in her knee extensors (compensatory passive locking of the knee), extensor mass synergy pattern, and/or poor recruitment and selective control.
4. Several factors may potentially contribute to her poor obstacle clearance. She has reduced foot clearance during gait and a reduced ability to modify step height. She has reduced balance, affecting stability during single limb stance. She is highly fearful of falling, and this also contributes to her poor performance.

Lab Activity 15-4

It is important to remember that there is no single correct way to train walking in Jean. It is essential that all aspects of gait be included in her rehabilitation program (e.g., progression, stability and adaptation) and that a range of tasks and conditions be used to help her develop a variety of gait strategies so that she is able walk safely in a wide diversity of tasks and conditions. The specific order, duration, and timing of each activity may vary from therapist to therapist.

We begin by determining Jean's main concern and goals related to her walking. She wants to increase the speed and distance that she is able to walk so that she can keep up with her friends when they walk in the community. She wants to improve her stability when she turns and steps over obstacles so she does not fall.

Therefore, our approach to training walking will focus both on improving underlying impairments (her weakness and reduced range of motion), improving movement patterns effective in achieving progression, stability and adaptation; and practicing functional mobility tasks under a variety of conditions.

Activities will be goal-directed, and progressively challenging, beginning with relatively simple challenges (e.g., walking on a firm flat surface with good lighting or standing up from a 17-in. chair with arms) to more complex (e.g., changing speeds, irregular terrains, with manual loads, increased attentional demands, or standing up from a lower-height chair, a chair without arms, or a rocking chair). In order to facilitate extended practice, we will perform locomotor training with body weight support on a treadmill system. We may also include circuit training, setting up stations in which she can practice complex walking tasks (see Table 15. 8 for treatment ideas for these stations).

We will incorporate motor learning principles into her training. Initially, we will have her practice functional tasks in a blocked manner (practicing each task for a time, before switching to a different task). As she improves, we will shift to a more random practice pattern (alternating the types of tasks she practices) and modifying the conditions under which she practices as well (variable practice). As she is reacquiring balance ability, we will vary the timing and extent of the external feedback she is given.

There is considerable research to support our clinical decision-making regarding a task-oriented approach to treatment. The following table presents some examples. What other research can you find to support your evidence-based mobility rehabilitation program?

Individual Component of Balance	Task or Activity	Environmental Conditions	Research Evidence
Motor: Strength	Progressive resistance strength training	Free weights, 60% of 1 RM	Ada et al, 2006; Duncan et al, 2003; Ouelette et al., 2004
Motor: Gait Pattern: Progression	Walking—part practice	Hip pull-off while standing in a diagonal leg position Push-off while standing with hemiparetic limb in a trailing limb position	Milot et al., 2008; Olney et al., 1991, 1994
Motor: Gait pattern	Walking—whole task practice	Treadmill and body weight support Manual and verbal cues related to gait pattern	Ada et al., 2003; Hesse et al., 1994, 1995, 1999; Sullivan et al., 2002
Motor: Gait pattern	Walking—whole task practice	Functional electrical stimulation to the plantar flexors and dorsiflexor	Kesar et al., 2009
Motor: Velocity and distance	Walking for progressively longer distances	Treadmill and Overground Vary distance and speed	Sullivan et al, 2002
Motor: Gait pattern, velocity	Walking	Lateral wedge insole	Chen et al., 2010
Motor: Complex walking tasks	Walking under varying task and environmental conditions	Task-oriented training of complex walking tasks using the eight environmental dimensions Circuit training	Bassile et al., 2003; Dean et al., 2000; Duncan et al., 2003; Mudge et al., 2009; Salbach et al., 2004
Sensory: Organization of Sensory Inputs for Balance	Walking	Eyes open, closed, while wearing opaque glasses Firm, foam surface Carpeted surfaces	Bayouk et al., 2006; Bonan et al., 2004; Smania et al., 2008
Cognitive: Dual-Task Balance Training	Walking Sit to stand	Practice tasks under dual-task conditions, adding secondary cognitive tasks	Silsupadol et al., 2009; Yang et al, 2007

RM = Repetition Max

PART IV

REACH, GRASP, AND MANIPULATION

Upper-extremity function is the basis for the fine motor skills important to activities such as feeding, dressing, and grooming. In addition, upper-extremity function plays an important role in gross motor skills such as crawling, walking, the ability to recover balance, and the ability to protect the body from injury when balance recovery is not possible.

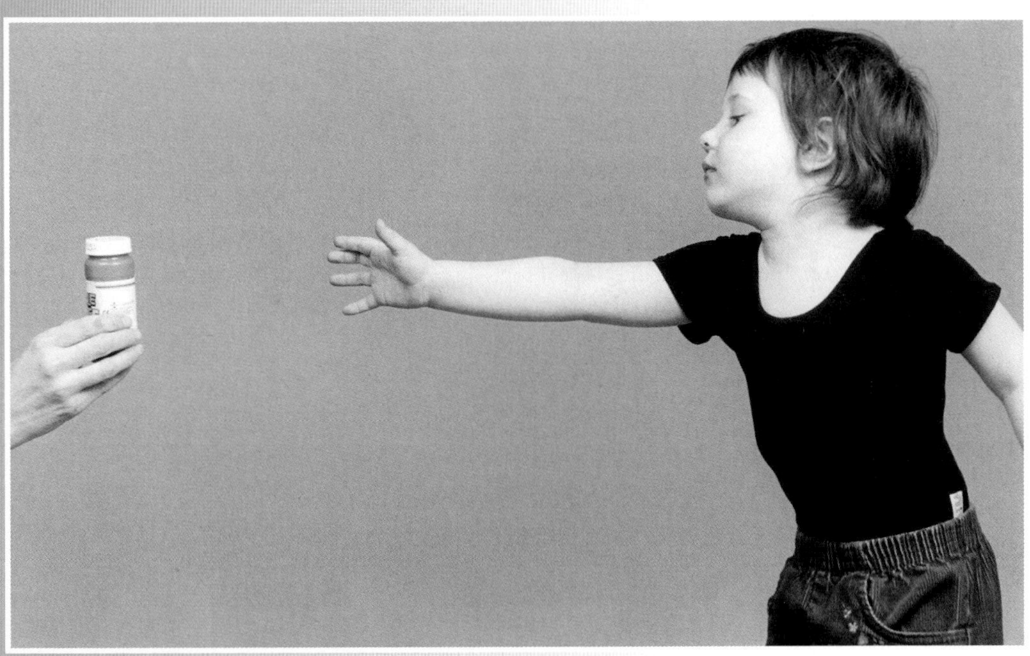

CHAPTER 16

NORMAL REACH, GRASP, AND MANIPULATION

LEARNING OBJECTIVES

Following completion of this chapter, the reader will be able to:

1. Describe the principle components of eye—head—trunk—hand coordination during reach and grasp skills.
2. Discuss the contributions of neural and musculoskeletal systems to reach and grasp skills, and predict the skill deficits that would occur with lesions to these systems.
3. Discuss the general principles of motor control of reach and grasp, including the way the nervous system plans movements, and different theories of the control of reach and grasp.

INTRODUCTION

How important is upper-extremity function to successfully moving through the activities of our day? Take a moment to scan the activities you completed within the first hour after waking up this morning. They probably included brushing your teeth, combing your hair, buttoning your clothes as you dressed, and using your spoon as you stirred your coffee or ate your breakfast. In reviewing the typical activities of our day, it becomes apparent that upper-extremity function is the basis for the fine motor skills important to activities such as feeding, dressing, and grooming.

In addition, although we may not be as consciously aware of it, upper-extremity function plays an important role in gross motor skills such as crawling, walking, the ability to recover balance, and the ability to protect the body from injury when balance recovery is not possible.

Because of this interweaving of upper-extremity control with both fine and gross motor skills, recovery of upper-extremity function is an important aspect of retraining motor control and thus falls within the purview of most areas of rehabilitation, including both occupational and physical therapy.

In upper-extremity control, as in balance and gait, three factors contribute to sensorimotor processing: (1) the constraints of the individual, including age, experience with the task, and presence or absence of pathology; (2) the type of task (e.g., to point at an object, to grasp and manipulate an object, or to grasp and throw an object); and (3) the specific environmental constraints, including the properties of the objects to be grasped.

How does the nervous system accomplish the complex process of upper-extremity control? Before we can answer this question, we need to understand the basic requirements of reach, grasp, and manipulation. This will provide a framework for discussing normal control and the effect of neurologic pathology on functional grasp and manipulatory skills. In addition, it will provide the structure for clinical management of upper-extremity dysfunction in patients with neurologic impairments.

We suggest that the following components could be considered key elements of upper-extremity reach, grasp, and manipulation skills: (a) locating a target also, called "visual regard," which requires the coordination of eye–head movements and is essential in guiding movements of the hand; (b) reaching, involving transportation of the arm and hand in space as well as postural support; (c) grasping, including grip formation, grasp and release; and (d) in-hand manipulation skills.

As we mentioned in earlier chapters, the systems theory of motor control predicts that there are specific neural and musculoskeletal subsystems that contribute to the control of the components of reach, grasp, and manipulation. Musculoskeletal components include joint range of motion, spinal flexibility, muscle properties, and biomechanical relationships among linked body segments. Neural components encompass: (a) motor processes, including the coordination of the eye, head, trunk, and arm movements and coordination of both the transport and grasp phases of the reach; (b) sensory processes, including the coordination of visual, vestibular, and somatosensory systems; (c) internal representations important for the mapping of sensation to action; and (d) higher-level processes essential for adaptive and anticipatory aspects of manipulatory functions.

In addition, control of manipulation involves both reflexive and voluntary movements and both feedback and feedforward processing. Voluntary movements also obey specific psychophysical principles (e.g., motor programs have invariant features, and movements show a lengthening of reaction time with increasing information to be processed) (Ghez & Krakauer, 2000).

We begin our discussion with a review of some general principles of movement control that apply equally to eye, head, and hand coordination during reaching. We then move to a discussion of components of reach, grasp, and manipulation, beginning with visual regard, which describes the manner in which the eyes and head are coupled during target location. We then discuss the components of reach and grasp, describing the role of the motor and sensory systems, and higher-level adaptive abilities. Finally, we review some of the theories of the control of reaching movements.

MOVEMENT CONTROL PRINCIPLES

Feedforward versus Feedback Control of Movement

In Chapters 7 and 12, on the control of posture and locomotion, we emphasized the importance of both feedback and feedforward (anticipatory) processes in movement control. Efficient reaching also involves both feedback and feedforward control processes. We learn to improve our reaching efficiency and accuracy with practice, as we both *anticipate* the requirements of the task and obstacles that might perturb the arm movement trajectory and *correct* for the effects of perturbations. An example of feedback control is shown in Fig. 16.1A. Feedback control involves input from the sensory systems (typically visual or somatosensory sensors) being compared to a reference signal, representing a desired state of the system (e.g., a position of the arm). The difference between the sensory input and the reference signal (error signal), is used to update the output of the system (e.g., the muscles controlling the arm, called "actuators"). For example, the goal may be to maintain the position of the arm while catching a ball. The reference signal would indicate the muscle contraction required to do this. Sensory information from proprioceptors or the visual system would provide feedback on the current position of the arm and the difference between the current arm position and the desired position would be used to activate arm muscles to maintain that position (Ghez & Krakauer, 2000).

Feedforward, or anticipatory, control takes advantage of previous experience to predict the consequences of sensory information that is received. This occurs before the feedback sensors are stimulated, and thus reduces the reliance on feedback control. For example, when catching a ball (Fig. 16.1B), we use visual information about the trajectory of the ball's movement to anticipate where to move the hand to catch it. This activates a feedforward controller (continuously updated through information from prior experience), and the controller activates the muscles at the correct level to catch the ball. After the ball hits the hand, feedback processes will also be used to react to the perturbation of hand position by the ball (Ghez & Krakauer, 2000).

These two mechanisms can be seen to contribute to the muscle activation patterns involved in catching a ball, as shown in Figure 16.2. The feedforward or anticipatory responses are indicated by the arrows and occur in the biceps, triceps, and flexor and extensor carpi radialis. After the ball hits the hand, feedback control consists of a short-latency reflex at about 50 msec after impact, in both flexor and extensor muscles. These same processes underlie the accurate movement of the eye, head, and hand toward a target, topics to be discussed below (Ghez & Krakauer, 2000).

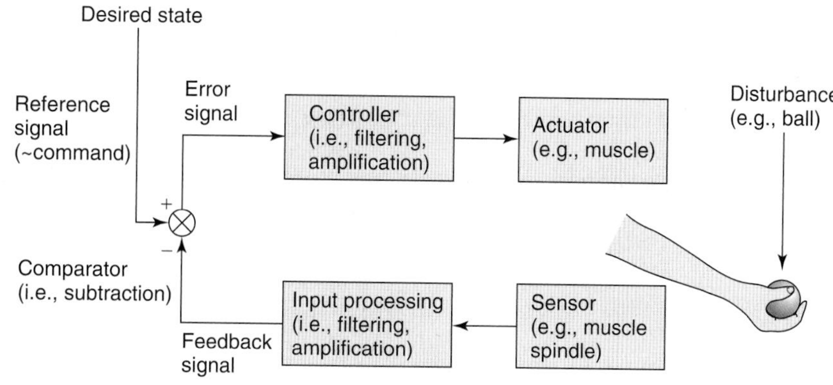

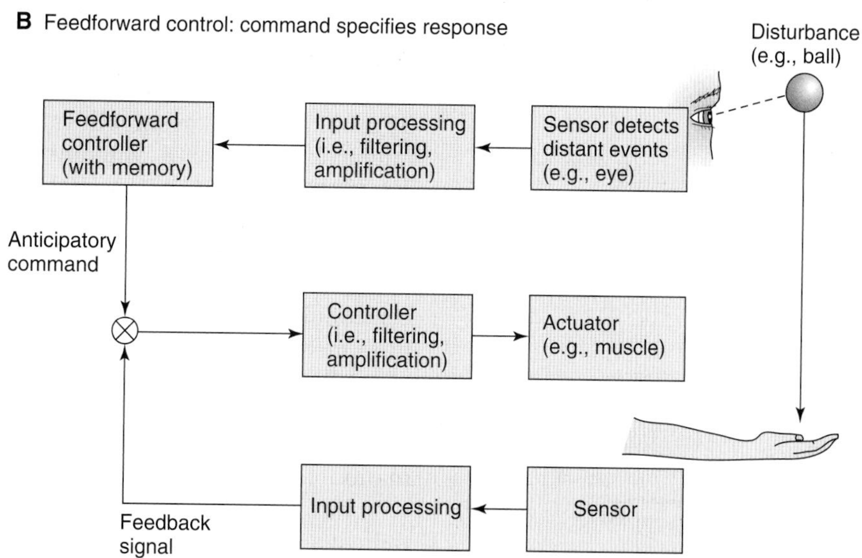

FIGURE 16.1 A, A feedback control circuit. In feedback control, a signal from the sensory systems (marked "Sensor" and typically visual or somatosensory sensors) is processed by higher centers (Input processing) and then compared with a reference signal, representing a desired state of the system (e.g., a position of the arm). The difference between the sensory input and the reference signal (Error signal), is used to update the output of the system, including the controller (e.g., motor cortex) and the actuator (e.g., the muscles controlling the arm). B, A feedforward control circuit for catching a ball. Information from a distance sensor (e.g., the eye) is processed (input processing) and then sent to the feedforward controller (with memory access to paths of previously thrown balls) to anticipate the path of the ball and the best response. The anticipatory command is sent to the controller and actuator (as for panel A). Feedback control is then used once the ball hits the hand and activates cutaneous and muscle receptors. (Reprinted with permission from Ghez C, Krakauer J. The organization of movement. In: Kandel E, Schwartz J, Jessel T, eds. Principles of neuroscience, 4th ed. New York: McGraw-Hill, 2000:655.)

LOCATING A TARGET

Eye–Head–Trunk Coordination

In order to reach for an object successfully, we must first locate the object in space. Normally, vision is used for object location and to guide the movements of the hand (for reach, grasp, and manipulation). Object location typically involves movement of the eyes alone, when the target is in our central visual field, or the eyes and head when the target is in our peripheral visual field.

How are reaching movements of the arm coordinated with the movements of the eye and head? Do we move our eyes first to a target, then our head, and finally our hand? Kinematic studies have shown that

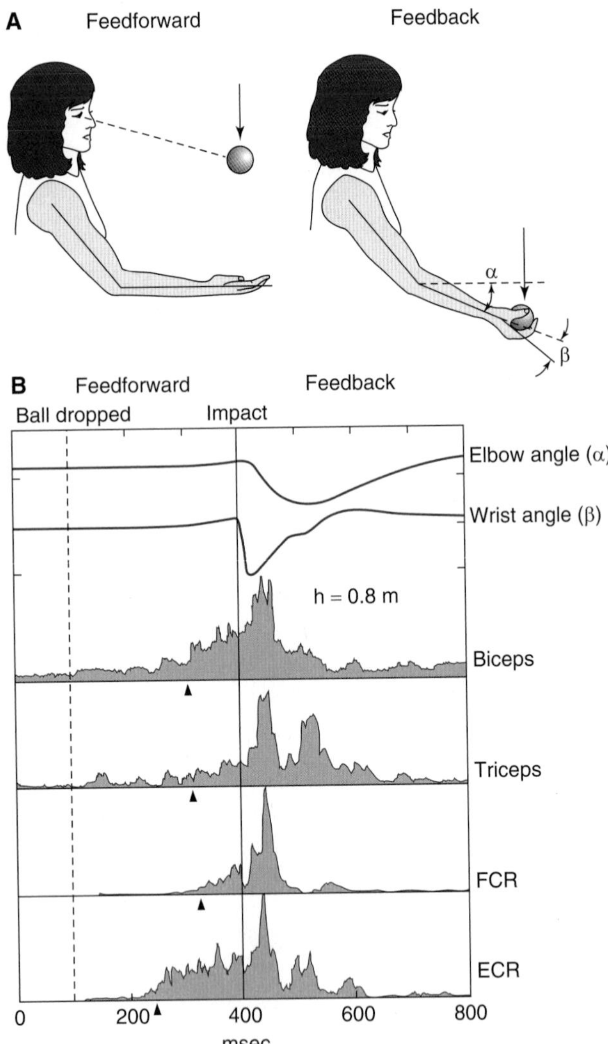

FIGURE 16.2 A, Experimental conditions for feedforward/feedback control experiments. Initial input is feedforward (using vision), while final input is feedback (using somatosensory inputs from the arm/hand). The ball is dropped from different heights. B, Angular changes in the elbow and wrist and muscle responses (rectified surface electromyograms) from the biceps, triceps, flexor carpi radialis (FCR), and extensor carpi radialis (ECR). Anticipatory (feedforward) responses are indicated by the arrows. Feedback responses occur after impact. (Reprinted with permission from Ghez C, Krakauer J. The organization of movement. In: Kandel E, Schwartz J, Jessel T, eds. Principles of neuroscience, 4th ed. New York: McGraw-Hill, 2000:656.)

when an object to be grasped appears in the peripheral visual field, there is normally the following sequence of movements. The eye movement onset has the shortest latency, so it begins first, even before the head. The eyes reach the target first because they move very quickly, so they focus on the target before the head stops moving (Jeannerod, 1990). EMG studies have shown that activation of neck muscles usually occurs 20 to 40 msec prior to activation of the muscles controlling eye movements. However, because the eyes have less inertia than the head, the eyes move first, even though the neural signal occurs first in the neck muscles.

When head movement is needed to look at an object, the amplitude of head movement is usually only about 60 to 75% of the distance to the target (Biguer et al., 1984; Gresty, 1974). However, when arm movements requiring great accuracy are performed, this behavior may be modified. It has been shown that people trained to throw with great accuracy make combined eye and head movements that go most of the distance to the target (Roll et al., 1986).

Reaching to objects located in the far visual field requires a combination of eye, head, and trunk movements. Because of this variability, researchers have argued that eye–head coordination is not controlled by a unitary mechanism, but rather emerges from an interaction of several different neural mechanisms. These could include one neural mechanism that subserves the ability to locate objects in the near periphery, requiring primarily eye movements; a second mechanism to locate objects in the further periphery, controlling combined eye–head movements; and a third mechanism to locate objects in the far periphery, controlling the movements of eye, head, and trunk together (Jeannerod, 1990).

What is the functional significance of this information to understanding and retraining a patient who has problems with functional grasp? Part of the patient's problems may relate to the coordination of eye–head movements needed for visual regard. Thus, when retraining, the clinician might focus on training the different control systems separately. For example, the clinician might begin by retraining eye movements to targets located within the central visual field, then progress to retraining eye–head movements to targets located in the peripheral visual field. Finally, movements involving eye, head, and trunk motions could be practiced as patients learn to locate targets oriented in the far periphery.

Interactions between Eye Movements and Hand Movements

There is evidence that eye and hand movements both interact with and influence each other. For example, when accompanied by eye movement, hand movements are more accurate. In addition, during smooth pursuit eye movements, there is an increase in gain if the hand is also following the target (Gauthier et al., 1988). Vercher and colleagues (1996) found that even in deafferented subjects, there was an increase in gain and reduction in latency for smooth pursuit when the hand was used to follow the target. Thus, they suggest it is the efference copy or corollary discharge about limb movement that helps the smooth pursuit system, rather than proprioceptive feedback from the hand movement.

Other research has shown that proprioceptive signals from the eye muscles do contribute to our ability to localize targets in extrapersonal space. Gauthier and colleagues (1990) performed an experiment in which they perturbed the movement of one eye, so it was deviated 30 degrees to the left while the subject was asked to point at a target located straight ahead. They found that the subjects mislocalized the targets in the leftward direction by 3 to 4 degrees.

BEHAVIORAL CHARACTERISTICS (KINEMATICS) OF REACH AND GRASP

It is interesting to note that the control of arm movements changes depending on the goal of the task. For example, when the arm is used to point to an object, all the segments of the arm are controlled as a unit. But when the arm is used to reach for and grasp an object, the hand appears to be controlled independently of the other arm segments, with the arm carrying out movements related to transport and the hand carrying out movements related to grasping the object. In this case, reaching for an object can be divided into two subcomponents—the reach component versus the grasp component—which appear to be controlled by separate areas of the brain.

In this section, we will first examine the kinematic characteristics of reaching movements and the way kinematics change depending on the task and the environment. We will then discuss the contributions of specific neural and musculoskeletal subsystems to the control of visual regard, reach, and grasp.

Studies have been performed to better understand the way that reach-and-grasp movements are affected by both task and environment. As you will see, this research suggests that the ability to adapt how we reach is a critical part of upper-extremity function, since reaching movements vary according to the goals and constraints of the task.

Researchers have shown that the velocity profiles and movement durations of a reach vary depending on the goal of the task. If the subject was asked to grasp the object, the movement duration of the reach was much longer than if the subject was asked to point and hit the target. Also, when preparing to grasp an object, the acceleration phase of the reaching movement was much shorter than the deceleration phase, but if the subject was asked to hit the target with the index finger, the acceleration phase was longer than

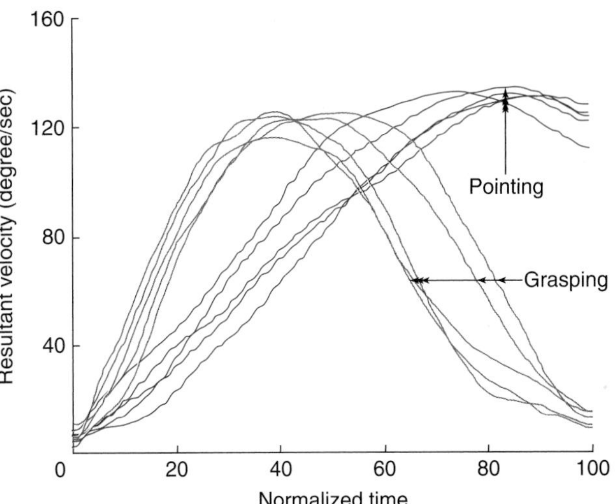

FIGURE 16.3 Velocity of the arm versus time (velocity profile) for a number of individual trials of both pointing and grasping movements. Note that in the grasp, the acceleration phase is shorter than the deceleration phase, while in the point, the reverse is true. (Reprinted with permission from Jeannerod M. The neural and behavioral organization of goal-directed movements, Oxford: Clarendon Press, 1990:19.)

the deceleration phase, with the subject hitting the target at a relatively high velocity (Marteniuk et al., 1987). This is shown in Figure 16.3, which shows the different velocity profiles for the arm over time for grasping versus pointing movements.

In addition, if the subject grasped the target, then either fit it in a small box or, alternatively, threw it, movement times and velocity profiles were also different. Movement times were shorter for grasp and throw versus grasp and fit. In addition, the acceleration phase of the movement was longer for grasp and throw than for grasp and fit. Clearly, the task constraints and goals affect the reaching phase of the movement. This finding has implications for the clinician engaged in retraining the patient with problems related to reach and grasp. Since movements used during reaching for an object vary depending on the nature of the task, reaching movements need to be practiced within a variety of tasks. For example, these tasks might include practicing reach during reach and point; reach and grasp; reach, grasp, and throw; and reach, grasp, and manipulate.

SYSTEMS CONTRIBUTING TO REACH AND GRASP

Research on both monkeys and humans has shown that in addition to sensory information, three areas of the cerebral cortex are critical to the control of reach and grasp. These include the primary motor cortex, premotor cortex, and areas of the posterior parietal lobe. In addition, the cerebellum is important for the control of both feedforward and feedback control of these skills. In the following sections we will discuss the contributions of each of these areas to reach and grasp.

Sensory Systems

What is the role of sensory information in controlling reach and grasp? You may recall that in Chapter 3, to better understand the function of the different levels of the nervous system, we took a specific upper-extremity function task and walked through the pathways of the nervous system that contributed to its planning and execution. We gave the example of being thirsty and wanting to pour some milk from the milk carton in front of you into a glass.

Sensory inputs come in from the periphery to tell you what is happening around you, where you are in space, and where your joints are relative to each other: they give you a map of your body in space. Sensory inputs from the visual system go through two parallel pathways involved in goal-directed reaching: one related to what is being reached for (perception and object recognition) and the other related to where the object is in extrapersonal space (localization) and the action systems involved in object manipulation. The perceptual pathway goes from visual cortex to temporal cortex, while the localization and action pathway goes from visual cortex to parietal lobe.

Higher centers in the cortex take this information (using, e.g., the parietal lobes and premotor cortex) and make a plan to act on it in relation to the goal: reaching for the carton of milk. You make a specific movement plan: you're going to reach over the box of corn flakes in front of you. This plan is sent to the motor cortex, and muscle groups are specified. The plan is also sent to the cerebellum and basal ganglia, and they modify it to refine the movement.

The cerebellum sends an update of the movement output plan to the motor cortex and brainstem. Descending pathways from the motor cortex and brainstem then activate spinal cord networks, spinal motor neurons activate the muscles, and you reach for the milk. If the milk carton is full, when you thought it was almost empty, spinal reflex pathways will compensate for the extra weight that you did not expect and activate more motor neurons. Then the sensory consequences of your reach will be evaluated, and the cerebellum will update the movement—in this case, to accommodate a heavier milk carton.

From this description, you can see that sensory information plays many roles during the control of reaching. Sensory information is used to correct errors during the execution of the movement itself, ensuring accuracy during the final portions of the movement. In addition, sensory information is used proactively in helping to make the movement plan.

In the following section we will discuss recent research exploring the role of specific visual pathways involved in reach and grasp.

Visual Pathways Related to Visual Regard, Reach, and Grasp

When we move our eyes to locate a stationary target we want to grasp, that object excites successive locations on the retina during the movement. In spite of this continual shift in input across the retina, we perceive a stable visual environment. How does the brain deal with the problem of transforming a sensory stimulus coded at the level of the retina into a motor output code for controlling reach and grasp motions? The relationships between eye, head, and hand movements can be best understood in relationship to the role of optimizing vision for the guidance of hand motion (Crawford et al., 2004). Research has shown that neurons in the parietal cortex use information about the intended eye movement to update the brain's representation of visual space. The neurons anticipate the retinal consequences of the intended eye movement and shift the cortical representation first. Then the eye catches up.

These neurons thus send a corollary discharge of the output to the eye muscles to other areas of the brain, allowing the visual world to be remapped with each eye movement into the coordinates of the current gaze location. Research (Duhamel et al., 1992a, b) has shown that these corollary discharge visual cells in the lateral intraparietal area (LIP) start to increase their firing rate about 80 msec before a saccade occurs.

The two visual pathways involved in reach and grasp include the dorsal stream pathway, going from the visual to the parietal cortex, and the ventral stream pathway, going from visual cortex to the temporal lobe. Research (Goodale & Milner, 1992; Goodale et al., 1991) suggests that the dorsal stream projection to the parietal cortex provides action-relevant information about all phases of the reaching movement, including object position, structure, and orientation, while ventral stream projections to the temporal lobe provide our conscious visual perceptual experience.

Goodale and Milner note that the dorsal and ventral stream visual pathways are different with respect to their access to consciousness. For example, a patient with "ventral stream" lesions had no conscious perception of the orientation or dimension of objects, but she could pick them up with great adeptness. Thus, it may be that information in the dorsal system can be processed without reaching conscious perception (Goodale & Milner, 1992).

Evidence supporting the concept of separate visual pathways for perception (ventral stream) and action (dorsal stream) in normal subjects comes from work by Haffenden and Goodale (1998). In this experiment, they used a visual illusion to separate perceptual judgments about an object's size and the ability to reach for it accurately. They used the Ebbinghaus illusion, in which two target circles of equal size are surrounded by an array of either smaller or larger circles. Subjects typically report that the circle surrounded by the smaller circles is larger than the one surrounded by larger circles. If the same pathway controlled perception and action, one would expect that both perception and grasp would be equally affected by the illusion.

In this experiment, subjects were asked to either reach for a disk placed in the center of one of the two sets of circles (hypothesized dorsal stream) or manually estimate the size of a disk (hypothesized ventral stream), as shown in Figure 16.4, A and B. Results showed that subjects manually estimated disk size as different, although they were the same. However, grip size was scaled to actual target size rather than apparent size. Figure 16.4C shows the difference in maximum grip aperture and manual estimation for the disks surrounded by either small or large circles. Note that maximum grip aperture is significantly greater for the large disks than small disks, though the subjects reported they were identical in size (left) and estimation of size of disks, which were perceptually identical, but physically different (right), was not significantly different (Haffenden & Goodale, 1998).

Thus, it appears that the ventral stream of projections to the temporal cortex play a major role in the perceptual identification of objects, while the dorsal stream projections to the parietal cortex mediates the required sensorimotor transformations for visually guided actions directed at those objects (Goodale & Milner, 1992).

There are a number of clinical implications of this research. This research suggests that clinicians should assess both perceptual and action components of visually guided reaching, because they are subserved by different neural components. Understanding the essential perceptual features of an object to be grasped is as important as the ability to modify grasp to accommodate those features. In addition, treatment should focus on training both perceptual and action components of the movement.

Posterior Parietal Cortex and Sensorimotor Transformations. It is interesting to note that most neurons in the dorsal stream area (in the posterior

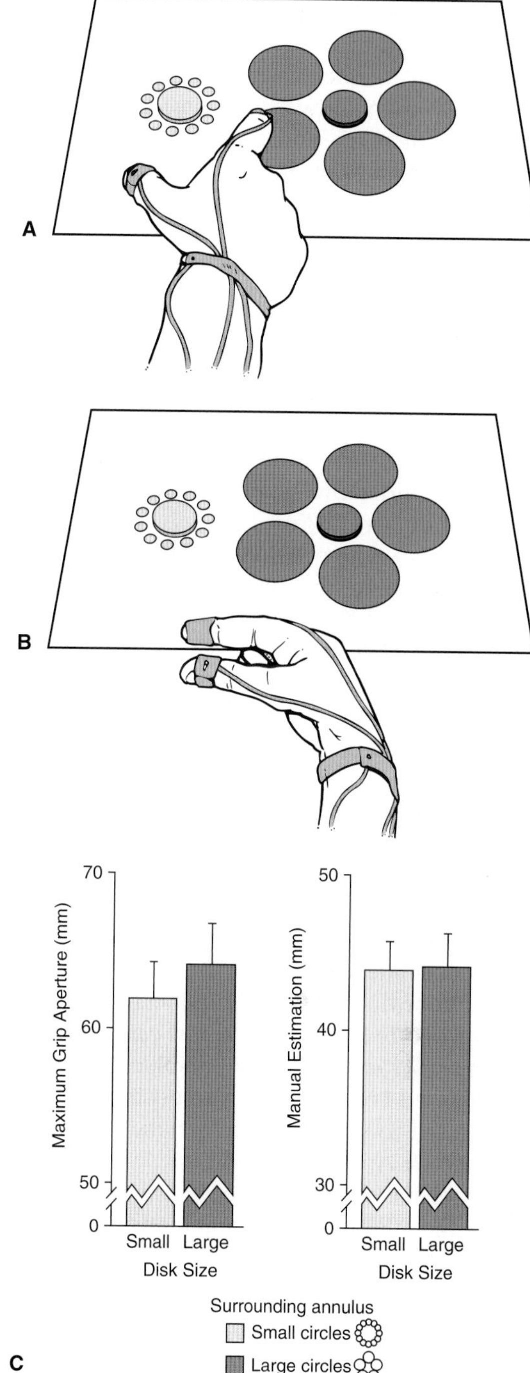

FIGURE 16.4 Reaching and manual-estimation tasks. Shown is both the subject's hand in the grasping task on the way to the target (A) and in the manual-estimation task (B). Also shown (C) are graphs of mean maximum grip aperture on trials in which subjects reported that the disks were identical in size, even though they were physically different (Left); and mean estimation of disk size on trials in which disks were perceptually identical, but physically different in size (Right). (Adapted with permission from Haffenden AM, Goodale MA. The effect of pictorial illusion on prehension and perception J Cogn Neurosci 1998;10:127, 128.)

parietal cortex, or PPC) show both sensory-related and movement-related activity and thus may be involved in sensorimotor transformation processes involved in both eye movements toward the object to be grasped and subsequent reach and grasp movements of the object as well. For example, the LIP serves as a sensorimotor processing area or interface for the production of saccadic eye movements toward an object. As is found in other sensory processing areas, the LIP governs both sensory attention (required for reaching for a specific object within the sensorimotor map) and eye movements. This interface is a shared boundary between the sensory and motor systems involved in reaching. The strongest eye-movement–related activity is typically found in the inferior parietal lobule, which includes Brodmann's area 7a and the LIP (Buneo & Andersen, 2005).

There is also evidence that the PPC plays the same role in the planning and control of arm movements. This activity is strongest in the superior parietal lobule, which includes Brodmann's area 5 and the parietal reach region (PRR).

What computations does the brain need to make in order to make an accurate reach? First of all, it needs to determine both the hand position and the target position. As shown in Figure 16.5, the target in this case is the door knob used to open the door. The brain can define these positions in terms of either an eye-centered coordinate system (represented by the red lines in Fig. 16.5) or with respect to a body-centered coorinate system (in Fig. 16.5, the black lines show the coordinates involving the right shoulder, for a right-handed person). Then it can compute the motor error, for example, the "displacement vector" in eye-centered coordinates or a "position vector" in hand-centered coordinates between the target and the hand (Buneo & Andersen, 2006).

Research has shown that some neurons in the PPC (those in the PRR) encode target position and current hand position in eye-centered coordinates, while other PPC neurons encode reach-related variables in limb-centered coordinates. A third group of neurons encodes these variables in both eye- and limb-centered coordinates; this suggests that they may play a crucial role in transforming spatial information between the two reference frames (Buneo & Andersen, 2006).

In fact, the PPC is involved in a number of different types of sensorimotor transformations, including: (1) movement planning or what could be called "intention" for the movement (the goal of the movement and the type of movement; e.g., "I wish to pick up my glass of milk"). This also includes decision making (a competition between different intentions), and the specifics of how to reach for and grasp the glass; (2) the formation of internal models; and (3) coordinate

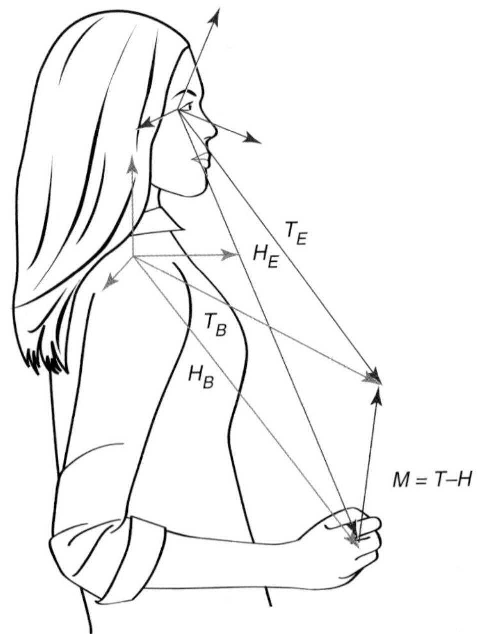

FIGURE 16.5 Drawing illustrating both an eye-centered representation for reaching (target and hand are coded with respect to the current point of visual fixation) and a body-centered representation (target and hand are coded with respect to a fixed position on the trunk). T = target position; H = hand position; B = body-centered coordinates; E = eye-centered coordinates; M = motor error. (Reprinted with permission from Buneo CA, Andersen RA. The posterior parietal cortex: sensorimotor interface for the planning and online control of visually guided movements. Neuropsychologia 2006;44:2594–2606.)

transformations as part of the process of carrying out the movement plan (Andersen & Cui, 2009).

Movement Planning and Intentional Maps. Research using functional magnetic resonance imaging (fMRI) in humans and single-unit recording in nonhuman primates suggests that there is a map related to movement planning or intention in the PPC. As shown in Figure 16.6, area LIP (lateral intraparietal cortex) is specialized for saccade planning; area MIP (medial intraparietal), also called the parietal reach region (PRR), is specialized for planning of a reach; area AIP (anterior intraparietal) is specialized for planning of a grasp; and area MST (medial superior temporal) is for planning smooth-pursuit eye movements. If area AIP, the grasp area, is reversibly inactivated in monkeys, there is a deficit in the shaping of the hand prior to grasping. This is similar to what is found in humans who have PPC damage (Andersen & Buneo, 2002).

For example, it has been shown that patients with lesions in the PPC, resulting in optic ataxia, have problems not only with reaching in the right direction, but

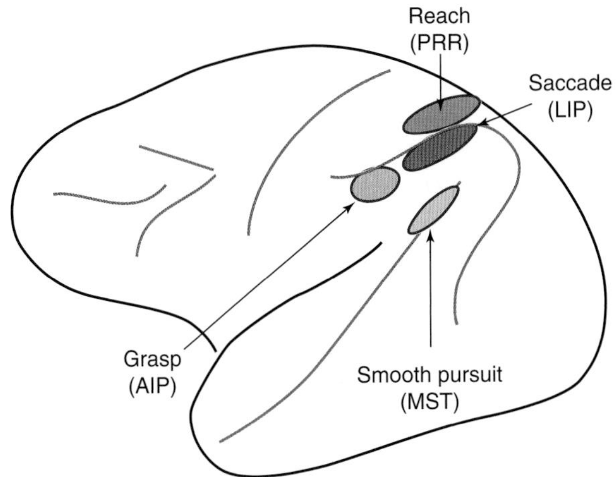

FIGURE 16.6 Map of intentional areas (involved in early plans for movement) in the posterior parietal cortex of a non-human primate. Area LIP (lateral intraparietal area) is specialized for saccade planning, area MIP (medial intraparietal area), the parietal reach reagion (PRR) for reaching, area AIP (anterior intraparietal area) for grasping, and area MST (medial superior temporal) for smooth-pursuit eye movements. (Reprinted with permission from Andersen & Buneo, Intentional maps maps in posterior parietal cortex. Annu Rev Neurosci 2002;25:199.)

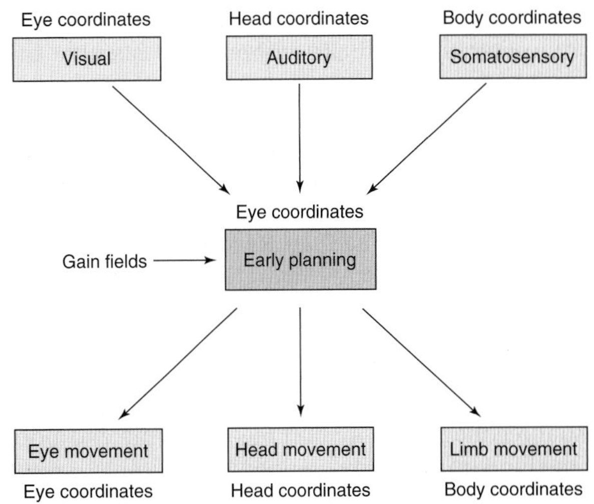

FIGURE 16.7 Model for multisensory integration and eye, head, and body coordinate transformations occuring within the posterior parietal cortex (PPC). (Reprinted with permission from Andersen RA, Buneo CA. Intentional maps in posterior parietal cortex. Annu Rev Neurosci 2002;25:207.)

also with positioning their fingers or adjusting the orientation of their hand when reaching toward an object. They also have trouble adjusting their grasp to reflect the size of the object they are picking up. Researchers have found that damage to the parietal lobe can impair the ability of patients to use information about the size, shape, and orientation of an object to control the hand and fingers during a grasping movement, even though this same information can be used to identify and describe objects. In particular, patients with superior parietal lesions have problems with scaling maximum grip aperture to the size of the object to be grasped. In addition, fMRI studies in humans have shown that the AIP along with premotor cortex, sensorimotor cortex, and other areas of the posterior parietal cortex are active during a precision grip in humans (Binkofski et al., 1998; Castiello, 2005; Goodale & Milner, 1992).

Coordinate Transformations. When we make a movement in response to a sensory stimulus, it is an amazingly complex feat, requiring that our brain solve a large number of difficult computational tasks. The first task that must be solved is that the different types of sensory inputs used to help us know where the body and the object are in space are coded in different reference frames. As shown in Figure 16.7, visual information is coded in eye-centered coordinates, auditory information in head-centered coordinates, and somatosensory information (e.g., touch) in body-centered coordinates (Andersen & Buneo, 2002). The central nervous system (CNS) needs to resolve these in some way, as all three systems may be needed to guide the movement. All of the coordinate frames must then be transformed into coordinates of the muscles to be used for the eye, head, and arm movements, which are the final execution systems for the movements. As shown in Figure 16.7, the nervous system solves this problem during the early planning process by using the eye-centered coordinate system as a common coordinate system. Using a common coordinate frame facilitates eye–hand coordination, and as vision is the most accurate of all the senses, it also improves movement accuracy (Andersen & Buneo, 2002).

The next problem to be solved is to convert the information into limb-centered coordinates for the reach itself. There is evidence to suggest that, at least in some contexts, this is solved by using a direct transformation scheme, using eye coordinates to subtract the current hand position from the current target position (this can be seen in Figure 16.5) and creating a motor vector in limb coordinates. Researchers have found that cells in Brodmann's area 5, a somatosensory-motor cortical area within the PPC, code the locations of targets in both eye-centered and limb-centered coordinates. The transformation process appears to involve simple gain changes in neuron responses (Andersen & Buneo, 2002).

A part of reach and grasp involves the complex and elegant transformation of objects perceived in a visual coordinate system to movements created in a body-centered coordinate system. It is possible that training the perceptual and action components of reach and grasp enhances the transformation among coordinate systems. However, reseasrch is needed to confirm this hypothesis.

Role of Visual Feedback in Reach and Grasp. The primary function of visual feedback in reaching appears to be related to the attainment of final accuracy. It has been hypothesized that the constancy of thumb position with relation to the wrist during reaching may be part of a strategy of providing clear visual feedback information regarding the end point of the limb (Wing & Frazer, 1983).

To determine the function of visual feedback in reaching, studies have been performed to compare reaches made with and without vision. Reaches with visual feedback showed a longer duration than those performed without feedback. Absence of visual feedback did not alter the grasp component of the reach (Jeannerod, 1990).

Can reaching still occur in the absence of visual cortex function? It is usually accepted that destruction of the visual cortex in humans produces total blindness, except for very poor visual perception of illumination changes. However, research on monkeys with visual-cortex lesions has shown some very interesting results related to visual-motor control. Although these monkeys appeared to be blind when their visual behavior was tested, they could still reach for objects that appeared in or moved across the visual field. It has been hypothesized that the superior colliculus in the midbrain contributes to this residual reaching behavior (Humphrey & Weiskrantz, 1969).

Since the studies in monkeys were performed, studies in humans have verified these results. In extending the studies in monkeys to humans, these researchers used a new experimental paradigm that had not been used before in humans. Instead of asking humans with visual-cortex lesions if they could see an object, they asked them to try to point to where they "guessed" the target would be. It was shown that subjects did not point randomly; there was a significant correlation between pointing and target position. However, subjects did show larger constant errors when reaching within their blind visual fields. They typically overshot targets when they were within 30 degrees of midline and undershot them when they were beyond 30 degrees (Perenin & Jeannerod, 1975; Weiskrantz et al., 1974).

Visually Controlled Reaches Across the Midline. Is visual processing more complex when reaching to the contralateral side of the body? Yes. Researchers have consistently found that reaching movements across the midline (toward targets in the visual hemifield of the opposite arm) are slower and less accurate than movements to targets on the same side as the arm. Ipsilateral (uncrossed) reaches in these studies were shorter in latency, made with higher maximum velocity, completed more quickly, and made significantly more accurately than contralateral (crossed) reaches (Fisk & Goodale, 1985).

Thus, even normal adults show decrements when reaching to the contralateral side of the body. This must be remembered when evaluating patients with reaching problems. In addition, when structuring a training program, one may wish to begin with reaching to objects placed on the ipsilateral side prior to progressing to objects placed on the contralateral side.

Somatosensory Contributions to Reach

Is somatosensory input essential for the production of reaching movements? Taub and Berman (1968) have shown that within 2 weeks of deafferentation, monkeys were able to perform adequate reach-and-grasp movements as long as vision was available. They noted that the monkeys' movements were awkward at first, with animals' only sweeping objects along the floor. Monkeys then developed a primitive grasp with four fingers together and no thumb, and finally redeveloped a crude pincer grasp a few months after the lesion was made.

Other experiments discussed later in this chapter have shown that deafferented monkeys can still make reasonably accurate single-joint pointing movements, even when vision of the arm is occluded, when the pointing task was learned before deafferentation (Polit & Bizzi, 1979). In this case, even displacing the arm before the movement did not substantially affect terminal accuracy, even though the monkeys could not see or feel their arm positions. Thus, it was concluded that monkeys are capable of using a central motor program to perform previously learned reaching movements and that kinesthetic feedback is not required for achieving reasonable accuracy when performing well-learned movements.

Experiments performed with humans with severe peripheral sensory neuropathy in all four limbs have shown similar results. One patient was able to perform a wide variety of hand movements, such as tapping movements and drawing figures in the air, even with the eyes closed. However, when he was asked to repeat the movement many times with the eyes closed, his performance deteriorated quickly. Thus, it appears that somatosensory information is not required for arm-movement initiation or execution, as long as the movements are simple or nonrepetitive. However, if subjects have to make complex movements requiring coordination of many joints, or repeat movements, without visual feedback, they are unable to update their central representations of body space and show considerable movement "drift" and problems with coordination (Rothwell et al., 1982).

These experiments suggest that certain movements may be carried out without somatosensory feedback. Nevertheless, considerable work has also shown the important contributions of sensory feedback to the fine regulation of movement.

Researchers originally thought that it was mainly joint receptors that controlled position sense during reaching. However, more recent research suggests that joint receptors are active mainly at the extremes of joint motion, but not at midposition. This would thus make it impossible for these receptors to signal limb position in the mid–working range of joints (Jeannerod, 1990).

More recent work has begun to build evidence for a strong role for muscle spindles in position sense. Experiments have been performed in which tendons were vibrated, specifically activating muscle spindle Ia afferents. Subjects consistently had the illusion that the joint was moving in the direction that it would have been moving if the muscle were being stretched. For example, when the biceps tendon was vibrated, it produced the illusion of elbow extension (Goodwin et al., 1972).

Cutaneous afferents are also important contributors to position sense. Mechanoreceptors in the glabrous area of the hand are strongly activated by isotonic movements of the fingers (Hulliger et al., 1979).

Interestingly, subjects who are recovering from paralysis report that when the muscle is still completely paralyzed, they have no feeling of heaviness in the limb. But as they begin to regain movement ability, they feel as if the limb is being held down by weights. These sensations of heaviness are reduced as movements become easier and strength increases. This could be due to an internal perception of the intensity of motor commands (Jeannerod, 1990).

Somatosensory Contributions to Grasping

Cutaneous afferent input is essential for the control of grip forces. If objects are slippery, cutaneous afferents will detect the slip and activate pathways to increase activity in finger muscles to increase the grip force and in shoulder and elbow muscles to slow the acceleration of the hand. When experiments were performed in which fingers were anesthetized to prevent cutaneous feedback, subjects used the strategy of increasing grip forces to compensate for lack of information, but coordination between grip and load forces was lost, even if the person had previous experience lifting the object (Witney et al., 2004).

In addition, the grip force declined significantly over a 20- to 30-second hold period, and 7 of 10 subjects dropped the object at least once. Adaptation to this loss of information did not occur, even with vision of the grasping hand. Patients with polysensory neuropathy (complete loss of primary afferent sensory inputs) also have been reported to have similar difficulty with the control of grip forces and to show little to no ability to adapt with time. However, those with moderately impaired sensation have shown no problems of this type (Augurelle et al., 2003; Monzee et al., 2003; Nowak et al., 2003; Witney et al., 2004).

Elegant studies have shown that the CNS areas critical for this control include the somatosensory cortex (SI). Studies inactivating the finger area of SI showed that this was correlated with uncoordinated grip and load forces and an increase in grip force (Brochier et al., 1999). Single-cell recording in SI during lift-and-hold tasks in primates has shown that rapidly adapting cells are briefly active at grip onset, slowly adapting cells show continuous activity during the holding phase, and both cells respond strongly to slip. They also receive input from movement-related areas of the brain and may play a role in the activation of responses when afferent input suddenly changes from its normal pattern (Salimi et al., 1999a, b).

Visual and Somatosensory Contributions to Anticipatory (Feedforward) Control of Reach and Grasp

An essential component of all reaching movements is proactive visual and somatosensory control, which is responsible for the correct initial direction of the limb toward the target and the initial coordination between limb segments. In addition, visual information about the characteristics of the object to be grasped is used proactively to preprogram the forces used in precision grip.

It has been hypothesized that visual and somatosensory information is also used to update proprioceptive and visual body maps that allow the accurate programming of reaching movements. To determine the influence of updated maps of the body workspace on the accuracy of a reaching movement, experiments were performed to manipulate visual information regarding hand and target positions prior to movement. It was shown that when a subject could not see the hand prior to movement, there were large errors in reaching the target. It was thus concluded that a proprioceptive map of the hand, by itself, was not adequate to appropriately code the hand position in the reaching workspace. This suggests that somatosensory inputs must be calibrated by vision in order for the proprioceptive map and the visual map to be matched (Jeannerod, 1990). No experiments have yet been performed to determine how often the proprioceptive map needs to be updated by visual inputs to ensure accurate movements.

Motor Systems

Premotor and Primary Motor Cortex Involvement

As noted above, in the section on visual contributions to reach and grasp, the PPC is involved in encoding goals for movement, such as the intended hand formation and orientation toward the object. Information is then sent to the premotor and primary motor cortex (Crawford et al., 2004; Castiello, 2005). Though we think of the parietal cortex as "sensory" and the premotor and motor cortexes as being involved with movement execution, there are both interesting similarities and differences related to activity in the PPC and in the premotor cortex. For example, neurons in both the AIP grasp area and the motor areas code for grasping actions that relate to the type of object that will be grasped (e.g., precision vs. power grip), but the AIP neurons represent the entire action, while the premotor neurons are concerned with a particular part of the action. In addition, the AIP codes objects in visual coordinates, while premotor cortex codes in body coordinates (as noted in the lower part of Figure 16.7, under eye movement, head movement, and limb movement) (Castiello, 2005; Andersen & Buneo, 2002).

Two separate descending pathways are also involved in reach and grasp, as described below.

Two Separate Descending Pathways for Reach and Grasp

During reaching, the arm movement carrying the hand to the target is performed in parallel with the preshaping of the fingers for grasping the object. There are many experiments that suggest that the respective motor systems contributing to reach and grasp involve separate descending motor pathways.

For example, reaching is observed in newborn infants, although grip formation develops later. Research has shown that 1-week-old infants may reach for and intercept moving objects and come into contact with them, but this is done with a hand that is wide open, with no grip formation. Grip formation appears to develop at about 10 to 22 weeks of age (Bruner & Koslowski, 1972).

This is also the case in monkeys. It has been shown that the appearance of the grasp component, at 8 months of age, is correlated with the maturation of connections between the corticospinal tract and the motor neurons (Kuypers, 1962). Thus, a successful grasp requires an intact primary motor cortex and corticospinal tract: if either of these areas has lesions, there is a clear problem with individual finger control for grasping. However, lesions here do not affect synergistic control of fingers for power grips. Interestingly, it has also been shown that motor cortex neurons that are active during fine movements, like a precision grip, become inactive during a power grip (Castiello, 2005; Muir & Lemon, 1983).

Children with pyramidal lesions show problems with the grasp component of reaching, although the transport component may be normal (Jeannerod, 1990). This suggests that midbrain and brainstem pathways such as the red nucleus and reticular nuclei may control the more proximal muscles involved in reaching movements, while pyramidal pathways are required for the fine control of grasping movements.

This same information from primary motor cortex to the spinal cord also is sent to the cerebellum (intermediate lobe). It has been shown that the cerebellum is also important for the control of hand movements during grasping: 93% of output neurons from the cerebellum were more active during reaching out and grasping than during simply gripping an object (Castiello, 2005; Gibson et al., 1994).

Experiments on monkeys performing a precision-grip versus a power-grip task (Fig. 16.8) have shown that there are neurons in the primary motor cortex that fire during the execution of a precision but not a power grip. This indicates that their connections are with intrinsic hand muscles rather than with forearm muscles. These neurons show a short-latency burst onset (approximately 11 msec) prior to muscle activation, which suggests they are monosynaptically connected to the motor neuron pools (Lemon et al., 1986; Muir & Lemon, 1983). Figure 16.8 shows the activity of a pyramidal-tract neuron and an interosseus muscle during a precision-grip task with light versus heavy force and during a power-grip task (grasping a cylinder). Note that the pyramidal-tract neuron is activated only during the precision-grip task at both force levels, but is not activated during the power-grip task. However, the interosseus muscle showed activity in all three tasks.

Musculoskeletal Contributions

Reaching also involves a complex interaction of musculoskeletal and neural systems. Musculoskeletal components include things such as joint range of motion, spinal flexibility, muscle properties, and biomechanical relationships among linked body segments. In

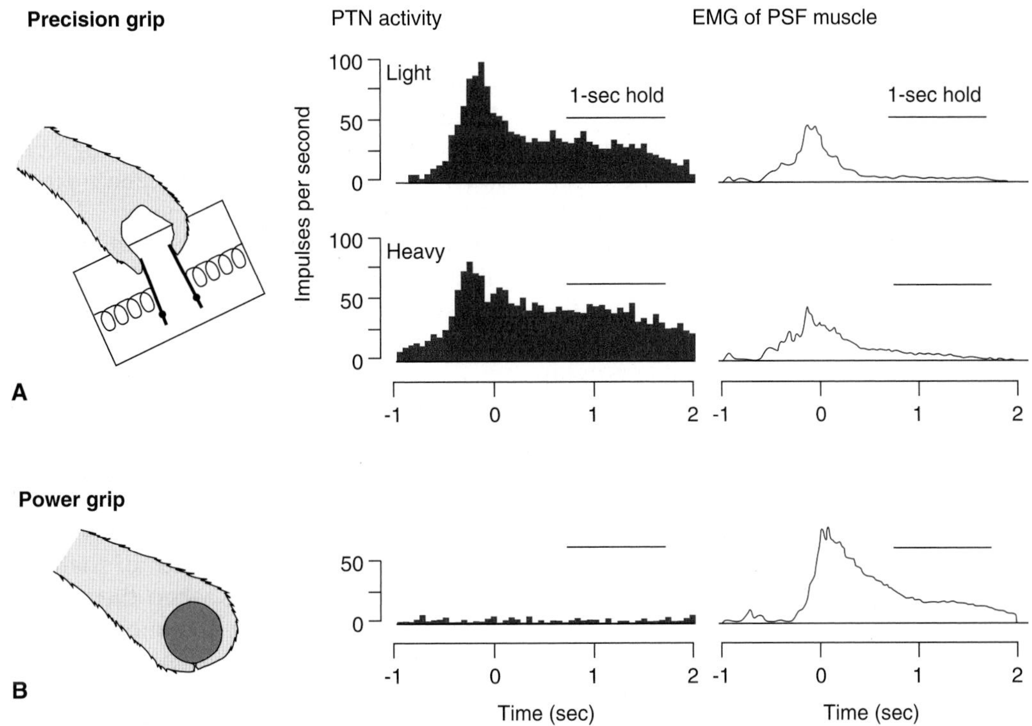

FIGURE 16.8 Graph of activity (impulses/sec) of a pyramidal-tract neuron (PTN) and an interosseus muscle (PSF) during two different tasks: (a) a precision-grip task executed with light versus heavy force (top two traces) and (b) a power-grip task (bottom trace). (Redrawn with permission from Muir RB, Lemon RM. Corticospinal neurons with a special role in precision grip. Brain Res 1983;261:312–316.)

particular, it has been suggested that the following types of joint motion are essential to the ability to move the arm normally: scapular rotation, appropriate movement of the humeral head, the ability to supinate the forearm, shoulder, and elbow flexion to approximately 100 to 120 degrees, the ability to extend the wrist to slightly beyond neutral, and sufficient mobility in the hand to allow grasp and release (Charness, 1994).

Motor aspects of reaching include appropriate muscle tone, muscle strength, and coordination. More specifically, this involves appropriate activation of muscles to stabilize the scapula, rib cage, and humeral head during upper-extremity reaching movements, and activation of muscles at the shoulder, elbow, and wrist joint for transport of the arm.

The work of Kaminski et al. (1995) provides evidence for coupling between the trunk, scapula, and arm when one reaches toward targets. The authors found motion of the trunk to make a significant contribution during arm transport, which affected both the velocity and the path of the hand. Specific evidence of coupling was documented during reaches for anteriorly placed targets, in that trunk rotation was countered by glenohumeral horizontal abduction and scapular retraction in order to keep the hand moving in a straight path.

In a patient with neurologic deficits, it is often not easy to determine the relative contribution of neural versus musculoskeletal problems to abnormal reaching. Motor control problems that affect the inertial characteristics of the system will give rise to coordination problems, even when the patterns of activation are normal. For example, an increase in stiffness will change the inertial characteristics of the head, arm, and/or trunk, making the initiation of motion more difficult. Thus, we see the important interaction between the biomechanics of movement and the neural control mechanisms.

Postural Support of Reaching

As was discussed in Chapter 7, postural control, defined as the ability to control the body's position in space for the purpose of stability and orientation, has a strong influence on upper-extremity function. The ability to control the body's position in space is essential to being able to move one part of the body, in this case one or both arms, without destabilizing the rest of the body.

Research has shown that a key brain structure involved in the learning of anticipatory postural adjustments during a bimanual task (e.g., holding an object in one hand and lifting it with the other) is the cerebellum. Studies of task efficiency in patients with cerebellar lesions showed that although well-learned anticipatory postural adjustments in this task were mainly intact, short-term adaptation of the adjustment was not possible. In addition, patients with cerebellar abnormalities were not able to learn to make an anticipatory postural adjustment for a task for which they had previously not been trained. The authors conclude that adaptation of these responses and the acquisition of novel anticipatory adjustments requires the cerebellum. They also found that patients with cerebellar damage showed poorly timed anticipatory adjustments, with responses beginning earlier than in normal adults (Diedrichsen et al., 2005).

Just as manipulatory control is task-dependent, postural requirements also vary according to the task. For example, postural requirements involved in a seated reaching task will be less stringent than those in a standing task and thus may require only muscles in the trunk. In contrast, postural demands during reaching while standing are greater, requiring more extensive activation of muscles in both the legs and the trunk to prevent instability. Postural demands can affect the speed and accuracy of an upper-extremity movement. When postural demands are decreased by providing external support, upper-extremity movements are faster, since prior postural stabilization is not necessary (Cordo & Nashner, 1982).

Helping a patient to regain sufficient postural control to meet the postural requirements inherent in a reaching task is essential to retraining that task. The reader is urged to review Chapters 7 to 11, which discuss postural control, its relationship to reaching, and issues related to retraining the patient with postural disorders.

GRASPING

Classification of Grasping Patterns

Grasping patterns vary as a function of location, size, and shape of the object to be grasped (Johansson, 1996). In 1956, Napier classified human grasping movements as either power or precision grips. He found that precision and power grips could be used alternatively or in combination for almost every type of object. He also believed that it was not solely the shape or size of the object that determined the grip pattern, but also the intended activity, since a cylindrical object could be used for writing (precision grip) or hammering (power grip) (Castiello, 2005; Jeannerod, 1996; Napier, 1956).

The anatomical difference between the two grips involves both the posture of the thumb and that of the fingers. In a power grip, the finger and thumb pads are directed toward the palm to transmit a force to an object. Power grips include a hook grasp (holding a handle of a suitcase), a spherical grasp (holding a softball), and a cylindrical grasp (holding a bottle). In contrast, during a precision grip, the forces are directed between the thumb and fingers. The two grips are used very differently in manipulative skills: the precision grip allows movements of the object relative to the hand and within the hand, while the power grip does not.

In addition to the power versus precision distinction, researchers have shown that subjects tend to classify objects into four broad categories according to prior knowledge about the object. These categories include four hand shapes: poke, pinch, clench, and palm. The boundaries between categories are determined by the pattern of hand movements used with these objects when they are grasped and manipulated. This differentiation of hand shape also appears during actual reaching in the preshaping of the grasp (Castiello, 2005; Jeannerod, 1996; Klatzky et al., 1987).

Two important requirements are necessary for successfully grasping an object. First, the hand must be adapted to the shape, size, and use of the object. Second, the finger movements must be timed appropriately in relation to transport so that they close on the object just at the appropriate moment. If they close too early or too late, the grasp will be inappropriate (Jeannerod, 1990). Most of the research related to grip formation has been on precision grip, and this will be discussed in the following section.

Anticipatory Control of Grasping Patterns: Precision Grip Formation

When reaching forward to grasp an object, the shaping of the hand for grasping occurs during the transportation component of the reach. Figure 16.9 shows changes in both hand movement velocity (16.9A, left) and grip size (16.9A, right) during a reach. This pregrasp hand shaping appears to be under visual control. What are the properties of an object that affect anticipatory hand shaping? Lab Activity 16.1 will help answer this question.

As you can see from the Lab Activity 16.1, there are two different categories of properties of objects that affect pregrasp hand shaping: intrinsic properties, such as the object's size, shape, and texture, and extrinsic or contextual properties, such as the object's orientation, distance from the body, and location with respect to the body (Jeannerod, 1984).

Remember that grip formation takes place during the transportation phase and is anticipatory of

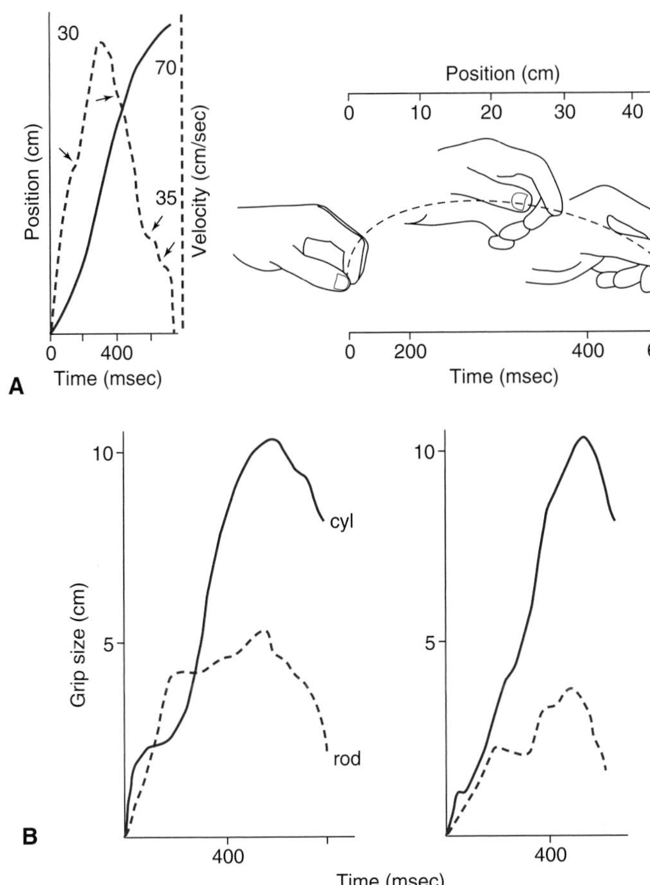

FIGURE 16.9 Characteristics of the transport phase of reaching. A, left, Changes in hand movement velocity (dotted line) and position (solid line) as a function of time during a reach. A, right, Drawing of hand movement changes, including grip opening, during reach. (Adapted from Brooks VB. The neural basis of motor control. New York: Oxford University Press, 1986:133.) B, Changes in grip size over time for two different subjects reaching for a 2-mm-diameter, 10-cm-long rod (dashed lines) versus a 55-mm-diameter, 10-cm-long cylinder (solid lines). Note that there are different grip sizes but similar curve shapes. (Reprinted with permission from Jeannerod M. The neural and behavioral organization of goal-directed movements. Oxford: Clarendon Press, 1990:61.)

the characteristics of the object to be grasped. The size of the maximum grip opening is proportional to the size of the object. This relationship is shown in Figure 16.9B, with a subject reaching for a 2-mm rod versus a 55-mm cylinder. Each increase of 1 cm in object size is associated with a maximum grip size increase of 0.77 cm (Marteniuk et al., 1990). When subjects change the grip opening, they do it almost entirely with finger movements, while the thumb stays in one place. When reaching for an object, as the arm is transported

LAB ACTIVITY 16-1

Objective: To examine how properties of the task affect reach-and-grasp movements.

Procedures: You will be working in pairs for this lab. You will need the following items: a pitcher of water, a glass, a quarter, a pencil, a block, and a plastic glass covered with oil. In the first part of the lab, observe the arm and hand movements of your partner while he or she picks up and sets down the glass, quarter, pencil, block, and plastic glass coated with oil. Next, set the glass upright next to the water pitcher. Observe your partner while he or she reaches for and pours a glass of water. Now, pour the water back in the pitcher and invert the glass next to the pitcher. Again observe your partner while he or she reaches for and pours a glass of water.

Assignment:

1. Describe the properties of the objects that affected how you reach for and grasp the various objects.
2. During the pouring task, how did changing the orientation of the glass affect the movement strategy used to pick up the glass?
3. When during the reach for an object did the hand begin to shape in preparation for grasp?
4. How did characteristics of the object affect anticipatory hand shaping?

forward, the fingers begin to stretch, and the grip size increases rapidly to a maximum and then is reduced to match the size of the object (Castiello, 2005; Jeannerod, 1990).

Subjects show differential hand shaping for different shapes of objects as well. The distance between the thumb and index finger is usually largest during the final-slow-approach phase. It has been shown that adults with prosthetic hands show this same relationship between grasp and transport phases (Fraser & Wing, 1981). Apparently, this relationship is not due to neural constraints, but may be the most efficient way to reach.

Grasp and Lift Tasks

The types of objects that are picked up during a given day may vary from a light pen to a heavy slick bottle of oil. The nervous system is capable of adapting precision grip so that it accommodates objects of many different weights and surface characteristics. The control mechanisms underlying these abilities have been carefully investigated. It has been shown that there are discrete phases to any lifting task. These phases are associated with responses in sensory receptors of the hand.

The first phase of a lift starts with contact between the fingers and the object to be lifted. When contact has been established, the second phase begins, with the grip force and the load force (load on the fingers) starting to increase. The third phase begins when the load force has overcome the weight of the object and it starts to move. The fourth phase occurs at the end of the lifting task, when there is a decrease in the grip and load force shortly after the object makes contact with the table (Johansson & Edin, 1992).

This type of an organizational control scheme has many advantages. For example, it allows great flexibility in lifting objects of different weights. Thus, the duration of the loading phase depends on the object's weight: heavier objects require higher load forces before they move. This also ensures that proper grip forces are used during the load phase. This scheme also requires limited sensory processing, since the end of one phase serves as the trigger for the next.

Once the object is grasped, the grip-to-load force ratio has to be above a certain level to ensure a safe grip; otherwise, slipping will occur. How does the nervous system choose the correct parameters for grip and load force? Two objects of the same weight will not necessarily require the same grip force, since one may be much more slippery than the other. The CNS appears to use both previous experience and afferent information during the task to choose correct grip parameters. If there is a mismatch between the expected and actual properties of an object, then receptors in the finger pads are activated. Pacinian corpuscles are very sensitive and capable of easily detecting that an object has started to move earlier than expected. In addition, visual and other types of cutaneous cues are important in determining the choice of grip parameters (Johansson & Edin, 1992).

The cerebellum appears to be a key system contributing to predictive control of grip forces. In studies in which monkeys were required to maintain their grip on an object during perturbations that simulated object slip, it was found that cerebellar interpositus nucleus and cortical neurons with inputs from cutaneous receptors were activated about 45 msec after the perturbation. The cerebellar neurons also showed anticipatory increases in activation along with grip force increases over repeated trials (Monzee & Smith, 2004). This indicates that the cerebellum plays a role in organizing predictive responses. Research indicates that primary, premotor, and supplementary motor areas do not show predictive responses of this type. This research is supported by work with patients with cerebellar lesions, who have poor predictive control of grip forces, especially related to timing of these forces. On the contrary, patients with hemiparesis have normal timing of predictive grip forces, but with reduced response amplitudes (Babin-Ratte et al., 1999; Boudreau & Smith, 2001; Wiesendanger & Serrien, 2001; Witney et al., 2004).

COORDINATION OF REACH AND GRASP

Although the neurophysiological and developmental research discussed above indicates that the two components, reach and grasp, are controlled by different motor systems, to be functionally effective they must be coordinated with each other. Thus, transport of the hand must be coordinated with the shaping of the fingers to ensure that reaching ends when the fingers come in contact with the object.

Researchers have used kinematics to determine whether there are invariant relationships between reach components and grasp components. It has been shown that there is a fixed ratio of maximum grip aperture to total movement time, such that it occurs at about 75 to 80% of movement time (Jeannerod, 1984; Wallace et al., 1990). This ratio was invariant across variations in movement time and speed and different initial finger postures and was preserved even in pathological conditions. This is a strong indication of functional coupling of the two components (Jeannerod, 1996).

Invariance related to the coordination of reach and grasp has also been studied by examining the effect of a perturbation of one component on the second component. For example, in order to perturb the transport (reach) component, researchers displaced the object to be grasped and found that this perturbation of reach also affected grasp, since there was a brief interruption in grip-aperture formation. In addition, when object size was changed in order to perturb the grip component, it affected the transport component. Thus, the two components were kinematically coupled during corrections for these perturbations (Paulignan et al., 1990). Although the two components are correlated, they appear to be only loosely coupled in time. Thus, they appear to be functionally linked, without stereotyped structural relationships (Jeannerod, 1996).

Based on this research, we could hypothesize that in the case of a patient who has upper-extremity paresis complicated by spasticity, both reach (transport) and grasp will be affected. We might predict, based on the neurophysiological research, that the patient will recover the reach phase earlier and more completely than the grasp phase (De Souza et al., 1980). While the two components are controlled separately, they require coordination to be functionally effective; thus, they will need to be trained both separately and together. For example, the patient may begin practicing the reach component by moving her hand toward an object but not actually grasping it. Because even the reach phase is task-dependent, it is important to practice reaching within the context of many different types of functional tasks, such as reach and point, reach in preparation for a grasp, reach in preparation for a grasp and lift, or grasp and move.

She may also work on grasp and release of an object close to her hand, alleviating the need for controlling reach. Finally, she may work on combining reach components and grasp components.

GENERAL PRINCIPLES OF NEURAL CONTROL OF REACH AND GRASP

Until now, we have described the biomechanical and neural contributions to the different components of reach and grasp. However, another approach to studying the control of reaching has come from the field of psychology, where researchers have focused on describing basic characteristics of reaching and formulated principles and theories about the neural control of reaching based on these characteristics.

Invariant Features of Movement: Motor Programs

In Chapter 1, we mentioned that most movements are performed with similar characteristics even when made with different body segments or limbs. Thus, you can write a word with your fingers, your left or right arm, or with the pen in your mouth and the word will have similar characteristics. This feature has been called "motor equivalence," and it predicts that most movements are represented in the brain in terms of abstract rules that can be used to activate any set of muscles, and are not represented solely at the level of muscle contractions or joint motions.

Reaction Times for Reach and Grasp

Reaction time (RT) is defined as the period between a stimulus and the beginning of a voluntary response (measured as the activation of muscle responses or movement). Voluntary movements require significantly more processing time than reflexes, with the fastest RTs being about 80 to 120 msec for a voluntary response to a somatosensory cue. In contrast, monosynaptic reflex responses are about 40 msec in response to similar cues. Visually initiated RTs are even longer, on the order of 150 to 180 msec, because of increased synaptic processing in the visual system (Ghez & Krakauer, 2000).

Reaction time also varies according to the amount of information to be processed in making the decision to move. RT is fastest if the subject knows in advance the response that is required and is increasingly slowed by adding choices (different cues indicating different movements to be made) or more complex tasks. Figure 16.10A shows how RT increases with the addition of response alternatives. This is called the "choice effect." It has led researchers to hypothesize that movement processing involves three general stages, including stimulus identification, response selection (varying with the number of choices to be made), and response programming (Fig. 16.10B). Although it has been hypothesized that movement processing involves three stages, it has also been shown that parallel processing of movement characteristics, such as movement direction and movement extent can occur, thus speeding movement processing. RT also decreases with learning, as shown in Figure 16.10C. If one group of subjects is given 10 blocks of 10 trials (pressing a key under one of four lights when it is illuminated) each with a repeated sequence and a second group is given a completely random set of responses, there is a substantial drop in RT in the first case, but not in the second (Ghez & Krakauer, 2000).

Fitts' Law

Some basic characteristics of arm movements that you may find intuitively obvious are that whenever arm-movement precision is increased or movement

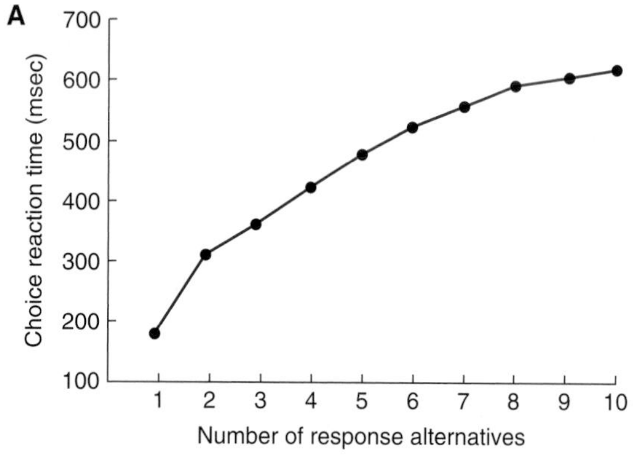

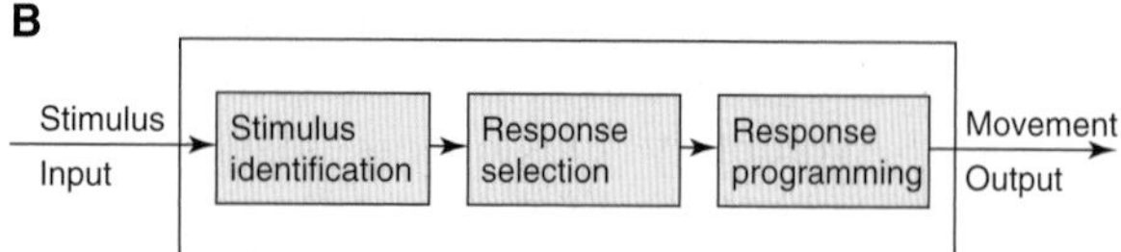

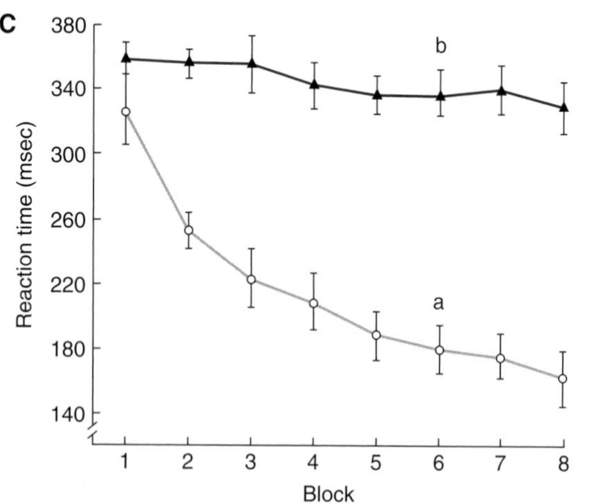

FIGURE 16.10 A, A comparison of reaction time (RT) and the number of response alternatives available. Note that RT increases nonlinearly with the number of response alternatives. B, Information-processing model with three stages between stimulus input and movement output. C, Comparison of RT during successive blocks of trials (10 trials/block) when responding to a predictable (a) versus a nonpredictable (b) stimulus. On each trial one of four lights flashed and participants pressed the key under the light. The same 10-trial sequence was given for each block in the predictable condition. Note that RT decreases with predictable stimuli (a), but does not change with successive blocks of nonpredictable (random) stimuli (b). (Reprinted with permission from Ghez C, Krakauer J. The organization of movement. In: Kandel E, Schwartz J, Jessel T, eds. Principles of neuroscience, 4th ed. New York: McGraw-Hill, 2000:662.)

distance is increased, movement time becomes longer. In the 1950s, Fitts quantified these characteristics in the following experiments. He asked subjects to move a pointer back and forth between an initial position and a target position as quickly as possible. In the set of experiments, he systematically varied the movement distance and the width of the target. He found that he could create a simple equation relating movement time to the distance moved and the target width. This equation, which has become known as Fitts' law, is shown below:

$$MT = a + b \log_2 2D/W$$

where a and b are empirically determined constants, MT is movement time, D is distance moved, and W is the width of the target. The term $\log_2 2D/W$ has been called the "index of difficulty." Movement time increases linearly with the index of difficulty; that is, the more difficult the task, the longer it takes to make the movement (Fitts, 1954; Keele, 1981).

This equation has come to be known as Fitts' law, because its ability to relate movement time to movement accuracy and distance applies to many different kinds of tasks, including discrete aiming movements, moving objects to insert them in a hole, moving a cursor on a screen, small finger movements under a microscope, and even throwing darts. Fitts' law has proven accurate in describing movements made by subjects of all ages, from infants to older adults (Keele, 1981; Rosenbaum, 1991).

What are the constraints of the individual and the task that lead to this particular law regarding movement? It has been suggested that movement time increases with distance and accuracy, due in part to the constraints of our visual system. It is difficult to translate our visual perception of the distance to be covered precisely into an actual movement; thus, as the hand approaches the target, time is needed to further update the movement trajectory (Keele, 1981). Lab Activity 16.2 gives you the opportunity to explore Fitts' law and the relationship between task difficulty and movement time.

How Does the Nervous System Plan Movements? Muscle Coordinate, Joint-Angle Coordinate, and End-Point–Coordinate Strategies

In Chapter 1, when we discussed theories of motor control, we mentioned Bernstein's contributions to systems theory. Remember that he proposed that a given nervous system program will produce different outcomes in different situations because the response of the body will depend on the initial position of the limbs and on outside forces such as gravity and inertia. When body segments act together, the nervous system must also take into account the forces they generate with respect to each other. Bernstein hypothesized that the

LAB ACTIVITY 16-2

Objective: To examine the effect of task difficulty on reaching (Fitts' law). Remember, Fitts defined task difficulty in terms of target size (*W*, which is the width of the target) and the distance to move (*D*, which is the distance between targets). He thus quantified task difficulty (which he called "index of difficulty" or simply, ID) by using the following equation: ID = $\log_2 2D/W$.

Procedure: For this lab, you will work in pairs. With a pencil, tap quickly and accurately between two targets that vary in width and distance. The objective is to make as many *accurate* tapping movements as possible in a 10-second period. Accuracy is important. Remember that there should be no more errors made in the most difficult task than in the easiest tasks. If the number of errors exceeds 5% of the pencil dots, the trial should be done again.

Two combinations of task difficulty will be used. The first and easiest task has *D* = 2 cm and *W* = 2 cm. Solving the equation for ID, that would be log (base 2) of (2 X 2)/2. This works out to the $\log_2$ of 2, which is 1. The most difficult task has *D* = 16 cm and *W* = 1 cm—that is, the $\log_2$ of (2 X 16)/1, which is 5.

Each person will perform three trials (10 seconds each) for the two task conditions. When you are the subject, your partner will time each trial and count and record the number of dots in each target. Your partner should tell you to "start" and "stop" on each 10-second trial. The rest interval between trials should be the amount of time needed to count and record the taps. After the three trials you can switch jobs with your partner.

Make a table and record the number of taps on each of the three trials for both the easy and difficult task. Calculate the mean and standard deviation as well. For each task, calculate the average movement time (in milliseconds) for a single movement of the tapping task. Do this by dividing each number of taps by 10, which will give you the number of taps per second during the 10-second trial. Record this value in the table as well. Next, take the inverse of this number (1/x, where x is the average number of taps). Then, multiply this number by 1000 to obtain the average movement time in milliseconds. Record this average movement time in the table.

Assignment:

1. What impact did the difficulty of the task have on movement time?
2. If you tried to maintain the same speed on the difficult task as you used on the easy task, how would this affect your accuracy?
3. Describe a functional task that has relatively low demands for accuracy and distance, versus a functional task that has relatively high demands for accuracy.
4. What impact will these differences in task difficulty have on your patient's performance?

nervous system possessed a central representation of the movement that was in the form of a "motor image," representing the form of the movement to be achieved, not the impulses needed to achieve it. He believed that proprioception was important to the final achievement of the movement, not in a reflex-triggering sense, but as it contributed to the central representation of the movement. He also suggested that one way to control the high number of degrees of freedom involved in any complex movement was to organize the actions in terms of synergies, or groups of muscles or joints that were constrained to act as a unit (Bernstein, 1967).

In fact, many researchers have now shown that hand movements are organized synergically or through coordinative structures. For example, it was shown that when subjects were asked to use their two hands to point at two separate targets, they moved their hands simultaneously, even if the pointing tasks were very different in difficulty (e.g., one was near and large and the other one was far away and small). Other researchers have noted this same tight bimanual coordination when subjects reached forward to manipulate an object with two hands. Thus, it has been suggested that independent body segments become functionally linked for the execution of a common task (Kelso et al., 1979; Jeannerod, 1990).

How does the nervous system control complex arm movements to reach targets with speed and elegant precision? This is an intricate problem that could be solved in different ways. For example, the nervous system could plan reaching movements with respect to the activation sequences of individual muscles; this has been referred to as a "muscle coordinate strategy." Alternatively, reaching could be planned in relationship to joint-angle coordinates—that is, planning the movements of shoulder, elbow, and wrist joints to arrive at the target. This would mean that the nervous system was planning the movement around a set of intrinsic coordinates of the body, expressed in terms of the joint angles. Finally, the nervous system could plan arm movements in terms of the final end-point coordinates, using extrinsic coordinates in space (Hollerbach, 1990).

Levels of planning could also be considered in terms of a hierarchy, with, for example, both kinematic and kinetic levels of planning. Kinematic levels of planning would be organized around geometry, such as joint-angle variables and end-point variables. Kinetic levels of planning would be organized around forces such as those of muscle activation and joint torques.

On the one hand, it seems intuitively obvious that we would need to use some variation of end-point–coordinate planning in order to do something like picking up a glass of water. If we plan a movement using intrinsic coordinates alone, without regard to the actual position of the object in space, the accuracy of the movement with respect to the end position needed is likely to be decreased. But when the nervous system plans according to end-point coordinates, it needs to make a complex mathematical transformation called an "inverse kinematics transformation," which would transform end-point coordinates into joint-angle coordinates. Then it has to create this trajectory by producing the appropriate muscle-activation patterns (Hollerbach, 1990).

It has also been proposed that movements are planned in terms of joint-angle coordinates, which has the advantage of not requiring an inverse kinematics transformation. This would mean that the organization of movement by the nervous system would be simplified. However, the nervous system would still have to do an inverse dynamics transformation that would transform joint-angle coordinates into muscle torques and muscle-activation patterns required to make the movement.

If trajectories were planned in terms of the muscle-activation pattern, this planning would have the advantage of simplifying the inverse kinematics and inverse dynamics problems. But as we have also mentioned, muscle-activation patterns are only indirectly related to final joint positions. Thus, programming movements in this manner could cause large inaccuracies (Hollerbach, 1990).

How does one go about answering the question of how the nervous system plans movements? In Hollerbach's (1990) excellent review of the research on arm-movement planning, he mentions that Bernstein (1967) actually made the following statement, which has guided modern physiologists in their experiments exploring the control of reaching movements:

> If the spatial shape of a trajectory is invariant irrespective of the muscle scheme or the joint scheme, then the motor plan must be closely related to the topology of the trajectory and considerably removed from joints and muscles.

Thus, experimenters have begun to look for invariant characteristics in different variables related to the reach. If invariances are found across different conditions, this could be considered evidence that the nervous system uses this variable to plan movements.

It has been shown that the path of the wrist in an arm movement is unaffected by movement speed or by load (weights held in the hand). In addition, the velocity profiles of a movement are also unaffected by movement speed or load. These findings support the concept that the nervous system uses kinematic variables for planning (Atkeson & Hollerbach, 1985).

Remember that there are two types of kinematic variables that could be used for movement planning: joint-angle coordinates and end-point coordinates. If the nervous system controls movements in joint-angle coordinates, the hand should move in a curved line, because the movements will be about the axis of a joint, as shown in Figure 16.11A. However, if it plans movements with respect to extrapersonal space or end-point coordinates, the hand would be expected to move in a straight line (Fig. 16.11B) (Hollerbach, 1990; Rosenbaum, 1991).

To answer this question, researchers (Morasso, 1981) asked subjects to point to different targets in two-dimensional space (on a surface) and recorded their hand trajectories (see Fig. 16.12A for the experimental setup for this type of experiment). They found that subjects tended to move the hand in straight lines, with hand-velocity characteristics having the same shape and scale in relation to the distance the hand moved. However, elbow and shoulder joints went through complex angular changes (see Fig. 16.12, B and C). Even when they were asked to draw curved lines, the subjects tended to draw a series of straight-line subunits. These results (straight hand path and similar velocity characteristics) support the concept that the CNS programs movements according to the hand and movement end-point coordinates (Ghez & Krakauer, 2000).

Other researchers have explored arm-movement control further and have shown that the nervous system can directly control the joints and still produce straight-line movements. This is done by varying the onset times for the joint movements, with all joints stopping at the same time. This method of control gives movements with almost straight-line paths. This suggests that straight-line trajectories can occur even when the CNS is using joint-angle coordinates to program movements. Thus, it is not clear whether the CNS programs movements exclusively by one method or the other (Hollerbach, 1990).

Russian researchers have shown that the elbow and wrist joints are controlled as a synergic unit. When subjects were asked to move the elbow and wrist joint congruently (flexing both together), the subjects

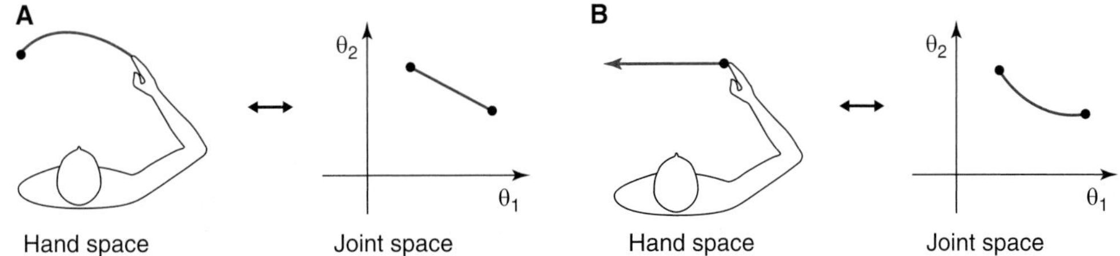

FIGURE 16.11 Different variables that can be used for planning arm movements. A, If movements are controlled in joint-angle coordinates, hand trajectories are curved. B, If movements are controlled in end-point coordinates, joint space is curved (a complex elbow and shoulder movement is required). (Adapted from Hollerbach JM. Planning of arm movements. In: Osherson DN, Kosslyn SM, Hollerbach JM, eds. Visual cognition and action: an invitation to cognitive science, vol. 2. Cambridge, MA: MIT Press, 1990:187.)

could perform this task with ease, with joint motions starting and stopping as a unit. When asked to move the joints incongruently (flexing one and extending the other), they performed the task with considerable difficulty, moving the joints much less smoothly. This is additional evidence for joint-based planning (Kots & Syrovegin, 1966).

A number of additional theories on the control of reaching will be described in the following section. The first group of theories tends to assume that the nervous system is programming distance in making movements, while the second group of theories suggests that final location is the parameter being programmed.

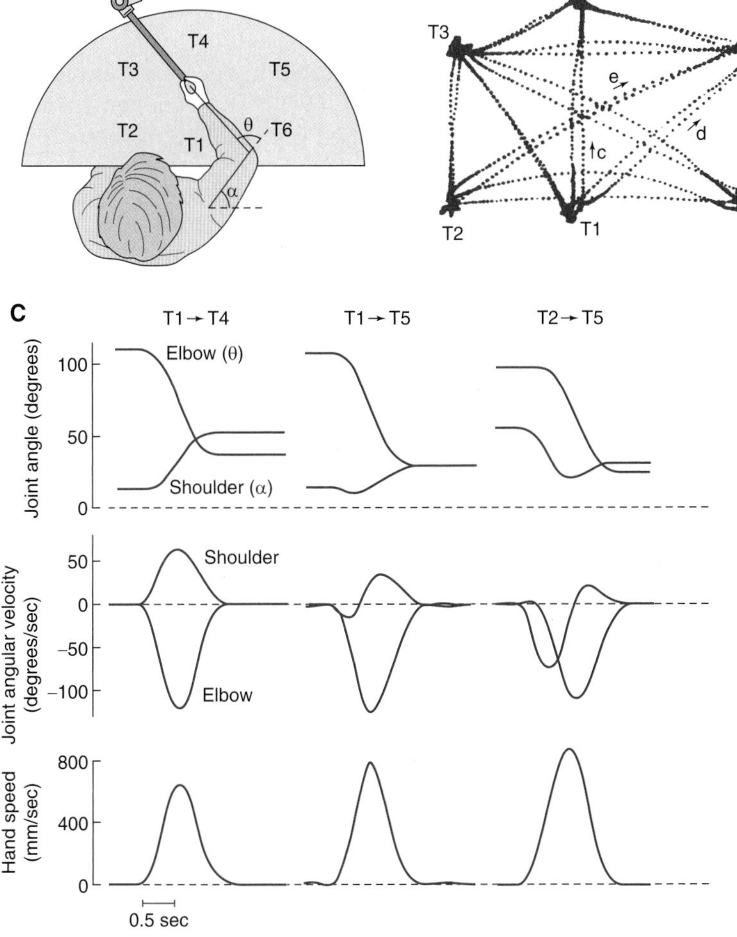

FIGURE 16.12 A, Subject sitting in front of a plate, grasping a handle, which can be moved to one of six positions. The two-jointed handle system records hand position. B, Hand-position paths of one participant when moving to different targets. C, Elbow- and shoulder-joint angle and joint angular velocity, in addition to hand speed when moving among three different targets. Elbow and shoulder angles differ for the three paths. Hand paths are approximately straight, and hand speed curves have similar shapes in proportion to distance between targets, suggesting that movement planning is made with reference to the hand. (Reprinted with permission from Ghez C, Krakauer J. The organization of movement. In: Kandel E, Schwartz J, Jessel T, eds. Principles of neuroscience, 4th ed. New York: McGraw-Hill, 2000:658.)

Distance versus Location Programming Theories

What do we mean by programming distance versus location? According to the distance programming theory, when making an arm movement toward a target, people visually perceive the distance to be covered. Then, they activate a particular set of agonist muscles to propel the arm the proper distance to the target. At a particular point, they turn off the agonist muscles and activate antagonist muscles at the joint in order to provide a braking force to stop the movement (Keele, 1986).

According to the location programming theory, the nervous system programs the relative balance of tensions (or stiffness) of two opposing (agonist and antagonist) muscle sets. According to this theory, every location in space corresponds to a family of stiffness relations between opposing muscles, as we explain later in the chapter. Let's first look at distance programming theories.

Distance Theories

Multiple-Corrections Theory. It has been shown repeatedly that accuracy of arm movements decreases when vision is absent. For example, when subjects were asked to make arm movements of different durations to a target, movements of 190 msec or less were unaffected by loss of vision, while movements of 260 msec or more were affected by loss of visual feedback (Keele & Posner, 1968). Thus, it appears that movement trajectories are corrected based on visual feedback, and that it takes about 200 to 250 msec for vision to be able to update a movement trajectory. Considering that some movement time must occur before the limb is close enough to the target to use visual feedback, one realizes that the visual processing time is slightly shorter. It has been shown (Carlton, 1981) that subjects need to see their hand for at least 135 msec during a movement to use vision to improve movement accuracy.

In the 1960s, researchers (Keele, 1968; Crossman & Goodeve, 1983) proposed that aiming movements consisted of a series of submovements, each responding to and reducing visual error. Thus, an initial movement, before any visual correction takes place, covers most of the distance to a target and is independent of final precision. This model predicts a constant b for Fitts' law, which is almost identical to the one that Fitts and Peterson calculated originally (Keele, 1981).

There are, however, some problems with this model. Typically, aiming movements to a target have only one correction, if any, and when corrections are made, they do not have constant durations or proportions of the distance to the target (Rosenbaum, 1991).

How might this theory be used to explain problems related to inaccurate reaching movements commonly found in patients with neurologic deficits? The multiple-corrections theory stresses the importance of visual feedback when making corrections during a movement to increase accuracy. Thus, inaccurate movements could be the result of loss of visual feedback. When retraining a patient using a multiple-corrections theory, the clinician could have the patient practice slow movements, requiring a high degree of accuracy, drawing the patient's attention to visual cues relating hand movement to target location.

Schmidt's Impulse Variability Model. Another way of explaining the characteristics of arm movement seen in Fitts' equation is to hypothesize that the initial phase of the movement, involving the generation of a force impulse, is more important than later phases of the movement dealing with ongoing control. This would be particularly true in cases in which the movement is too fast to use visual feedback to aid in accuracy.

Schmidt performed research in which subjects were asked to make fast movements over a fixed distance. These movements required large amounts of force, since high-velocity movements require large forces to generate the movement. He showed that the size of the subject's error increased in proportion to the magnitude of the force used. Thus, when he asked subjects to make a fast but accurate movement, the large forces required caused increased force variability. This increased variability resulted in decreased movement accuracy (Schmidt et al., 1979). These movement characteristics were described in the following equation:

$$W_e = a + b\ D/MT$$

where W_e is variation in movement end point expressed in standard deviation units, D is distance moved, and MT is movement time. This equation is similar to Fitts' law. It indicates that simply taking into account the fact that faster movement requires more force can explain Fitts' law, without having to factor in a need for visual feedback for movement accuracy (Keele, 1981).

This theory alone cannot be used to explain aiming movements, since as we have seen above, many movements, particularly those lasting longer than 250 msec, do use visual feedback for accuracy.

Nonetheless, this theory does have relevance for the clinician involved in retraining upper-extremity control. It suggests the importance of practicing fast movements of varying amplitudes during therapy sessions. In this way, patients learn to program forces appropriately for quick and accurate movements.

Hybrid Model: Optimized Initial Impulse Model. The previous two models deal with two extremes of movement control: (a) the use of visual feedback to improve accuracy during ongoing portions of slower movements, and (b) very fast movements that cannot easily use visual feedback, and thus are controlled only through the amplitude of the initial impulse. In an attempt to create a model to explain the entire range of possible aiming movements, more recent studies (Meyer et al., 1988) have described a hybrid model that combines elements of both of these models. This hybrid model is referred to as the "optimized initial impulse model."

Researchers involved in studying this model hypothesized that a subject makes a first movement toward a target, which, if successful, is the sole movement. However, if it is inaccurate (e.g., if it undershoots or overshoots the target), another movement will be required involving visual feedback during ongoing movement control. Clearly, the subject needs to find a balance between moving quickly, which requires a large initial force, and moving slowly enough to allow corrections to the ongoing movement, thereby ensuring accuracy.

It was found that an equation taking these issues into account was similar to Fitts' law:

$$T = a + b\,(n(D/W)^{1/n})$$

where T is movement time, D is distance, and W is width of the target, and n is the number of submovements used to reach the target (Rosenbaum, 1991).

Since functional activities require a variety of movements, both fast and slow, with varying degrees of accuracy, it is important to retrain a patient's ability to perform a continuum of movements that vary in both speed and accuracy.

Location Programming Theories

As we mentioned above, the nervous system could program arm movements in one of two ways: distance programming or programming the end-point location of the movement (Keele, 1981; Feldman, 1974). The example of a cafe-door swinging on springs has sometimes been used to explain the location programming model (Keele, 1986). Figure 16.13A shows the door in a closed position. The movement of the cafe door is described as occurring when there is a reduction in the length of one spring and the lengthening of the other spring. When the door is released, the imbalance between the springs causes the door to return to its closed position, in which the springs are at their resting length. If you want to keep the door open, you can simply change one spring for another of a different stiffness, and then it will have a new resting position (Fig. 16.13B).

It has been suggested that the agonist/antagonist muscle pairs at the joints are like the springs of the cafe door. We can change the position of the joint simply by changing the relative stiffness of the two muscles, through higher or lower relative activation levels. Although this may sound like an unusual way for the nervous system to program reaching movements, experiments have shown that this occurs in many circumstances.

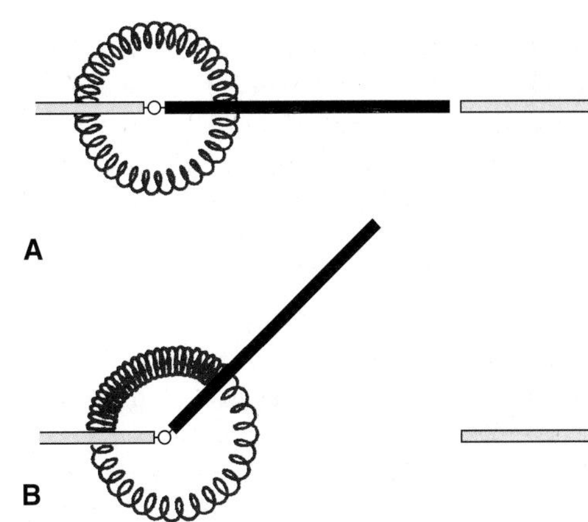

FIGURE 16.13 The cafe-door model. Simplified explanation of the mass-spring model of motor control. A, When a cafe door is at rest, it resembles a joint at midpoint, with both muscles at midlength. B, When one spring of a cafe door is shortened and the other is lengthened, the door is open, analogous to one muscle contracting and the other relaxing to allow the joint to flex.

For example, experiments performed on monkeys (Polit & Bizzi, 1979) suggest that many movements may be controlled through location rather than distance programming. In these experiments, the monkeys were trained to make elbow movements to different targets whenever lights above those targets were turned on, as shown in Figure 16.14D. The monkeys wore a large collar that blocked sight of the arm, eliminating visual feedback. In addition, in certain experiments, the dorsal roots of the spinal cord were severed, eliminating kinesthetic feedback from the arm. The accuracy of the monkeys' arm movements was measured with and without visual and kinesthetic feedback. Researchers found that the monkeys' reaching was normal, despite a loss of visual and kinesthetic feedback (Fig. 16.14A).

The investigators then gave a perturbation to the deafferented monkey's arm, moving it from its original position, just after the target light was turned on but before the monkey began to move. Remember that the monkeys could not feel or see the arm position when it was perturbed. Nevertheless, the monkeys reached for the target with reasonable accuracy (Fig. 16.14, B and C). If the monkeys were using distance programming for reaching, this would have been impossible, because they would have applied a fixed-force pulse in the elbow muscles to move the arm to the new position. Since the arm had already been perturbed, they should have ended up in the wrong place.

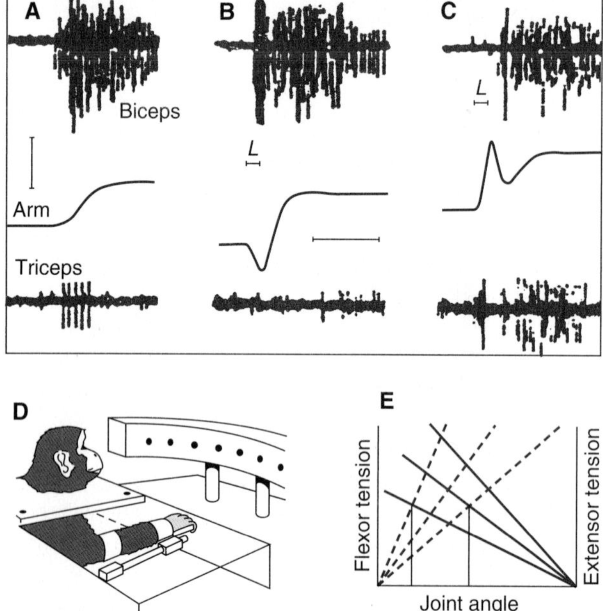

FIGURE 16.14 Experimental setup to test the mass-spring model of control. The deafferented monkey is pointing to a target but is unable to see its hand (see panel D). A, The monkey flexes the arm at the elbow to move to the target in a control trial. Biceps, triceps, and arm position traces are shown. Note that the biceps muscle is predominantly active, with little activity in the triceps. B, The hand is moved by a torque motor to a new position further from the target after the target is illuminated, but before the hand starts to move. Note that the biceps muscle is active and the triceps silent. C, The hand is moved by a torque motor to a new position past the target after the target is illuminated but before the hand starts to move. Note that now the triceps muscle also shows considerable activity, since the monkey must extend the arm slightly. As shown in the movement traces, the monkey was able to successfully point to the target, even when the unseen deafferented hand was perturbed. For A, B, C: Time calibration, 1 sec; vertical bar, 15 deg. L incidates timing and duration of load application. Target light is on during actual pointing. Initial forearm position was different from trial to trial. E, A graph showing different flexor (dotted lines) and extensor (solid lines) muscle tension levels that would move the arm to different joint angles. The intersection of two curves on the x-axis shows the resultant joint angle produced by two combined tensions (left vertical line = greater angle of flexion, next line to right = great extension). (Reprinted with permission from Brooks VB. The neural basis of motor control. New York: Oxford University Press, 1986:138.)

The only way these results can be explained is through the use of end-point-location programming. In this case, what the nervous system would program is the stiffness (or background activity level) settings on the agonist and antagonist muscles of the arm. For example, if the arm was originally in a flexed position, there would be high background activity levels in the elbow flexors and low levels in the extensors. To move the arm precisely to the new location (increased extension angle), the background activity (stiffness) levels would simply change so that the spring constant of the elbow flexors was at a lower level, and that of the extensors was at a higher level. This is shown graphically in Figure 16.14E. Once this new spring setting was made, it would not matter where the limb was perturbed, because, just like the cafe door, the limb would swing to its new spring setting. Thus, the monkey did not have to know its starting point in order to go to the correct end point.

It is interesting that in these experiments, the monkeys were not able to continue to make accurate movements when the shoulder position was changed. It appears that without visual or somatosensory feedback from the arm, they could not update a central reference concerning shoulder position changes. These changes then threw off the elbow location programming (Polit & Bizzi, 1979).

Work by Kelso and Holt (1980) with humans produced similar results. In this study, subjects were blindfolded, and their fingers were anesthetized by using a pressure cuff. Before testing began, they were trained to move their fingers to a specific position in space. They were then given brief finger perturbations during the course of their finger movement. With complete loss of finger sensation, there was very little difference in terminal error between the perturbed and unperturbed movements.

These results suggest that the nervous system is able to encode the location of body segments in space, in relation to a base body position as varying activation levels of agonist and antagonist muscles. What does this mean? It has been suggested that this could explain why we can perform a skill (such as reaching for a cup or throwing a ball) hundreds of times without repeating exactly the same movement. According to classic programming theory, one would have to make a new program for each movement variation, but according to the mass-spring model, all one would have to do is program the appropriate muscle activity ratios and the limb would move appropriately to its final position (Keele, 1986).

Do these results suggest that distance programming is wrong? No. Most likely, both strategies are used for arm movements, depending on the task and the context. For example, it has been shown that when humans make rapid elbow-flexion movements (Hallett et al., 1975), they show a triphasic burst of contraction: first, the biceps is activated, followed by the triceps (braking the movement), and then the biceps again. This same pattern was found in patients with loss of kinesthetic sensation. However, when subjects were asked to move more slowly and smoothly, they showed continuous biceps activity and no triceps activity. This has led some researchers to argue that the subjects are using mass-spring or location programming for slow movements, and a combination of distance programming and location programming for faster movements. There are also limitations to the mass-spring model. The model holds only with single-joint, one-plane movements. Most movements involve many joints, are carried out in three-dimensional space, and have to take gravity into account (Keele, 1981).

Ghez (1979) has also proposed a pulse-step model for arm-movement control, in which an initial pulse of force is followed by a step change in force levels. He states that the initial pulse component is required to overcome the constraints imposed by mechanical properties of the muscle and limb. This again could be considered a combined distance/location type of movement control.

In summary, research studies appear to indicate that single-joint movements that are shorter than 0.25 second are too short to take advantage of visual feedback, while those longer than 0.25 second involve visual feedback in the homing-in phase. Slower movements may involve location programming, while faster movements may involve a combination of distance and location programming.

This model would suggest that the capacity to modulate stiffness levels between the agonist and antagonist muscles is an important part of retraining accurate upper extremity movements.

SUMMARY

1. From a kinematic perspective, coordination in reaching is characterized by the sequential activation of eye, head, and then hand movements. However, muscle responses in these segments tend to be activated synchronously, not sequentially. Thus, inertial characteristics play an important part in the final movement characteristics.
2. Reach and grasp represent two distinct components that appear to be controlled by different neural mechanisms. Thus, patients with motor control problems can have difficulties in one or both aspects. This has implications for retraining.
3. Certain aspects of the grasp component, such as force of the grasp, are based on the person's perception of the characteristics of the object to be grasped, and thus are programmed in advance.
4. Visual and somatosensory information is also used reactively for error correction during reach and grasp.
5. Fitts' law expresses the relationship between movement time, distance, and accuracy, stating that when the demands for accuracy increase, movement time will also increase.
6. There are two theories regarding the neural control of reaching: distance programming and location theories.
7. According to the distance programming theory, when people make an arm movement toward a target, they visually perceive the distance to be covered, and then they activate a particular set of agonist muscles to propel the arm the proper distance to the target. At a particular point, they turn off the agonist muscles and activate antagonist muscles at the joint to provide a braking force to stop the movement.
8. According to the location programming theory, the nervous system programs the relative balance of tensions (or stiffness) of two opposing (agonist and antagonist) muscle sets. According to this theory, every location in space corresponds to a family of stiffness relations between opposing muscles.
9. It is probably the case that both strategies are used for arm movements, depending on the task and the context.

ANSWERS TO LAB ACTIVITY ASSIGNMENTS

Lab Activity 16-1

1. The properties that affect reach/grasp include the object's size, shape, and surface texture (including its slipperiness) as well as the object's orientation, distance from the body, and location with respect to the body.
2. The orientation of the hand was opposite for the two glass orientations (glass right side up: thumb up; glass upside down: thumb down, so that the hand/glass orientation would be the same for the final upright position of the glass.
3. Almost from the beginning of the reach.
4. It was wider for larger objects.

Lab Activity 16-2

1. Movement time was longer.
2. Accuracy would decrease.
3. Functional task with low demands for accuracy/ distance: Placing a coffee cup on a nearby shelf. High demands: Fitting a screwdriver in a small screw head at arm's length.
4. Either accuracy or movement time will go down in the task with high distance/accuracy demands.

CHAPTER 17

REACH, GRASP, AND MANIPULATION: CHANGES ACROSS THE LIFE SPAN

LEARNING OBJECTIVES

Following completion of this chapter, the reader will be able to:

1. Discuss the developmental changes in neural and musculoskeletal systems involved in reach and grasp skills across the lifespan.
2. Describe the changes in reach and manipulation skills that occur with each stage of development up to adulthood and any decrements that occur as part of the aging process; discuss the underlying subsystem changes contributing to these changes in skill.

INTRODUCTION

The development of reach, grasp, and manipulation skills is complex and actually involves the development of many behaviors, each of which emerges progressively over time in association with maturation of different parts of the nervous and musculoskeletal systems and with experience. For example, the infant's ability to transport the arm toward an object precedes the ability to grasp. The ability to grasp emerges at 4 to 5 months of age, preceding the infant's ability to explore objects, which does not emerge until about the first year of life. Thus, the development of mature upper-extremity function, including reach, grasp, and manipulation occurs gradually over the first few years of life.

This chapter explores research on the development of reaching abilities in infants and children as well as the changes in reaching abilities that occur in older adults. We first discuss some of the early hypotheses concerning the development of reaching, which propose that reaching results either from the inhibition of primitive reflexes or from the integration of those reflexes into voluntary movement (Twitchell, 1970). We also discuss the relative contributions of genetics versus experience to the emergence of reaching in the neonate. We then review more recent studies that come from newer theories of motor control such as the ecological and systems approaches.

Role of Reflexes in Development of Reaching Behaviors

Is early reaching reflexly controlled? This is a question that has been debated in the developmental literature for many years. Early theories of the development of reaching argued that reflexes provide the physiological substrate for complex voluntary movements such as reaching (Twitchell, 1970). According to these theories, the transition from reflexes to voluntary reaching is a continuous process, with newborn reflexes gradually being incorporated into a hierarchy of complex coordinated actions (McDonnell, 1979). A review of eye–hand coordination development mentions that early developmental theoreticians may have overlooked another possibility regarding the development of reaching: that eye–hand coordination may emerge concurrently with the maturation of reflex function rather than emerging from the modification of reflex function (McDonnell, 1979). Thus, reflexes such as the grasp reflex may develop separately from the eye–hand coordination system, and may underlie different functions.

Reaching Behaviors: Innate or Learned?

A second question that has intrigued researchers concerns the extent to which the integration of sensory and motor systems underlying eye–hand coordination is genetically predetermined and/or experientially determined.

If the integration of eye–hand coordination were completely genetically predetermined, it would imply that the nervous system has a ready-made map of visual space and one of manipulative space laid out in a one-to-one correspondence. Thus, just by seeing an object, an infant would know exactly where to reach. In contrast, if eye–hand coordination were completely experientially determined, experience would be required to "map" visual space onto motor space or to learn to transform arm spatial coordinates into coordinates of the object.

The first hypothesis implies that once the nervous system's sensory and motor pathways for visually guided reaching have matured, the infant will be able to reach accurately for an object, with little or no prior experience. The second hypothesis predicts that a learning period is required in development, during which the infant creates, through trial and error, the visual map or perceptual rules that overlay the motor map or actions required for reaching.

In the 1950s, Piaget's research on child development led him to believe that although nervous system maturation is a requirement for the appearance of a behavior, experience is responsible for its coordination with the senses. He believed that only through repeatedly and simultaneously looking at and touching an object would the visual and manipulative impressions be associated (Piaget, 1954).

Other researchers gave further support to this concept when they noted that neonates showed both visual and manual activity in the first few weeks after birth, but these movements were apparently unrelated (White et al., 1964). Thus, in the 1960s, many researchers in development supported the theory that visual and hand control systems are unrelated at birth.

In the 1970s, a group of scientists (Bower et al., 1970a, b) presented interesting evidence that they believed supported the opposite concept: that there was clear coordination of eye and hand in the newborn. They reported that infants between 7 and 14 days of age showed arm movements that were clearly directed toward an object in the visual field. They said a significant proportion of reaches were within 5 to 10 degrees of the object and that in 30 to 40% of the reaches, the hand closed around the object. They also observed that infants differentiated between objects that could be grasped (small object) from those that could not (large objects at large distances): they reached for the first but not the second.

Many researchers initially had difficulty replicating these experiments, and thus the results were questioned (Dodwell et al., 1976). However, later studies indicated that an early form of eye–hand coordination does exist in the neonate, although reaching does not seem to be as accurate or as coordinated as originally indicated (Vinter, 1990; von Hofsten, 1982).

In 1980, Amiel-Tison and Grenier, two researchers from France, wrote a surprising article on neonatal abilities. They reported that when the heads of neonates were stabilized, giving them postural support, amazing coordination of other behaviors was seen. For example, they reported that chaotic movements of the arms became still and the infants appeared to be able to reach forward toward objects, as shown in Figure 17.1. Their article is one example of research that supports the hypothesis that infants are born with certain innate abilities or behaviors, which have sometimes been termed "prereaching behaviors."

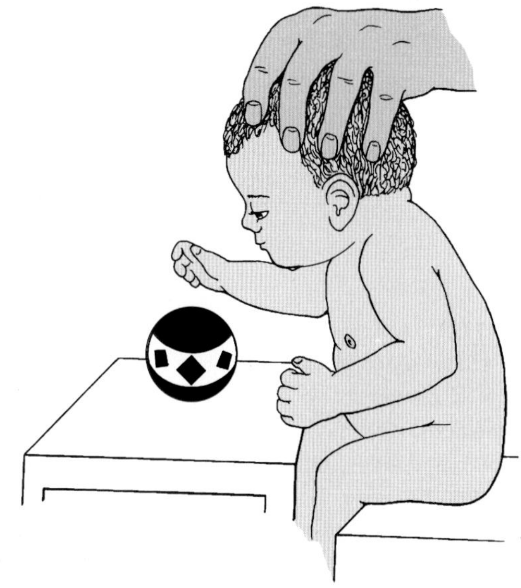

FIGURE 17.1 The release of reaching movements in a neonate by stabilizing the head. (Modified from Amiel-Tison C, Grenier A. Evaluation neurologique du nuveau-ne et du nourrisson. Paris: Masson, 1980:95.)

In the late 1970s and 1980s, von Hofsten (1984, 1993) began exploring the development of eye–hand coordination in the neonate. He placed infants in an infant seat and moved an object in front of them, as shown in Figure 17.2, and carefully documented the number and accuracy of reaches that he observed. He showed that the number of extended movements performed when the infants were visually fixating on the object was twice as high as when the infants did not fixate on the object. The reaching movements were not very accurate. However, those that were made while the infants fixated on the target were aimed within an average of 32 degrees laterally and 25 degrees vertically toward the target, while those that were made without fixation were only within 52 degrees laterally and 37 degrees vertically. Although these reaching movements were not as accurate as had previously been postulated, they were clearly aimed at the target, since they were significantly more accurate than the nonvisually fixated movements. These results thus showed a clear effect of vision on reaching movements. von Hofsten noted that the system works from hand to eye as well. Several times, the infant accidentally touched the object and immediately turned the eyes toward it. Neonates also have proprioceptive control of hand movements: they reach toward their mouth without vision, in a goal-directed way.

Van der Meer et al. (1995) recorded the arm-waving movements of newborn infants as they lay supine, with the head facing to the side. They were either given vision of the arm they were facing, vision of the opposite arm through a monitor, or vision of neither arm. They found that the infants would counteract small forces applied to the wrist in order to keep the limb up and moving if they could see it, but did not do this if they could not see it. This also suggests that infants have visual control of arm movements shortly after birth (Gordon, 2001).

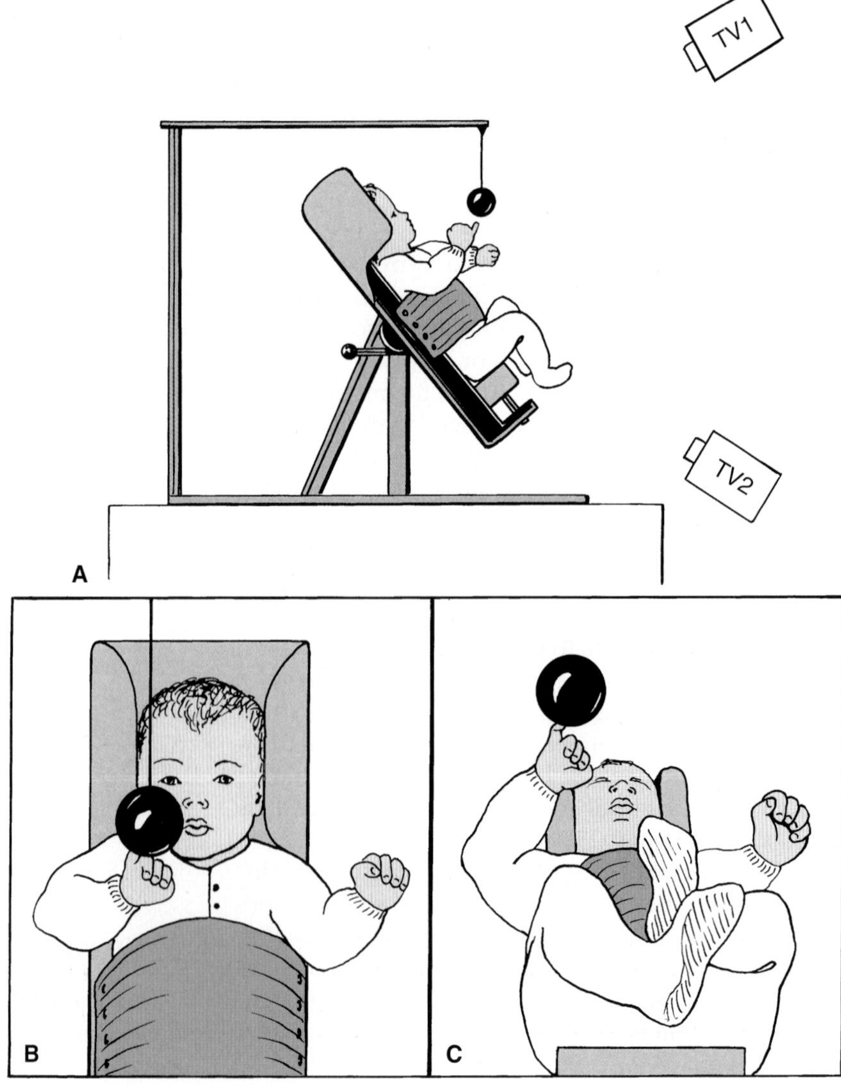

FIGURE 17.2 A, Experimental setup used to study reaching in neonates. The infant is placed in an infant seat (50-degree angle) that has head support on the back and sides, but allows the arms freedom to move. B, Diagram of the outline of the infant as it touched the object, taken from single frames from the two video cameras seen in panel A. (Adapted with permission from von Hofsten C. Eye–hand coordination in the newborn. Dev Psychol 1982;18:452.)

Thus, this research suggests that some aspects of reaching, in particular the ability to locate objects in space and transport the arm, may be present in rudimentary form (prereaching behaviors) at birth, while other components, such as grasp, develop later in the first year of life. These findings suggest support for the hypothesis that at least some aspects of reaching are innate.

In the next sections, we follow the progression of the development of reaching and manipulation skills through infancy and childhood, exploring the emergence of various aspects of reaching and manipulation behaviors. We have already seen that location of an object in space is possible in the neonate and that the ability to transport the arm toward the object in a rudimentary way is also available at birth. However, as you will see, more accurate reaching and the grasp component of reaching do not develop until 4 to 5 months of age, with pincer grasp developing at 9 to 13 months. Higher cognitive aspects of reaching begin to emerge at about 1 year of age. Throughout development, there appears to be a repetitive shift between visually triggered (or proactively guided reaching) and visually guided (or feedback-controlled) reaching.

LOCATING A TARGET: EYE–HEAD COORDINATION

In order to reach for a target, the infant must first locate the target in space. If the target is moving, this requires that the infant stabilize the gaze on the moving target and move the gaze at the same speed as the image of the target. This may involve eye movements alone or eye and head movements in combination, and control of these movements involves visual, vestibular, and proprioceptive information. How do infants develop the coordination of head and eye movements for gaze control? To do this, they need to master two tasks: moving the eyes to specific targets and stabilizing gaze on the targets. This is done with saccadic eye movements (moving the eye to the target) and smooth pursuit movements (stabilizing the eye on the target) (von Hofsten, 2003; 2007).

Shifting Gaze

The control of saccadic eye movements develops before that of smooth pursuit. In fact, saccadic movements are present in the neonate. Tracking targets is done with saccadic eye movements at this age. To shift gaze, the infant needs to shift attention from the current object of fixation to a new object. This ability is also present at birth. However, as attention matures, it goes through a period in which the infant has difficulty looking away from a target (called "obligatory attention"). At about 4 months of age, infants become able to disengage attention and examine new objects at will (von Hofsten, 2003).

Tracking Object Movements

Limited smooth pursuit tracking ability is present in the neonate. Researchers have shown that neonates can follow visual objects covering a wide angle of visual space (about 16 degrees or more) moving slowly (10 degrees per second or less) with smooth eye movements, but eye movements become jerky for a small target (Aslin, 1981). Rosander and von Hofsten (2002) also observed that 1-month-old infants followed large moving vertical gratings more smoothly than small objects. But they found that when the saccades were subtracted from the recordings, the remaining smooth tracking was not different for the two targets. This suggests that the reason the pursuit of the small objects appears jerky is because the infants are making many catch-up saccades to stay with the small target, which they do not need to do for the larger target. von Hofsten (2003) proposes that this is because a wide-angle pattern of vertical stripes allows the eyes to always be on the target, however they move.

By about 6 weeks of age, smooth pursuit of objects begins to improve quickly (Shea & Aslin, 1990). In addition, 1-month-olds show a substantial lag (180 msec) in following a moving stimulus (sinusoid), which is reduced with age. By about 3 months of age, infants can keep the eyes on target most of the time, and by 5 months of age they show predictive abilities and thus are able to lead the sinusoidal motion of a target (von Hofsten, 2003; 2007; von Hofsten & Rosander, 1996, 1997).

Is head motion involved in the early use of smooth pursuit? Yes, it is present even in 1-month-olds and increases with age through at least 5 months. However, its lag is always large (250 msec). In spite of this lag, the infants are able to finely coordinate head and eye movements to track moving targets accurately. Figure 17.3 shows the eye and head tracking ability of infants of 2 to 5 months of age. Note that head involvement is not substantial until 5 months. As its involvement increases, the contribution of eye movement naturally goes down. Note that gaze, which is the combination of head and eye movements, tracks the target almost perfectly, taking into account head-movement lag, as well as the relative contribution of eye and head movements to total gaze (Rosander & von Hofsten, 2000; von Hofsten & Rosander, 1997).

von Hofsten and Rosander's results support the concept that one system is responsible for smooth tracking of large and small objects. They note that

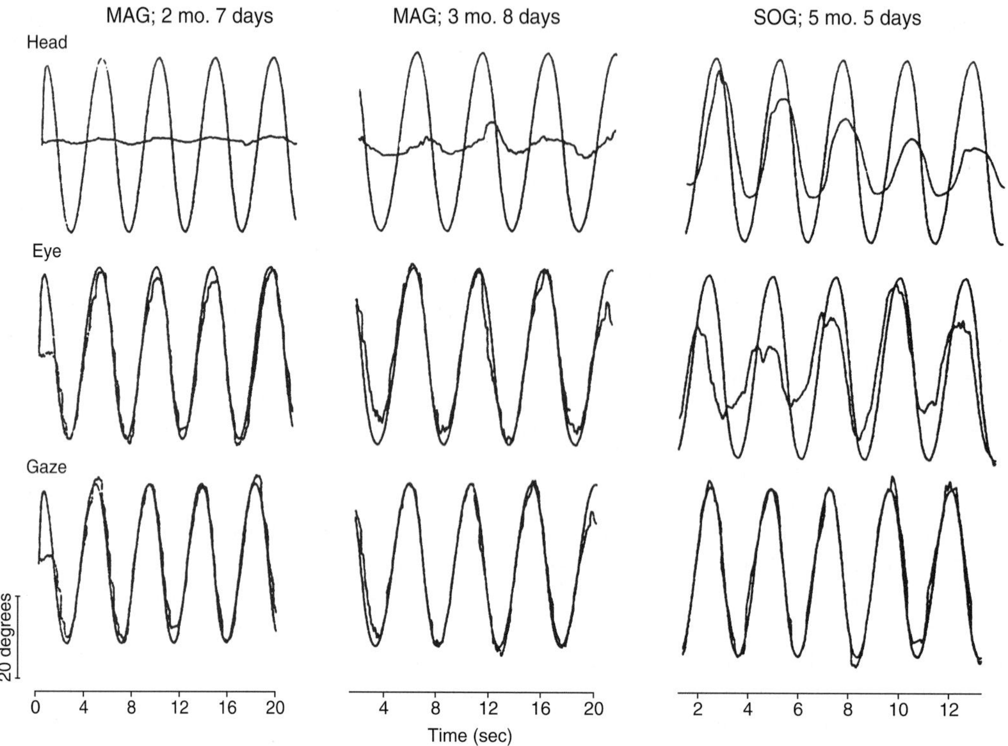

FIGURE 17.3 Examples of pursuit tracking of a sinusoidal motion by infants of 2 (left), 3 (middle) and 5 (right) months of age. Movement of the head (upper trace), eye (middle trace), and gaze (lower trace) is shown. Note that head involvement is not substantial until 5 months of age. As its involvement increases, the contribution of eye movement naturally goes down. Note that gaze, which is the combination of head and eye movements, tracks the target almost perfectly, taking into account head movement lag, as well as the relative contribution of eye and head to total gaze. MAG, SOG = codes for subjects. (Reprinted with permission from von Hofsten C, Rosander K. Development of smooth pursuit tracking in young infants. Vision Res 1997;13:1803.)

both the visual areas of MT (medial temporal cortex) and MST (medial superior temporal cortex) are involved in smooth tracking and that their function improves quickly after 6.5 weeks. Research suggests that the gain of the smooth pursuit system is set in the frontal cortex, which develops rapidly during this period. The smooth-pursuit gain improves gradually from 6.5 to 15 weeks, in agreement with this research (von Hofsten, 2003; 2007; von Hofsten & Rosander, 1997; Rosander and von Hofsten, 2002).

Development of Visual Pathways for Reaching

In Chapter 16 we discussed the Ebbinghaus illusion, in which adults typically misjudge the physical size of a central disk surrounded by smaller disks, yet open their hand aperture to its actual size and suggested that separate processing in the ventral versus the dorsal stream visual pathways for perception and action underlies this phenomenon. In a study of the development of this dissociation between perception and action, Hanisch et al. (2001) asked children between the ages of 5 and 12 years to both estimate the size of the central disk in the Ebbinghaus test and to grasp the disk. They found that when children of all ages were asked to estimate the size of the object without grasping it, they experienced the same illusion as adults. However, when asked to estimate the size and then grasp the disk, the younger (5 to 7 years) children's perceptual judgments were unreliable, although adults still showed the effect of the illusion for 80% of the trials. In addition, the younger children were more affected by the illusion created by the surround when making their grasp opening. They grasped disks of the same size with a smaller grasp opening when the disks were surrounded by smaller disks, although they perceived the central disks as being larger. The younger children also had the largest safety margin during grasping, with a larger grasp opening than required. The researchers conclude that ventral- and dorsal-stream pathways may not to be functionally segregated in early and middle childhood, with children using both of the visual processing streams during perceptual as well as visuomotor tasks.

Eye–Head–Hand Coordination Development

In Chapter 16, we mentioned that the eye, head, and hand are coordinated when adults reach, such that the eyes move first, followed by the head, and then the arm. How does eye, head, and hand coordination develop in children?

At 2 months, head–arm movements become coupled very strongly as the infant gains control over the neck muscles (von Hofsten, 1984, 1993). Over the next 2 months, there is an increased uncoupling of head and arm movements, which allows more flexibility in eye–head–hand coordination. At about 4 months, infants begin to gain trunk postural stability, so they have a more stable base for reaching movements.

A number of developmental changes thus converge at about 4 months of age, all of which are essential for the emergence of successful reaching. This supports the concept that the emergence of successful reaching is not due to the maturation of a single system, but to contributions of multiple maturing systems (Bertenthal & von Hofsten, 1998; von Hofsten, 1984, 1993).

REACH AND GRASP

Motor Components

Early Development

During the first year of life, there are a number of clear transitions in the infant's reach-and-grasp motor abilities. As mentioned earlier, rudimentary "pre-reaching" movements can be observed in infants at birth. Until about 2 months of age, whenever the infant extends the arm, the hand opens in extension at the same time, so that it is difficult to grasp an object. At about 2 months of age, the first motor transformation in reaching occurs (von Hofsten, 1984). At this age (about 7 weeks) the amount of reaching is substantially reduced and the hand becomes fisted instead of remaining open during arm extension toward the object. von Hofsten (1984) has hypothesized that the reduction in reaching at this age is due to an inhibition that is associated with the development of the corticospinal pathway; he proposed that it is not yet synchronized with the brainstem pathways, involving whole-arm extension and flexion synergies. After this short period of about 1 to 2 weeks, the proportion of fisted reaches decreases again, and the arm becomes controlled in a more functional fashion so that only when the infant fixates on an object does the hand open in preparation for intentionally grasping and manipulating the object. Thus, an intentional reach begins to emerge, with the extension synergy being broken up, so that the fingers flex as the arm extends toward the desired object (von Hofsten, 1984, 1993).

At about 4 months, infants enter a new developmental phase, involving integration of the newly developed skill of reaching. Reaches of 4-month-olds typically consist of several steps (often called "movement units"), and the final approach toward the object is crooked and awkward. In the next 2 months, the approach path straightens and the number of steps in the reach are reduced in number, with the first part of the reach getting longer and more powerful. The largest movement units in a reach move closer to the beginning of the reach with age. Studies show that at the age of 2 years, 75% of trials show a velocity profile with a single peak (von Hofsten, 1984; 1991; 1993).

More recently, researchers have performed longitudinal studies examining reaching in infants from 2 months to 3 years of age. Figure 17.4 shows examples of sagittal hand paths of one infant reaching at four different developmental times. As you see, infant reaches are curved at early ages and become much straighter by 2 to 3 years of age. This has been defined by the "straightness ratio," which is about 2 at reach onset and decreases to 1.3 to 1.4 by 2 to 3 years of age, still less straight than for adults, who have a ratio of about 1. This is accompanied by an increase in smoothness (or decrease in jerk) of the movements. In addition, maximum hand speed during the reach occurs closer to the beginning of the reach with development, being at 0.35 to 0.5 of the reach in the earliest ages and moving to 0.2 to 0.4 of the reach by 2 to 3 years of age. However, average reaching speed does not increase during this time period.

Laboratories have begun to use a dynamic systems approach to exploring the development of reaching. In one set of studies, the transition to the development of reaching was explored in infants from the age of 3 weeks through 1 year (Thelen et al., 1993, 1996). Thelen and colleagues noted that the four infants studied entered the transition to reaching at different ages and with different activity levels and preferred movement patterns. They suggest that the process of learning to reach is one of discovering the match between intrinsic dynamics (the opportunities and constraints of their bodies) and their intention to bring the hand (using proprioceptive and/or visual cues) to the toy (using visual cues). They believe that the infants chose the patterns for executing a reach in a flexible way, in relation to their dynamic resources and the demands of the task, rather than from a preexisting motor program.

For example, at the time of reach onset, each infant had characteristic intrinsic dynamics, including preferred postures, movements, and energy levels. They noted that two of the infants had higher energy levels and energized their muscles with large coactive phasic bursts, often rhythmically. Movements looked like

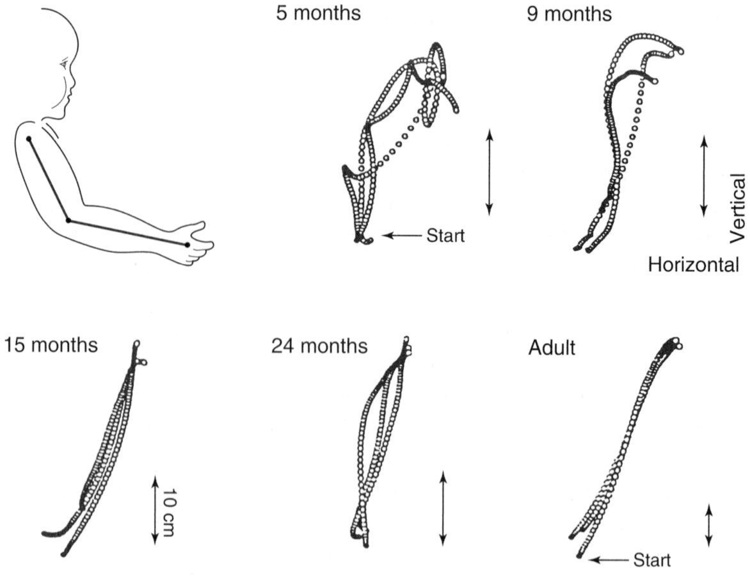

FIGURE 17.4 Example of hand paths used by one infant at four different ages, recorded in the sagittal plane. Three different reaches are shown for each age. Note the progression toward the smoothing of the end-point motion. The time interval between successive points is 10 msec. (Reprinted with permission from Konczak J, Dichgans J. The development toward stereotypic arm kinematics during reaching in the first 3 years of life. Exp Brain Res 1997; 117:348.)

bilateral flapping (described as similar to limit cycle oscillators). When they reached for the toy, they converted these oscillations into a task-specific movement (described as a point attractor), by damping down their oscillations and stiffening the arm with coactivation of the muscles.

The second two infants were quieter and thus needed to lift their arms against gravity and move them forward. These movements were slow and sustained, with limbs relatively compliant, and without perturbations from motion-dependent forces from connected segments. The authors conclude that smooth trajectories and coupling of joints were a byproduct of particular levels of force and arm stiffness or compliance (Thelen et al., 1993).

They also noted that infants acquired stable head control several weeks before reaching onset. Reaching onset involved a reorganization of muscle patterns in trapezius and deltoid muscles, serving to stabilize the head and shoulders and provide a stable base for reaching (Thelen & Spencer, 1998).

The authors state that their results support mass-spring (or equilibrium-point) models of motor control in which the trajectory of the hand, joint angles, and muscle patterns are not explicitly planned in advance. Instead, the central nervous system (CNS) sets up new spring constants for the muscles at the involved joints that bring the joint to the desired position (Hogan et al., 1987).

Additional research by Konczak and colleagues (1995, 1997), studying nine infants longitudinally from 4 to 15 months of age, has shown that there are two developmental phases in hand-trajectory formation: a first phase between 16 and 24 weeks involved rapid improvements, including reductions in movement time and number of movement units. This was followed by a second phase (28 to 64 weeks) involving fine-tuning of the sensorimotor system, in which there were more gradual changes in end-point kinematics. They noted that early reaching was not limited by lack of ability to generate adequate levels of muscle torques. This suggests that, as for postural and locomotion development, muscle strength is not the limiting factor for the onset of reaching. However, there were significant increases in their production of muscle flexor torque with time, with early reachers using a combination of flexion and extension torque, and mature reachers using only adult-like flexor torques. These mature reachers, like adults, thus took advantage of motion-dependent and gravitational forces to extend the arm.

In addition, relative timing of muscle- and motion-dependent torque peaks showed a systematic development toward adult profiles with increasing age. They suggested that control problems of proximal joint torque generation could account for the segmented hand paths seen in early reaching. They concluded that the development of stable patterns of interjoint coordination does not occur simply by regulating torque amplitude, but also by modulating the correct timing of force production and by the system's use of reactive forces (Konczak et al., 1995, 1997). Like Thelen and colleagues, they also noted variability in the longitudinal profiles of each infant, indicating that each child followed his or her own strategy to explore the internal and external forces that are the basis of coordinated movements.

In a longitudinal study of reaching development in 12 infants during varying periods from reaching onset to 20 months of age, Berthier & Keen (2006) found a gradual slowing of reach speed and a more rapid reduction in movement jerk with development (probably similar to the second phase of reaching development described by Konczak and colleagues, 1997 [see above]). Infants first learning to reach primarily used the shoulder muscles to extend the hand to the target. The use of the elbow gradually increased after the onset of reaching and reached a plateau at about 6 months of age. The increase in use of the elbow coincides with the rapid or active phase of learning, observed by Konczak et al. (1995) and Thelen et al. (1996). These developmental changes in reaching support Bernstein's (1967) hypothesis that early in skill development there is a fixing of the degrees of freedom of a limb, with a gradual release of these degrees of freedom with skill acquisition (Berthier & Keen, 2006; Konczak & Dichgans, 1997; Thelen et al., 1996). Thus, there are probably a number of developmental changes that contribute to this improvement, including development of trunk postural control.

Early reaches are often bimanual, with both mirror movements and nondifferentiated movements of both limbs being typical of the infant's early reaching behavior. By 6 months of age, unilateral reaching begins to dominate. It has been suggested that the early mirror movements could be due to crossed corticospinal projections from the right and left hemispheres, which are reduced during development (Gordon, 2001).

Researchers believe that the development of the cortiocospinal tract contributes to the emergence of independent finger movements. However, it is also possible that the maturation of the tract depends on the use of the hands and fingers. In fact, animal studies have shown that the formation of normal patterns of corticospinal tract development depends on neural activity in the sensorimotor cortex in early postnatal development and that blocking this activity results in the inability to create normal reaching movements (Martin, 1999; 2000). This suggests that there may be an early critical period for the development of reaching, in which practice in manipulative activity shapes the development of corticospinal circuits (Gordon, 2001).

von Hofsten (2007) emphasizes this issue in noting that the neural starting point of development in the neonate is not a set of reflexes that are triggered by sensory stimuli but a set of action systems activated by the infant. This creates a dynamic system in which the development of the nervous system and the development of action each influence the other through activity and the infant's experience. He notes that infants have a number of endogenous skills present at birth, including visually controlling their arms in space, and that these skills give activity-dependent input to the sensorimotor and cognitive systems. This allows the infant to explore the relationship between commands and movements and between the different sensory modalities (vision, somatosensation, etc.) and to discover all the possibilities of their actions and the ways their actions are constrained by the environment. We must remember that a key driving force for all these actions is exploration and social interaction.

Clinical implications for this research are that it is important to work with children with developmental disabilities to allow them active exploration of their environment as well as to initiate social interactions with others. These are key factors in habilitation of the nervous system.

Development in Childhood

A study by Schneiberg et al. (2002) further examined the development of coordination during reaching in children from 4 to 11 years of age. They asked children to reach from the seated position with the dominant arm and to grasp a cone placed in front of them. Kinematic data from markers placed on the arm, head, and trunk showed that younger children used immature patterns of reaching, characterized by increased variability. With increasing age, hand trajectories became smoother and less variable while interjoint coordination became more consistent. Finally, trunk displacement and variability also decreased with age. By 8 to 10 years of age children showed variability similar to that in adults.

A second study (Kuhtz-Buschbeck et al., 1998) examined the kinematics and coordination of reaching and grasping for a cylindrical target in children 4 to 12 years of age. Across this age range, movement duration and normalized peak spatial velocity of the reaching hand did not change significantly. However, the authors found that the hand path became straighter and the coordination between hand path and grip formation improved, creating smooth predictable kinematic trajectories at the age of 12 years. They noted that younger children opened their grip relatively wider than older children, using a higher safety margin. In addition, the children showed a decrease in the use of visual control with development. Thus, only the oldest children were able to scale the grip opening appropriately to object size, when vision of the object was not available during the reach. The authors concluded that the development of control of manipulation skills continues through about 10 to 12 years of age.

Development of Force Adaptation during Reaching

In order to be able to reach accurately in many different contexts, children need to learn to adapt the forces used during reaching to task and environmental demands. It has been hypothesized that humans learn to make reaching movements in a variety of contexts by creating an internal motor model of their limb dynamics. In order to determine the gradual time course of development of inverse dynamics models for reaching in children, Konczak et al. (2003) examined the movement characteristics of children (4 to 11 years of age) as they adapted to changes in arm dynamics.

The children were asked to make goal-directed forearm movements while different external damping forces were applied. The researchers found that all children showed after-effects from the previous condition in response to changes in damping, which suggests that their neural control systems did not rapidly adapt to changes in damping forces. However, they found that with increasing age there was a reduction in the number of trials required for adaptation, although it did not reach adult levels by 11 years of age. The youngest children showed the most difficulty compensating for damping forces, with the path of the forearm most perturbed and most variable when making reaches under these conditions. These findings suggest that the neural representations of limb dynamics are less precise and less stable in young children. The researchers propose that this instability might be a cause of the high kinematic variability seen in children during many motor tasks.

Sensory Components

Visually Triggered versus Visually Guided Reaching

Early Development. Remember from Chapter 16 that reaching movements in adults have two different phases: the transport phase and the grasp phase. It has been hypothesized that the beginning of the reach is visually triggered—that is, visual location of the target is used to initiate the movement. Thus, the position of the object is defined visually, while the position of the arm is defined proprioceptively. In contrast, the last part of the reach is considered visually guided. In this case, the position of the arm is defined visually with reference to the target, allowing precise adjustments to be made to ensure the accuracy of the reach (Paillard, 1982).

Newborns seem able to use the visually triggered mode reasonably well, since they are able to initiate a reach aimed toward the target (von Hofsten, 1982). However, they do not appear to be proficient in the visually guided mode, since they are still very inaccurate in their reaches. Visually guided reaching requires the ability to attend to the hand as it moves toward the object, as well as the ability to attend to the object. It also requires the ability to anticipate possible errors.

Research indicates that the visually guided mode of reaching emerges between the fourth and the fifth month of life, just as trunk control and arm coordination are also improving (McDonnell, 1979; von Hofsten, 1984).

In order to study the development of visually guided reaching in infants, researchers have fitted infants with special glasses with prism lenses to give an apparent lateral shift in the target position as the infants reached for small toys (McDonnell, 1979). By 5 1/2 months of age, when the infant's hand comes into view, he or she is able to perceive the discrepancy between hand position and target position and correct the trajectory. This suggests that by 5 1/2 months, visually guided reaching is evident in most infants.

Visually guided reaching, or the ability to make corrections to a trajectory based on visual information, peaks at around 7 months of age, and then is gradually replaced by a ballistic style of reaching, although infants can still use visual guidance when needed. In a ballistic style of reaching, corrections are made at the end of the movement instead of during the ongoing movement. Once the movement is completed, the error between hand position and target position is used to correct the position of the hand in space.

Development in Childhood. To determine whether there are continued developmental changes in children's use of visual feedback in making reaching movements, studies were performed in which children from 4 to 11 years of age were asked to make movements with or without visual feedback. Hay (1978) has shown that there are interesting changes in the use of visual information by children between 4 and 11 years of age. Children between 4 and 6 years of age can make movements without visual feedback with reasonable accuracy, as shown in Figure 17.5. (Note that, although 5-year-olds may appear to be more accurate than adults, there are no significant differences between these groups.) However, at age 7, there is an abrupt reduction in this ability, as seen in the increased errors made in reaching without visual feedback. The accuracy then begins to increase again, reaching adult levels by 10 to 11 years of age. As we describe in the next section, this reduction in accuracy is reflected in an increased dependence on visual feedback at the age of 7 years. This is one piece of research to support the hypothesis that the age of 7 is a transition time in the development of reaching (Dellen & Kalverboer, 1984; Hay, 1990).

Other studies analyzing the kinematics of reaching movements without visual feedback in children ages 5 to 11 also support this hypothesis. Figure 17.6 shows that 5-year-olds produce mainly ballistic movements, with sharp decelerations at the end of the movement (1—dark bars), while this pattern shows a sharp decrease at age 7. At this age, a ramp-and-step

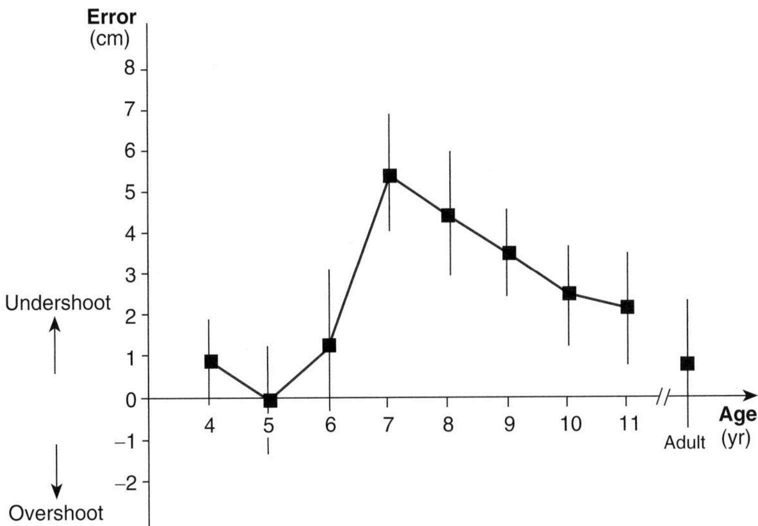

FIGURE 17.5 Graph showing pointing errors when visual feedback was not present for children from 4 to 11 years of age, as compared with adults. Note that large errors appear at 7 years of age, indicating reliance on visual feedback for reaching. These gradually are reduced in subsequent years, as children restrict feedback to the homing-in phase of the reach. (Adapted with permission from Hay L. Developmental changes in eye–hand coordination behaviors: preprogramming versus feedback control. In: Bard C, Fleury M, Hay L, eds. Development of eye–hand coordination across the lifespan. Columbia: University of South Carolina Press, 1990:228.)

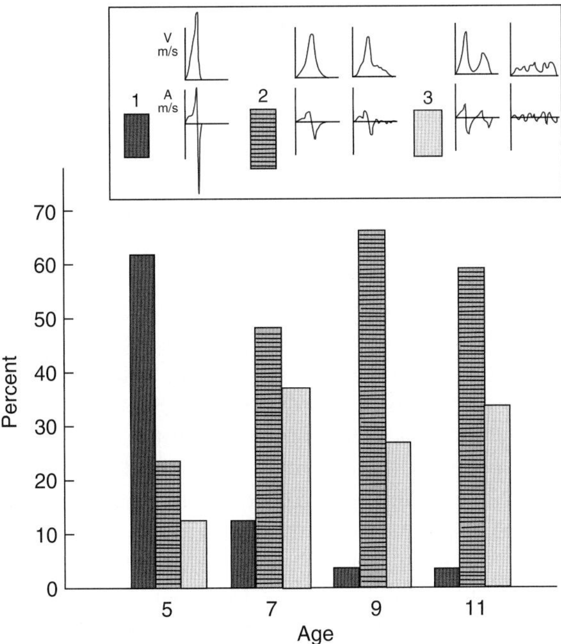

FIGURE 17.6 Percentage of time three different reaching movement patterns were seen in children from 5 to 11 years of age. 1 = ballistic pattern with sharp accelerations/decelerations; 2 = ballistic patterns with smooth decelerations; 3 = step-and-ramp patterns. Note that the 5-year-olds used the highest levels of ballistic patterns, while the 7-year-olds used high levels of step-and-ramp patterns, indicating increased reliance on vision. Children 9 to 11 years old used the highest levels of ballistic patterns, with smooth decelerations, indicating primary use of visual feedback at the end of the movement. V = velocity; A = acceleration. (Adapted with permission from Hay L. Developmental changes in eye–hand coordination behaviors: preprogramming versus feedback control. In: Bard C, Fleury M, Hay L, eds. Development of eye–hand coordination across the lifespan. Columbia: University of South Carolina Press, 1990:231.)

movement pattern increases (3—light bars). At the same time, ballistic patterns with a smooth deceleration at the end of the movement increase and continue to increase through 9 years of age (2—striped bars). It has been hypothesized that this could be due to the increased use of proprioceptive feedback control in 7-year-olds and the progressive restriction of feedback control to the final homing-in phase in older children, possibly the result of increased efficiency of the movement braking system (Hay, 1979).

For a closer look at developmental changes in the use of visual feedback in reaching movements in children, experiments were performed in which children ages 5 to 11 were asked to make reaches while wearing prismatic lenses, which make an illusory shift in the image of the object. These experiments are similar to those described earlier, examining the use of visual feedback in reaching in neonates and infants. As shown in the upper part of Figure 17.7, as the children make a reach, the kinematics of the hand movement show a curved, rather than a straight-line trajectory toward the object. This occurs as the hand shifts from an initially incorrect path, due to the shift in the visual image caused by the prismatic lenses, to a correct path when the hand comes into view, based on visual information of the relative hand and target positions. The length of the visually corrected path indicates the amount of visual feedback used in the movement (Hay, 1979).

As evident in the bottom half of Figure 17.7, 5-year-old children corrected the movement late in its trajectory, and in fact, the majority of these children did not make a correction until they reached the virtual target, indicating minimal use of visual feedback. Thus, in this age group, visual control occurs mainly after, rather than during, reaching movements. This

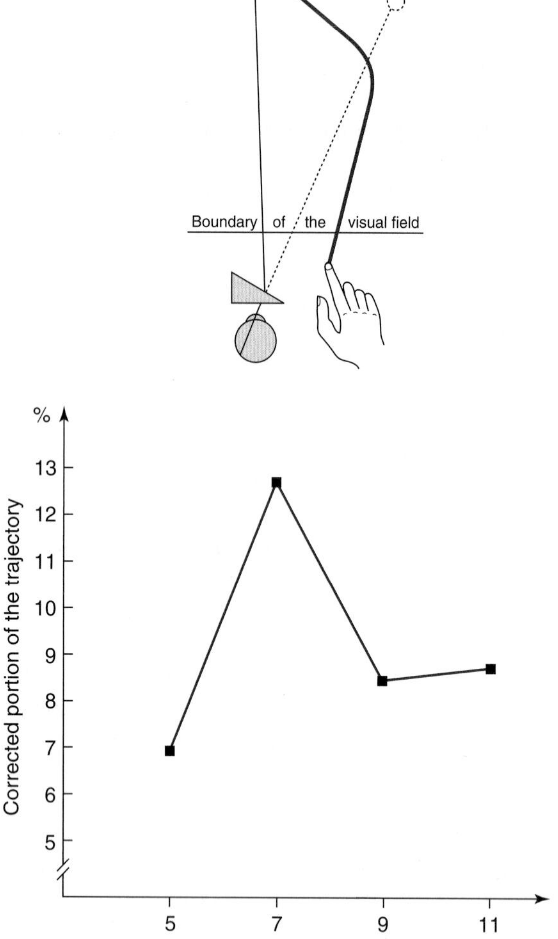

FIGURE 17.7 Top, Diagram of reaching movements of children who wore prismatic lenses, displacing the apparent position of the target in the visual field. Bottom, Corrected portion of the reaching trajectory for 5-, 7-, 9-, and 11-year-olds. Note that 7-year-olds correct the reaching movement much earlier than the other age groups, indicating increased use of visual feedback. (Adapted from Hay L. Spatial-temporal analysis of movements in children: motor programs versus feedback in the development of reaching. J Mot Behav 1979;11:196, 198.)

is correlated with highly stereotyped movement times seen in this age group.

The 7-year-old children corrected the movements earlier than any other group, indicating a strong use of visual feedback. While this gives rise to an increased flexibility in reaching behavior, it is coupled with increased variability in movement times and decreased accuracy when visual feedback is not present.

The 9- and 11-year-olds showed an intermediate level of trajectory correction, indicating a shift in the use of visual control toward the final phase of the movement trajectory. Thus, between 5 and 9 years of age there appears to be a reorganization in the programming of reaching movements from mainly feedforward or anticipatory activation of reaching, to predominantly feedback control, and finally to an integration of the feedforward and feedback control, resulting in fast, accurate movements by 9 years of age.

Grasp Development

Emergence of Hand Orientation

In the neonatal period, infants show reflexive grasping patterns. What transitional changes occur as these patterns are transformed into effective grasping patterns? In order to answer this question, researchers made video recordings of the spontaneous hand and finger movements made by infants during their first 5 months. They found that during this period, spontaneous hand and digit movements gradually changed from the predominant occurrence of fist postures to nearly continuous random movements and finally to self-directed grasping movements. They noted that voluntary grasp movements can be observed at about 2 to 3 months of age (Wallace & Whishaw, 2003).

Reseachers found four grasping patterns during the first 5 months of life, defined as fists, pre-precision grasps associated with numerous digit postures, precision grips including the pincer grasp, and self-directed grasps. They proposed that the wide range of independent digit movements and grasp patterns during this time suggests that some direct connections of the pyramidal tract may be functional relatively early in infancy. They also suggest that "hand babbling," defined as first random and then self-directed movements, is part of the preparatory process for the emergence of accurate reaching (Wallace & Whishaw, 2003).

When do infants first begin to orient their hands to the position and shape of the object? To answer this question, researchers placed brightly colored rods either horizontally or vertically in front of the infant and recorded the characteristics of their reaching movements, as shown Figure 17.8. Preparatory adjustments of hand orientation (vertical vs. horizontal, depending on object orientation) occurred when infants first began to grasp objects, as early as 4 1/2 to 5 months of age (von Hofsten & Fazel-Zandy, 1984). However, the adjustments of the hand to the orientation of the object became more precise with age. Adjustments of the hand were often done before or

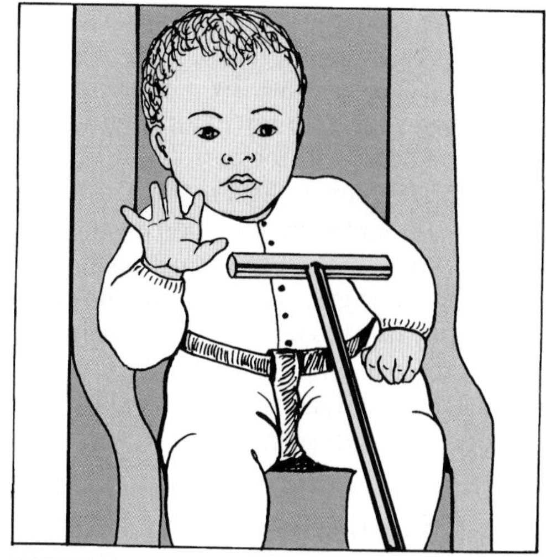

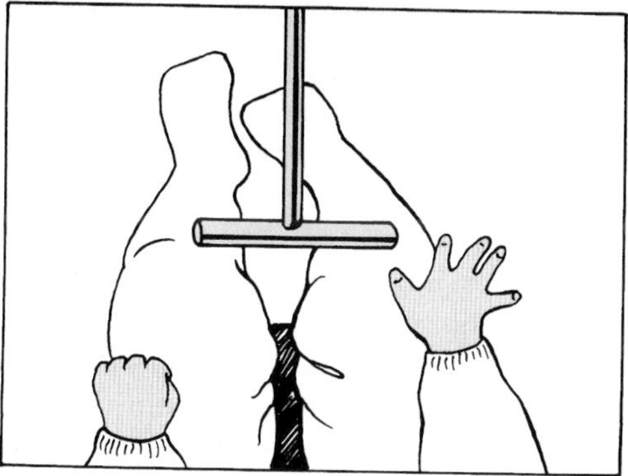

FIGURE 17.8 Two video camera views of an infant reaching for a horizontally oriented bar. Note that the infant uses correct hand orientation for grasping the bar. (Adapted from von Hofsten C, Fazel-Zandy S. Development of visually guided hand orientation in reaching. J Exp Child Psychol 1984;38:210.)

during the early part of the reach, although they could also be seen during the approach phase. Infants are also able to use predictive control to reach for a rotating rod; they prepare to grasp it by creating a hand orientation that is aligned with the future orientation of the rod (von Hofsten, 2007).

To reach smoothly for an object, the infant must time the grasp appropriately with relation to encountering the object. If the hand closes too late, the object will bounce off the palm, and if the hand closes too early, the object will hit the knuckles. This type of planning requires visual control, since tactile control would not allow the hand to close until after touching the object (von Hofsten & Fazel-Zandy, 1984).

In experiments in which the kinematics of reaching in 5-, 6-, 9-, and 13-month-olds were compared with those of adults, it was shown that infant grasping was visually controlled as early as 5 to 6 months of age, with the hand starting to close in anticipation of reaching the object. Also, the opening of the hand was related to the size of the object for the 9- and 13-month-olds, but not in the younger group. Finally, the 13-month-olds initiated the grasp farther away from the target than the younger groups, with timing of the grasp similar to that seen in adults. The grasp component of the reach is still not mature in 13-month-olds, however, since, unlike adults, they do not yet correlate the onset of closing of the hand with the size of the object to be grasped (von Hofsten & Ronnqvist, 1988).

Development of the Pincer Grasp

There are two different ways that objects can be grasped—in a power grip, using the palm and palmar surface of the fingers, with the thumb reinforcing this grip, or in a precision grip, between the terminal pads of the finger and the thumb. The precision grip requires that the fingers be moved independently, and is a prerequisite for accurate and skilled movement of objects (Forssberg et al., 1991; Napier, 1956).

In the first months after birth, infant grasping movements are controlled by tactile and proprioceptive reflexes. Thus, when an object contacts the palm, the fingers close. Also, when the arm flexes, the hand closes, as part of a flexor synergy. At about 4 months of age, with the onset of functional reaching, the infant uses the palmer grasp exclusively. With subsequent development, first the thumb and then the fingers begin to operate independently, and at about 10 months of age, pincer grasp (with opposition of the thumb) develops (Forssberg et al., 1991).

Developmental changes related to reaching and grasping skills correlate well with research performed on the anatomic development of the primate motor system. In primates, it has been shown that neural pathways controlling movements of the arm are different from those that control the fine movements of the fingers and hand. The two systems develop at different times. Arm control, which appears to be coordinated mainly at the brainstem level, develops earlier than hand and finger control, which appears to be coordinated at the cortical level (Kuypers, 1962, 1964).

Researchers found that infant monkeys show arm movements toward objects early in development, but do not show independent finger and hand movements until they are 3 months old (Lawrence & Hopkins, 1972). It has also been shown that at about 9 to 13 months of age, with the development of the pyramidal tract, infants are able to control fractionated finger movements and thus develop more difficult grasping skills such as the pincer grasp (von Hofsten, 1984, 2007).

Experiments have followed the development and refinement of precision grasp in human infants and children ranging in age from 8 months to 15 years. Remember from Chapter 16 that when an adult is asked to lift an object, as soon as his or her fingers touch the object, cutaneous receptors activate a centrally programmed response that consists of an increase in grip forces and load forces, designed to lift the object without letting it slip through the fingers. In adults, these two forces are always programmed in parallel, to prevent slips and to avoid squeezing the object too hard (Forssberg et al., 1991).

This parallel programming of grip and load forces was not found in human infants. In fact, until 5 years of age, the children pushed the object into the table as they increased the grip force, showing a reversed coordination between the two forces. In these children, the grip force had to be very high before the load force increase occurred. In addition, the timing and sequencing of the different phases of lifting were much longer in the infants. For example, the time between first and second finger contact was three times as long in 10-month-olds and two times as long in children up to 3 years of age, as compared with adults. It was common in the younger children to have several touches by the thumb and index finger before the object was properly gripped. Also, any finger could be the first to contact the object (Forssberg et al., 1991).

In a similar study (Pare & Dugas, 1999), distinct developmental milestones were found for the maturation of precision grip from 2 to 9 years of age. For the grasps of 2-year-old children, the peak vertical acceleration of the object during lifting was negatively correlated with peak grip force. By 3 years of age, peak acceleration and peak grip force during lifting became positively correlated, and the correlation continued to strengthen up to 9 years of age. By 4 years of age, children controlled both the acceleration and deceleration of the lifting movement in a symmetrical pattern and used a single burst of grip force to grasp the object, suggesting that they had begun to use an anticipatory control strategy for grasping. To explore for yourself the ages at which children refine control in the grasping of different types of objects complete Lab Activity 17.1.

When Do Children Start Using Anticipatory Control in Grasping and Lifting Objects?

In the study by Pare & Dugas (1999), it was noted that children younger than 2 years of age did not increase grip and load forces in parallel, but used a sequential force activation with grip force increases occurring prior to load force increases. They also showed force increases in steps, indicating a feedback strategy, since the forces were not scaled in one force rate pulse. In a second study, Forssberg and colleagues (1992) further examined the development of this anticipatory control of precision grip, exploring how weight from the previous lift is used to scale current forces. They found that anticipatory control of isometric force output

LAB ACTIVITY 17-1

Objective: To examine how properties of the task affect reach-and-grasp movements in children of different ages.

Procedures: For this lab, you will find one child from at least two of the following age groups—8–12 mo, 12–18 mo, 2–3 yr, and 4–6 yr—in your community and observe them performing the following tasks. Bring with you when you work with the children the following items (you can vary the size of the items so they are appropriate to the size of the child): two small plastic glasses (one with water in it and one without), a small block (small square shape), a crayon (something long and narrow), and a second small plastic glass or cylinder that you have coated with oil. In the first part of the lab, observe the arm and hand movements of the children while they pick up the empty plastic glass, block, crayon, plastic glass with water, and plastic glass coated with oil. For the older children, place the two cups (one with water and one without) next to each other. Ask the child to pour you a cup of water. Then try it again, but invert the empty glass and place it near the glass with water.

Assignment:

1. Describe how the children of the different age groups reached for and grasped the various objects.
2. When during the reach for an object did the hand begin to shape in preparation for grasp? How did characteristics of the object affect anticipatory hand shaping?
3. For the older children, how did changing the orientation of the glass affect hand orientation? Were they able to modify the orientation of the hand so they did not have to pour the water in multiple steps?
4. Compare the data from the children to your own or other adult reach/grasp characteristics from Lab Activity 16.1. Do your results agree with those of von Hofsten and Forssberg et al., on developmental changes in anticipatory hand shaping and in lifting objects?

during lifts with precision grip emerges during the second year. The youngest children, those younger than 18 months of age, showed no or very small differences in force rates for lifts using different weights, while children older than 18 months showed this ability. This anticipatory control develops gradually, with large changes occurring between 1 and 4 years of age and more gradual changes occurring from 4 to 11 years, with adult levels being reached at about 11 years of age.

Forssberg and colleagues (1995) also noted that the younger children used a high grip-to-load-force ratio, particularly in trials with nonslippery objects (sandpaper). This showed their use of a large safety margin against slips, indicating an immature capacity to adapt to the frictional condition. The safety margin decreased during the first 5 years of life, along with a lower variability in the grip force and a better adaptation to the current condition.

They found that by 18 months of age children could adapt grip forces to a surface condition when the same surface was presented in blocks of trials, but failed when the surface was unexpectedly changed. They suggest that this may indicate a poor capacity to form a sensorimotor memory representation of the friction. These memory abilities increased gradually with age, with older children requiring only a few lifts and adults only one lift to update their force coordination to a new surface friction.

Adaptation of Grip Forces

One aspect of adaptation of grasping is the ability to increase or decrease grip forces smoothly within a single trial—for example, if an object begins to slip during lifting. In order to study the development of grip-force adaptation, Blank et al. (2000) asked children from 3 to 6 years of age to use visual feedback to increase or decrease isometric forces on a small cylindrical sensor using a pinch grip. There were clear developmental changes in the precision of force tracking. For children up to 4 years of age, there was a tendency to overshoot the target force change by "jumping and waiting." The older children overshot the target only when there was a slow target force decrease. In contrast, adults used small amounts of undershooting as they followed the target change in all conditions, suggesting that they used a continuous "following" strategy. These results suggest that there is a developmental strategy change for the adaptation of grip forces from a feedforward strategy with intermittent use of sensorimotor feedback toward parallel and integrated feedback and feedforward processing, with a critical transition period at 5 to 6 years of age.

Learning to Grasp Moving Objects (Catching)

Studies have also been performed to determine the emergence of the ability of infants to reach for and grasp a moving object; this could be considered a rudimentary form of catching behavior. Researchers have shown that by the time infants could reach successfully for nonmoving objects, they were also successful at reaching for moving objects. Infants as young as 18 weeks could catch objects moving at 30 cm/sec. Fifteen-week-olds could intercept the object, but were not yet able to grasp it. These results suggest that infants are able to predict where the object will be at a future point in time because they must start reaching early to intercept it in its path. It was noted that the infants did not automatically reach toward every object that passed by. Rather, they seemed to be able to detect in advance whether they had a reasonable chance to reach it (von Hofsten & Lindhagen, 1979).

Cognitive Components: Emergence of Object Exploration

When do infants first begin to change their manipulative activities in relation to the characteristics of the objects grasped? During the first year, the actions infants perform with objects tend to be mouthing, waving, shaking, or banging. Rigid objects tend to be banged, while spongy objects are squeezed or rubbed (Gibson & Walker, 1984). In studies on 6-, 9-, and 12-month-olds, it was noted that mouthing activity decreased with age and that object rotation, transferring the object between hands and looking at and fingering the object, increased (Corbetta & Mounoud, 1990; Ruff, 1984).

At about 1 year of age, infants begin to acquire the understanding of how to use objects, but even before this age, they can discover simple functional relationships if these require little precision. Thus, an infant first uses a spoon for banging or shaking before using it for eating. The infant establishes the relationships between spoon and hand, spoon and mouth, and spoon and plate as subroutines before putting them together for the act of eating, in which the spoon is filled at the plate and transported to the mouth with an anticipatory opening of the mouth (Connolly, 1979).

If infants are given a spoon to grasp when they are young (in the first year) they tend to ignore the handle orientation and grasp it with the preferred hand even if this creates an awkward grasp. However, in their second year they begin to understand the task and grasp the handle of the spoon with the approprate hand using an efficeint grip (McCarty et al., 1999).

At about 14 to 16 months of age, the infant develops the ability to adapt reaching to the weight of objects, using shape and size as indicators of weight (Corbetta & Mounoud, 1990). At about 16 to 19 months of age, infants begin to understand that certain objects go together culturally, such as a cup in a saucer. Finally, at the end of the second year, they begin to perform symbolic actions like pretending to eat or drink (Corbetta & Mounoud, 1990).

After 1 year of age, infants begin to develop skills requiring more precision of movement and closer relationships between objects, such as fitting one object into another. At 13 to 15 months, infants begin piling two cubes on top of each other; at 18 months, three cubes; at 21 months, five cubes; and at 23 to 24 months, six cubes. This shows that the infant is gradually developing coordinated reaching and manipulation, so that objects can be placed and released carefully (Bayley, 1969; Corbetta & Mounoud, 1990). One of the most complex hand skills—in-hand manipulation of objects—develops over a number of years. This allows the development of activities of daily living such as eating, handwriting, buttoning clothes, and brushing the teeth (Gordon, 2001).

A study to examine the onset of manipulation abilities encouraged infants to insert elongated objects of various shapes into snuggly fitting holes. Infants who were younger than 18 months understood the task, tried hard, but had little concept of how to do it. They simply pressed the object against the hole without regard to orientation. Children who were 22 months old, however, systematically raised the horizontally placed objects when transporting them to the hole, and the 26-month-old children turned the objects before arriving at the hole, so that they were oriented appropriately. The authors state that a pure feedback strategy (used by the 18-month-olds) would not work for this task and that infants needed to acquire and master a variety of skills, including motor competence, perception of the spatial relationship between the object and the hole it fit into, and mental rotation of the object (Örnkloo & von Hofsten, 2006; von Hofsten, 2007).

THE ROLE OF EXPERIENCE IN THE DEVELOPMENT OF EYE–HAND COORDINATION

Remember that in humans, reaching behavior has two aspects, a visually triggered portion and a visually guided portion. These two aspects of eye–limb coordination are also found in cats. Elegant studies on the development of these two aspects of eye–limb coordination have shown that movement-produced visual feedback experience is essential for the visually guided portion to develop (Hein & Held, 1967).

In these experiments, kittens were raised in the dark until 4 weeks of age and then allowed to move freely for 6 hours each day in a normal environment. But during this time, they wore lightweight opaque collars that kept them from seeing their limbs and torso. This is shown in Figure 17.9A. For the rest of the day, they remained in the dark. After 12 days of this treatment, the animals were tested for the presence of visually triggered versus visually guided placing reactions. This was accomplished by lowering the kitten toward a continuous surface (requires only visually triggered placing, since accuracy is not required) versus a discontinuous surface, made up of prongs (requires visually guided placing to hit the prong). All animals showed a visually triggered placing reaction, in which they automatically extended the forelimb toward a continuous surface. But they showed no greater than chance hits for a placing reaction to a pronged surface (Fig. 17.9B). However, after removal

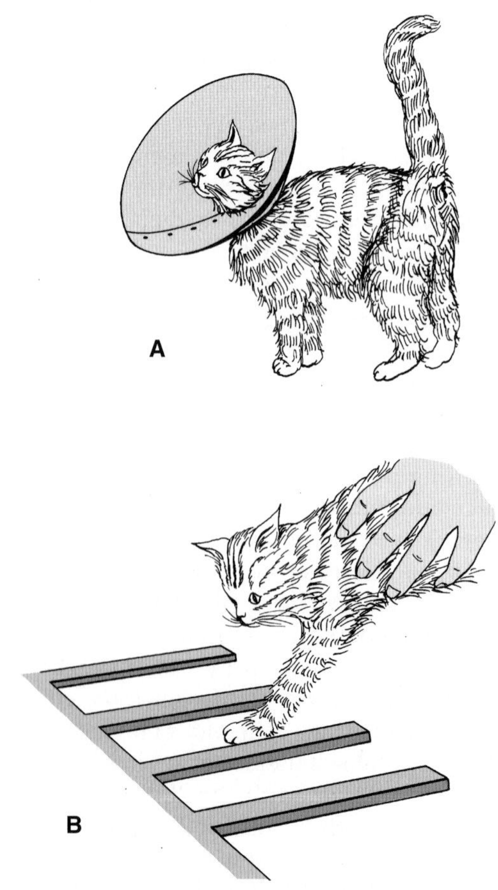

FIGURE 17.9 A, Experimental collar worn by kittens to block the view of their paws during early development. B, Pronged apparatus for testing visually guided reaching. (Adapted with permission from Hein A, Held R. Dissociation of the visual placing response into elicited and guided components. Science 1967;158:391.)

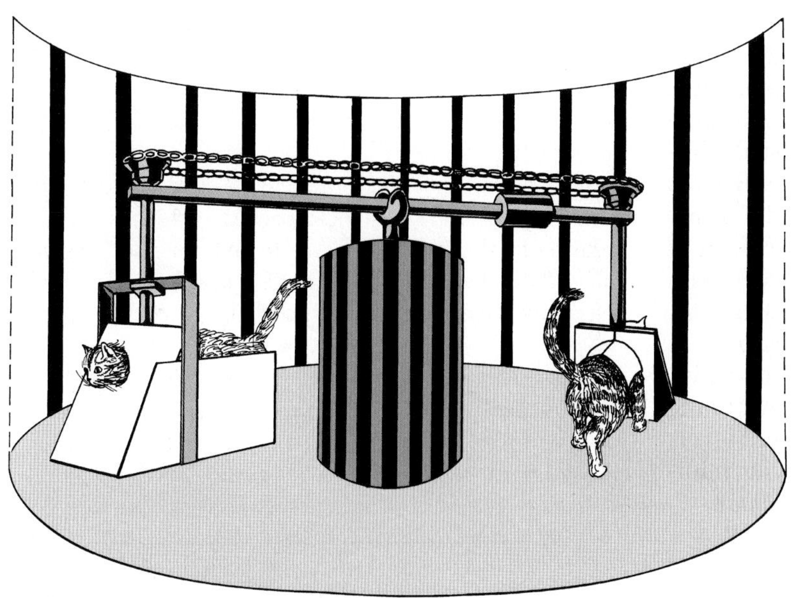

FIGURE 17.10 Experimental apparatus in which one cat actively pulls a second cat, which is passively pulled in the gondola. (Adapted from Held R, Hein A. Movement-produced stimulation in the development of visually guided behavior. J Comp Physiol Psychol 1963;56:873.)

of the collar, the animals required only 18 hours in a normal environment before showing visually guided placing. It was thus concluded that visually triggered paw extension develops without sight, but visually guided paw placing requires prolonged viewing of the limbs (Hein & Held, 1967).

The researchers then asked: What kind of contact with the environment is important for visually guided behavior? Is passive contact sufficient, or must it be active? To answer this question, they tested 10 pairs of kittens. One kitten of each pair was able to walk freely in a circular room, pulling a gondola, and the other kitten was placed in the gondola and was passively pulled around the room. This is shown in Figure 17.10. Thus, both kittens had similar visual feedback and motion cues, but for the kittens who walked, the cues were active, and for the kittens who rode, they were passive.

The kittens had experience with the apparatus for 3 hours a day. At the end of the experiment, the active animals showed normal visually guided placing reactions and responses to a visual cliff test (in which a normal animal does not walk out over an illusory cliff) but the passive animals did not. Thus, the researchers concluded that self-produced movement is necessary for the development of visually guided behavior. However, once again, after 48 hours in a normal environment, the passive group of animals showed normal visually guided paw placement (Held & Hein, 1963).

REACTION-TIME REACHING TASKS

A great deal of research has been performed on developmental changes in reaction-time (RT) tasks. In general, it has been shown that for simple RT tasks, reaction times become faster as children mature. The greatest changes occur until about 8 to 9 years of age, with slower changes occurring subsequently, until reaction times reach adult levels at 16 to 17 years. However, when children are asked to perform more complex movements as part of the RT task, these developmental changes vary according to the task. For example, in a study in which 2- to 8-year-old children were asked to make target-aiming movements, a decrease in RT was observed from 2 to 5 years of age, followed by a stabilization in RT (Brown et al., 1986; Favilla, 2005; Hay, 1990).

Movement time in most RT tasks also changes as a function of age. Remember from Chapter 16 that movement time depends on the accuracy and distance requirements of a task. Strategies for programming movements also vary, depending on whether the movement requires an accurate stop. If an accurate stop is required, the individual must use a braking action controlled by antagonist muscles. Alternatively, if the movement can be stopped automatically by hitting a target, antagonist muscle activation is not required.

Studies analyzing movement time in children from 6 to 10 years of age, for either type of movement, have shown a reduction in movement time with increased age. As might be expected, movements that require an accurate stop are slower at all ages. However, the difference between the speed of the two types of movements is about three times higher at 6 years of age than at 8 to 10 years of age. It has been hypothesized that this could be due to a difficulty experienced by the 6-year-olds in modulating the braking action of the antagonist muscle system (Hay et al., 1986).

In a slightly different cross-sectional study of children 6 to 9 years of age (in addition to a single child tested longitudinally across this period), participants were asked to reach as quickly and accurately as possible to a visual target, thus minimizing visual feedback corrections after the movement began. Results showed that RTs decreased between 6 and 7 years of age. Accuracy decreased temporarily at 7 years of age, followed by an increase at age 8. By age 9, both accuracy and RT reached approximately adult levels. Movement times were similar in all age groups. It is possible that the differences in this study as compared with earlier studies (lack of change in movement time with age and RTs being approximately at adult levels by age 9) relate to the conditions used, involving minimizing visual feedback corrections (Favilla, 2005).

Fitts' Law

Remember from Chapter 16 that Fitts' law shows a specific relationship between the time to make a movement and the amplitude and accuracy of that movement. The difficulty of the task is related both to the accuracy and the amplitude requirements, and is represented by the following equation:

$$ID = \log_2 2D/W$$

where D = distance of the movement; W = width of the target, and ID = index of difficulty (Fitts, 1954).

Studies testing the extent to which Fitts' law applies to children have found that movement time decreases with age. This decrease is in general a linear change, except for a regression, which appears to occur at about 7 years of age. Remember that in the development of postural control, there is also a regression, as indicated by an increase in postural response latencies, between 4 and 6 years of age. A study examining 5- to 9-year-olds has shown that these developmental decreases and regressions in movement time are not related to any changes in biomechanical factors, such as growth of the bones of the arm (Kerr, 1975; Rey, 1968; Shumway-Cook & Woollacott, 1985).

Using Fitts' law, one can plot movement time as a function of index of difficulty for different age groups. This relationship is shown in Figure 17.11. The intercept of the line with the y-axis reflects the general efficiency of the motor system, while the slope of the line reflects the amount of information that can be processed per second by the motor system. Almost all studies have shown that the y-intercept decreases with age, indicating increased efficiency. However, age-related improvements in slope appear to depend on the task involved, and appear to be more evident in discrete rather than serial movements (Hay, 1990; Sugden, 1980). To examine the effect of age on the ability of children to perform a reciprocal tapping task and how Fitts' Law applies to these movements in children, complete Lab Activity 17.2.

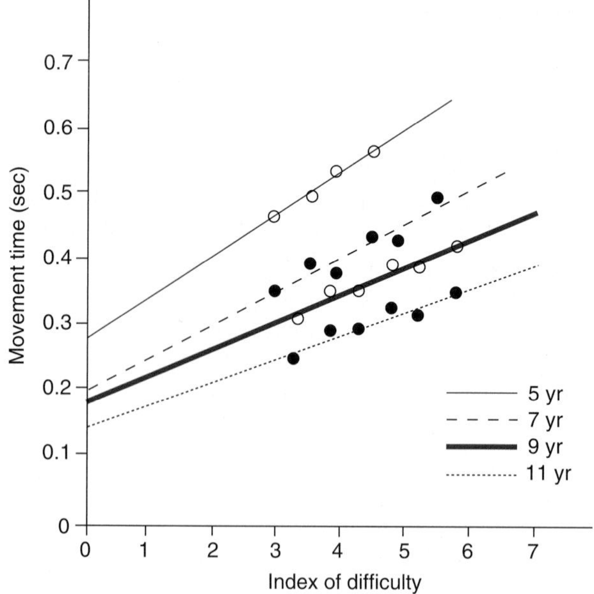

FIGURE 17.11 Graph showing the relationship between movement time and the index of difficulty of a task, for four age groups of children. The intercept of the line with the y-axis reflects the general efficiency of the motor system, while the slope of the line reflects the amount of information that can be processed per second by the motor system. Almost all studies have shown that the y-intercept decreases with age, indicating increased efficiency. (Adapted with permission from Hay L. Developmental changes in eye–hand coordination behaviors: preprogramming versus feedback control. In: Bard C, Fleury M, Hay L, eds. Development of eye–hand coordination across the lifespan. Columbia, SC: University of South Carolina Press, 1990:227.)

In summary, the emergence of reach, grasp, and manipulation occurs gradually during development and is characterized by changes in many systems. With the emergence and refinement of these skills, one sees changes in timing, coordination, and modulation of forces used for reach and grasp. We now turn to examine age-related changes in reach, grasp, and manipulation.

CHANGES IN OLDER ADULTS

As we have noted in our previous chapters on age-related changes in postural control and mobility skills, there are specific changes in these skills with age. These can be divided into: (a) time-related changes, such as slowing of onset latencies for postural

LAB ACTIVITY 17-2

Objective: To examine the effect of age on the ability of children to perform a reciprocal tapping task. Remember, Fitts defined task difficulty in terms of target size (*W*, which is the width of the target) and the distance to move (*D*, which is the distance between targets). He thus quantified task difficulty (which he called "index of difficulty" or simply, ID) by using the following equation: $ID = \log_2 2D/W$.

Procedure: For this lab, find a child of at least two of the following ages—5 yr, 7 yr, 9 yr, 11 yr—in your community and observe them performing the following task. When you work with the child, bring with you a pencil and six pieces of paper, one for each of the three trials in each task. They should be already marked with appropriate target sizes and distances (see below). Ask the children to tap quickly and accurately between two targets that vary in width and distance. The objective is to make as many *accurate* tapping movements as possible in a 10-second period. Accuracy is important. Remind the children that there should be no more errors made in the most difficult task than in the easiest tasks. If the number of errors exceeds more than 5% of the pencil dots, the trial should be done again.

Two combinations of task difficulty will be used. The first and easiest task has $D = 2$ cm and $W = 2$ cm. Solving the equation for *ID*, that would be log (base 2) of (2 × 2)/2. This works out to the $\log_2$ of 2, which is 1. The most difficult task has $D = 16$ cm and $W = 1$ cm. That is, the $\log_2$ of (2 × 16)/1, which is 5.

Each child will perform three trials (10 sec each) for the two task conditions. You will time each trial and count and record the number of dots in each target. You should verbally tell the child when to start and stop each 10-sec trial (use a watch with a second hand). The rest interval between trials should be the amount of time needed to count and record the taps.

Assignment:

1. Make a table with a record of the number of taps on each of the three trials for both the easy and difficult tasks for each child. Calculate the mean and standard deviation as well. For each task, calculate the average movement time (in milliseconds) for a single movement of the tapping task. Do this by dividing each number of taps by 10, which will give you the number of taps per second during the 10-sec trial. Record this value in the table as well. Next, take the inverse of this number (1/*x*, where x is the average number of taps). Then, multiply this number by 1000 to obtain the average movement time in milliseconds. Record this average movement time in the table for each child. What impact did the difficulty of the task have on movement time for children in the different age groups? How did the children's performance change with increasing age? Compare your results with those of others in the class. Did you find a regression (slowing) in movement time for 7-year-olds as compared with the younger and older children?

response or decreased movement speed in locomotion; (b) coordination factors, related to changes in movement or muscle activation patterns; and (c) changes in the use of feedback and feedforward control of both postural and mobility skills. We will find that these same factors are important to consider in examining age-related changes in reaching and grasping skills.

Reaching: Changes with Age

Changes in Reaching Movement Time with Age

A review of studies examining changes in the speed of reaching movements with age has shown that discrete reaching movements show a range of 30 to 90% reduction in velocity with aging, depending on the ages compared and the task performed. For example, one study examining changes in the speed of discrete arm movements showed a 32% reduction between the ages of 50 and 90 years, while another showed a reduction in movement speed of 90% when comparing subjects from 20 to 69 years performing a repetitive tapping task (Welford, 1982; Williams, 1990).

What are some of the age-related changes in different systems of the body that might contribute to this slowing in reaching movements? Different systems that could contribute to the slowing include: (a) sensory and perceptual systems, such as the visual system's ability to detect the target, (b) central processing systems, (c) motor systems, and (d) arousal and motivational systems (Welford, 1982). For a review of changes in individual sensory, motor and cognitive subsystems that could contribute to these changes, see Chapter 9.

Welford performed an experiment to determine whether changes in central mechanisms contribute to the slowing in reaching speed in older adults. In these experiments, subjects were asked to keep a pointer

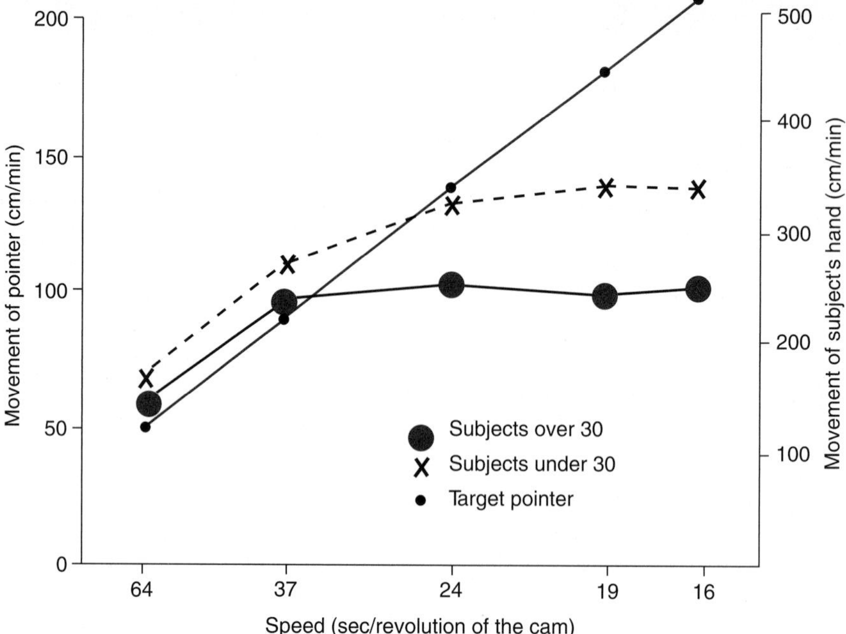

FIGURE 17.12 The ability of young versus older adults to follow unpredictable target movements of different speeds. Note that older adults have more problems following the target movements at higher speeds. (Adapted with permission from Welford AT. Motor skills and aging. In: Mortimer JA, Pirozzolo FJ, Maletta GJ, eds. The aging motor system. New York: Praeger, 1982:159.)

(which they could move with a handle) in line with a target that continuously moved from side to side, in an irregular sinusoidal fashion, with the movement varying in both speed and extent. He found that as the speed of the target movement was increased, the subjects could follow it less easily, until at some point it was impossible to follow.

However, there was a difference between the older and younger subjects. As shown in Figure 17.12, the ability to follow the movements dropped off sooner in the older adults than in the young adults. Welford (1977) hypothesized that the limitation in the performance of the older adults was not due to problems with the motor system, because they could move faster if they were not following the target. He theorized that the limitation was not sensory because the older adults could easily see the target. Therefore, he concluded that the limitation was in central processing abilities—i.e., in the older adults' ability to match the target and pointer and react quickly to changes in target direction. This implies that the time spent in actual movement itself slows little as compared with the time taken to make decisions about the next part of the movement sequence.

Changes in Reaching Coordination with Age

Motion analysis of the trajectories of older adults performing rapid aiming movements has indicated that they spend more time in the target-approach, or deceleration, phase than do young adults (Fradet et al., 2008). This is the period of sensory processing that ensures accuracy in reaching the target. A number of studies have explored possible contributing factors to this slowing in the target-approach phase. A study by Pohl et al. (1996) compared the movements of young (mean age, 25 years) and older (mean age, 71 years) adults in a reciprocal tapping task with different accuracy requirements (8-cm-wide vs. 2-cm-wide targets, 37 cm apart). They noted that the older adults showed significantly more movement adjustments coupled with a longer absolute adjustment time and a longer reversal time when moving between the two targets. The authors suggest that the young adults used more online and feedforward processes in achieving the goals of speed and accuracy in movement, while the older adults relied more on slower feedback processes.

Other researchers have suggested that the increased submovements during the deceleration phase of the reach are not necessarily related to corrective adjustments, but may also be due to velocity fluctuations caused by the lower movement speed at the end of the reach observed with aging. Young adults also have increased submovements at lower movement speeds; however, the velocity fluctuations in older adults are even greater than those seen in young adults. This may be attributed to a reduction in motor units in older adults, which results in a reduced ability to generate smooth muscle forces, especially at low force levels (Fradet et al., 2008).

Additional studies of movement kinematics in young versus older adults used a task that required drawing a line to 5-, 10-, and 20-mm targets (a digitizing tablet was used) and compared subjects at similar

LAB ACTIVITY 17-3

Objective: To examine the effect of aging on the ability to perform a reciprocal tapping task.

Procedure: Repeat the procedure from Lab Activity 17.2, but with an older adult (70 yr or older) from your community.

Assignment:

1. Repeat the assignment from Lab Activity 17.2, with the following changes in questions. What impact did the difficulty of the task have on movement time for the older adult, as compared with your own or other young adult times, from Lab Activity 17.2?
2. Did you notice any additional movement or hesitancy in making the movements? Do you think that the fitness level of the older adult would affect performance on the task?

movement speeds (Morgan et al., 1994). Older adults showed comparable overall accuracy on the tasks but again showed more hesitancy and submovements, implying possible increased reliance on visual guidance. The authors concluded that this indicates a central deficit in motor coordination. Other research has examined changes in force production during reaching movements in older adults and shown similar discontinuities in their movement trajectories (Vrtunski & Patterson, 1985). It is interesting to remember that increased submovements were characteristic of early reaching patterns in normal infants (von Hofsten, 1993). Like older adults, these submovements in infants are often associated with higher reliance on visual feedback during reaching (Hay, 1979).

It has also been shown that hand steadiness decreases with age during reaching tasks (Williams, 1990). When older adults were asked to insert a small stylus in slots of different diameters (1/2- to 1/8-in.), steadiness dropped by 77%, from 50 to 90 years of age. Steadiness deteriorated faster in the nonpreferred hand than in the preferred hand.

Based on the literature, there appears to be little change in performance speed for reaching movements with age, if subjects are asked to repeat the same simple action, like tapping a pencil between two targets, or performing a simple reaction time task (Welford, 1977, 1982). In this case, the slowing may be as little as 16%. But if the complexity of the task is increased, by making the target smaller, using successive targets, or using a choice reaction time task, then slowing can range from 86 to 276%. To observe changes in reciprocal movement patterns found in old adults under a variety of conditions and how Fitts' Law applies to their movement patterns, perform Lab Activity 17.3.

Table 17.1 gives examples of differences in the slowing of the performance of reaching movements in older adults with the complexity of the task. The largest slowing in performance was in tasks involving symbolic translations (using a code to relate a stimulus to a response) or spatial transpositions (e.g., a light cue on the left requiring a reach to the right). Although decrements have been found in performance on many RT tasks, one study has also shown that when older adults are not instructed to worry about accuracy on such a task, they demonstrate no decrease in reaching speed (Williamson et al., 1993).

The primary source of the slowing in complex RT tasks is in the first phase of performance, the time to observe the signals and relate them to action, rather than in the second phase, the time to execute the movement (Welford, 1977, 1982). When performing more continuous tasks, the second phase, that of movement execution, can overlap to some extent with the first. For example, a person may process the information relating to the next signal while making the first response. This type of task appears to be more difficult for older adults, possibly because they need more time to monitor their responses, and thus have difficulty processing other signals simultaneously (Welford, 1982).

For example, older adults (63 to 76 years) were compared with younger adults (19 to 29 years) on a task in which they moved as quickly as possible to one of two end points, with one farther away than the other, in the same direction (Rabbitt & Rogers, 1965). The younger subjects could overlap the time required to choose the end point with the initial stages of the movement itself, while the older subjects were less able to do this. Although there is no evidence that the time taken for monitoring increases with age, older adults seem less able to suppress monitoring.

What reasons might there be for this lack of suppression? It has been hypothesized that suppression of monitoring occurs when the outcome of a task is certain; thus, if there is a possibility of error, monitoring will be more probable. In addition, suppression of monitoring may be possible when movement subunits are coordinated into higher units of performance

TABLE 17.1 Age-Related Slowing in the Performance of Reaching Movements as a Function of Task Complexity

Task	Age Groups Compared	Percentage Increase*
Simple key press or release to light or sound		
Average of 11 studies listed by Welford	20s, with 60s	16%
Ten-choice (Birren, Riegel, & Morrison, 1962)	18–33 with 65–72	
Straightforward relationship		27
With numerical code, mean of 5 studies		50
With verbal code, mean of two studies		45
With color code		94
With part color and part letter code		86
Ten-choice (Kay, 1954, 1955)	25–34 with 65–72	
a. Signal lights immediately above response keys		−13 (no error made)
b. Signal lights 3 ft from keys		26 (−43)
c. As b, but signal lights arranged so that leftmost responded to with rightmost key, and so forth		46 (−19)
d. With numerical code		56 (+138)
e. The difficulties of d and b combined		299 (+464)

*Percentage changes of errors are shown in parentheses. Adapted from Welford AT. Motor skills and aging. In: Mortimer JA, Pirozzolo FJ, Maletta GJ, eds. The aging motor system. New York: Praeger, 1982:163.

(Welford, 1982). However, to do this often requires that the subject hold the movement subunits together in working memory while performing the task.

A study tested this ability in older (60 to 81 years) versus young (17 to 28 years) adults. Subjects were asked to perform two serial key pressing tasks, one that had few subunits (12, 12, 12, etc.) and one that was more complex (1234, 32, 1234, etc.). The investigators found that the older adults were slower than the young adults, particularly with the second series (Rabbitt & Birren, 1967).

Grasping: Changes with Age

One of the problems faced by older adults is a decrease in manual dexterity, which becomes apparent in tasks such as tying shoelaces and fastening buttons. For example, the time required to manipulate a small object increases 25 to 40% by 70 years of age. These age-related changes have been explored by measuring the fingertip forces used to grip and lift objects, in experiments similar to those performed with young children, described earlier. Figure 17.13 shows the experimental apparatus often used to measure grip forces in older adults. It is known that tactile sensation is reduced in older adults, and this may affect their ability to detect how strongly they are holding an object (Agnew et al., 1982; Cole, 1991; Keogh et al., 2006).

Studies by Cole and colleagues have shown that older adults (mean age, 81 years) used grasp forces that were, on average, twice as large as those of young adults, with some older adults producing forces that were many times larger than the young adult mean. Figure 17.14 shows examples of grasp-force records for a young versus an older adult for the third trial picking up a nonslippery object (covered with sandpaper) and the first and third trials picking up a slippery object (covered with rayon). Note that the older subject shows much larger grasp forces and takes longer to adapt to the final grasp force for the rayon object than the young adult. A portion of the increased force was due to increased skin slipperiness. In addition, the older adults simply produced a higher margin of safety against object slippage. Variability of grip forces was also much higher across trials and the direction of fingertip forces was not aligned with vertical in

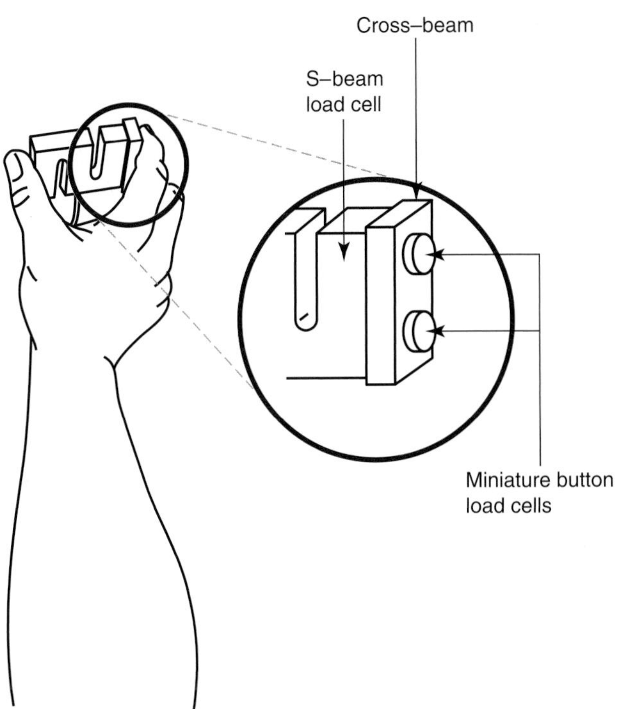

FIGURE 17.13 Experimental apparatus used for the recording of digit forces during finger pinch tasks. The magnified area shows the positions of the load cells for measuring finger forces (Reprinted with permission from Keogh J, Morrison S, Barrett R. Age-related differences in inter-digit coupling during finger pinching. Eur J Appl Physol 2006;97:79.)

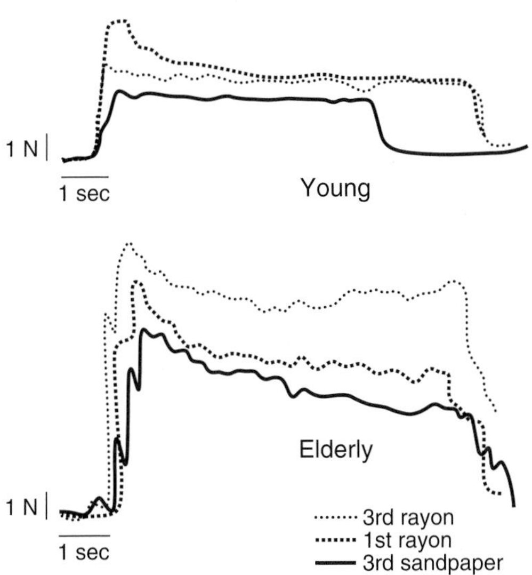

FIGURE 17.14 Grasp force traces from a young subject and an older adult showing typical grasp force patterns when lifting an object with a nonslippery (sandpaper) versus a slippery (rayon) surface. Traces represent the third lift with sandpaper followed by the first and third rayon trials. N = newtons. (Reprinted with permission from Cole KJ. Grasp force control in older adults. J Motor Behav 1991;23:255.)

the older as compared with the young adults. It is hypothesized that this may contribute to clumsiness in older adults during fine manipulation (Cole, 1991, 2006; Cole et al., 1999).

Additional experiments have examined whether this increased safety margin is due to decreased tactile sensation or decreased ability to encode skin–object frictional properties (Cole & Rotella, 2001; Cole et al., 1998, 1999). Results suggest that declining cutaneous afferent function contributes to safety margin increases after about 60 years of age. Researchers noted that grip-force adjustments to new surfaces were delayed about 100 msec in older adults as compared with young adults. They also found that when a grasped handle was pulled unexpectedly, older adults (mean age, 78 years) showed a twofold increase in the force required to evoke a response, showed delays in response onsets, and showed significantly larger resulting fingertip forces than young adults. Previous research has shown that friction is signaled locally by fast-adapting afferents, which decrease in number with age; thus, this could account for the delays in force adjustments.

In a separate set of experiments Cole et al. (1998) hypothesized that if age-related tactile changes were the cause of decreased manual dexterity, then performing a grip-and-lift task in the dark would cause a disproportionate increase in the duration of the grip-and-lift task in older as compared with younger adults. Their results showed that the grip–lift duration in the no-vision condition was equally increased for the young (mean age, 45 years) and older (mean age, 74 years) adult groups, with ratios of 2.1 and 2.3 for the duration in the vision and no-vision conditions for the respective groups. The authors conclude that these results fail to support the hypothesis that age-related declines in dexterity were due predominantly to changes in availability of tactile information.

In additional experiments, Kinoshita and Francis (1996) attempted to determine whether there are age-related changes in the control of precision grip force during the lifting and holding of objects with different surface textures (slippery [silk] and nonslippery [sandpaper]). They compared the performance of two groups of active older adults (69 to 79 years and 80 to 93 years) and a group of young adults (18 to 32 years) in a grasp-and-lift task. They found that the older adults (especially the 81-to-93-year-old group) had increased fluctuations in the grip-force rate curve and longer force application time than the younger subjects during lifting. They also noted that prior experience with one surface had less effect on the performance with the next surface in the older adults. The authors conclude that this indicates a decrease in the capacity to program force production with aging. As noted previously, they found that the fingers of the elderly subjects were more slippery and they used a larger grip-force safety margin than younger adults. The overall results demonstrated that the capacity for precision-grip-force control declines with advancing age.

The age-associated decrease in force control during lifting is believed to be related to decreased motor unit control. For example, older adults show increases in average motor unit force, motor unit force variability, and modulation of motor unit firing rate. In addition, older adults show a reduced coupling between the force output of the fingers of the hand when grasping (Keogh et al., 2006).

One possible reason that older adults have difficulty lifting objects efficiently is that aging impairs the ability to learn the visual-motor associations needed to set appropriate fingertip forces for handling familiar objects. Cole and Rotella (2002) tested the ability of young (mean age, 22 years) versus older (mean age, 77 years) adults to use visual color cues about the texture (sandpaper vs. acetate) or weight (200 g vs. 400 g) of an object to control fingertip forces during a grasp-and-lift task. Objects to be lifted were color-coded according to the weight or slipperiness in the "visual cue" condition, and these properties changed unpredictably across trials in the "no visual cue" condition. When object texture was visually cued, grip forces of young adults were 24% smaller; however, grip forces for older adults did not vary in response to the visual cues, although they accurately reported the surface colors prior to lifts. Similar results were found for prior cueing concerning object weights to be lifted (older adults did not use cueing information), although old and young adults each used approximately a 2-N grip force when lifting the 200-g object.

The researchers concluded that the older adults' inability to adjust grip force to object properties when the color cue was present was not due to a general inability or unwillingness to use a low grip force when handling objects, but that aging affects the associative learning linking visual identification of objects with fingertip forces required to efficiently lift the object. In contrast to these results, the grip force of older and young adults was affected by the prior lifting, suggesting that more than one internal representation contributes to predictive control of forces during grasp and lift tasks (Cole & Rotella, 2002).

Reach–Grasp Adaptation: Changes with Age

Do older adults have more difficulty adapting to unexpected changes in object size? In order to answer this question, Bennett and Castiello (1995) compared the movement trajectories of older (60 to 70 years) and younger (20 to 26 years) adults in response to a perturbation of object size during a reach-to-grasp movement. In most trials (80 of 100), participants reached for and grasped an illuminated cylinder of small (0.7 cm) or large (8.0 cm) diameter. In 20 trials, a visual perturbation (switching from one to the other cylinder) occurred at the onset of the reach, requiring a switch from precision to power grip or vice versa. Although the older group successfully adapted to these changes, they used a more conservative strategy, involving a longer approach time to the object and the use of the standard coordination pattern between transport and manipulation components. Younger adults, instead, used a new pattern, with a decrease of temporal coordination between the components. The authors suggest that the more rigid movement pattern of older adults with regard to the unexpected changes in grip requirements could contribute to a higher incidence of accidents during manipulation tasks. To examine how properties of a task affect reach-and-grasp movements in older adults, perform Lab Activity 17.4.

LAB ACTIVITY 17-4

Objective: To examine how properties of a task affect reach-and-grasp movements in older adults.

Procedures: For this lab, you will repeat Lab Activity 17.1, but now you will find an older adult (70 yr or older) in your community and observe him or her performing the same tasks as described in Lab Activity 17.1.

Assignment:

1. Describe how the older adult reached for and grasped the various objects.
2. When during the reach for an object did the hand begin to shape in preparation for grasp? How did characteristics of the object affect anticipatory hand shaping?
3. Compare the data from the older adult to young adult reach-and-grasp characteristics from Lab Activity 17.1. Do your results agree with those of Cole (1991) regarding ability to change lift forces easily with changing object surface characteristics?

Compensation and Reversibility of Decrements in Reaching Performance

Although decrements in reaching performance may be found in older adults under experimental conditions, they are often not observed in the workplace or in activities of daily living. It has been suggested that performance is preserved because many compensatory strategies are used to improve reach-and-grasp skills. Many of these compensatory strategies used by older adults appear to be unconscious, automatic processes. For example, older adults may increase the effort they put into the movement. In the workplace, they may work more continuously with fewer brief pauses. They may also prepare for movements that require speed and accuracy in advance, thus allowing anticipatory processes to aid in performance. In many tasks, they may also make a trade-off between speed and accuracy. Finally, it has also been shown that older adults set higher criteria for responding to RT signals in sensory-discrimination tasks (Welford, 1982).

Can the changes in reaching skills that occur with aging be counteracted by practice or training? Yes. This can occur with training at both the impairment level (muscle strength training) and at the functional level (eye–hand coordination skill training). Keogh et al. (2007) compared the performance of a group of older adults (70 to 80 years) who underwent upper-limb strength training (2 times per week for 6 weeks) with that of a control group of older adults (70 to 80 years) on finger-pinch-force control. They found that the strength-training group showed significantly greater reductions in force variability and target error and well as greater increases in finger-pinch force than did the control group. This suggests the importance of upper-limb strength to high-level performance on precision-grip tasks.

In addition, clear improvement with practice has been reported for eye–hand coordination skills in older adults (Falduto & Baron, 1986). The greatest improvement is seen in more complex tasks. Interestingly, older adults show more improvement with practice than do younger adults on performance of RT tasks (Jordan & Rabbitt, 1977). This may occur because young adults are closer to their ceiling of performance when starting to learn the task. However, practice does not eliminate the age differences in the performance of these tasks.

Practice also improves performance in older adults with regard to the perceptual processes involved in eye–hand coordination tasks, such as visual acuity, signal detection, and auditory discrimination. In addition, the effects of practice remain high, even 1 month after practice on eye–hand coordination tasks has ended. One study compared the performance of young (19 to 27 years) and older (62 to 73 years) adults on a task that involved fine movements of the hands, signal detection, memory scanning, visual discrimination, and anticipation timing, called "space trek." Subjects were given 1-hour practice sessions, 51 over a period of 2 to 5 months. One month after training ended, there was only a small decrease in performance levels (Welford, 1982).

In another study, older adults (57 to 83 years) were given practice in eye–hand coordination skills by playing video games. These games involved making fast decisions about changes in the speed and direction of hand movements. Over a 7-week period, scores tripled on the task. In addition, practice on the video games transferred over to other RT tasks that required subjects to select a motor response quickly (Clark et al., 1987).

Many older adults have additional slowing or error production as compared with young adults when asked to perform two tasks simultaneously because attentional resources must be shared between the two tasks. Can motor practice improve this decrease in performance under dual-task conditions? To answer this question, researchers asked young and older adults to perform a precision grip sine-wave force-tracking and a working memory task simultaneously before and after 100 motor-training trials. Results showed that motor practice improved force tracking in both groups. Younger adults showed higher performance at both pretraining and posttraining than older adults, but older adults reached the younger adult pretraining performance levels after extended practice. Interestingly, this training did not prevent the decline in motor performance in the older adult group when going from the single- to the dual-task condition. After training, however, the cognitive task performance was improved in older adults (Voelcker-Rehage & Alberts, 2005, 2007).

Most of these studies suggest that older adults learn as much, if not more, with practice as young adults and that they retain the learned skills as well as young adults do. However, it appears that motor training does not eliminate completely the decrements in dual-task performance seen in older as compared with younger adults. In addition, the way subjects improved with practice was similar for the young and older adults; however, the older adults simply learned more slowly. This slower rate of learning of eye–hand coordination skills in older subjects may be due to material taking longer to register in long-term memory (Welford, 1982).

What does this mean in terms of determining the best strategies for teaching eye–hand coordination skills to older adults? Since the time required for registering information in long-term memory lengthens with age, learning needs to be unhurried. Otherwise extra information to be processed during the time required to register information in longer-term memory will simply disrupt the memory process.

In teaching eye–hand coordination skills, there are sometimes problems in translating verbal instruction into motor performance. To avoid this, one can use demonstrations. However, in this case, the pace of the demonstration should be under the learner's control. Thus, using slow-motion, self-paced videos in training may help (Welford, 1982).

Active decision making is also an important factor in learning at any age. In a maze study with adults, it was shown that learning took place much faster if the correct pathway was marked, but the subject had to make an active choice. This helped subjects of all ages, but it especially helped older adults (Wright, 1957).

It was also shown that using a mixture of mental practice and physical practice when learning a pursuit rotor task was as good as physical practice alone for 65-to-69- and 80-to-100-year-olds (Surberg, 1976).

Thus, learning of eye–hand coordination tasks by older adults can be facilitated by using a type of discovery learning, which involves demonstrations that can be self-paced, active learning, and a combination of physical and mental practice (Welford, 1982).

During development, the emergence of mature reach-and-grasp behavior is characterized by a reduction in reaction time, a decrease in safety margins during grip and lift, and a reduction in the number of subunits during the reaching movement, resulting in a smoother trajectory. Similarly, a decline in reach and grasp with aging is characterized by an increase in reaction time, an increase in safety margins, and an increase in the number of subunits contributing to a reaching movement. Multiple factors may be contributing to these characteristic changes across the lifespan. These include both primary deficits in the nervous and musculoskeletal systems and secondary strategies used to compensate for these deficits.

A CASE STUDY APPROACH TO UNDERSTANDING AGE-RELATED CHANGES IN REACH, GRASP AND MANIPULATION

Bonnie B is a 90-year-old woman with impaired balance and gait resulting in multiple falls. Like many older adults Bonnie has impaired upper-limb function resulting from age-related changes in reach, grasp and manipulation. With respect to her participation, Bonnie is limited in both IADLs and ADLs, and has a home health aide three days per week to help with cooking, cleaning, and laundry. Bonnie cannot stand and walk without the use of a walker, limiting her ability to carry objects; thus she requires assistance when shopping as well.

Bonnie's functional movements are slowed and she has reduced end-point accuracy when reaching for targets or picking up small objects. Reach and grasp problems are often worse when Bonnie is performing multiple tasks simultaneously. Researchers have found that age-related changes in reach, grasp and manipulation include time-related changes, such as slowed reaction and movement times, coordination factors related to changes in multijoint movements and muscle activation patterns, and changes in the use of feedback and feedforward control. In addition, older adults demonstrate velocity fluctuations resulting from a reduction in motor units that affect the ability to generate and coordinate muscle forces, particularly those used in precision grip. Among older adults, reduced ability to allocate attentional appropriately can reduce upper-limb function under dual-task conditions. Researchers have found that many older adults like Bonnie have a reduced ability to adapt reach and grasp forces to unexpected changes in task and environmental demands, which contributes to a higher incidence of accidents during manipulation tasks (Bennett & Castiello, 1995).

Bonnie demonstrates age-related decreases in manual dexterity affecting her ability to perform tasks such as writing, tying shoelaces and fastening buttons. Her movements are slow and accuracy is reduced, increasing the time required to perform common daily tasks.

Like many older adults, Bonnie has age-related changes in motor, sensory and cognitive systems; thus many impairments contribute to her functional limitations and restricted participation. Motor impairments include reduced range of motion and strength in her upper-extremities. She has reduced multijoint coordination affecting the coordination of reach and grasp. Bonnie has deficits in multiple sensory systems. She has age-related changes to vision, including reduced contrast sensitivity, problems with depth perception, and reduced visual acuity. She also has somatosensory changes including reduced vibratory sense, proprioception, and light touch sensation. Reduced somatosensation in her hands contributes to a reduced ability to regulate fingertip forces during grip and lift tasks. Bonnie also has reduced vestibular function associated with a history of Meniere's disease. Finally, Bonnie has some cognitive deficits, including problems with short-term memory and mildly impaired executive function, which contribute to impaired upper-limb functions.

Bonnie's impaired balance plays a significant role in her reduced upper-limb function. In addition to reduced steady state postural control in standing, Bonnie has significantly impaired anticipatory postural control, which makes it difficult for her to maintain stability during the performance of many upper-limb tasks, such as reaching, lifting, and leaning over to pick up objects from the floor. In addition, impairments in reactive balance control limit her ability to recover stability and avoid a fall when she performs these tasks.

Practice would most likely improve Bonnie's upper-limb function. Researchers have found that practice can reduce, though not eliminate, many age-related changes in reach and grasp skills (Clark et al., 1987; Falduto & Baron, 1986; Keogh et al., 2007; Voelcker-Rehage & Alberts, 2007).

SUMMARY

1. Infants as young as a week old show prereaching behaviors, in which they reach toward objects that are in front of them. These reaches are not accurate, and the infants do not grasp the object, since an extension synergy controls the arm and hand movements. When the arm is extended, the hand is open. But the reaches are clearly aimed at the object, since they are significantly more accurate than arm movements in which the eyes are not fixated on the object.
2. At about 2 months, the extension synergy is broken up, so that the fingers flex as the arm extends. At this time, head–arm movements become coupled as the infant gains control over the neck muscles.
3. At about 4 months, infants begin to gain trunk stability, along with a progressive uncoupling of head–arm–hand synergies. These changes allow the emergence of functional reach-and-grasp behavior.
4. From 4 months onward, reaching becomes more refined, with the approach path straightening and the number of segments of the reach being reduced.
5. Visually triggered reaching is dominant in the newborn, changing to visually guided reaching at about 5 months of age, and returning to visually triggered reaching by 1 year of age, although guided reaching is still available.
6. The development of hand orientation begins to occur at the onset of successful reaching, at about 5 months of age.
7. The pincer grasp develops at about 9 to 10 months of age, along with the development of the pyramidal tract.
8. Reaction time shows a progressive reduction with age, with sharper changes occurring up to 8 to 9 years, followed by slower changes up to 16 to 17 years.
9. Children from 4 to 6 years of age make predominantly visually triggered (feedforward) movements, using little visual feedback. At 7 to 8 years, visual feedback is dominant, leading to poor reaching in the dark, but more accurate reaching with vision present. By 9 to 11 years, there is an integration between feedforward and feedback movements.
10. Older adults show a slowing in reaching movements, with much of this due to central processing slowing. The slowing in performance on reaching movements is greater for more complex tasks.
11. Part of the slowing may result from an inability to suppress monitoring of movements, due to either uncertainty concerning the accuracy of the movement or an inability to integrate movement subunits into larger chunks in working memory.
12. Older adults are less efficient than young adults when performing grip-and-lift tasks, using higher grip forces (a larger safety margin) and showing more variability in grip-and-lift forces and a longer time to attain the final grip force.
13. Most age-related decrements in reaching performance can be improved with training. Training effects remain high for at least a month after training has ended and also transfer to other reaching tasks.

ANSWERS TO LAB ACTIVITY ASSIGNMENTS

Lab Activity 17-1

1. Hand closes in anticipation of reaching object.
2. 8–12 mo: child may use palmer grasp for everything if about 8 mo, but will shift to pincer grasp at about 9–10 mo for block (if small enough) and crayon. Opening of hand is related to size of object from 9 mo of age. Cannot adapt to sudden changes in friction of object (slippery glass).

   12–18 mo: Use pincer grasp for block and crayon, palmer grasp for glass. Opening of hand is related to size of object. They initiate the grasp farther from the target than 8- to 12-month-olds. Cannot adapt to change in friction of object.

2–3 yr: Like 12- to 18-month–olds, with the addition that arm movements are smoother than in the younger age groups. Can adapt to unexpected changes in friction when given in blocks of trials, but not when suddenly changed (slippery glass)

4–6 yr: Use pincer grasp, smooth arm movement, adapt to changes in friction (slippery glass) with just a few practice trials. May be able to orient hand to glass being upside down, to make single smooth movement.

3. To be determined by student's observed data.
4. To be determined by student's observed data.

Lab Activity 17-2

1. With increased age there will be a decrease in movement time for the tasks. Increased difficulty of the task should increase movement time more in the younger children than in the older children. There may be a slight slowing in movement in the 7-year-olds as compared with the other children.

Lab Activity 17-3

1. Depending on the age and health of the older adult you may find that increasing the difficulty of the task increased movement time more than for a young adult.
2. Again, you may find that a very old adult or one who has low fitness levels will have lower performance levels than a fit older adult or a young adult.

Lab Activity 17-4

1. Healthy older adults would be expected to grasp objects like young adults. The very old or unfit older adults would possibly show slowing and hesitation in reaching, causing increased movement units in the reach and decreased smoothness of the trajectory.
2. To be determined by student's observed data.
3. Most healthy and fit older adults would show results similar to young adults.
4. To be determined by student's observed data.

CHAPTER 18

ABNORMAL REACH, GRASP, AND MANIPULATION

LEARNING OBJECTIVES

Following completion of this chapter, the reader will be able to:

1. Discuss the effect of central nervous system (CNS) pathology on reach and grasp.
2. Discuss the role of sensory deficits on reach and grasp.
3. Compare and contrast deficits in reach and grasp in persons with poststroke hemiparesis, Parkinson's disease, cerebellar pathology, and cerebral palsy.

INTRODUCTION

Normal upper-extremity function, including the ability to reach for, grasp, and manipulate objects, is the basis for fine-motor skills important to activities such as feeding, dressing, grooming, and handwriting. In addition, upper-extremity function plays an important role in gross motor skills such as crawling, walking, the ability to recover balance, and the ability to protect the body from injury when recovery is not possible. Because upper-extremity control is intertwined with both fine and gross motor skills, development and recovery of upper-extremity function is an important aspect of training and retraining the patient with impaired motor control, and falls within the purview of most areas of rehabilitation, including both occupational and physical therapy.

This chapter focuses on understanding problems related to reach, grasp, and manipulation in patients with neurologic pathology. We first review problems related to the key components of upper-extremity control, incorporating a discussion of sensory, motor, and higher-level problems that affect the key components, including: (a) locating a target, involving the coordinated movement of the eyes, head, and trunk; (b) reaching, involving transportation of the arm and hand in space as well as postural support; (c) grasp, including grip formation, grasp, and release; and (d) in-hand manipulation skills. We then use a case study approach to explore the types of upper-extremity problems found in patients with specific types of neurologic diagnoses.

TARGET-LOCATION PROBLEMS

A critical aspect of manipulatory function is the ability to locate a target and maintain gaze on that target preceding a reach. Depending on the task, target (or object) localization requires some combination of eye, head, and trunk motion, depending on the eccentricity of the target. Thus, neural pathology affecting the ability to coordinate eye, head, trunk, and hand movements can affect the ability to locate targets or objects in space. In addition, gaze stabilization problems can result from: (a) oculomotor system pathology disrupting visually driven eye movements; (b) damage to the vestibular system, which disrupts vestibulo-ocular reflex control of eye movements in response to head movements; and (c) inability to adapt the vestibulo-ocular reflex to changes in task demands because of cerebellar damage (Martin et al., 1993). All of these types of problems affect the patient's ability to stabilize gaze on an object when moving the head. However, in this chapter, we focus primarily on problems related to visually driven eye movements that affect the ability to locate targets or objects to be reached. In addition, we review research on problems affecting the ability to coordinate and integrate eye movements with head and hand movements for tasks such as pointing to a target or reaching for an object.

Visual Deficits and Object Localization

Central lesions affecting the processing of visual signals will impair the ability to locate a target or object in space. Visual-field deficits following a stroke, such as homonymous hemianopsia, restrict a person's ability to "see" objects in half the visual field, affecting reach and grasp in the contralesional hemifield (Jeannerod, 1990). More than 50% of children with spastic hemiplegic cerebral palsy have homonymous hemianopsia; many compensate with atypical head postures in order to improve visual acuity and binocular vision (Porro et al., 2005; Prayson & Hanahoe, 2004). Visual neglect and visual extinction are often the consequence of damage to the right cerebral hemisphere. Individuals with visual neglect show a profound lack of awareness of the contralesional side of personal and external space, while those with visual extinction are unable to detect a stimulus in the contralesional field under conditions of bilateral stimulus presentation. It is unclear whether neglect and extinction are related to sensory, attentional, or other factors.

In both visual neglect and visual extinction, the relative location of the target appears to influence the patient's ability to detect an object or target in space. Smania et al. (1998) examined the spatial distribution of visual attention in subjects with right hemispheric damage and either hemineglect or extinction. Subjects were required to press the space bar of a computer keyboard after the appearance of a light flash in one of four positions (10, 20, 30, or 40 degrees along the horizontal meridian) presented in either the left or right visual field. Both the neglect and the extinction groups were less able to detect targets presented in their left hemifield. In addition, impairments in detecting targets increased with target eccentricity. This study reminds us that patients with right hemisphere damage who also have left unilateral neglect will have difficulty reaching for objects presented on the left side of the body because of difficulty in locating objects presented in the left visual field. In addition, the more eccentric the target, the more difficulty the patient will have in reaching.

Experiments have been performed on subjects with hemianopsia due to a hemispherectomy on one side (Perenin & Jeannerod, 1975). Patients with hemianopsia were asked to point to the target when it appeared in either the normal visual field or the affected field. When it was in the affected field, they were asked to "guess" where it was and to point there, as patients said that they could not see it. Again, pointing positions in the hemianopsic field were definitely correlated with the target positions. Although subjects were initially very poor at reaching for objects in this manner, their performance improved with training. If they were simply told that the target would appear at a different location for each trial, with practice they showed a clear and rapid improvement in their abilities (Zihl & Werth, 1984).

Individuals with parietal lesions also show problems with eye movements when these movements are a part of exploratory visual searches or reaching behavior. They may have problems breaking visual fixation (Balint's syndrome) or in optic ataxia; they also may have slowed reaction times for saccades, with the saccades subdivided into staircase patterns (Balint, 1909; Waters et al., 1978).

Visual deficits also impact the planning and execution of reach and grasp. Experiments with healthy young adults, in which the field of view was reduced to 11 degrees (an absence of peripheral vision), affected the planning and execution of both reach and grasp (González-Alvarez et al., 2007). In patients with reduced binocular vision, the reach phase of movement was significantly slower as compared with individuals with intact vision, particularly during the end phase of reaching, which was characterized by a prolonged final approach, more velocity corrections, and poorer coordination during object contact. In addition, during the grasp phase, reduced visual information resulted in increased reliance on somatosensory inputs, with a subsequent increase in the number of grip adjustments after contact had been made with the object to be grasped (Melmoth et al., 2009).

Finally, problems in the visual system can affect perceptual aspects of object identification and localization. In Chapter 16, we discussed the two visual pathways involved in reach and grasp, including the dorsal stream pathway going from the visual to the parietal cortex, which provides critical information for all phases of a reach, and the ventral stream pathway, going from visual cortex to the temporal lobe, which provides conscious visual perceptions (Goodale & Milner, 1992; Goodale et al., 1991). Thus, a patient with "ventral stream" lesions will have no conscious perception of the orientation or dimension of objects, but will show great skill in picking them up, while the opposite may be true for a patient with a "dorsal stream" lesion.

PROBLEMS WITH EYE–HEAD–HAND COORDINATION

Remember from Chapters 16 and 17 that some target location tasks require eye movements alone, while others require a combination of eye and head movement, and still others require a combination of eye, head, and trunk movements, depending on the eccentricity of the target in space. This has led researchers to suggest that eye–head coordination is not controlled by a single mechanism, but rather, emerges from an interaction of several different neural mechanisms (Jeannerod, 1990).

Problems coordinating eye, head, and hand movements contributing to impaired reaching abilities have been reported in a number of neurologic populations, including cerebral palsy (Saavedra et al., 2009), developmental coordination deficits (Wilmut et al., 2006), stroke, and cerebellar pathology (Van Donkelaar & Lee, 1994). Saavedra and colleagues (2009) compared the coordination of eye, head, and hand movements during seated reaches in 10 children with cerebral palsy (CP), 6 to 16 years of age, with that in typically developing children. The children made eye and hand movements either together or in isolation with different levels of external postural support. Children with CP had a reduced ability to isolate eye, head and hand movements, suggesting that inappropriate coupling of eye, head and hands contributes to impaired reach and grasp in children with CP. Interestingly providing external postural support to the children with CP did not affect eye or head movements, but did affect the initiation and execution of hand movements. This is consistent with other research demonstrating that providing additional postural support at the trunk improves performance on reach and grasp in children with CP (Van der Heide et al., 2005; Van Roon et al., 2005).

Van Donkelaar and Lee (1994) examined the interaction between eye and hand movements in patients with cerebellar pathology. They compared kinematic output of the eye and hand motor systems in both controls and subjects with cerebellar pathology during the performance of two tasks: (1) while tracking a moving target with the hand, and (2) while performing a pointing movement to intercept a target. As one might expect, the subjects with cerebellar damage were slower to begin tracking the visual target and had more inaccurate and variable hand movements as compared with the control subjects. Interestingly, a large amount of the increased variability in hand movements occurred just prior to and after each corrective eye movement (ocular saccade) made to track the object. The increased variability in hand movements could be decreased when vision of the hand was restricted. This is shown in Figure 18.1. Figure 18.1A shows that in a normal control subject, variability of hand velocity does not change in the three visual conditions: normal, visual fixation, and restricted vision (e.g., the individual cannot see his or her hand). In contrast, Figure 18.1B indicates that hand velocity in a subject with cerebellar damage is greatest under unrestricted visual conditions (normal) and is reduced when vision is restricted. The authors conclude that there is a reciprocal interaction

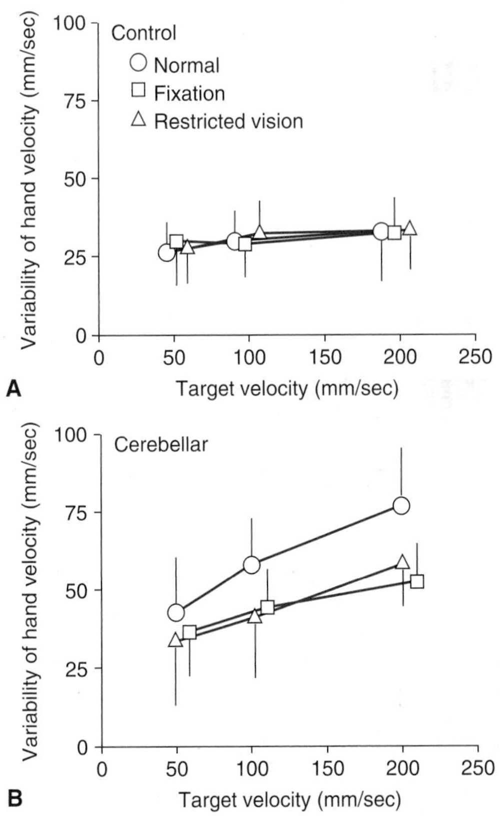

FIGURE 18.1 A comparison of hand-velocity variability produced in a tracking task during normal visual conditions (Normal), when eye motion is restricted (Fixation), or when vision of the hand is restricted (Restricted vision) in a healthy control and a subject with cerebellar pathology. (Redrawn with permission from Van Donkelaar P, Lee RG. Interactions between the eye and hand motor systems: disruptions due to cerebellar dysfunction. J Neurophysiol 1994;72:1679.)

between the eye and hand motor systems. In addition, in cerebellar subjects, problems affecting the output of one system adversely affect the other, so that inaccuracies in hand movements are influenced by inaccuracies in eye movements, and vice versa.

PROBLEMS WITH REACH AND GRASP

As we mentioned earlier, reaching is controlled by a different neural mechanism from that for grasping; hence, patients can have impaired reach but intact grasp, or vice versa. For many patients who are neurologically impaired, however, both reach and grasp are affected, reflecting dysfunction in the multiple systems controlling upper-extremity function. Separating the two, while artificial, makes it easier to analyze problems in each. However, it is important to remember that because of their close coordination and synchronization, pathology affecting reach most often disrupts grasp as well.

Impairments of Reach

Remember that during normal reaching, movement trajectories involving more than one joint tend to be straight and smooth and to have bell-shaped velocity profiles (Hogan & Flash, 1987). In contrast, movement trajectories in patients with neurologic pathology are often characterized by loss of coordinated coupling between synergistic muscles and joints. Disruptions in the coordination of movements can affect the timing and trajectory of movements.

Motor Problems

Timing Problems. Studies on reach and grasp have consistently shown delayed movement times in most types of neural pathology. For example, a number of researchers have reported that after stroke, reaching movements are slower, less accurate, and not as well coordinated as those made by healthy controls (Beer et al., 2000; Cirstea et al., 2003; Dewald & Beer, 2001; Levin, 1996; Reisman & Scholz, 2003). In addition, the ability to adapt reach to changing task demands is also impaired after stroke; patients have difficulty adjusting reach extent and tend to overshoot closer targets and undershoot the more distant targets (van Vliet & Sheridan, 2009).

Similarly, children with CP also have difficulty making coordinated reaching movements to point at or grasp objects (Mackey et al., 2006; Petrarca et al., 2009; Ronnqvist & Rosblad, 2007; Saavedra et al., 2009; Verrel et al., 2008). Reaches in children with CP are characterized by slower reaction times (Petrarca et al., 2009; Saavedra et al., 2009; van Thiel et al., 2000; Utley & Sugden, 1998), slower movement times, and increased submovements (Chang et al., 2005; Mutsaarts et al., 2006; Saavedra et al., 2009; van der Heide et al., 2005). In addition, underlying patterns of muscle activity used for reaching are more variable in children with CP as compared with typically developing children (Zaino & McCoy, 2008). Differences are more apparent in the affected versus the unaffected arms in children with hemiplegia (Hung et al., 2004; Mackey et al., 2006; Ronnqvist & Rosblad, 2007; Steenbergen et al., 1998). For example, children with spastic hemiparetic CP use more trunk movement when reaching with the impaired arm as compared with the nonimpaired arm (Ricken et al., 2005). This is similar to research in adults with poststroke hemiplegia who have been shown to use increased trunk movement when reaching as compared with controls (van Der Heide et al., 2004; Van Thiel & Steenbergen, 2001).

Interestingly, several researchers have shown that despite their motor impairments, children with CP were able to accurately reach for and grasp even quickly moving targets. These researchers found that the children aimed their reaches well ahead of the moving targets, suggesting that when planning a reaching movement, the children were able to compensate for the movement deficits that resulted in their slowed movement times (Forsstrom & von Hofsten, 1982; Ricken et al., 2005).

Reaching in individuals with cerebellar dysfunction is also characterized by delayed movement times (Rand et al., 2000; Van Donkelaar & Lee, 1994). Van Donkelaar and Lee (1994) found that both response (reaction) and movement times were prolonged when reaching to moving targets. They suggest that delays in timing may be due to the patient's need for more time to determine target velocity.

Delayed reaching times have been shown in person's with Parkinson's disease (PD) (Bertram et al., 2005; Kelly et al., 2002; Negrotti et al., 2005; Wang et al., 2006). Kelly et al. (2002) examined the effect of medication (levodopa) and external cueing on voluntary reaching in nine people with PD (tested on and off medication) and nine age-matched controls. Subjects were asked to reach to a target under speed constraints versus accuracy constraints and in one of two cue conditions: noncued (self-initiated) versus cued (triggered by a light). Results showed that persons with PD had slower reaching times under all conditions as compared with controls. Levodopa and cueing both increased the velocity of reaching movements of subjects with PD; however, these factors were not additive. Levodopa increased movement speed more when reaches were self-initiated as compared with cued, and it improved accurate (self-paced) reaches more than fast reaches. In a related study, these researchers also examined the effect of levodopa on the modulation of muscle activity (e.g., the ability to activate agonist muscles and inhibit antagonist muscles) during reaching movements (Kelly & Bastian, 2005). As had been reported previously, medication improved the speed of reaches in persons with PD and improved the ability to activate agonist muscle activity, but it did not improve the ability to inhibit antagonist muscle activity. Instead, the activity of both agonist and antagonist muscles increased with levodopa; thus, the medication, while improving the speed of movement, did not improve muscle modulation during voluntary reaching.

Delayed movement times, then, are a common feature of reaching in patients with a wide variety of neural pathologies. One factor implicated in prolonged movement times is a disruption to the coordination of multijoint movements.

Problems with Interjoint Coordination. Normally, elbow- and shoulder-joint angles change smoothly and at synchronized rates related to one another to produce a smooth reaching movement with a fairly straight trajectory. Children develop this coordination gradually during the first years of reaching (Konczak et al., 1995, 1997). In contrast, many studies have reported that in patients with a variety of neural pathologies, reaching movements are characterized by multijoint incoordination, leading to abnormal movement trajectories.

For example, Bastian and colleagues (1996, 2000, 2002) studied movement trajectories in adult subjects with cerebellar pathology. Movement trajectories were characterized by either undershooting or overshooting the target (dysmetria) and decomposition (moving one joint at a time). This can be seen in Figure 18.2. In Figure 18.2, A and B, the data from a normal control subject are shown. The wrist trajectories associated with a slow accurate (A) and a fast accurate (B) reach are smooth and straight. In addition, the movements are quite accurate; this can be seen by comparing the position of the fingertip (shown as an open circle) to the target (shown as a shaded circle). In contrast, the wrist trajectories and finger-point accuracy for a cerebellar patient are shown in Figure 18.2C (slow accurate conditions) and 18.2D (fast accurate conditions). For both the slow and the fast movements, wrist trajectories show decomposition—that is, an initial vertical movement (primarily related to shoulder flexion), followed by a horizontal movement (related to elbow

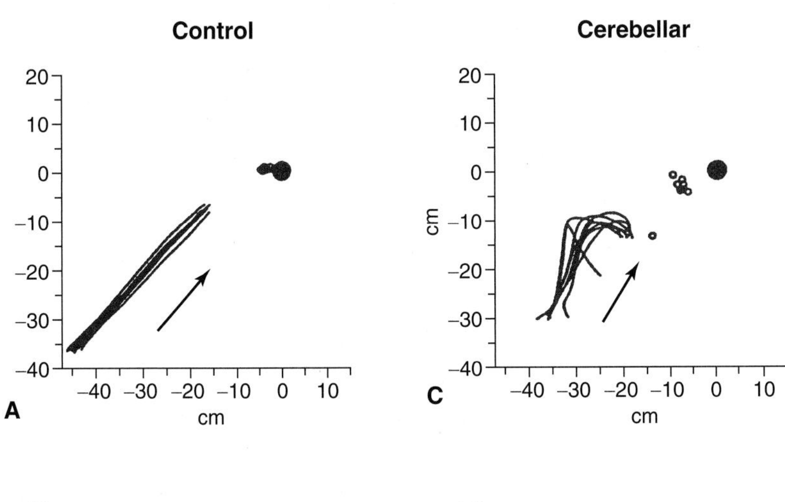

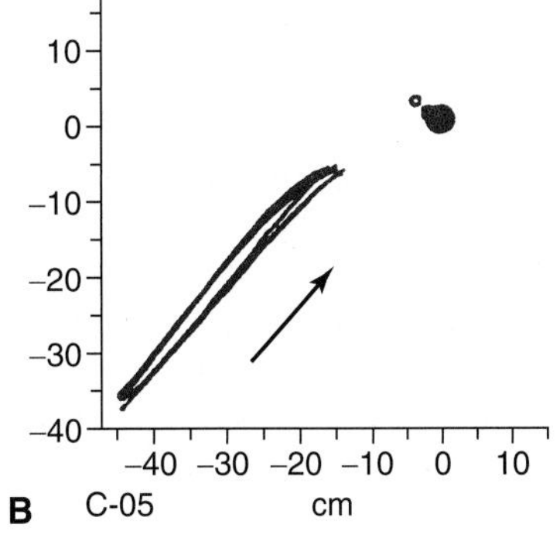

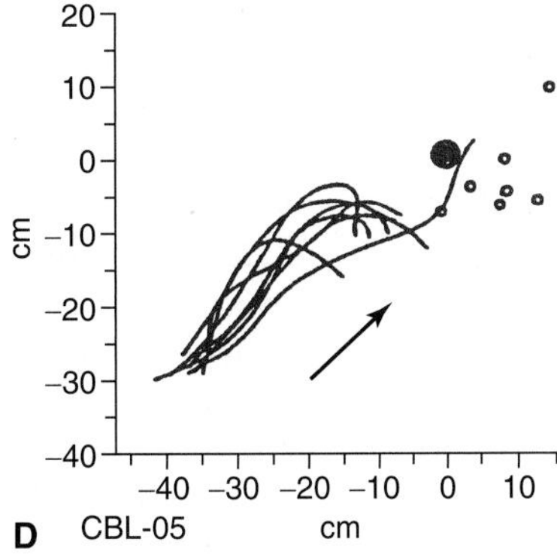

FIGURE 18.2 A comparison of wrist path in a control (A and B) versus a subject with cerebellar pathology (C and D) moving in slow accurate (A and C) and fast accurate (B and D) conditions. Arrows indicate the direction of movement. The shaded circle indicates the location of the target. Open circles indicate the position of the tip of the index finger at the end of the movement. (Redrawn with permission from Bastian AJ, Martin TA, Keating JG, Thach WT. Cerebellar ataxia: abnormal control of interaction torques across multiple joints. J Neurophysiol 1996;76:497.)

extension) during the latter half of the reach. In addition, slow movements were associated with hypometric reaches (undershooting), while the fast movements were hypermetric (overshooting). Control subjects initiated shoulder and elbow motion within 73 msec of one another. In contrast, the subjects with cerebellar pathology initiated shoulder flexion approximately 296 msec before the onset of elbow extension (Bastian et al., 1996).

Bastian and colleagues hypothesized that impaired multijoint coordination reflects the role of the cerebellum in anticipating and controlling interaction torques generated during multijoint movements. An interaction torque reflects the effect of movement at one joint (e.g., the elbow) on another joint (e.g., the shoulder). They examined multijoint coordination between the shoulder and elbow during a pointing task requiring elbow flexion (Fig. 18.3) when the shoulder was free to move (Fig. 18.3A) versus constrained (Fig. 18.3D). Eight individuals with cerebellar pathology and eight age-matched controls were tested. Control subjects (Fig. 18.3, B and E) made few end-point errors in either condition. In contrast, subjects with cerebellar pathology made large end-point errors in the free condition (Fig. 18.3C) but not in the constrained condition (Fig. 18.3F). Elbow movements were near normal in the constrained condition (when the movement was performed at a single joint). In contrast, multijoint movements were associated with excessive shoulder flexion and an inability to control interactive torques, and this resulted in large end-point errors (Bastian, 2002).

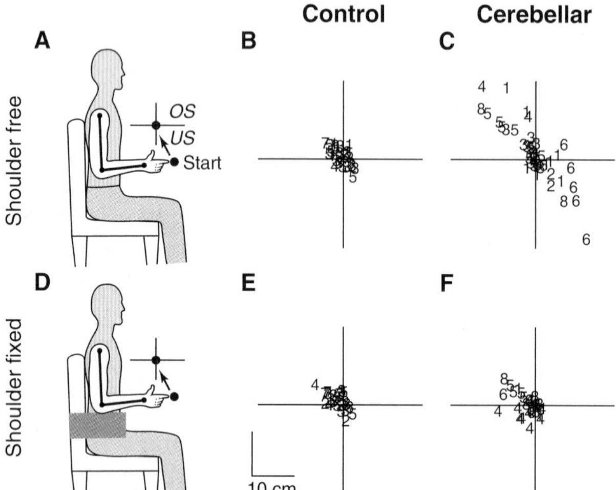

FIGURE 18.3 Experimental method used to study multijoint coordination between the shoulder and elbow during a pointing task requiring elbow flexion under two conditions: when the shoulder was free to move (A) and when it was constrained (D). Control subjects (B and E) made few end-point errors in either condition. Individuals with cerebellar pathology made large end-point errors in the free condition (C) but not in the constrained condition (F). (Reprinted with permission from Bastian AJ. Cerebellar limb ataxia: abnormal control of self generated and external forces. Ann NY Acad Sci 2002;978:18.)

Impaired multijoint coordination has also been reported in several studies examining upper-extremity movements in individuals with PD (Bertram et al., 2005; Teulings et al., 1997; Wang et al., 2006; Wiesendanger & Serrien, 2001). Tuelings et al. (1997) used handwriting-like tasks to study upper-extremity control in individuals with PD. They found that many of the fine motor control problems (as shown by their handwriting-like tasks) in persons with PD were caused by a reduced ability to coordinate wrist and finger movements and by a reduced ability to control wrist flexion. Researchers have also reported that individuals with PD have difficulty coordinating arm, hand, and trunk motion during tasks that require trunk-assisted reaching (Bertram et al., 2005; Wang et al., 2006). Bertram et al. (2005) examined multisegmental coordination in persons with PD and healthy aged-matched controls during a prehension task that involved reaching for a glass of water with and without a cover, placed beyond the reach of the outstretched arm. The task required coordinated movement of the arm and trunk. Movement times in persons with PD were comparable to those in healthy controls when reaching for a covered glass of water, but were significantly slower when reaching for an uncovered glass. In addition, there was a difference in the strategy used when reaching for the uncovered cup, with individuals with PD using less trunk motion during forward reaches than did age-matched controls.

Levin (1996) used pointing movements to study upper-extremity control in 10 hemiparetic and 6 control subjects to determine the relationship between functional upper-extremity limitations and underlying impairments such as abnormal synergies and spasticity. Subjects were seated in front of a horizontal surface and made reaching movements to four targets located in front of them (200 and 400 mm) and in the ipsilateral and contralateral workspace (Fig. 18.4). The targets were arranged so that moving toward the ipsilateral target: (1) required an out-of-synergy movement (e.g., a combination of shoulder horizontal abduction and elbow extension), (2) required that movement to the contralateral target could be performed with an extensor synergy (e.g., shoulder adduction and elbow extension), and (3) required that movement to the near and far targets needed a combination of flexor and extensor synergies in order to move the arm forward. Kinematic data were used to study coordination of finger, wrist, elbow, and shoulder joints to the four targets. In addition, subjects underwent clinical

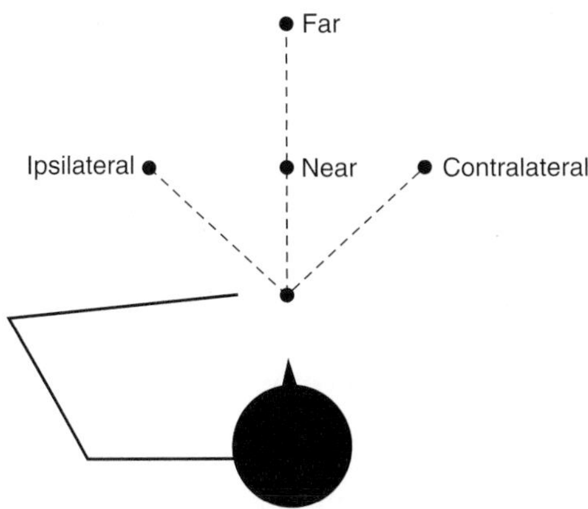

FIGURE 18.4 A diagram of the target positions (black circles) for reaching movements made on a horizontal surface. (Reprinted with permission from Levin MF. Interjoint coordination during pointing movements is disrupted in spastic hemiparesis. Brain 1996;119:283.)

evaluation to assess spasticity (modified Ashworth scale) and sensorimotor function (Fugl–Meyer scale).

For all subjects with hemiparesis, movement times were significantly longer and movement amplitudes smaller in the affected arm as compared with the less affected arm. In the affected arm, trajectories were characterized by segmented movements, increased variability, and disrupted interjoint coordination. This can be seen in Figure 18.5, which compares end-point trajectory and interjoint coordination to all four targets in the less affected arm and the affected arm of one of the subjects with hemiparesis. As can be seen in Figure 18.5, in the less affected arm the trajectories are smooth and continuous, with good coordination of movement in the elbow and shoulder joints.

In contrast, the subject could not produce smooth end-point trajectories in the affected arm (left panels), and movement to the contralateral target is segmented and poorly coordinated. Movement segmentation resulted from a lack of coordination between shoulder- and elbow-joint movements, reminiscent of the findings from studies on reaching in subjects with cerebellar pathology. This disruption of interjoint coordination led to a limitation in active range of elbow- and shoulder-joint motion, resulting in hypometric movements that undershot the target.

Poor coordination was obvious for both movements made within the extensor synergy (to the contralateral target) and those requiring out-of-synergy movements (to near and far targets). Thus, the disruption to movements was not strictly linked to the presence of pathologic movement synergies. Finally, severity of spasticity was correlated with both movement time and amplitude, but not with interjoint coordination measures. The author suggests that

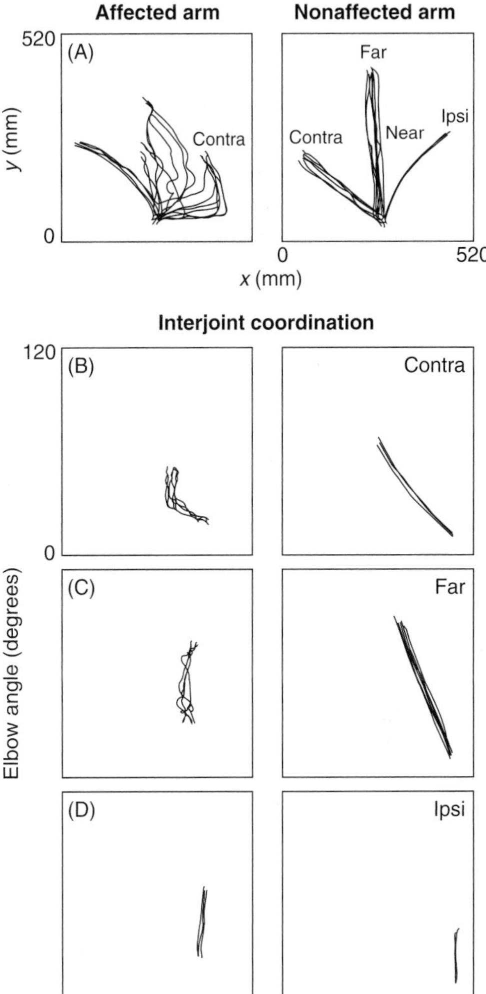

FIGURE 18.5 A comparison of end-point trajectories (A) in spatial coordinates and interjoint coordination (B, C, and D) in angular coordinates for the affected left arm (left panels) and the nonaffected arm (right panels) for a subject with hemiparesis and severe spasticity. Diagrams show movements made from the starting position to the target positions. Trajectories shown in panel A are for movements made to the contralateral (contra), far, near, and ipsilateral (Ipsi) targets. Interjoint coordination (elbow- vs. shoulder-angle diagrams) for the movements in A are shown for the contralateral (B), far (C), and ipsilateral (D) targets. (Redrawn with permission from Levin MF. Interjoint coordination during pointing movements is disrupted in spastic hemiparesis. Brain 1996;119:285.)

regardless of the location of the lesion, following a stroke, the CNS may not be able to determine the optimal set of relationships between muscles and segments to perform smooth coordinated reaching movements (Levin, 1996).

Various researchers have documented deficits in interjoint coordination in children with hemiplegic cerebral palsy. In their study of reaching toward a stationary and a moving ball, Ricken and colleagues (2005) found greater variability and joint segmentation in the coordination patterns between the elbow, shoulder, and trunk in the affected limb. The children tended to show more trunk motion, perhaps in an effort to compensate for the reduction in shoulder and elbow excursion. Others have also provided evidence of greater joint segmentation, describing the reaching pattern in the affected limb as one of increased movement units (Chang et al., 2005; van der Heide et al., 2005). Problems with coordination during reach and grasp have also been reported in children with developmental coordination disorder (DCD). Astill and Utley (2006) studied the kinematics of reach and grasp during a catching task in 10 children with DCD and found that during reach, initiation and movement times were slower, the grasp phase of the movement occurred earlier, and was more variable as well. The authors suggest that during reach and grasp, children with DCD use a decomposition strategy to simplify the movement control of the transport and grasp phases of a catch (Astill & Utley, 2008).

Synergies, Loss of Movement Individuation, and Global Synkinesis. Atypical movement patterns, specifically the presence of abnormal synergies and difficulty with selective movement, are commonly observed in individuals who have had a stroke. Synergies have been defined as fixed patterns of movement involving an entire extremity, with an inability to isolate movements outside the synergy pattern (Twitchell, 1951). Historically, clinicians have characterized recovery from stroke relative to movements both within and outside synergy patterns, with the highest level of recovery associated with the ability to make isolated movements in individual joints (Brunnstrom, 1966; Twitchell, 1951).

However, researchers have demonstrated that upper-extremity movements in healthy subjects are characterized by fixed relationships among upper limb segments—a "synergy" between shoulder and elbow joints. In these studies the term *synergy* means "acting together" and is a characteristic of normal limb movement (Micera et al., 2005). Micera and colleagues describe a synergy as a rule that establishes a relationship among individual joints and shifts control of multijoint movements to a higher level as compared with control of individual joints, thus decreasing the number of variables controlled by the CNS. They examined interjoint arm synergies during 12 different reaching movements in subjects with hemiparesis and healthy controls. Motion analysis was used to examine upper-extremity kinematics, specifically the synergistic relationship between shoulder and elbow angular velocity profiles during different reaching movements. While angular trajectories for the shoulder and elbow were very consistent in the healthy control subjects (strong synergistic coupling), they varied significantly in the hemiparetic group. Thus, in the hemiparetic group there was a disruption to the normal synergistic coupling between shoulder and elbow motion during reaching movements.

While many researchers have examined the role of upper-extremity synergistic relationships to reaching, others have focused on examining the ability to make isolated motions of individual joints or body segments, referred to as "individuation" (Zackowski et al., 2004). Poor individuation results in excessive and unintended motion at linked body segments (Beer et al., 2000; Lang & Schieber, 2004). Studies have shown abnormal coupling between elbow and shoulder torques in the paretic limbs of subjects with hemiparetic stroke that closely parallel abnormal movement synergies characteristic of upper-extremity movement following stroke (Dewald et al., 1999). Abnormal torque coupling makes it difficult for a person with stroke to extend the elbow while simultaneously flexing the shoulder.

Zackowski et al. (2004) studied the impact of impaired joint individuation during reaching in people with chronic hemiparesis. In this study, 18 subjects with chronic hemiparesis and 18 age- and gender-matched controls were evaluated while either reaching up (requiring flexion at both the shoulder and elbow) or reaching out (flexion at the shoulder and extension at the elbow). In addition, subjects performed three upper-extremity individuation movements, shoulder individuation (shoulder flexion with the remaining limb segments in extension), elbow individuation (elbow flexion with no associated movement at the shoulder or wrist), and wrist individuation (wrist extension without associated movement at the elbow and shoulder). Other impairments tested in this study included strength (using a handheld dynamometer), spasticity (response to passive movements using the modified Ashworth scale), and fine touch sensation using a monofilament test.

Results indicated that while both types of reaches were abnormal in the hemiparetic group, performance was worse on the reach-out versus the reach-up task. In addition, the ability to individuate movement at shoulder, elbow, and wrist was significantly impaired. Abnormal individuation is shown in Figure 18.6, which compares individuation at the shoulder (top traces), elbow (middle traces), and wrist (lower traces) in a control subject (A) compared with two subjects with hemiparesis (B and C). The control subject was able to flex the shoulder 73 degrees, with less than 8 degrees of combined motion at the wrist and elbow, resulting in an individuation index of 0.97. Individuation was similarly good at both the elbow and the

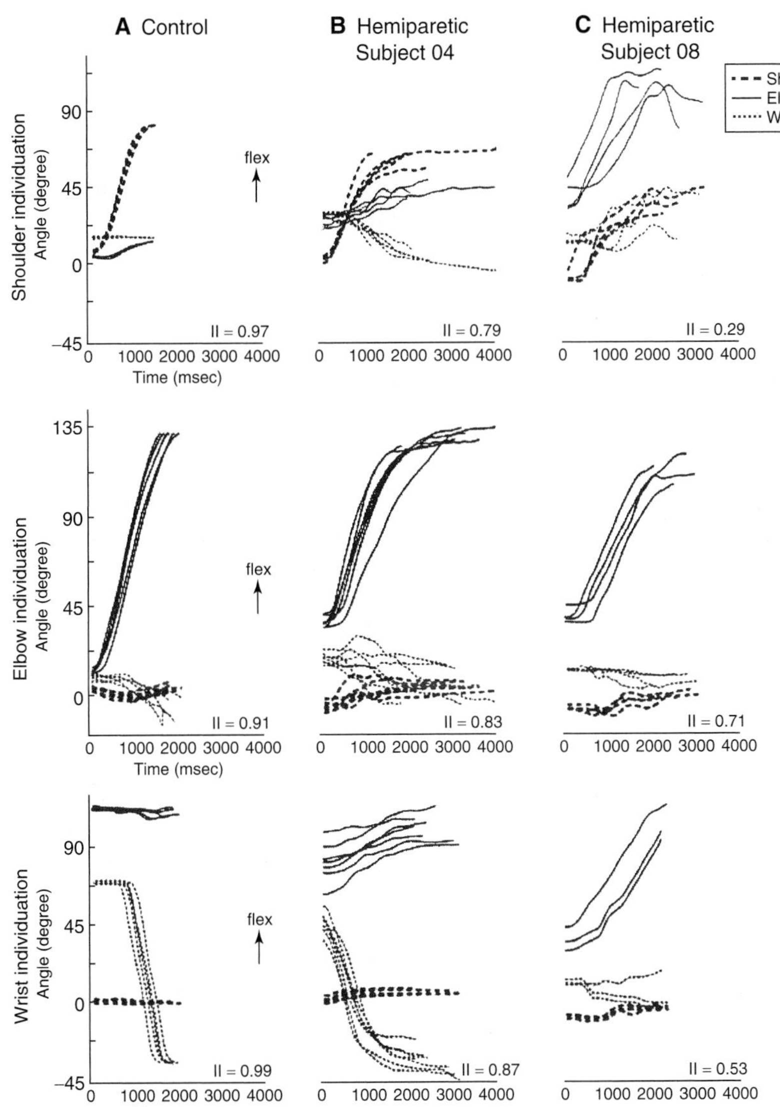

FIGURE 18.6 Abnormal individuation at the shoulder (top traces), elbow (middle traces), and wrist (lower traces) in a control subject (A) and two subjects with hemiparesis (B and C). Bold dashed lines are shoulder angular excursion, narrow solid lines are elbow angular excursion, and narrow dashed lines are wrist angular excursion. Note that in the control subject, individuated motion at the shoulder (top trace) is associated with minimal motion at the elbow and wrist. This is also true for elbow and wrist motion (middle and bottom panels). In contrast, in both subjects with hemiparesis (B and C), motion at the shoulder is associated with significant motion at the elbow and wrist. This is also true when the primary movement is at the elbow (middle panels) and wrist (lower panels). II = individuation index. (Reprinted with permission from Zackowski KM, Dromerick AW, Sahrmann SA, et al. How do strength, sensation, spasticity and joint individuation relate to the reaching deficits of people with chronic hemiparesis? Brain 2004;127:1041.)

wrist. In contrast, both subjects with hemiparesis had difficulty making individuated movements, with subject 04 (Fig. 18.6B) showing mild deficits as compared with subject 08 (Fig. 18.6C). For the subject with mild hemiparesis (subject 04), shoulder flexion to 70 degrees was associated with 15 degrees of elbow flexion and 20 degrees of wrist extension, for an individuation index of 0.79. Similar patterns were also present in the elbow and wrist individuation tasks (middle and lower traces). For the subject with severe hemiparesis, shoulder flexion of 40 degrees was associated with 65 degrees of elbow motion and 20 degrees of wrist motion, resulting in a 0.29 individuation index.

Finally, these researchers used regression analysis to determine which combination of impairments best explained deficits in reaching, including reach trajectories and end-point error and found that individuation explained most of the variance. Sensation also contributed, while strength and spasticity did not. Strength did explain variance in reaching velocity. They conclude that deficits in joint individuation are the primary problem affecting impaired reaching in persons who have had a stroke.

In contrast to Zackowski et al., who did not find strength a major factor in reaching trajectories and end-point error, McCrea and colleagues (2005) argue that insufficient force generation in paretic arm muscles results in the compensatory activation of additional arm muscles, which contributes to atypical movement trajectories during reaching movements following stroke. McCrea and colleagues (2005) compared patterns of muscle recruitment in paretic and nonparetic limbs during a forward reaching movement in 20 individuals who had had a stroke and 10 healthy age-matched controls. They hypothesized that paretic arm muscles would be maximally activated (e.g., saturated) during a sagittal-plane reach, thus requiring compensatory recruitment of other muscles, and this would result in out-of-plane movement trajectories.

Results indicated that muscle recruitment and arm trajectories in the nonparetic arm of the stroke subjects were similar to those in control subjects; however, in the paretic limb, there was increased activation of all muscles, especially the lateral deltoid and anterior deltoid. This pattern of muscle activation resulted in shoulder abduction, segmented interjoint movement, and indirect hand motion. They suggest that the inability to generate sufficient force in paretic arm muscles involved in a forward reach task results in the recruitment of additional muscles in order to successfully complete the task (McCrea et al., 2005).

The studies by McCrea and Zackowski and their colleagues have examined excessive and atypical recruitment of muscles within a paretic limb during a reaching task. Another characteristic of movement following stroke is referred to as global synkinesis or motor irradiation, described as the involuntary and unintentional movement of one limb when the opposite limb is active. Neuroimaging has suggested that global synkinesis results from the bilateral excitation of the motor cortex and a loss of inhibitory influence on the opposite hemisphere via transcallosal fibers (Meyer et al., 1995; Schnitzler et al., 1996).

Hwang and colleagues (2005) used surface electromyography (EMG) to characterize motor irradiation in the paretic upper extremity during flexion movements of the nonparetic contralateral limb in 20 persons with poststroke hemiparesis, classified into one of two groups according to severity of involvement, and 20 healthy controls. In subjects with poststroke hemiparesis, muscle activation in the nonparetic limb was associated with widespread activation of muscles in the paretic limb—global synkinesis. Interestingly, increased levels of global synkinesis were associated with better motor recovery. While control subjects did show some level of global synkinesis (primarily in the elbow flexors), the pattern of muscle recruitment was significantly different in the two patient groups (primary recruitment of shoulder adductors) as compared with the control group.

All of these studies are consistent in reporting excessive activation of muscles within both the paretic and the contralateral limb during upper-extremity movements. There is, however, disagreement as to whether atypical patterns of muscle recruitment represent a primary problem related to stroke or a compensatory mechanism designed to improve functional performance of upper-extremity tasks. In addition, there is a clear difference in the way the term *synergy* is being used.

Many clinicians use the term *synergy* to represent an abnormal coupling of muscles and limb segments during voluntary movements in patients with poststroke hemiparesis. Good recovery is characterized by a reduction in synergistic movements and an increase in individual control of muscles and joints. In contrast, many researchers use the term *synergy* to describe the normal interjoint coupling that is characteristic of higher levels of CNS control. From this perspective, hemiparetic movements are characterized by a decrease in normal synergistic coupling between limb segments. Careful definition of terms by clinicians and researchers alike is necessary to reduce confusion regarding deficits in interjoint coordination affecting reaching movements in patients with CNS pathology.

Sensory Problems

The ability to adapt reaching movements to changes in task and environmental demands is an essential component of normal upper-extremity control. Sensory information is critical to adapting movements and is used to correct errors during the execution of upper-extremity movement, ensuring accuracy during the final portions of the movement.

Effect of Visual Deficits on Visually Guided Reach. The primary function of visual feedback in reaching appears to be related to the attainment of final accuracy. It has been hypothesized that the constancy of thumb position with relation to the wrist during reaching may be part of a strategy of providing clear visual feedback information regarding the end point of the limb (Wing & Frazer, 1983).

Lesions on either side of the posterior parietal area in humans can cause marked eye–hand coordination impairment, or optic ataxia. Optic ataxia is defined as the inability to reach for objects in extrapersonal space, in the absence of extensive motor, visual, or somatosensory deficits (Jeannerod, 1990). Patients with optic ataxia are impaired in their ability to reach and grasp, although they retain the ability to describe objects. In contrast, patients with bilateral occipitotemporal cortex lesions have impaired shape perception (visual-form agnosia) but retain the ability to reach and grasp for objects, although they cannot describe them (Rossetti et al., 2005).

Optic ataxia was first described by Balint in 1909, using the term *visual disorientation*. He noted that the patient could reach normally with his left hand, but when asked to reach with his right hand, he made mistakes in all directions, until he eventually bumped into the object with his hand. He found that the problem was related to visual control of that hand, because if he asked the patient to first point to the object with his left hand, then he could reach accurately with his right hand. On autopsy, it was found that the patient had a lesion in the posterior parietal areas, including the angular gyrus and the anterior occipital lobe on both sides of the brain (Jeannerod, 1990).

There are specific motor disorganization problems in these patients as well. It has been hypothesized that their problems relate to programming visually guided goal-directed movements. It has been shown that the deceleration phase of reaching is much longer than that in the normal hand, with many small peaks. In addition, these patients have problems with grasp formation. Figure 18.7 shows a reach of a patient with optic ataxia with his normal hand (A), with his affected hand, with visual feedback (B), and (C) without vision. Note that even with visual feedback, the affected hand did not begin to close until the last moment and the terminal grip size was too big. Without visual feedback, grasp formation did not occur (Jeannerod, 1990). Thus, it has been suggested that optic ataxia results from a specific problem with eye–hand coordination mechanisms responsible for adjusting finger posture to the shape of the object (Jeannerod, 1990).

Visual motor problems in reaching to a target in individuals with optic ataxia were also described by Rossetti et al. (2005). In this experiment, patients with optic ataxia reached for a target under congruent and incongruent conditions. In the congruent condition, the target was presented at the same location prior to and after a delay during which the target was not visible. In the incongruent task condition, the target was displayed at one location, then after a delay subjects reached for a target that was presented at a different location. Results are shown in Figure 18.8. The control subject (Fig. 18.8A) demonstrated smooth and efficient

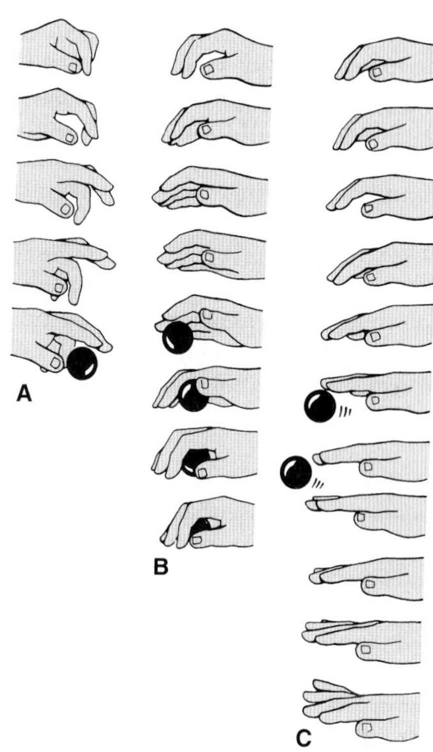

FIGURE 18.7 Grip patterns of a patient with optic ataxia. A, Normal hand. B, Affected hand, visual feedback. C, Affected hand, no visual feedback. (Reprinted with permission from Jeannerod M. The neural and behavioral organization of goal-directed movements. Oxford: Oxford University Press, 1990:225.)

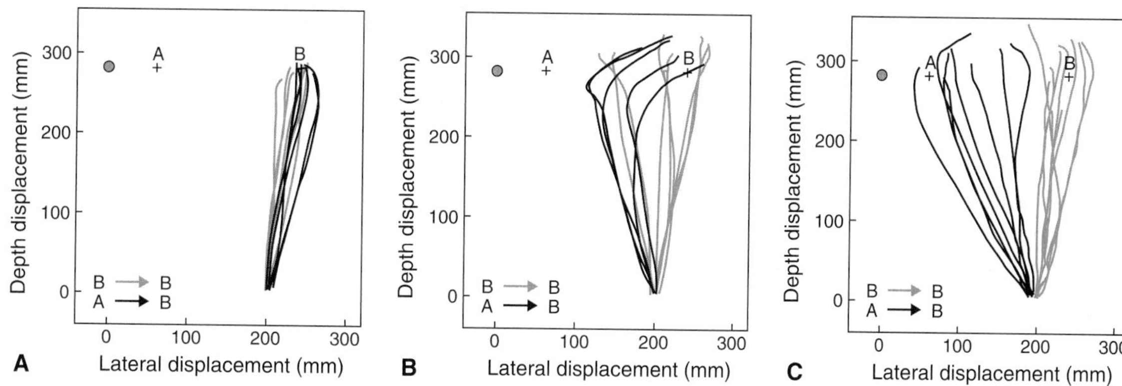

FIGURE 18.8 Reaching trajectories made in congruent (dark lines) and incongruent (light lines) conditions in a healthy control (A) and two subjects with optic ataxia (B and C). The control subject (A) demonstrates smooth and efficient reaching trajectories to point B under both congruent (target placement at point B both before and after the delay) and incongruent (before delay target at point A, after delay target at point B) conditions. Both subjects with optic ataxia (B and C) show impaired trajectories in both conditions. During the incongruent trials, patients initially reach toward the remembered target (located at position A) rather than the actual target (located at position B). (Reprinted with permission from Rossetti Y, Revol P, McIntosh R, et al. Visually guided reaching: bilateral posterior parietal lesions cause a switch from fast visuomotor to slow cognitive control. Neuropsychologia 2005;43:171.)

reaching trajectories to point B under both congruent (target placement at point B both before and after the delay) and incongruent (before delay target at point A, after delay target at point B) conditions. Both subjects with optic ataxia (B and C) show impaired trajectories in both conditions. During the incongruent-condition trials, patients reach initially toward the remembered target (located at position A) rather than the actual target (located at position B). The authors suggest that individuals with optic ataxia rely more on remembered information (slow cognitive control) rather than on online visual information (fast visuomotor control) when reaching (Rossetti et al., 2005).

Effect of Somatosensory Deficits on Reach. Is somatosensory input essential for the production of reaching movements? As noted in earlier chapters, experiments by Sherrington in the late 1800s showed that monkeys that were deafferented on one side of the spinal cord stopped using the affected limb. He thus concluded that sensory feedback was critical to movement control. In contrast, researchers who deafferented both limbs of animals showed that the animals recovered motor function. Movements were initially awkward, but improved within as little as 2 weeks, as long as visual feedback was available (Taub & Berman, 1968).

Interestingly, recovery starts with the animals being able to only sweep the object across the floor. Then, a coarse grasp with all four fingers develops, and then a pincer grasp reappears (Taub, 1976). It has been suggested that when unilateral deafferentation occurs, the animals may learn not to use the deafferented limb, or may even develop inhibition of the deafferented arm (Taub, 1976). This "learned disuse" hypothesis is supported by the fact that unilaterally deafferented animals recover movement coordination as well as bilaterally deafferented animals if their nonaffected limb remains immobilized so that they have to use the deafferented limb (Jeannerod, 1990).

Also, remember from Chapter 16 that experiments on deafferented monkeys showed that, when making single-joint movements, they could reach targets with relative accuracy, even when they could not see the hand. Displacing the forearm just prior to movement onset during a reach also did not significantly disturb pointing accuracy in these deafferented animals. It was thus concluded that single-joint movements depend on changes in muscle activation levels that are programmed prior to movement onset and that no feedback is required for reasonably accurate execution of these movements (Polit & Bizzi, 1979).

In addition, experiments on humans after pathological deafferentation have confirmed the results from experiments on monkeys (Rothwell et al., 1982). One patient had suffered a severe peripheral sensory neuropathy, so that there was loss of sensation in both the arms and the legs. Light touch, vibration, and temperature sensation were impaired or totally absent in both hands. Tests showed that in spite of these problems, the patient could perform many motor tasks, even without vision. For example, the patient could tap, do fast alternating flexion and extension movements, and draw figures in the air, using only the wrist and fingers (Jeannerod, 1990; Rothwell et al., 1982).

It was also noted that EMG activity during flexion and extension of the thumb was similar to that seen in normal subjects. The subject could also learn new thumb positions with vision and then reproduce those positions without vision. Thus, motor learning was also possible. However, the patient's performance rapidly deteriorated when asked to repeat the movement many times with the eyes closed.

In a second study on patients with peripheral sensory neuropathy, patients could perform repetitive flexion and extension movements of the wrist, with normal EMG activity, as long as the movements were not too fast. At a certain point, however, the intervals between the EMG bursts tended to disappear. It was hypothesized that this was due to the higher level of cocontraction of agonist and antagonist muscles seen in these patients (Sanes et al., 1985). Patients could also hold a steady posture with their deafferented limb as long as they had visual feedback. However, without visual feedback, large errors were made, and the limb drifted back to its initial position, as shown in Figure 18.9 (Sanes et al., 1985). This was further supported in work by Sainburg and colleagues (1993, 1995), who compared patients with proprioceptive deafferentation with controls during a pantomimed task of slicing bread. This task required sharp joint reversals in movement direction. They found that without visual feedback, controls exhibited synchronous movements of the shoulder and elbow at the reversal, exploiting the interaction torques. However, patients showed timing errors at shoulder- and elbow-joint reversals, resulting in large trajectory errors. The authors concluded that without proprioception, patients were unable to control the interaction torques, disrupting the interjoint coordination necessary to perform this multijoint task with ease. Performance improved significantly with vision.

What does this information tell us about the role of kinesthetic feedback in reaching? It appears that it is not required for movement initiation and execution. However, it is still important for accurate reaching involving multiple joints. Researchers testing humans with peripheral sensory neuropathy found that patients were able to make accurate movements only if they involved single joints or if they were

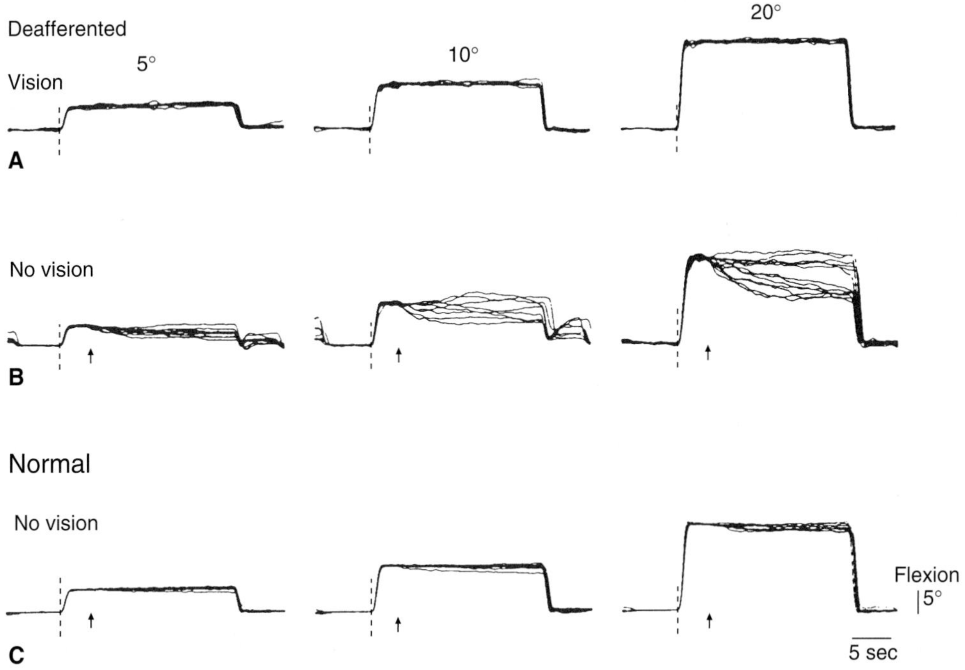

FIGURE 18.9 Recordings of wrist position of a patient with peripheral sensory neuropathy. The patient was asked to rotate the wrist to reach positions of 5, 10, and 20 degrees against an elastic load. A, With vision, the patient had no problems. B, When the visual cue related to the position to be maintained was removed (shown by the up-pointing arrow), the position drifted back in the direction of the load. C, A normal subject's performance showing that even when the visual position cue is removed, wrist position is fairly well maintained. (Redrawn with permission from Sanes JN, Mauritz KH, Dalakas MC, Evarts EV. Motor control in humans with large-fiber sensory neuropathy. Hum Neurobiol 1985;4:101.)

able to compensate using vision. They showed great problems in performing natural movements used in everyday life (Sanes et al., 1985).

Problems with Grasp

In addition to problems with reach, many studies have reported deficits in grasp in a wide variety of patients with neurologic pathology. For example, a number of researchers have described deficits in grasp following stroke, including slower and less accurate finger and hand movements, poorly modulated fingertip forces, and a reduced ability to control individual fingers (Hermsdörfer et al., 2003; Lang & Schieber, 2004; van Vliet & Sheridan, 2007). Not surprisingly, the degree of deficit shown is highly dependent on the severity of stroke. For example, among individuals with less severe paresis, the ability to scale grip aperture to object size for different grasp types is retained; however, timing deficits—including slowed movement times, prolonged deceleration times, and earlier time to maximal grip aperture—remain (Michaelsen et al., 2009).

Because the greatest proportion of inputs from the corticospinal tract is to motor neuron pools of the distal upper segments, it has been reported that the severity of hemiparesis following stroke is most often greatest in the distal as compared with the proximal muscles (Colebatch & Gandevia, 1989). This has led to the hypothesis that after stroke, deficits in grasp, which rely on distal limb segments, are greater than those in reach, which rely on proximal segment motion. Lang et al. (2005) found that among persons with acute hemiparesis, the ability to perform a purposeful movement with the distal segments was not clearly more disrupted than movements made with the proximal segments.

In examining the recovery of reach and grasp following stroke, these researchers reported that the majority of recovery in both reach and grasp occurred by the 90-day time point, with little change occurring between the 90-day and 1-year time points. Movement speed improved over time for both reach and grasp, as did deficits in accuracy in both components. In contrast, deficits in efficiency did not recover, and they were greater in grasp than reach (Lang et al., 2006).

Reach and grasp deficits may vary as a function of the side of the lesion, since hemispheric specialization appears to contribute to differential reach and grasp impairments following stroke. Tretriluxana and colleagues (2008, 2009) investigated the role of hemispheric specialization in visuomotor transformation of grasp preshaping and the coordination between transport and grasp in individuals after stroke. Components of grasp preshaping, including changes in aperture velocity and peak aperture relative to three different object dimensions, were measured in patients with right versus left hemiparesis. There were significant differences between the groups. Movement times were prolonged for the right- but not the left-stroke group. In addition, for the right-stroke group, grasp preshaping began earlier but was less coordinated as compared with the left-stroke group, whose primary deficit was in scaling grasp preshaping. The authors suggest that the left hemisphere is specialized for the visuomotor transformation of grasp preshaping, while the right hemisphere specialization is related to transport-grasp coordination (Tretriluxana et al., 2009).

Bradykinesia contributes to slowing in both the reach and grasp components in individuals with Parkinson's disease, though the degree of slowing may be task-dependent (Majsak et al., 2008; Rand et al., 2006, 2009). Majsak et al. (2008) reported that among persons with PD, slowing was present when reaching for a stationary object, but movement times were comparable to those of controls when reaching for moving objects (Majsak et al., 2008). In addition, disease progression appears to affect grasp components more than reach components. Grasp was characterized by slower velocity of hand opening and closing, a smaller maximal aperture, a longer time to maximal aperture as compared with healthy subjects (Majsak et al., 2008), and increased variability in aperture timing and scaling (Alberts et al., 2000). Interestingly, even in a relatively advanced stage of the disease, persons with PD retain the ability to modify reach and grasp in response to object properties (Weiss et al., 2009; Negrotti et al., 2005). Medications, such as L-dopa, appear to improve the kinematics of reach more than grasp (Negrotti et al., 2005; Schettino et al., 2006), leading to the hypothesis that slowed reach in PD is in part a strategy used to compensate for deficiencies in the grasp component of the task (Negrotti et al., 2005).

Studies have examined the reach-and-grasp behavior of developmentally disabled children, including those with cerebral palsy (Cole et al., 1998; Eliasson et al., 1991; Jeannerod, 1986; Kearney & Gentile, 2003; Mackey et al., 2006; Petrarca et al., 2009; Ronnqvist & Rosblad, 2007; Saavedra et al., 2009; Verrel et al., 2008). In some cases of mild impairment, hemiplegia is not readily identified until about 40 weeks, when the infant first begins to use the pincer grasp and manipulate objects (Jeannerod, 1990). In a 23-month-old child, the hand with hemiplegia was used only when the normal hand was immobilized, and even then, it was with great difficulty that the child grasped objects. Figure 18.10, adapted from film records, illustrates the child reaching for a prong from a pegboard with the normal hand and the affected hand, with visual feedback. Note that the normal hand did not anticipate the shape of the object well, but a finger extension/flexion pattern was used. Also, contact of the hand with the object caused the fingers to close around the object, giving an accurate grasp. However, the hemiplegic hand showed an exaggerated opening during the entire movement, with no anticipatory grasp formation. There was a very slight closing of the hand after contact with the object, giving a very clumsy grasp (Jeannerod, 1990).

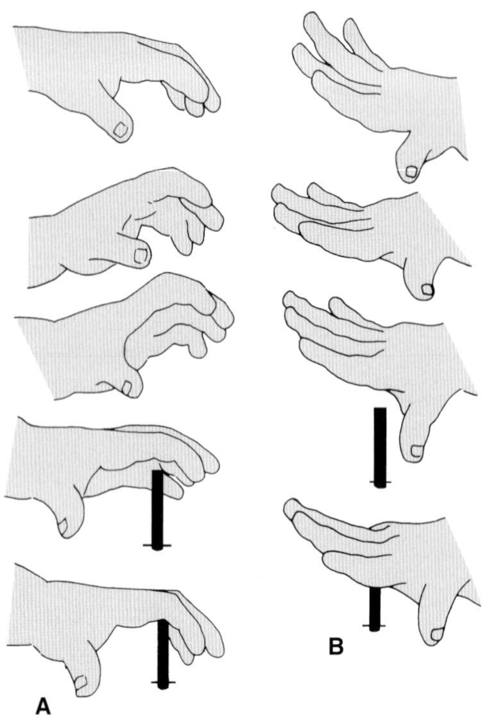

FIGURE 18.10 Drawing from film records of the reaches of a 23-month-old child with hemiplegia reaching for a prong from a pegboard with the nonaffected hand (A) and the affected hand (B). (Redrawn with permission from Jeannerod M. The neural and behavioral organization of goal-directed movements. Oxford: Oxford University Press, 1990:72.)

In a second child, 5 years of age, the hemiplegic hand showed more normal reaches and grasp movements. The authors suggest that more normal movement patterns may be the result of many years of rehabilitation training (Jeannerod, 1990). Figure 18.11 depicts film records of her reaching movements with her normal hand (A) and her hemiplegic hand (B, C, and D). Note that reaching with the hemiplegic hand was affected only in relation to the pattern of grip formation. Finger shaping was abnormal, with the index finger extended in an exaggerated manner, and then flexing only slightly, if at all, before contacting the

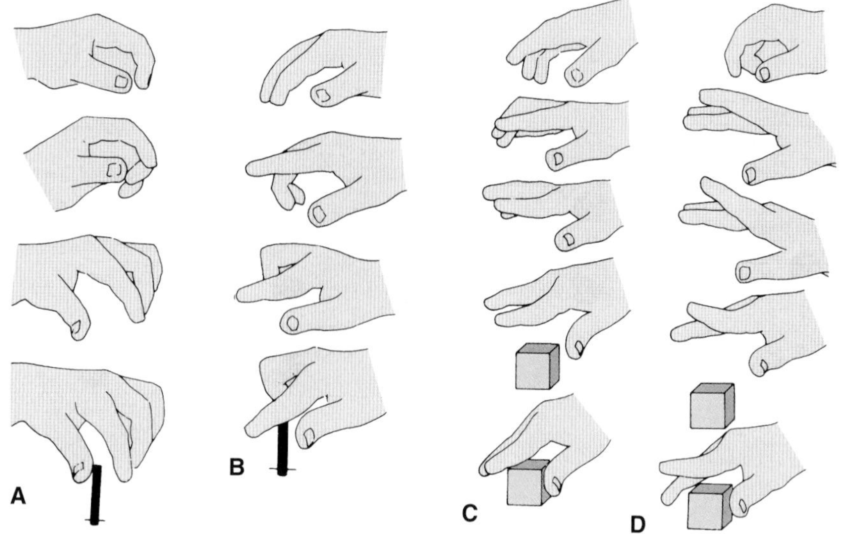

FIGURE 18.11 Drawing from film records of the reaches of a 5-year-old child with hemiplegia after many years of rehabilitation reaching with the non-affected hand (A) and the affected hand (B, C, and D). (Redrawn with permission from Jeannerod M. The neural and behavioral organization of goal-directed movements. Oxford: Oxford University Press, 1990:73.)

object. Because of these problems, the objects were sometimes dropped during the grasp (Jeannerod, 1990).

Hanna and colleagues (2003) also examined changes in hand function (Peabody fine motor scores) and upper-extremity movement using the Quality of Upper Extremity Skills Test (QUEST, DeMatteo et al., 1992) in 51 children with cerebral palsy (29 boys and 22 girls; mean age, 36 months) studied prospectively four times over 10 months. Results found that hand function developed differently from overall upper-extremity function. Figure 18.12 compares Peabody fine motor scores in children with cerebral palsy as a function of children's ages. At 16 months of age, children had a mean hand function score of 101.9 points, and showed a positive improvement, on average, of 2.36 points per month. This average rate of improvement was slower in the older children, while interindividual variation increased. In contrast to the hand function measures, measures of upper-extremity movement using QUEST scores demonstrated significant interindividual variability across all ages.

Experiments have been performed in which the reach-and-grasp skills of patients with lesions in the somatosensory pathways at brainstem levels and at parietal-cortex levels were examined. In the patient with the lesion at the brainstem level, the hand ipsilateral to the lesion was affected. When vision was

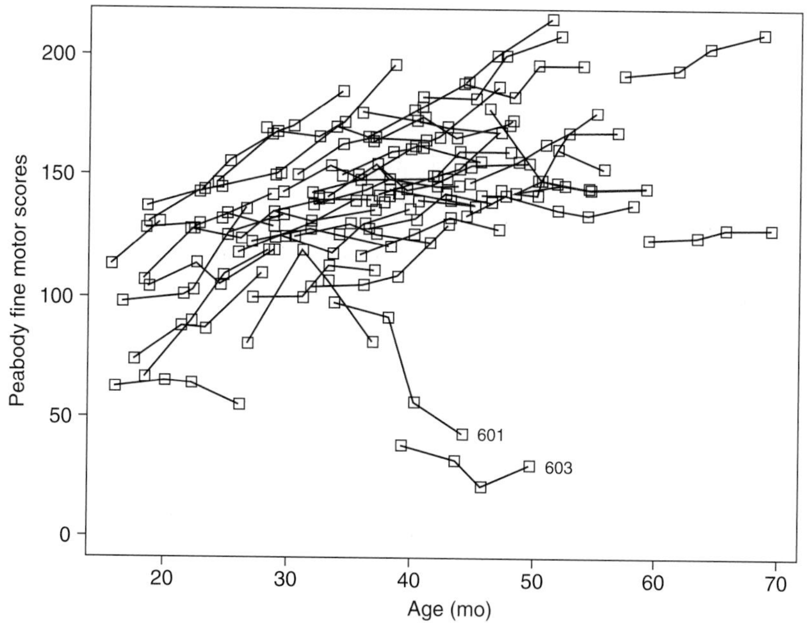

FIGURE 18.12 Changes in hand function in children with cerebral palsy studied four times over a 10-month period. Shown are observed Peabody fine motor scores as a function of children's ages. Numbers 601 and 603 indicate the study numbers of children with atypical patterns of change. (Reprinted with permission from Hanna SE, Law MC, Rosenbaum PL, et al. Development of hand function among children with cerebral palsy: growth curve analysis for ages 16 to 70 months. Dev Med Child Neurol 2003;45:449.)

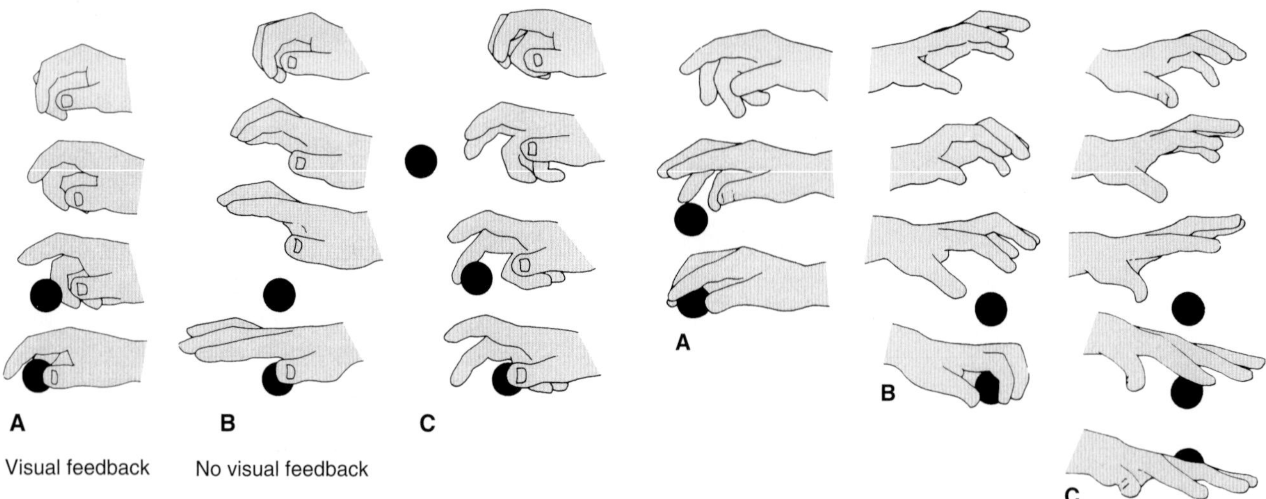

FIGURE 18.13 Drawing from film records of the grip patterns of a patient with a lesion of the somatosensory pathway at the brainstem level. A, With vision, grasp was normal. B and C, Without vision, grasp was absent or incomplete. (Redrawn with permission from Jeannerod M. The neural and behavioral organization of goal-directed movements. Oxford: Oxford University Press, 1990:205.)

FIGURE 18.14 Drawing of the grip patterns of a patient with a parietal lobe lesion. A, Normal hand, visual feedback. B, Affected hand, visual feedback. C, Affected hand, no visual feedback. (Redrawn with permission from Jeannerod M. The neural and behavioral organization of goal-directed movements. Oxford: Oxford University Press, 1990:208.)

present, grasp formation was normal, as shown in Figure 18.13A, except that it was longer in duration than it was in the normal hand. However, without vision, the grasping movements were critically changed (Fig. 18.13, B and C). Finger grip was either absent altogether, or incomplete. In the first reach the patient made with no visual feedback, there was no grip formation at all, while in the second reach, there was incomplete grip formation (Jeannerod, 1990).

Patients with lesions to the parietal lobe, particularly the postcentral gyrus and the supramarginal gyrus, show patterns for reach and grasp that are similar to those of patients with peripheral sensory problems. In a detailed study on the recovery of reach and grasp in a patient with a parietal lobe lesion, researchers found that the patient did not use her right hand spontaneously immediately following her lesion, but later used it in many actions, as long as she had visual feedback. Without visual control, her movements were very awkward. For example, she could not sustain repetitive tapping movements unless she could see or hear her fingers moving (Jeannerod, 1990).

In contrast to patients with peripheral deafferentation, who could grip normally as long as visual feedback was present, grip formation was impaired in the patient with a parietal lesion, even with visual feedback present (Jeannerod, 1990). Figure 18.14A shows the grasp component of a reach with the patient's normal hand, while B and C show the grasp of the affected hand both with and without visual feedback. When the patient had visual feedback while reaching with the affected hand, she made grasps using the whole palm of the hand. Without visual feedback, only the initial part of the transportation phase was normal. Then the hand seemed to "wander above the object, without a grasp" (Jeannerod, 1990, p. 207). Thus, loss of sensory information results in abnormal grip and lift forces, and problems in the control of fine movements of the hand.

Problems with Precision Grip and Lift

The ability to produce and regulate force is an important aspect of tasks in which an object has to be grasped and lifted. Tactile sensation from the fingertips is particularly important when lifting objects with a precision grip in order to adjust the amplitude of forces used to grip and lift. If grip force is too tight, the object cannot be manipulated; if it is too loose, the object will be dropped. In a precision grip, forces for gripping and lifting are generated simultaneously and appear to be very dependent on cutaneous input.

Impairments in the regulation of forces for precision grip-and-lift tasks have been reported in a wide variety of patients with neural pathology. For example, disruptions to the initiation and sequencing of grip-and-lift forces have been reported in patients with PD. Grip forces in persons with PD are much greater than those of healthy controls, and force development is slower (Rand et al., 2009;

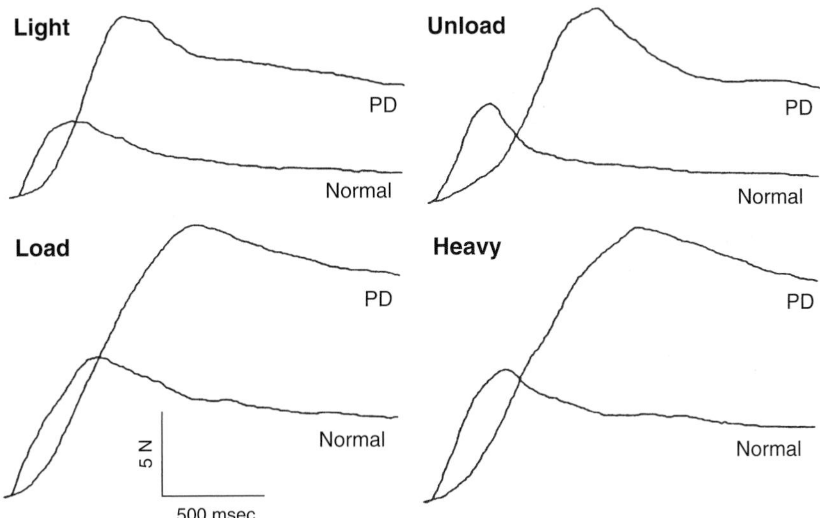

FIGURE 18.15 Mean grip force curves for a person with PD and an age-matched control, obtained from five lifts performed under four conditions (expecting and lifting a light load [Light], expecting and lifting a heavy load [Heavy], expecting a heavy load and lifting a light load [Unload], and expecting a light load and lifting a heavy load [Load]. As expected, for both subjects with PD and normal controls, peak grip force values were higher for the heavier loads as compared with values for lighter loads (compare "Heavy" traces with "Light"). Subjects with PD tended to produce inappropriately high grip forces compared with normal controls in all conditions. 5 N = 5 Newtons. (Redrawn with permission from Fellows SJ, Noth J, Schwarz M. Precision grip and Parkinson's disease. Brain 1998;121:1776.)

Weiss et al., 2009). Despite these deficits, individuals with PD were able to adapt grip force to load conditions (Weiss et al., 2009). Ingvarsson and colleagues (1997) reported frequent oscillations and fluctuations in the force profiles associated with grip-and-lift movements in subjects with PD, while "off" medication. The amplitude of oscillations decreased when subjects were "on" medication, suggesting the oscillations were due to action tremor superimposed on the force trajectories.

Fellows et al. (1998) investigated force development in 16 individuals with PD and 12 age-matched controls. Subjects performed a grip-and-lift task under conditions in which the weight of the object was altered both with and without warning. Results for the grip-and-lift task under the four conditions are shown in Figure 18.15. The subjects with PD, like the control subjects, lifted the unpredictable load using grip-force parameters they had used in the preceding lift. Both groups were able to modulate grip forces to the new load during the lift. However, subjects with PD required a significantly longer time to develop grip force as compared with the healthy controls in all conditions. In addition, they showed significantly higher levels of grip force during the lift phase of the movement, indicating a higher safety margin than seen in control subjects. However, individuals with PD were capable of modulating grip forces to match changes in the object weight.

A study examining grasp and lift in children with cerebral palsy (CP) documented the presence of excessive and oscillatory grip forces (Eliasson et al., 1991). Eliasson et al. also found that in contrast to healthy control children, children with CP did not coordinate grip and lift forces simultaneously, but sequentially. The authors suggest that these excessive grip forces, establishing a high safety margin against slips, may be compensatory to unstable motor output. This type of safety margin has been reported in older adults and in young healthy children under the age of 5, who also show oscillations in force control. What are some of the other factors that contribute to impairments in force regulation during grip-and-lift tasks? A number of studies suggest sensory deficits as a primary cause.

Sensory Deficits and Precision Grip. How does loss of somatosensation affect precision grip? It appears that both impaired somatosensation and deficits in force production contribute to reduced hand function following stroke (Blennerhassett et al., 2007; Robertson & Jones, 1994). In individuals with poststroke hemiparesis, reduced somatosensation, specifically impaired friction-discrimination ability, contributed to altered timing and force adjustment during tasks that required a precision pinch grip (Blennerhassett et al., 2007). In addition, reduced somatosensation (pressure sensitivity and two-point discrimination) significantly affected the regulation of grip-and-lift forces.

Surprisingly, despite impaired somatosensation, the ability to adapt forces to changes in the weight and surface properties of the object being held correlated with poor performance on object-recognition tests; it did not predict performance on functional hand tests, such as the Jebsen–Taylor hand function test (Robertson & Jones, 1994).

Lesions of the anterior parietal lobe result in somatosensory deficits that limit precision grip and in-hand manipulation skills (Jeannerod, 1996). Pause et al. (1989) referred to these motor impairments due to central sensory deficits as "tactile apraxia." Lesions of the posterior parietal area produce spatial disorientation and misreaching. Lesions in this area affect the ability to shape the hand according to object size and configuration. Deficits are more severe in the absence of visual feedback from the limb (Jeannerod, 1996). Damage to posterior parietal areas produces a disconnection between visual and proprioceptive inputs, so that limb and object positions in space are no longer matched with each other. Thus, the importance of the posterior parietal lobe is in organizing object-oriented action. Sakata et al. (1985) suggest that neurons in this area are able to integrate visual and motor signals related to object-oriented action, thus linking sensory information on object properties with corresponding motor commands.

Impaired Anticipatory Control of Precision Grip. As discussed in Chapters 16 and 17, the development of precision grip and manipulation depends on the availability of both tactile information (from both slow- and fast-adapting afferents, which convey information on texture) and weight-related information (from muscles spindles and tactile afferents) (Johansson, 1996). During an ongoing lift, small slips between the skin and the object result in activation of cutaneous receptors, which causes the grip force to be increased. Sensory information is also used in the development of internal representations about an object's physical characteristics. During subsequent lifts, expectations based on internal representations of the object are used to preprogram grip-and-lift forces. Thus, scaling of forces is performed prior to the lift and is dependent on both sensorimotor memory (internal representations) and current sensory (visual and tactile) information (Gordon et al., 1997). Anticipatory control emerges with development. By 6 to 8 years of age, anticipatory control of fingertip forces (both pinch and vertical lift) is adult-like (Forssberg et al., 1992; Gordon et al., 1992).

Gordon and Duff (1999a) studied anticipatory grip-and-lift forces in 15 children, ages 8 to 14 years, with spastic hemiplegic CP. They found that children with CP were initially impaired in their ability to scale forces during the first few trials of a grip-and-lift task. However, they eventually learned to use anticipatory control of load forces based on the texture and weight of an object, but only after extended practice with the object.

Duff and Gordon (2003) also investigated the effects of practice on anticipatory aspects of grasp in children with hemiparetic CP who were learning to grasp novel objects. In this study, 18 children with hemiparetic CP practiced lifting three novel objects of varying weight but constant volume 27 times using either a blocked or random practice schedule. Children with CP were able to form and retain internal representation of novel objects for anticipatory control of grasp, but anticipatory control was not as well differentiated in the children with CP as compared with age-matched typically developing children. They also reported that while blocked practice was superior during the acquisition of novel grasp tasks, retention was comparable in both practice types, leading the authors to conclude that for children with hemiparetic CP, the amount of practice is more important than the type of practice when learning to grasp novel objects.

What is the basis for the deficits found in children with CP in initial ability to scale the rate of force to the weight of the object to be lifted? Gordon and Duff (1999a) report no clear relationship between degree of spasticity and anticipatory control of grip and lift in children with CP, suggesting that spasticity, while present, was not the major factor related to impaired grip and lift. In addition, they found that sensory information from the less affected hand could transfer to improve anticipatory scaling of forces by the contralateral (affected) hand in subsequent manipulations (Gordon et al., 1999a). These two findings suggest that sensory deficits account for many problems related to precision grip and lift.

The assumption that sensory deficits are a major factor in impaired precision grip in children with CP is supported by results from a study by Eliassson & Gordon (2000), who found impaired tactile regulation of isometric fingertip forces during grasping in these children. They suggest that children with CP who have sensory impairments may not be able to extract enough information during initial manipulatory experiences to form internal representations of the object's properties. Instead they appear to require considerable practice to form accurate internal representations of objects.

Impaired Adaptation. Daily life activities require us to continually modify and adapt how we reach and grasp to changing task conditions. Objects to be picked up and manipulated vary in size, shape, and weight. This requires the ability to adjust to changing

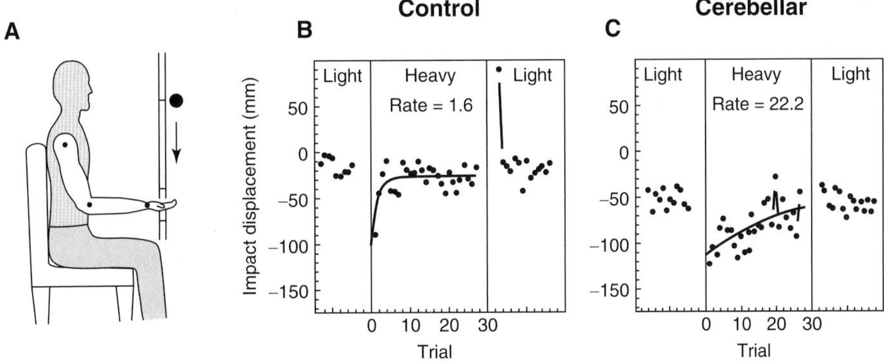

FIGURE 18.16 Experimental setup for adaptation of a catching task. Subjects sit and catch a ball, which is dropped vertically (A). Impact-displacement values are plotted as a function of trials. A control subject (B) catches a light ball initially (left panel), then adapts within two trials to catching a heavy ball (middle panel). When the light ball is reintroduced (right panel), the subject shows a large negative impact displacement on the first trial. In contrast, the subject with cerebellar pathology (C) requires 22 trials to adapt to the heavy ball (middle panel) and has no negative impact displacement on the first trial when the light ball is reintroduced (right panel). (Adapted from Bastian AJ. Cerebellar limb ataxia: abnormal control of self generated and external forces. Ann NY Acad Sci 2002;978:23, 24.)

conditions, and this is done through practice. Cerebellar pathology reduces a person's ability to adjust to novel loads through trial-and-error practice (Bastian, 2002; Lang & Bastian, 1999, 2001). Bastian and colleagues used a catching task to examine adaptation to a novel load (light vs. heavy ball). The experimental setup is shown in Figure 18.16. Subjects caught a ball dropped vertically. Adaptation was determined from measures of impact displacement, and the rate of adaptation was defined by how quickly impact displacement changed after exposure to a new ball. Figure 18.16 compares impact displacement in a control subject (B) and a person with cerebellar pathology (C) as subjects initially caught a light ball (left panel), adapted to a heavy ball (middle), then were reintroduced to the light ball (right). As can be seen in the middle panel, when learning to catch a heavy ball after exposure to a light ball, the subject with cerebellar pathology adapted much more slowly as compared with the control subject. Control subjects adapted rapidly (average, 1.6 trials) as compared with participants with cerebellar pathology (average, 24.6 trials). In addition, when the light ball was reintroduced, the control subjects showed a large aftereffect (large impact displacement in the first trial of the right panel), while the subjects with cerebellar pathology did not. These results support the hypothesis that the cerebellum is important in the ability to adapt movements to changing task demands through practice.

Problems with In-Hand Manipulation

In typically developing individuals, prehension and in-hand manipulation are associated with a complex interaction between the fingers in order to isolate motion (Hager-Ross & Schieber, 2000; Schieber, 1995) and coordinate forces (Scholz et al., 2002). While mechanical coupling may be responsible for limitations in finger independence in typical individuals (Lang & Schieber, 2004), after a subcortical stroke, adults show greater deficits in finger individuation (Raghaven, 2007), perhaps stemming from disruptions in corticomotoneuronal loops. In contrast, persons with Down syndrome (DS) show a less complex pattern of interfinger coordination in which forces within individual fingers are not independently modifiable; rather, force control among the fingers is linked (Latash et al., 2002). However, finger coordination in those with DS can be modified with variable practice as shown by Latash and colleagues (2002). In a related experiment Latash and colleagues (2002) reported that variable practice was superior to constant practice during the acquisition of an interfinger force coordination grasp task in persons with DS.

Problems with Release

Gordon and colleagues (1997) studied task-dependent problems during release of an object in subjects with PD, both on and off medication. Results showed that impairments in grasping and releasing objects were dependent on the task condition. Coordination of grip and load forces in subjects with PD approximated those of normal subjects during object replacement and release at preferred speeds. In contrast, when instructed to move as quickly as possible, release was significantly slower as compared with age-matched controls (Gordon et al., 1997). These findings were consistent with those of Kunesch and colleagues (1995), who also found that impaired release of an isotonic force was impaired in subjects with PD.

Eliasson and Gordon (2000) examined object release in children between 8 and 14 years of age who had hemiplegic CP. They found that these children tended to replace objects abruptly as compared with controls, and they took a longer time to release objects from finger contact. In a follow-up study (Gordon et al., 2003) the speed (self-paced and as fast as possible) and accuracy requirements (stable and unstable release surface) of the task were altered. The authors found that the impairments in temporal coordination of replacement and release of the novel object were greater and significantly different from those of controls when the speed and accuracy requirements were higher. Interestingly, impairments in release were also found in the less-affected hand.

Interlimb Coupling and Bimanual Tasks

Researchers have studied the effect of coupling the paretic and nonparetic limbs during bimanual reaching in individuals with hemiparesis in order to determine whether paretic arm reaching improves under the bilateral condition as compared with the unilateral condition (Harris et al., 2005; Rose & Winstein, 2004; Utley & Sugden, 1998; Wu et al., 2008). Rose and Winstein (2004) compared unimanual to bimanual aiming in individuals with hemiparesis secondary to a cerebrovascular accident (CVA) and found that during bimanual reaches the less-affected limb extended its movement time to allow nearly simultaneous target contact. When the bimanual condition was compared with the unimanual condition, peak velocity decreased for the less-affected limb and increased for the affected limb. Similarly, Utley and Sugden (1998) reported that during bimanual reaches in children with CP, the affected limb sped up and the less-affected slowed down during bimanual reaching tasks, resulting in greater coupling between limbs.

Wu et al. (2008) examined the ability to adapt movements to objects of different sizes during a bimanual prehension task in 14 patients with left CVAs and 13 healthy controls. Movement kinematics were used to characterize both intralimb and interlimb coordination while participants reached to grasp a large and a small jar with the affected hand and to open the cap with the other hand. Participants with stroke were able to adapt reach and grasp in both their affected and nonaffected limbs to changes in object size, though timing was altered in the affected limb.

Speed may play a role in coordination during bimanual tasks. Hung et al. (2004) examined the coordination of involved and noninvolved hands during a bimanual task in children with hemiplegic CP (mean age, 13 years) and 10 age-matched typically developing children. Children were asked to reach forward and open a drawer with one hand and then activate a light switch inside the drawer with the contralateral hand. The children with hemiplegic CP were slower and less coordinated than the typically developing children. Interestingly, when asked to complete the task as fast as possible, the faster speed facilitated better bimanual coordination.

Reach and Grasp in the Ipsilesional Nonhemiparetic Limb

Traditionally, researchers have maintained that unilateral cerebral lesions manifest in the limb contralateral to the lesions. Now researchers are also finding subtle deficits affecting the ability to reach on the nonhemiparetic side or ipsilesional limb (Giulliani et al., 1993; Gordon et al., 1999; Haaland et al., 2004; Nowak et al., 2007; Quaney et al., 2005; Sunderland, 2000). For example, a study examining motor problems in the ipsilesional nonhemiparetic limb has suggested that weakness is a contributing factor in reaching problems in this limb as well as the hemiparetic limb (Giulliani et al., 1993). Other studies have found that problems in reaching in the ipsilesional nonhemiparetic arm following unilateral hemispheric lesion may involve other factors as well.

Gordon et al. (1999) studied the coordination of fingertip forces during object manipulation in both affected and nonaffected hands of children with hemiplegic CP. They found subtle deficits in sequencing of grip-and-lift movements in the nonaffected hand. Sunderland (2000) studied dexterity and apraxia in the ipsilesional hands of 24 patients with an acute stroke. All patients showed initial deficits in the ipsilesional hand on tests of dexterity and apraxia; however, most had recovered by 6 months after the stroke. Seven patients, all of whom had left hemispheric damage, continued to show persistent problems related to dexterity and apraxia in the ipsilesional hand.

Bilateral impairments in hand function found in both children with CP and in adult patients who had had a unilateral stroke are not surprising, considering that 10 to 30% of fibers in the lateral corticospinal tract are uncrossed. These data support an anatomical substrate for bilateral impairment in hand function in individuals with lesions affecting one hemisphere.

APRAXIA

In the preceding sections, our discussion of abnormal reach and grasp has related to the examination of problems in each of the constituent components: visual regard, reach, grasp, manipulation, and release. However, the use of the upper extremity in the performance of simple everyday tasks is more than the simple summation of these components. It requires the integration of these components into an action plan. An action plan specifies the conceptual content of the action, along with its hierarchical and sequential organization (Poizner et al., 1990). The left cerebral cortex includes structures specialized for higher-order motor programming or the formation of action plans (Schwartz et al., 1991).

One way researchers have studied the nature of these motor programs is by analyzing the types of errors made by patients with left hemispheric damage. Disorders that result from dysfunction of this specialized left hemisphere have been termed "apraxias." One type of apraxia that has been studied extensively is ideational apraxia, also referred to as "frontal apraxia" (Luria, 1966) or "frontal lobe executive disorder" (Wilkens et al., 1987). This is a disorder of the execution of movement that cannot be attributed to weakness, incoordination or sensory loss, or poor language comprehension or inattention to commands.

To understand this disorder, it is helpful to first appreciate what occurs when a normal adult decides to perform a task. It is hypothesized that the first step involves formulating the intention to perform the task and then formulating an action plan. The essential requirement of an action plan is that it specifies the goal of the action along with the hierarchical and sequential organization of nested actions that are required to achieve the ultimate goal. Intentions, as defined by activated action plans, are an integral feature of all purposeful behavior. It has been hypothesized that the core of the intentional disorder of frontal apraxia is a weakening of the top-down formulation of action plans—that is, an inability to sustain the intent to the completion of the action plan (Schwartz et al., 1991).

As a result, irrelevant objects exert a strong influence on the action plan, and this leads to numerous performance errors. Researchers have begun to develop a system for coding performance errors based on this concept of hierarchically organized units of action within an action plan. These studies have enumerated examples of errors during the performance of common activities of daily living, including buttering hot coffee, putting clothes on backward or inside-out, drinking from an empty cup, skipping key steps during activities such as shaving, tooth brushing, or hair brushing, using a fork to eat cereal, putting toothpaste on a razor, scrubbing the upper lip and chin with a toothbrush, eating toothpaste, and applying arm deodorant over a shirt (Schwartz et al., 1991). In a classic paper, Luria (1966) describes the behavior of a patient with frontal apraxia who would light a candle and put it in his mouth to perform the habitual movements of smoking a cigarette.

Haaland and colleagues (Wetter et al., 2005) examined dexterity using the Jebsen–Taylor hand function test in adults with left and right hemispheric damage and after stroke. They found similar dexterity impairments in those with both types of damage. However, patients with left hemispheric damage and apraxia exhibited greater impairments than those with left hemispheric damage but without apraxia. The authors recommend that screening for apraxia in patients with left hemispheric damage should be done regularly.

A CASE STUDY APPROACH TO UNDERSTANDING UPPER-EXTREMITY DISORDERS

Jean J: Reach-and-Grasp Problems Following Cerebrovascular Accident

Upper-extremity impairment is common following a stroke, with 85% of individuals in the acute phase showing functional deficits affecting the upper extremity, while 40% of persons with chronic stroke continue to have these impairments (Parker et al., 1986). However, the type of problem will depend on the location of the lesion. In the case of Jean J, the reach-and-grasp movements in her right hemiparetic arm are characterized by decreased movement speed and a lack of smoothness and coordination in movement trajectories due to abnormal patterns of muscle activity. Deficits in coordinated arm movements are most evident in the limb contralateral to her lesion, and occur together with spasticity, muscle weakness, and stereotypic movement patterns. When Jean reaches with her affected arm, the movement trajectory is segmented, with increased variability due to impaired interjoint coordination. She has very impaired grasp due to a limited ability to extend her fingers, and she shows fluctuations in force due to impairments in her ability to regulate forces.

Though Jean does not, many patients with stroke have visual problems such as field deficits (homonymous hemianopsia), visual neglect, and extinction, which will affect the ability to reach and grasp objects presented in the contralesional hemifield. Jean does have other sensory impairments within the somatosensory system, which significantly impair her precision grip.

Jean had several complications that interfered with her early recovery of upper-extremity function, including pain and swelling in her hemiparetic arm.

Approximately 15% of patients who have had a stroke also have a shoulder–hand syndrome, which includes pain when moving and loss of range of motion in both the shoulder and the hand. In severe cases, there is pain at rest. If the shoulder–hand syndrome is prolonged, it can lead to a "frozen" shoulder. There is no agreement concerning the underlying cause of shoulder pain following stroke, nor is there agreement on methods for treatment (Cailliet, 1980; Davies, 1985; Partridge et al., 1990; Roy, 1988).

Mike M: Reach-and-Grasp Problems in Parkinson's Disease

Bradykinesia, or slowed movement, is a classic symptom of Parkinson's disease (PD) and has a significant impact on upper-extremity function in Mike. His movements are slower than expected for someone his age. However, his impairments in reach and grasp are task-dependent. For example, when he is performing fast, accurate movements, reaching impairments related to force regulation are most apparent. In contrast, in simple motor tasks, or during slow movements where speed and accuracy are not important, he shows much better control of both reach and grasp.

Mike is less impaired when performing a reach-and-grasp movement at his preferred speed, or when the movement amplitude is small. In addition, his ability to adjust to external perturbations during reach and grasp are less impaired than adjustments to self-generated perturbations. Across all tasks, however, he shows a reduced capability for coordinating multiple joints. In addition, tremor results in a disrupted force trajectory. Mike takes longer to develop grip force, and uses excessive forces when lifting an object to ensure that it does not slip. However, surprisingly Mike retains the ability to modulate forces to match changes in object weight. Finally, he has difficulty when releasing an object. The medication he takes improves his ability to reach, although not grasp. On medication, the speed of his movements increases, and this is most apparent in self-generated movements and movements that require increased accuracy. His tremor significantly interferes with his upper-extremity function, especially as his medication wears off.

John C: Reach-and-Grasp Problems Following Cerebellar Pathology

Cerebellar damage results in dysmetria, which is characterized by errors in the direction, amplitude, velocity, and force of movement. John has ataxia; thus, during reach-and-grasp tasks, his movements are slower and less accurate and there is increased variability in the movement trajectory. When reaching for an object, or pointing to a target, he either undershoots (if he is moving slowly) or overshoots (if he is moving quickly) the target. In addition, his movements are segmented (decomposition of movement), with movements at multiple joints occurring sequentially rather than synchronously. Both eye and hand movements are inaccurate when John is reaching for a stationary object. In addition, when reaching for moving objects, he is unable to match the target velocity, and thus demonstrates inaccuracies when reaching or tracking.

Thomas: Reach and Grasp Problems in Cerebral Palsy

In addition to lower-extremity problems affecting postural control and mobility functions, Thomas our 7-year-old child with spastic diplegia, has impairments in upper-extremity function, In children with cerebral palsy, the level of hand function depends on a number of factors, including: severity of motor impairments such as paresis, spasticity, and dyscoordination, as well as the extent of sensory loss, (Ohata et al., 2008). Brændvik et al. (2009) reported that the combination of limited active supination range at the wrist and elbow in conjunction with reduced muscle strength in the elbow, forearm, and grip explained 74% of the variance in actual use of the hands in bimanual activities in children with hemiplegic or diplegic forms of cerebral palsy.

What kinds of problems with reach and grasp do we see in Thomas? First, his movement times are delayed during reach and grasp. Thomas has particular difficulty reaching for a moving target, since when altering his trajectory of reach he quickly loses his balance. He has poor anticipatory grasp formation during reaches. In addition, his grip and load forces are uncoordinated. He uses excessive grip forces when lifting an object to compensate for poor motor control. Thomas has difficulty when first learning to perform a task that requires precision grip. However, with practice he improves significantly, as he develops better internal representations of the object.

Both sensory and motor impairments contribute to impaired reach, grasp, and manipulation in Thomas as in other children with cerebral palsy. Neuromuscular impairments include weakness, spasticity, abnormal synergies, muscle imbalance, and incoordination. Sensory problems include impaired stereognosis, two-point discrimination, and position sense.

SUMMARY

1. Problems with reach, grasp, and manipulation are a common finding in most individuals with neural pathology.
2. Understanding the causes of these problems is complex because of the many interactions between neural substrates affecting reach, grasp, and manipulation skills.
3. A critical aspect of reach and grasp is the ability to locate a target and maintain one's gaze on that target preceding a reach. Problems affecting target localization and gaze stabilization include: (a) disruption of visually driven eye movements because of damage within the oculomotor system; (b) damage to the vestibular system, which disrupts vestibulo-ocular reflex control of eye movements in response to head movements; and (c) inability to adapt the vestibulo-ocular reflex to changes in task demands, because of cerebellar damage.
4. Visual deficits affecting target localization also appear to have an impact on hand motor function because of the reciprocal interaction between the eye and hand motor systems.
5. Impaired interjoint coordination is common in many types of neural pathology and affects both the timing and the trajectory of movements made during reach and grasp. In addition, most patients with neural pathology show delayed movement times.
6. Sensory impairments can also affect reach, grasp, and manipulation. Sensory impairments can affect the regulation of forces in response to the slip of a lifted object during an ongoing grip-and-lift task. In addition, sensory impairments can affect the formation of internal representations, which is important to regulating forces in subsequent lifts.
7. It appears that each hemisphere has a specialized role in the control of goal-directed voluntary movements. The right hemisphere appears to have a role in processing visual feedback for movement adjustments affecting control of aiming movements in tasks with high demands for accuracy. In contrast, the left hemisphere appears to have a role in some aspects of motor programming, including the timing and sequencing of movement phases specifically related to the ballistic components of the reaching movement.
8. Traditionally, researchers have maintained that unilateral cerebral lesions manifest in the limb contralateral to the lesions. Now researchers are also finding subtle deficits affecting the ability to reach on the nonhemiparetic side.
9. Damage to the left hemisphere may cause apraxia, a disorder of the execution of movement that cannot be accounted for by weakness, incoordination, sensory loss, poor language comprehension, or inattention to commands. The core of this disorder may be a weakening of the top-down formulation of action plans (i.e., an inability to sustain the intent to the completion of the action plan). As a result, irrelevant objects exert a strong influence on the action plan, leading to performance errors.

CHAPTER 19

CLINICAL MANAGEMENT OF THE PATIENT WITH REACH, GRASP, AND MANIPULATION DISORDERS

Sue V. Duff, EdD, PT, OTR/L, CHT*
Anne Shumway-Cook, PhD, PT
Marjorie Woollacott, PhD

LEARNING OBJECTIVES

Following completion of this chapter, the reader will be able to:

1. Describe a task-oriented approach to evaluating prehension, including tests and measures used to quantify functional skills, underlying strategies, and impairments constraining function. Discuss approaches to determining the effect of upper-extremity problems on participation.
2. Discuss a task-oriented approach to treating functional prehensile limitations, including reach, grasp, and manipulation skills.
3. Review the evidence for prehensile training in neurologic populations.

*Susan V. Duff, EdD, PT, OTR/L, CHT

Associate Professor
Physical and Occupational Therapy
Thomas Jefferson University
Philadelphia, PA 19107

Clinical Specialist
Occupational Therapy
Children's Hospital of Philadelphia
Philadelphia, PA 19104s

Hospital of Philadelphia
Child Development & Rehabilitation
Philadelphia, PA 19104

INTRODUCTION

Problems with reach, grasp, and manipulation have an impact on participation in life roles and activities performed in daily life, such as dressing, eating, and grooming. As such, they are a major focus of intervention for clinicians involved in the rehabilitation of persons with neurologic pathology. This chapter focuses on the clinical management of problems related to reach, grasp, and manipulation in individuals with neurologic pathology. The first section will review examination methods pertinent to upper-extremity function from a task-oriented approach. As described throughout this book, our task-oriented approach is based on both the International Classification of Functioning, Disability and Health (ICF) and systems framework. The three-level examination attempts to answer the following questions:

1. To what degree can the patient consistently perform functional tasks that engage one or both upper extremities? What is the extent and quality of use of one or both limbs as they are engaged in functional tasks? Does upper-extremity dysfunction have an impact on the ability of the patient to engage in life roles?

2. What strategies and movement elements does the patient take advantage of during task performance? Does he or she have the ability to adapt these strategies to changing task conditions and are the movements efficient?
3. What cognitive, visual-perceptual, musculoskeletal, sensory, or other impairments constrain how the patient performs tasks? Can these impairments be altered through intervention, thereby enhancing the patient's capabilities?

The second half of the chapter uses a task-oriented approach to review intervention options aimed at: (1) improving underlying impairments constraining upper-extremity function, (2) developing effective and efficient strategies and components of movement used to perform functional tasks that require one or both hands, and (3) improving functional abilities, including the ability to adapt performance of functional tasks to changing task and environmental demands in order to increase participation in daily activities and life roles. Evidence for the effectiveness of specific clinical treatments will be included within this section.

Two case studies will be used to illustrate a task-oriented approach to assessment and treatment of upper-extremity function. The first case, Jean J, is our patient who sustained a stroke in the left hemisphere several weeks ago and has been referred for therapy to deal with deficits in activities of daily living (ADLs) and inadequate use of her right arm Initially, after her stroke, her right arm movements were confined to a flexion synergy. Now she is beginning to develop isolated arm movement, although the movements appear weak and uncoordinated. The second case features a child with underdeveloped prehension. Tim is a 4.5-year-old boy mainstreamed in a regular preschool who has been referred to therapy by his teacher because of her concerns about his fine motor skills. Tim was born prematurely at 28 weeks of gestation and has a history of retinopathy of prematurity. He prefers his right hand for fine motor tasks and holds a crayon with a cross-thumb grasp. He has difficulty tracing shapes, and while he has begun to copy letters and numbers from a visual model, he often reverses select letters and uses varying sizes. He also has difficulty securing fasteners, tying his shoes, and performing other manual tasks.

A TASK-ORIENTED APPROACH TO EXAMINATION

In a top-down approach to examination, the clinician examines upper-extremity function, including the effect of impaired reach, grasp, and manipulation on the person's ability to participate in life roles. A functional assessment uses tests and measures to determine the person's abilities in his or her actual living environment ("performance" in the ICF framework), and in a standard (clinical) environment ("capacity" in the ICF framework). Examination also includes evaluation of strategies used to accomplish the underlying components of upper-extremity function, including visual regard, reach, grasp, manipulation, and release. Finally the underlying impairments of body structure and function that potentially constrain functional movement skills are examined.

The following section reviews a wide range of standardized tests available to clinicians when evaluating upper-extremity function in both adults and children. Are these tests categorized as measures of activities, participation, capacity, or performance? In many instances, classifying a test within the ICF framework can be difficult and often controversial. Many tests include items considered an activity within the ICF (e.g., a task performed by an individual), as well as items related to participation (e.g., the societal level of functioning). When a test is performed in a standardized clinical environment it measures the ICF's concept of capacity, and it may or may not predict actual performance in the person's own environment (ICF concept of performance). In this book, a test is classified as a measure of participation (performance) when it gathers information about the person's actual behavior (self-reported or observed) in his or her environment. We classify tests and measures performed in a clinical (standardized) environment as measures of activity (capacity). We recognize that not everyone will agree with this approach and that many may disagree with the way a specific test or measure is classified. Though subject to interpretation and error, we think that it is important to create a consistent framework for the presentation of these materials.

Evaluating Participation (Performance)

Understanding the effect of upper-extremity limitations on elements of participation can be based on objective information or subjective information obtained during the initial interview of the patient and family. Difficulty with upper-extremity control can have a significant impact on one's ability to take part in life roles (e.g., student or homemaker) and should be considered first in an examination because of the personal importance they hold (Trombly, 1993).

Along with medical and social information, the initial interview is directed toward gathering information on current symptoms and primary areas of patient concern. Within the interview, information about any restrictions in tasks and activities that the individual has difficulty performing can be obtained, as well as perceptions regarding satisfaction with the ability to participate and beliefs regarding the underlying cause of the problem (e.g., weakness). Information on family and cultural values that influence task performance should also be investigated, as they may have an impact on treatment outcome. For example, a child who ties his or her shoes at school may not carry this over at home because of time constraints when getting ready for school or parental values related to functional independence. An interview also allows clinicians to gain a general sense of an individual's cognitive status and can help them structure and establish priorities for the formal examination.

Standardized Measures of Participation

Most measures of participation rely on self-report (by the individual or his or her proxy) to determine the degree to which upper-extremity function interferes with performance of social roles and daily life activities. Limitations in participation can be determined through observation of the individual performing tasks in his or her home or community environment. However, direct observation is time-consuming and not easily performed as part of a clinical assessment. Alternatively, many clinical facilities have simulated home (or community) environments that facilitate observing performance of daily life activities.

Adult Measures. Many scales that examine participation are not exclusive to upper-extremity function. The Canadian Occupational Performance Measure (COPM) (Carswell et al., 2004; Law et al., 2005) is an outcomes assessment based on a structured interview and obtains measures of performance and satisfaction on client-identified problem areas. The COPM has been found to be a valid and reliable way to identify key areas of concern and measure improvement following intervention within various pediatric and adult neurologic populations (Cup et al., 2003; Donovan et al., 2005; Kaiser et al., 2005). It is also being used more frequently as an outcome measure for context-based training studies involving participation (Combs et al., 2010; Graham et al., 2010).

The Stroke Impact Scale (SIS) (Duncan et al., 2002) is a 59-item scale that measures eight domains of self-reported function in adults: strength, hand function, mobility, ADLs, emotion, memory, communication, and social participation. The clients rate the impact of the stroke on a 5-point scale for each section.

The Motor Activity Log (MAL) was developed to determine the amount and quality of hemiparetic arm use after stroke (Taub & Wolf, 1997). The MAL incorporates two separate Likert scales that range from 1 to 5 and measure the amount of use and quality of use in the affected limb based on observation or interview. The MAL can be tailored to the most pertinent activities in the daily life of each individual, as has been done for research purposes with adults after a stroke (Blanton & Wolf, 1999) and children with hemiplegic cerebral palsy (Charles et al., 2001) (see Assessment Tool 19.1 for a sample MAL for children). The log can be used to document baseline and progressive use of the limb. It has been shown to be reliable and valid (Uswatte et al., 2006).

There are numerous published adult ADL assessments that focus on self-care capabilities (Keith et al., 1987; Mahoney & Barthel, 1965). Areas of primary concern in adults include bathing, dressing, grooming, toileting, feeding, mobility, and continence. Two popular basic ADL scales include the Functional Independence Measure (FIM) (Keith et al., 1987) and the Barthel Index (Mahoney & Barthel, 1965). The Barthel Index is an older but commonly used test, which is designed to assess function based on 10 tasks rated on a 2- or 3-point ordinal scale and weighted to achieve a maximum score of 100. Granger and colleagues (1979) determined that a score of 60 or below indicates that the individual is dependent in self-care. Because the Barthel Index has been found to have a ceiling effect in the later stages of recovery from stroke (Hsueh et al., 2001; van der Putten et al., 1999) a scale that measures higher-level function should be used during that period.

Standardized instrumental ADL scales offer an approach to assessing higher-level upper-extremity function by examining skills that require environmental interactions (e.g., telephone usage, traveling, shopping, preparing meals, housework, and finances). For instance, the Assessment of Motor and Process Skills (Fisher, 1994) can be used to identify deficits in functional performance and examine underlying causes based on observation. This interval scale has been found to have good reliability and validity.

Pediatric Measures. The number of pediatric scales continues to expand rapidly. Two pediatric measures of participation used in children from 6 to 21 years of age, introduced in Chapter 6 are the Children's Assessment of Participation and Enjoyment (CAPE) and the Preferences for Activities of Children (PAC) (King et al., 2004; Law et al., 2005).

The Pediatric Evaluation of Disability Inventory (PEDI; Haley et al., 1992) is standardized for children 6 months to 7.5 years of age, and evaluates the skills a child can perform independently and with assistance. Areas of assessment include self-care, mobility, and social functioning as measured through three separate scales (functional skills, caregiver assistance, and modifications required for function). The PEDI has established reliability and validity (Nichols & Case-Smith, 1996).

Assessment Tool 19-1

Motor Activity Log*

This assessment was adapted from a scale designed for use with patients who have had a stroke and is intended for use with the parents of children with hemiplegia.

Instruction: I am going to read a list of activities to you. After each activity, I would like you to use the scales in front of you to tell me about the use that your son/daughter (or you) has in his/her affected arm for each activity listed. We will go over the activities list twice. First, I will ask you to think about the amount of use of your son/daughter's affected arm 1 year ago and then we will go through the list again thinking about the quality of use in the affected arm 1 week ago.

Amount of Use (AOU) Scale

0 = Did (does) not use the affected arm.

1 = Occasionally tried (tries) to use the affected arm.

2 = Used (uses) affected arm, but did (does) most of the activity with less-affected arm.

3 = Used (uses) affected arm about half as much as normal or half as often as less-affected arm.

4 = Used (uses) affected arm almost as much as normal.

5 = Used (uses) affected arm as much as normal.

Quality of Movement (QOM) Scale

0 = The affected arm was (is) never used for this activity.

1 = The affected arm moved (moves) during the activity, but was (is) of very little use (very poor).

2 = The affected arm was (is) of some use during that (this) activity, but needed (needs) some help from the stronger arm. It moved (moves) very slowly, or with difficulty (poor).

3 = The affected arm was (is) used for the purpose indicated, but movements were (are) slow or were (are) made only with some effort (fair).

4 = The movements made by the affected arm were (are) almost normal, but not quite as fast or accurate as normal.

5 = The ability to use the affected arm for this activity was equal to the ability to use the less-affected arm (normal).

Sample Activities YES, NO, **N/A AOU QOM**

1. Uses two hands to hold a book for reading.
2. Uses both hands to towel dry face or other body part.
3. Carries an object in the affected hand while using the less-affected hand to perform a task
4. Uses both hands for dressing (e.g., holds shirt or trousers and pulls garments over head or hips using both hands).
5. Carries an object in the less-affected hand while using the affected hand to perform a task such as opening the refrigerator.
6. Eats finger food such as popcorn, potato chips, etc. with the affected hand.
7. Uses both hands to play video games that require both hands. Uses both hands to button or zip an article of clothing.
9. Uses both hands in sports such as baseball, basketball, etc.

*Adapted with permission from Charles J, Lavinder G, Gordon A. Effects of constraint-induced therapy on hand function in children with hemiplegic cerebral palsy. Pediatric Phys Ther 2001;13:68–76.

The School Functional Assessment (Costner et al., 1998) is normalized for children in kindergarten to sixth grade (Assessment Tool 19.2). It was designed to identify strengths and limitations related to the performance of school-related functional tasks. It is divided into three separately rated parts: participation, task supports, and activity performance. Part 3 includes physical and cognitive/behavioral activity performance, and rates task execution on a scale of 1 to 4. Part 3 is the most useful test of functional performance involving the upper extremity. The validity and reliability of the SFA have been established (Davies et al., 2004).

Another functional scale for children, adapted from the adult FIM (Braun & Granger, 1991), is the WeeFIM (Guide for the Functional Independence Measure for Children, 1993). It can be administered by interview or observation (Sperle et al., 1997). Norms are available for infants and children 6 months to 7 years of age (Msall et al., 1994). The six subscales, scored on a 7-point ordinal scale (1 = total assistance to 7 = complete independence) focus on self-care,

Assessment Tool 19-2

School Functional Assessment*

THREE PARTS OF ASSESSMENT WITH ADAPTATIONS CHECKLIST

1. Participation
2. Task supports
3. Activity performance
   a. Physical tasks
   b. Cognitive/behavioral tasks

SAMPLE: ACTIVITY PERFORMANCE—PHYSICAL TASKS

1. Travel
2. Maintaining and changing positions
3. Recreational movement
4. Using materials
5. Setup and cleanup
6. Eating and drinking
7. Hygiene
8. Clothing management
9. Up/down stairs
10. Written work
11. Computer and equipment use

RATING FOR ACTIVITY PERFORMANCE

1. Does not perform
2. Partial performance
3. Inconsistent performance
4. Consistent performance

TASKS WITHIN "CLOTHING MANAGEMENT"

Task				
1. Removes hat	1	2	3	4
2. Removes front-opening garment top (e.g., coat)	1	2	3	4
3. Puts on hat	1	2	3	4
4. Puts on front-opening garment top (e.g., coat)	1	2	3	4
5. Lowers garment bottoms from waist to knees and pulls up from knees to waist (e.g., for toileting).	1	2	3	4
6. Zips and unzips, not including separating/hooking zipper	1	2	3	4
7. Removes pullover garment top (e.g., sweatshirt)	1	2	3	4
8. Removes shoes/boots	1	2	3	4
9. Hangs clothing on hook or hanger	1	2	3	4
10. Puts on pullover garment top (e.g., sweater)	1	2	3	4
11. Puts on and removes socks	1	2	3	4
12. Puts on shoes/boots (do not consider tying closures)	1	2	3	4
13. Secures shoes by tying or using Velcro	1	2	3	4
14. Separates and hooks zippers	1	2	3	4
15. Buttons a row of buttons with one-to-one correspondence	1	2	3	4
16. Fastens a belt buckle	1	2	3	4
17. Buttons small buttons (less than 1 in.)	1	2	3	4

*Reprinted with permission from Costner W, Deeney T, Haltiwanger J, Haley S. School Function Assessment (SFA). San Antonio: The Psychological Corporation of Harcourt Brace & Co., 1998.

sphincter control, transfers, locomotion, and cognition. This tool has been found to be reliable and valid for children with neurodevelopmental disorders (Msall et al., 1996; Ottenbacher et al., 1997).

The Manual Abilities Classification Scheme (MACS) was designed for children 4 to 18 years of age who have cerebral palsy, to quantify typical hand use in everyday activities (Eliasson et al., 2005b). This ordinal scale (Assessment Tool 19.3) resembles the Gross Motor Function Classification System (GMFCS) (Palisano et al., 1997) used to classify typical gross motor performance in children with cerebral palsy. This observational tool rates the child's manual ability on a five-level ordinal scale from handling objects easily and successfully in Level I, to severe limitations in the ability to handle objects and perform simple actions in Level V. As with the GMFCS, the classification scheme of the MACS can be used to identify service needs and assess longitudinal improvements. The reader is referred to www.macs.nu for more details on this classification scheme. The MACS has been shown to be reliable and valid (Eliasson et al., 2006).

Assessment Tool 19-3
Manual Abilities Classification System (MACS)

This assessment tool is intended for use with children 4 to 18 years of age who have cerebral palsy. The therapist observes the child performing everyday manual tasks. The child's typical manual ability is graded on a five-level scale:

Level I: Handles objects easily and successfully. Limitations only in speed and accuracy of manual performance, not ADLs.

Level II: Handles most objects but with somewhat reduced quality and/or speed of achievement. Performs tasks as in Level I, but with reduced quality and speed. Certain tasks may be avoided, or achieved with difficulty. ADL independence is maintained.

Level III: Handles objects with difficulty: needs help to prepare and/or modify activities. Independent with setup or adaptations. Performance may be slow or achieved with limited success in terms of quality and quantity.

Level IV: Handles a limited selection of easily managed objects in adapted situations. Requires continuous support, partial assistance, or adaptive equipment in all activities just to achieve partial success.

Level V: Does not handle objects and has severely limited ability to perform even simple actions. Requires total assistance. Participates best if given simple tasks, such as pushing a button.

Reprinted with permission from Elliason A-C, Rösblad B, Beckung E, et al. Development and reliability of a system to classify hand function in children with cerebral palsy. Manual Ability Classification System (MACS). Workshop presented at the American Academy for Cerebral Palsy and Developmental Medicine, Orlando, FL, 2005.

Standardized Measures of Functional Activities (Capacity)

A number of standardized tests have been designed to examine upper-extremity function in both adults and children.

Shriners Hospitals for Children Upper Extremity Evaluation (SHUEE)

The Shriners Hospitals for Children Upper Extremity Evaluation (SHUEE) is a video-based assessment of upper-extremity function with established reliability and validity (Davids et al., 2006). It has two primary sections. Section 1 evaluates impairments and Section 2 evaluates spontaneous use of the upper extremity, segmental alignment, and grasp-and-release ability. Each section and subtest has slightly different scoring criteria. The total score for each section is tabulated and reported as a percentage.

Quality of Upper Extremity Skills Test (QUEST)

The Quality of Upper Extremity Skills Test (QUEST) (Dematteo et al., 1993; Hickey & Ziviani, 1998) was designed for children 18 months to 8 years of age. The purpose of this tool is to assess the quality of upper-extremity movement in children with cerebral palsy in four domains: dissociated movement, grasp, protective extension, and weight bearing. This outcome measure has established reliability and validity (DeMatteo et al., 1994).

Assisting Hand Assessment (AHA)

Krumlinde-Sundholm and Eliasson (2003) introduced the standardized criterion-referenced Assisting Hand Assessment (AHA). The AHA is intended to determine the degree to which the affected limb of a child with unilateral disability is engaged in bimanual tasks (Krumlinde-Sundholm et al., 2005). It is designed for infants and children 18 months to 12 years of age and scores 22 items on a 4-point scale from a videotape. The AHA has been found to have reliability, construct validity, and internal consistency based on Rasch analysis and was found to be sensitive to change following intervention (Holmefur et al., 2009; Krumlinde-Sundholm et al., 2007).

Wolf Motor Function Test (WMFT)

The Wolf Motor Function Test (WMFT) (Wolf et al., 1989a) is a timed test that quantifies single- or multiple-joint upper-extremity movement (Items 1–6) and functional tasks (Items 7–15). The tasks are arranged from proximal to distal in order of complexity (Wolf et al., 2001) (see Assessment Tool 19.4). It has been found to have high interrater reliability, internal consistency, test–retest reliability, and adequate stability (Morris et al., 2001; Wolf et al., 2001). It has

Assessment Tool 19-4

Wolf Motor Function Test

The tasks listed below are performed as quickly as possible while being timed. Maximal time for each task is 120 sec.

TASKS:

1. Forearm to table (side): Subject attempts to place forearm on the table by abduction at shoulder.
2. Forearm to box (side): Subject attempts to place forearm on the box by abduction at shoulder.
3. Extend elbow (side): Subject attempts to reach across the table by extending the elbow (to side).
4. Extend elbow (to the side), with weight: Subject attempts to push the sandbag against outer wrist joint across the table by extending the elbow.
5. Hand to table (front): Subject attempts to place affected hand on the table.
6. Hand to box (front): Subject attempts to place hand on the box.
7. Reach and retrieve (front): Subject attempts to pull 1-lb weight across the table by using elbow flexion and cupped wrist.
8. Lift can (front): Subject attempts to lift can and bring it close to lips with a cylindrical grasp.
9. Lift pencil (front): Subject attempts to pick up pencil by using three-jaw chuck grasp.
10. Pick up paper clip (front): Subject attempts to pick up paper clip by using a pincer grasp.
11. Stack checkers (front): Subject attempts to stack checkers onto the center checker.
12. Flip cards (front): Using the pincer grasp, patient attempts to flip each card over.
13. Turning the key in lock (front): Using pincer grasp, while maintaining contact, patient turns key fully to the left and right.
14. Fold towel (front): Subject grasps towel, folds it lengthwise, and then uses the tested hand to fold the towel in half again.
15. Lift basket (standing): Subject picks up basket by grasping handles and placing it on bedside table.

Reprinted with permission from Wolf SL, McJunkin JP, Swanson ML, Weiss PS. Pilot normative database for the Wolf Motor Function Test. Arch Phys Med Rehabil. 2006;87(2):443–445.

also been shown to discriminate between higher- and lower-functioning individuals with subacute stroke across different research sites (Wolf et al., 2005).

Action Research Arm Test (ARAT)

The Action Research Arm Test (ARAT), shown in Assessment Tool 19.5, was developed to examine upper-extremity function in adults with neurologic dysfunction, including those who have had a stroke (Lyle, 1981). The ARAT has four subscales: (1) grasp; (2) grip; (3) pinch; and (4) gross movement. The 19 test items are scored on a 4-point ordinal scale as follows: 0 = can perform no part of the test; 1 = performs test partially; 2 = completes test but takes an abnormally long time or has great difficulty; and 3 = performs test normally. The ARAT has been found to correlate with the upper limb portion of the Fugl-Meyer Scale (r = 0.94) (De Weerdt & Harrison, 1985).

Chedoke Upper Limb and Hand Activity Inventory

The Chedoke Upper Limb and Hand Activity Inventory (CAHAI) was designed to assess functional recovery of the arm and hand after a stroke (Barreca et al., 2004, 2006). As shown in Assessment Tool 19.6, it contains 13 functional tasks that the individual performs while being timed. The item number can be reduced in level of difficulty yet still scored (CAHAI-7; CAHAI-8; CAHAI-9; and CAHAI-13). Clients are scored as follows: 1 = needs total assistance, and weak upper limb performs <25% of the task; 2 = needs maximal assistance, and weak upper limb performs 25 to 49% of the task. There are no signs of arm or hand manipulation, only stabilization; 3 = needs moderate assistance, and weak upper limb performs 50 to 74% of the task. Begins to show signs of arm or hand manipulation; 4 = needs minimal assistance (light touch), and the weak upper limb performs more than 75% of the task; 5 = requires supervision, coaxing, or cueing; 6 = requires use of assistive devices or requires more than reasonable time, or there are safety concerns; and 7 = total independence in completing the task. The CAHAI (CAHAI-9 and CAHAI-13) correlated with the ARAT (r = 0.93, 1 month after stroke; and r = 0.95, 3 months after stroke) (Barreca et al., 2005). The CAHAI also correlates with the Fugl-Meyer Scale (r = 0.95) and the FIM (r = 0.79) (Gowland et al., 1993).

Assessment Tool 19-5

Action Research Arm Test

Scoring: 0-3 points on 19 items in four subtests with 57 total possible points. If the subject passes the first item in a subtest, no more need be administered, and he or she scores top marks for that subtest. If the subject fails the first item and fails the second item in a subtest, he or she scores 0, and again no more tests need to be performed in that subtest. Otherwise, he or she needs to complete all tasks within the subtest.

Scale:

0 = can perform no part of the test
1 = performs test partially
2 = completes test but takes an abnormally long time or has great difficulty
3 = performs test normally

Subtests:

Grasp (6) Attempt to pick up the following per directions above:

1. 10-cm wood block (If score = 3, total = 18 and go to Grip)
2. 2.5-cm wood block (If score = 0, total = 0 and go to Grip)
3. 5-cm wood block
4. 7.5-cm wood block
5. Ball (cricket), 7.5-cm diameter
6. Stone, 10 × 2.5 × 1 cm

Grip (4) Attempt the following per directions above:

1. Pour water from glass to glass (If score = 3, total = 12, and go to Pinch)
2. Pick up 2.25-cm tube (If score = 0, total = 0 and go to Pinch)
3. Pick up tube, 1 × 16 cm
4. Place washer (3.5-cm diameter) over bolt

Pinch (6) Attempt to pick up the following per directions above:

1. Ball bearing, 6 mm, third finger and thumb (If score = 3, total = 18 and go to Gross Movements)
2. Marble, 1.5 cm, index finger and thumb (If score = 0, total = 0 and go to Gross Movements)
3. Ball bearing, second finger and thumb
4. Ball bearing, first finger and thumb
5. Marble, second finger and thumb
6. Marble, first finger and thumb

Gross Movements (3) Attempt the following:

1. Place hand behind head
2. Place hand on top of head
3. Hand to mouth

Reprinted with permission from Lyle RC. A performance test for assessment of upper limb function in physical rehabilitation treatment and research. Int J Rehabil Res 1981;4:483–492.

Jebsen-Taylor Hand Function Test

The Jebsen–Taylor Hand Function test (JHFT) was designed to simulate hand function common to many ADL tasks (Jebsen et al., 1969). It contains seven timed subtests: writing, card turning, picking up small items, simulated feeding, stacking checkers, picking up light cans, and picking up heavy cans (Fig. 19.1) and requires that both hands be tested (nondominant first). The test takes 10 to 15 minutes to administer. In addition, it has established norms for adults (Jebsen et al., 1969) and children (Taylor et al., 1973). The JHFT generally has excellent test–retest reliability, with the exception of writing and feeding subtests, which tend to show practice effects (Stern, 1992).

Manual Ability Measure (MAM)

The Manual Ability Measure (MAM-16) is a task-oriented, patient-focused outcome measure (Chen et al., 2005). This two-part tool uses self-reports to assess unimanual and bimanual function. The first part documents demographics, and the second part evaluates function on 16 task items (Assessment Tool 19.7). Using Rasch analysis (Wright & Masters, 1982), the MAM-16 was found to have good validity and reliability. It may be best used as a screening tool or in conjunction with other hand-function assessments.

Handwriting

Analysis of specialized functional tasks, such as handwriting, is sometimes warranted. Dysfunctional behaviors observed during handwriting may include an unstable grip on the pen or pencil, poor wrist stabilization, or failure to secure the paper when writing. Formal tests typically measure global legibility, writing speed, pencil management, and specific subcomponents such as near- and far-point copying. Sample pediatric tools include: (1) Developmental Skill Observations of the "K" & "1" Child Observations for Cursive Writing Skills Training (Benbow, 1992); and (2) the Evaluation Tool of Children's Handwriting (Amundson, 1995). To confirm the influence of other factors, formal tests should be coupled with

Assessment Tool 19-6

Chedoke Inventory of Hand and Arm Inventory

This assessment tool was designed to measure response to change in hand and arm function in adults after a stroke.

Scale:

1. Total assist (weak upper limb < 25%)
2. Maximal assist (weak upper limb = 25–49%)
3. Moderate assist (upper limb = 50–74%)
4. Minimal assist (weak > 75%)
5. Supervision
6. Modified independence (device)
7. Complete independence (timely, safely)

SUBTESTS AFFECTED LIMB SCORE

1. Open jar of coffee _____holds jar _____holds lid _____
2. Call 911 _____holds receiver _____dials phone _____
3. Draw a line with a ruler _____holds ruler _____ holds pen _____
4. Put toothpaste on toothbrush _____holds toothpaste _____holds brush _____
5. Cut median consistency putty _____holds knife _____holds fork _____
6. Pour a glass of water _____holds glass _____holds pitcher _____
7. Wring out washcloth _____
8. Clean a pair of eyeglasses _____holds glasses _____ wipes lenses _____
9. Zip up the zipper _____holds zipper _____ holds zipper pull _____
10. Do up five buttons
11. Dry back with towel _____reaches for towel _____ grasps towel end _____
12. Place container on table _____
13. Carry bag up stairs _____

Reprinted with permission from Barreca S. Gowland CK, Stratford P, Huijbregts M, Griffiths J, Torresin W, Dunkley M, Miller P, Masters L. Development of the Chedoke Arm and Hand Activity Inventory: theoretical constructs, item generation, and selection. Top Stroke Rehabil 2004;11(4):31–42.

analysis of motor strategies and resources such as attention, visual skills, or hand strength. For example, handwriting parameters displayed by children with left hemiplegic cerebral palsy have been found to correlate with many other factors, such as speed and dexterity, bilateral coordination, visual and spatial perception and visual-motor organization (Bumin & Kavek, 2010).

Some handwriting problems, such as difficulty copying from the blackboard or copying small text may require referral to a specialist such as an optometrist. Because of the potential for discrepancies between formal testing and classroom performance in children (Sudsawad et al., 2001), it is important to obtain an opinion from the teacher in addition to reviewing the results from formal testing.

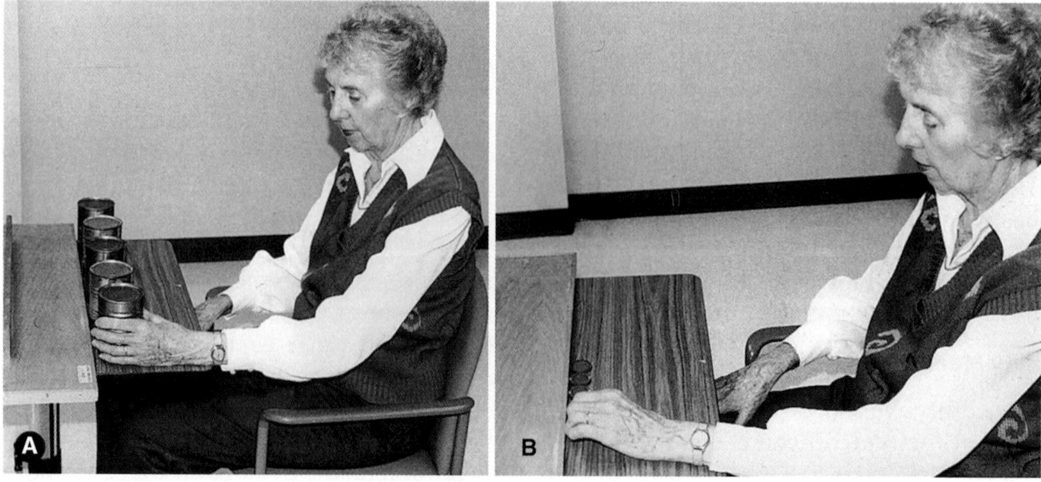

FIGURE 19.1 Jebsen-Taylor hand function test. Two items from this seven-item test are shown: A, lifting light cans, and B, stacking checkers.

Assessment Tool 19-7

Manual Ability Measure (MAM-16)

Please choose one response from the scale, regarding how difficult it is for you to perform the following activities:

Scale:

(4) Easy
(3) A little hard
(2) Very hard
(1) Cannot do
(0) Almost never do

A little hard = Compared with the time before I had the disabilities (due to injuries or illness), it takes me more time, or causes me discomfort, or it tires me out to do the activity. However, I would usually do it. Very hard = Unless absolutely necessary, I prefer others to do it for me. Almost never do = I just never do the activity, because I cannot.

_____ **1.** Eat a sandwich.
_____ **2.** Pick up a half-full water pitcher.
_____ **3.** Use a spoon or fork.
_____ **4.** Cut meat on my plate with a knife.
_____ **5.** Squeeze toothpaste onto a toothbrush.
_____ **6.** Brush my teeth.
_____ **7.** Wring a towel.
_____ **8.** Zip my jacket.
_____ **9.** Button my shirt or clothes.
_____ **10.** Use a telephone.
_____ **11.** Turn a key to open a door.
_____ **12.** Open a wide-mouth jar (jam, pickle) previously opened.
_____ **13.** Open a medication bottle with child-proof cap.
_____ **14.** Count money (bills and coins).
_____ **15.** Take things out of my billfold (ID, credit card, bills).
_____ **16.** Write three to four sentences legibly.

Reprinted with permission from Chen CC, Granger CV, Peimer CA, Moy OJ, Wald S. Manual Ability Measure (MAM-16): a preliminary report on a new patient-centred and task-oriented outcome measure of hand function. J Hand Surg Br 2005;30:207–216.

Examination at the Strategy Level

Although an individual may perform a functional task successfully, his or her repertoire of movement strategies may be limited, restricting performance over a range of conditions. Examination at the strategy level involves key elements of prehension, including: (a) visual regard, (b) reach-and-grasp formation, (c) grasp, (d) manipulation, and (e) release. Deficits in any one of these areas can significantly limit function even if the individual has adequate resources (e.g., strength). The patient's ability to adapt each element to task and context changes should be assessed (Wu et al., 1994, 1998).

Visual Regard

Examination of eye–head coordination, which underlies localization of an object to be grasped, requires the assessment of three components (Herdman, et al., 2001; Jeannerod, 1990; Shumway-Cook & Horak, 1990). First, the patient's ability to locate and maintain a stable gaze on either a fixed or moving target, presented in the central and or near peripheral visual field is examined and graded on a 3-point scale: intact, impaired, or unable. The patient is asked to keep the head still and to move only the eyes. Both saccadic eye movements to fixed targets and smooth pursuit eye movements used to track moving targets are tested. Figure 19.2 shows a patient making saccadic eye movements to a still target located in the near peripheral field. Subjective reports related to blurred or unstable vision, dizziness, or nausea are recorded. In examining Jean J, our patient with an acute stroke, you might note that she has difficulty making accurate eye movements to targets in her left visual field and tracking moving targets.

Next, the patient's ability to locate and stabilize gaze on targets presented in the far peripheral visual field is examined (Fig. 19.3) and graded as previously described. Patients should be able to localize a target with the eyes and maintain a stable gaze on that target while the head is moving. Finally, the patient's ability to make eye–head–trunk movements necessary to locate targets oriented in the far periphery is examined. Patients are tested initially while seated; yet, if they are capable, eye–head coordination may also be tested in standing and during walking (Shumway-Cook & Horak, 1990).

Reach and Grasp

Reaching and reach-to-grasp behaviors have distinct features that may reveal underlying problems with

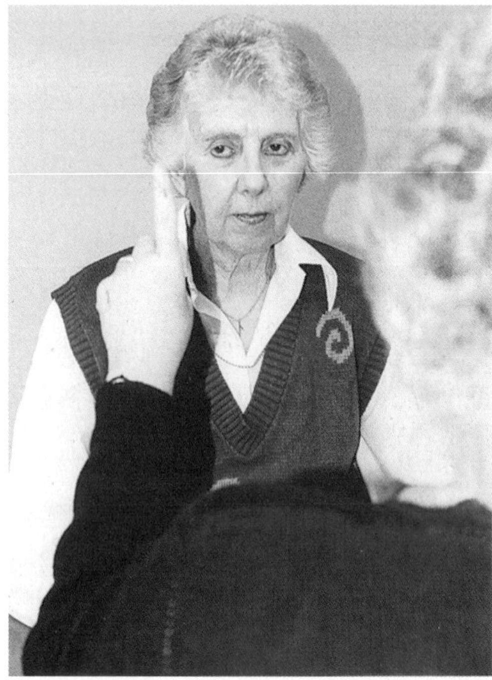

FIGURE 19.2 Testing eye-head coordination. Shown is the patient's ability to make saccadic eye movements to locate and maintain gaze on a target located in the near peripheral field.

planning and anticipatory control. Grip formation, or hand shaping, typically begins in the last part of the reach (transport) in anticipation of object size and contour and incorporates finger opening and closure (Jeannerod, 1986) (Fig. 19.4). Kinematic measures of reach-to-grasp ability provide excellent information; yet they are expensive and time-consuming. Thus, examination of reaching or reach-to-grasp behaviors can be done simply by videotaping functional performance and/or using a stopwatch to time movements. Videotaping allows the clinician to analyze movement components by repeated viewing at segments of interest; a stopwatch may allow for the capture of temporal features of the movement, such as total movement time (initiation of reach to object contact) or timing of maximum finger opening.

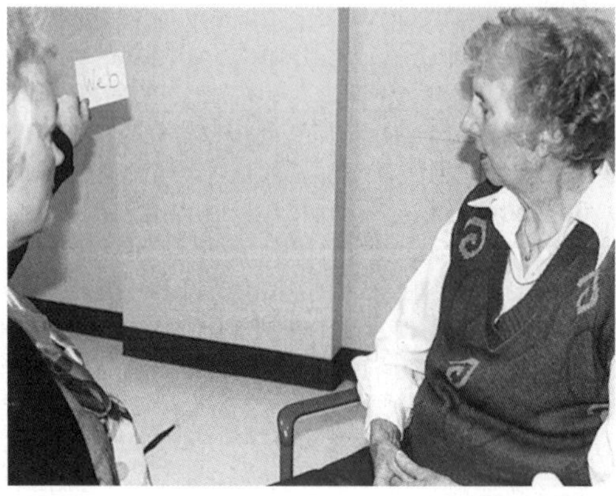

FIGURE 19.3 Testing eye-head coordination. The patient's ability to make coordinated eye-head movements to locate a target in the far peripheral visual field is shown.

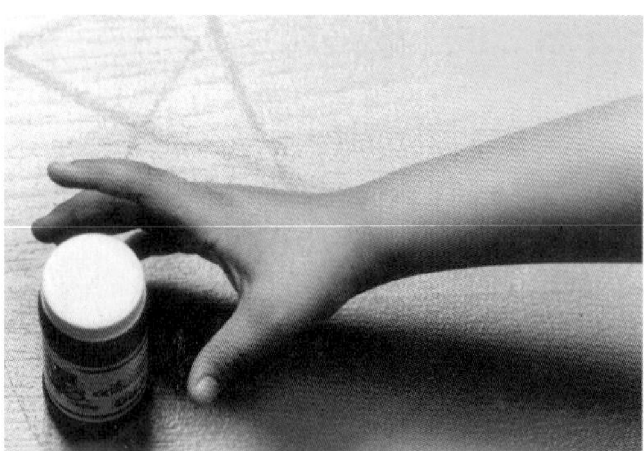

FIGURE 19.4 The development of grip formation during transport in anticipation of object size and contour.

Tasks that incorporate pointing or reach-to-grasp behaviors in different parts of the workspace demand that the individual use a range of movement strategies. To assess a patient's repertoire of strategies, targets or objects could be placed ipsilateral and contralateral to the reaching arm, within arm's reach or at the extreme ends of the workspace (requiring trunk motion). During testing it is important to remember Fitts' law, or the relationship between movement speed and accuracy (Fitts, 1954). If accuracy demands are high (fragile or unstable target object) subjects typically slow down (decelerate) during the final phase of the reach.

Two problems you might expect to see in patients who have underdeveloped or impaired reach are increased movement time and an inefficient hand trajectory. Problems with grip formation include: (a) impaired hand shaping during reaching, resulting in inaccurate closure around the target object (e.g., web space contacts the object before the fingers), (b) premature finger closure, resulting in unstable grasp points on the object, and (c) insufficient finger opening for objects of different shapes and sizes due to associated impairments (e.g., weak finger extension). Thus, during observations it is important to note the trajectory of the reach, the orientation of the hand and the shape of the fingers relative to the thumb. Specifically, one may determine the point in the trajectory at which the hand opens maximally and then begins to close in preparation for object contact, observing whether the thumb remains in a stable position throughout the movement, thereby serving as a reference point for the reach to grasp motion.

The trunk should be analyzed not only for its role as a postural stabilizer (see Massion, 1992, for review) during reach–to-grasp movements but also

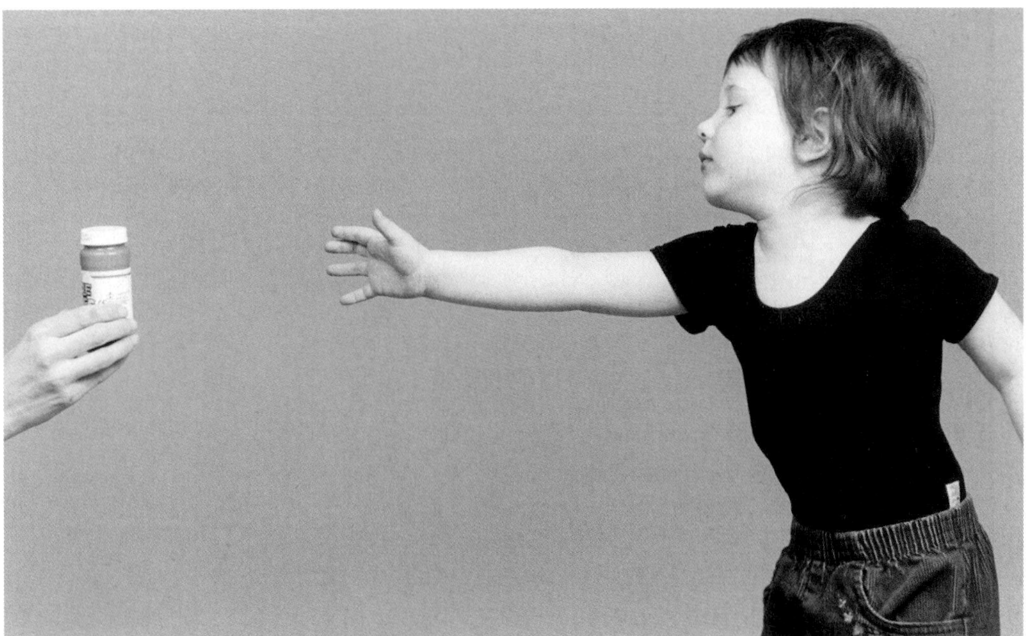

FIGURE 19.5 The importance of coupling movements between the trunk, glenohumeral joint, and scapula during reaching for anteriorly placed targets.

for its role in the terminal stage of hand transport. As shown by Kaminski and colleagues (1995), when reaching for anteriorly placed targets, trunk rotation is countered by glenohumeral horizontal abduction and scapular retraction to keep the hand moving in a straight path (Fig. 19.5). Levin and colleagues (2002) examined trunk motion during forward reaching and found that the trunk made a greater contribution and was used earlier in the reach in adults with hemiparesis than in controls. Based on its importance, trunk motion should be analyzed during reach-and-grasp tasks, particularly during reaches for objects placed at the terminal end of the workspace. Observations from different viewpoints (lateral, posterior, and anterior) can provide an estimate of trunk involvement during reaches in various locations. An overhead video camera may help capture trunk and arm coordination.

Anticipatory Control of Grasp. In preparation for grasp, relevant object features (e.g., texture, weight) are identified. We draw on previously formed internal representations and body awareness to plan movements and forces in advance. If anticipatory force scaling is impaired, one must wait for sensory feedback to modify fingertip forces, which is often too late and could result in object slippage or crushes unless compensatory strategies are used.

Behavioral signs of impaired anticipatory control include: (1) repeatedly knocking over objects because of insufficient finger opening (underestimated aperture), (2) contacting objects with the web space first instead of the fingertips (delay in finger closure), (3) denting or crushing lightweight objects after grasping (exaggerated grip force), and (4) difficulty raising heavy but liftable objects off a table (underestimated load force rate). If one or more signs are evident, the clinician should determine the reason for the impaired anticipatory control (e.g., distorted internal representation stemming from diminished sensibility).

Because anticipatory grip formation and final object contact depend on accurate identification of object location and properties, remember to examine the patient's ability to use visual information for this end. Inaccurate grip formation may also be due to poor visual stabilization on the object.

Grasp Stabilization. Prehension patterns vary with the configuration of the target object. An individual's repertoire of grasp patterns can be ascertained easily using Sollerman's (1984) grasp-and-lift test during an observation or a review of a videotaped session. The nine test items require the use of various patterns such as a spherical grip to open a jar and a three-jaw chuck to open a tube of toothpaste. Following each lift the examiner rates the pattern exhibited on a scale of 1 to 4 (see Assessment Tool 19.8). This assessment can be used to establish a baseline and document progress.

Numerous tasks, such as handwriting, require a sustained grip posture on a utensil or tool. Weakness due to hemiplegia or dystonia (writer's cramp) may contribute to an awkward grip posture and limited endurance for sustained writing tasks, and thus

Assessment Tool 19-8

Sollerman's Grips

Each activity listed is videotaped and scored using the following criteria:

- 0 = Cannot grip the object
- 1 = Grips the object but cannot complete the task
- 2 = Grips the object using an awkward grip and motion but completes the task
- 3 = Grips the object using a slightly deviant grip and motion but completes the task
- 4 = Grips the object using a normal grip and motion and completes the task.

GRIP	ACTIVITY	SCORE
Transverse grip	Grasp a 2.5-cm diameter horizontal bar in midair and place it on the table	
Transverse grip	Move a 2.5-cm diameter vertical bar from one pegboard position to another	
Transverse grip	Lift a glass and pretend to drink	
Diagonal grip	Hold a knife and cut paste into pieces	
Five-finger pinch (modified spherical grip)	Pull a sleeve on and off of the less-affected arm	
Tripod pinch (three-jaw chuck)	Unscrew a 2-cm cylindrical cap from a toothpaste tube	
Tripod pinch (three-jaw chuck)	Unscrew a 7-cm cylindrical lid from a jar	
Lateral pinch	Grasp a vertically oriented plate (5 x 5 x 1 cm)	
Palmar pinch (pad-to-pad pinch)	Pick up a small cube and touch the chin with it	

warrants close examination. Ten pencil and crayon grips, typically observed during development, compiled from various authors are shown in Figure 19.6 (Schneck & Henderson, 1990). These grip postures can be used as a guide when analyzing pencil grip in children and adults. Although children younger than 4 years of age use a variety of grip patterns, the ones most commonly used among typical children, older than 6.6 years, are the dynamic tripod (Fig. 19.6J) and lateral tripod (Fig. 19.6I) (Schneck & Henderson, 1990). Bergmann (1990) found that 88% of adults used the dynamic tripod, while 9% used a lateral tripod grip.

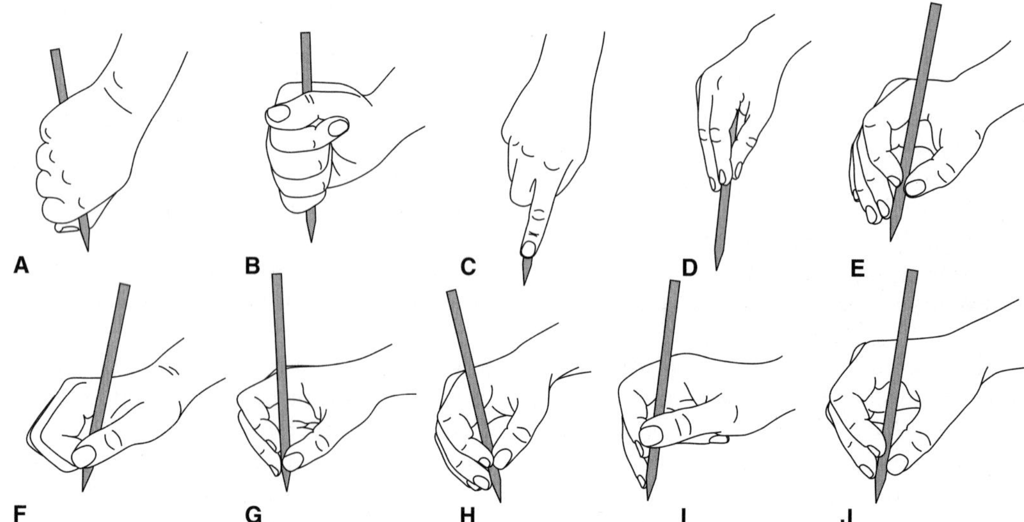

FIGURE 19.6 Ten pencil and crayon grips observed during development (Redrawn with permission from Schneck CM, Henderson A. Descriptive analysis of the developmental progression of grip position for pencil and crayon control in nondysfunctional children. Am J Occup Ther 1990;44:895.)

Adults and children with neurologic dysfunction such as upper-limb hemiplegia often display awkward pencil grips that may or may not be efficient. Once a consistent grip pattern has been identified, its efficiency during writing can be determined through timed copying tests at near and far points.

Manipulation and Release

Once an object is secured it can either be stabilized or manipulated. Stabilization requires sustained isometric fingertip forces to prevent object slippage. Manipulation is the movement of an object in space, or with reference to another object (Corbetta & Mounoud, 1990). It includes several types of tasks, such as tool use (e.g., pencils, scissors), dressing (buttoning), eating (use of a knife), or money handling (Swanson et al., 1978). Performance of these manipulation skills requires various hand movements with reference to an object, including pushing, pulling, shaking, throwing, transferring, and releasing.

Modulation of fingertip force during object manipulation and release has been shown to be impaired in individuals with neurologic impairment (Duff & Gordon, 2003; Gordon et al., 2003; Muratori et al., 2006; Nowak et al., 2003; Quaney et al., 2005). Fingertip force modulation of stable objects is often measured using small force transducers. However, this lab-based assessment is expensive and not feasible to use in the clinic. To clinically examine fingertip force modulation without using force transducers requires keen observation of task performance during grasp, lift, and release of objects of different sizes, shape, weight, and texture (Fig. 19.7). For example, patients may be asked to grasp and lift, grasp and throw, or grasp and place (into various objects). Observation of the patient's performance should include determining whether the grip pattern is modified appropriately to accommodate changes in object properties. Specifically, is there evidence of errors in anticipatory force scaling such as excessive squeeze (grip) force for objects of varying weight, slips when lifting heavy/large objects, or overshoots during successive lifts with lightweight objects? Also, how much voluntary control/range does the individual display through the wrist, finger, and thumb extensors to allow him or her to release large objects? What is the release pattern used (e.g., wrist flexion to extend the fingers)? Can the individual place one object on top of another, or grade release? Observations can also be made during functional tasks, dexterity testing, or in-hand manipulation tests, because many of those components require variable distal movements.

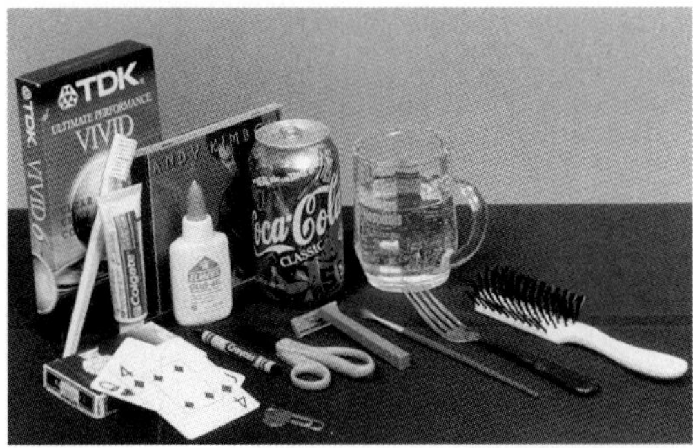

FIGURE 19.7 Objects of varied size, shape, weight and texture can be used to roughly estimate available prehension patterns, the ability an individual has to form an anticipatory grip pattern and scale the fingertip forces during object manipulation.

Jean J our acute stroke patient makes frequent errors in programming fingertip forces, and objects frequently slip from her grasp when she is trying to lift them. For instance, she typically uses too much force when grasping and lifting a paper cup, causing compression of the sides of the cup and spilling of the liquid inside. This suggests significant errors in anticipatory scaling of the grip and load force.

A test has been developed to examine the ability an individual has to manipulate unstable objects, entitled The Strength-Dexterity test or SD test (Valero-Cuevas et al., 2002; Vollmer et al., 2010). This task requires control of fingertip force direction during compression of a series of springs attached to a grip device. The goal is to compress the spring without buckling it. Calibration for the series of springs varies across a continuum of difficulty level based on the *strength index* (force required to compress it) and *dexterity index* (tendency of the spring to buckle). Three attempts are allowed for each spring presented, and performance is scored as either a success (1) or failure (0). The test allows for classification based on individual ability. Further testing is being conducted with neurologic populations (Vollmer et al., 2010).

Dexterity and Fine Motor Tests

Dexterity is the ability to manipulate various objects using different prehension patterns quickly and efficiently. Examinations of dexterity differ by age and diagnosis. It is important to keep in mind that patients with apparent unilateral involvement in the limb contralateral to the central lesion often exhibit ipsilateral control problems as well (Gordon et al., 1999a, b; Haaland et al., 2004; Pohl & Winstein, 1999). Hence, the clinician should examine skill levels for the affected and less-affected sides. Some commonly used tests of hand dexterity and manipulation skills that have normative data for different ages and clinical populations include the 9-Hole Peg test (Mathiowetz et al., 1985; Oxford et al., 2003; Poole et al., 2005), the Purdue Pegboard test (Mathiowetz et al., 1986; Tiffin, 1968), the Minnesota

Rate of Dexterity test (Desrosiers et al., 1997; Surrey et al., 2003), and the Box and Block test (Desrosiers, et al., 1994; Platz et al., 2005; Mathiowetz et al., 1985).

Developmental Fine Motor Tests. The fine motor section of developmental tests is often used to evaluate prehensile skill. Commonly used tests normalized for infants and young children include the Peabody Fine Motor Scale (up to 7 years) (Folio & Fewell, 1983), the Gesell Developmental Schedules (up to 2.5 years) (Gesell et al., 1940), the Bayley Scale of Infant Development (0 to 30 months) (Bayley, 1969), and the Erhardt Developmental Prehension Assessment (up to 6 years) (Erhardt, 1984). The fine motor section of the Bruininks–Oseretsky Motor Development Scale (Bruininks, 1978) and its second edition (Bruininks & Bruininks, 2005) contain both unimanual and bimanual items and are normed for children 4.5 to 14.5 years of age. Finally, the Movement Assessment Battery for Children, second edition (Movement ABC-2) is a widely used test of motor function and coordination with a section on manual dexterity and a section on ball skills (Henderson & Sugden, 2007). It is normed for children from 3 to 16.11 years of age.

In-Hand Manipulation. In-hand manipulation is the process of adjusting an object within one hand after grasping it (Exner, 1989; Pehoski, 1995). As shown in Figure 19.8, elements of in-hand manipulation include: (a) *translation,* moving an object from the fingers to the palm and back, as when picking up a coin and moving it to the palm; (b) *shift,* defined as adjusting the position of an object held near the distal interphalangeal joints of the fingers with the thumb opposed (e.g., moving a pen so it is held closer to the point, for writing); (c) *rotation* (simple or complex), involving rotation then stabilization of an object (e.g., turning a spoon so it can be used after it has been picked up).

Given its strong association with fine motor coordination and handwriting (Case-Smith, 1996; Cornhill & Case-Smith, 1996), evaluation of in-hand manipulation may provide further insight into dexterity and handwriting problems and serve as a method to document improvement. Methods to quickly examine translation, shift, and rotation include: (1) placing a pencil in a subject's palm and asking the individual to adjust it for use, and (2) placing a quarter in a subject's palm and asking the individual to use the fingers to place it into the coin slot of machine.

The In-Hand Manipulation Test designed by Exner and colleagues (Breslin & Exner, 1999) objectively examines all three components of in-hand manipulation, and has been found to have content and construct validity (Breslin & Exner, 1999; Exner, 1993), yet has not been widely distributed. The Test of In-Hand Manipulation (Case-Smith, 1996; Pont et al., 2008) uses the nine-hole peg test to assess two components of in-hand manipulation in children from 3 to 6 years of age. The two components are translation with stabilization, and rotation. The Test of In-Hand Manipulation was recently shown to be reliable and valid (Pont et al., 2008).

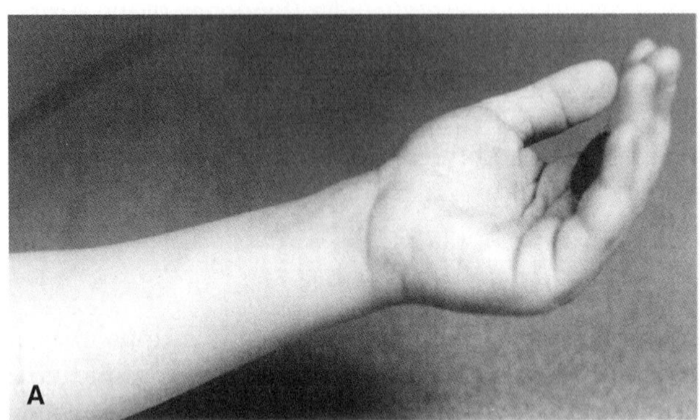

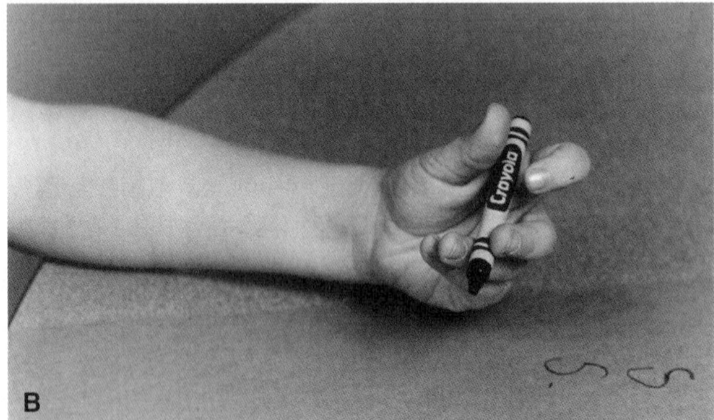

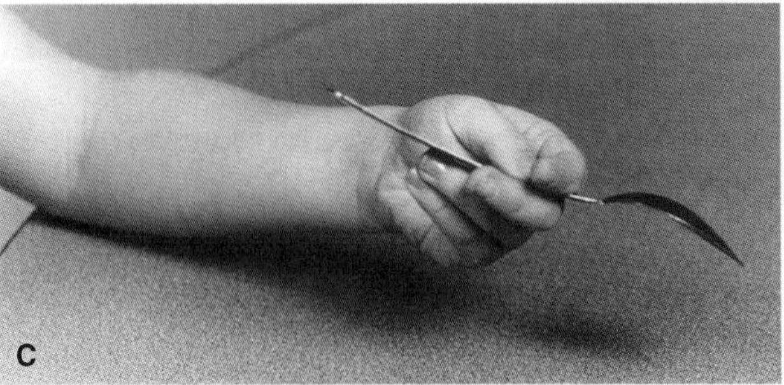

FIGURE 19.8 Elements of in-hand manipulation include: (a) translation, (b) shift, and (c) rotation (simple or complex).

Bilateral Coordination

Bilateral or bimanual tasks can be symmetrical, with both limbs performing the same action, or asymmetrical, in which one limb stabilizes an object or item while the other limb performs an action on it. Common symmetrical tasks that can be used to assess performance are ball throwing and catching and towel folding. Many ADL tasks are asymmetrical, and thus could be used for assessment. These include holding a toothbrush with one hand and squeezing toothpaste onto the brush with the other hand. Some standardized tools such as the Bruininks–Oseretsky Test of Motor Proficiency, second edition, contain specific items designed to test bilateral coordination in children (Bruininks & Bruininks, 2005).

Bilateral task performance can easily be examined for efficiency by using a stopwatch. However, to better quantify bilateral coordination, videotaping or the use of kinematic analysis is best. Wiesendanger and colleagues (Kazennikov et al., 2002) designed a clever test of asymmetrical bimanual skill entitled the "drawer-pulling" task that has been used in conjunction with videotape or kinematic analysis to examine performance at different ages and in various neurologic populations (Hung et al., 2004, 2010; Serrien & Wiesendanger, 2000; Serrien et al., 2001).

Examination at the Impairment Level

The third level of examination identifies factors that limit or enhance an individual's performance and strategic planning of task-specific movements. In the ICF framework, these factors reflect examination of body structure and function.

Perception and Cognition

Impairments in this category relevant to upper-extremity dyscontrol include selective attention, visual neglect, planning, sequencing, apraxia/dyspraxia, and visual perception. Deficits in any of these areas can significantly influence hand and arm function. For example, research has shown that apraxia and deficits in sequencing can significantly affect hand and upper-extremity function in adults after stroke and in children with hemiplegic cerebral palsy (Gordon et al., 1999; Wetter et al., 2005). See Chapter 5 for a full review.

Musculoskeletal and Neuromuscular Factors

One's ability to move may be restricted by available joint motion, weakness, or the inability to make isolated movements with or without spasticity. To obtain a clear picture of musculoskeletal impairments it is important to assess all three areas.

Range of Motion (ROM). The American Society of Hand Therapists (ASHT) has established procedural guidelines aimed at enhancing the reliability of ROM measures (see Adams et al., 1992). Factors that will affect reliability include the size and placement of the goniometer (or ruler), the amount of passive force used during measurement, and the method of documentation. Variations in traditional techniques used to measure wrist and forearm ROM have been proven to be reliable (Flowers et al., 2001; LaStayo & Wheeler, 1994). A composite measure of total active motion or total passive motion through a single digit (finger or thumb) can be made following guidelines published by the ASHT (Adams et al., 1992). Total motion is the sum of flexion measurements of the metacarpophalangeal and interphalangeal joints minus the extension deficits of the same joints. Composite finger flexion and hook fist flexion can also be measured using the centimeter ruler of a finger goniometer, taken as the distance between the fingertip and the proximal palmar crease (composite) and the fingertip and the distal palmar crease (hook) (Gilliam & Barstow, 1997). Thumb carpometacarpal joint opposition can also be measured with the ruler from the volar thumb interphalangeal joint to the third metacarpal. Normative data associated with typical adult upper-extremity function are available (American Society of Orthopedic Surgeons, 1965; Gilliam & Barstow, 1997). Variability in normative values may exist depending on the diagnosis or age of the individual (Chaparro et al., 2000).

Strength. The ability to generate sufficient force (strength) is essential to active upper-extremity movement and function. However, as described in previous chapters, strength testing in those with neurologic lesions is controversial. The primary methods to evaluate strength use dynamometers and manual muscle testing scales. Handheld dynamometers provide an objective measure of large muscle strength as well as grip and pinch strength (Wadsworth & Krishman, 1987). For instance, the grip dynamometer shown in Figure 19.9 adjusts for various hand widths (Jamar Dynamometer, Asimow Engineering, Los Angeles) (Bechtol, 1954; Fess, 1992). The ASHT recommends the use of a calibrated grip dynamometer and a static position of 90 degrees of elbow flexion with the forearm and wrist in neutral, recording the mean of three trials in kilograms or pounds (Fess, 1987, 1992). Use of all five handle positions should reveal a skewed bell-shaped curve (when plotted) with maximal strength in the second or third handle position. Although grip strength is typically measured in the static position, measurement of dynamic grip strength, in which the wrist and forearm are allowed to move into different positions, may be a better measure of functional grip strength (LaStayo & Hartzel, 1999).

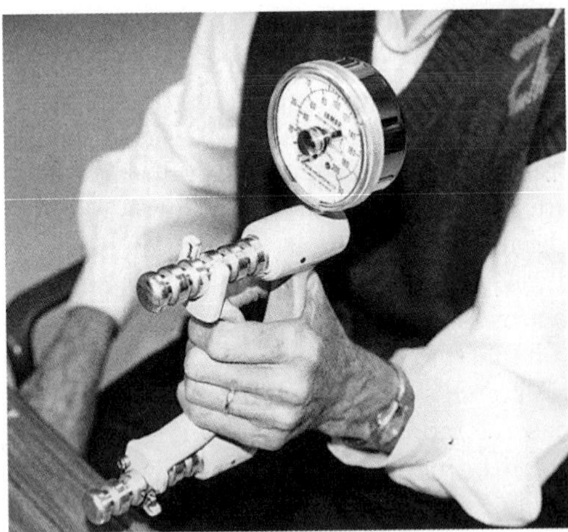

FIGURE 19.9 A Jamar dynamometer yields an objective measure of grip strength.

In cases of weak grip or an inability to grasp the handle, a bulb dynamometer, or a blood pressure cuff rolled to 5 cm and inflated to 5 mm Hg can be used to measure grip strength. Change in the millimeters of mercury is recorded as the power of grip (Fess, 1990). Pinch strength can be evaluated using electronic pinch meters (Pinch Gauge, B & L Engineering, Santa Fe Springs, CA) (Fess, 1990). Usually, three types of pinch are assessed using a pinch meter (Fig. 19.10): (a) *tip-to-tip* (thumb tip to index finger tip), (b) *three-jaw chuck* (thumb pulp to index and long finger pulp), and (c) key or lateral pinch (thumb pulp to lateral aspect of index finger). Typically, three measurements are taken and compared to normative data (Mathiowetz et al., 1983, 1986) or against baseline measures.

Variability in muscle strength and grip and pinch exists across different diagnoses and ages (Desrosiers et al., 1995; Hughes et al., 1999a, b; Jansen et al., 2008; Lee-Valkov et al., 2003; Surrey et al., 2001; Yim et al., 2003). In neurologic populations pinch strength may be more closely associated with fine-motor skill than is grip strength (Chen et al., 2007).

Spasticity. The Modified Ashworth Scale measures spasticity on a scale of 0 to 4 point (Bohannon & Smith, 1987). It has established interrater reliability. See Chapter 5 for more details on this tool.

Edema. Upper-extremity edema affects many patients with neurologic impairments and can be attributed to insufficient pumping mechanisms acting on the venous/lymphatic systems and a disruption in normal tissue physiology (Zarro, 1986). Because edema expands the size of the wrist and hand, active motion can be significantly limited, leading to disuse.

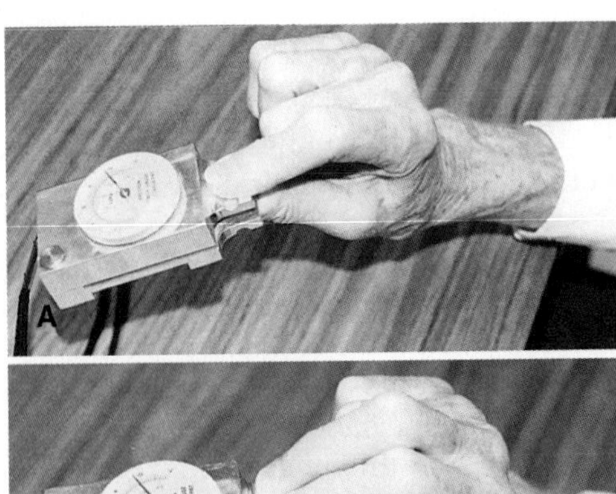

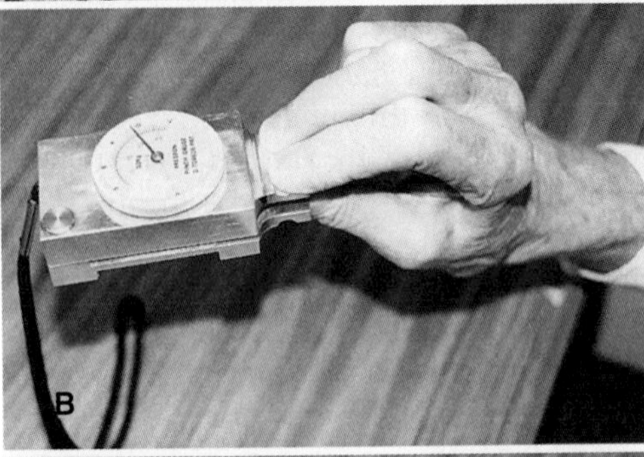

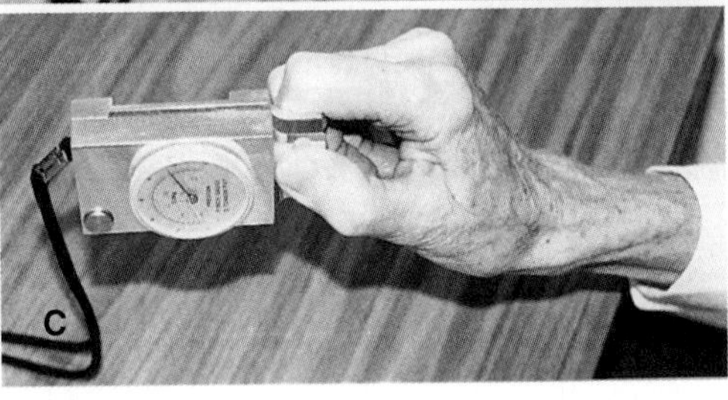

FIGURE 19.10 Use of a pinch meter to measure precision grip strength. Three types of pinch are examined: A, Tip-to-tip; B, Three-jaw chuck; C, Key or lateral grip.

Poststroke edema has been found to be associated with arm and hand dysfunction (Boomkamp-Koppen et al., 2005).

Edema can be evaluated by measuring limb/hand circumference at reproducible anatomic landmarks or by volumetric measurement (Waters et al., 1978). Volumetric assessment measures the water displaced when a limb is immersed; it has been found to have high reliability (Farrell et al., 2003). Because there are significant differences between the dominant and nondominant hands, clinicians should not compare volume measurement of the affected and the less-affected arms in those with hemiplegia. Instead, volume of the affected extremity should be compared to itself over time (Waters et al., 1978). Because volumes are lower while sitting than while standing, a consistent testing position should always be used.

Sensibility. Upper-extremity sensibility tests focus primarily on the hands and fingertips, and are thus quite important to understanding impairments affecting

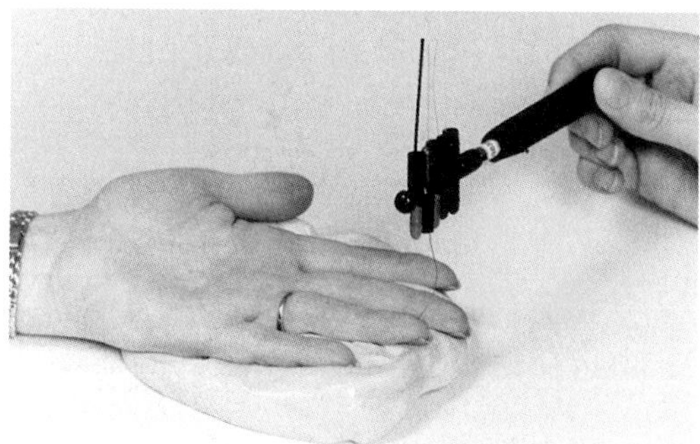

FIGURE 19.11 The use of the Weinstein Enhanced Sensory Test to examine touch pressure sensibility.

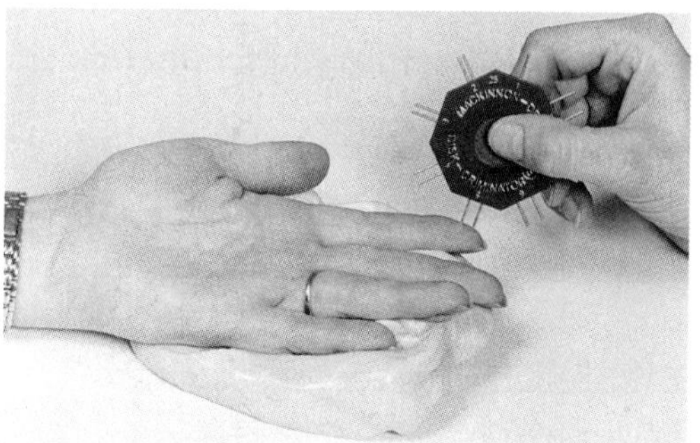

FIGURE 19.12 Examination of two-point discrimination using the DiskCriminator, a commercially available testing instrument.

upper-extremity control (see Figs. 19.11 and 19.12). See Chapter 5 for a full review. A detailed description of tests and norms may be found in the ASHT evaluation manual (Stone, 1992).

Pain. Another complication that reduces participation and recovery of upper-extremity function is pain, because of its association with unpleasant sensory and emotional experiences (Aras et al., 2004; Merskey et al., 1986). Subjective pain information can be obtained through history, interviews and questionnaires, body diagrams, or pain rating scales (Maurer & Jezek, 1992). The McGill Pain Questionnaire (Melzack, 1975) uses a descriptive word list from which patients can choose the quality and intensity of pain. Body diagrams allow the individual to visually describe the location and type of pain. Rating scales such as the Visual Analog Scale and the Faces Pain Rating Scale (Wong & Baker, 1988) have good predictive and high concurrent validity in adults (Price et al., 1983) and children (Jedlinsky et al., 1999). The Face, Legs, Activity, Cry and Consolability (FLACC) behavioral scale is a measure of pain, validated for use with infants and young children from 2 months to 7 years of age (Merkel et al., 2002). Responses for each of the five categories are scored between 0 and 2, for a maximum score of 10, based on a 5-minute observation. The FLACC scale has also been validated to measure pain in children with cognitive impairment (Malviya et al., 2006; Voepel-Lewis et al., 2002).

In summary, when examining upper-extremity control, it is necessary to examine performance at all three levels: (1) function, which includes tests and measures that determines functional capability both in a standardized environments like the clinic (measuring capacity in the ICF) and in the person's actual environment (measuring performance and participation in the ICF); (2) strategies used to accomplish the key components of upper-extremity function, and (3) underlying impairments (body structure and function in the ICF). Because the list of possible tests and measures is extensive, it is important to focus on the areas that seem to restrict upper-extremity function as relevant to the execution of life roles and participation in social and community activities. Tables 19.1 and 19.2 summarize evaluation profiles for both Jean J and Tim. The brief list highlights key areas of function, including participation, underlying components and impairments, with specific tests that could be used for assessment.

TRANSITION TO TREATMENT

Developing therapeutic strategies to retrain upper-extremity control in patients with neurologic dysfunction begins with the identification of patient strengths and weaknesses at all three levels of performance, including functional capability (frequency and independence in activities performed in context [participation]), strategies used to achieve function, and impairments. In addition, understanding contextual factors, including both environmental and personal, that impact treatment decisions is important. Personal factors, include things such as age, gender, ethnicity, educational level, personal interests and desires, self-efficacy and outcomes expectation can all impact goals, choice of therapeutic strategies, and response to intervention. Environmental factors, including social support, available technology and other factors also impact treatment.

Long-Term Goals

As proposed in Chapter 6, long-term goals should be objective and measurable, and they should be expressed in terms of participation in self-care, work, or leisure activities executed to fulfill role expectations. For example, a long-term goal for Jean J could be, "Jean will be able to prepare a morning

TABLE 19-1 Summary of Evaluation Profile for Mrs. Jean J.

Function (Capacity and Performance)	Strategy	Impairments of Body Structure
1. Documentation of frequency of social participation	Qualitative Movement: • Eye-head coordination, • Anticipatory reach to grasp • Prehension patterns available • Grading of fingertip forces • In-hand manipulation ability	• Cognition: Mini-Mental Status Examination • Visual-perception (MVPT) • Musculoskeletal: ROM, strength, • Isolated finger movement available • Spasticity in RUE • Sensibility in RUE • Edema in RUE • Pain at rest and with sustained grip
2. Level of self-care independence: dressing, grooming, bathing, toileting		
3. Level of independence in cooking and self-feeding		
4. Level of mobility with an assistive device		
5. Level of independence in handwriting	• Pencil grip • Efficiency of near and far copying without assistive device	

MVPT = Motor Free Visual Test; RUE = right upper extremity.

TABLE 19-2 Summary of Evaluation Profile for Tim

Function (Capacity and Performance)	Strategy	Impairments (Body Structure and Function)
1. Documentation of frequency of play interaction during class-room activities UE play tasks at recess	Manipulation skills: • Prehension patterns frequently used, • Pencil grip, • In-hand manipulation skill • Efficiency of prehension (task duration)	• Cognition: Visual/auditory memory ABCs & numbers, visual perception • Perception: VMI (Beery & Butenica, 1997), TVPS-R (Gardner, 1996) • Musculoskeletal: Strength, isolated movement of fingers and thumb, core muscle strength • Sensibility through both hands • Pain after prolonged hand use (endurance)
2. Level of self-care independence: don/doff coat with, shoe tying/untying, hand washing, toileting		
3. Level of independence in manipulation of materials: pencils, scissors, glue, tape, others		
4. Level of independence in handwriting	• Efficiency of near and far copying skill (task duration) • Method used to hold paper steady	

VMI = Visual Motor Integration; TVPS-R = Test of Visual Perceptual Skills, Revised.

meal independently (in order to fulfill her homemaker role)." A long-term goal for Tim could be, "Tim will be able to independently and efficiently don outdoor clothing for recess (to fulfill his student role)."

Short-Term Goals

Short-term goals should also be objective and measurable. They may be described with regard to resolving impairments and recovery of key motor strategies. They may also include movement planning, sequencing, and the ability to adapt strategies so that functional tasks can be performed in changing environments. In addition, they may be described as interim steps to achieving independence in a functional task. Tables 19.3 and 19.4 illustrate how the identification of problems progresses to the formation of goals and treatment planning in our two case studies. The examples are not considered all-inclusive yet allow the concepts to be examined more closely.

Patient-Identified Goals

In this era of client-centered practice, clinicians are more inclined to focus on goals set by the patient or parent. This can be done objectively using the Canadian Occupational Performance Measure (COPM) (Carswell et al., 2004; Donovan et al., 2005; Kaiser et al., 2005; Law et al., 2005), introduced above. The tool has successfully been used to document improvement in hand function in children with tetraplegia and to document improvements in self-identified goals and a reduction in disability in adults with mild to moderate brain injury (Mulcahey et al., 2004a, b; Trombly et al., 2002). Use of the COPM may help clinicians to direct intervention toward patients' or parents' goals and to objectively assess treatment outcomes.

TASK-ORIENTED APPROACH TO INTERVENTION

A task-oriented approach to intervention focuses on all levels in which deficits are exposed. For example, in the case of Jean J, interventions within a single session could include strengthening her wrist and finger extensors (impairment level), grasp and release of various objects requiring different prehension patterns (strategy), and practice of a task that incorporates all features (functional activities and participation), such as grasping and placing plastic glasses from the countertop into a kitchen cabinet. This task could be practiced in context by unloading a dishwasher or cleaning the counter in a simulated kitchen or, if one is working in home health care, the tasks could be conducted in the patient's home. The relationship between underlying impairments and hand function may be task-dependent (Gordon & Duff, 1999b). Thus, if the context in which the individual typically performs is not considered, intervention may focus on impairments or strategies that are irrelevant to functional activity and participation in life roles.

Intervention at the Impairment Level

Treatment strategies aimed at modifying sensory and motor impairments were presented in Chapter 5; thus, only a brief discussion of treatment suggestions are presented below.

Cognition and Perception

As emphasized in Chapter 5, cognitive and perceptual impairments can significantly restrict functional movement and are a major factor in lack of progress in those with neurologic insults (Berspang et al., 1989; Sea et al., 1993; Titus et al., 1991; Warburg, 1994). See Table 5.3 for a review of perceptual and cognitive impairments.

Attention and Unilateral Neglect. To promote the identification of an object's characteristics, patients can be encouraged to explore objects visually and haptically, drawing their attention to relevant object features used to shape their hand correctly and to scale fingertip forces. Before patients grasp objects, they can be asked about their perceptions regarding the essential characteristics. For example, the clinician could ask: "Do you think that object is heavy or light?" "Is it slippery or not?" "Can you open your hand wide enough to secure the object?" Research suggests that retraining perceptual aspects of grip is important to the recovery of control (Desanghere & Marotta, 2008).

In patients who have had a stroke, and exhibit unilateral neglect (neglect of one side of the body or extrapersonal space), the clinician can promote movement into that workspace by placing target objects in the area these patients tend to avoid, then asking them to find those objects. Modeling or mirror training could also be used to promote movement in the affected arm by having the patient perform tasks with the less-affected arm in a mirror or through observation of another person. Mirror neurons found in the premotor and parietal cortex and more recently in the primary motor cortex (M1) have been found to be active during motor actions and observation of actions (Bonaiuto & Arbib, 2010; Dushanova & Donoghue, 2010). Thus, viewing action causes

TABLE 19-3 Problems, Goals, and Methods Appropriate for Mrs. Jean J

Level	Problems	Long-Term Goals	Short-Term Goals	Methods
1: Function (Capacity & Performance)	1. Mrs. J. is unable to prepare meals for herself and her husband. 2. Mrs. J is unable to hold kitchen utensils. 3. Mrs. J. is unable to perform self-grooming.	1. Mrs. J. will be able to prepare 3, 2-person meals independently, using utensils. 2. Mrs. J. will be able to groom herself in preparation for guests or outings.	1. Mrs. J. will prepare a simple one- person 3 step meal independently. 2. Mrs. J. will manage utensils, a hairbrush, a toothbrush, and a toothpaste tube independently or with adaptive devices.	1. Provide written step-by-step directions 2. Modeling, task-specific practice, intrinsic/extrinsic variable feedback 3. Adapt tools such as adding foam to handles of: utensils hairbrush, toothbrush to gross allow her to use a gross grasp or a lateral pinch.
2: Strategy	1. Mrs. J. can achieve a gross grasp only in her affected hand 2. Mrs. J. seems to wait until she contacts objects before closing her fingers (poor anticipatory control).		1. Mrs. J. will grasp objects of various sizes and shapes using gross grasp and other pinch patterns. 2. Mrs. J. will prepare for object contact during reaches by opening & partly closing her hand	1. Practice reaching for objects of various objects requiring a gross grasp and progress to to elicitation of a lateral pinch. 2. During reaches, provide variable verbal cues to open then close fingers to prepare for object contact. 3. Replay videotaped practice and talk through action in advance.
3: Impairments (Body, structure, & function)	1. Mrs. J. has visual & auditory memory deficits. 2. Mrs. J. is unable to sequence tasks greater than 2 steps in length. 3. Mrs. J. has incomplete isolated movement of thumb and fingers. 4. Mrs. J. has weak wrist and finger extensors. 5. Sensibility is impaired in volar fingers & thumb		1. Mrs. J. will be verbally state the 3-step sequence of one meal preparation 2. Mrs. J. will read sequence of one meal preparation independently. 3. Mrs. J. will isolate her thumb adductors to achieve a lateral pinch. 4. Mrs. will increase active wrist extension to 25 degrees and MP extension to −10 deg. 5. Mrs. J. will identify objects given tactile & proprioceptive cues.	1. Verbal rehearsal of of meal preparation sequence prior to task-specific practice. 2. Replay of video-taped sessions, discussing steps taken during performance. 3. Place & hold thumb on a small object in a lateral pinch. 4. Biofeedback or FES and resistive equipment such as 1- to 3-lb weights, Theraputty and Velcro boards (finger extension), Biometrics Exercise Kit®. 5. Place familiar small objects on the table and have her practice identifying them with and without vision.

FES = functional electrical stimulation; MP = metacarpophalangeal.

TABLE 19-4 Problems, Goals, and Methods Appropriate for Tim

Level	Problems	Long-Term Goals	Short-Term Goals	Methods
1: Function	1. Tim takes too long donning his coat & boots limiting his play time with friends as recess. 2. Tim requires moderate assistance to complete art projects that require scissor usage.	1. Tim will don his outdoor gear independently and efficiently allowing him to attend full recess. 2. Tim will complete art projects requiring use of scissors independently.	1. Tim will increase his effeciency for donning his coat and boots by reducing the task duration 25% per week. 2. Tim will trace a circle, cut it out, and paste it on paper as described in the directions.	1a. Therapist/peer modeling 1b. Timed task-specific practice donning coat/boots, & securing buttons 1c. Variable intrinsic/ extrinsic. 1d. Button-hook or large boots. 2. Introduce scissors with smaller finger openings to enhance stability. 3. Peer modeling with variable verbal feedback.
2: Strategy	1. Tim has difficulty solving motor problems such as learning to secure fasteners on new jacket. 2. Tim's in-hand manipulation skills are limited.		1. Tim will secure and open a range of coat fasteners using a range of solutions in 2 mos. 2. Tim will shift a pencil among his fingerpads to write & erase within one hand in one month.	1a. Teacher/peer modeling 1b. Task-specific practice with a different fasteners from various types of jackets 1c. Variable intrinsic/ extrinsic feedback on solutions used. 2. Task specific practice moving different writing utensils one hand.
3: Impairments	1. Tim has weak intrinsic hand muscles, reducing his pinch/grip strength.		1. Tim will increase his pinch strength by 1/2 lb in 2 mo. (lateral pinch, 3-jaw chuck).	1. Therapeutic putty exercises at school and at home. 2. Construction of objects using Legos.

enough activity to help predict the direction and trajectory of observed movement online. Clinicians may be able to take advantage of the mirror neuron system to promote active movement in neurologic populations such as individuals with stroke (Garrison et al., 2010).

Problem-Solving and Apraxia. Learning to solve movement problems is a major step toward the development or recovery of motor skills (Adolph, 1994). To promote this, the clinician can ask the patient to demonstrate "how to hold the fork in order to get the potatoes on it" or offer a verbal solution to the problem. In clients without perceptual deficits, modeling of an alternative strategy may allow for easy success. If they have perceptual problems, such as poor spatial relations, one may need to model the task and then provide verbal or manual cues to initiate or guide them through the appropriate movement(s). Whenever manual assistance is given, the therapist (or helper) becomes part of the movement solution. Therefore, any manual assistance should be immediately followed by independent task practice to give patients the opportunity to plan and perform the movement themselves.

Treatment methods that require the patient to solve movement problems can lead to greater motor learning. Two clinical examples are robotic training in adults after stroke and training using the mobile paradigm in infants. Patton and colleagues (2005) used robotic training in 18 patients after stroke. Patients were trained to reach in a force field that pushed the limb clockwise or counterclockwise in proportion to its speed and perpendicular to its direction of motion. All subjects showed evidence of adaptation to the force field through measurable after-effects. However, after-effects were not correlated with clinical impairment measures. Interestingly, improvements were primarily observed when the forces for training magnified the original errors, suggesting that error-enhancing therapy fostered learning.

Galloway and colleagues (Heathcock et al., 2004) proposed that the mobile paradigm might be one way to assess the learning and memory abilities of infants. The mobile-conjugate reinforcement paradigm introduced by Rovee-Collier and Sullivan (1980) engages young infants by associating movement of the mobile with kicking or reaching behaviors, due to tethering of the mobile to either the leg or arm of the infant. The efficacy for using the mobile paradigm for training infants with upper-extremity movement disorders has also been examined. Duff and colleagues (2004) had three infants with brachial plexus birth palsy participate in 1 month of movement training (unilateral, bilateral, or unspecified) through interaction with an overhead mobile along with standard care. All infants displayed improved motion/strength based on the Active Movement Scale (Curtis et al., 2002) immediately after training and 2 months after training. Although reaching improved in the involved limb, reach-to-grasp skill, as measured by toy contact, was better in the noninvolved limb at follow-up. Interestingly, passive shoulder flexion improved, yet, external rotation (ER) in the involved limb was more limited at 2 months of follow-up, suggesting that a loss in ER may coincide with reaching onset, habitual recruitment of internal rotators, and changes in glenohumeral joint alignment.

Training to Improve Musculoskeletal and Neuromuscular System Characteristics

Numerous methods are available to enhance ROM and strength, reduce the effects of spasticity, and increase isolated movement. For example, passive and active exercises, myofascial release (Manheim & Lavett, 1989), the Feldenkrais method (Apel, 1992), Tai Chi (Hogan, 2005; Venglar, 2005), yoga, and related approaches (Wanning, 1993) can be used to mobilize structures essential to upper-extremity control. Participation in enjoyable recreational activities such as Tai Chi has been found to increase not only physical function but also cognitive skills (Hogan, 2005).

Manual Techniques. Many sources describe in detail approaches to mobilizing the trunk and upper-extremity structures and enhancing movement in patients with neurologic dysfunction (Bobath, 1970; Boehme, 1988; Carr & Shepard, 1987; Davies, 1985; Duncan & Badke, 1987; Voss et al., 1985). While passive stretching techniques are useful, active movement should follow it to promote carryover. For example, in patients with hemiplegia who habitually hold the affected upper extremity in a mass flexion pattern, tightness of the hand and wrist flexors typically develops, limiting the development or return of active movement. Thus, in treatment, after the distal flexors have been passively stretched, the clinician can ask the patient to attempt to open the hand to touch or grasp (depending on skill) stable objects placed on the table within reach and at the far end of the workspace to promote elbow extension.

Splints. Approaches to the remediation of musculoskeletal tightness and shortening of arm and hand structures often include the use of plaster casts, splints, and orthoses (Cannon, 1985; Cruickshank & O'Neill, 1990; Cusick & Sussman, 1982; Fess et al., 2005; Lindholm, 1985; Malick, 1980; Neuhaus et al., 1981; Smith & Harris, 1985; Yasukawa, 1992). Sustained low-load stretch to muscle and joint structures, accomplished through splinting, has been found to increase the number of muscle sarcomeres and change the length of the noncontractile tissue (joint capsule, ligaments) (Blanchard et al., 1985; Tardieu et al., 1988).

The use of splints that minimize joint restriction and allow functional hand use is optimal. But, in cases of flaccidity or inactive hand movement, positions that minimize the potential development of undesirable contractures associated with immobility are preferred. For example, the intrinsic plus position of the hand (Fig. 19.13A) places the thumb in partial abduction and the fingers in metacarpophalangeal joint flexion and interphalangeal joint extension to ensure that the ligaments are taut and the joints adequately positioned. If a patient displays excessive wrist flexion that interferes with active grasp, a semiflexible splint (Fig. 19.13B) may be useful; this allows partial wrist movement within the individual's active joint

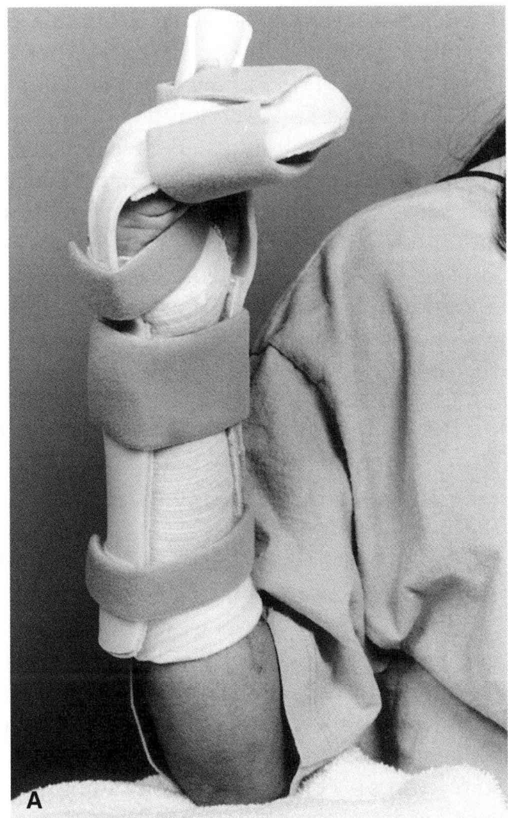

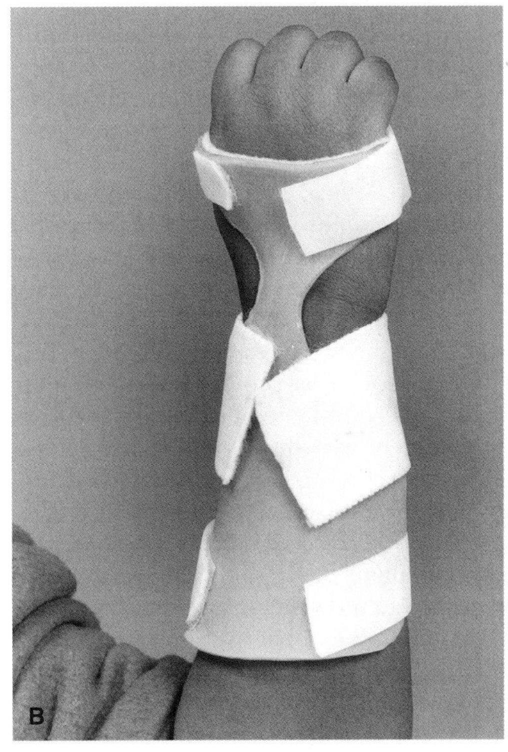

FIGURE 19.13 Splints used to influence hand and wrist position, including an intrinsic plus splint (A) and a semiflexible wrist splint (B).

excursion, yet prevents extreme wrist flexion, which limits grasp function. Although hand splinting does provide support and prevent contractures, nonaffected structures should be allowed to move freely, to prevent secondary impairments due to immobility.

Augmented Motion and Feedback. Various methods are available to augment motion and provide feedback to reduce impairments and expand resources. These include robotic training, biofeedback, electrical stimulation, transcranial motor stimulation (TMS), and sensory reeducation. We will now review the efficacy of a few forms of augmented motion feedback.

Robotic Training. To augment passive/active training provided by therapists, researchers have begun to explore the use of robotic training. Hogan and colleagues (Fasoli et al., 2004; Stein et al., 2004) have compared the effect of robotic training in the form of progressive resistive exercise (PRE) versus active assistive (AA) training on functional and motor recovery performed three times per week for 6 weeks. Results from 46 individuals revealed improvements in Fugl-Meyer scores and maximal force output (Stein et al., 2004). However, there was no difference between the PRE and AA groups, with the exception that those with better motor control before treatment made the most gains with PRE robotic training based on the Fugl-Meyer score.

Fasoli and colleagues (2004) further examined the long-term effects of robotic training with tests 4 months after the end of therapy. The authors found significant improvements based on the Modified Ashworth, the Fugl-Meyer, and the Motor Status Scales from time of admission to follow-up sessions. Robotic training also seems to have an effect on improving muscle activation during reaching after stroke (Lum et al., 2004). Lum and colleagues (2004) had 13 subjects with chronic stroke practice with robotic training for twenty-four 1-hour sessions over an 8-week period. The authors found that following training, subjects improved both muscle activation when reaching against gravity and overall work output.

Some studies have found that the effects from robotic therapy are comparable to those achieved with conventional therapy. Reinkensmeyer and colleagues (2009) examined the basis of motor recovery after stroke. The authors found that 4 to 5 weeks of either robotic training or nonrobotic training resulted in improved strength, speed, and coordination.

Based on this study and others (i.e., Masiero et al., 2007), robotic therapy may best be used to complement conventional therapy or other methods such as virtual reality (Eng et al., 2007). Robotic training may also be most useful if it requires error correction from patients for movements that are off target versus only providing active assistance to minimize errors (Patton et al., 2006).

Biofeedback and Neuromuscular Electrical Stimulation. Biofeedback and neuromuscular electrical stimulation (NMES) or functional electrical stimulation (FES) can provide support and enhance movement in those with reduced upper-extremity function. Electrical stimulation can be provided through surface, percutaneous, or implanted electrodes. Because timelines for treatment vary depending on the nature of the dysfunction, clinical judgment will have to guide schedules for biofeedback and NMES. The positive outcomes from research studies support the integration of both biofeedback and NMES into clinical practices related to the development and recovery of active movement in the upper extremities in adults and children.

How effective is biofeedback and NMES in the recovery of upper-extremity function, and do outcomes differ in adults and children and in different neurologic populations? A number of studies have examined the effect of NMES used to improve upper-extremity function. Alon and colleagues (2003) used a home-based self-administered program of NMES to improve hand function in 77 subjects with chronic stroke. After training, subjects showed a significant reduction in performance on timed dexterity tests based on the Jebsen–Taylor hand-function test, the Box and Block Test, and the Nine-Hole Peg Test. Furthermore, a reduction in spasticity and pain was reported after training.

Scheker and colleagues (1999) combined FES 1 hour a day (to triceps and wrist/finger extensors) with dynamic bracing (assisted metacarpophalangeal extension, biceps strengthening aimed at supination) in children with hemiplegic cerebral palsy and found a reduction in spasticity and improved hand function. Wright and Granat (2000) applied 30 minutes of FES to the wrist extensors of children (mean age, 10 years) with hemiplegic cerebral palsy for 6 weeks, and found that active wrist extension and hand function improved with treatment and was maintained at 6 weeks follow-up.

Sullivan and Hedman (2004) used a single case study design to study the effects of 18 weeks of home-based sensory amplitude electrical stimulation (SES) and NMES on upper-extremity performance in an adult patient who had sustained a stroke. The first 6 weeks of training involved 2 hours of SES to the volar forearm (just above the level of perception) and 15 minutes of NMES to the left wrist extensors during grasp and lift of an aluminum can. The amplitude of the NMES was self-adjusted based on the amount of stimulation needed to lift the can. From 6 to 18 weeks, SES treatment continued, but the NMES stimulation site was changed to the finger extensors because the subject could actively engage the wrist extensors, allowing for a wider grip aperture. After 18 weeks, the subject showed significant improvements on both the ARAT and the STREAM tests and reported that he could now fasten buttons, use a knife and fork, and tie simple fishing knots. The authors concluded that many factors contributed to these improvements and recommended further study to separate the effects of SES and NMES.

A 3-week training program that included NMES in combination with a wrist splint (HANDS) was found to improve upper-extremity motor function and reduce spasticity in 20 adults with chronic stroke immediately and after a 3-month follow-up (Fujiwara et al., 2009). Other studies have found that training using electromyography-triggered NMES contributed to recovery of arm function, although the effects were small or based on other factors, such as contributions from muscle groups other than those receiving NMES (Barker et al., 2009; Bello et al., 2009).

The benefits of cortical stimulation for recovery of arm and hand movement have been examined through implanted electrode methods and external transcranial magnetic stimulation (TMS). Cortical implanted, stimulation has been examined for use in recovery of arm function after stroke (Huang et al., 2009). A 6 month follow-up from that training study revealed significant differences as compared with controls based on the Upper Extremity Fugl-Meyer scores and the Box and Block test. The benefits of cortical stimulation after stroke were found to be enhanced if they were combined with task-oriented training (Bravi & Stoykov, 2007). A pilot study with 10 patients examined the benefits of transcranial direct stimulation in combination with robotic therapy and found significant improvement in a small number of patients and little change in the remaining patients (Hesse et al., 2007). The authors concluded that the techniques were safe but required further examination.

Sensory Reeducation

It is uncertain just how much functional sensibility can be improved following a peripheral or central lesion. Does sensory reeducation teach patients how to use the remaining sensibility to their advantage, or does it actually alter the physiologic basis for sensation? Investigators involved in training and retraining of sensory function report that improvement is highly dependent on the individual's motivation as well as the training. Patients who were willing to use the affected limb were better able to recover function.

A safe guideline to follow for sensory training is related to the patient's level of performance on the Semmes–Weinstein Monofilaments test (refer to Chapter 5 for a discussion of this test of sensory function). If an individual is unable to detect a 4.83 pressure rating, he or she is considered to have absent or significantly impaired protective sensation. In those cases, treatment should focus on teaching strategies to protect the limb from harmful stimuli (Brand, 1980). Table 19.5 summarizes a series of guidelines aimed at protecting the hand and arm from injury. As dictated by returning or developing sensibility (once protective sensation is intact or touch pressure is above a pressure rating of 4.83), treatment can focus on the detection and localization of moving and stationary light touch stimuli. As patients learn to perceive constant and moving touch, sensory reeducation can shift to stereognosis (e.g., size/shape discrimination, object recognition).

A large part of sensory reeducation makes use of higher cortical functions, including attention, learning, and memory, to facilitate sensory detection, recognition, and localization (Dellon et al., 1974). Tactile retraining generally is done with and without vision. For example, because it is known that moving stimuli are easier to detect than stationary stimuli, the patient can be taught to move the hand to follow a moving stimulus, and thus improve the chances for sensory awareness. Vision can be used to compensate for deficits in tactile sensation; thus, the patient can be taught to look at the hand when reaching for or grasping an object (Bell-Krotoski et al., 1993).

Sensory stimulation may also be an effective method to enhance motor function. Rosen and Lundborg (2003) examined the use of artificial sensibility in the form of vibrotactile cues to replace the absence of sensibility following median and ulnar nerve injury in a single case study. Specifically, they placed microphones on the tips of a sensor glove to pick up friction information during object manipulation. The functional outcome at 6 and 12 months showed higher performance levels than usual for this type of surgical intervention. Lundborg and colleagues (2005) used functional magnetic resonance imaging to verify that typical adults trained in vibrotactile input using the sensor glove were able to integrate the audio-tactile information provided. The authors demonstrated that trained subjects showed greater activation of the somatosensory cortex than untrained adults.

TABLE 19.5 Summary of Guidelines Aimed at Protecting the Hand and Arm from Injury

1. Avoid exposure to thermal extremes and sharp objects.
2. Do not use excessive force when gripping a tool or object.
3. Build up small handles to distribute force and avoid localized increase in pressure.
4. Avoid tasks that require the use of a uniform grip over long periods.
5. Change tools frequently to alter grip pattern and to rest tissues.
6. Observe skin for signs of excess pressure.
7. Treat blisters and lacerations quickly and with care to avoid infection.
8. Maintain daily skin care, including soaking and oil massage to maintain optimal skin condition.

Adapted from Brand PW. Management of sensory loss in the extremities. In: Omer E, Spinner M, eds. Management of peripheral nerve problems. Philadelphia: Saunders, 1980:862–872.

Edema and Pain

To reduce hand edema, one or more of the following strategies can be used: compression (through the use of gloves made of stretchable material), ice, elevation above the level of the heart, or active muscle pumping. The effectiveness of any method can be verified using volume or circumference measurement. Reduction in edema with an increase in active movement may also assist in pain reduction. Other methods to reduce pain include the use of heat or cold or transcutaneous electrical nerve stimulation (TENS) (Mannheimer & Lampe, 1984). Depending on the characteristics of the pain, TENS may be appropriate for rest periods after exercise or during active movement.

Intervention at Strategy Level

A task-oriented approach to retraining involves more than just the resolution of impairments constraining performance of functional tasks and participation in social roles. Yet, alleviating underlying impairments allows for the possibility of using previously developed strategies for upper-extremity control. When permanent impairments make the resumption of previously used strategies impossible, patients will need to be guided in the recovery (or development of) sensory and motor strategies that are effective in performing the key components of upper-extremity control.

Key movement components such as a smooth hand path and anticipatory grip formation may be best elicited if real tasks are used instead of simulated ones (Wu et al., 1998). Because research has shown that development of key components such as reach and grasp are driven by the nature and context of the activity, retraining these key components must be done within the context of purposeful tasks and real-life situations as much as possible.

Eye-Head Coordination

An important part of upper-extremity control is training or retraining eye–head coordination, which is essential to locating and stabilizing gaze on a target or an object to be grasped. Problems that affect the ability to locate objects and stabilize gaze potentially affect the accuracy and precision of reaching movements. Because different control mechanisms underlie the movements of eyes, head, and trunk, these systems need to be trained both separately and in combination.

A progression of exercises for retraining eye–head coordination and gaze stabilization in patients with vestibular dysfunction has been proposed by Susan Herdman, a physical therapist, and David Zee, M.D. (Herdman, 2001; Zee, 1985). These exercises have been used successfully to retrain eye–head coordination problems in patients with central neurologic disorders (Herdman, 2001; Zee, 1985).

This approach is reviewed in Table 19.6 and begins with exercises to retrain saccadic and smooth-pursuit eye movements while the head is still. Progressive exercises are given to retrain coordinated eye movements in conjunction with head movements to targets located in the periphery. Also practiced are exercises to maintain a stable gaze on an object moving in phase with the head. Finally, movements involving eye, head, and trunk motions are practiced as patients learn to locate targets oriented in the far periphery. Exercises are practiced while sitting, standing, and walking (Herdman, 2001; Zee, 1985).

Research in the field of training/retraining visual perception in patients with central neural lesions is just beginning. Strategies to assist patients with visual-field deficits, such as homonymous hemianopsia, involve teaching them to consciously scan the space represented by the impaired visual field (see earlier suggestions regarding treatment strategies for visual neglect in this and other chapters).

Reach and Grasp

Reach-to-grasp movements require the ability to move the arm in all directions. They involve transporting the hand to an object to be grasped, forming the grip appropriately, stabilizing or manipulating the object, and possibly moving the object to a new location.

Facilitation of Active Motion. Training or retraining control of upper-extremity movement in cases of congenital or acquired paresis often begins with therapeutic strategies used to facilitate active motion by the patient. Several authors have laid out a progression of activities for retraining arm function, which includes training or retraining control of arm movements underlying the transport phase of upper-extremity function (Bobath, 1970; Boehme, 1988; Carr & Shepard, 1986; Davies, 1985; Duncan & Badke, 1987; Voss et al., 1985). Most of the suggestions are directed toward practicing control of isolated joint movements through "place-and-hold" techniques in supine, sitting, and standing positions. These exercises are based on the assumption that practicing activation of isolated muscles will carry over to functional tasks. For example, retraining active control of arm movements is often begun in the supine position with the shoulder flexed and the elbow extended (Fig. 19.14A). This position minimizes the amount of force the patient must generate to move the arm actively against gravity. However, based on what we know about the difficulty of transferring tasks learned in isolation to task performance in context, these suggestions must be examined more closely.

The inclusion of target objects in upper-extremity movement activities often engages the patient more successfully than movement alone, because it makes the task more goal-directed. The target objects used should vary depending on grasp capabilities and program goals. For example, in individuals without grasp, simply pointing to pictures with the whole hand or engaging in tasks such as knocking down blocks or pushing balls will suffice. As grasp improves, task complexity and the type of objects used can be expanded.

In cases of weakness, it may be best to require movement in the gravity-eliminated plane. For example, shoulder horizontal abduction and elbow extension can be practiced while sitting by asking the individual to knock over a series of cardboard blocks with the dorsum of the hand, initially providing table support under the arm and progressing to performance of the same movement without arm support.

In some cases, gravity can assist motion. For example, as shown in Figure 19.14B, when the

TABLE 19-6 Exercises to Retrain Saccadic and Smooth-Pursuit Eye Movements While the Head is Still

Stage I. Eye Exercises
A. Exercises to improve visual following (smooth pursuit)
1. Sit in a comfortable position; do not move your head.
2. Hold a small target (about 2 × 2 inches, like a matchbook cover) containing written material at arm's length in front of you.
3. Keep your head still.
4. Move your arm slowly from side to side about 45 degrees. Try to keep the words in focus as you move.
5. Move your arm to the left, then right, then center. Rest for 3 seconds. Repeat 5 times.
6. Move your arm up and down about 30 degrees. Move your arm up, then down, then center. Rest for 3 seconds. Repeat 5 times.
B. Exercises to improve gaze redirection (saccade)
1. Sit in a comfortable position; do not move your head.
2. Hold two small targets (2 inches × 2 inches), one in each hand, about 12 inches apart in front of you.
3. Move your eyes only from one target to the other.
4. Move right; move left. Stop and rest.
5. Repeat 5 times.
6. Hold the two targets in front of you vertically, above and below the midline. Keep your head still; move your eyes only from one target to the other.
7. Move eyes up, eyes down. Stop and rest.
8. Repeat 5 times.
Stage II. Head Exercises
A. Move head, object still
1. Side-to-side movements: Hold at arm's length a small target, such as a matchbook. Try to keep the words in clear focus; move your head slowly from side to side. Move head to the right, move head left, move head to the center. Rest. Repeat 5 times.
2. Up and down movements: Repeat, but move your head up and down while keeping your eyes on the target held in front of you. Move head up; move head down; come to the center. Stop and rest. Repeat 5 times.
3. To progress, move your head faster and faster until you can no longer read the words. Repeat using a target that is attached to the wall 6 feet away.
4. Practice steps 1 and 2 with your eyes closed. Try to visualize the target in your mind and focus on it as if your eyes were open.
Stage III. Eye-Head Exercises
A. Move eyes and head to stationary objects
1. Side-to-side movements: Hold two small targets (2 inches × 2 inches), one in each hand, about 36 inches apart in front of you. Move your head and eyes to look first at one target, then at the other. Try to clearly focus on the words on each target each time you move your head and eyes. Look left; look right; then rest. Repeat 5 times.

(*continued*)

TABLE 19-6 Exercises to Retrain Saccadic and Smooth-Pursuit Eye Movements While the Head is Still

2. Up-and-down movements: Hold the two targets in front of you vertically, above and below the midline, about 36 inches apart. Move your head and eyes to look first at one target, then at the other. Try to focus clearly on the words on each target each time you move your head and eyes. Look left; look right; then rest. Repeat 5 times.
3. To progress, repeat steps 1 and 2, moving your head at faster and faster speeds until you can no longer read the words. Repeat using a target that is attached to the wall 6 feet away.
B. Move eyes, head, and object in phase together
1. Side-to-side movements: Hold a small target (about 2 inches × 2 inches, like a matchbook cover) containing written material at arm's length in front of you. Move your arm and head together from side to side. Try to keep the words in clear focus while you move your arm and head together slowly from side to side (about 45 degrees). Move left; move right; move center; rest. Repeat 5 times.
2. Up-and-down movements: Hold a small target (about 2 inches × 2 inches, like a matchbook cover) containing written material at arm's length in front of you. Move your arm and head together up and down. Try to keep the words in clear focus while you move your arm and head together slowly up and down about 30 degrees. Move up; move down; move center; rest. Repeat 5 times.
3. To progress, repeat steps 1 and 2, moving your head at faster and faster speeds until you can no longer read the words. Repeat using a target which is attached to the wall 6 feet away.

Reprinted with permission from Zee DS. Vertigo. In Johnson RT. Current Therapy in Neurological Diseases. St. Louis: C.V. Mosby, 1985:8–13.

supine patient is asked to touch his hand to his nose (or shoulder or head), gravity assists elbow flexion, while he eccentrically activates his triceps to slow the descent of the hand (this may be combined with NMES). As isolated control improves, transport activities (e.g., tapping a suspended ball or retrieving a beanbag from the ipsilateral shoulder and throwing it toward the feet) may be used (possibly in conjunction with NMES). These activities activate the triceps both concentrically and eccentrically.

Retraining Task-Dependent Characteristics of Reach. Because the characteristics of the transport phase vary with the task, it is important to structure intervention so that the patient learns to modify the movements used to transport the arm and hand in space

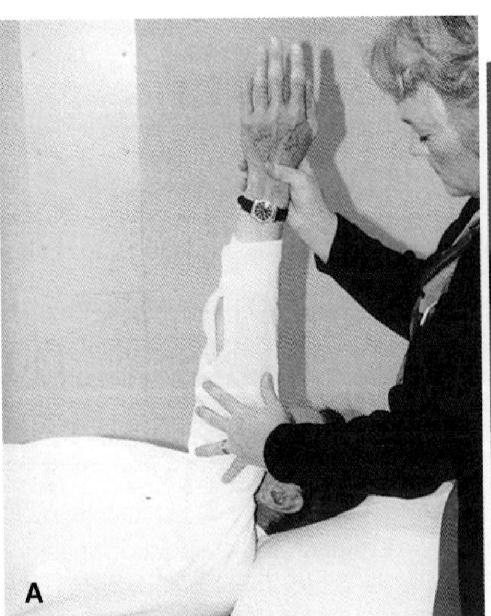

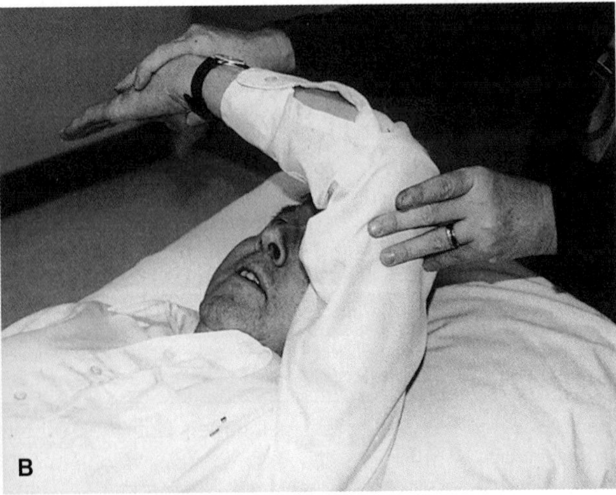

FIGURE 19.14 Exercises to assist active movement in the upper extremity. Use of the supine position can allow gravity to assist movement. In this case, the patient is asked to touch his nose. Gravity assists elbow flexion while the triceps work eccentrically to slow the descent of the hand.

in a task-dependent way. The following are potential ways to train and retrain reaching based on research examining the characteristics of transport during upper-extremity tasks. As with other suggestions made throughout this chapter, these suggestions require validation through research.

1. Because the transport phase of movements such as pointing, reaching and grasping, and grasping and manipulating an object have very different characteristics, training needs to be specific to each type of task.
2. To help patients become proficient in scanning for relevant cues before movement onset, the clinician can provide cues on target location and characteristics of the object to be grasped. Initially, it may be advantageous to have the patient practice slower movements, drawing the attention to visual cues relating to hand movement, particularly thumb position in relation to target location.
3. Research also suggests that the ability to reach to a new position in space without visual feedback is also important. Without vision, proprioceptive information provides cues to allow for the modulation of stiffness in agonist and antagonist muscles surrounding joints (refer to the section on location programming in Chapter 15). To facilitate performance, one might place the patient at a table where he or she could locate the target visually but not be allowed to see his or her hands. Reaching accuracy would provide the clinician with outcome information regarding the patient's ability to modulate the stiffness of agonist and antagonist muscles through proprioceptive cues only.
4. To facilitate force modulation during reaching, the clinician could ask the patient to reach slowly, then quickly, to targets placed at various reaching distances and locations in the workspace. In this way, the patient learns to program forces appropriately for both slow and fast movements, and in addition to movements requiring increased accuracy.
5. To reduce the development of compensatory strategies and facilitate greater extent and speed of reaching movements in the affected limb of adult patients who have had a stroke, it has been recommend that trunk movement be restricted during reach-to-grasp training (Michaelsen et al., 2006; Thielman et al., 2008).
6. As reviewed earlier, modeling or mental rehearsal (self-initiated or verbalized by the therapist) may take advantage of the Mirror Neuron System to enhance movement strategies (Garrison et al., 2010). These strategies conducted prior to active movement may allow for longer processing and preparation time.

Verbal and Vibrotactile Cues. Fasoli and colleagues (2002) studied the impact of verbal instructions on functional reach in individuals with stroke. They found that the reaches of those given externally focused or task-related instructions were shorter and exhibited a higher peak velocity for all three tasks than the group who received internally focused or movement-related instructions. The effect of using visual cueing to enhance movement in those with Parkinson's disease (PD) has been well documented; less is known about the impact of auditory cueing. Nowak and colleagues (2005) trained individuals with PD on a grasp-modulation task using auditory cues or stimulation of the subthalamic nucleus (SN). They found that use of the auditory cues was more effective than SN stimulation at improving akinesia. Interestingly, SN stimulation caused subjects to use excessive grip force during self-paced and externally paced conditions. More research is needed on the impact of different schedules of verbal and auditory cueing during treatment in neurologic populations.

Postural Training. Stoykov and colleagues (2005) used postural activities to improve prehensile function in the ataxic upper limb. The intervention involved 4 weeks of 1-hour treatments, three times per week. Improvements were supported by significant change in Fugl-Meyer scores and modest increases in the PASS. The authors suggest that treatment focused on improving postural control contributed to recovery of upper extremity function; however, further research is needed.

What is the effect of constraining trunk motion on reach-and-grasp abilities? Two studies by Michaelsen and colleagues and one study by Thielman and colleagues examined the effect of restraining the trunk on upper-extremity recovery in individuals with chronic stroke. Michaelsen and Levin (2004) had participants perform a reach-to-grasp training task for 60 trials over a 1-day session. Participants were randomly divided into a trunk-restrained (TR) group or a control group and asked not to move the trunk during reaches. The results indicated that the TR group used less trunk motion after training than controls. While elbow extension increased in both groups it was larger in the TR group at retention. The authors used a Temporal Coordination Index (TCI) to examine interjoint coordination. The TCI is the calculated difference between elbow- and shoulder-phase angles (velocity against angle) at each moment in time (phase angle against time) throughout movement. Multiple small peaks in the TCI provide evidence for a disruption in temporal coordination. TCI amplitude (TCI plotted against time) was found to correlate with performance as measured on the Fugl-Meyer Scale.

A follow-up study (Michaelsen et al., 2006) involved a double-blind, randomized, controlled trial comparing TR against a control group. The supervised home program was carried out with 30 patients three times per week for 5 weeks. Baseline, immediate, and 1-month follow-up results were compared using the upper extremity Fugl-Meyer test, the Upper Extremity Performance Assessment (TEMPA), isometric force, manual dexterity (Box and Block Test), and reaching kinematics. Follow-up results indicated that TR training generally showed greater improvement than those in the control group, based on the Fugl-Meyer and TEMPA tests, particularly those with moderate hemiparesis. Kinematic results at follow-up also revealed a greater reduction in trunk displacement and elbow extension in those with moderate hemiparesis. Conversely, the control group demonstrated an increase in compensatory trunk displacement and a decrease in elbow extension. These studies suggest that treatment aimed at reducing compensatory strategies in the trunk may lead to better upper limb reaching strategies and subsequent function.

Thielman and colleagues (2008) compared task-related training (TRT) and resistive exercise (RE) in 11 adults after stroke for twelve 4-week sessions. For both groups, the trunk was restrained during training. Outcome measures included the Fugl-Meyer, the WMFT, and kinematic reaching to unilateral, midline, and contralateral targets. Findings showed that after training the hand path was straighter for the TRT group but not for the RE group. Also, trunk flexion decreased after both TRT and RE, yet arm flexion increased in all subjects in the TRT group and only at midline and contralateral targets. After scores improved on the Fugl-Meyer in both groups, but was no change on the WMFT.

Adaptive Positioning. Adaptive seating is a frequently used intervention aimed at improving upper-extremity function by enhancing postural control. Seating programs are based on three assumptions: (1) adaptive seats will reduce abnormal muscle tone; (2) improved muscle tone will improve postural stability; and (3) increased postural stability will enhance upper-extremity control (Kluzik et al., 1990; McPherson et al., 1991; Shellenkens et al., 1983; Waksvik & Levy, 1979). Several studies have examined the effect of altered seat angles on arm movements in children with and without cerebral palsy (CP). While one study showed that arm movements in children with CP were faster with a backrest set at 90 degrees (Nwaobi et al., 1983), most kinematic studies have not found seating posture to make a difference on immediate reaching movements (McPherson et al., 1991; Seeger et al., 1984). These results do not rule out a long-term effect of altered seating posture on reaching skills.

Retraining Anticipatory Aspects of Reach and Grasp. Despite the importance of planning movement trajectory and forces in advance, it is difficult to teach anticipatory control. However, therapists can encourage its development by enhancing underlying resources and by providing opportunities to grasp and manipulate diverse objects in various locations with and without preparatory cues and feedback.

What can be done to assist patients who underestimate or overestimate the location and size of target objects? First, related components such as vision and sensibility in the hand can be examined. We rely on sensory feedback to develop and strengthen our internal representations of object properties and distances, which we use for anticipatory control of grip formation and force scaling during object manipulation. If there are deficits in either vision or sensation in the hand, the potential for improvement in these components should be determined first. With an estimate of the potential for improvement, visual and/or sensory reeducation techniques may be implemented (reviewed above). Until hand sensibility improves, or if the potential for improvement is low, patients should be allowed extended practice or be taught compensatory techniques. With extended practice, patients with underdeveloped or impaired anticipatory control demonstrate significant improvement (Dawson et al., 2010; Duff & Gordon, 2003; Gordon & Duff, 1999a). Interlimb transfer has also been found to improve anticipatory force scaling in adults and children with hemiplegia (Gordon et al., 1999; Raghavan et al., 2006).

Grasp and Manipulation

Training and retraining grasp function in patients with paresis and dyscontrol often begins with the establishment of a power grip (Erhardt, 1982). The power grip uses simultaneous finger flexion to allow for a cylindrical hold on objects with wrist stabilization. It is probably best to retrain power grip first, because finger fractionation (used with precision grips) may be limited. Second, power grip plays an important role in holding/manipulating assistive mobility devices.

When retraining power grasp, patients can be assisted in molding the hand to cylindrical objects of different sizes in a pattern of finger flexion and

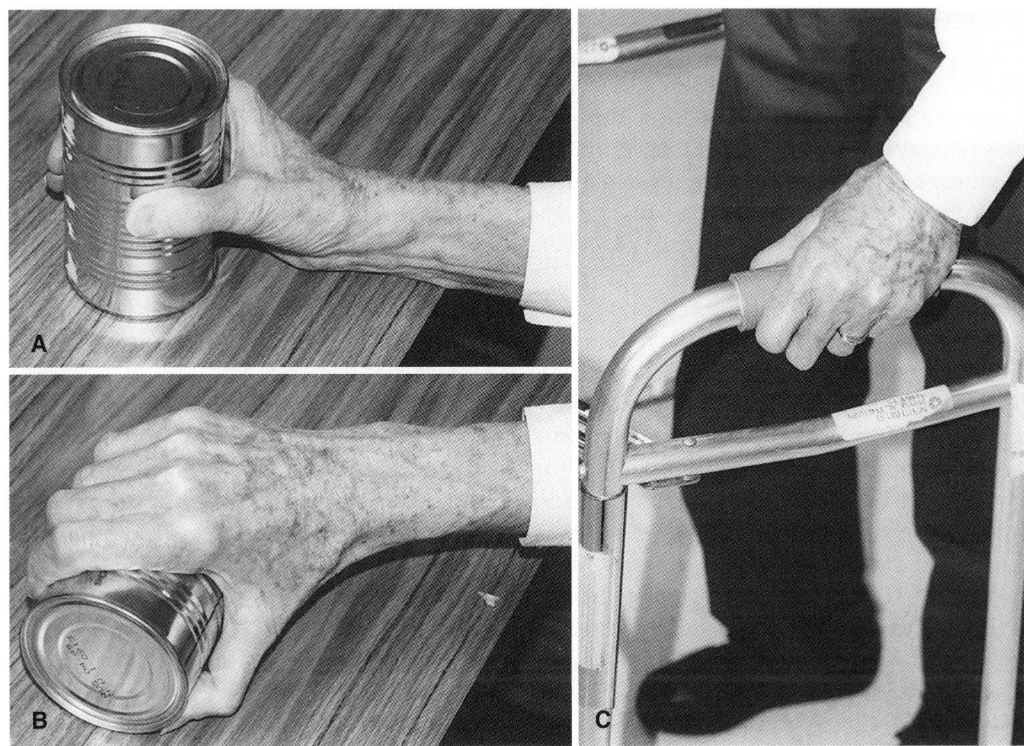

FIGURE 19.15 Retraining power grasp. Power grasp used: A, to pick up an object oriented vertically; B, to pick up an object oriented horizontally; or C, to hold an assistive device used for gait.

thumb opposition. Once achieved, the power grasp can be practiced in the vertical and horizontal planes to encourage various forearm and wrist orientations (Fig. 19.15). Grasp retraining should progress to teaching patients a succession of precision grip patterns (as corticomotoneuronal connections and subsequent isolation of the fingers allow). These patterns include a lateral pinch (thumb to lateral index finger), three-jaw chuck (thumb opposed to radial two fingers), and a pincer grasp (index to thumb opposition, tip to tip or pad to pad) (Erhardt, 1994). Figure 19.16 depicts a child with hemiplegic CP attempting a pincer grasp.

Research has shown that many of the elements of grasp are planned in advance of object contact. Thus, hand orientation, shape, and force characteristics are determined based on our previous experience grasping objects, in conjunction with our ability to perceive relevant cues about the target object (Fisk, 1990; Forssberg et al., 1991; Jeannerod, 1986; Westling & Johansson, 1984). Errors in grasp control, including gripping too loosely and letting objects slip or gripping too tightly and crushing them, result from impairments in grading or scaling grip or fingertip forces. However, it may be difficult to determine whether errors are the result of poor muscle control, or due to impaired perception of target object characteristics, leading to inaccurate force scaling.

Elements of skilled grasp and manipulation include: (1) control over extrinsic and intrinsic hand muscles, (2) discrimination of perceptual cues critical to anticipatory hand shaping and force scaling, and (3) accurate gradation of grip and fingertip forces. Thus, retraining of grasp control should address strength, coordination, and perceptual aspects of the task. Training and strengthening the intrinsic hand muscles is best accomplished with resistive therapeutic putty. In addition, other activities, such as lacing

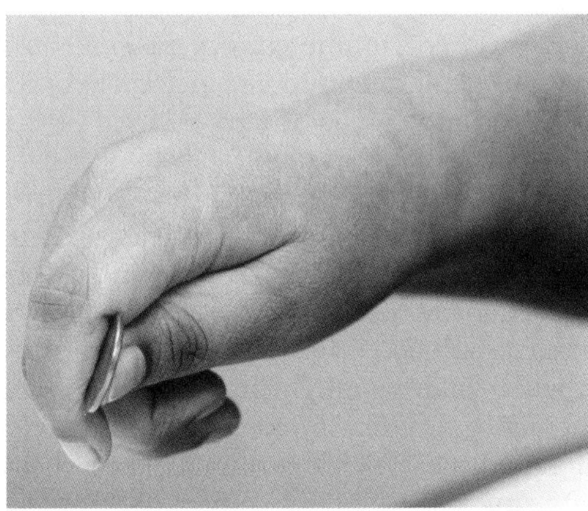

FIGURE 19.16 A child with hemiplegic CP attempting a pincer grasp.

cardboard or leather with pipe cleaners or plastic laces may be useful. One could train fingertip force control by having the patient drop a selected number of water drops from an eyedropper or pick up and replace objects such as polystyrene/paper cups without denting them. To gain or regain functional upper-extremity control sufficiently, one must learn to modify grasp strategies to changing task demands through practice.

Contextual Interference. To examine the impact of contextual interference on learning, researchers have separated practice into blocked, random (contextual interference), and mixed schedules. Hanlon (1996) measured retention of a five-step functionally oriented movement sequence in the affected limb of 24 patients who had had a stroke. The patients practiced a task in either a blocked or a random manner or were placed in a control group. The results revealed greater improvement in the random-practice group on the first and second retention tests, supporting the positive effects of contextual interference on learning in this population.

Duff and Gordon (2003) studied the effect of blocked versus random practice on improving anticipatory force scaling for grasp control in children with hemiplegic CP. While better performance was observed for the blocked group during acquisition, they found similar immediate and delayed retention between the two forms of practice. They postulated that the children may have needed more practice time to better determine which schedule would ultimately lead to better retention. A study by Cauraugh and Kim (2003) found that blocked and random practice during a FES program were both effective at improving hand function.

Finger Fractionation and In-Hand Manipulation. Many individuals with neurologic deficits have lost or never had intact corticomotoneuronal mechanisms (Rothwell, 1994), thus limiting finger fractionation (isolated finger and thumb movements) and therefore making it difficult to manipulate objects in one hand. The ability to move objects in one hand, or in-hand manipulation, is an important feature of hand function. Individuals are candidates for in-hand manipulation training if they exhibit basic grasp-and-release patterns using the fingers and/or the pads of the fingers and exhibit at least some finger movement (Exner & Henderson, 1995).

In-hand manipulation practice in individuals with hemiplegia or fine motor delays can be graded, beginning with easy tasks, using objects of high friction and multiple points of contact and progressing to difficult tasks, using slippery objects with minimal points of contact. Progressively, the size and shape of the objects can be varied as well as the cues and difficulty of the practice conditions. For instance, one child may be able to begin training at the level of object rotation while another must begin with finger-to-palm translation. Activities that often coincide with in-hand manipulation training include sensory reeducation and intrinsic muscle strengthening.

Treatment over multiple sessions could focus on all three forms of in-hand manipulation (translation, rotation, and shift) using small manipulatives, such as coins (Exner, 1990). For example, one could have a child pick up pennies one at a time, move them to the palm, and hold them in the ulnar side of the hand. Alternatively, pennies could be placed one at a time into a child's palm with the instruction that each penny be translated to the fingertips and then shifted to the thumb and index pads. Rotation and shift could be practiced by placing a pencil into the palm of a child's hand with the instruction to rotate and adjust it to rest between the pads of the thumb, index, and long fingers. The two sides of the hand can be encouraged to develop separate roles while practicing tasks that require the power (ulnar) side to stabilize and the skill (radial) side to manipulate. One such task requires the individual to roll putty between the thumb and index finger while the ring and small fingers hold a small object. Another task requires squeezing the trigger of a spray bottle with the index and long fingers while the ring and small fingers hold the neck of the bottle. As skill improves, the complexity of tasks can increase.

Individuals with focal hand dystonia often lose motor control of one or more fingers stemming from highly repetitive, intensive hand use and atypical learning (Byl, 2003). The usual individual finger representation found in the somatosensory cortex changes. For instance, in musicians with dystonia the distance between representations of the fingers is reduced and often begins to blend (Elbert, 1998), resulting in an inability to localize light pressure or move the fingers in isolation. Sensory and motor training programs for this group have been studied as a method of fostering change. Zeuner and colleagues (2005) had 10 patients with focal hand dystonia undergo a 4-week motor training program to increase finger individuation with an emphasis on decreasing the abnormal overflow of movement to fingers not involved in selected tasks. After training there was a trend toward better handwriting and improvements on the Fahn dystonia scale. However, no changes were found in cortical excitability based on electroencephalography and TMS.

Release

To manipulate objects, patients not only must be able to grasp them, but they must also be able to release them. For many patients with neurologic lesions, a power grasp is accomplished by using a mass flexion pattern. Although this pattern is successful in grasping objects, the patient may be unable to actively extend the fingers to release the object without the assistance of the other hand (Lang et al., 2009). Thus, a patient may use wrist flexion to passively extend the fingers to accomplish release (Boehme, 1988; Erhardt, 1982). Even if a patient can release objects actively, the process may be inefficient. Gordon and colleagues (Eliasson & Gordon 2000; Gordon et al., 2003) found that while children with hemiplegic CP can release objects successfully, they often do so abruptly, with minimal gradation to the movement. Addressing the process of release in treatment may enhance prehension capabilities.

Rhoda Erhardt, an occupational therapist, has published an extensive assessment that describes a developmental sequence for releasing objects (Erhardt, 1982). This sequence has been used as the basis for a program to train or retrain release in individuals with a neurologic impairment (Boehme, 1988). The suggested sequence begins with learning to release an object that is externally stabilized and progresses to release without external stabilization. This approach is based on the observation that children learn to release an object externally stabilized on a supporting surface prior to learning to release objects in space (Boehme, 1988). Patients also practice releasing an object using a pattern of finger extension with the wrist in neutral, as opposed to release resulting from wrist flexion, producing a mechanical extension of the fingers (tenodesis). As release improves, practice can progress to the release of objects into a container and stacking objects.

Training Proximal and Distal Function: Should One Precede the Other?

One issue that has concerned both researchers and clinicians is whether proximal function such as reaching must be trained prior to distal functions such as grasp and manipulation. Development of the trunk and proximal upper-limb neuromuscular system precedes that of the distal component (Kuypers, 1981). This developmental feature likely contributes to the predominance of the trunk and proximal muscle activation in early reaching in infants (Berthier et al., 1999). However, because control over proximal body segments is not a necessary precursor to distal hand function, the two can be addressed simultaneously in treatment, rather than sequentially. In essence, one should not wait for proximal control to emerge before working on hand function.

It is possible that select areas of the CNS can substitute for injured regions (see Chapter 4; Merzenich & Jenkins, 1993; Merzenich et al., 1983b). Proximal functions involving the transport phase and/or shoulder stability may be easily substituted with the use of alternative neural pathways. In contrast, corticomotoneuronal lesion or damage to the corticospinal tract (CST) often results in profound loss of precision movements of the hand because alternative pathways are not as readily available (Rothwell, 1994). Therefore, recovery of isolated thumb and finger movement and precision grip may be limited following lesions of the CST (Lang & Schieber, 2004; Raghavan et al., 2005).

Interventions at the Functional Level

A task-oriented approach to intervention requires that gains made in resolving impairments and improving key components of upper-extremity skills be extended into improving the performance of functional activities. Because the ability to adapt functional skills to changing environmental conditions is important to the recovery of participation, the context under which functional tasks are practiced should be controlled and modified. As functional abilities improve, the ability to resume life roles (e.g., homemaker, student) increases, and recovery of participation is facilitated.

Task-Specific Training of Functional Activities

An important part of a task-oriented approach to treatment is task-specific practice of functional activities under changing environmental and task demands. Dunn and colleagues (1994) designed a therapeutic framework for practice—*The Ecology of Human Performance* (EHP)—that considers the effect of context. This model stems from the theory that ecology, or the interaction between person(s) and the environment, affects human behavior and performance. This framework is discussed and applied to our case study, Mrs. J., in Assessment Tool 19.9.

Integrating familiar or enjoyable tasks into the therapeutic practice environment aids the recovery of many aspects of function in both adults and children. In their review, Ma and Trombly (2002) reported that cognitive function improved to a greater degree following intervention strategies that incorporated functional tasks and activities familiar and enjoyable to the individual. For example, many homemaking tasks, such as doing the laundry, incorporate both upper limbs and simple cognitive/perceptual skills. Sorting clothes prior to washing requires classification and identification of fabric color and texture. Loading clothes into the washer/dryer and folding them afterward incorporates bimanual coordination, trunk stabilization, and large proximal and distal movements activating related muscle groups. While adults may

Assessment Tool 19-9

Dunn's Framework of Ecology of Human Performance

This framework considers the interaction between the person, the environment, and human task performance. This framework can be applied to retraining upper-extremity control in Mrs. J. in her role as a homemaker. The activities used during treatment depend on the goal of the intervention and the status of the person's recovery. Note the different example activities used below.

Goal	Interpretation	Activity Example
Establish/restore	Improve person's skills and experiences	Introduce tasks/exercises that strengthen finger flexors and wrist (remediate) extensors. With greater strength, Mrs. J. may be able to expand the use of her affected hand during bimanual tasks (e.g., hold a bowl with her affected hand while stirring the contents with the less-affected hand).
Alter	Select context that enables performance. Place person in different setting.	Have Mrs. J. assist in meal preparation by setting the dining room table in her own home, using her affected hand and arm to hold extra items while placing them strategically on the table with her less-affected hand.
Adapt	Change aspects of context and/or tasks to allow person to perform task	Introduce tools with large handles that allow Mrs. J. to hold them with her affected hand (e.g., stir bowl contents using her affected hand while the less-affected hand holds the bowl).
Prevent	Change course of events based on predictions of barriers to performance	Because Mrs. J.'s affected upper limb tends to fatigue and her balance is only fair, have her prepare meals while sitting at a table with her elbows supported.
Create	Provide enriched contextual and task experiences to enhance performance	Have Mrs. J. prepare a lunch for her family members that requires the use of her affected hand to manipulate pots, pans, dishes, and utensils unimanually and bimanually. The items could be retrieved from their original locations in cupboards etc. to expand reach-and-grasp demands as well as trunk and balance requirements.

be quite motivated to work on ADLs, children often require the added element of integrating practice into games to make ADLs more enjoyable.

Task-Related Training Versus Exercise. Thielman and colleagues (2004) compared the effect of two 4-week training programs on reaching in patients with chronic stroke (>6 months after stroke). Participants were placed in either a low- or high-level group based on the Motor Assessment Scale and randomly assigned to one of the two treatment groups. One program involved task-related training (TRT), while the other required progressive resistive exercise (PRE) in the form of therapeutic tubing in the planes and distances similar to TRT activities. The kinematic results for the low-level group revealed an increase in trunk use during ipsilateral targeted reaching following TRT and for midline and contralateral targeted reaching following PRE. With TRT, hand paths straightened only in the low-level group, suggesting better interjoint coordination. Subjects in the high-level group showed the most change following PRE training, revealing less-compensatory movement and trunk use, signifying gains in the extent of the reach.

Winstein and colleagues (2004) compared the immediate and long-term benefits of two upper-extremity protocols for stroke, functional task practice (FT) and strength training (ST) with standard care (SC). The authors categorized 64 patients by severity using the Orpington Prognostic Scale, then, randomly assigned them to one of three treatment groups. All subjects participated in the 4-to-6-week inpatient and outpatient program, while the FT and ST groups received 20 hours of treatment beyond SC.

Performance measures included the Fugl-Meyer Scale, isometric torque strength, and the Functional Test of the Hemiparetic Upper Extremity (FTHUE).

Subjects in the less severe category showed the most improvement in Fugl-Meyer scores, isometric torque strength, and FTHUE immediately after treatment for both the FT and ST groups. However, at 6 months, improvement in isometric muscle torque in the FT group progressed significantly beyond that of the ST group. Winstein and colleagues reached conclusions similar to those reported by Duncan et al. (2003)—that both task specificity and severity of stroke are important factors to consider during upper-extremity rehabilitation in the acute phase following stroke. Furthermore, while strength training and task-specific training are both beneficial in the short-term, the long-term benefits of task-specific training seem to be greater.

Learning to Sequence Complex Functional Tasks. Modeling and verbal/mental rehearsal may be the most effective methods to improve sequencing of complex functional tasks (McCullagh et al., 1989). For example, Jean J has difficulty sequencing the steps associated with meal preparation. During therapy sessions throughout a given week, the therapist could model the multistep process, such as making a sandwich and preparing a cup of tea, while giving simple verbal cues along the way. Before Jean attempts to repeat the same task, she could be asked to verbalize the sequence (declarative or explicit learning), and then imagine herself performing the sequence (mental rehearsal). During practice, the therapist may initially coach the patient through the task as needed (verbally and/or manually). Treatment could progress to practice from a written list (given intact vision) to practice without verbal or written cues.

Tim's sequencing problems may center on classroom art projects. In those situations, peer modeling may be effective only if the child is able to filter out irrelevant cues and focus only on those that are important to sequence the task correctly (Exner & Henderson, 1995; Vygotsky, 1978). It is possible that Tim is unable to carry out task sequences for a number of reasons (impaired visual perception, distractibility when given verbal instructions/visual demonstrations, and/or constructional apraxia, among others).

If peer modeling of task sequences is ineffective, Tim may need individual coaching on sequencing as in the case of Jean J, which may include visual modeling and verbal rehearsal prior to performing the task (Vygotsky, 1978). For example, during the construction of an art project, one could begin by showing him the end product and have him verbally state how to complete it step by step. If he fails to give a correct response the therapist can verbally interject, reviewing the correct step(s). Once the project is complete, the therapist may need to model the task sequence. It may be reinforcing for him to verbally repeat the task sequence to the therapist or to teach a fellow student how to complete the same task by demonstration and verbal cueing.

Practicing Functional Activities in Virtual Environments. Virtual environments have been used to promote learning of functional tasks in various neurologic populations. Virtual reality in isolation or in combination with other therapies has been found to aid movement recovery in adults and children with neurologic disorders (Broeren et al., 2004; Connelly et al., 2009; Eng et al., 2007; Golomb et al., 2010; Holden et al., 2001; Qiu et al., 2009). Holden and colleagues (2001) trained four individuals 3 to 18 years of age following an acquired brain injury in real-world tasks through the use of virtual-world pouring tasks. Subjects imitated the "teacher" on a screen while holding a "real" cup during training sessions (trained 1 hour, three times per week, totaling 16 sessions). In three of the four subjects, the trajectories of the pouring movement were smoother, straighter, and more accurate after training. Two subjects demonstrated transfer of the pouring trajectory into a novel part of the workspace.

Golomb and colleagues (2010) conducted a pilot study to examine the benefit of a home-based video-game program that was remotely monitored, for three children with hemiplegic CP. All subjects participated 5 days per week for 3 months. To monitor use, all subjects wore a sensor glove on the affected hand. Findings showed that all subjects improved range of motion, hand and arm function, and bone density of the radius and had an expansion in the spatial extent of activation after treatment.

Qiu and colleagues (2009) conducted a pilot study of virtual reality combined with robotic training in two children with CP. Both children participated in the clinic-based training three times per week for 3 weeks. Both subjects improved performance on the outcome measures including the Melbourne Assessment of Unilateral Upper Limb, active range of motion, grip and pinch strength, and arm kinematics during a virtual reality reaching task (smoothness, hand path length and duration).

Broeren and colleagues (2004) combined training in a virtual environment and the use of a haptic device to improve motor function in a single subject with left hemiparesis over the course of twelve 90-minute sessions and documented improvements in manual dexterity, grip force, and motor control. Connelly and colleagues (2009) used a pneumatic glove to assist finger extension during a 6-week training program combined with a virtual reality setup in seven subjects with poststroke chronic hand impairment. After training they found an improvement on the Fugl-Meyer Scale (primarily the hand-wrist component), which was maintained 1 month after training.

Housman and colleagues (2009) compared the benefit of a computer-based virtual reality system combined with a robotic device to a table-top exercise program in 28 adults with chronic stroke. The findings showed that all subjects made improvements on the Fugl-Meyer Scale, active range-of-reaching motion, and the Motor Activity Log, which remained 6 months after training. However, improvements on the Fugl-Meyer Scale at 6 months were greater for the experimental group. Because of the benefits of virtual reality, affordable home-based programs have been developed and are being marketed (King et al., 2010).

Dominance Training or Retraining. Bilateral upper-limb tasks are either symmetrical or asymmetrical. During symmetrical tasks, both arms and hands attempt to perform the same function as when throwing a ball or folding a large towel. During asymmetrical tasks, one arm and hand stabilizes an object while the other performs some form of manipulation or action on the object. For example, when chopping an onion, the nondominant limb may stabilize the onion while the other uses a knife to chop it. The nondominant or stabilizing limb acts to control impedance while the dominant controls the limb trajectory during a reach or the manipulative component of an action (Sainburg, 2005). A child who fails to develop a strong dominance or an adult who suffers a stroke and loses substantial control of the dominant limb may benefit from dominance training or retraining.

Rehabilitation strategies should focus on training both the affected and less-affected limbs. As reviewed earlier, the dominant limb seems specialized for trajectory (reach) control while the nondominant limb seems specialized for positional or impedance control (Sainburg, 2002). Therefore, if a right-handed individual suffers a left hemisphere stroke, the dominant right limb will be affected and often must take on the role of the nondominant limb while the less-affected nondominant left limb must take on the role of the dominant limb. In essence, years of practice performing asymmetrical bimanual tasks one way must now be relearned. To promote retraining therapists, could design activities to allow the right limb to practice impedance control by stabilizing objects while the left limb practices trajectory control while performing actions on those objects (Sainburg & Duff, 2006). Sample tasks could include: (1) holding a glass with the right hand while pouring water from a pitcher with the left; (2) stabilizing a piece of paper with the right while drawing using the left; and (3) holding a bagel while cutting it in half with the left. Future research should be directed at uncovering the best methods to enhance dominant and nondominant limb performance during development and following neurologic injury.

Ipsilesional Limb Training. Although many studies have examined the affected limb of adults who have had a stroke or children with hemiplegic CP, because of its functional importance, researchers are now closely examining the less-affected limb. Pohl and Winstein (1999) studied the effects of reaching practice with the ipsilesional limb in 10 right-handed subjects who had had a stroke and 10 age-matched controls. The protocol varied the target width and the distance between targets, resulting in an easy and complex aiming task. After practice, subjects who had had a stroke were slower than controls; however, movement times for all subjects were faster in both conditions. Peak velocity during reaches increased only in the easy condition. The authors concluded that motor performance in the less-affected limb can improve with practice and recommended further study to ascertain whether the changes are generalizable.

Byl and Mckenzie (2000) examined the effect of clinic- and home-based treatment aimed at reducing symptoms and increasing function in 12 individuals with occupation-related focal hand dystonia. All subjects were asked to stop performing the target task for the duration of the study. Clinical treatment included: (1) sensory training with and without biofeedback; and (2) instructions in stress-free hand use, mirror imagery, mental rehearsal, and mental practice techniques designed to stop the abnormal movements and facilitate typical hand motor control. The home program attempted to reduce neural tension, improve posture, facilitate relaxation, and promote aerobic capacity. Follow-up, 3 to 6 months after treatment, revealed functional improvements from baseline, including independence in ADL; 11 of 12 subjects had returned to work. Performance measures also revealed improvements in motor control, motor accuracy, sensory discrimination, and physical performance. Thus, sensory and motor programs do seem to facilitate recovery in those with focal hand dystonia.

Training Handwriting. Training in handwriting may be needed for young children with underdeveloped skills or children or adults with neurologic disorders. Adaptive writing implements or splints may be essential to maximize function for adults or children with neurologic dysfunction to help them maintain a sustained hold on a writing implement. Although manipulating writing implements can be awkward, performance usually improves with practice.

For children with underdeveloped handwriting skills, there are well-designed manuscript and cursive handwriting programs that can be successfully used in school-based therapy programs or classroom curriculums. Two such programs are Benbow's "Loops and Other Groups," (1991) and Olsen's "Handwriting Without Tears" (1998). Benbow's program teaches cursive handwriting from a kinesiologic perspective through creative clustering of letters into "kites" and other subgroups with subsequent practice. Its success lies in the ease of instruction and ample practice time suggested for each grouping. Olsen's program emphasizes multisensory experiences and features gray blocks and simple line structure to visually guide printing and cursive writing. Pencil grips or writing utensils can aid function (Fig. 19.17, A and B).

Handwriting is one functional task that has subcomponents such as legibility, that can effectively be addressed separately. Case-Smith (2002) compared the effects of a year-long occupational therapy intervention versus no intervention for twenty-nine 7- to 10-year-old students with poor handwriting legibility. Intervention primarily addressed visual-motor skills and handwriting practice. She found that those in the intervention group demonstrated a 14.2% improvement in legibility, versus a 5.8% improvement in the no-treatment group. Although scores on in-hand manipulation and visual perceptual tests increased significantly, there was no increase in handwriting speed. In an alternate study, Sudsawad and colleagues (2002) studied the effect of kinesthetic training on the performance of handwriting in first-graders. The 4-week program divided 45 students into three groups: kinesthetic training, handwriting practice, and no treatment. While there was a subjective improvement in handwriting legibility in all groups, standardized assessment did not indicate improvement. The authors suggested that the study may have been too short and the standardized assessment might not have been sensitive to change in relevant variables. Comparing the two studies, it seems that longer treatment time is needed to show changes in handwriting.

Interventions to Increase Frequency of Arm and Hand Use

There are several therapeutic methods designed to enhance the frequency of arm and hand use, which often have a positive effect on the frequency of participation and independence in ADL tasks. These methods include Constraint-Induced Movement Therapy, Bimanual Training, and Interlimb Transfer.

Constraint-Induced Movement Therapy. Constraint-induced movement therapy (CIMT) is a form of massed practice designed to improve function in individuals with hemiplegia by constraining the less-affected limb

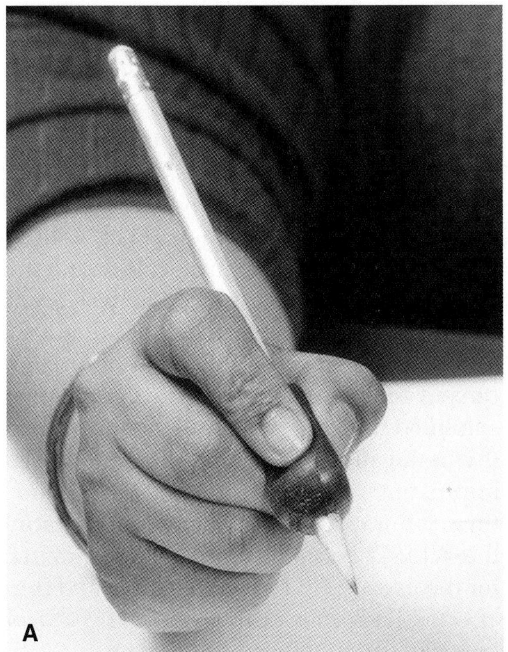

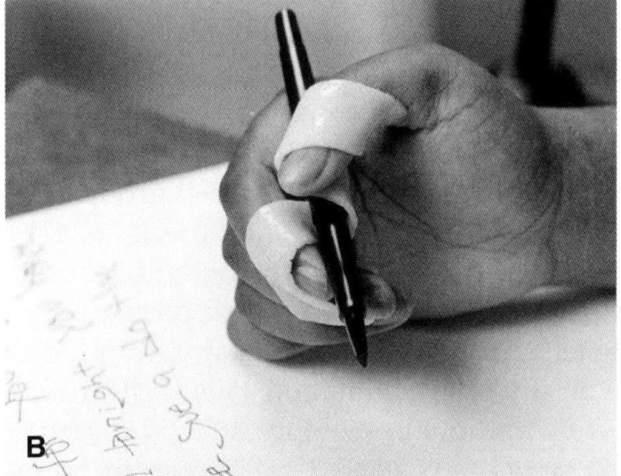

FIGURE 19.17 Assistive devices such as a pencil grip (A) and a custom-made writing utensil (design by Bobbie Ciocco, OTR/L) (B) used for handwriting.

and eliciting shaping behaviors in the affected limb. The efficacy of CIMT has been studied in adults after stroke (Kunkel et al., 1999; Miltner et al., 1999; Pierce et al., 2003; Schaechter et al., 2002; Taub et al., 1993; Wolf et al., 1989b, 2006), in children with hemiplegic CP (Charles et al., 1999, 2001; Crocker et al., 1997; Dromerick et al., 2009; Eliasson et al., 2005a; Gordon et al., 2005; Lavender & Gentile, 1998; Pierce et al., 2002; Taub et al., 2004; Yasukawa, 1990), and in those with traumatic brain injury (Karman et al., 2003).

Wolf and colleagues (1989b) studied, for 14 days-25 adults who had had a hemiplegic stroke or a head injury and wore slings to restrain the less-affected arm during waking hours. During follow-up, the investigators found that task execution speed in the affected limb improved for most functional tasks, for up to 1 year after intervention. Taub and colleagues (1993) compared CIMT (treatment group) with an attention-comparison group (controls) in patients with chronic hemiplegic stroke. The treatment group had their less-affected limb restrained during the waking hours for 14 days. For 10 weekdays of those 14 days, the treatment group spent 6 hours a day practicing tasks that required upper extremity function with the affected limb (e.g., eating, writing, pushing a broom), while the control group was instructed to focus attention on the affected limb and received placebo and ROM exercises. The results showed that motor ability and ADL skills improved significantly following intervention, as compared with controls; these improvements were sustained for 1 to 2 years after intervention.

Wolf and colleagues (Winstein et al., 2003; Wolf et al., 2005, 2006, 2008) conducted a multisite study of CIMT, entitled the EXCITE trials, to compare the effect of a 2-week program of CIMT versus usual and customary care on upper-extremity function 3 to 9 months after stroke. Findings taken immediately, 1 year, and 2 years after training showed greater improvements in the CIMT group versus controls on performance time for the Wolf Motor Function Test and the amount of use on the Motor Activity Log. Furthermore, after training the score for self-perceived hand function difficulty from the Stroke Impact Scale was lower in the CIMT group than in the control group. In a separate analysis Alberts and colleagues (2004) found that hand function improved more in the CIMT group than in controls, as documented by greater precision grip strength, enhanced regulation of forces, and reduced force rate variability during precision grip tasks.

The benefit of very early constraint-induced movement in stroke rehabilitation (VECTORS) was compared with traditional therapy in 52 adults after stroke (Dromerick et al., 2009). CIMT and traditional therapy were found to be equally beneficial during inpatient treatment. However, at 3 months the CIMT group had less motor improvement, suggesting that higher doses of therapy early may not be beneficial.

CIMT has been found to be effective in children with hemiplegic cerebral palsy (Gordon et al., 2005, 2006, 2007; Pierce et al., 2002; Taub et al., 2004). Gordon and colleagues (2005) adapted the CIMT program for use with children based on intervention with 37 children 4 to 14 years of age. The protocol involved restraining the less-affected limb in a sling 6 hours a day for 10 days. Shaping activities and repetitive practice were conducted in groups of two to three children to allow socialization and encouragement; the ratio of interventionist to child was 1:1. The joint movements emphasized were individualized based on deficits and the potential for improvement. In essence, modifications made to the adult program were well tolerated by the children. Findings revealed an improvement in dexterity and coordination and the amount of use and quality of use of the affected limb. In a follow-up study 1 year later, in this same group of children further improvement on the outcome measures were found (Gordon et al., 2007). Using a single case study, Pierce and colleagues (2004) used a 3-week home-based CIMT, including six 2-hour outpatient occupational and physical therapy sessions. At follow-up, there was a reduction in mean completion time on the Wolf Motor Function Test (WMFT) and significant improvements in functional use as documented with the Assessment of Motor and Process Skills (Fisher, 1994). Taub and colleagues (2004) also studied the effect of 21 days of CIMT in this group, including 6 hours of shaping per day. They found evidence of an improved amount and quality of use in the affected extremity immediately after treatment and 6 months later.

Modified CIMT Programs. Some studies have modified CIMT programs in an attempt to replicate outpatient treatment schedules. Page and Levine (2003) used CIMT to study improvements in three individuals with traumatic brain injury (TBI) with documented learned nonuse. Their protocol included restraint of the affected limb five times per week 5 hours a day for 10 weeks during periods of frequent use, with the addition of shaping activities in the context of physical and occupational therapy. After treatment, subjects exhibited improvements in the amount and quality of use in the affected limb based on the MAL, functional improvements based on the ARAT, and decreased time and improved task performance rating based on the WMFT. This study provides preliminary support for the use of CIMT to enhance use and function in the affected limb after TBI.

Pierce and colleagues (2003) had 17 patients with chronic stroke and 1 with subacute stroke engage in home forced use in addition to seven outpatient occupational and physical therapy sessions of 1 hour per session per discipline over a 2- to 3-week period. At follow-up, completion time for 12 of 17 subtests on the WMFT were reduced. The results suggest that modified forced use may have a positive effect on function and is easy to implement outside the clinic.

Studies have examined the effects of interventions aimed at reducing impairments and enhancing sensory and motor function. Byl and colleagues (2003) examined the treatment effect of an upper-extremity crossover training program in 21 patients who were stable after having had a stroke. The 8-week program (4 weeks for sensory and 4 weeks for motor training) required placing a glove on the less-affected limb and using shaping, in the form of attended, graded, repetitive sensory and motor activities. The results revealed a 20% improvement in functional independence, fine motor function, sensory discrimination, and musculoskeletal performance.

Despite the promising results on the use of CIMT to improve hand function in those with hemiparesis, Charles and Gordon (2005) caution that more studies need to be conducted before CIMT can be promoted for general clinical use. Criteria need to be established with patients for whom this approach might be appropriate. Many patients are excluded from this type of treatment because of imbalance and the need to use the less-affected upper extremity for balance control and to prevent falls. One encouraging aspect of CIMT training studies is the awareness that motor improvements are possible even in chronically impaired patients at 1 to 5 years after the onset of the impairment or in those with congenital hemiplegia.

Bimanual Training. Bilateral or bimanual training engages both limbs simultaneously to encourage interlimb coordination and motion in a hemiparetic limb. Bilateral training is in direct contrast to CIMT, which actively restrains use of the intact arm, forcing the use of the affected extremity in functional tasks. Types of bilateral training vary from asymmetrical tapping to symmetrical reaching or asymmetrical performance (Hung et al., 2004; Luft et al., 2004; McCombe-Waller & Whitall, 2004; Mudie & Matyas, 2000, 2001; Whitall et al., 2000). It is possible that after stroke, the bilateral approach is appropriate early in recovery, when rapid reorganization of the cortex is occurring and new networks controlling movement are being formed. CIMT may then be appropriate in ensuring that new networks are used, avoiding the development of learned disuse. Further research is needed to determine the efficacy of this type of sequence for training.

Bilateral/bimanual training in those with hemiplegia has been found to improve interlimb coordination as well as coordination in the affected limb. McCombe-Waller and Whitall (2004) used the fine motor control task of unilateral and bimanual tapping to measure the effect of 6 weeks of bilateral arm training with rhythmic auditory cuing, conducted three times per week. Daily training involved 20 minutes (four 5-minute periods) of bilateral in-phase and antiphase push/pull of T-bar handles, paced with a metronome, while sitting. The results showed few training effects in the affected hand, yet, improved control in the less-affected hand. The authors concluded that bilateral arm training might have a positive effect on interlimb coordination.

Bilateral training has also been found to improve coordination in the affected limb of individuals with central or peripheral unilateral impairment (Cauraugh et al., 2005; Luft et al., 2004; Mudie & Matyas, 2000; Whitall et al., 2000). Mudie and Matyas (2000) reported data from 12 controlled single-case experiments (patients with hemiparesis after stroke) using a multiple-baseline design across three reach-and-grasp activities. All 12 patients showed significant improvements in the hemiplegic arm following simultaneous bilateral training, as compared with either unilateral movement training, or use of the less-affected arm to guide the affected arm. The improvements were specific to the task trained and were well maintained even 6 months after the training period. The authors suggest that following stroke, the undamaged hemisphere might provide a template of appropriate neural responses for a restored neural network. The template is available through transcortical communications that are no longer inhibited during bilateral simultaneous isokinematic performance.

Cauraugh and colleagues (2005) compared the effect of unilateral and bilateral training on three groups: (1) a coupled bilateral group (concurrent wrist/finger movements on less-affected limb coupled with electromyographically triggered active stimulation of wrist and finger extensors on the affected limb); (2) unilateral group (active stimulation of affected wrist/fingers); and (3) control group. The program consisted of 4 days of 90 minutes of training per week for 2 weeks. Posttraining kinematic results revealed an increase in peak velocity and shorter deceleration times during bimanual reaching only for the bimanual training group, while the unilateral group increased peak velocity during the unilateral reach and produced longer deceleration times during the bimanual reach. Furthermore, the results supported the hypothesis that coupled bilateral training of distal joints of both limbs would transfer to proximal joints better than unilateral training.

A program of hand–arm bimanual intensive training program was designed for use with children with hemiplegic CP by Charles and Gordon (2006). As in

CIMT, children practice tasks for 6 hours per day for 10 days, except that all of the tasks are bimanual. The outcomes support the benefit of bimanual training in terms of improved dexterity, hand and arm function and the amount of use in the affected arm and hand.

Despite reported positive effects from bilateral training studies, some studies reveal few differences in functional outcomes between usual treatment and bilateral practice (Desrosiers et al., 2005) or bimanual versus unimanual training (Gordon et al., 2008). Perhaps more research is needed to examine the effect of combining bimanual training with other rehabilitation methods or to examine when in treatment (early or late development/recovery) bilateral training is most effective.

Interlimb Transfer. Intuitively, therapists have patients perform tasks with the less-affected limb first in an attempt to promote more frequent use of the affected limb. The efficacy of this approach for the improvement of movement and function in the affected limb of those with hemiparesis will likely depend on the side of the lesion and the task under consideration.

Interlimb transfer of visuomotor learning and novel force conditions during targeted planar reaching tasks have been found for typical young adults (Criscimagna-Hemminger et al. 2003; Malfait & Ostry, 2004; Sainburg & Wang, 2002; Wang & Sainburg, 2004a, b, 2006a, b). However, the specifics of the transfer depend on workspace location and handedness. Research has begun to support the efficacy of interlimb transfer as a method to improve prehension in those with unilateral dyscontrol.

As introduced earlier, interlimb transfer has also been found to improve anticipatory force scaling during grasp and manipulation in adults and children with hemiplegia (Dawson et al., 2010; Gordon et al., 1999; Raghavan et al., 2006). Gordon and colleagues (1999, 2008) have shown that if children with hemiplegic CP lift objects with the less-affected hand first and then with the affected hand, they exhibit evidence of anticipatory scaling of fingertip forces during the first lift of a grip device. Interestingly, in the later study the authors also found interlimb transfer of anticipatory scaling from the involved to the noninvolved hand, also on the first lift, which they postulated to be the result of an inability to integrate sensory information with the motor command in the involved hand.

Camus and colleagues (2009) examined the neurophysiological mechanisms of interlimb transfer in typical young adults with TMS to characterize changes from the left to the right primary motor cortex (M1) during a sequential pinch force task. All subjects were right-handed and practiced the task only with the right hand. After practice, the ability of the left hand to perform the task was measured. The authors found task speed and accuracy improved in the right trained hand and in the left untrained hand. These changes coincided with an increase in recruitment curves in the left M1 and decreased short intracortical inhibition in the left and right M1 based on TMS.

Lab Activity 19.1 will help you practice applying a task-oriented approach to treating a patient with upper-extremity problems. In this lab, you will develop a treatment plan for Jean, our acute stroke patient, and identify the research evidence that supports your treatment choices.

SUMMARY

1. Retraining upper-extremity control is important to most areas of rehabilitation, including physical and occupational therapy. While both therapy areas retrain upper-extremity control, physical therapists tend to focus on postural and mobility aspects of upper-extremity function, while occupational therapists tend to focus on ADL aspects, including the recovery of prehensile skills.
2. A task-oriented approach to assessment of upper-extremity function requires a battery of tests that measure: (a) function, including both capacity (behavior in a standardized environment) and performance (participation in real-world contexts); (b) strategies or the qualitative components of function, including eye–head coordination, transport, grasp and release, and manipulation; and (c) underlying sensory, motor, and cognitive impairments, including range of motion, strength, sensibility, edema, and pain.
3. Clinical research has begun to support the use of a task-oriented approach to treatment of neurologic disorders by itself and in combination with other therapies. However, the degree of integration of research findings into current clinical practice has yet to be investigated.
4. Preparing treatment plans to retrain upper-extremity control requires the identification of a comprehensive list of patient problems, including the limitations in function and strategies, as well as the specific impairments that constrain function. From this list, short- and long-term treatment goals are established, and therapeutic strategies are developed to meet those goals.

LAB ACTIVITY 19-1

Individual Component of Reach, Grasp, & Manipulation	Task or Activity	Environmental Conditions	Research Evidence
Motor: Frequency of affected hand use	Massed practice—shaping tasks	Constraint-induced movement therapy—three times a week in an outpatient program	Pierce et al., 2003; Taub et al., 1993; Winstein et al., 2003; Wolf et al., 2005, 2006, 2008

Objective: Apply a task-oriented approach to retrain reach, grasp and manipulation in a patient with post-stroke hemiparesis. To identify the research evidence to support clinical decisions regarding specific treatment interventions.

Procedure: Reread the case study presented in Assessment Tool 19.1. Review the list of functional problems, strategies, and impairments outlined.

Assignment: Create a table identifying the various treatments you will use to improve hand function in Jean. List the specific individual system to be targeted (column 1), the task or activity to be practiced (column 2), the environmental conditions under which practice will occur (column 3), and the research evidence that supports this aspect of treatment (column 4). For example, you may select to do theraputty exercises with Jean because weakness is an underlying impairment contributing to her impaired hand function.
The individual component listed in the table is Motor: Frequency of hand use, the task is massed practice, the specific environmental conditions you choose may be constraint-induced movement therapy. Several research studies supports your decision to use constraint-induced movement therapy with Jean, including the EXCITE trials by Wolf and colleagues. Is increasing frequency alone enough to ensure recovery of hand function? What other aspects of hand function will you train? What research supports your decision?

5. A task-oriented approach to retraining upper-extremity control seeks to minimize impairments, while maximizing the patient's capacity for function and participation. Retraining involves the development of therapeutic strategies to: (a) remediate as many sensory, motor, and cognitive impairments as possible; (b) generate strategies to improve qualitative and quantitative upper-extremity control; and (c) develop the capacity to perform functional tasks in a variety of environmental contexts to allow satisfactory social participation.
6. Research suggests that the development of control over proximal body segments is not a necessary precursor to the emergence of distal hand function. Proximal and distal segments of the upper extremities appear to be controlled separately, and therefore can be retrained simultaneously, rather than sequentially.
7. Hand function requires the ability to grasp, release, and manipulate objects, as well as the capacity to adapt how we grasp in response to characteristics of the target object. Many elements of grasp, including hand shape and force characteristics, use the internal representation we hold of an object's physical properties. Thus, retraining hand function requires attention to both motor and perceptual aspects of the task.
8. Sensory reeducation programs focus on protective or discriminative sensibility. It is unclear whether sensory reeducation teaches the patient how to use the remaining sensibility to their advantage, or whether it actually alters the physiological basis for sensation. It is certain, however, that the capacity to adapt to impaired sensibility is dependent on the patient's motivation as well as training. Studies have shown that patients who were willing to use the affected limb were better able to recover function.
9. A major constraint to recovery of arm function may be the unwillingness of patients to use an affected upper extremity when the less-affected extremity is available. However, bilateral, unilateral, and interlimb transfer training may be effective methods to promote usage either separately or in a planned sequence of intervention. Further research is needed to determine when in recovery each type of training would be most beneficial.
10. Hand dominance may play a key role in the rehabilitation of unimanual and bimanual skills. Research suggests that the dominant

limb has an advantage for reach or trajectory control and the nondominant limb for positional or impedance control. Because of the impact these advantages may have on upper-extremity skill, they should be given consideration during intervention. Further research is needed to determine methods of enhancing skill during development or after injury given the interlimb asymmetries.

ANSWER TO THE LAB ACTIVITIES

Lab Activity 19-1

It is important to remember that there is no single correct way to train upper-extremity function in Jean. It is essential that all aspects of arm and hand motor control be included in her rehabilitation program, and that a range of tasks and conditions be used to help her develop a variety of strategies so that she is able to grasp and manipulate a variety of objects in a wide diversity of tasks and conditions. The specific order, duration, and timing of each activity may vary from therapist to therapist.

We begin by determining Jean's main concern and goals related to hand function. She expresses concern that she be able to perform ADL activities using her hands (brushing her teeth, cooking, etc.) without dropping items and without the assistance of her spouse. She is confident in her ability to use her less-affected hand, but some activities, such as brushing her teeth or holding kitchen items may be difficult.

So our approach to training hand function will focus both on improving underlying impairments (her weakness and sensibility deficits) and on practicing functional ADL tasks in context.

We will try to incorporate principles of participation and motor learning into her program. Initially, we will have her participate in a constraint-induced movement therapy program that is offered three times per week to increase use of her affected hand. As the frequency of use of her affected hand improves, we will shift to interlimb transfer tasks in which she will grasp and lift objects with the less-affected hand first followed by lifts with the affected hand. The physical properties of the objects will be varied. At the same time we will attempt to strengthen her hand through finger exercises using resistive foam progressing to Theraputty. We will also incorporate methods to improve sensory discrimination in her hand and memory through tactile discrimination tasks and stereognosis activities. Finally, in an attempt to improve her participation in ADL tasks and sequencing we will practice simple three-step kitchen tasks in the simulated therapy kitchen.

Research to support our clinical decision making regarding this approach to treatment is steadily increasing. The following table presents some examples. What other research can you find to support your evidence-based rehabilitation program to improve hand function?

Individual Component of Upper-Extremity Function	Task or Activity	Environmental Conditions	Research Evidence
Motor: Frequency of affected hand use	Massed practice—shaping tasks	Constraint induced movement therapy—three times a week in an outpatient program	Pierce et al., 2003; Taub et al., 1993; Winstein et al., 2003; Wolf et al., 2005, 2006, 2008
Motor: Anticipatory force scaling	Grasp and lift of stationary objects.	Interlimb Transfer—Lift various objects first with less-affected hand followed by affected hand	Camus et al., 2009; Dawson et al., 2010; Gordon et al., 1999; Raghavan et al., 2006
Motor: Wrist and finger extension activation and strength	Wrist and finger extension used to preshape hand before grasping	NMES to wrist and finger/thumb extensors used in conjunction with grasp and release activities with objects of various sizes	Fujiwara et al., 2009; Hara et al., 2008; Lang et al., 2009
Motor: Sustained grip	Grasp and hold utensils	Blocked and random practice employing different grooming utensils in context	Trombly & Ma, 2002; Dunn et al., 1994
Cognitive and Sensory: Memory and tactile discrimination	Tactile discrimination tasks and object identification tasks	Eyes open, closed, five textures used for identification; identify objects first with eyes open then after placed in a box	Byl et al., 2003; Decker, 2010
Cognitive: Memory and sequencing	Simple 3-step meal preparation	Making a cup of tea given written directions at first progressing to independence	Trombly & Ma, 2002; Dunn et al., 1994

REFERENCES

A

Abbruzzese G. The medical management of spasticity. Eur J Neurol 2002;9:1–9.

Abrams TW, Kandel ER. Is contiguity detection in classical conditioning a system or a cellular property? Learning in Aplysia suggests a possible molecular site. Trends Neurosci 1988;11:128–135.

Ada L, Dean CM, Hall JM, et al. A treadmill and overground walking program improves walking in persons residing the community after stroke: a placebo controlled randomized trial. Arch Phys Med Rehabil 2003;84: 1486–1491.

Ada L, Dorsch S, Canning CG. Strengthening interventions increase strength and improve activity after stroke: a systematic review. Aust J Physiother 2006;52:241–248.

Adams JA. A closed-loop theory of motor learning. J Motor Behav 1971;3:111–150.

Adams LS, Greene LW, Topoozian E. Range of motion. In: Casanova JS, ed. Clinical assessment recommendations, 2nd ed. Chicago: American Society of Hand Therapists, 1992:55–70.

Adkin AL, Bloem BR, Allum JH. Trunk sway measurements during stance and gait tasks in Parkinson's disease. Gait Posture 2005;22: 240–249.

Adolph KE. Learning to solve the problem of moving: Exploration, experience, and control. Paper presented at The Annual Conference in The Movement Sciences: Development of Skill in Infancy and Early Childhood, Teacher's College, Columbia University, New York, 1994.

Adolph KE, Berger SE. Motor development. In: Damon W, Lerner R, series eds.; Kuhn D, Siegler RS, vol. eds. Handbook of child psychology, vol. 2. Cognition, perception, and language, 6th ed. New York: Wiley, 2006:161–213.

Agnew PJ, Dip OT, Maas F. Hand function related to age and sex. Arch Phys Med Rehabil 1982;63:269–271.

Aguayo AJ, Clarke DB, Jelsma TN, et al. Effects of neurotrophins on the survival and regrowth of injured retinal neurons. In: Growth factors as drugs for neurological and sensory disorders. Chicester, England: Wiley, Ciba Foundation Symposium, 1996:135–148.

Ahmed S, Mayo NE, Higgins J, et al. The Stroke Rehabilitation Assessment of Movement (STREAM): a comparison with other measures used to evaluate the effects of stroke and rehabilitation. Phys Ther 2003;83:617–660.

Alberts JL, Butler AJ, Wolf SL. The effects of constraint-induced therapy on precision grip: a preliminary study. Neurorehabil Neural Repair 2004;18:250–258.

Alberts JL, Saling M, Adler CH, Stelmach GE. Disruptions in the reach-to-grasp actions of Parkinson's patients. Exp Brain Res 2000; 134:353–362.

Alexander GE, Crutcher MD. Functional architecture of basal ganglia circuits: neural substrates of parallel processing. Trends Neurosci 1990;13:266–271.

Alexander NB, Mollo JM, Giordani B, et al. Maintenance of balance, gait patterns and obstacle clearance in Alzheimer's disease. Neurology 1995;45:908–914.

Alexander NB, Schultz AB, Warwick DN. Rising from a chair: effect of age and functional ability on performance biomechanics. J Gerontol 1991;46:M91–M98.

Alexander RM. Optimization and gaits in the locomotion of vertebrates. Physiol Rev 1989;69:1199–1227.

Allet L, Leemann B, Guyen E, et al. Effect of different walking aids on walking capacity of patients with poststroke hemiparesis. Arch Phys Med Rehabil 2009;90:1408–1413.

Allison L. Balance disorders. In: Umphred DA, ed. Neurological rehabilitation. St. Louis: Mosby Year Book, 1995:802–837.

Allum JH, Carpenter MG, Honegger F. Directional aspects of balance corrections in man. IEEE Eng Med Biol Mag 2003;22:37–47.

Allum JHJ, Honegger F, Schicks H. The influence of a bilateral vestibular deficit on postural synergies. J Vestib Res 1994;4:49–70.

Allum JHJ, Pfaltz CR. Visual and vestibular contributions to pitch sway stabilization in the ankle muscles of normals and patients with bilateral peripheral vestibular deficits. Exp Brain Res 1985;58:82–94.

Almli RB, Finger S. Toward a definition of recovery of function. In: Le Vere TE, Almli RB, Stein DG, eds. Brain injury and recovery: theoretical and controversial issues. New York: Plenum, 1988:1–4.

Alon G, Sunnerhagen KS, Geurts AC, Ohry A. A home-based self-administered stimulation program to improve selected hand functions in chronic stroke. Neurorehabilitation 2003;18:215–225.

Alzghoul MB, Gerrard D, Watkins BA, Hannon K. Ectopic expression of IGF-I and Shh by skeletal muscle inhibits disuse-mediated skeletal muscle atrophy and bone osteopenia in vivo. FASEB J 2004;18:221–223.

Amaral D. The anatomical organization of the central nervous system. In: Kandel ER, Schwartz JH, Jessell TM, eds. Principles of neural science, 4th ed. New York: McGraw-Hill, 2000:317–336.

American Physical Therapy Association. Guide to physical therapy practice, 2nd ed. Phys Ther 2003;81:9–746.

American Society of Orthopedic Surgeons. Joint motion: method of measuring and recording. Chicago: American Academy of Orthopedic Surgeons, 1965.

Amiel-Tison C, Grenier A. Evaluation neurologique du nouveau-né et du nourrisson. [Neurological evaluation of the human infant.] New York: Masson, 1980:81–102.

Amundsen, LR, ed. Muscle strength testing: Instrumented and non-instrumented systems. New York: Churchill Livingstone, 1990: 123–150.

Amundson S. Evaluation Tool of Children's Handwriting (ETCH). Morganville, NJ: ETCH Administration, 1995.

Anacker SL, DiFabio RP. Influence of sensory inputs on standing balance in community dwelling elders with a recent history of falling. Phys Ther 1992;72:575–584.

Andersen RA, Buneo CA. Intentional maps in posterior parietal cortex. Annu Rev Neurosci 2002;25:189–220.

Andersen RA, Cui H. Intention, action planning, and decision making in pareital-frontal circuits. Neuron 2009;63:568–583.

Andersen RA. In: Mountcastle VB, Plum F, Geiger SR, eds. Higher functions of the brain, part 2: The nervous system, vol. 5, Handbook of physiology, section 1. Bethesda, MD: American Physiological Association, 1987:483–518.

Anderson JB, Sinkjaer T. Stretch reflex variations during gait. In: Pedotti A, Ferrarin M, Quintern J, Riener R, eds. Neuroprosthetics. Berlin: Springer, 1996:45–50.

Anderson JL, Terzis G, Kryger A. Increase in the degree of coexpression of myosin heavy chain isoforms in skeletal muscle fibers of the very old. Muscle Nerve 1999;22:449–454.

Andersson G, Hagman J, Talianzadeh R, et al. Effect of cognitive load on postural control. Brain Res Bull 2002;58:135–139.

Andersson G, Magnusson M. Neck vibration causes short-latency electromyographic activation of lower leg muscles in postural reactions of the standing human. Acta Otolaryngol 2002;122:284–288.

Andrews AW. Hand-held dynamometry for measuring muscle strength. J Hum Muscle Perform 1991;1:35–50.

Andrews AW, Bohannon RW. Distribution of muscle strength impairments following stroke. Clin Rehabil 2000;14:79–87.

Andriacchi TP, Oagle JA, Galante JO. Walking speed as a basis for normal and abnormal gait measurements. J Biomech 1977;10:261–268.

Aniansson A, Grimby F, Gedberg A. Muscle function in old age. Scand J Rehabil Med 1978;6(Suppl):43–49.

Aniansson A, Hedberg M, Henning G, et al. Muscle morphology, enzymatic activity and muscle strength in elderly men: a follow up study. Muscle Nerve 1986;9:585–591.

Antal A, Nitsche MA, Kincses TZ, et al. Facilitation of visuo-motor learning by transcranial direct current stimulation of the motor and extrastriate visual areas in humans. Eur J Neurosci 2004;19(10):2888–2892.

Apel U. The Feldenkrais method: awareness through movement. WHO Reg Publ Eur Ser 1992;44:324–327.

Aras MD, Gokkaya NK, Comert D, et al. Shoulder pain in hemiplegia: results from a national rehabilitation hospital in Turkey. Am J Phys Med Rehabil 2004;83:713–719.

Arce FI, Katz N, Sugarman H. The scaling of postural adjustments during bimanual load-lifting in traumatic brain-injured adults. Hum Move Sci 2004;22:749–768.

Arshavsky Yu I, Berkinblit MB, Fukson OI, et al. Recordings of neurones of the dorsal spinocerebellar tract during evoked locomotion. Brain Res 1972a;43:272–275.

Arshavsky Yu I, Berkinblit MB, Gelfand IM, et al. Activity of the neurones of the ventral spino-cerebellar tract during locomotion. Biophysics 1972b;17:926–935.

Aruin AS, Almeida LH. Organization of a simple two joint synergy in individuals with Down Syndrom. Am J Ment Retard 1996;101:256–268

Arutyunyan GH, Gurfnkel VS, Mirskii ML. Organization of movements on execution by man of an exact postural task. Biophysics 1969; 14:1162–1167.

Asai H, Fujiwara K, Tachino K. Limiting factor for moveable range of the center of foot pressure in backward direction. In: Taguchi K, Igarashi M, Mori S, eds. Vestibular and neural front. Amsterdam: Elsevier Science B.V., 1994:525–528.

Asanuma H, Keller A. Neuronal mechanisms of motor learning in mammals. Neuroreport 1991;2:217–224.

Ashburn A, Hyndman D, Pickering R, et al. Predicting people with stroke at risk of falls. Age Ageing 2008;37:270–276.

Ashburn A, Stack E. Fallers and non-fallers with Parkinson's disease (PD): the influence of a dual task on standing balance. Mov Disord 2000;15(Suppl 3):78. [abstract].

Ashburn A, Stack E, Pickering RM, Ward CD. A community dwelling sample of people with Parkinson's disease: characteristics of fallers and non-fallers. Age Ageing 2001;30:47–52.

Ashmead DH, Hill EW, Talor CR. Obstacle perception by congenitally blind children. Percept Psychophys 1989;46:425–433.

Aslin RN. Development of smooth pursuit in human infants. In: Fisher DF, Monty RA, Senders JW, eds. Eye movements: cognition and visual perception. Hillsdale, NJ: Erlbaum, 1981.

Assaiante C, Amblard B. An ontogenetic model for the sensorimotor organization of balance control in humans. Hum Move Sci 1995;14: 13–43.

Assaiante C, Mallau S, Viel S, et al. Development of postural control in healthy children: a functional approach. Neural Plast 2005;12:109–118.

Assaiante C, Woollacott M, Amblard B. Development of postural adjustment during gait initiation: kinematic and EMG analysis. J Motor Behav 2000;32:211–226.

Astill S, Utley A. Coupling of the reach and grasp phase during catching in children with developmental coordination disorder. J Motor Behav 2008;40:315–323.

Atkeson CG, Hollerbach JM. Kinematic features of unrestrained vertical arm movements. J Neurosci 1985;5:2318–2330.

Augurelle AS, Smith AM, Lejeune T, Thonnard JL. Importance of cutaneous feedback in maintaining a secure grip during manipulation of handheld objects. J Neurophysiol 2003;89:665–671.

Ayres AJ. Sensory integration and learning disorders. Los Angeles: Western Psychological Services, 1972.

B

Baars BJ. How does a stream of consciousness that is relatively simple, serial, and limited in capacity emerge from a brain that is largely unconscious, complex, and massively parallel? In: Marsh E, ed. Ciba Symposium on Experimental and Theoretical Foundations of Consciousness (#174). London: Wiley Interscience, 1993.

Babin-Ratte S, Sirigu A, Gilles M, Wing A. Impaired anticipatory finger grip-force adjustments in a case of cerebellar degeneration. Exp Brain Res 1999;128:81–85.

Bach-y-Rita P, Balliet R. Recovery from stroke. In: Duncan P, Badke MB, eds. Stroke rehabilitation: the recovery of motor control. Chicago: Year Book, 1987:79–107.

Badell-Ribera A. Cerebral palsy: postural-locomotor prognosis in spastic diplegia. Arch Phys Med Rehabil 1985;66:614–619.

Badke MB, DiFabio RP. Balance deficits in patients with hemiplegia: considerations for assessment and treatment. In: Duncan P, ed. Balance: proceedings of the APTA Forum. Alexandria, VA: American Physical Therapy Association, 1990:73–78.

Baer HR, Wolf SL. Modified Emory Functional Ambulation Profile: an outcome measure for the rehabilitation of poststroke gait dysfunction. Stroke 2001;32:973–979.

Bailey CH, Chen M. Morphological basis of long-term habituation and sensitization in Aplysia. Science 1983;220(4592):91–93

Bailey CH, Kandel ER. Synaptic growth and the persistence of long-term memory: a molecular perspective. In: Gazzaniga, MS, ed. The cognitive neurosciences, 3rd ed. Cambridge, MA: MIT Press, 2004.

Bair WN, Kiemel T, Jeka JJ, Clark JE. Development of multisensory reweighting for posture control in children. Exp Brain Res 2007;183:435–446.

Baker MP, Hudson JE, Wolf SL. A "feedback" cane to improve the hemiplegic patient's gait. Phys Ther 1979;59:170–171.

Baker PS, Bodner EV, Allman RM. Measuring life space mobility in community-dwelling older adults. J Am Geriatr Soc 2003;51:1610–1614.

Bakker M, Verstappen CCP, Bloem BB, Toni I. Recent advances in functional neuroimaging of gait. J Neural Transm 2007;114:1323–1331.

Balint R. Seelenhamung des "Schauens," optische Ataxie, raumlische Storung des Aufmersamkeit. Monatshr Psychiatr Neurol 1909;25:51–81.

Ballard CG, Shaw F, Lowery K, et al. The prevalence, assessment and associations of falls in dementia with Lewy bodies and Alzheimer's disease. Dement Geriatr Cogn Disord 1999;10(2):97–103.

Baloh RW. Dizziness, hearing loss and tinnitus: the essentials of neurotology. Philadelphia: FA Davis, 1984.

Balzini L, Vannucchi L, Benvenuti F, et al. Clinical characteristics of flexed posture in elderly women. J Am Geriatr Soc 2003;51:1419–1426.

Barbeau H. Locomotor training in neurorehabilitation: emerging rehabilitation concepts. Neurorehabil Neural Repair 2003;17:3–11.

Barclay-Goddard RE, Stevenson TJ, Poluha W, et al. Force platform feedback for standing balance training after stroke. Cochrane Database Syst Revi 2004;4:D004129.

Barker RN, Brauer S, Carson R. Training-induced changes in the pattern of triceps to biceps activation during reaching tasks after chronic and severe stroke. Exp Brain Res 2009;196:483–496.

Barnes MR, Crutchfield CA, Heriza CB. The neurophysiological basis of patient treatment. vol. II: Reflexes in motor development. Morgantown, WV: Stokesville, 1978.

Barra J, Oujamaa L, Chauvineau V, et al. Asymmetric standing posture after stroke is related to a biased egocentric coordinate system. Neurology 2009;72;1582–1587.

Barreca S, Gowland CK, Stratford P, et al. Development of the Chedoke Arm and Hand Activity Inventory: theoretical constructs, item generation, and selection. Top Stroke Rehabil 2004;11(4):31–42.

Barreca SR, Stratford PW, Lambert CL, et al. Test-retest reliability, validity, and sensitivity of the Chedoke arm and hand activity inventory: a new measure of upper-limb for survivors of stroke. Arch Phys Med Rehabil 2005;86:1616–1622.

Barreca SR, Stratford PW, Masters LM, et al. Comparing 2 versions of the Chedoke Arm and Hand Activity Inventory with the Action Research Arm Test. Phys Ther 2006;86: 245–253.

Bartlett D, Birmingham T. Validity and reliability of a pediatric reach test. Pediatr Phys Ther 2003;15:84–92.

Bartolic A, Pirtosek Z, Rozman J, Ribaric S. Postural stability of Parkinson's disease patients is improved by decreasing rigidity. Eur J Neurol 2005;12:156–159.

Basford JR, Chou LS, Kaufman KR, et al. An assessment of gait and balance deficits after traumatic brain injury. Arch Phys Med Rehabil 2003;84:343–349.

Basler H, Luckmann J, Wolf U, Quint S. Fear-avoidance beliefs, physical activity, and disability in elderly individuals with chronic low back pain and healthy controls. Clin J Pain 2008;24:604–610.

Basmajian JV, De Luca CJ. Muscles alive: their functions revealed by electromyography, 5th ed. Baltimore: Williams & Wilkins, 1985.

Basmajian JV, Kukulka CG, Narayan MD, Takebe K. Biofeedback treatment of foot-drop after stroke compared with standard rehabilitation technique: effects on voluntary control and strength. Arch Phys Med Rehabil 1975;56: 231–236.

Bassile CC, Dean C, Boden-Albala B, Sacco R. Obstacle training programme for individuals post stroke: feasibility study. Clin Rehabil 2003;17:130–136.

Bastian AJ. Cerebellar limb ataxia: abnormal control of self generated and external forces. Ann NY Acad Sci 2002;978:16–27.

Bastian AJ, Martin TA, Keating JG, Thach WT. Cerebellar ataxia: abnormal control of interaction torques across multiple joints. J Neurophysiol 1996;76:492–509.

Bastian AJ, Zackowski KM, Thach WT. Cerebellar ataxia: torque deficiency or torque mismatch between joints? J Neurophysiol 2000;83: 3019–3030.

Bateni H, Heung E, Zettel J, et al. Can use of walkers or canes impede lateral compensatory stepping movements? Gait Posture 2004a;20: 74–83.

Bateni H, Maki BE. Assistive devices for balance and mobility: benefits, demands, and adverse consequences. Arch Phys Med Rehabil 2005;86:134–145.

Bateni H, Zecevic A, McIlroy WE, Make BE. Resolving conflicts in task demands during balance recovery: does holding an object inhibit compensatory grasping? Eve Brain Res 2004b;157:49–58.

Bates D, Pruess K, Souney P, Platt R. Serious falls in hospitalized patients;correlates and resource utilization. Am J Med 1995;99:137–143.

Bayley N. Bayley Scales of Infant Development. San Antonio, TX: Psychological, 1969.

Bayouk JF, Boucher JP, Leroux A. Balance training following stroke: effects of task-oriented exercises with and without altered sensory input. Int J Rehabil Res 2006;29:51–59.

Bean JF, Kiely DK, Herman S, et al. The relationship between leg power and physical performance in mobility-limited older people. J Am Geriatr Soc 2002;50:461–467.

Bean JF, Leveille SG, Kiely DK, et al. A comparison of leg power and leg strength within the InCHIANTI study: which influences mobility more? J Gerontol Med Sci 2003;58A: 728–733.

Beauchet O, Dubost V, Herrmann FR, Kressig RW. Stride-to-stride variability while backward counting among healthy young adults. J Neuroeng Rehabil 2005;2:26.

Bechtol CO. Grip test use of dynamometer with adjustable hand spacing. JAMA 1954;36: 820–824.

Beer RF, Dewald JP, Rymer WZ. Deficits in the coordination of multijoint arm movements in patients with hemiparesis: evidence for disturbed control of limb dynamics. Exp Brain Res 2000;131:305–319.

Beery KE, Butenica NA, Beery NA. Beery-Butenica Developmental Test of Visual-Motor

Integration, 5th ed. Minneapolis, MN: NCS Pearson, 2004.

Behrman AL, Bowden MG, Nair PM. Neuroplasticity after spinal cord injury and training: an emerging paradigm shift in rehabilitation and walking recovery. Phys Ther 2006;86:1406 -1425

Behrman AL, Lawless-Dixon AR, Davis SB, et al. Locomotor training progression and outcomes after incomplete spinal cord injury. Phys Ther 2005;85:1356–1371.

Beilock SL, Carr TH, MacMahon C, Starkes JL. When paying attention becomes counterproductive: Impact of divided versus skill-focused attention on novice and experienced performance of sensorimotor skills. J Exp Psychol Appl 2002;8:6–16.

Beldarrain MG, Gafman J, deVelasco IR, et al. Prefrontal lesions impair the implicit and explicit learning of sequences on visualmotor tasks. Exp Brain Res 2002;142:529–538.

Belen'kii VY, Gurfinkel VS, Paltsev YI. Elements of control of voluntary movements. Biofizika 1967;12:135–141.

Bell-Krotoski J, Weinstein S, Weinstein C. Testing sensibility, including touch-pressure, two-point discrimination, point localization, and vibration. J Hand Ther 1993;2:114–123.

Bello AI, Rockson BE, Olaogun MO. The effects of electromyographic-triggered neuromuscular electrical muscle stimulation on the functional hand recovery among stroke survivors. Afr J Med Med Sci 2009;38(2):184–191.

Benbow M. Loops and other groups: a kinesthetic writing system, instructor's ed. Randolph, NJ: OT Ideas, 1991.

Benbow M, Hanft B, Marsh D. Handwriting in the classroom: improving written communication. In: Royeen C, ed. Classroom applications for school-based practice from the American Occupational Therapy Association Self Study Series. Rockville, MD: American Occupational Therapy Press, 1992.

Benda BJ, Riley PO, Krebs DE. Biomechanical relationship between center of gravity and center of pressure during standing. IEEE Trans Rehab Eng 1994;2:3–10.

Bennett KM, Castiello U. Reorganization of prehension components following perturbation of object size. Psychol Aging 1995;10:204–214.

Bensoussan L, Viton JM, Schieppati M, et al. Changes in postural control in hemiplegic patients after stroke performing a dual task. Arch Phys Med Rehabil 2007;88:1009–1015.

Bentzel K. Evaluation of sensation. In: Trombly CA, ed. Occupational therapy for physical dysfunction, 4th ed. Baltimore: Williams & Wilkins, 1995.

Berardelli A, Sabra AF, Hallett M. Physiological mechanisms of rigidity in Parkinson's disease. J Neurol Neurosurg Psychiatry 1983;46: 45–53.

Berg K. Measuring balance in the elderly: validation of an instrument. Dissertation. Montreal: McGill University, 1993.

Berg K, Wood-Dauphinee S, Williams J, Gayton D. Measuring balance in the elderly: preliminary development of an instrument. Physiother Can 1989;41:304–308.

Berg K, Wood-Dauphinee SL, Willimans JT. Measuring balance in the elderly: validation of an instrument. Can J Public Health 1992;83: S9–S11.

Berger SE, Adolph KE. Learning and development in infant locomotion. Prog Brain Res 2007;164: 237–255.

Berger W, Altenmueller E, Dietz V. Normal and impaired development of children's gait. Hum Neurobiol 1984a;3:163–170.

Berger W, Horstmann GA, Dietz VL. Tension development and muscle activation in the leg during gait in spastic hemiparesis: the independence of muscle hypertonia and exaggerated stretch reflexes. J Neurol Neurosurg Psychiatry 1984b;47:1029–1033.

Berger W, Quintern J, Dietz V. Stance and gait perturbations in children: developmental aspects of compensatory mechanisms. Electroencephalogr Clin Neurophysiol 1985;61: 385–395.

Bergmann K. Incidence of atypical pencil grasps among nondysfunctional adults. Am J Occup Ther 1990;44:736–740.

Bernspang B, Fugl–Meyer AR, Viltanen M. Perceptual function in the elderly and after stroke. Scand J Caring Sci 1988;2:75–99.

Bernspang B, Vitanin M, Eriksson S. Impairments of perception and motor functions: their influence on self care ability 4 to 6 years after a stroke. Occup Ther J Res 1989;9:27–37.

Bernstein N. The coordination and regulation of movement. London: Pergamon, 1967.

Bertenthal B, von Hofsten C. Eye, head and trunk control: the foundation of manual development. Neurosci Biobehav Rev 1998;22: 515–520.

Bertenthal BI, Rose JL, Bai DL. Perception-action coupling in the development of visual control of posture. J Exp Psychol 1997;23:1631–1643.

Bertera EM, Bertera RL. Fear of falling and activity avoidance in a national sample of older adults in the United States. Health Social Work, 2008;33:54–62.

Berthier NE, Clifton RK, McCall DD, Robin DJ. Proximodistal structure of early reaching in human infants. Exp Brain Res 1999;127: 259–269.

Berthier NE, Keen R. Development of reaching in infancy. Exp Brain Res 2006;169:507–518.

Berthoz A, Pozzo T. Head and body coordination during locomotion and complex movements. In: Swinnen SP, Heuer H, Massion J, Casaer P, eds. Interlimb coordination: neural, dynamical and cognitive constraints. San Diego: Academic, 1994:147–165.

Bertram CP, Lemay M, Stelmach GE. The effect of Parkinson's disease on the control of multi-segmental coordination. Brain Cogn 2005;57:16–20.

Beuter A, Hernández R, Rigal R, et al. Postural sway and effect of levodopa in early Parkinson's disease Can J Neurol Sci 2008;35:65–68.

Bhatt T, Wening JD, Pai YC. Adaptive control of gait stability in reducing slip-related backward loss of balance. Exp Brain Res 2006;170: 61–73.

Biernaskie J, Chernenko G, Corbett D. Efficacy of rehabilitative experience declines with time after focal ischemic brain injury. J Neurosci 2004 Feb 4;24(5):1245–1254.

Biguer B, Prablanc C, Jeannerod M. The contribution of coordinated eye and head movements in hand pointing accuracy. Exp Brain Res 1984;55:462–469.

Bilodeau EA, Bilodeau IM, Schumsky DA. Some effects of introducing and withdrawing knowledge of results early and late in practice. J Exp Psychol 1959;58:142–144.

Binkofski F, Dohle C, Posse S, et al. Human anterior intraparietal area subserves prehension. Neurology 1998;50:1253–1259.

Birren JE, Cunningham W. Research on the psychology of aging: principles, concepts and theory. In: Birren JE, Schaie KW, eds. Handbook of the psychology of aging, 2nd ed. New York: Van Nostrand Reinhold, 1985:3–34.

Birren JE, Riegel KF, Morrison DF. Age differences in response speed as a function of controlled variations of stimulus conditions: evidence of a general speed factor. Gerontologia 1962; 6:1–18.

Bishop B. Neurophysiology of motor responses evoked by vibratory stimulation. Phys Ther 1974;54:1273–1282.

Bishop M, Brunt D, Pathare N, et al. Changes in distal muscle timing may contribute to slowness during sit to stand in Parkinsons disease. Clin Biomech (Bristol, Avon). 2005;20(1):112–117.

Bjorklund A. Long distance axonal growth in the adult central nervous system. J Neurol 1994;241:S33–S35.

Black FO, Nashner LM. Postural disturbance in patients with benign paroxysmal positional nystagmus. Ann Otol Rhinol Laryngol 1984a; 93(6 Pt 1):595–599.

Black FO, Nashner LM. Vestibulo-spinal control differs in patients with reduced versus distorted vestibular function. Acta Otolaryngol (Stockh) Suppl 1984b;406:110–114.

Black FO, Nashner LM. Postural control in four classes of vestibular abnormalities. In: Igarashi M, Black FO, eds. Vestibular and visual control of posture and locomotor equilibrium. Basel: Karger, 1985:271–281.

Black FO, Shupert C, Horak FB, Nashner LM. Abnormal postural control associated with peripheral vestibular disorders. In: Pompeiano O, Allum J, eds. Vestibulospinal control of posture and movement. Progress in brain research, vol. 76. Amsterdam: Elsevier Science, 1988:263–275.

Black K, Zafonte R, Millis S, et al. Sitting balance following brain injury: doe sit predict outcome? Brain Inj 2000;14:141–152.

Black P, Markowitz RS, Cianci SN. Recovery of motor function after lesions in motor cortex of monkeys. Ciba Found Symp 1975;34:65–83.

Blanchard O, Cohen-Solal L, Tardieu C, et al. Tendon adaptation to different long term stresses and collagen reticulation in soleus muscle. Connect Tissue Res 1985;13(3):261–267.

Blank R, Heizer W, von Voss H. Development of externally guided grip force modulation in man. Neurosci Lett 2000;286:187–190.

Blanton S, Wolf AL. An application of upper-extremity constraint-induced movement therapy in a patient with subacute stroke. Phys Ther 1999;79:847–853.

Bleck EE. Locomotor prognosis in cerebral palsy. Dev Med Child Neurol 1975;17:18–25.

Blennerhassett JM, Matyas TA, Carey LM. Impaired discrimination of surface friction contributes to pinch grip deficit after stroke. Neurorehabil Neural Repair 2007;21:263–272.

Bliem BR, Grimbergen YA, Cramer M, et al. Prospective assessment of falls in Parkinson's disease. J Neurol 2001;248:950–958.

Blin O, Ferrandez AM, Pailhous J, Serratrice G. Dopa-sensitive and dopa-resistant gait parameters in Parkinson's disease. J Neurol Sci 1991;103:51–54.

Blin O, Ferrandez AM, Serratrice G. Quantitative analysis of gait in Parkinson patients: increased variability of stride length. J Neurosci 1990;98:91–97.

Bliss TVP, Lomo T. Long-lasting potentiation of synaptic transmission in the dentate area of the anaesthetized rabbit following stimulation of the perforant path. J Physiol (Lond) 1973;232:331–356.

Bloem BR, Beckley DJ, van Dijk JG. Are automatic postural responses in patients with Parkinson's disease abnormal due to their stooped posture? Exp Brain Res 1999;124:481–488.

Bloem BR, Grimbergen YA, van Dijk JG, Munneke M. The 'posture second" strategy: a review of wrong priorities in Parkinson's disase. J Neurol Sci 2006;248:196–204.

Bloem BR, Grimbergen YAM, Cramer M, et al. "Stops Walking When Talking" does not predict falls in Parkinson's disease. Ann Neurol 2000;48:268.

Bobath B. Abnormal postural reflex activity caused by brain lesions. London: Heinemann, 1965.

Bobath B. Adult hemiplegia: evaluation and treatment. 3rd ed. London: Heinemann, 1990.

Bobath B. Adult Hemiplegia: Evaluation and Treatment. London: William Heinemann Medical Books, 1978.

Bobath B, Bobath K. Motor development in different types of cerebral palsy. London: Heinemann, 1975.

Bobath K, Bobath B. The neurodevelopmental treatment. In: Scrutton D, ed. Management of the motor disorders of cerebral palsy. Clinics in Developmental Medicine, no. 90. London: Heinemann, 1984.

Boehme R. Improving upper body control. Tucson: Therapy Skill Builders, 1988.

Boenig DD. Evaluation of a clinical method of gait analysis. Phys Ther 1977;7:795–798.

Bogataj U, Gros N, Malezic M, et al. Restoration of gait during two to three weeks of therapy with multichannel electrical stimulation. Phys Ther 1989;69:319–327.

Bohannon RW. Hand-held compared with isokinetic dynamometry for measurement of static knee extension torque (parallel reliability of dynamometers). Clin Phys Physiol Meas 1990; 11:217–222.

Bohannon RW. Comfortable and maximum walking speed of adults aged 20–79 years: reference values and determinants. Age Ageing 1997;26:15–19.

Bohannon RW, Andrews AW. Correlation of knee extensor muscle torque and spasticity with gait speed in patients with stroke. Arch Phys Med Rehabil 1990;71:330–333.

Bohannon RW, Smith MB. Interrater reliability of a Modified Ashworth Scale of muscle spasticity. Phys Ther 1987;67(2):206–207.

Bohannon RW, Walsh S. Nature, reliability, and predictive value of muscle performance measures in patients with hemiparesis following stroke. Arch Phys Med Rehabil 1992;73: 721–725.

Bonaiuto J, Arbib MA. Extending the mirror neuron system model, II: what did I just do? A new role for mirror neurons. Biol Cybern 2010;102(4):341–359.

Bonan IV, Colle FM, Guichard JP, et al. Reliance on visual information after stroke. Part I. Balance on dynamic posturography. Arch Phys Med Rehabil 2004;85:268–273.

Bonan IV, Guettard E, Leman MC, et al. Subjective visual vertical perception relates to balance in acute stroke. Arch Phys Med Rehabil 2006;87:642–646.

Boomkamp-Koppen HGM, Visser-Meily JMAMA, Post MWM, Prevo AJH. Poststroke hand swelling and oedema: prevalence and relationship with impairment and disability. Clin Rehabil 19:552–559.

Booth FW. Effect of limb immobilization on skeletal muscle. J Appl Physiol 1982;52: 1113–1118.

Borst MJ, Peterson CQ. Overcoming topographical orientation deficits in an elderly woman with right cerebrovascular accident. Am J Occup Ther 1993;47:551–554.

Bortz WM IV, Bortz WM II. How fast do we age? Exercise performance over time as a biomarker. J Gerontol A Biol Sci Med Sci 1996;51: M223–M225.

Boudreau MJ, Smith AM. Activity in rostral motor cortex in response to predictable force-pulse perturbations in a precision grip task. J Neurophysiol 2001;86:1079–1085.

Bouisset S, Zattara M. A sequence of postural movements precedes voluntary movement. Neurosci Lett 1981;22:263–270.

Bovend'Eerdt TJ, Newman M, Barker K, et al. The effects of stretching in spasticity: a systematic review. Arch Phys Med Rehabil 2008;89: 1395–13406.

Bowen A, Wenman R, Mickelborough J, et al. Dual-task effects of talking while walking on velocity and balance following a stroke. Age Ageing 2001;30:319–323.

Bower TGR, Broughton JM, Moore MK. The coordination of visual and tactual input in infants. Percept Psychophys 1970a;8:51–53.

Bower TGR, Broughton JM, Moore MK. Demonstration of intention in the reaching behavior of neonate humans. Nature 1970b;228:679–681.

Boyd LA, Winstein CJ. Implicit motor sequence learning in humans following unilateral stroke: the impact of practice and explicit knowledge. Neurosci Lett 2001;298:65–69.

Boyd LA, Winstein CJ. Impact of explicit information on implicit motor sequence learning following middle cerebral artery stroke. Phys Ther 2003;83:976–989.

Brach JS, Berlin JE, Van Swearingen JM, et al. Too much or too little step width variability is associated with a fall history in older persons who walk at or near normal gait speed. J Neuroeng Rehabil 2005;2:21.

Bradley NS, Bekoff A. Development of locomotion: animal models. In: Woollacott MH, Shumway-Cook A, eds. Development of posture and gait across the lifespan. Columbia: University of South Carolina, 1989:48–73.

Bradley NS, Smith JL. Neuromuscular patterns of stereotypic hindlimb behaviors in the first two postnatal months. I. Stepping in normal kittens. Dev Brain Res 1988;38:37–52.

Brændvik SM, Elvrum AK, Vereijken B, Roeleveld K. Relationship between neuromuscular body functions and upper extremity activity in children with cerebral palsy. Dev Med Child Neurol 2010;52:29–34.

Brand PW. Management of sensory loss in the extremities. In: Omer E, Spinner M, eds. Management of peripheral nerve problems. Philadelphia: Saunders, 1980:862–872.

Brandstater M, deBruin H, Gowland C, et al. Hemiplegic gait: analysis of temporal variables. Arch Phys Med Rehabil 1983;64:583–587.

Brandt T, Daroff RB. The multisensory physiological and pathological vertigo syndromes. Ann Neurol 1979;7:195–197.

Brandt T, Wenzel D, Dichgans J. Die Entwicklung der visuellen Stabilisation des aufrechten Standes bein Kind: Ein Refezeichen in der Kinderneurologie (Visual stabilization of free stance in infants: a sign of maturity). Arch Psychiatr Nervenkr 1976;223:1–13.

Brashear A, Zafonte R, Corcoran M, et al. Inter- and intrarater reliability of the Ashworth scale and the Disability Assessment Scale in patients with upper limb post stroke spasticity. Arch Phys Med Rehabil 2002;83:1349–1354.

Brauer S. Mediolateral postural stability: changes with age and prediction of fallers. Doctoral dissertation, University of Queensland, June 1998.

Brauer SG, Broome A, Stone C, et al. Simplest tasks have greatest dual task interference with balance in brain injured adults. Hum Move Sci 2004;23:489–502.

Brauer SG, Woollacott M, Shumway-Cook A. The interacting effects of cognitive demand and recovery of postural stability in balance-impaired elderly. J Gerontol Med Sci 2001;56: 489–496.

Brauer SG, Woollacott M, Shumway-Cook A. The influence of a concurrent cognitive task on the compensatory stepping response to a perturbations in balance-impaired and healthy elders. Gait Posture 2002;15:83–93.

Braun JJ, Meyer PM, Meyer DR. Sparing of a brightness habit in rats following visual decortication. J Comp Physiol Psychol 1986;61:79–82.

Braun S, Granger CV. A practical approach to functional assessment in pediatrics. Occup Ther Pract 1991;2:46–51.

Bravi L, Stoykov ME. New directions in occupational therapy: implementation of the task-oriented approach in conjunction with cortical stimulation after stroke. Top Stroke Rehabil 2007;14(6):68–73.

Breniere Y, Bril B. Development of postural control of gravity forces in children during the first 5 years of walking. Exp Brain Res 1998;121: 255–262.

Breniere Y, Do MC, Sanchez J. A biomechanical study of the gait initiation process. J Biophys Med Nucl 1981;5:197–205.

Breniere Y, Do MC. When and how does steady state gait movement induced from upright posture begin? J Biomech 1986;19:1035–1040.

Bril B, Breniere Y. Posture and independent locomotion in childhood: learning to walk or learning dynamic postural control? In: Savelsbergh GJP, ed. The development of coordination in infancy. Amsterdam: North-Holland, 1993: 337–358.

Brochier T, Boudreau MJ, Pare M, Smith AM. The effects of muscimol inactivation of small regions of motor and somatosensory cortex on independent finger movements and force control in the precision grip. Exp Brain Res 1999;128:31–40.

Brod M, Mendelsohn GA, Roberts B. Patients' experiences of Parkinson's disease. J Gerontol B Psychol Sci Soc Sci 1998;53:213–222.

Broderick MP, Newell KM. Coordination patterns in ball bouncing as a function of skill. J Motor Behav 1999;31:165–189.

Broeren J, Rydmark M, Sunnerhagen KS. Virtual reality and haptics as a training device for movement rehabilitation after stroke: a single-case study. Arch Phys Med Rehabil 2004;85:1247–1250.

Brogren E, Forssberg H, Hadders-Algra M. Influence of two different sitting positions on postural adjustments in children with spastic diplegia. Dev Med Child Neurol 2001;43: 534–546.

Brogren E, Hadders-Algra M, Forssberg H. Postural control in children with spastic diplegia: muscle activity during perturbations to sitting. Dev Med Child Neurol 1996;38:379–388.

Brogren E, Hadders-Algra M, Forssberg H. Postural control in sitting children with cerebral palsy. Neurosci Biobehav Rev 1998;22:591–596.

Bronstein AM, Guerraz M. Visual-vestibular control of posture and gait: physiological mechanisms and disorders. Curr Opin Neurol 1999; 12:5–11.

Brooks VB. The neural basis of motor control. New York: Oxford University Press, 1986.

Brown DM, Cullers CM, McMonigal LL, et al. The use of neuromuscular electrical stimulation for facilitation of task-oriented exercise in the upper extremity to achieve functional improvement in an individual with chronic post-stroke hemiparesis: a case study. Neurol Rep 2000;24:198–199.

Brown JK. Science and spasticity. Dev Med Child Neurol 1993;35:471–472.

Brown JV, Sepehr MM, Ettlinger G, Skreczek W. The accuracy of aimed movements to visual targets during development: the role of visual information. J Exp Child Psychol 1986;41: 443–460.

Brown LA, McKenzie NC, Doan JB. Age-dependent differences in the attentional demands of obstacle negotiation. J Gerontol 2005;60A:924–927.

Brown LA, Shumway-Cook A, Woollacott MH. Attentional demands and postural recovery: the effects of aging. J Gerontol 1999;54A: M165–M171.

Brown M, Dijkers M, Gordon WA, et al. Participation objective, participation subjective: a measure of participation combining outsider and insider perspectives. J Head Trauma Rehabil 2004;19:459–481.

Brown TG. The intrinsic factors in the act of progression in the mammal. Proc R Soc Lond B 1911;84:308–319.

Bruce MF. The relation of tactile thresholds to histology in the fingers of the elderly. J Neurol Neurosurg Psychiatry 1980;43:730.
Bruininks RH, Bruininks BD. Bruininks-Oseretsky test of motor proficiency, 2nd ed. Circle Pines, MN: American Guidance Service, 2005.
Bruininks RH. Bruininks-Oseretsky Test of motor proficiency. Circle Pines, MN: American Guidance Service, 1978.
Bruner JS, Koslowski B. Visually pre-adapted constituents of manipulatory action. Perception 1972;1:3–14.
Brunnstrom S. Motor testing procedures in hemiplegia: based on sequential recovery stages. Phys Ther 1966;46:357–375.
Brunnstrom S. Movement therapy in hemiplegia: a neurophysiological approach. New York: Harper & Row, 1970.
Buchner DM, DeLateur BJ. The importance of skeletal muscle strength to physical function in older adults. Ann Behav Med 1991;13:1–12.
Buchner DM, Larson EB. Falls and fractures in patients with Alzheimer-type dementia. JAMA 1987;257:1492–1495.
Buchner DM, Larson EB, Wagner EH, et al. Evidence for a non-linear relationship between leg strength and gait speed. Age Ageing 1996;25:386–391.
Bullinger A. Cognitive elaboration of sensorimotor behaviour. In: Butterworth G, ed. Infancy and epistemology: an evaluation of Piaget's theory. London: Harvester, 1981:173–199.
Bullinger A, Jouen F. Sensibilite du champ de detection peripherique aux variations posturales chez le bebe. Arch Psychol 1983;51:41–48.
Bumin G, Kavak ST. An investigation of the afactors affecting handwriting skill in children with hemiplegic cerebral palsy. Disabil Rehabil 2010;32:692–703.
Buneo CA, Andersen RA. The posterior parietal cortex: sensorimotor interface for the planning and online control of visually guided movements. Neuropsychologia 2006;44:2594–2606.
Burgess PR, Clark FJ. Characteristics of knee-joint receptors in the cat. J Physiol Lond 1969;203:317–325.
Bürkle A, Brabeck C, Diefenbach J, Beneke S. The emerging role of poly(ADP-ribose) polymerase-1 in longevity. Int J Biochem Cell Biol 2005 May;37(5):1043–1053.
Burridge JH, Wood DE, Hermens HJ, et al. Theoretical and methodological considerations in the measurement of spasticity. Disabil Rehabil 2005;27:69–80.
Burtner PA, Woollacott MH, Qualls C. Stance balance control with orthoses in a select group of children with and without spasticity. Dev Med Child 1999;41:748–757.
Busse ME, Pearson OR, Van Deursen R, Wiles CM. Quantified measurement of activity provides insight into motor function and recovery in neurological disease. J Neurol Neurosurg Psychiatry 2004;75:884–888.
Bütefisch C, Khurana V, Kopylev L, Cohen LG. Enhancing encoding of a motor memory in the primary motor cortex by cortical stimulation. J Neurophysiol 2004;91:2110–2116.
Butland RJA, Pang J, Gross ER, et al. Two-, six-, and 12-minute walking tests in respiratory disease. BMJ 1982;284:1607–1608.
Butterworth G, Cicchetti D. Visual calibration of posture in normal and motor retarded Down's syndrome infants. Perception 1978;7: 513–525.
Butterworth G, Hicks L. Visual proprioception and postural stability in infancy: a developmental study. Perception 1977;6:255–262.
Butterworth G, Pope M. Origine et fonction de la proprioception visuelle chez l'enfant. In: de Schonen S, ed. Le developpement dans la premiere année. Paris: Presses Universitaires de France, 1983:107–128.
Byl N, Roderick J, Mohamed O, et al. Effectiveness of sensory and motor rehabilitation of the upper limb following the principles of the upper limb following the principles of neuroplasticity: patients stable poststroke. Neurorehabil Neural Repair 2003;17(3):176–191.
Byl NN, McKenzie A. Treatment effectiveness for patients with a history of repetitive hand use and focal hand dystonia: a planned, prospective follow-up study. J Hand Ther 2000;13: 289–301.

C

Cahill BM, Carr JH, Adams R. Inter-segmental coordination in sit-to-stand: an age cross-sectional study. Physiother Res Int 1999;4:12–27.
Cailliet R. The shoulder in hemiplegia. Philadelphia: FA Davis, 1980.
Cameron DM, Bohannon RW, Garrett GE, et al. Physical impairments related to kinetic energy during sit-to-stand and curb-climbing following stroke. Clin Biomech (Bristol, Avon) 2003;18(4):332–340.
Cameron M, Horak FB, Herndon RR, Bourdette D. Imbalance in multiple sclerosis: a result of slowed spinal somatosensory conduction. Somatosens Motor Res 2008;25:113–122.
Camicioli R, Howieson D, Lehman S. Talking while walking: the effects of a dual task on aging and Alzheimer's disease. Neurology 1997;48:955–958.
Camicioli R, Licis L. Motor impairment predicts falls in specialized Alzheimer care units. Alzheimer Dis Assoc Disord 2004;18: 214–218.
Campbell AJ, Borrie MJ, Spears GF. Risk factors for falls in a community-based prospective study of people 70 years and older. J Gerontol 1989;44:M112–M117.
Campbell AJ, Reinken J, Allen BC, Martiniz GS. Falls in old age: a study of frequency and related clinical factors. Age Ageing 1981;10: 264–279.
Campbell AJ, Robertson MC. Rethinking individual and community fall prevention strategies: a meta-regression comparing single and multifactorial interventions. Age Ageing 2007 Nov;36(6):656–662.
Campbell C, Rowse J, Ciol MA, Shumway-Cook A. The effect of attentional demands on the Timed Up and Go test in older adults with and without Parkinson's disease. Neurol Rep 2003;3:2–7.
Campbell C, Rowse J, Ciol MA, Shumway-Cook A. The effect of attentional demands on the timed up and go test in older adults with and without Parkinson's disease. Neurol Rep 2003;3:2–7.
Campbell SK. Are models of disability useful in real cases? Pediatric case examples realized in research, clinical practice, and education. Phys Ther 2006;86:881–887.
Campbell SK. Measurement of motor performance in cerebral palsy. In: Forssberg H, Hirschfeld H, eds. Movement disorders in children. Basel: Karger, 1991:264–271.
Campbell SK, Kolobe THA, Osten ET, et al. Construct validity of the Test of Infant Motor Performance. Phys Ther 1995;75:585–596.
Campbell SK, Wilhelm IJ. Development from birth to 3 years of age of 15 children at high risk for central nervous system dysfunction. Phys Ther 1985;65:463–469.
Camus M, Ragert P, Vandermeeren Y, Cohen LG. Mechanisms controlling motor output to a tranfer hand after learning a sequential pinch force skill with the opposite hand. Clin Neurophysiol 2009;120:1859–65.
Cannon N. Manual of hand splinting. New York: Churchill Livingstone, 1985.
Cantin JF, McFadyen BJ, Doyon J, et al. Can measures of cognitive function predict locomotor behavior in complex environments following a traumatic brain injury? Brain Inj 2007;21: 327–334.
Carey L, Matyas T, Oke L. Sensory loss in stroke patients: effective training of tactile and proprioceptive discrimination. Arch Phys Med Rehabil 1993;74:602–611.
Carlsoo A. The initiation of walking. Acta Anat 1966;65:1–9.
Carlton LG. Processing visual feedback information for movement control. J Exp Psychol Hum Percept 1981;7:1019–1030.
Carpenter MG, Allum JH, Honegger F. Vestibular influences on human postural control in combinations of pitch and roll planes reveal differences in spatiotemporal processing. Exp Brain Res 2001;140:95–111.
Carpenter MG, Allum JHJ, Adkin AL, Bloem BR. Postural abnormalities to multidirectional stance perturbations in Parkinson's disease. J Neurol Neurosurg Psychiatry 2004;75: 1245–1254.
Carr JH, Shepherd RB. Motor relearning programme for stroke, 2nd ed. Rockville, MD: Aspen, 1992.
Carr JH, Shepherd RB. Neurologic rehabilitation: optimizing motor performance. Oxford: Butterworth and Heinemann, 1998.
Carswell A, McColl MA, Baptiste S, et al. The Canadian Occupational Performance Measure: a research and clinical literature review. Can J Occup Ther 2004;71(4):210–222.
Case-Smith J. Effectiveness of school-based occupational therapy intervention on handwriting. Am J Occup Ther 2002;56(1): 17–25.
Case-Smith J. Fine motor outcomes in preschool children who receive occupational therapy services. Am J Occup Ther 1996;50(1):52–61.
Cass SP, Borello-France D, Furman JM. Functional outcome of vestibular rehabilitation in patients with abnormal sensory organization testing. Am J Otol 1996;17:581–594.
Castiello U. The neuroscience of grasping. Nat Rev Neurosci 2005;6:726–736.
Catalano JF, Kleiner BM. Distant transfer and practice variability. Percept Mot Skills 1984; 58:851–856.
Catena RD, van Donkelaar P Chou LS. Altered balance control following concussion is better detected with an attention test during gait. Gait Posture 2007;25:406–411.
Catena RD, van Donkelaar P, Chou LS. Different gait tasks distinguish immediate vs. long-term effects of concussion on balance control. J Neuroeng Rehabil. 2009;7:25–30.
Cattaneo D, DeNuzzo C, Fascia T, et al. Risks of falls in subjects with multiple sclerosis. Arch Phys Med Rehabil 2002;83:864–867.
Cattaneo D, Jonsdottir J. Sensory impairments in quiet standing in subjects with multiple sclerosis. Mult Scler 2009;15:59–67.
Cauraugh JH, Kim SB. Stroke motor recovery: active neuromuscular stimulation and repetitive practice schedules. J Neurol Neurosurg Psychiatry 2003;74:1562–1566.
Cauraugh JH, Kim SB, Duley A. Coupled bilateral movements and active neuromuscular stimulation: intralimb transfer evidence during bimanual aiming. Neurosci Lett 2005;382 (1–2):39–44.
Cavagna GA, Franzetti P. The determinants of the step frequency in walking in humans. J Physiol (Lond) 1986;373:235–242.
Cavanagh PR, Gregor RJ. Knee joint torques during the swing phase of normal treadmill walking. J Biomech 1975;8:337–344.
Cernak K, Stevens V, Price R, Shumway-Cook A. Locomotor training using body-weight support on a treadmill in conjunction with ongoing physical therapy in a child with severe cerebellar ataxia. Phys Ther 2008;88: 88–97.

Cham R, Redfern MS. Changes in gait when anticipating slippery floors. Gait Posture 2002;15:159–171.

Chambers AJ, Cham R. Slip-related muscle activation patterns in the stance leg during walking. Gait Posture 2007;25:565–572.

Chambers HG. The surgical treatment of spasticity. Muscle Nerve 1997;(Suppl 6):S121–S125.

Chandler JM, Duncan PW, Studenski SA. Balance performance on the postural stress test: comparison of young adults, healthy elderly, and fallers. Phys Ther 1990;70:410–415.

Chandler JM, Hadley EC. Exercise to improve physiologic and functional performance in old age. In: Studenski S. Clinics in geriatric medicine: gait and balance disorders, vol. 12. Philadelphia: Saunders, 1996:761–784.

Chandler LS, Skillen M, Swanson MW. Movement assessment of infants, a manual. Rolling Bay, WA: Authors, 1980.

Chang HA, Krebs DE. Dynamic balance control in elders: gait initiation assessment as a screening tool. Arch Phys Med Rehabil 1999;80: 490–494.

Chang JJ, Wu TI, Wu WL, Su FC. Kinematical measure for spastic reaching in children with cerebral palsy. Clin Biomech 2005;20:381–388.

Chaparro A, Rogers M, Fernandez J, et al. Range of motion of the wrist: implications for designing computer input devices for the elderly. Disabil Rehabil 2000;22:633–637.

Chapman SB, McKinnon L. Discussion of developmental plasticity: factors affecting cognitive outcome after pediatric traumatic brain injury. J Commun Disord 2000;33:333–344.

Chari VR, Kibry RL, Lower limb influence on sitting balance while reaching forward. Arch Phys Med Rehabil 1986;67:730–733.

Charles J, Gordon AM. A critical review of constraint-induced movement therapy and forced use in children with hemiplegia. Neural Plast 2005;12:245–261.

Charles J, Gordon AM. Constraint-induced therapy in children with hemiplegic cerebral palsy. Poster presented at the Combined Sections Meeting of The American Physical Therapy Association, Seattle, Washington, 1999.

Charles J, Gordon AM. Develoment of hand-arm bimanual intensive training (HABIT) for improving bimanual coordination in children with hemiplegic cerbral palsy. Dev Med Child Neurol 2006;48:931–936.

Charles J, Lavinder G, Gordon A. Effects of constraint-induced therapy on hand function in children with hemiplegic cerebral palsy. Pediatr Phys Ther 2001;13:68–76.

Charness A. Stroke/head injury: a guide to functional outcomes in physical therapy management. Rockville, MD: Aspen, 1986.

Charness AL. Management of the upper extremity in the patient with hemiplegia. Course syllabus for the annual meeting of the Washington Physical Therapy Association, 1994.

Chemerinski E, Robinson RG, Kosier JT. Improved recovery in activities of daily living associated with remission of poststroke depression. Stroke 2001;32:113–117.

Chen CC, Granger CV, Peimer CA, et al. Manual Ability Measure (MAM-16): a preliminary report on a new patient-centered and task-oriented outcome measure of hand function. J Hand Surg [Br] 2005;30:207–216.

Chen CC, Kasven N, Karpatkin HI, Sylvester A. Hand strength and perceived manual ability among patients with multiple sclerosis. Arch Phys Med Rehabil 2007;88:794–797.

Chen CH, Lin KH, Lu TW, et al. Immediate effect of lateral-wedged insole on stance and ambulation after stroke. Am J Phys Med Rehabil 2010;89:48–55.

Chen CL, Chen HC, Tang SF, et al. Gait performance with compensatory adaptations in stroke patients with different degrees of motor recovery. Am J Phys Med Rehabil 2003;82: 925–935.

Chen G, Patten C. Joint moment work during the stance to swing transition in hemiparetic subjects. J Biomech 2008;41:877–883.

Chen H, Ashton-Miller JA, Alexander NB, Schultz AB. Stepping over obstacles: gait patterns of healthy young and old adults. J Gerontol 1991;46:M196–M203.

Chen HC. Factors underlying balance restoration after tripping: biomechanical model analyses. Doctoral dissertation, University of Michigan, 1993.

Chen HC, Schultz AB, Ashton-Miller JA et al. Stepping over obstacles: dividing attention impairs performance of old more than young adults. J Gerontol 1996;51(3):M116–M122.

Chen LC, Metcalfe JS, Chang TY, et al. The development of infant upright posture: sway less or sway differently? Exp Brain Res 2008;186:293–303.

Chen R, Cohen LG, Hallett M. Nervous system reorganization following injury. Neuroscience 2002;4:761–773.

Cheng PT, Chen CL, Wang CM, Hong WH. Leg muscle activation patterns of sit-to-stand movement in stroke patients. Am J Phys Med Rehabil 2004;83:10–16.

Cheng PT, Liaw MY, Wong MK, et al. The sit-to-stand movement in stroke patients and its correlation with falling. Arch Phys Med Rehabil 1998;79:1043–1046.

Cherng RJ, Su FC, Chen JJ, Kuan TS. Performance of static standing balance in children with spastic diplegic cerebral palsy under altered sensory environments. Am J Phys Med Rehabil 1999;78:336–343

Cho B, Scarpace D, Alexander NB. Tests of stepping as indicators of mobility, balance and fall risk in balance-impaired older adults. J Am Geriatr Soc 2004;52:1168–1173.

Chong R, Horak F, Woollacott M. Parkinson's disease impairs the ability to change set quickly. J Neurol Sci 2000;175:57–70.

Chong RKY, Horak FB, Frank J, Kaye J. Sensory organization for balance: specific deficits in Alzheimer's but not in Parkinson's disease. J Gerontol A Biol Sci Med Sci 1999;54:M122–M128.

Chou L-S, Kaufman KR, Brey RH, Drafanich LF. Motion of the whole body's center of mass when stepping over obstacles of different heights. Gait Posture 2001;13:17–26.

Chou L-S, Kaufman KR, Hahn ME, Brey RH. Medio-lateral motion of the center of mass during obstacle crossing distinguishes elderly patients with imbalance. Gait Posture 2003;18:125–133.

Chou LS, Kaufman KR, Walker-Rabatin AE, et al. Dynamic instability during obstacle crossing following traumatic brain injury. Gait Posture 2004;20:245–254.

Cirstea MC, Mitnitski AB, Feldman AG, Levin MF. Interjoint coordination dynamics during reaching in stroke. Exp Brain Res 2003;151: 289–300.

Clark J, Lanphear A, Riddick C. The effects of videogame playing on the response selection processing of elderly adults. J Gerontol 1987;42:82–85.

Clark JE, Whitall J. Changing patterns of locomotion: from walking to skipping. In: Woollacott MH, Shumway-Cook A, eds. Development of posture and gait across the lifespan. Columbia: University of South Carolina, 1989:128–151.

Claverie P, Alexandre F, Nichol J, et al. L'activité tonique reflexe du nourisson. Pediatrie 1973;28: 661–679.

Cockburn J, Haggard P, Cock J, Fordham C. Changing patterns of cognitive-motor interference (CMI) over time during recovery from stroke. Clin Rehabil 2003;17:167–173.

Cohen H, Blatchly CA, Gombash LL. A study of the clinical test of sensory interaction and balance. Phys Ther 1993;73:346–351.

Cohen LG, Bandinelli S, Findlay TW, Hallett M. Motor reorganization after upper limb amputation in man: a study with focal magnetic stimulation. Brain 1991;114:615–627.

Cole KJ. Grasp force control in older adults. J Mot Behav 1991;23:251–258.

Cole KJ. Age-related directional bias of fingertip force. Exp Brain Res 2006;175:285–291.

Cole KJ, Rotella DL. Old age affects fingertip forces when restraining an unpredictably loaded object. Exp Brain Res 2001;136:535–542.

Cole KJ, Rotella DL. Old age impairs the use of arbitrary visual cues for predictive control of fingertip forces during grasp. Exp Brain Res 2002;143:35–41.

Cole KJ, Rotella DL, Harper JG. Tactile impairments cannot explain the effect of age on a grasp and lift task. Exp Brain Res 1998;121: 263–269.

Cole KJ, Rotella DL, Harper JG. Mechanisms for age-related changes of fingertip forces during precision gripping and lifting in adults. J Neurosci 1999;19:3228–3247.

Colebatch JG, Gandevia SC. The distribution of muscular weakness in upper motor neuron lesions affecting the arm. Brain 1989;112: 749–763.

Collen FM, Wade DT, Bradshaw CM. Mobility after stroke: reliability of measures of impairment and disability. Int Disabil Studies 1990;12:6–9.

Collen FM, Wade DT, Robb GF, Bradshaw CM. The Rivermead Mobility Index: a further development of the Rivermead Motor Assessment. Int Disabil Studies 1991;13:50–54.

Collignon O, Davare M, De Volder AG, et al. Time-course of posterior parietal and occipital cortex contribution to sound localization. J Cogn Neurosci 2008;20:1454–1463.

Collignon O, Voss P, Lassonde M, Lepore F. Cross-modal plasticity for the spatial processing of sounds in visually deprived subjects. Exp Brain Res 2009;192:343–358.

Colman RJ, Anderson RM, Johnson SC, et al. Caloric restriction delays disease onset and mortality in rhesus monkeys. Science. 2009;325(5937):201–204.

Colon-Emeric CS, Sloane R, Hawkes WG, et al. The risk of subsequent hip fracture in community-dwelling men and male veterans with hip fracture. Am J Med 2000;109:324–326.

Combs SA, Kelly SP, Barton R, et al. Effects of an intensive, task-specific rehabilitation program for individuals with chronic stroke: a case series. Disabil Rehabil 2010;32:669–678.

Connelly L, Stoykov ME, Jia Y, et al. Use of a pneumatic glove for hand rehabilitation following stroke. Conf Proc IEEE Eng Med Biol Soc 2009; 2009:2434–2437.

Connolly KJ. The development of competence in motor skills. In: Nadeau CH, Halliwell WR, Newell KM, Roberts GC, eds. Psychology of motor behavior and sport. Champaign, IL: Human Kinetics, 1979:229–250.

Cook T, Cozzens B. Human solutions for locomotion: 3. The initiation of gait. In: Herman RM, Grillner S, Stein PSG, Stuart DG, eds. Neural control of locomotion. New York: Plenum, 1976:65–76.

Coppin AK, Shumway-Cook A, Saczynski JS, et al. Association of executive function and performance of dual-task physical tests among older adults: analyses from the InChianti study. Age Ageing 2006;35:619–624.

Corbetta D, Mounoud P. Early development of grasping and manipulation. In: Bard C, Fleury M, Hay L, eds. Development of eye-hand coordination across the lifespan. Columbia: University of South Carolina Press, 1990: 188–213.

Cordo P, Nashner L. Properties of postural adjustments associated with rapid arm movements. J Neurophysiol 1982;47:287–302.

Corriveau H, Prince F, Hebert R, et al. Evaluation of postural stability in elderly with diabetic neuropathy. Diabetes Care 2000;23:1187–1191.

Corriveau H, Hebert R, Prince F, Raiche M. Postural control in the elderly: an analysis of test-retest and interrater reliability of the COP-COM variable. Arch Phys Med Rehabil 2001;82: 80–85.

Coryell J, Henderson A. Role of the asymmetrical tonic neck reflex in hand visualization in normal infants. Am J Occup Ther 1979;33: 255–260.

Costner W, Deeney T, Haltiwanger J, Haley S. School Function Assessment (SFA). San Antonio: The Psychological Corporation of Harcourt Brace & Co., 1998.

Cote L, Crutcher MD. The basal ganglia. In: Kandel E, Schwartz JH, Jessell TM, eds. Principles of neuroscience, 3rd ed. New York: Elsevier, 1991.

Craik R. Changes in locomotion in the aging adult. In: Woollacott MH, Shumway-Cook A, eds. Development of posture and gait across the lifespan. Columbia: University of South Carolina, 1989:176–201.

Craik RL. Recovery processes: maximizing function. In: Contemporary management of motor control problems. Proceedings of the II Step Conference. Alexandria, VA: American Physical Therapy Association, 1992:165–173.

Craik RL, Cozzens BA, Freedman W. The role of sensory conflict on stair descent performance in humans. Exp Brain Res 1982;45:399–409.

Crawford JD, Medendorp WP, Marotta JJ. Spatial transformations for eye-hand coordination. J Neurophysiol 2004;92:10–19.

Creath R, Kiemel T, Horak F, et al. A unified view of quiet and perturbed stance: simultaneous co-existing excitable modes. Neurosci Lett 2005;377:75–80.

Crenna P. Spasticity and "spastic" gait in children with cerebral palsy. Neurosci Biobehav Rev 1998;22:571–578.

Crenna P, Inverno M. Objective detection of pathophysiological factors contributing to gait disturbance in supraspinal lesions. In: Fedrizzi E, Avanzini G, Crenna P, eds. Motor development in children. New York: Libbey, 1994:103–118.

Criscimagna-Hemminger SE, Donchin O, Gazzaniga MS, Shadmehr R. Learned dynamics of reaching movements generalize from dominant to nondominant arm. J Neurophysiol 2003;89:168–176.

Crisostomo EA, Duncan PW, Propst MA, et al. Evidence that amphetamine with physical therapy promotes recovery of motor function in stroke patients. Ann Neurol 1988;23:94–97.

Crocker MD, Mackay-Lyons M, McDonnell E. Forced use of the upper extremity in cerebral palsy: a single case design. Am J Occup Ther 1997;51:824–833.

Crossman ERFW, Goodeve PJ. Feedback control of hand-movement and Fitts' law. Q J Exp Psychol 1983;35A:251–278.

Crow JL, Harmeling-van der Wel BC. Hierarchical properties of the motor function sections of the Fugl-Meyer Assessment Scale for people after stroke: a retrospective study. Phys Ther 2008;88:1554–1567.

Crowe TK, Dietz JC, Richardson PK, Atwater SW. Interrater reliability of the pediatric clinical test of sensory interaction for balance. Phys Occup Ther Pediatr 1990;10:1–27.

Cruickshank DA, O'Neill DL. Upper extremity inhibitive casting in a boy with spastic quadriplegia. Am J Occup Ther 1990;6:552–555.

Cruz TH, Dhaher YY. Impaired lower limb muscle synergies post-stroke. Conf Proc IEEE Eng Med Biol Soc 2009;2009:3956–3959.

Cuoco A, Callahan DM, Sayers S, et al. Impact of muscle power and force on gait speed in disabled older men and women. J Gerontol A Biol Sci Med Sci 2004;59:1200–1206.

Cup EH, Scholte op Reimer WJ, Thijssen MC, van Kuyk-Minis MA. Reliability and validity of the Canadian Occupational Performance Measure in stroke patients. Clin Rehabil 2003;17: 402–409.

Cupps C, Plescia MG, Houser C. The Landau reaction: a clinical and electromyographic analysis. Dev Med Child Neurol 1976;18:41–53.

Curtis C, Stephens D, Clarke HM, Andrews D. The active movement scale: an evaluative tool for infants with obstetrical brachial plexus palsy. J Hand Surg Am 2002;27:470–478.

Cusick B, Sussman MD. 'Short leg casts: their role in the management of cerebral palsy. Phys Occup Ther Pediatr 1982;2:93–110.

Cyarto EV, Myers AM, Tudor-Locke C. Pedometer accuracy in nursing home and community-dwelling older adults. Med Sci Sports Ex 2004; 36:205–209.

D

Daley K, Mayo N, Wood-Dauphinee S. Reliability of scores on the Stroke Rehabilitation Assessment of Movement (Stream). Phys Ther 1999;79(1):8–19.

Damiano DL, Abel MF. Functional outcomes of strength training in spastic cerebral palsy. Arch Phys Med Rehabil 1998;79:119–125.

Damiano DL, Arnold AS, Steele KM, Delp SL. Can strength training predictably improve gait kinematics? a pilot study on the effects of hip and knee extensor strengthening on lower-extremity alignment in cerebral palsy. Phys Ther 2010;90:269–279.

Damiano DL, Quinlivan JM, Owen BF, et al. What does the Ashworth scale really measure and are instrumented measures more valid and precise? Dev Med Child Neurol 2002;44:112–118.

Daniels GL, Newell KM. Attentional focus influences the walk-run transitions in human locomotion. Biol Psychol 2003;63:163–178.

Dannenbaum R, Dykes R. Sensory loss in the hand after sensory stroke: therapeutic rationale. Arch Phys Med Rehabil 1988;69:833–839.

Dargent-Molina P, Favier F, Grandjean H. Fall-related factors and risk of hip fracture: The EPIDOS prospective study. Lancet 1996;348:145–149.

Darrah J, Loomis J, Manns P, et al. Role of conceptual models in a physical therapy curriculum: application of an integrated model of theory, research, and clinical practice. Physiother Theory Pract 2006;22:239–50.

Das P, McCollum G. Invariant structure in locomotion. Neuroscience 1988;25:1023–1034.

Davids JR, Peace LC, Wagner LV, et al. Validation of the Shriners Hospital for Children Upper Extremity Evaluation (SHUEE) for children with hemiplegic cerebral palsy. J Bone Joint Surg Am 2006;88:326–333.

Davies P. Aging and Alzheimer's disease: new light on old problems. Presented at the annual meeting of the Neuroscience Society, New Orleans, 1987.

Davies PL, Soon PL, Young M, Clausen-Yamaki A. Validity and reliability of the school function assessment in elementary school students with disabilities. Phys Occup Ther Pediatr 2004;24(3):23–43.

Davies PM. Steps to follow. New York: Springer Verlag, 1985.

Dawson AM, Buxbaum LJ, Duff SV. The impact of left hemisphere stroke on force control with familiar and novel objects: neuroanatomic substrates and relationship to apraxia. Brain Res 2010;1317:124–136.

Day BL, Steiger MJ, Thompson PD, Marsden CD. Effect of vision and stance width on human body motion when standing: implications for afferent control of lateral sway. J Physiol 1993;469:479–499.

De Haart M, Geurts AC, Huidekoper SC, et al. Recovery of standing balance in postacute stroke patients: a rehabilitation cohort study. Arch Phys Med Rehabil 2004;85:886–895.

De Luca PA, Perry JP, Ounpuu S. The fundamentals of normal walking and pathological gait. AACP and DM Inst. Course 2, London: Mac Keith Press, 1992.

De Quervain IA, Simon SR, Leurgans S, et al. Gait pattern in the early recovery period after stroke. J Bone Joint Surg Am 1996;78:1506–1514.

De Souza LH, Hewer RL, Miller S. Assessment of recovery of arm control in hemiplegic stroke patients. 1. Arm function tests. Int Rehab Med 1980;2:3–9.

De Vries JIP, Visser GHA, Prechtl HFR. The emergence of fetal behavior: 1. Qualitative aspects. Early Hum Dev 1982;7:301–322.

De Weerdt W, Harrison MA. Measuring recovery of arm-hand function in stroke patients: a comparison of the Brunnstrom-Fugl-Meyer test and the Action Research Arm test. Physiother Canada 1985;37:65–70.

Dean CM, Richards CL, Malouin F. Task-related circuit training improves performance of locomotor tasks in chronic stroke: a randomized, controlled pilot trial. Arch Phys Med Rehabil 2000;81:409–417.

Dean CM, Richards CL, Malouin F. Walking speed over 10 meters overestimates locomotor capacity after stroke. Clin Rehabil 2001;15:415–421.

Dean CM, Shepherd RB. Task-related training improves performance of seated reaching tasks after stroke: a randomized controlled trial. Stroke 1997;28:722–728.

Deane KH, Jones D, Playford ED, et al. Physiotherapy for patients with Parkinson's Disease: a comparison of techniques. Cochrane Database Syst Rev 2001;(3):CD002817.

DeBolt LS, McCubbin JA. The effects of home-based resistance exercise on balance, power and mobility in adult with multiple sclerosis. Arch Phys Med Rehabil 2004;85:290–297.

Decety J, Sjoholm H, Ryding E, et al. The cerebellum participates in mental activity: tomographic measurements of regional cerebral blood flow. Brain Res 1990;535:313–317.

Decker SL. Tactile measures in the structure of intelligence. Can J Exp Psychol 2010;64(1): 53–59.

DeFabio R, Badke MB. Relationship of sensory organization to balance function in patients with hemiplegia. Phys Ther 1990;70:542–560.

Dehaene S, Changeux, J-P. Neural mechanisms for access to consciousness. In: Gazzaniga MS, ed. The cognitive neurosciences III. Cambridge, MA: MIT Press, 2004:1145–1157.

DeJersey MC. Report on a sensory programme for patients with sensory deficits. Aust J Phyiother 1979;25:165–170.

DeKleijn A. Experimental physiology of the labyrinth. J Laryngol Otol 1923;38:646–663.

Del Rey P, Whitehurst M, Wood J. Effects of experience and contextual interference on learning and transfer. Percept Mot Skills 1983;56: 581–582.

Delacour J. Neurobiology of consciousness: an overview. Behav Brain Res 1997;85:127–141.

Delbaere K, Crombez G, Vanderstraeten G, et al. Fear-related avoidance of activities, falls and physical frailty: a prospective community-based cohort study. Age Ageing 2004;33: 368–373.

Dellen TV, Kalverboer AF. Single movement control and information processing, a developmental study. Behav Brain Res 1984;12:237–238.

Dellon A, Kallman C. Evaluation of functional sensation in the hand. J Hand Surg 1983;8: 865–870.

Dellon AL, Curtis RM, Edgerton MT. Reeducation of sensation in the hand following nerve injury. Plast Reconstr Surg 1974;53:297–305.

Delong, M. The basal ganglia. In: Kandel ER, Schwartz JH, Jessell TM, eds. Principles of neural science, 4th ed. New York: Elsevier, 2000: 853–867.

DeMatteo C, Law M, Russell D, et al. Quality of Upper Extremity Skill Test. Ontario: Neurodevelopmental Clinical Research Unit, 1992.

DeMatteo C, Law M, Russell D, et al. The reliability and validity of Quality of Upper Extremity Skills Test. Phys Occup Ther Pediatr 1993; 13:1–18.

Den Otter AR, Geurts ACH, Mulder T, Duysens J. Gait recovery is not associated with changes in the temporal patterning of muscle activity during treadmill walking in patients with post stroke hemiparesis. Clin Neurophysiol 2006; 117:4 –15.

Desanghere L, Marotta JJ. The specificity of learned associations in visuomotor and perceptual processing. Exp Brain Res 2008;187:595–601.

Deshpande N, Metter E, Lauretani F, et al. Activity restriction induced by fear of falling and objective and subjective measures of physical function: a prospective cohort study. J Am Geriatr Soc 2008;56:615–620.

Desrosiers J, Bourbonnais D, Bravo G, et al. Performance of the unaffected upper extremity of elderly stroke patients. Stroke 1996;27: 1564–1570.

Desrosiers J, Bourbonnais D, Corriveau H, et al. Effectiveness of unilateral and symmetrical bilateral task training for arm during the subacute phase after stroke: a randomized controlled trial. Clin Rehabil 2005;19:581–593.

Desrosiers J, Bravo G, Gerbert R, et al. Validation of the box and block test as a measure of dexterity of elderly: reliability, validity and norms study. Arch Phys Med Rehabil 1994;75: 751–755.

Desrosiers J, Bravo G, Hebert R, Dutil E. Normative data for grip strength of elderly men and women. Am J Occup Ther 1995;49:637–644.

Desrosiers J, Noreau L, Robichaud L, et al. Validity of the Assessment of Life Habits in older adults. J Rehabil Med 2004;36:177–182.

Desrosiers J, Noreau L, Rochette A, et al. Predictors of handicap situations following post-stroke rehabilitation. Disabil Rehabil 2002;24:774–785.

Desrosiers J, Rochette A, Hebert R, Bravo G. The Minnesota Manual Dexterity Test: reliability, validity and reference values studies with healthy elderly people. Can J Occup Ther 1997;64:270–276.

Deuschl G, Bain P, Brin M. Consensus statement of the Movement Disorder Society on tremor. Mov Disord 1998;13:2–23.

Devita P, Hortobagyi T. Age causes a redistribution of joint torques and powers during gait. J Appl Physiol 2000;88:1804–1811.

Dewald JP, Beer RF, Given JD, et al. Reorganization of flexion reflexes in the upper extremity of hemiparetic subjects. Muscle Nerve 1999;22:1209–1221.

Dibble LE, Lange M. Predicting falls in individuals with Parkinson disease: a reconsideration of clinical balance measures. J Neurol Phys Ther 2006;30:60–67.

Dichgans J, Fetter M. Compartmentalized cerebellar functions upon the stabilization of body posture. Rev Neurol (Paris) 1993;149:654–664

Dicken DC, Rose DJ. Sensory organization abilities during upright stance in late onset Alzheimer's-type dementia. Exp Aging Res 2004;30:373–e90.

Dickstein R, Peterka RJ, Horak FB. Effects of light fingertip touch on postural responses in subjects with diabetic neuropathy. J Neurol Neurosurg Psychiatry 2003;74:620–626.

Dickstein R, Shefi S, Marcovitz E, Villa Y. Anticipatory postural adjustments in selected trunk muscles in post stroke hemiparetic patients. Arch Phys Med Rehabil 2004;85:261–267.

Dickstein R, Shupert CL, Horak FB. Fingertip touch improves postural stability in patients with peripheral neuropathy. Gait Posture 2001;14:238–247.

Diedrichsen J, Verstynen T, Lehman S, Ivry R. Cerebellar involvement in anticipating the consequences of self-produced actions during bimanual movements. J Neurophysiol 2005;93: 801–812.

Diener HC, Dichgans J, Bacher M, Gompf B. Quantification of postural sway in normals and patients with cerebellar diseases. Electroencephalogr Clin Neurophysiol 1984a;57: 134–142.

Diener HC, Dichgans J, Bruzek W, Selinka H. Stabilization of human posture during induced oscillations of the body. Exp Brain Res 1982;45:126–132.

Diener HC, Dichgans J, Guschlbauer B, Mau H. The significance of proprioception on postural stabilization as assessed by ischemia. Brain Res 1984b;296:103–109.

Dierick F, Lefebvre C, van den Hecke A, Detrembleur C. Development of displacement of centre of mass during independent walking in children. Dev Med Child Neurol 2004;46:533–539.

Dietz V, Ketelsen UP, Berger W, Quintern J. Motor unit involvement in spastic paresis: relationship between leg muscle activation and histochemistry. J Neurol Sci 1986;75:89–103.

Dietz V, Schmidtbleicher D, Noth J. Neuronal mechanisms of human locomotion. J Neurophysiol 1979;42:1212–1222.

Dietz V, Schubert M, Discher M, Trippel M. Influence of visuoproprioceptive mismatch on postural adjustments. Gait Posture 1994;2: 147–155.

Dietz V, Trippel M, Horstmann GA. Significance of proprioceptive and vestibulo-spinal reflexes in the control of stance and gait. In: Patla AE, ed. Adaptability of human gait. Amsterdam: Elsevier, 1991:37–52.

Dietz V. Locomotor recovery after spinal cord injury. Trends Neurosci 1997;20:346–347.

DiFabio FP, Badke MB, Duncan PW. Adapting human postural reflexes following a localized cerebrovascular lesion: analysis of bilateral long latency responses. Brain Res 1986;363: 257–264.

DiFabio R, Badke MB. Relationship of sensory organization to balance function in patients with hemiplegia. Phys Ther 1990;70:543–552.

DiFabio RP, Badke MB. Stance duration under sensory conflict conditions in patients with hemiplegia. Arch Phys Med Rehabil 1991;72: 292–295.

Dimitrova D, Horak FB, Nutt JG. Postural muscle responses to multidirectional translations in patients with Parkinson's disease. J Neurophysiol 2004a;91:489–501.

Dimitrova D, Nutt J, Horak FB. Abnormal force patterns for multidirectional postural responses in patients with Parkinson's disease. Exp Brain Res 2004b;156:183–195.

Dion L, Malouin F, McFadyen B, Richards CL. Assessing mobility and locomotor coordination after stroke with the rise-to-walk task. Neurorehabil Neural Repair. 2003;17:83–92.

Divani AA, Vazquez G, Barrett AM, et al. Risk factors associated with injury attributable to falling among elderly population with history of stroke. Stroke 2009;40:3286–3292.

Dobkin BH. Neurologic rehabilitation. Philadelphia: FA Davis, 1996.

Dobrossy MD, Dunnett SB. The influence of environment and experience on neural grafts. Nat Rev Neuroscience 2001;2:871–879.

Dobson F, Morris ME, Baker R, Graham HK. Gait classification in children with cerebral palsy: a systematic review. Gait Posture 2007;25: 140–152.

Dodd KJ, Taylor NF, Damiano DL. A systematic review of the effectiveness of strength-training programs for people with cerebral palsy. Arch Phys Med Rehabil. 2002;83:1157–1164.

Dodwell PC, Muir D, Difranco D. Responses of infants to visual presented objects. Science 1976;194:209–211.

Dombovy, Duncan P, Badke MB. Stroke rehabilitation: the recovery of motor control. Chicago: Year Book, 1987.

Donker SF, Roerdink M, Greven AJ, Beek PJ. Regularity of center-of-pressure trajectories depends on the amount of attention invested in postural control. Exp Brain Res 2007;181:1–11.

Donoghue D, Stokes EK. How much change is true change? The minimum detectable change of the Berg Balance Scale in elderly people. J Rehabil Med 2009;41:343–346.

Donoghue JP. Plasticity of adult sensorimotor representations. Curr Opin Neurobiol 1995;5: 749–754.

Donovan JM, VanLeit BJ, Crowe TK, Keefe EB. Occupational goals of mothers of children with disabilities: influence of temporal, social, and emotional contexts. Am J Occup Ther 2005;59:249–261.

Doumas M, Smolders C, Krampe RT. Task prioritization in aging: effects of sensory information on concurrent posture and memory performance. Exp Brain Res 2008 February 14. [Epub ahead of print.]

Dowling JE. The retina: an approachable part of the brain. Cambridge, MA: Belknap, 1987.

Drillis R. The influence of aging on the kinematics of gait: the geriatric amputee. Washington, DC: National Academy of Science, National Research Council, 1961. Publication 919.

Dromerick AW, Lang CE, Birkenmeier RL, et al. Very early constraint-induced movement during stroke rehabilitation. Neurology 2009;73:195–201.

Dubost V, Beauchet O, Manckoundia P, et al. Decreased trunk angular displacement during sitting down: an early feature of aging. Phys Ther 2005;85:404–412.

Duff SV, Charles J. Enhancing prehension in infants and children: fostering neuromotor strategies. Phys Occup Ther Pediatr 2004;24:129–172.

Duff SV, Gordon AM. Learning of grasp control in children with hemiparetic cerebral palsy. Dev Med Child Neurol 2003;45:746–757.

Duffy CJ, Wurtz RH. Medial superior temporal area neurons respond to speed patterns in optic flow. J Neurosci 1997;17:2839–2851.

Duhamel JR, Colby CL, Goldberg ME. The updating of the representation of visual space in parietal cortex by intended eye movements. Science 1992a;255:90–92.

Duhamel JR, Goldberg ME, Fitzgibbon EJ, et al. Saccadic dysmetria in a patient with a right frontoparietal lesion. Brain 1992b;115:1387–1402.

Duncan P, Badke MB. Stroke rehabilitation: the recovery of motor control. Chicago: Year Book, 1987.

Duncan P, Richards L, Wallace D, et al. A randomized, controlled pilot study of a home-based exercise program for individuals with mild and moderate stroke. Stroke 1998;29:2055–2060.

Duncan P, Studenski S, Chandler J, Prescott B. Functional reach: a new clinical measure of balance. J Gerontol 1990;45: M192–M197.

Duncan P, Studenski S, Richards L, et al. Randomized clinical trial of therapeutic exercise in subacute stroke. Stroke 2003;34:2173–2180.

Duncan PW, Chandler J, Studenski S, et al. How do physiological components of balance affect mobility in elderly men? Arch Phys Med Rehabil 1993;74:1343–1349.

Duncan PW, Lai SM, Tyler D, et al. Evaluation of proxy responses to the stroke impact study. Stroke 2002; 33:2593–99.

Duncan PW, Propst M, Nelson SG. Reliability of the Fugl-Meyer assessment of sensorimotor recovery following cerebrovascular accident. Phys Ther 1983;63:1606–1610.

Duncan PW, Weiner DK, Chandler J, Studenski S. Functional reach: a new clinical measure of balance. J Gerontol 1990;45:M192–M197.

Dunn W, Brown C, McGuigan A. The ecology of human performance: a framework for considering the effect of contex. Am J Occup Ther 1994;48:595–607.

Duong TT, Englander J, Wright J, et al. Relationship between strength, balance and swallowing deficits and outcome after traumatic brain injury: a multicenter analysis. Arch Phys Med Rehabil 2004;85:1291–1297.

Dupont Salter AC, Richmond FJ, Loeb GE. Effects of muscle immobilization at different lengths on tetrodotoxin induced disuse atrophy. IEEE Trans Neural Syst Rehabil Eng 2003;11:209–217

Dushanova J, Donoghue J. Neurons in primary motor cortex engaged during action observation. Eur J Neurosci 2010;31:386–398.

E

Earhart GM, Bastian AJ. Selection and coordination of human locomotor forms following cerebellar damage. J Neurophysiol 2001;85: 759–769.

Ebersbach G, Dimitrijevic MR, Poewe W. Influence of concurrent tasks on gait: a dual-task approach. Percept Mot Skills 1995;81:107–113.

Edwards AS. Body sway and vision. J Exp Psychol 1946;36:526–535.

Edwards JM, Elliott D, Lee TD. Contextual interference effects during skill acquisition and transfer in Down's syndrome adolescents. Adapt Physical Activity Q 1986;3:250–258.

Eichhorn J, Orner J, Rickard K, Craik R. Aging effects on dual-task methodology using walking and verbal reaction time. Issues Aging 1998;21:8–12.

Einkauf DK, Gohdes ML, Jensen GM, Jewell MJ. Changes in spinal mobility with increasing age in women. Phys Ther 1987;67:370–375.

Einspieler C, Prechtl HFR. Prechtl's assessment of general movements: a diagnostic tool of the functional assessment of the young nervous system. Ment Retard Dev Disabil Res Rev 2005;11:61–67.

Elbert T, Candia V, Altenmuller E, et al. Alteration of digital representations in somatosensory cortex in focal hand dystonia. Neuroreport 1998;9:3571–3575.

Elble RJ, Leffler K. Pushing and pulling with the upper extremities while standing: the effects of mild Alzheimer's dementia and Parkinson's disease. Mov Disord 2000;15:255–268.

Eliasson AC, Gordon AM, Forssberg H. Basic coordination of manipulative forces in children with cerebral palsy. Dev Med Child Neurol 1991;134:126–154.

Eliasson AC, Gordon AM. Impaired force coordination during object release in children with hemiplegic cerebral palsy. Dev Med Child Neurol 2000;42:228–234.

Eliasson A-C, Krumlinde-Sundholm L, Rösblad B, et al. The Manual Ability Classification System (MACS) for children with cerebral palsy: scale development and evidence of validity and reliability. Dev Med Child Neurol 2006;48:549–554.

Elliason AC, Krumlinde-Sundholm L, Shaw K, Wang C. Effects of constraint-induced movement therapy in young children with hemiplegic cerebral palsy: an adapted model. Dev Med Child Neurol 2005a;47:266–275.

Elliason AC, Rösblad B, Beckung E, et al. Development and reliability of a system to classify hand function in children with cerebral palsy. Manual Ability Classification System (MACS). Workshop presented at the American Academy for Cerebral Palsy and Developmental Medicine, Orlando, FL, 2005b.

Elovic E, McGuire J, Simpson D. Traditional pharmacological treatments for spasticity. Part II. General and regional treatments. Muscle Nerve 1997;6:S92–S120.

Eng JJ, Winter DA, Patla AE. Strategies for recovery from a trip in early and late swing during human walking. Exp Brain Res 1994;102:-339–349.

Eng JJ, Winter DA, Patla AE. Intralimb dynamics simplify reactive control strategies during locomotion. J Biomech 1997;30:581–588.

Eng JJ, Winter DA. Kinetic analysis of the lower limbs during walking: what information can be gained from a three-dimensional model? J Biomech 1995;28:753–758.

Eng K, Siekierka E, Pyk P, et al. Interactive visuomotor therapy system for stroke rehabilitation. Med Biol Eng Comput 2007;45:901–907.

Enoka R. Neuromechanics of human movement, 3rd ed. Champaign, IL: Human Kinetics, 2002.

Era P, Schroll M, Ytting H, et al. Postural balance and its sensory-motor correlates in 75-year-old men and women: a cross-national comparative study. J Gerontol Med Sci 1996;51A:53–63.

Erhardt RP. Developmental hand dysfunction: theory, assessment and treatment. Tucson: Therapy Skill Builders, 1982.

Erhardt RP. Erhardt Developmental Prehension Assessment (EDPA). Tuscon, AZ: Therapy Skill Builders, 2nd ed. 1994.

Evarts EV. Relation of pyramidal tract activity to force exerted during voluntary movement. J Neurophysiol 1968;31:14–27.

Exner C. In-hand manipulation skills in normal young children: a pilot study. Occup Ther Pract 1990;1(4):63–72.

Exner CE, Henderson A. Cognition and motor skill. In: Henderson A, Pehoski C, eds. Hand function in the child: foundations for remediation. Philadelphia: Mosby, 1995.

Exner CE. Development of hand functions. In: Pratt PN, Allen AS, eds. Occupational therapy for children. St. Louis: CV Mosby, 1989.

Eyring EJ, Murray WR. The effect of joint position on the pressure of intra-articular effusion. J Bone Joint Surg Am 1964;46:1235–1241.

F

Fahn S, Marsden CD. The treatment of dystonia. In: Marsden CD, Fahn S, eds. Movement disorders 2. London: Butterworth, 1987.

Fahn S, Marsden CD, Caine DB. Classification and investigation of dystonia. In: Marsden CD, Fahn S, eds. Movement disorders 2. London: Butterworth, 1987.

Fahn S. An open trial of high-dosage antioxidants in early Parkinson's disease. Am J Clin Nutr 1991;53(1 Suppl):380S–382S.

Fahn S. The freezing phenomenon in parkinsonism. Adv Neurol 1995;67:53–63.

Fait P, McFadyen BJ, Swaine B, Cantin JF. Alterations to locomotor navigation in complex environment at 7 and 30 days following a concussion in an elite athlete. Brain Inj 2009;23:362–369.

Falduto L, Baron A. Age-related effects of practice and task complexity on card sorting. J Gerontol 1986;41:659–661.

Faria CD, Teixeira-Salmela LF, Nadeau S. Effects of the direction of turning on the timed up & go test with stroke subjects. Top Stroke Rehabil 2009;16:196–206.

Farin E, Fleitz A, Frey C. Psychometric properties of an International Classification of Functioning, Disability and Health (ICF)-oriented, adaptive questionnaire for the assessment of mobility, self-care and domestic life. J Rehabil Med 2007;39:537–546.

Farley CT, Ferris DP. Biomechanics of walking and running: center of mass movements to muscle action. Exerc Sport Sci Rev 1998;26:253–85.

Farley CT, Taylor CR. A mechanical trigger for the trot-gallop transition in horses. Science 1991;253:306–308.

Farrell K, Johnson A, Duncan H, Offenbacker T, Curry C. The intertester and intratester reliability of hand volumetrics. J Hand Ther 2003;16(4):292–299.

Fasoli SE, Krebs HI, Stein J, et al. Robotic therapy for chronic motor impairments after stroke: follow-up results. Arch Phys Med Rehabil 2004;85:1106–1111.

Fasoli SE, Trombly CA, Tickle-Degnen L, Verfaellie MH. Effect of instructions on functional reach in persons with and without cerebrovascular accident. Am J Occup Ther 2002;56:380–390.

Faulkner KA, Redfern MS, Cauley JA, et al. Multitasking: association between poorer performance and a history of recurrent falls. J Am Geriatr Soc 2007;55:570–576.

Favilla M. Reaching movements in children: accuracy and reaction time development. Exp Brain Res 2005;21:1–4.

Feeney DM. Pharmacological modulation of recovery after brain injury: a reconsideration of diaschisis. J Neurol Rehabil 1991;5:113–128.

Feeney DM, Baron JC. Diaschisis. Stroke 1986;17:817–830.

Feeney DM, Gonzalez A, Law WA. Amphetamine restores locomotor function after motor cortex injury in the rat. Proc West Pharmacol Soc 1981;24:15–17.

Feeney DM, Gonzalez A, Law WA. Amphetamine haloperidol and experience interact to affect the rate of recovery after motor cortex injury. Science 1982;217:855–857.

Feeney DM, Sutton RL, Boyeson MG, et al. The locus-coeruleus and cerebral metabolism: recovery of function after cortical injury. Physiol Psychol 1985;13:197–203.

Feeney DM, Sutton RL. Pharmacology for recovery of function after brain injury. Crit Rev Neurobiol 1987;3:135–185.

Feigin L, Sharon B, Czaczkes B, Rosin AJ. Sitting equilibrium 2 weeks after stroke can predict walking ability after 6 months. Gerontology 1996;42:348–353.

Feldman AB, Haley SM, Coryell J. Concurrent and construct validity of the Pediatric Evaluation of Disability Inventory. Phys Ther 1990;70: 602–610.

Feldman AG. Change in the length of the muscle as a consequence of a shift in equilibrium in the muscle-load system. Biofizika 1974;19:534–538.

Fellows SJ, Noth J, Schwarz M. Precision grip and Parkinson's disease. Brain 1998;121:1171–1184.

Fentress JC. Development of grooming in mice with amputated forelimbs. Science 1973;179:704.

Ferber-Viart C, Ionescu E, Morlet T, et al. Balance in healthy individuals assessed with Equitest: maturation and normative data for children and young adults. Int J Pediatr Otorhinolaryngol 2007;71:1041–1046.

Fernie GR, Gryfe CI, Holliday PJ, Llewellyn A. The relationship of postural sway in standing: the incidence of falls in geriatric subjects. Age Ageing 1982;11:11–16.

Ferris DP, Louie M, Farley CT. Running in the real world: adjusting leg stiffness for different surfaces. Proc Biol Sci 1998;265:989–994.

Fess E. Assessment of the upper extremity: instrumentation criteria. Occup Ther Pract 1990;1:1–11.

Fess EE, Gettle K, Phillips C, Janson JR. Hand and upper extremity splinting principles and Methods, 3rd ed. Elsevier/Mosby, 2005.

Fess EE. A method for checking Jamar dynamometer calibration. J Hand Ther 1987;1:28–32.

Fess EE. Grip strength. In: Casanova JS, ed. Clinical assessment recommendations, 2nd ed. Chicago: American Society of Hand Therapists, 1992:41–45.

Fetter M. Vestibular system disorders. In: Herdman S, ed. Vestibular rehabilitation, 2nd ed. Philadelphia: FA Davis, 2000:91–102.

Fiatarone MA, Marks EC, Ryan ND, et al. High-intensity strength training in nonagenarians: effects on skeletal muscle. JAMA 1990;263: 3029–3034.

Fiatarone MA, O'Neill EF, Ryan ND, et al. Exercise training and nutritional supplementation for physical frailty in very elderly people. N Engl J Med 1994;330:1769–1775.

Fiez, JA, Petersen SE, Cheney, MK, Raichle, ME. Impaired non-motor learning and error detection associated with cerebellar damage. Brain 1992;115:155–178.

Finch L, Barbeau H, Arsenault B. Influence of body weight support on normal human gait: development of a gait retraining strategy. Phys Ther 1991;71:842–856.

Finlayson ML, Peterson EW, Cho CC. Risk factors for falling among people aged 45 to 90 years with multiple sclerosis. Arch Phys Med Rehabil 2006;87:1274–1279.

Finley FR, Cody KA. Locomotive characteristics of urban pedestrians. Arch Phys Med Rehabil 1970;51:423–426.

Finley FR, Cody KA, Finizie RV. Locomotion patterns in elderly women. Arch Phys Med Rehabil 1969;50:140–146.

Fisher AG. Assessment of motor and process skills manual. Fort Collins, CO: Colorado State University, 1994.

Fishkind M, Haley SM. Independent sitting development and the emergence of associated motor components. Phys Ther 1986;66:1509–1514.

Fisk JD. Sensory and motor integration in the control of reaching. In: Bard C, Fleury M, Hay L, eds. Developmental of eye-hand coordination across the lifespan. Columbia: University of South Carolina Press, 1990:75–98.

Fisk JD, Goodale MA. The organization of eye and limb movements during unrestricted reaching to targets in contralateral and ipsilateral visual space. Exp Brain Res 1985;60:159–178.

Fitts PM. The information capacity of the human motor system in controlling the amplitude of movement. J Exp Psychol 1954;47:381–391.

Fitts PM. Perceptual-motor skill learning. In: Melton AW, ed. Categories of human learning, New York: Academic Press, 1964:243–285.

Fitts PM, Posner MI. Human performance. Belmont, CA: Brooks/Cole, 1967.

Flansbjer U, Miller M, Downham D, Lexell J. Progressive resistance training after stroke: effects on muscle strength, muscle tone, gait performance and perceived participation. J Rehabil Med 2008;40:42–48.

Floel A, Cohen LG. Translational studies in neurorehabilitation: from bench to bedside. Cogn Behav Neurol 2006;19(1):1–10.

Florence SL, Kaas JH. Large–scale reorganization at multiple levels of the somatosensory pathway follows therapeutic amputation of the hand in monkeys. J Neurosci 1995;15: 8083–8095.

Flowers KR, Stephens-Chisar J, LaStayo P, Galante BL. Intrarater reliability of a new method and instrumentation for measuring passive supination and pronation: a preliminary study. J Hand Ther 2001;14(1):30–35.

Floyer-Lea A, Matthews PM. Changing brain networks for visuomotor control with increased movement automaticity. J Neurophysiol 2004;92:2405–2412.

Foerster O. The motor cortex in man in the light of Hughlings Jackson's Doctrines. In: Payton OD, Hirt S, Newman, R, eds. Scientific bases for neurophysiologic approaches to therapeutic exercise. Philadelphia: FA Davis, 1977:13–18.

Folio RM, Fewell RR. Peabody Developmental Motor Scales. Allen TX: DLM Teaching Resources, 1983.

Folstein MF, Folstein SE, McHugh PR. Mini-mental state: a practical method for grading the cognitive states for the clinician. J Psychiatr Res 1975;12:188–198.

Ford-Smith CD, VanSant AF. Age differences in movement patterns used to rise from a bed in subjects in the third through fifth decades of age. Phys Ther 1992;73:300–309.

Forlander DA, Bohannon RW. Rivermead Mobility Index: a brief review of research to date. Clin Rehabil 1999;13:97–100.

Forssberg H. Motor learning: a neurophysiological review. In: Berg K, Eriksson B, eds. Children and exercise, vol. 9. Baltimore: University Park Press, 1980:13–22.

Forssberg H. Ontogeny of human locomotor control: I. Infant stepping, supported locomotion, and transition to independent locomotion. Exp Brain Res 1985;57:480–493.

Forssberg H, Eliasson AC, Kinoshita H, et al. Development of human precision grip. I. Basic coordination of forces. Exp Brain Res 1991;85:451–457.

Forssberg H, Eliasson AC, Kinoshita H, et al. Development of human precision grip. IV. Tactile adaptation of isometric finger forces to the frictional condition. Exp Brain Res 1995;104:323–330.

Forssberg H, Grillner S, Rossignol S. Phase dependent reflex reversal during walking in chronic spinal cats. Brain Res 1975;85:103–107.

Forssberg H, Grillner S, Rossignol S. Phasic gain control of reflexes from the dorsum of the paw during spinal locomotion. Brain Res 1977;132:121–139.

Forssberg H, Hirschfeld H. Postural adjustments in sitting humans following external perturbations:

Forssberg H, Kinoshita H, Eliasson AC, et al. Development of human precision grip. II. Anticipatory control of isometric forces targeted for object's weight. Exp Brain Res 1992;90:393–398.

Forssberg H, Nashner L. Ontogenetic development of postural control in man: adaptation to altered support and visual conditions during stance. J Neurosci 1982;2:545–552.

Forsstrom A, von Hofsten C. Visually directed reaching in children with motor impairments. Dev Med Child Neurol 1982;24:653–661.

Forster A, Young J. Incidence and consequences of falls due to stroke: a systematic inquiry. BMJ 1995;311:83–86.

Foster E, Sveistrup H, Woollacott MH. Transitions in visual proprioception: a cross-sectional developmental study of the effect of visual flow on postural control. J Motor Behav 1996;28:101–112.

Foudriat BA, Di Fabio RP, Anderson JH. Sensory organization of balance responses in children 3–6 years of age: a normative study with diagnostic implications. Int J Pediatr Otorhinolaryngol 1993;27:255–271.

Fox MD, Delp SL. Contributions of muscles and passive dynamics to swing initiation over a range of walking speeds. J Biomech 2010;43:1450–1455.

Fradet L, Lee G, Dounskaia N. Origins of submovements in movements of eldelry adults. J Neuroeng Rehabil 2008;5:28.

Fraizer EV, Mitra S. Methodological and interpretive issues in posture-cognition dual- tasking in upright stance. Gait Posture 2008;27(2): 271–279.

Franchignoni F, Horak F, Godi M, et al. Using psychometric techniques to improve the Balance Evaluation System's Test: the mini-BESTest. J Rehabil Med 2010;42:323–331.

Franchignoni FP, Tesio L, Ricupero C, Martino MT. Trunk control test as an early predictor of stroke rehabilitation outcome. Stroke 1997;28:1382–1385.

Franjoine MR, Gunther JS, Taylor MJ. Pediatric balance scale: a modified version of the Berg balance scale for the school-age child with mild to moderate motor impairment. Pediatr Phys Ther 2003;15:114–128.

Frank JS, Patla AE, Brown JE. Characteristics of postural control accompanying voluntary arm movement in the elderly. Soc Neurosci Abstr 1987;13:335.

Frascarelli M, Mastrogregori L, Conforti L. Initial motor unit recruitment in patients with spastic hemiplegia. Electromyogr Clin Neurophysiol 1998;38:267–271.

Fraser C, Wing A. A case study of reaching by a user of a manually-operated artificial hand. Prosthet Orthot Int 1981;5:151–156.

Fredericks CM, Saladin LK. Clinical presentations in disorders of motor function. In: Fredericks CM, Saladin LK, eds. Pathophysiology of the motor systems: principles and clinical presentations. Philadelphia: FA Davis, 1996.

Friel KM, Nudo RJ. Recovery of motor function after focal cortical injury in primates: compensatory movement patterns used during rehabilitative training. Somatosens Motor Res 1998; 15:173–189.

Fries JF. Successful aging: an emerging paradigm of gerontology. Clin Geriatr Med 2002;18:371–382.

Fries W, Danek A, Scheidtmann K, Hamburger C. Motor recovery following capsular stroke: role of descending pathways from multiple motor areas. Brain 1993;116:369–382.

Frontera WR, Hughes VA, Fielding RA, et al. Aging of skeletal muscle: a 12 yr longitudinal study. J Appl Physiol 2000;88:1321–1326.

Fugl-Meyer AR, Jääskö L, Leyman I, et al. The post-stroke hemiplegic patient 1. A method for evaluation of physical performance. Scand J Rehabil Med 1975;7:13–31.

Fuhrer MJ, Keith RA. Facilitating patient learning during medical rehabilitation: a research agenda. Am J Phys Med Rehabil 1998;77: 557–561.

Fujiwara T, Kasashima Y, Honaga K, et al. Motor improvement and corticospinal modulation induced by hybrid assistive neuromuscular dynamic stimulation (HANDS) therapy in patients with chronic stroke. Neurorehabil Neuroal Repair 2009;23(2):125–132.

Fujiwara T, Sonoda S, Okajima Y, Chino N. The relationship between trunk function and findings of transcranial magnetic stimulation among patients with stroke. J Rehabil Med 2001;33:249–255.

Fukuyama H, Ouchi Y, Matsuzaki S, et al. Brain functional activity during gait in normal subjects: a SPECT study. Neurosci Lett 1997;228:183–186.

Fuster JM. The prefrontal cortex: anatomy, physiology and neuropsychology of the frontal lobe, 2nd ed. New York: Raven, 1989.

G

Gabell A, Nayak USL. The effect of age on variability in gait. J Gerontol 1984;39:662–666.

Gabell A, Simons MA, Nayak USL. Falls in the healthy elderly: predisposing causes. Ergonomics 1985;28:965–975.

Gage JR. Gait analysis. An essential tool in the treatment of cerebral palsy. Clin Orthop Relat Res 1993;288:126–134.

Gagnon I, Swaine B, Forget R. Exploring the comparability of the Sensory Organization Test and the Pediatric Clinical Test of Sensory Interaction for Balance in children. Phys Occup Ther Pediatr 2006;26:23–41.

Gagnon I, Swaine B, Friedman D, Forget R. Children show decreased dynamic balance after mild traumatic brain injury. Arch Phys Med Rehabil 2004;85:444–452.

Gahery Y, Massion J. Coordination between posture and movement. Trends Neurosci 1981;4:199–202.

Gallahue DL. Understanding motor development: infants, children, adolescents. Indianapolis: Benchmark, 1989.

Galletly R, Brauer SG. Does the type of concurrent task affect preferred and cued gait in people with Parkinson's disease? Aust J Physiother 2005;51:175–180.

Gallichio JE. Pharmacologic management of spasticity following stroke. Phys Ther 2004;84: 973–981.

Galna B, Peters A, Murphy AT, Morris ME. Obstacle crossing deficits in older adults: a systematic review. Gait Posture 2009;30: 270–275.

Gan SM, Tung LC, Tang YH, Wang CH. Psychometric properties of functional balance assessment in children with cerebral palsy. Neurorehabil Neural Repair 2008;22: 745–753.

Gard SA, Childress DS. The effect of pelvic list on the vertical displacement of the trunk during normal walking. Gait Posture 1997;5:233–238.

Gard SA, Childress DS. The influence of stance-phase knee flexion on the vertical displacement of the trunk during normal walking. Arch Phys Med Rehabil 1999;80:26–32.

Gardner EP, Kandel ER. Touch. In: Kandel ER, Schwartz JH, Jessell TM, eds. Principles of neural science, 4th ed. New York: McGraw-Hill, 2000:451–471.

Gardner EP, Martin JH, Jessell TM. The bodily senses. In: Kandel ER, Schwartz JH, Jessell TM, eds. Principles of neural science, 4th ed. New York: McGraw-Hill, 2000:430–450.

Gardner MF. Test of visual-perceptual skills (n-m) revised. Hydesville, CA: Ann Arbor Publishers, 1996.

Garland SJ, Willems DA, Ivanova TD, Miller KJ. Recovery of standing balance and functional mobility after stroke. Arch Phys Med Rehabil 2003;84:1753–1759.

Garraghty PE, Hanes DP, Florence SL, Kaas JH. Pattern of peripheral deafferentation predicts reorganizational limits in adult primate somatosensory cortex. Somatosens Motor Res 1994;11:109–117.

Garrison KA, Winstein CJ, Aziz-Zadeh L. The mirror neuron system: a neural substrate for methods in stroke rehabilitation. Neurorehabil Neural Repair 2010;24:404–412.

Gatev P, Thomas S, Lou JS, et al. Effects of diminished and conflicting sensory information on balance in patients with cerebellar deficits. Mov Disord 1996;11:654–664.

Gatts SK, Woollacott MH. Neural mechanisms underlying balance improvement with short term Tai Chi training. Aging Clin Exp Res 2006;18:7–19.

Gatts SK, Woollacott MH. How Tai Chi improves balance: biomechanics of recovery to a walking slip in impaired seniors. Gait Posture 2007;25:205–214.

Gauthier GM, Vercher JL, Ivaldi FM, Marchetti E. Oculo-manual tracking of visual targets: control learning, coordination control and coordination model. Exp Brain Res 1988;73:127–137.

Gehlsen GM, Whaley MH. Falls in the elderly: Part I, gait. Arch Phys Med Rehabil 1990;71: 735–738.

Geldhof E, Cardon G, Bourdeaudhuij ID, et al. Static and dynamic standing balance: test-retest reliability and reference values in 9 to 10 year old children. Eur J Pediatr 2006;165: 779–786.

Genthon N, Rougier P, Gissot AS, et al. Contribution of each lower limb to upright standing in stroke patients. Stroke 2008;39:1793–1799.

Gentile A. Skill acquisition: action movement, and neuromotor processes. In: Carr J, Shepherd R, Gordon J, ed. Movement science: foundations for physical therapy in rehabilitation. Rockville, MD: Aspen, 1987.

Gentile AM. Movement organization and delayed alternation behavior of monkeys following selective ablation of frontal cortex. Acta Neurobiol Exp (Wars) 1972;32(2):277–304.

Georgiou N, Iansek R, Bradshaw JL, et al. An evaluation of the role of internal cues in the pathogenesis of Parkinsonian hypokinesia. Brain 1993;116:1575–1587.

Georgopoulos AP, Kalaska JF, Caminiti R, Massey JT. On the relations between the direction of two-dimensional arm movements and cell discharge in primate motor cortex. J Neurosci 1982;2:1527–1537.

Gesell A. The ontogenesis of infant behavior. In: Carmichael L, ed. Manual of child psychology. New York: Wiley, 1946:335–373.

Gesell A. Behavior patterns of fetal-infant and child. In: Hooker D, Kare C, eds. Genetics and inheritance of neuropsychiatric patterns. Res Publ Assoc Res Nerv Ment Dis 1954;33:114–126.

Gesell A, Amatruda CS. Developmental diagnosis, 2nd ed. New York: Paul B. Hoeber, 1947.

Gesell A, Halverson HM, Thompson H, et al. The first five years of life. New York: Harper & Row, 1940.

Geurts AC, de Haart M, van Nes IJ, Duysens J. A review of standing balance recovery from stroke. Gait Posture 2005;22:267–281.

Geurts AC, Mulder TW, Nienhuis B, Rijken RA. Dual-task assessment of reorganization of postural control in persons with lower limb amputation. Arch Phys Med Rehabil 1991;72(13):1059–1064.

Ghafouri M, McIlroy WE, Maki BE. Initiation of rapid reach-and-grasp balance reactions: is a pre-formed visuospatial map used in controlling the arm trajectory? Exp Brain Res 2004;155:532–536.

Ghez C. Contributions of central programs to rapid limb movement in the cat. In: Asanuma H, Wilson VJ, eds. Integration in the nervous system. Tokyo: Igaku-Shoin, 1979:305–320.

Ghez C. The cerebellum. In: Kandel E, Schwartz JH, Jessell TM, eds. Principles of neuroscience, 3rd ed. New York: Elsevier, 1991:633.

Ghez C, Krakauer J. The organization of movement. In: Kandel E, Schwartz J, Jessel T, eds. Principles of neuroscience, 4th ed. New York: McGraw-Hill, 2000:653–673.

Ghez C, Thatch WT. The cerebellum. In: Kandel E, Schwartz J, Jessel T, eds. Principles of neuroscience, 4th ed. New York: McGraw-Hill, 2000:832–852.

Gibson AR, Horn KM, Van Kan PLE. Grasping cerebellar function. In: Bennett KMB, Castiello U, eds. Insights into the reach to grasp movement. Amsterdam: Elsevier, 1994:129–150.

Gibson E, Walker AS. Development of knowledge of visual-tactual affordance of substance. Child Dev 1984;55:453–460.

Gibson JJ. The senses considered as perceptual systems. Boston: Houghton Mifflin, 1966.

Giladi N, Kao R, Fahn S. Freezing phenomenon in patients with parkinsonian syndromes. Mov Disord 1997;12:302–305.

Gilbert PFC, Thatch WT. Purkinje cell activity during motor learning. Brain Res 1977;128: 309–328.

Gilchrist AL, Cowan N, Naveh-Benjamin M. Working memory capacity for spoken sentences decreases with adult aging: recall of fewer, but not smaller chunks in older adults. Memory 2008;16:773–787.

Gill-Body KM, Popat RA, Parker SW, Krebs DE. Rehabilitation of balance in two patients with cerebellar dysfunction. Phys Ther 1997;77: 534–552.

Gillespie LD, Robertson MC, Gillespie WJ, et al. Interventions for preventing falls in older people living in the community Cochrane Database Syst Rev 2009;2:CD007146.

Gilliam J, Barstow IK. Joint range of motion. In: Van Deusen J, Brunt D, eds. Assessment in occupational and physical therapy. Philadelphia: Saunders, 1997:49–77.

Gilman S. The spinocerebellar ataxias. Clin Neuropharmacol 2000;23:296–303.

Gioux M, Petit J. Effects of immobilizing the cat peroneus longus muscle on the activity of its own spindles. J Appl Physiol 1993;75:2629–2635.

Giuliani CA. Dorsal rhizotomy for children with cerebral palsy: support for concepts of motor control. Phys Ther 1991;71:248–259.

Giuliani C, Genova PA, Purser KE, Light KE. Limb trajectory in non-disabled subjects under two conditions of external constraint compared with the non-paretic limb of subjects with hemiparesis. Neurosci Abs 1993;19:990.

Gladstone DJ, Danells CJ, Black SE. The Fugl-Meyer Assessment of Motor Recovery after Stroke: a critical review of its measurement properties. Neurorehabil Neural Repair 2002;16:232–240.

Godges JJ, MacRae PG, Engelke KA. Effects of exercise on hip range of motion, trunk muscle performance and gait economy. Phys Ther 1993;73:468–477.

Goldberg ME, Hudspeth AJ. The vestibular system. In: Kandel ER, Schwartz JH, Jessell TM, eds. Principles of neural science, 4th ed. New York: McGraw-Hill, 2000:801–815.

Goldstein LB. Pharmacology of recovery after stroke. Stroke 1990;21(Suppl III):139–142.

Goldstein LB. Basic and clinical studies of pharmacologic effects on recovery from brain injury. J Neural Transplant Plast 1993;4:175–192.

Goldstein LB. Neuropharmacology of TBI-induced plasticity. Brain Injury 2003;17:685–694.

Goldstein LB, Davis JN. Physician prescribing patterns after ischemic stroke. Neurology 1988;38:1806–1809.

Gollhofer A, Schmidtbleicher D, Quintem J, Dietz V. Compensatory movements following gait perturbations: changes in cinematic and muscular activation patterns. Int J Sports Med 1986;7:325–329.

Golomb MR, McDonald BC, Warden SJ, et al. In-home virtual reality videogame telerehabilitation in adolescents with hemiplegic cerebral palsy. 2010;9:1-8e1.

Gomes MM, Barela JA. Postural control in Down syndrome: the use of somatosensory and visual information to attenuate body sway. Motor Control 2007;11:224–234.

Gonshor A, Melville-Jones G. Short-term adaptive changes in the human vestibulo-ocular reflex arc. J Physiol (Lond) 1976;256:361–379.

González-Alvarez C, Subramanian A, Pardhans S. Reaching and grasping with restricted peripheral vision. Ophthalmic Physiol Opt 2007;27:265–274.

Goodale MA, Milner AD. Separate visual pathways for perception and action. Trends Neurosci 1992;15:20–25.

Goodale MA, Milner AD, Jakobson LS, Carey DP. A neurological dissociation between perceiving objects and grasping them. Nature 1991;349:154–156.

Goode SL. The contextual interference effect in learning an open motor skill. Unpublished doctoral dissertation. Baton Rouge: Louisiana State University, 1986.

Goodwin GM, McCloskey DI, Matthews PBC. The contribution of muscle afferents to kinaesthesia shown by vibration induced illusions of movement and by the effects of paralysing joint afferents. Brain 1972;95:705–748.

Goodwin RD, Devanand DP. Stroke, depression, and functional health outcomes among adults in the community. J Geriatric Psychiatry Neurol 2008;21:41–46.

Gordon AM. Development of hand motor control: handbook of brain and behavior in human development. Boston: Kluwer, 2001:513–537.

Gordon AM, Charles J, Duff SV. Fingertip forces during object manipulation in children with hemiplegic cerebral palsy. II. Bilateral coordination. Dev Med Child Neurol 1999;41:176–185.

Gordon AM, Charles J, Steenbergen B. Fingertip force planning during grasp is disrupted by impaired sensorimotor integration in children with hemiplegic cerebral palsy. Pediatr Res 2006;60:587–591.

Gordon AM, Charles J, Wolf SL. Methods of constraint-induced movement therapy for children with hemiplegic cerebral palsy: development of a child-friendly intervention for improving upper-extremity function. Arch Phys Med Rehabil 2005;86(4):837–844.

Gordon AM, Chinnan A, Gill S, et al. Both constraint-induced movement therapy and bimanual training lead to improved performance of upper extremity function in children with hemiplegia. Dev Med Child Neurol 2008;50:957–958.

Gordon AM, Duff SV. Fingertip forces during object manipulation in children with hemiplegic cerebral palsy. I. Anticipatory scaling. Dev Med Child Neurol 1999a;41:166–175.

Gordon AM, Duff SV. Relationships between clinical measures and fine manipulative control in children with hemiplegic cerebral palsy. Dev Med Child Neurol 1999b;41:586–591.

Gordon AM, Forssberg H, Johansson RS, et al. Development of human precision grip. III. Integration of visual size cues during the programming of isometric forces. Exp Brain Res 1992;90:399–403.

Gordon AM, Ingvarsson PE, Forssberg H. Anticipatory control of manipulative forces in Parkinson's disease. Exp Neurol 1997;145: 477–488.

Gordon AM, Lewis S, Eliasson AC, Duff SV. Object release under varying task constraints in children with hemiplegic cerebral palsy. Dev Med Child Neurol 2003;45:240–248.

Gordon J. Assumptions underlying physical therapy intervention: theoretical and historical perspectives. In: Carr JH, Shepherd, RB, Gordon J, et al., eds. Movement sciences: foundations for physical therapy in rehabilitation. Rockville, MD: Aspen, 1987:1–30.

Gordon J. Motor control workshop for physical therapists, Umea, Sweden, June 1997.

Gordon J, Ghez C. Muscle receptors and spinal reflexes: the stretch reflex. In: Kandel E, Schwartz JH, Jessell TM, eds. Principles of neuroscience, 3rd ed. New York: Elsevier, 1991: 564–580.

Gormley ME, O'Brien CF, Yablon SA. A clinical overview of treatment decisions in the management of spasticity. Muscle Nerve 1997;Suppl 6:S14–S20.

Gottschall J, Kram R. Energy cost and muscular activity required for propulsion during walking. J Appl Physiol 2003;94:1766–1772.

Gowland C, deBruin H, Basmajian JV, et al. Agonist and antagonist activity during voluntary upper-limb movement in patients with stroke. Phys Ther 1992;72:624–633.

Gowland C, Stratford P, Ward M, et al. Measuring physical impairment and disability wit the Chedoke-McMaster Stroke Assessment. Stroke 1993;24:58–63.

Graci V, Elliott DB, Buckley JG. Peripheral visual cues affect minimum-foot-clearance during overground locomotion. Gait Posture 2009;30: 370–374.

Graci V, Elliott DB, Buckley JG. Utility of peripheral visual cues in planning and controlling adaptive gait. Optom Vis Sci 2010;87:21–27.

Gracies JM. Pathophysiology of spastic paresis. I: Paresis and soft tissue changes. Muscle Nerve 2005a;31:535–551.

Gracies JM. Pathophysiology of spastic paresis. II: Emergence of muscle overactivity. Muscle Nerve 2005b;31:552–571.

Gracies JM, Elovic E, McGuire J, Simpson D. Traditional pharmacological treatments for spasticity: 1. Local treatments. Muscle Nerve 1997a;Suppl 6:S61–S83.

Gracies JM, Elovic E, McGuire J, Simpson D. Traditional pharmacological treatments for spasticity: 2. General and regional treatments. Muscle Nerve 1997b;Suppl 6:S92–S97.

Graham F, Rodger S, Ziviani J. Enabling occupational performance of children through coaching parents: three case reports. Phys Occup Ther Pediatr 2010;30(1):4–15.

Granger CV, Albrecht GL, Hamilton BB. Outcome of comprehensive medical rehabilitation: measurement of PULSES profile and the Barthel index. Arch Phys Med Rehabil 1979;60: 145–154.

Grasso R, Assaiante C, Prevost P, Berthoz A. Development of anticipatory orienting strategies during locomotor task in children. Neurosci Biobehav Rev 1998;22:533–539.

Gray DB, Hollingsworth HH, Stark SL, Morgan KA. Participation Survey/mobility: psychometric properties of a measure of participation for people with mobility impairments and limitations. Arch Phys Med Rehabil 2006;87:189–197.

Gray P, Hildebrand K. Fall risk factors in Parkinson's disease. J Neurosci Nurs 2000;32: 222–228.

Green LN, Williams K. Differences in developmental movement patterns used by active vs sedentary middle-aged adults coming from a supine position to erect stance. Phys Ther 1992;72:560–568.

Gregson JM, Leathley M, Moor AP, et al. Reliability of the Tone Assessment Scale and the Modified Ashworth Scale as clinical tools for assessing poststroke spasticity. Arch Phys Med Rehabil 1999;80:1013–1016.

Gresty MA. Coordination of head and eye movements to fixate continuous and intermittent targets. Vision Res 1974;14:395–403.

Grillner S, Deliagnina T, Ekebuerg O, et al. Neural networks that co-ordinate locomotion and body orientation in lamprey. Trends Neurosci 1995;18:270–280.

Grillner S, Halbertsma J, Nilsson J, Thorstensson A. The adaptation to speed in human locomotion. Brain Res 1979;165:177–182.

Grillner S, Rossignol S. On the initiation of the swing phase of locomotion in chronic spinal cats. Brain Res 1978;146:269–277.

Grillner S, Zangger P. On the central generation of locomotion in the low spinal cat. Exp Brain Res 1979;34:241–261.

Grillner S. Control of locomotion in bipeds, tetrapods, and fish. In: Brooks VB, ed. Handbook of physiology: the nervous system, vol. 2. Motor control. Baltimore: Williams & Wilkins, 1981:1179–1236.

Grillner S. Locomotion in the spinal cat. In: Stein RB, Pearson KG, Smith RS, Redford JB, eds. Control of posture and locomotion. New York: Plenum, 1973:515–535.

Gronley JK, Perry J. Gait analysis techniques: Rancho Los Amigos Hospital gait laboratory. Phys Ther 1984;64:1831–1837.

Grossman GE, Leigh RJ. Instability of gaze during locomotion in patients with deficient vestibular function. Ann Neurol 1990;27:528–532.

Guadagnoli MA, Lee TD. Challenge point: a framework for conceptualizing the effects of various practice conditions in motor learning. J Motor Behav 2004;36:212–224.

Guarrera-Bowlby PL, Gentile AM. Form and variability during sit-to-stand transitions: children versus adults. J Motor Behav 2004;36:104–114.

Guccione AA. Physical therapy diagnosis and the relationship between impairments and function. Phys Ther 1991;71:499–504.

Guide for the Functional Independence Measure for Children (WeeFIM) of the Uniform Data System for Medical Rehabilitation. Version 4.0. Buffalo: State University of New York at Buffalo, 1993.

Guralnik JM, Ferrucci L, Pieper CF, et al. Lower extremity function and subsequent disability: consistency across studies, predictive models, and value of gait speed alone compared with the Short Physical Performance Battery. J Gerontol A Biol Sci Med Sci 2000;55: M221–M231.

Guralnik JM, LaCroix AZ, Abbott RD, et al. Maintaining mobility in late life: Demographic characteristics and chronic conditions. Am J Epidemiol 1993;127:845–857.

Guralnik JM, LaCroix AZ, Everett DF, Kovar MG. Aging in the eighties: the prevalence of comorbidity and its association with disability. Vital Health Stat 1989;170:1–8.

Guralnik JM, Simonsick EM, Ferrucci L, et al. A short physical performance battery assessing lower extremity function: association with self-reported disability and prediction of mortality and nursing home admission. J Gerontol A Biol Sci Med Sci 1994;49:M85–M94.

Gurfinkel VS, Levik YS. Sensory complexes and sensorimotor integration. Fiziolog Cheloveka 1978;5:399–414.

Gurfinkel VS, Levick YS. Perceptual and automatic aspects of the postural body scheme. In: Paillard J, ed. Brain and space. New York: Oxford Science, 1991.

Gurfinkel VS, Lipshits MI, Popov KE. Is the stretch reflex the main mechanism in the system of regulation of the vertical posture of man? Biophysics 1974;19:761–766.

H

Haaland KY, Prestopnik JL, Knight RT, Lee RR. Hemispheric asymmetries for kinematic and positional aspects of reaching. Brain 2004; 127(Pt 5):1145–1158.

Hadders-Algra, M, Brogren E, Forssberg H. Training affects the development of postural adjustments in sitting infants. J Physiology 1996;493:289–298.

Hadders-Algra M, Gramsberg A. Discussion on the clinical relevance of activity-dependent plasticity after an insult to the developing brain. Neurosci Biobehav Rev 2007;31: 1213–1219.

Haffenden AM, Goodale MA. The effect of pictorial illusion on prehension and perception. J Cogn Neurosci 1998;10:122–136.

Häger-Ross C, Schieber MH. Quantifying the independence of human finger movements: comparisons of digits, hands, and movement frequencies. J Neurosci 2000;20:8542–8550.

Hahn ME, Chou L-S. Can motion of individual body segments identify dynamic instability in the elderly? Clin Biomech 2003;18:737–744.

Hahn ME, Chou L-S. Age-related reduction in sagittal plane center of mass motion during obstacle crossing. J Biomech 2004;37:837–844.

Haken H. Principles of brain functioning: A synergetic approach to brain activity, behavior and cognition. Berlin: Springer. 1996.

Haley SM, Coster WJ, Ludlow LH, et al. Pediatric Evaluation of Disability Inventory (PEDI). Boston: New England Medical Center Hospitals, 1992.

Haley SM, Jette AM, Coster WJ, et al. Late life function and disability instrument. II. Development and evaluation of the disability component. J Gerontol A Biol Sci Med Sci 2002;57A: M217–M222.

Hall CD, Herdman SJ. Reliability of clinical measures used to assess patients with peripheral vestibular disorders J Neurol Phys Ther 2006;30:74–81.

Hall KM, Bushnik T, Lakisic-Kazazic B, Wright J, Cantagallo A. Assessing traumatic brain injury outcome measures for long-term follow-up of community-based individuals. Arch Phys Med Rehabil 2001;82:367–374.

Hallemans A, Dhanis L, De Clercq D, Aerts P. Changes in mechanical control of movement during the first 5 months of independent walking: a longitudinal study. J Motor Behav 2007;39:227–233.

Hallett M. Overview of human tremor physiology. Mov Disord 1998;13:43–48.

Hallett M. Physiology of basal ganglia disorders: an overview. Can J Neurol Sci 1993;20: 177–183.

Hallet M. Transcranial magnetic stimulation and the human brain. Nature 2000;406:147–150.

Hallett M, Shahani BT, Young RR. EMG analysis of stereotyped voluntary movements in man. J Neurol Neurosurg Psychiatry 1975;38: 1154–1162.

Hammer A, Nilsagard Y, Wallquist M. Balance training in stroke patients—a systematic review of randomized, controlled trials. Adv Physiother 2008;10:163–172.

Hanakawa T, Katsumi Y, Fukuyama H, et al. Mechanisms underlying gait disturbance in Parkinson's disease: a single photon emission computed tomography study. Brain 1999;122:1271–1282.

Hanisch C, Konczak J, Dohle C. The effect of the Ebbinghaus illusion on grasping behaviour of children. Exp Brain Res 2001;137:237–245.

Hanlon RE. Motor learning following unilateral stroke. Arch Phys Med Rehabil 1996;77: 811–815.

Hanna SE, Law MC, Rosenbaum PL, et al. Development of hand function among children with cerebral palsy: growth curve analysis for ages 16 to 70 months. Dev Med Child Neurol 2003;45:448–455.

Hara Y, Ogawa S, Tsujiuchi K, Muraoka Y. A home-based rehabilitation program for the hemiplegic upper extremity by power-assisted functional electrical stimulation. Disabil Rehabil 2008;30(4):296–304.

Harbourne R, Stergiou N. Movement variability and the use of nonlinear tools: principles to guide physical therapist practice. Phys Ther 2009;89:267–282.

Harbourne RT, Deffeyes JE, DeJong SL. Nonlinear variables can assist in identifying postural control deficits in infants. J Sport Exerc Psychol (Suppl). 2007;29:S9.

Harbourne RT, Giuliani C, MacNeela, J. A kinematic and electromyographic analysis of the development of sitting posture in infants. Dev Psychobiol 1993;26:51–64.

Harbourne RT, Stergiou N. Nonlinear analysis of the development of sitting postural control. Dev Psychobiol 2003;42:368–377.

Hardy SE, Perera S, Roumani YF, et al. Improvement in usual gait speed predicts better survival in older adults. J Am Geriatr Soc 2007;55:1727–1734.

Harley C, Boyd JE, Cockburn J, et al. Disruption of sitting balance after stroke: influence of spoken output. J Neurol Neurosurg Psychiatry 2006;77:674–676.

Harris JE, Eng JJ, Marigold DS, et al. Relationship of balance and mobility to fall incidence in people with chronic stroke. Phys Ther 2005;85: 150–158.

Harris ML, Polkey MI, Bath PM, Moxham J. Quadriceps muscle weakness following acute hemiplegic stroke. Clin Rehabil 2001;15: 274–281.

Hase K, Stein RB. Turning strategies during human walking. J Neurophysiol 1999;81:2914–2922.

Hass G, Diener HC. Development of stance control in children. In: Amblard B, Berthoz A, Clarac F, eds. Development, adaptation and modulation of posture and gait. Amsterdam: Elsevier, 1988:49–58.

Hass G, Diener HC, Bacher M, Dichgans J. Development of postural control in children: short-, medium-, and long-latency EMG responses of leg muscles after perturbation of stance. Exp Brain Res 1986;64:127–132.

Hauer K, Lamb SE, Jorstad EC, et al. Systematic review of definitions and methods of measuring falls in randomised controlled fall prevention trials. Age Ageing 2006;35:5–10.

Hauer K, Pfisterer M, Weber C, et al. Cognitive impairment decreased postural control during dual tasks in geriatric patients with a history of severe falls. J Am Geriatr Soc 2003;51:1638–1644.

Haugh AB, Pandyan AD, Johnson GR. A systematic review of the Tardieu Scale for the measurement of spasticity. Dis Rehabil 2006;28: 899–907.

Hausdorff JM. Gait dynamics, fractals and falls: finding meaning in the stride-to-stride fluctuations of human walking. Hum Mov Sci 2007;26:555–589.

Hausdorff JM, Cudkowicz ME, Firtion R, et al. Gait variability and basal ganglia disorders: stride-to-stride variations of gait cycle timing in Parkinson's disease and Huntington's disease. Mov Disord 1998;13: 428–437.

Hausdorff JM, Edelberg HK, Mitchell SL, et al. Increased gait unsteadiness in community-dwelling elderly fallers. Arch Phys Med Rehabil 1997;78:278–283.

Hausdorff JM, Rios DA, Edelberg HK: Gait variability and fall risk in community-living older adults: a 1-year prospective study. Arch Phys Med Rehabil 2001;82:1050–1056.

Hay L. Accuracy of children on an open-loop pointing task. Percept Motor Skills 1978;47: 1079–1082.

Hay L. Spatial-temporal analysis of movements in children: motor programs versus feedback in the development of reaching. J Motor Behav 1979;11:189–200.

Hay L. Developmental changes in eye-hand coordination behaviors: Preprogramming versus feedback control. In: Bard C, Fleury M, Hay L, eds. Development of eye-hand coordination across the lifespan. Columbia: University of South Carolina Press, 1990:217–244.

Hay L, Bard C, Fleury M. Visuo-manual coordination from 6 to 10: specification, control and evaluation of direction and amplitude parameters of movement. In: Wade MG, Whiting HTA, eds. Motor development in children: aspects of coordination and control. Dordrecht: Martinus Nijhoff, 1986.

Hayes KC, Riach CL. Preparatory postural adjustments and postural sway in young children. In: Woollacott MH, Shumway-Cook A, eds. Development of posture and gait across the life span. Columbia: University of South Carolina, 1989:97–127.

Heathcock JC, Bhat AN, Lobo MA, Galloway JC. The performance of infants born preterm and full-term in the mobile paradigm: learning and memory. Phys Ther 2004;4:8–21.

Hedberg A, Carlberg EB, Forssberg H, Hadders-Algra M. Development of postural adjustments in sitting position during the first half year of life. Dev Med Child Neurol 2005;47: 312–320.

Hedberg A, Forssberg H, Hadders-Algra M. Postural adjustments due to external perturbations during sitting in 1-month-old infants: evidence for the innate origin of direction specificity. Exp Brain Res 2004;157:10–17.

Hein A, Held R. Dissociation of the visual placing response into elicited and guided components. Science 1967;158:390–392.

Heitmann DK, Gossman MR, Shaddeau SA, Jackson JR. Balance performance and step width in non-institutionalized elderly female fallers and nonfallers. Phys Ther 1989;69: 923–931.

Helbostad JL. Treadmill training and/or body weight support may not improve walking ability following stroke: commentary. Aust J Physiol 2003;49:278.

Held JM. Environmental enrichment enhances sparing and recovery of function following brain damage. Neurol Rep 1998;22:74–78.

Held JM. Recovery of function after brain damage: theoretical implications for therapeutic intervention. In: Carr JH, Shepherd, RB, Gordon J, et al., eds. Movement sciences: foundations for physical therapy in rehabilitation. Rockville, MD: Aspen, 1987:155–177.

Held JM, Gordon F, Gentile AM. Environmental influences on locomotor recovery following cortical lesions in rats. Behav Neurosci 1985; 99:678–690.

Held R, Hein A. Movement-produced stimulation in the development of visually guided behavior. J Comp Physiol Psychol 1963;56:872–876.

Hellstrom K, Lindmark B, Wahlberg B, Fugl-Meyer AR. Self-efficacy in relation to impairments and activities of daily living disability in elderly patients with stroke: a prospective investigation. J Rehabil Med 2003;35:202–207.

Henderson SE, Sugden DA. Movement Assessment Battery for Children—Second Edition (Movement ABC). Upper Saddle River, NJ: Pearson, 2007.

Henry SM, Fung J, Horak FB. EMG responses to maintain stance during multidirectional surface translations. J Neurophysiol 1998;80: 1939–1950.

Herdman SJ, ed. Vestibular rehabilitation, 3rd ed. Philadelphia: FA Davis, 2007.

Herdman SJ, Schubert MC, Tusa RJ. Role of central preprogramming in dynamic visual acuity with vestibular loss. Arch Otolaryngol Head Neck Surg 2001;127:1205–1210.

Herman R. Augmented sensory feedback in control of limb movement. In: Fields WS, ed. Neural organization and its relevance to prosthetics. New York: Intercontinental Medical Book, 1973.

Herman R, Cook T, Cozzens B, Freedman W. In: Stein RB, Pearson KG, Smith RS, Redford JB, eds. Control of posture and locomotion. New York: Plenum, 1973:363–388.

Herman S, Grillner R, Ralston HJ, et al., eds. Neural control of locomotion. New York: Plenum, 1976:675–705.

Herman T, Inbar-Borovsky N, Brozgol M, et al. The Dynamic Gait Index in healthy older adults: the role of stair climbing, fear of falling and gender. Gait Posture 2009;29:237–241.

Hermsdörfer J, Blankenfeld H, Goldenberg G. The dependence of ipsilesional aiming deficits on task demands, lesioned hemisphere, and apraxia. Neuropsychologia 2003;41: 1628–1643.

Hermsdorfer J, Laimgruber K, Kerkhoff G, et al. Effects of unilateral brain damage on grip selection, coordination, and kinematics of ipsilesional prehension. Exp Brain Res 1999;128(1–2):41–51.

Hess JA, Woollacott M. Effect of high-intensity strength-training on functional measures of balance ability in balance-impaired older adults. J Manipulative Physiol Ther 2005;28:582–590.

Hess JA, Woollacott M, Shivitz N. Ankle force and rate of force production increase following high intensity strength training in frail older adults. Aging Clin Exp Res 2006;18:107–115.

Hesse S, Bertelt C, Jahnke MT, et al. Treadmill training with partial body weight support compared with physiotherapy in non ambulatory hemiparetic patients. Stroke 1995;26: 976–981.

Hesse S, Bertelt C, Schaffrin A, et al. Restoration of gait in non ambulatory hemiparetic patients by treadmill training with partial weight support. Arch Phys Med Rehabil 1994;75:1087–1093.

Hesse S, Konrad M, Uhlenbroch D. Treadmill walking with partial body weight support versus floor walking in hemiparetic subjects. Arch Phys Med Rehabil 1999;80:421–427.

Hesse S, Reiter F, Jahnke M, et al. Asymmetry of gait initiation in hemiparetic stroke subjects. Arch Phys Med Rehabil 1997;78:719–724.

Hesse S, Werner C, Schonhardt EM, et al. Combined transcranial direct current stimulation and robot-assisted arm training in subacute stroke patients: a pilot study. Restor Neurol Neurosci 2007;25(1):9–15.

Hickey A, Ziviani J. A review of the quality of upper extremities skills test (QUEST) for children with cerebral palsy. Phys Occup Ther Pediatr 1998;18(3/4):123–135.

Hidler J, Nichols D, Pelliccio M, et al. Multicenter randomized clinical trial evaluating the effectiveness of the Lokomat in subacute stroke. Neurorehabil Neural Repair 2009;23:5–13.

Higgens JR, Spaeth RA. Relationship between consistency of movement and environmental conditions. Quest 1979;17:65.

Higgins C-I, Campos J-J, Kermoian R. Effect of self-produced locomotion on infant postural compensation to optic flow. Dev Psychol 1996;32:836–841.

Hird JS, Landers DM, Thomas JR, Horan JJ. Physical practice is superior to mental practice in enhancing cognitive and motor task performance. J Sport Exer Psychol 1991;13: 281–293.

Hirschfeld H. On the integration of posture, locomotion and voluntary movement in humans: normal and impaired development. Dissertation. Karolinska Institute, Stockholm, 1992.

Hirschfeld H, Forssberg, H. Epigenetic development of postural responses for sitting during infancy. Exp Brain Res 1994;97:528–540.

Hirvansalo, M., Rantanen, T., & Heikkinen E. Mobility difficulties and physical activity as predictors of mortality and loss of independence in the community-living older population. J Am Ger Soc 2000;48:493–498.

Hodges PW, Gurfinkel VS, Brumagne S, et al.. Coexistence of stability and mobility in postural control: evidence from postural compensation for respiration. Exp Brain Res 2002;144:293–302.

Hoehn MM, Yahr MD. Parkinsonism: onset, progression and mortality. Neurology 1967;17: 433–450.

Hoffer MM, Feiwell E, Perry R, et al. Functional ambulation in patients with myelomeningocele. J Bone Joint Surg Am 1973;55:137–148.

Hogan M. Physical and cognitive activity and exercise for older adults: a review. Int J Aging Hum Dev 2005;60:95–126.

Hogan N, Bizzi E, Mussa-Ivaldi FA, Flash T. Controlling multijoint motor behavior. Exerc Sport Sci Rev 1987;15:15–90.

Holbein MA, Redfern MS. Functional stability limits while holding loads in various positions. Int J Ind Ergon 1997;19:387–395.

Holden MK, Dettwiler A, Dyar T, et al. Retraining movement in patients with acquired brain injury using a virtual environment. Stud Health Technol Inform 2001;81:192–8.

Holden MK, Gill KM, Magliozzi MR, et al. Clinical gait assessment in the neurologically impaired: reliability and meaningfulness. Phys Ther 1984;64:35–40.

Hollerbach JM. Planning of arm movements. In: Osherson DN, Kosslyn SM, Hollerbach JM, eds. Visual cognition and action: an invitation to cognitive science, vol. 2. Cambridge, MA: MIT Press, 1990:183–211.

Holmefur M, Aarts P, Hoare B, Krumlinde-Sundholm L. Test-retest and alternate forms reliability of the assisting hand assessment. J Rehabil Med 2009;41(11):886–891.

Hong M, Earhart GM. Effects of medication on turning deficits in individuals with Parkinson's disease. J Neurol Phys Ther 2010;34:11–16.

Horak F. Assumptions underlying motor control for neurologic rehabilitation. In: Contemporary management of motor control problems. Proceedings of the II Step Conference. Alexandria, VA: American Physical Therapy Association, 1991:11–27.

Horak F. Clinical measurement of postural control in adults. Phys Ther 1987;67:1881–1885.

Horak F, Diener HC, Nashner LM. Influence of central set on human postural responses. J Neurophysiol 1989a;62:841–853.

Horak F, Diener HC. Cerebellar control of postural scaling and central set in stance. J Neurophysiol 1994;72:479–493.

Horak F, Jones-Rycewicz C, Black FO, Shumway-Cook A. Effects of vestibular rehabilitation on dizziness and imbalance. Otolaryngol Head Neck Surg 1992;106:175–180.

Horak F, Moore S. Lateral postural responses: the effect of stance width and perturbation amplitude. Phys Ther 1989;69:363.

Horak F, Nashner L. Central programming of postural movements: adaptation to altered support surface configurations. J Neurophysiol 1986;55:1369–1381.

Horak F, Shumway-Cook A, Black FO. Are vestibular deficits responsible for developmental disorders in children? Insights Otolaryngol 1988;3:2.

Horak F, Shumway-Cook A. Clinical implications of postural control research. In: Duncan P, ed. Balance: proceedings of the APTA Forum. Alexandria, VA: American Physical Therapy Association, 1990:105–111.

Horak F, Shupert C, Mirka A. Components of postural dyscontrol in the elderly: a review. Neurobiol Aging 1989;10:727–745.

Horak F, Shupert C. The role of the vestibular system in postural control. In: Herdman S, ed. Vestibular rehabilitation. New York: Davis, 1994:22–46.

Horak FB. Comparison of cerebellar and vestibular loss on scaling of postural responses. In: Brandt T, Paulus IO, Bles W, et al., eds. Disorders of posture and gait. Stuttgart: George Thieme Verlag, 1990:370–373.

Horak FB. Adaptation of automatic postural responses. In: Bloedel JR, Ebner TJ, Wise SP, eds. The acquisition of motor behavior in vertebrates. Cambridge MA: MIT Press, 1996:57–85.

Horak FB, Anderson M, Esselman P, Lynch K. The effects of movement velocity, mass displaced and task certainty on associated postural adjustments made by normal and hemiplegic individuals. J Neurol Neurosurg Psychiatry 1984;47:1020–1028.

Horak FB, Dimitrova D, Nutt JG. Directional-specific postural instability in subjects with Parkinson's disease. Exp Neurology 2005;193:504–521.

Horak FB, Earhart GM, Dietz V. Postural responses to combinations of head and body displacements: vestibular and somatosensory interactions. Exp Brain Res 2001;141:410–414.

Horak FB, Hlavacka F. Somatosensory loss increases vestibulospinal sensitivity. J Neurophsyiol 2001;86:575–585.

Horak FB, Macpherson JM. Postural orientation and equilibrium. In: Shepard J, Rowell L, eds. Handbook of physiology, section 12. Exercise: regulation and integration of multiple systems. New York, Oxford University, 1996:255–292.

Horak FB, Nashner LM, Diener HC. Postural strategies associated with somatosensory and vestibular loss. Exp Brain Res 1990;82: 167–177.

Horak FB, Nutt JG, Nashner LM. Postural inflexibility in parkinsonian subjects. J Neurol Sci 1992;111:46–58.

Horak FB, Shupert CL, Dietz V, Horstmann G. Vestibular and somatosensory contributions to responses to head and body displacements in stance. Exp Brain Res 1994;100:93–106.

Horak FB, Wrisley DM, Frank J. The Balance Evaluation Systems test (BESTest) to differentiate balance deficits. Phys Ther 2009; 89:484–498.

Hore J, Wild B, Diener HC. Cerebellar dysmetria at the elbow, wrist, and fingers. J Neurophysiol 1991;65:563–571.

Hornby TG, Campbell DD, Kahn JH, et al. Enhanced gait-related improvements after therapist-versus robotic-assisted locomotor training in subjects with chronic stroke: a randomized controlled study. Stroke 2008;39:1786–1792.

Horowitz L, Sharby N. Development of prone extension postures in healthy infants. Phys Ther 1988;68:32–39.

Housman SJ, Scott KM, Reinkensmeyer DJ. A randomized controlled trial of gravity-supported, computer-enhanced arm exercise for individuals with severe hemiparesis. Neurorehabil Neural Repair 2009;23(6):505–514.

Hovda DA, Feeney DM. Haloperidol blocks amphetamine induced recovery of binocular depth perception after bilateral visual cortex ablation in the cat. Proc West Pharmacol Soc 1985;28:209–211.

Howe TE, Rochester L, Jackson A, et al. Exercise for improving balance in older people. Cochrane Database Syst Rev 2007;4:CD004963.

Hoy MG, Zernicke RF, Smith JL. Contrasting roles of inertial and muscle moments at knee and ankle during paw-shake response. J Neurophysiol 1985;54:1282–1294.

Hoy MG, Zernicke RF. Modulation of limb dynamics in the swing phase of locomotion. J Biomech 1985;18:49–60.

Hoy MG, Zernicke RF. The role of intersegmental dynamics during rapid limb oscillations. J Biomech 1986;19:867–877.

Hoyle G. Muscles and their neural control. New York: Wiley, 1983.

Hoyt DF, Taylor CR. Gait and energetics of locomotion in horses. Nature 1981;292:239–240.

Hreljac A. Determinants of the gait transition speed during human locomotion: kinetic factors. Gait Posture 1993a;1:217–223.

Hreljac A. Preferred and energetically optimal gait transition speeds in human locomotion. Med Sci Sports Exerc 1993b;25:1158–1162.

Hreljac A. Determinants of the gait transition speed during human locomotion: kinematic factors. J Biomech 1995a;28: 669–677.

Hreljac A. Effects of physical characteristics on the gait transition speed during human locomotion. Hum Mov Sci 1995b;14:205–216.

Hsieh CL, Cheu CF, Hsueh IP, Wang CH. Trunk control as an early predictor of comprehensive activities of daily living function in stroke patients. Stroke 2002;33:2626–2630.

Hsieh Y, Hsueh I, Chou Y, et al. Development and validation of a short form of the Fugl-Meyer Motor Scale in patients with stroke. Stroke 2007;38:3052–3054.

Hsueh IP, Lee MM, Hsieh CL. The psychometric characteristics of the Barthel ADL index in stroke patients. J Formos Med Assoc 2001;100:526–532.

Hu M, Woollacott M. Multisensory training of standing balance in older adults. 1. Postural stability and one-leg stance balance. J Gerontol 1994a;49:M52–M61.

Hu M, Woollacott M. Multisensory training of standing balance in older adults. 2. Kinetic and electromyographic postural responses. J Gerontol 1994b;49:M62–M71.

Huang H, Fetters L, Hale J, McBride A. Bound for success: a systematic review of constraint-induced movement therapy in children with cerebral palsy supports improved arm and hand use. Phys Ther 2009;89(11):1126–1141.

Hubel DH. Eye, brain and vision. New York: Scientific American, 1988.

Hubel DH, Wiesel TN. Receptive fields of single neurones in the cat's striate cortex. J. Physiol Lond 1959;148:574–591.

Hudson CC, Krebs DE. Frontal plane dynamic stability and coordination in subjects with cerebellar degeneration. Exp Brain Res 2000;132:103–113.

Hughes RE, Johnson ME, O'Driscoll SW, An KN. Age-related changes in normal isometric shoulder strength. Am J Sports Med 1999a;27: 651–657.

Hughes RE, Johnson ME, O'Driscoll SW, An KN. Normative values of agonist-antagonist shoulder strength ratios of adults aged 20 to 78 years. Arch Phys Med Rehabil 1999b;80:1324–1326.

Hughes VA, Frontera WR, Wood M, et al. Longitudinal muscle strength changes in older adults: influence of muscle mass, physical activity and health. J Gerontol Biol Sci 2001;56A:B209–B217.

Hugon M, Massion J, Wiesendanger M. Anticipatory postural changes induced by active unloading and comparison with passive unloading in man. Pflugers Arch 1982;393: 292–296.

Hulliger M, Nordh E, Thelin AE, Vallbo AB. The responses of afferent fibers from the glabrous skin of the hand during voluntary finger movements in man. J Physiol 1979;291:233–249.

Humm JL, Kozlowski DA, Bland ST, et al. Progressive expansion of brain injury by extreme behavior pressure: is glutamate involved? Exp Neurol 1999;157:349–358.

Hummel F, Celnik P, Giraux P, et al. Effects of non-invasive cortical stimulation on skilled motor function in chronic stroke. Brain 2005;128:490–499.

Humphrey NK, Weiskrantz L. Vision in monkeys after removal of the striate cortex. Nature 1969;215:595–597.

Hung YC, Charles J, Gordon AM. Bimanual coordination during a goal-directed task in children with hemiplegic cerebral palsy. Dev Med Child Neurol 2004;46:746–753.

Hung Y-C, Charles J, Gordon AM. Influence of accuracy constraints on bimanual coordination during a goal-directed task in children with hemiplegic cerebral palsy. Exp Brain Res 2010;201:421–428.

Husemann B, Müller F, Krewer C, et al. Effects of locomotion training with assistance of a robot-driven gait orthosis in hemiparetic patients after stroke: a randomized controlled pilot study. Stroke 2007;38:349–354.

Huxham F, Baker R, Morris ME, Iansek R. Head and trunk rotation during walking turns in Parkinson's disease. Mov Disord 2008;23: 1391–1397.

Huxhold O, Li S-C, Schmiedek F, Lindenberger U. Dual-tasking postural control: aging and the effects of cognitive demand in conjunction with focus of attention. Brain Res Bull 2006;69:294–305.

Hwang I, Tung L, Yang J, et al. Electromyographic analyses of global synkinsesis in the paretic upper limb after stroke. Phys Ther 2005;85: 755–765.

Hyndman D, Ashburn A. "Stops Walking When Talking" as a predictor of falls in people with stroke living in the community. J Neurol Neurosurg Psychiatry 2004;75:994–997.

Hyndman D, Ashburn A. People with stroke living in the community: attention deficits, balance, ADL ability, and falls. Disabil Rehabil 2003;25:817–822.

Hyndman D, Pickering RM, Ashburn A. Reduced sway during dual task balnace performance among people with stroke at 6 and 12 months after discharge from hospital. Neurorehabil Neural Repair 2009;23:847–854.

I

Ikai T, Kamikubo T, Takehara I, et al. Dynamic postural control in patients with hemiparesis. Am J Phys Med Rehabil 2003;82:463–469.

Imms FJ, Edholm OG. Studies of gait and mobility in the elderly. Age Ageing 1981;10:147–156.

Inglin B, Woollacott MH. Age-related changes in anticipatory postural adjustments associated with arm movements. J Gerontol 1988;43:M105–M113.

Inglis JT, Horak FB, Shupert CL, Rycewicz C. The importance of somatosensory information in triggering and scaling automatic postural responses in humans. Exp Brain Res 1994;101:159–164.

Ingvarsson PE, Gordon AM, Forssberg H. Coordination of manipulative forces in Parkinson's disease. Exp Neurol 1997;145:489–501.

Inkster LM, Eng JJ, MacIntyre DL, Stoessl AJ. Leg muscle strength is reduced in Parkinson's disease and relates to the ability to rise from a chair. Mov Disord 2003;18:157–162.

Inkster LM, Eng JJ. Postural control during a sit-to-stand task in individuals with mild Parkinson's disease. Exp Brain Res 2004;154:33–38.

Inman VT, Ralston H, Todd F. Human walking. Baltimore: Williams & Wilkins, 1981.

Isles RC, Choy NL, Steer M, Nitz JC. Normal values of balance tests in women aged 20–80. J Am Geriatr Soc 2004;52:1367–1372.

Ito M. The cerebellum and neural control. New York: Raven, 1984.

Ito M, Araki A, Tanaka H, et al. Muscle histopathology in spastic cerebral palsy. Brain Dev 1996; 18:299–303.

Ivanenko YP, Dominici N, Cappellini G, et al. Development of pendulum mechanism and kinematic coordination from the first unsupported steps in toddlers. J Exp Biol 2004; 207:3797–3810.

Ivanenko YP, Dominici N, Cappellini G, Lacquaniti F. Kinematics in newly walking toddlers does not depend upon postural stability. J Neurophysiol 2005;94:754–763.

Ivry R. Representational issues in motor learning: phenomena and theory. In: Keele S, Heuer H, eds. Handbook of perception and action: motor skills. New York: Academic, 1997.

Ivry RB, Keele SW. Timing functions of the cerebellum. J Cogn Neurosci 1989;1:136–152.

J

Jackson RT, Epstein CM, De L'Amme WR. Abnormalities in posturography and estimations of visual vertical and horizontal in multiple sclerosis. Am J Otol 1995;16:88–93.

Jansen CW, Niebuhr BR, Coussirat DJ, et al. Hand force of men and women over 65 years of age as measured by maximum pinch and grip force. J Aging Phys Act 2008;16(1):24–41.

Jeannerod M. The timing of natural prehension movements. J Motor Behav 1984;16:235–254.

Jeannerod M. The formation of finger grip during prehension: a cortically mediated visuomotor pattern. Behav Brain Res 1986;19:99–116.

Jeannerod M. The neural and behavioral organization of goal-directed movements. Oxford: Clarendon Press, 1990.

Jeannerod M. Reaching and grasping: parallel specification of visuomotor channels. In: Handbook of perception and action, vol. 2. London: Academic Press, 1996:405–460.

Jeannerod M, Arbib MA, Rizzolatti G, Sakata H. Grasping objects: the cortical mechisms of visuomotor transformation. Trends Neurosci 1995;18:314–320.

Jebsen RH, Taylor N, Trieschmann RB, et al. An objective and standard test of hand function. Arch Phys Med Rehabil 1969;50:311–319.

Jedlinsky BP, McCarthy CF, Michel TH. Validating pediatric pain measurement: sensory and affective components. Ped Phys Ther 1999;11:83–88.

Jeka J, Lackner JR. Fingertip contact influences human postural control. Exp Brain Res 1994:100:495–502.

Jeka J, Oie KS, Kiemel T. Multisensory information for human postural control: integrating touch and vision. Exp Brain Res 2000;134:107–125.

Jeka JJ, Easton RD, Bentzen BL, Lackner JR. Haptic cues for orientation and postural control in sighted and blind individuals. Percept Psychophys 1996;58:409–423.

Jeka JJ, Lackner JR. The role of haptic cues from rough and slippery surfaces in human postural control. Exp Brain Res 1995;103:267–276.

Jeka JJ. Light touch contact as a balance aid. Phys Ther 1997;77:477–487.

Jenkins WM, Merzenich MM. Reorganization of neocortical representations after brain injury: a neurophysiological model of the bases of recovery from stroke. Progr Brain Res 1987;71:249–266.

Jenkins, WM, Merzenich MM, Och MT, et al. Functional reorganization of primary somatosensory cortex in adult owl monkeys after behaviorally controlled tactile stimulation. J Neurophysiol 1990;63:82–104.

Jensen JL, Bothner KE, Woollacott MH. Balance control: the scaling of the kinetic response to accommodate increasing perturbation magnitudes. J Sport Exer Psychol 1996;18:S45.

Jensen JL, Thelen E, Ulrich BD, et al. Adaptive dynamics of the leg movement patterns in human infants: Age-related differences in limb control. J Motor Behav 1995;27:366–374.

Jette AM. Diagnosis and classification by physical therapists: a special communication. Phys Ther 1989;69:967–969.

Jette AM. Physical disablement concepts for physical therapy research and practice. Phys Ther 1994;74:380–386.

Jette AM. Assessing disability in studies on physical activity. Am J Prev Med 2003;25(3 Suppl 2):122–128.

Jette AM, Assmann SF, Rooks D, et al. Interrelationships among disablement concepts. J Geron Med Sci 1998; 20:M395–M404.

Jette AM, Haley SM, Coster WJ, et al. Late life function and disability instrument: II. Development and evaluation of the function component. J Gerontol A Biol Sci Med Sci 2002;57A: M209–M216.

Jette DU, Bacon K, Batty C, et al. Evidence-based practice: beliefs, attitudes, knowledge, and behaviors of physical therapists. Phys Ther 2003;83:786–805.

Jims C. Foot placement pattern, an aid in gait training: suggestions from the field. Phys Ther 1977;57:286.

Johansson BB. Brain plasticity in health and disease. Keio J Med 2004;53:231–246.

Johansson RS. Sensory control of dexterous manipulation in humans. In: Wing AM, Haggard P, Flanagan J, eds. Hand and brain: the neurophysiology and psychology of hand movements. New York: Academic Press, 1996:381–414.

Johansson RS, Edin BB. Neural control of manipulation and grasp. In: Forssberg H, Hirschfeld H, eds. Movement disorders in children. Basel: Karger, 1992:107–112.

Johansson S, Ytterberg C, Claesson IM, et al. High concurrent presence of disability in multiple sclerosis. Associations with perceived health. J Neurol 2007;254:767–773.

Johnson GR. Outcome measures in spasticity. Eur J Neurol 2002;9:10–16.

Johnston M, Nissim EN, Wood K, et al. Objective and subjective handicap following spinal cord injury: interrelationships and predictors. J Spinal Cord Med 2002;25:11–22.

Johnston MV, Goverover Y, Dijkers M. Community activities and individual's satisfaction with them: quality of life in the first year after traumatic brain injury. Arch PMR 2005;86: 735–745.

Jonkers I, Delp S, Patten C. Capacity to increase walking speed is limited by impaired hip and ankle power generation in lower functioning persons post stroke. Gait Posture 2009;29: 129–137.

Jonsdottir J, Cattaneo D. Reliability and validity of the dynamic gait index in persons with chronic stroke. Arch Phys Med Rehabil 2007;88: 1410–1415.

Jordan T, Rabbitt P. Response times to stimuli of increasing complexity as a function of ageing. Br J Psychol 1977;68:189–201.

Jorgensen L, Crabtree NJ, Reeve J, Jacobsen BK. Ambulatory level and asymmetrical weight bearing after stroke affects bone loss in the upper and lower part of the femoral neck differently: bone adaptation after decreased mechanical loading. Bone 2000;27:701–707.

Jouen F. Visual-vestibular interactions in infancy. Infant Behav Dev 1984;7:135–145.

Jouen F. Early visual-vestibular interactions and postural development. In: Bloch H, Bertenthal BI, eds. Sensory-motor organizations and development in infancy and early childhood. Dordrecht, the Netherlands: Kluwer, 1990: 199–215.

Jouen F. Titres et travaux en vue de l'habilitation a diriger des recherches. State doctoral thesis, Universite Paris IV Paris, 1993:104.

Jouen F, Lepecq J-C, Gapenne O, Bertenthal BI. Optic flow sensitivity in neonates. Infant Behav Dev 2000;23:271–284.

Judge J, Whipple R, Wolfson L. Effects of resistive and balance exercises on isokinetic strength in older persons. J Am Geriatr Soc 1994;42: 937– 946.

Judge JO, Underwood M, Gennosa T. Exercise to improve gait velocity. Arch Phys Med Rehabil 1993;74:400–406.

K

Kaas JH, Florence SL, Jain N. Reorganization of sensory systems of primates after injury. Neuroscientist 1997; 3:123–130.

Kabat H, Knott M. Proprioceptive facilitation therapy for paralysis. Physiotherapy 1954;40:171–176.

Kaiser ML, Braun M, Rhyner C. [Utilization of the Canadian Occupational Performance measure (COPM) among children and their parents: a Swiss experience] [in French]. Can J Occup Ther 2005;72(1):30–36.

Kalisch T, Ragert P, Schwenkreis P, et al. Impaired tactile acuity in old age is accompanied by enlarged hand representations in somatosensory cortex. Cereb Cortex 2009;19:1530–1538.

Kallin K, Gustafson Y, Sandman PO, Karlsson S. Factors associated with falls among older, cognitively impaired people in geriatric care settings: a population based study. Am J Geriatr Psychiatry 2005;13:501–509.

Kaminski T, Bock C, Gentile AM. The coordination between trunk and arm motion during pointing movements. Exp Brain Res 1995;106:457–466.

Kamm K, Thelen E, Jensen J. A dynamical systems approach to motor development: In: Rothstein JM, ed. Movement science. Alexandria, VA: American Physical Therapy Association, 1991:11–23.

Kandel ER. Cellular basis of behavior: an introduction to behavioral neurobiology. San Francisco: Freeman, 1976.

Kandel ER. Genes, nerve cells, and the remembrance of things past. J Neuropsychiatry 1989;1:103–125.

Kandel ER. Cellular mechanisms of learning and the biological basis of individuality. In: Kandel ER, Schwartz JH, Jessell TM, eds. Principles of neuroscience, 3rd ed. New York: Elsevier, 1991.

Kandel ER. Cellular mechanisms of learning and the biological basis of individuality. In: Kandel ER, Schwartz JH, Jessell TM, eds. Principles of neural science, 4th ed. New York: McGraw-Hill, 2000a:1247–1279.

Kandel ER. The brain and behavior. In: Kandel ER, Schwartz JH, Jessell TM, eds. Principles of neural science, 4th ed. New York: McGraw-Hill, 2000b:5–17.

Kandel ER, Schwartz JH. Molecular biology of learning: modulation of transmitter release. Science 1982;218:433–443.

Kandel ER, Kupfermann I, Iversen S. Learning and memory. In: Kandel ER, Schwartz JH, Jessell TM, eds. Principles of neural science, 4th ed. New York: McGraw-Hill, 2000:1231.

Kandel ER, Schwartz JH, Jessell TM, eds. Principles of neuroscience, 3rd ed. New York: Elsevier, 1991.

Kandel ER, Schwartz JH, Jessell TM, eds. Principles of neuroscience, 4th ed. New York: Elsevier, 2000

Kandel ER, Siegelbaum SA. Synaptic integration. In: Kandel ER, Schwartz JH, Jessell TM, eds. Principles of neural science, 4th ed. New York: McGraw-Hill, 2000: 207–228.

Kapteyn TS. Afterthought about the physics and mechanics of postural sway. Agressologie 1973;14:27–35.

Karasik D, Demissie S, Cupples A, Kiel D. Disentangling the genetic determinants of human aging: biological age as an alternative to the use of survival measures. J Gerontol Biol Sci 2005;60A:574–587.

Karman N, Maryles J, Baker RW, et al. Constraint-induced movement therapy for hemiplegic children with acquired brain injuries. J Head Trauma Rehabil 2003;18(3):259–267.

Karst GM, Venema DM, Roehrs TG, Tyler AE. Center of pressure measures during standing tasks in minimally impaired persons with multiple sclerosis. J Neurol Phys Ther 2005;29:170–180.

Katz R, Rymer Z. Spastic hypertonia: mechanisms and measurement. Arch Phys Med Rehabil 1989;70:144–155.

Katz RT, Rovai GP, Brait C, Rymer WZ. Objective quantification of spastic hypertonia: correlation with clinical findings. Arch Phys Med Rehabil 1992;73:339–347.

Katz S, Downs TD, Cash JR, Grotz RC. Progress in development of the index of ADL. Gerontologist 1970:20–30.

Katz-Leurer M, Fisher I, Neeb M, et al. Reliability and validity of the modified functional reach test at the sub-acute stage post-stroke. Disabil Rehabil 2009;31:243–248.

Katzman WB, Sellmeyer DE, Stewart AL, et al. Changes in flexed posture, musculoskeletal impairments, and physical performance after group exercise in community-dwelling older women. Arch Phys Med Rehabil 2007;88: 192–199.

Kavounoudias A, Gilhodes JC, Roll R, Roll JP. From balance regulation to body orientation: two goals for muscle proprioceptive information processing? Exp Brain Res 1999;124: 80–88.

Kavounoudias A, Roll R, Roll JP. Foot sole and ankle muscle inputs contribute jointly to human erect posture regulation. J Physiol 2001;532:869–878.

Kay H. The effects of position in a display upon problem solving. Quart J Exper Psychol 1954; 6:155–169.

Kay H. Some experiments on adult learning. In Old Age in the Modern World: Report of the third Congress of the International Association of Gerontology, London 1954, pp. 259–267. Edinburgh: Livingstone, 1955.

Kazennikov O, Perrig S, Wiesendanger M. Kinematics of a coordinated goal-directed bimanual task. Behav Brain Res 2002;134(1–2): 83–91.

Kearney K, Gentile AM. Prehension in young children with Down syndrome. Acta Psychol (Amst) 2003;112(1):3–16.

Keele S. Movement control in skilled motor performance. Psychol Bull 1968;70:387–403.

Keele S, Ivry R. Does the cerebellum provide a common computation for diverse tasks? A timing hypothesis. In: Diamond A, ed. Developmental and neural bases of higher cognitive function. New York: New York Academy of Sciences, 1990:179–207.

Keele SW. Behavioral analysis of movement. In: Brooks VB, ed. Handbook of physiology: I. The nervous system, vol. 2. Motor control, part 2. Baltimore: Williams & Wilkins, 1981: 1391–1414.

Keele SW. Motor control. In: Kaufman L, Thomas J, Boff K, eds. Handbook of perception and performance. New York: Wiley, 1986:1–30.

Keele SW, Posner MI. Processing visual feedback in rapid movement. J Exp Psychol 1968;77: 155–158.

Keenan MA, Perry J, Jordan C. Factors affecting balance and ambulation following stroke. Clin Orth Rel Res 1984;182:165–171.

Keith RA, Granger CV, Hamilton BB, Sherwin FS. The functional independence measure: a new tool for rehabilitation. In: Eisentberg MG, Grzesiak RC, eds. Advances in clinical rehabilitation, vol. 1. New York: Springer Verlag, 1987:6–18.

Kelly VE, Bastian AJ. Antiparkinson medications improve agonist activation but not antagonist inhibition during sequential reaching movements. Mov Disord 2005;20:694–704.

Kelly VE, Hyngstrom AS, Rundle MM, Bastian AJ. Interaction of levodopa and cues on voluntary reaching in Parkinson's disease. Mov Disord 2002;17(1):28–44.

Kelso JA, Holt KG, Rubin P, Kugler PN. Patterns of human interlimb coordination emerge from the properties of non-linear, limit cycle oscillatory processes: theory and data. J Motor Behav 1981;13:226–261.

Kelso JAS, Holt KG. Exploring a vibratory systems analysis of human movement production. J Neurophysiol 1980;43:1183–1196.

Kelso JAS, Southard DL, Goodman D. On the coordination of two-handed movements. J Exp Psychol Hum Percept 1979;5:229–238.

Kelso JAS, Tuller B. A dynamical basis for action systems. In: Gazanniga MS, ed. Handbook of cognitive neuroscience. New York: Plenum, 1984:321–356.

Kembhavi G, Darrah J, Magill-Evans J. Using the Berg Balance Scale to distinguish balance abilities in children with cerebral palsy. Pediatr Phys Ther 2002;14:92–99.

Kendall FP, McCreary EK. Muscles: testing and function, 3rd ed. Baltimore: Williams & Wilkins, 1983.

Kennard MA. Relation of age to motor impairment in man and in sub-human primates. Arch Neurol Psychiatry 1940;44:377–398.

Kennard MA. Cortical reorganization of motor function: studies on a series of monkeys of various ages from infancy to maturity. Arch Neurol Psychiatr 1942;48:227–240.

Kenshalo DR. Aging effects on cutaneous and kinesthetic sensibilities. In: Han SS, Coons DH, eds. Special senses in aging. Ann Arbor: University of Michigan, 1979.

Keogh J, Morrison S, Barrett R. Age-related differences in inter-digit coupling during finger pinching. Eur J Appl Physol 2006;97:76–88.

Keogh J, Morrison S, Barrett R. Strength training improves the tri-digit finger-pinch force control of older adults. Arch Phys Med Rehabil 2007;88:1055–1063.

Kepple T, Siegel KL, Stanhope SJ. Relative contributions of the lower extremity joint moments to forward progression and support during gait. Gait Posture 1997;6:1–8.

Kerns K, Mateer CA. Walking and chewing gum: the impact of attentional capacity on everyday activities. In: Sbordone RJ, Long CJ, eds. Ecological validity of neuropsychological testing. Delray Beach, FL: GR Press, 1996.

Kerr B, Condon SM, McDonald LA. Cognitive spatial processing and the regulation of posture. J Exp Psychol 1985;11:617–622.

Kerr C, Parkes J, Stevenson M, et al. Energy efficiency in gait, activity, participation, and health status in children with cerebral palsy. Dev Med Child Neurol 2008;50:204–210.

Kerr R. Movement control and maturation in elementary-grade children. Percept Motor Skills 1975;41:151–154.

Kerr R, Booth B. Skill acquisition in elementary school children and schema theory. In: Landers DM, Christina RW, eds. Psychology of motor behavior and sport, vol. 2. Champaign, IL: Human Kinetics, 1977.

Kerse N, Parag V, Feigin VL, et al. Falls after stroke: results from the Auckland regional Community Stroke (ARCOS) study, 2002 to 2003. Stroke 2008;39:1890–1893.

Kesar TM, Perumal R, Reisman DS, et al. Functional electrical stimulation of ankle plantarflexor and dorsiflexor muscles: effects on poststroke gait. Stroke 2009;40:3821–3827.

Kessler RM, Hertling D. Management of common musculoskeletal disorders. Philadelphia: Harper & Row, 1983.

Ketelaar M, Vermeet A, Helders P. Functional motor abilities of children with CP: a systematic literature review of assessment measures. Clin Rehabil 1998;12:369–380.

Kim CM, Eng JJ. The relationship of lower extremity muscle torque to locomotor performance in people with stroke. Phys Ther 2003;83: 49–57.

King G, Law M, King S, et al. Children's Assessment of Participation and Enjoyment (CAPE) and Preferences for Activities of Children (PAC). San Antonio: Harcourt Assessment, 2004.

King GA, Law M, King S, et al. Measuring children's participation in recreation and leisure activities: construct validation of the CAPE and PAC. Child Care Health Dev 2006;33: 28–39.

King LA, Horak FB. Lateral stepping for postural correction in Parkinson's disease. Arch Phys Med Rehabil 2008;89:492–499.

King M, Hale L, Pekkari A, et al. An affordable, computerized, table-based exercise system for stroke survivors. Disabil Rehabil Assist Techno 2010; 5:288–293.

Kinoshita H, Francis PR. A comparison of prehension force control in young and elderly individuals. Eur J Appl Physiol Occup Physiol 1996;74:450–460.

Kinsella S, Moran K. Gait pattern categorization of stroke participants with equinus deformity of the foot. Gait Posture 2008;27:144–151.

Kirshenbaum N, Riach CL, Starkes JL. Non-linear development of postural control and strategy use in young children: a longitudinal study. Exp Brain Res 2001;140:420–431.

Klatzky RL, McCloskey B, Doherty S, et al. Knowledge about hand shaping and knowledge about objects. J Motor Behav 1987;19: 187–213.

Kleim JA, Cooper NR, VandenBerg PM. Exercise induces angiogenesis but does not alter movement representations within rat motor cortex. Brain Res 2002;934:1–6.

Kleim JA, Jones TA, Schallert T. Motor enrichment and the induction of plasticity before or after brain injury. Neurochem Res 2003;28: 1757–1769.

Kleim JA, Jones TA. Principles of experience-dependent neural plasticity: implications for rehabilitation after brain damage. J Speech Lang Hear Res 2008;51:S225–S239.

Kleim JA, Swain RA, Armstrong K, et al. Selective synaptic plasticity within the cerebellar cortex following complex motor skill learning. Neurobiol Learn Mem 1998;69:274–289.

Kleim JA, Vij K, Ballard DH, Greenough WT. Learning dependent synaptic modifications in the cerebellar cortex of the adult rat persist for at least four weeks. J Neurosci 1997;17: 717–771.

Kluzik J, Fetters L, Coryell J. Quantification of control: a preliminary study of effects of neurodevelopmental treatment on reaching in children with spastic cerebral palsy. Phys Ther 1990;2:65–78.

Kluzik J, Horak FB, Peterka RJ. Differences in preferred reference frames for postural orientation shown by after-effects of stance on an inclined surface. Exp Brain Res 2005;162:474–489.

Kluzik, J, Peterka RJ, Horak FB. Adaptation of postural orientation to changes in surface inclination. Exp Brain Res 2007;178:1–17.

Knutsson E. An analysis of Parkinsonian gait. Brain 1972;475–486.

Knutsson E. Gait control in hemiparesis. Scand J Rehabil Med 1981;13:101–108.

Knutsson E. Can gait analysis improve gait training in stroke patients? Scand J Rehab Med Suppl 1994;30:73–80.

Knutsson E, Richards C. Different types of disturbed motor control in gait of hemiparetic patients. Brain 1979;102:405–430.

Kobayashi M, Hutchinson S, Theoret H, et al. Repetitive TMS of the motor cortex improves ipsilateral sequential simple finger movements. Neurology 2004;62:91–98.

Koester J, Siegelbaum SA. Membrane potential. In: Kandel ER, Schwartz JH, Jessell TM, eds. Principles of neural science, 4th ed. New York: McGraw-Hill, 2000:125–139.

Kollen B, Kwakkel G, Lindeman E. Time dependency of walking classification in stroke. Phys Ther 2006;86:618–625.

Kollen B, Port I, Lindeman E, et al. Predicting improvement in gait after stroke. Stroke 2005;36:2576–2680.

Kolobe THA, Bulanda M, Susman L. Predicting motor outcome at preschool age for infants tested at 7, 30, 60, and 90 days after term age using the Test of Infant Motor Performance. Phys Ther 2004;84:1144–1156.

Konczak J, Dichgans J. The development toward stereotypic arm kinematics during reaching in the first 3 years of life. Exp Brain Res 1997;117:346–354.

Konczak J, Borutta M, Dichgans J. The development of goal-directed reaching in infants: 2. Learning to produce task-adequate patterns of joint torque. Exp Brain Res 1997;113:465–474.

Konczak J, Jansen-Osmann P, Kalveram KT. Development of force adaptation during childhood. J Motor Behav 2003;35:41–52.

Konczak J, Borutta M, Topka H, Dichgans J. The development of goal-directed reaching in infants: hand trajectory formation and joint torque control. Exp Brain Res 1995;106: 156–168.

Kosnik W, Winslow L, Kline D, et al. Visual changes in daily life throughout adulthood. J Gerontol 1988;43:P63–P70.

Kots YM, Syrovegin AV. Fixed set of variants of interactions of the muscles to two joints in the execution of simple voluntary movements. Biophysics 1966;11:1212–1219.

Kozlowski DA, James DC, Schallert T. Use-dependent exaggeration of neuronal injury after unilateral sensorimotor cortex lesions. J Neurosci 1996;16:4776–4786.

Krakauer J, Ghez C. Voluntary movement. In: Kandel ER, Schwartz JH, Jessell TM, eds. Principles of neural science, 4th ed. New York: McGraw-Hill, 2000:756–779.

Kram R, Domingo A, Ferris D. Effect of reduced gravity on the preferred walk-run transition speed. J Exp Biol 1997;200:821–826.

Kramer AF, Erickson KI, Colcombe SJ. Exercise, cognition and the aging brain. J Appl Physiol 2006;101:1237–1242.

Kramer PL, Heiman GA, Gasser T, et al. The DYT1 gene on 9q34 is responsible for most cases of early limb-onset idiopathic torsion dystonia in non-Jews. Am J Hum Genet 1994;55(3):468–475.

Krebs DE, Edelstein JE, Fishman S. Reliability of observational kinematic gait analysis. Phys Ther 1985;65:1027–1033.

Krebs DE, Jette AM, Assmann SF. Moderate exercise improves gait stability in disabled elders. Arch Phys Med Rehabil 1998;79:1489–1495.

Krishnamoorthy V, Latash ML, Scholz JL, Zatsiorsky VM. Muscle synergies during shifts of the center of pressure by standing persons. Exp Brain Res 2003;152:281–292.

Kristinsdottir EK, Fransson PA, Magnusson M. Changes in postural control in healthy elderly subjects are related to vibration sensation, vision and vestibular asymmetry. Act Otolaryngol 2001;121:700–706.

Krumlinde-Sundholm L, Eliasson AC. Development of the assisting hand assessment: a Rasch-built measure intended for children with unilateral upper limb impairments. Scand J Occup Ther 2003;10(1):16–26.

Krumlinde-Sundholm L, Holmefur M, Eliasson AC. The assisting hand assessment: evidence of validity, reliability and responsiveness to change. Workshop presented at the American Academy for Cerebral Palsy and Developmental Medicine, Orlando, FL, 2005.

Krumlinde-Sundholm L, Holmefur M, Kottorp A, Eliasson AC. The Assisting Hand Assessment: current evidence of validity, reliability, and responsiveness to change. Dev Med Child Neurol 2007;49(4):259–264.

Kugler PN, Kelso JAS, Turvey MT. On the concept of coordinative structures as dissipative structures: 1. Theoretical line. In: Stelmach GE, Requin J, eds. Tutorials in motor behavior. Amsterdam: North-Holland, 1980:3–37.

Kugler PN, Kelso JAS, Turvey MT. On the control and coordination of naturally developing systems. In: Kelso JAS, Clark JE, eds. The development of movement control and coordination. New York: Wiley, 1982:5–78.

Kugler PN, Turvey MT. Information, natural law and self assembly of rhythmic movement. Hillsdale, NJ: Erlbaum, 1987.

Kuhtz-Buschbeck JP, Stolze H, Johnk K, et al. Development of prehension movements in children: a kinematic study. Exp Brain Res 1998;122:424–432.

Kunesch E, Schnitzler A, Tyercha C, et al. Altered force release control in Parkinson's disease. Behav Brain Res 1995;67:43–49.

Kung UM, Horlings CG, Honegger H, et al. Postural instability in cerebellar apraxia: correlations of knee, arm and trunk movements to center of mass velocity. Neuroscience 2009;159:390–404.

Kunkel A, Kopp B, Müller G, et al. Constraint-induced movement therapy for motor recovery in chronic stroke patients. Arch Phys Med Rehabil 1999;80:624–628.

Kuo AD, Zajac FE. A biomechanical analysis of muscle strength as a limiting factor in standing posture. J Biomech 1993;26:137–150.

Kuo AD, Speers RA, Peterka RJ, Horak FB. Effect of altered sensory conditions on multivariate descriptors of human postural sway. Exp Brain Res 1998;122:185–195.

Kupfermann I. Localization of higher cognitive and affective functions: the association cortices. In: Kandel E, Schwartz JH, Jessell TM, eds. Principles of neuroscience, 3rd ed. New York: Elsevier, 1991:823–838.

Kurtzke JF. Rating neurologic impairment in multiple sclerosis: an expanded disability status scale (EDSS). Neurology 1983;33:1444–1452.

Kuypers HGJM. Anatomy of the descending pathways. In: Brookhart JM, Montcastle VB, eds. Handbook of physiology: the nervous system, part II. Bethesda, MD: American Physiological Society, 1981.

Kuypers HGJM. Corticospinal connections: postnatal development in rhesus monkey. Science 1962;138:678–680.

Kuypers HGJM. The descending pathways to the spinal cord, their anatomy and function. In: Eccles JC, ed. Organization of the spinal cord. Amsterdam: Elsevier, 1964.

Kwakkel G, de Goede CJ, van Wegen EE. Impact of physical therapy for Parkinson's disease: a critical review of the literature. Parkinsonism Relat Disord 2007;13(Suppl 3):S478–S487.

Kwakkel G, Wagenaar RC, Kollen BJ, Lankhorst GJ. Predicting disability in stroke: a critical review of the literature. Age Ageing 1996;25:479–489.

L

Lackner JR, DiZio P. Visual stimulation affects the perception of voluntary leg movements during walking. Perception 1988;17:71–80.

Lackner JR, DiZio P. Sensory-motor calibration processes constraining the perception of force and motion during locomotion. In: Woollacott MH, Horak FB, eds. Posture and gait: control mechanisms. Eugene, OR: University of Oregon, 1992:92–96.

Lafortune MA, Hennig EM, Lake MJ. Dominant role of interface over knee angle for cushioning impact loading and regulating initial leg stiffness. J Biomech 1996;29:1523–1529.

Lajoie K, Drew T. Lesions of area 5 of the posterior parietal cortex in the cat produce errors in the accuracy of paw placement during visually guided locomotion. J Neurophysiol 2007;97:2339–2354.

Lajoie Y, Teasdale N, Bard C, Fleury M. Attentional demands for static and dynamic equilibrium. Exp Brain Res 1993;97:139–144.

Lamb SE, Ferrucci L, Volapto S, et al. Risk factors for falling in home-dwelling older women with stroke: the Women's Health and Aging Study. Stroke 2003;34:494–501.

Lamontagne A, Malouin F, Richards CL, Dumas F. Mechanisms of disturbed motor control in ankle weakness during gait after stroke. Gait Posture 2002;15:244–255.

Lance JW. Symposium synopsis. In: Feldman RG, Young RR, Koella WP, eds. Spasticity: disordered motor control. Chicago: Year Book, 1980.

Lang CE, Bastian AJ. Cerebellar subjects show impaired adaptation of anticipatory EMG during catching. J Neurophysiol 1999;82: 2108–2119.

Lang CE, Bastian AJ. Additional somatosensory information does not improve cerebellar adaptation during catching. Clin Neurophysiol 2001;112:895–907.

Lang CE, DeJong SL, Beebe JA. Recovery of thumb and finger extension and its relation to grasp performance after stroke. J Neurophysiol 2009;102(1):451–459.

Lang CE, Schieber MH. Reduced muscle selectivity during individuated finger movements in humans after damage to the motor cortex or corticospinal tract. J Neurophysiol 2004;91: 1722–1733.

Lang CE, Wagner JM, Bastian AJ, et al. Deficits in grasp versus reach during acute hemiparesis. Exp Brain Res 2005;166:126–136.

Lang CE, Wagner JM, Edwards DF, et al. Recovery of grasp versus reach in people with hemiparesis poststroke. Neurorehabil Neural Repair 2006;20:444–454.

Lang W, Obrig H, Lindinger G, et al. Supplementary motor area activation while tapping bimanually different rhythms in musicians. Exp Brain Res 1990;79:504–514.

Larson MA, Lee SL, Vasque DE. Comparison of ATNR presence and developmental activities in 2–4 month old infants. Alexandria, VA: American Physical Therapy Association conference proceedings, June, 1990.

Lashley KS. Brain mechanism and intelligence. Chicago: University of Chicago, 1929.

LaStayo P, Hartzel J. Dynamic versus static grip strength: how grip strength changes when the wrist is moved, and why dynamic grip strength may be a more functional measurement. J Hand Ther 1999;12(3):212–218.

LaStayo PC, Wheeler DL. Reliability of passive wrist flexion and extension goniometric measurements: a multicenter study. Phys Ther 1994;74(2):162–174.

Latash ML. The Bernstein problem: how does the central nervous system make its choices? In Latash ML, Turvey MT, eds, Dexterity and its development, Mahwah, NJ: Lawrence Erlbaum, 1996:277–304.

Latash ML. Motor coordination in Down syndrome: the role of adaptive changes. In: Weeks DJ, Chua R, Elliott D, eds. Perceptual-motor behavior in Down syndrome. Champaign IL: Human Kinetics, 2000:199–223.

Latash ML, Anson JG. Synergies in health and disease: relations to adaptive changes in motor coordination. Phys Ther 2006;86:1151–1160.

Latash ML, Aruin AS, Neyman I, Nicholas JJ. Anticipatory postural adjustments during self inflicted and predictable perturbations in Parkinson's disease. J Neurol Neurosurg Psychiatry 1995;58(3):326–334.

Latash ML, Gelfand IM, Li ZM, Zatsiorsky VM. Changes in the force-sharing pattern induced by modifications of visual feedback during force production by a set of fingers. Exp Brain Res 1998; 123(3):255–262.

Latash ML, Krishnamoorthy V, Scholz J, Zatsiorsky VM. Postural synergies in development. Neural Plasticity 2005;12:119–130.

Latash ML, Kang N, Patterson D. Finger coordination in persons with Down syndrome: atypical patterns of coordination and the effects of practice. Exp Brain Res 2002;146:345–355.

Latash ML, Scholz JP, Schöner G. Motor control strategies revealed in the structure of motor variability. Exerc Sport Sci Rev 2002;30:26–31.

Latash ML, Scholz JP, Schöner G. Toward a new theory of motor synergies. Motor Control 2007;11:276–308.

Laufer Y. Effect of age on characteristics of forward and backward gait at preferred and accelerated walking speed. J Gerontol 2005;60A:627–632.

Laufer Y, Ashkenazi T, Josman N. The effects of a concurrent cognitive task on the postural control of young children with and wiout developmental coordination disorder. Gait Posture 2008;27:347–351.

Lavender G, Gentile AM. Constraint-induced therapy in children with hemiplegic cerebral palsy. Poster presentation at the annual conference, Teacher's College, Columbia University, New York, 1998.

Lavery JJ. Retention of simple motor skills as a function of type of knowledge of results. Can J Psychol 1962;16:300–311.

Law LS, Webb CY. Gait adaptation of children with cerebral palsy compared with control children when stepping over an obstacle. Dev Med Child Neurol 2005;47:321–328.

Law M, Baptiste S, Carswell A, et al. Canadian Occupational Performance Measure, 4th ed. Ottawa, ON: Canadian Association of Occupational Therapists, 2005.

Law M, King G, King S, et al. Patterns of participation in recreational and leisure activities among children with complex physical disabilities. Dev Med Child Neuro 2006;48:337–342.

Lawrence DG, Hopkins DA. Developmental aspects of pyramidal motor control in the rhesus monkey. Brain Res 1972;40:117–118.

Lawton MP. The functional assessment of elderly people. J Am Geriatr Soc 1971;19:465–481.

Lebiedowska MK, Syczewska M. Invariant sway properties in children. Gait Posture 2000;12:200–204.

Ledebt A, Bril B, Breniere Y. The build-up of anticipatory behavior: an analysis of the development of gait initiation in children. Exp Brain Res 1998;120:9–17.

Ledebt A, Bril B, Wiener-Vacher S. Trunk and head stabilization during the first months of independent walking. Neuroreport 1995;6:1737–1740.

Lee DN, Aronson E. Visual proprioceptive control of standing in human infants. Percept Psychophys 1974;15:529–532.

Lee DN, Lishman R. Visual proprioceptive control of stance. J Hum Mov Studies 1975;1:87–95.

Lee DN, Young DS. Gearing action to the environment. Experiments in Brain Research, Series 15. Berlin: Springer Verlag, 1986:217–230.

Lee HJ, Chou LS. Balance control during stair negotiation in older adults. J Biomech 2007;40:2530–2536.

Lee I, Manson J, Hennekens C, Paffenbarger R. Body weight and mortality: a 27 year follow up of middle aged men. JAMA 1993;270:2623–2628.

Lee RG, van Donkelaar P. Mechanisms underlying functional recovery following stroke. Can J Neurol Sci 1995;22:257–263.

Lee TD. Transfer-appropriate processing: a framework for conceptualizing practice effects in motor learning. In: Meijer OG, Roth K, eds. Complex movement behavior: the motor-action controversy. Amsterdam: North-Holland, 1988.

Lee W, Buchanan T, Rogers M. Effects of arm acceleration and behavioral conditions on the organization of postural adjustments during arm flexion. Exp Brain Res 1987;66:257–270.

Lee-Valkov PM, Aaron DH, Eladoumikdachi F, et al. Measuring normal hand dexterity values in normal 3-,4-, and 5-year-old children and their relationship with grip and pinch strength. J Hand Ther 2003;16(1):22–28.

Leicht AS, Crowther RG. Influence of non-level walking on pedometer accuracy. J Sci Med Sport 2009;12:361–365.

Leicht AS, Crowther RG. Pedometer accuracy during walking over different surfaces. Med Sci Sports Exerc 2007;39:1847–1850.

Lekhel H, Marchand AR, Assaiante C, et al. Cross-correlation analysis of the lateral hip strategy in unperturbed stance. Neuroreport 1994;5:1293–1296.

Lemon RN, Mantel GWH, Muir RB. Corticospinal facilitation of hand muscles during voluntary movements in the conscious monkey. J Physiol 1986;381:497–527.

Lemsky C, Miller CJ, Nevitt M, Winograd C. Reliability and validity of a physical performance and mobility examination for hospitalized elderly. Soc Gerontol 1991;31:221.

Leonard CT, Sandholdt DY, McMillan JA, Queen S. Short- and long-latency contributions to reciprocal inhibition during various levels of muscle contraction of individuals with cerebral palsy. J Child Neurol 2006;21:240–246.

Lerner-Frankiel MB, Vargas S, Brown MB, et al. Functional community ambulation: what are your criteria? Clin Manage 1990;6:12–15.

Levin MF. Interjoint coordination during pointing movements is disrupted in spastic hemiparesis. Brain 1996;119(Pt 1):281–293.

Levin MF, Horowitz M, Jurrius C, et al. Trajectory formation and interjoint coordination of drawing movements in normal and hemiparetic subjects. Neurosci Abstr 1993;19:990.

Levin MF, Michaelsen SM, Cirstea CM, Rob-Brami A. Use of the trunk for reaching targets placed within and beyond the reach in adult hemiparesis. Exp Brain Res 2002;143(2): 171–180.

Lewald J. More accurate sound localization induced by short-term light deprivation. Neuropsychologia 2007;45:1215–1222.

Lewek MD, Hornby TG, Dhaher YY, Schmit BD. Prolonged quadriceps activity following imposed hip extension: a neurophysiological mechanism for stiff-knee gait? J Neurophysiol 2007;98:3153–3162.

Lewis C, Bottomly J. Musculoskeletal changes with age. In: Lewis C, ed. Aging: health care's challenge, 2nd ed. Philadelphia: Davis, 1990:145–146.

Lewis GN, Byblow WD. Bimanual coordination dynamics in post stroke hemiparetics. J Motor Behav 2004;36:174–186.

Lezak MD. Neuropsycholoigcal assessment. New York: Oxford University Press, 1976.

Li S-C, Huxhold O, Schmiedek F. Aging and attenuated processing robustness. Gerontology 2004;50:28–34.

Liao HF, Hwang AW. Relations of balance function and gross motor ability for children with cerebral palsy. Percept Motor Skills 2003;96 (3 Pt 2):1173–1184.

Lieber RL, Runesson E, Einarsson F, Friden J. Inferior mechanical properties of spastic muscle bundles due to hypertrophic but compromised extracellular matrix material. Muscle Nerve 2003;28:464–471.

Lieber RL, Steinman S, Barash IA, Chambers H. Structural and functional changes in spastic skeletal muscle. Muscle Nerve 2004;29:615–627.

Liebesman JL, Carafelli E. Physiology of range of motion in human joints: a critical review. Crit Rev Phys Med Rehabil 1994;6:131–160.

Liepert J, Miltner WH, Bauder H, et al. Motor cortex plasticity during constraint-induced movement therapy in stroke patients. Neurosci Lett 1998;250:5–8.

Lin S-I, Woollacott MH. Differentiating postural responses following dynamically changing balance threats in young adults, healthy older adults and unstable older adults: electromyography. J Motor Behav 2002;34:37–44.

Lin S-I, Woollacott MH, Jensen J. Differentiating postural responses following dynamically changing balance threats in young adults, healthy older adults and unstable older adults: kinematics and kinetics. Aging Clin Exp Res 2004;16:369–374.

Lindenberger U, Marsiske M, Baltes PB. Memorizing while walking: increase in dual-task costs from young adulthood to old age. Psychol Aging 2000;15:417–436.

Lindholm L. Weight-bearing splint: a method for managing upper extremity spasticity. Phys Ther Forum 1985;5:3.

Lipsitz LA, Jonsson PV, Kelley MM, Koestner JS. Causes and correlates of recurrent falls in ambulatory frail elderly. J Gerontol 1991;46: M114–M122.

Liu W, Lipsitz LA, Montero-Odasso M, et al. Noise-enhanced vibrotactile sensitivity in older adults, patients with stroke, and patients with diabetic neuropathy. Arch Phys Med Rehabil 2002;83:171–176.

Liu-Ambrose T, Katarynych LA, Ashe MC, et al. Dual-task gait performance among community-dwelling senior women: the role of balance confidence and executive functions. J Gerontol A Biol Sci Med Sci 2009;64:975–982.

Livingstone M, Hubel D. Segregation of form, color, movement and depth: anatomy, physiology, perception. Science 1988;240:740–749.

Lloyd DG. Environmental requirements for elderly people to have stability underfoot while walking. Proceedings of the National Forum on Prevention of Falls and Injuries amongst Older People. Sydney, Australia, 1990.

Lockhart TE, Woldstad JC, Smith JL. Effects of age-related gait changes on the biomehcanics of slips and falls. Ergonomics 2003;46:1136–1160.

Loewen SC, Anderson BA. Predictors of stroke outcomes using objective measurement scales. Stroke 1990;21:78–81.

Lomaglio MJ, Eng JJ. Muscle strength and weight-bearing symmetry relate to sit-to-stand performance in individuals with stroke. Gait Posture 2005;22:126–131.

Lord S, Rochester L. Measurement of community ambulation after stroke: current status and future developments. Stroke 2005;36:1457–1461.

Lord S, Sherrington C, Menz HB. Falls in older people. Cambridge: Cambridge University Press, 2001:68.

Lord S, Ward J, Williams P, Anstey K. An epidemiological study of falls in older community dwelling women: the Randwick falls and fracture study. Aust J Public Health 1993;17: 240–245.

Lord SE, Halligan PW, Wade DT. Visual gait analysis: the development of a clinical assessment and scale. Clin Rehabil 1998;12:107–119.

Lord SE, McPherson K, McNaughton HK, et al. Community ambulation after stroke: how important and obtainable is it and what measures appear predictive? Arch Phys Med Rehabil 2004;86:234–239.

Lord SE, Rochester L, Weatherall M, et al. The effect of environment and task on gait parameters after stroke: A randomized comparison of measurement conditions. Arch Phys Med Rehabil 2006;87:967–973.

Lord SR, Lloyd DG, Li SK. Sensorimotor function, gait patterns and falls in community-dwelling women. Age Ageing 1996;25:292–299.

Lovejoy CO. Evolution of human walking. Sci Am 1988;5:121.

Lovely RG, Gregor RJ, Edgerton VR. Effects of training on the recovery of full-weight-bearing stepping in the adult spinal cat. Exp Neurol 1986;92:421–435.

Lu TW, Yen HC, Chen HL, et al. Symmetrical kinematic changes in highly functioning older patients post-stroke during obstacle-crossing. Gait Posture 2010;March 16. 2010;31:511–516.

Lu T, Pan Y, Kao SY, et al. Gene regulation and DNA damage in the ageing human brain. Nature, 2004;429:883–891.

Luft AR, Waller S, Forrester L, et al. Lesion location alters brain activation in chronically impaired stroke survivors. Neuroimage 2004;21:924–935.

Lum PS, Burgar CG, Shor PC. Evidence for improved muscle activation patterns after retraining of reaching movements with the MIME robotic system in subjects with post-stroke hemiparesis. IEEE Trans Neural Syst Rehabil Eng 2004;12(2):186–194.

Lundborg G, Bjorkman A, Hansson T, et al. Artificial sensibility of the hand based on cortical audiotactile interaction: a study using functional magnetic resonance imaging. Scand J Plast Reconstr Surg Hand Surg 2005;39(6):370–372.

Lundgren-Lindquist B, Aniansson A, Rundgren A. Functional studies in 79 year olds: 3. Walking performance and climbing ability. Scand J Rehabil Med 1983;12:107–112.

Lundin-Olsson L, Nyberg L, Gustafson Y. Stops walking when talking as a predictor of falls in elderly people. Lancet 1997;349:617.

Luria AR. Higher cortical functions in man. New York: Basic, 1966.

Ly DH, Lockhart DJ, Lerner RA, Schultz PG. Mitotic misregulation and human aging. Science 2000;287:2486–2492.

Lyle RC. A performance test for assessment of upper limb function in physical rehabilitation treatment and research. Int J Rehabil Res 1981;4:483–492.

M

Ma HI, Trombly CA. A synthesis of the effects of occupational therapy for persons with stroke, Part II: Remediation of impairments. Am J Occup Ther 2002;56(3):260–274.

MacKay DG. The problem of flexibility, fluency, and the speed- accuracy trade-off in skilled behavior. Psychol Rev 1982; 89:48–506.

MacKay-Lyons M. Variability in spatiotemporal gait characteristics over the course of the L-dopa cycle in people with advanced Parkinson disease. Phys Ther 1998;78:1083–1094.

Mackey AH, Walt SE, Stott NS. Deficits in upper-limb task performance in children with hemiplegic cerebral palsy as defined by 3-dimensional kinematics. Arch Phys Med Rehabil 2006;87:207–215.

Macpherson J. The neural organization of postural control: do muscle synergies exist? In: Amblard B, Berthoz A, Clarac F, eds. Posture and gait: development, adaptation and modulation. Amsterdam: Elsevier, 1988:381–390. Massion J, Woollacott M. Normal balance and postural control. In: Bronstein AM, Brandt T, Woollacott M. Clinical aspects of balance and gait disorders. London: Edward Arnold, 2004.

Macpherson JM, Fung J, Jacobs R. Postural orientation, equilibrium and the spinal cord. In: Seil FJ, ed. Advances in neurology, vol. 72. Neuronal regeneration, reorganization, and repair. Philadelphia: Lippincott-Raven, 1997:227–232.

Macpherson JM, Fung J. Weight support and balance during postural stance in the chronic spinal cat. J Neurophysiol 1999;82:3060–3081.

Maddox WT, Ashby FG. Dissociating explicit and procedural-learning based systems of perceptual category learning. Behav Proc 2004;66: 309–332.

Magee DJ. Orthopedic physical assessment. Philadelphia: Saunders, 1987.

Magill RA, Hall KG. A review of the contextual interference effect in motor skill acquisition. Hum Mov Sci 1990;9:241–289.

Magnus R. Animal posture (Croonian lecture). Proc R Soc Lond 1925;98:339.

Magnus R. Some results of studies in the physiology of posture. Lancet 1926;2:531–585.

Magnusson M, Enbom H, Johansson R, Wiklund J. Significance of pressor input from the human feet in lateral postural control: the effect of hypothermia on galvanically induced body-sway. Acta Otolaryngol 1990;110:321–327.

Mahoney FI, Barthel DW. Functional evaluation: the Barthel Index. Md State Med J 1965;14: 61–65.

Majsak MJ, Kaminski T, Gentile AM, Gordon AM. Effects of a moving target versus a temporal constraint on reach and grasp in patients with Parkinson's disease. Exp Neurol 2008;210: 479–488.

Mak MK, Hui-Chan CW. Switching of movement direction is central to parkinsonian bradykinesia in sit-to-stand. Mov Disord 2002;17:1188–1195.

Mak MK, Levin O, Mizrahi J, Hui-Chan CW. Joint torques during sit-to-stand in healthy subjects and people with Parkinson's disease. Clin Biomech (Bristol, Avon) 2003;18:197–206

Mak MK, Patla A, Hui-Chan C. Sudden turn during walking is impaired in people with Parkinson's disease. Exp Brain Res 2008;190:43–51.

Maki B, Holliday PJ, Topper AK. Fear of falling and postural performance in the elderly. J Gerontol 1991;46:M123–M131.

Maki B, McIlroy W, Perry S. Compensatory responses to multi-directional perturbations. In: Taguchi K, Igarashi M, Mori S, eds. Vestibular and neural front. Amsterdam: Elsevier, 1994b:437–440.

Maki BE, McIlroy WE. Control of rapid limb movements for balance recovery: age-related changes and implications for fall prevention. Age Ageing 2006;35-S2:ii12–ii18.

Maldonado M, Allred RP, Felthauser EL, Jones TA. Motor skill training, but not voluntary exercise, improves skilled reaching after unilateral ischemic lesions of the sensorimotor cortex in rats. Neurorehabil Neural Repair 2008;22:250–261.

Malfait N, Ostry DJ. Is interlimb transfer of force-field adaptation a cognitive response to the sudden introduction of load? J Neurosci 2004;24:8084–8089.

Malick M. Manual on static hand splinting. Pittsburgh: Harmarville Rehab Center, 1980.

Malouin F, McFadyen B, Dion L, Richards CL. A fluidity scale for evaluating the motor strategy of the rise to walk task after stroke. Clin Rehabil 2003;17:674–684 [appendix].

Malouin F, Pichard L, Bonneau C, et al. Evaluating motor recovery early after stroke: comparison of the Fugl-Meyer Assessment and the Motor Assessment Scale. Arch Phys Med Rehabil 1994;75:1206–1212.

Malviya S, Voepel-Lewis T, Burke C, et al. The revised FLACC observational pain tool: improved reliability and validity assessment in children with cognitive impairment. Paediatr Anaesth 2006;16(3):258–265.

Man'kovskii NB, Mints AY, Lysenyuk VP. Regulation of the preparatory period for complex voluntary movement in old and extreme old age. Hum Physiol Moscow 1980;6:46–50.

Manchester D, Woollacott M, Zederbauer-Hylton N, Marin O. Visual, vestibular and somatosensory contributions to balance control in the older adult. J Gerontol 1989;44:M118–M127.

Mancini M, Rocchi l, Horak FB, Chiari L. Effects of Parkinson's disease and levodopa on functional limits of stability. Clin Biomech 2008;23:450–458.

Manheim CJ, Lavett DK. The myofascial release manual. Thorofare, NJ: Slack, 1989.

Mann RA, Hagy JL, White V, Liddell D. The initiation of gait. J Bone Joint Surg Am 1979;61: 232–239.

Mannheimer JS, Lampe GN. Clinical transcutaneous electrical nerve stimulation. Philadelphia: Davis, 1984.

Manns PJ, Baldwin E. Ambulatory activity of stroke survivors: measurement options for dose, intensity, and variability of activity. Stroke 2009;40:864–867.

Marchese R, Bove M, Abbruzzese G. Effect of cognitive and motor tasks on postural stability in Parkinson's disease: a posturographic study. Mov Disord 2003;18:652–658.

Marchetti GF, Whitney SL, Blatt PJ, et al. Temporal and spatial characteristics of gait during performance of the Dynamic Gait Index in people with and people without balance or vestibular disorders. Phys Ther 2008;88:640–651.

Margaria R. Biomechanics and energetics of muscular exercise. Oxford: Clarendon, 1976:67–74.

Marigold DS, Eng JJ, Dawson AS, et al. Exercise leads to faster postural reflexes, improved balance and mobility, and fewer falls in older persons with chronic stroke. J Am Geriatr Soc 2005;53:416–423.

Marigold DS, Eng JJ, Tokuno CD, Donnelly CA. Contribution of muscle strength and integration of afferent input to postural instability in persons with stroke. Neurorehabil Neural Repair 2004;18(4):222–229.

Marigold DS, Eng JJ. Altered timing of postural reflexes contributes to falling in persons with chronic stroke. Exp Brain Res 2006;171: 459–468.

Marigold DS, Misiaszek JE. Whole-body responses: neural control and implications for rehabilitation and fall prevention. Neuroscientist 2009;15:36–46.

Marigold DS, Patla AE. Strategies for dynamic stability during locomotion on a slippery surface: effects of prior experience and knowledge. J Neurophysiol 2002;88:339–353.

Marque P, Felez A, Puel M, et al. Impairment and recovery of left motor function in patients with right hemiplegia. J Neurol Neurosurg Psychiatry 1997;62:77–81.

Marsden CD, Merton PA, Morton HB. Anticipatory postural responses in the human subject. J Physiol 1977;275:47P–48P.

Marsden CD, Quinn NP. The dystonias. BMJ 1990;300:139–144.

Marsden CD. Slowness of movement in Parkinson's disease. Mov Disord 1989;4:26–37.

Marteniuk RG, Leavitt JL, Mackenzie CL, Athenes S. Functional relationships between grasp and transport components in a prehension task. Hum Mov Sci 1990;9:149–176.

Marteniuk RG, Mackenzie CL, Jeannerod M, et al. Constraints on human arm movements trajectories. Can J Psychol 1987;41:365–368.

Martin JH, Donarummo L, Hacking A. Impairments in prehension produced by early postnatal sensory motor cortex activity blockage. J Neurophysiol 2000;83:895–906.

Martin JH, Kably B, Hacking A. Activity-dependent development of cortical axon terminations in the spinal cord and brain stem. Exp Brain Res 1999;125:184–199.

Martin JP. The basal ganglia and posture. London: Pitman, 1967.

Martin TA, Keating JG, Goodkin HP, et al. Storage of multiple gaze-hand calibrations. Neurosci Abstr 1993;19:980.

Masiero S, Celia A, Rosati G, Armani M. Robotic-assisted rehabilitation of the upper limb after acute stroke. Arch Phys Med Rehabil 2007;88(2):142–149.

Massion J. Movement, posture and equilibrium: interaction and coordination. Prog Neurobiol 1992;38(1):35–36.

Massion J. Role of motor cortex in postural adjustments associated with movement. In: Asanuma H, Wilson VJ, eds. Integration in the nervous system. Tokyo: Igaku-Shoin, 1979:239–260.

Mathias S, Nayak U, Issacs B. Balance in elderly patients: the "Get-up and Go" test. Arch Phys Med Rehabil 1986;67:387–389.

Mathiowetz V, Bolding DJ, Trombly CA. Immediate effects of positioning devices on the normal and spastic hand measured by electromyography. Am J Occup Ther 1983;37(4):247–254.

Mathiowetz V, Rogers SL, Dowe-Keval M, et al. The Purdue Pegboard: norms for 14- to 19-year olds. Am J Occup Ther 1986;40(3):174–179.

Mathiowetz V, Weber K, Kashman N, Volland G. Adult norms for the Nine Hole Peg Test of finger dexterity. Occup Ther J Res 1985;5: 24–38.

Matsuda PN, Bamer A, Shumway-Cook A, et al. Falls in multiple sclerosis: incidence, risk factors and provider response(Abstract). 61st Annual Meeting of the American Academy of Neurology 2009; Seattle, Washington, USA.

Maurer GL, Jezek SM. Pain assessment in clinical assessment recommendations, 2nd ed. Chicago: American Society of Hand Therapists, 1992.

Mauritz KH, Dichgans J, Hufschmidt A. Quantitative analysis of stance in late cortical cerebellar atrophy of the anterior lobe and other forms of cerebellar ataxia. Brain 1979;102:461–482.

May D, Nayak US, Isaacs B. The life space diary: a measure of mobility in old people at home. Int Rehabil Med 1985;7:182–186.

Mayer NH, Esquenazi A, Childers MK. Common patterns of clinical motor dysfunction. Muscle Nerve 1997;6:S21–S35.

Mayer NH. Clinicophysiologic concepts of spasticity and motor dysfunction in adults with upper motoneuron lesion. Muscle Nerve 1997;6(Suppl):S1–S13.

Mayo NE, Goldberg MS, Levy AR, Danys I, Korner-Bitensky N. Changing rates of stroke in the province of Quebec Canada: 1981–1988. Stroke 1991;22:590–595.

Mayston M. The Bobath concept: evolution and application. In: Forssberg H, Hirschfeld H, eds. Movement disorders in children. Medicine and sport science, vol. 36. Basel: S. Karger, 1992:1–6.

McCarty ME, Clifton RK, Collard RR. Problem solving in infancy: the emergence of an action plan. Devel Psychol 1999;35:1091–1101.

McChesney JW, Woollacott MH. The effect of age-related declines in proprioception and total knee replacement on postural control. J Gerontol 2000;55:658–666.

McCombe-Waller S, Whitall J. Fine motor control in adults with and without chronic hemiparesis: baseline comparison to nondisabled adults and effects of bilateral arm training. Arch Phys Med Rehabil 2004;85:1076–1083.

McConvey J, Bennett SE. Reliability of the dynamic gait index in individuals with multiple sclerosis. Arch Phys Med Rehabil 2005;86: 130–133.

McCoy AO, VanSant AF. Movement patterns of adolescents rising from a bed. Phys Ther 1993;73:182–

McCrea DA, Rybak IA. Organization of mammalian locomotor rhythm and pattern generation. Brain Res Rev 2008;57:134–146.

McCrea PH, Eng JJ, Hodgson AJ. Saturated muscle activation contributes to compensatory reaching strategies after stroke. J Neurophysiol 2005;94:2999–3008.

McCullagh P, Weiss MR, Ross D. Modeling considerations in motor skill acquisition and performance: an integrated approach. Exer Sport Sci Rev 1989;17:475–513.

McCulloch K. Attention and dual-task conditions: physical therapy implications for individuals with acquired brain injury. J Neurol Phys Ther 2007;31:104–118.

McDonnell PM. Patterns of eye-hand coordination in the first year of life. Can J Psychol 1979;33:253–267.

McDowell BC, Kerr C, Kelly C, et al. The validity of an existing gait classification system when applied to a representative population of children with hemiplegia. Gait Posture 2008;28:442–447.

McFadyen BJ, Malouin F, Dumas F. Anticipatory locomotor control for obstacle avoidance in mid-childhood aged children. Gait Posture 2001;13:7–16.

McFadyen BJ, Winter DA. An integrated biomechanical analysis of normal stair ascent and descent. J Biomech 1988;21:733–744.

McGavin CR, Gupta SP, McHardy GJR. Twelve minute walking test for assessing disability in chronic bronchitis. BMJ 1976;1:822–823.

McGough E. A comparison of clinical reasoning strategies used by expert versus novice physical therapists during gait analysis, unpublished Master's thesis, University of Washington, 2005.

McGraw M. The neuromuscular maturation of the human infant. New York: Hafner Press, 1945.

McGraw MB. From reflex to muscular control in the assumption of an erect posture and ambulation in the human infant. Child Dev 1932;3:291.

McIlroy W, Maki B. Do anticipatory adjustments precede compensatory stepping reactions evoked by perturbation? Neurosci Lett 1993;164:199–202.

McKee KJ, Orbell S, Austin CA, et al. Fear of falling, falls efficacy, and health outcomes in older people following hip fracture. Disabil Rehabil 2002;24(6):327–333.

McKinnon CD, Winter DA. Control of body balance in the frontal plane during human walking. J Biomech 1993;26:633–644.

McLellan DL. Co-contraction and stretch reflex in spasticity during treatment with baclofen. Neurol Neurosurg Psychiatry 1973;40:30–38.

McMahon TA. Muscles, reflexes and locomotion. Princeton, NJ: Princeton University, 1984.

McNevin NH, Shea CH, Wulf G. Increasing the distance of an external focus of attention enhances learning. Psychol Res 2003;67:22–29.

McNevin NH, Wulf G, Carlson C. Effects of attentional focus, self-control, and dyad training on motor learning: implications for physical rehabilitation. Phys Ther 2000;80:373–385.

McNevin NH, Wulf G. Attentional focus on suprapostural tasks affects postural control. Hum Mov Sci 2002;21:187–202

McPherson J, Schild R, Spaulding SJ, et al. Analysis of upper extremity movement in four sitting positions: a comparison of persons with and without cerebral palsy. Am J Occup Ther 1991;2:123–129.

McVea DA, Pearson KG. Object avoidance during locomotion. Adv Exp Med Biol 2009;629: 293–315.

Medina JJ. The clock of ages. New York: Cambridge University Press, 1996.

Meier A. Rehabilitation following falls of undetermined etiology: results of an intervention study. Schweiz Rundsch Med Prax 1992;81: 1405–1410.

Melmoth DR, Finlay AL, Morgan MJ, Grant S. Grasping deficits and adaptations in adults with stereo vision losses. Invest Ophthalmol Vis Sci 2009;50:3711–3720.

Melville-Jones G, Mandl G. Neurobionomics of adaptive plasticity: integrating sensorimotor function with environmental demands. In: Desmedt JE, ed. Motor control mechanisms in health and disease. Adv Neurol 1983;39: 1047–1071.

Melzack R. The McGill Pain Questionnaire: major properties and scoring methods. Pain 1975;1:277–299.

Mercer VS, Freburger JK, Change S, Pursure JL. Step test scores are related to measures of activity and participation in the first 6 months after stroke. Phys Ther 2009;89:1061–1071.

Merkel S, Voepel-Lewis T, Malviva S. Pain assessment in infants and young children: the FLACC scale. Am J Nurs 2002;102(10):55–58.

Merskey H, Lindblom U, Mumford JM, et al. Classification of chronic pain: descriptions of chronic pain syndromes and definitions of pain terms. Pain 1986;Suppl 3:S215–S221.

Merzenich MM, Jenkins WM. Reorganization of cortical representation of the hand following alterations of skin inputs induced by nerve injury, skin island transfers & experience. J Hand Ther 1993;6(2):89–104.

Merzenich MM, Kaas JH, Wall J, et al. Topographic reorganization of somatosensory cortical areas 3b and 1 in adult monkeys following restricted deafferentation. Neuroscience 1983a;8: 33–55.

Merzenich MM, Kaas JH, Wall JT, et al. Progression of change following median nerve section in the cortical representation of the hand in areas 3b and 1 in adult owl and squirrel monkeys. Neuroscience 1983b;10:639–665.

Messier S, Bourbonnais D, Desrosiers J, Roy Y. Dynamic analysis of trunk flexion after stroke. Arch Phys Med Rehabil 2004;85:1619–1624.

Metaxiotis D, Accles W, Siebel A, Doederlein L. Hip deformities in walking patients with cerebral palsy. Gait Posture 2000;11:86–91.

Meyer DE, Abrams RA, Kornblum S, et al. Optimality in human motor performance: ideal control of rapid aimed movements. Psychol Rev 1988;95:340–370.

Meyer JS, Obara K, Muramatsu K, et al. Cognitive performance after small strokes correlates with ischemia, not atrophy of the brain. Dementia 1995;6:312–322.

Micera S, Carpaneto J, Posteraro F, et al. Characterization of upper arm synergies during reaching tasks in able-bodied and hemiparetic subjects. Clin Biomech 2005;20:939–946.

Michael KM, Allen JK, Macko RF. Reduced activity after stroke: the role of balance, gait, and cardiovascular fitness. Arch Phys Med Rehabil 2005;86:1552–1556.

Michaelsen SM, Dannenbaum R, Levin MF. Task-specific training with trunk restraint on arm recovery in stroke: randomized control trial. Stroke 2006;37:186–192.

Michaelsen SM, Jacobs S, Roby-Braimi, Levin MF. Compensation for distal impairments of grasping in adults with hemiparesis. Exp Brain Res 2004;157:162–173.

Michaelsen SM, Levin MF. Short-term effects of practice with trunk restraint on reaching movements in patients with chronic stroke: a controlled trial. Stroke 2004;35:1914–1919.

Michaelsen SM, Magdalon EC, Levin MF. Grip aperture scaling to object size in chronic stroke. Motor Control 2009;13:197–217.

Middleton FA, Strick PL. Anatomical evidence for cerebellar and basal ganglia involvement in higher cognitive function. Science 1994;266:458–461.

Milani-Comparetti A, Gidoni EA. Pattern analysis of motor development and its disorders. Dev Med Child Neurol 1967;9:625–630.

Milczarek JJ, Kirby RL, Harrison ER, MacLeod DA. Standard and four-footed canes: their effect on the standing balance of patients with hemiparesis. Arch Phys Med Rehabil 1993;74:281–285.

Miller PH. Theories of developmental psychology, 4th Edition. New York: Worth Publishers, 2002.

Millington PJ, Myklebust BM, Shambes GM. Biomechanical analysis of the sit-to-stand motion in elderly persons. Arch Phys Med Rehabil 1992;73:609–617.

Milner AD, Goodale MA. Visual pathways to perception and action. Prog Brain Res 1993;95: 317–337.

Milner AD, Ockleford EM, Dewar W. Visuo-spatial performance following posterior parietal and lateral frontal lesions in stumptail macaques. Cortex 1977;13:350–360.

Milner B. Amnesia following operation on the temporal lobes. In: Whitty CWM, Zangwill OL, eds. Amnesia. London: Butterworths, 1966: 109–133.

Milot MH, Nadeau S, Gravel D, Bourbonnais D. Effect of increases in plantarflexor and hip flexor muscle strength on the levels of effort during gait in individuals with hemiparesis. Clin Biomech (Bristol, Avon) 2008;23:415–423.

Miltner W, Bauder H, Sommer M, et al. Effects of constraint-induced movement therapy on patients with chronic motor deficits after stroke. Stroke 1999;30:586–592.

Milton JG, Small SS, Solodkin A. On the road to automatic: dynamic aspects in the development of expertise. J Clin Neurophysiol 2004; 21:134–143.

Mirbagheri MM, Barbeau H, Ladouceur M, Kearney RE. Intrinsic and reflex stiffness in normal and spastic, spinal cord injured subjects. Exp Brain Res 2001;141:446–459.

Mishkin M, Ungerleider LG. Contribution of striate inputs to the visuospatial functions of parieto-preoccipital cortex in monkeys. Behav Brain Res 1982; 6:57–77

Miszko TA, Cress ME, Slade JM, et al. Effect of strength and power training on physical function in community-dwelling older adults. J Gerontol A Biol Sci Med Sci 2003;58:171–175.

Miyai I, Fujimoto Y, Yamamoto H, et al. Long term effect of body weight supported treadmill training in Parkinson's disease: a randomized controlled trial. Arch Phys Med Rehabil 2002;83:1370–1373.

Moberg E. The unsolved problem—how to test the functional value of hand sensibility. J Hand Ther 1991;4:105–110.

Mochon S, McMahon TA. Ballistic walking. J Biomech 1980;13:49–57.

Mockford M, Caulton JM. Systematic review of progressive strength training in children and adolescents with cerebral palsy who are ambulatory. Pediatr Phys Ther 2008;20(4):318–333.

Mok NW, Brauer SG, Hodges PW. Hip strategy for balance control in quiet standing is reduced in people with low back pain. Spine 2004;29:E107–E112.

Molen HH. Problems on the evaluation of gait. Dissertation, Free University, Institute of Biomechanics and Experimental Rehabilitation, Amsterdam,1973.

Molinari M, Leggio MG, Solida A. Cerebellum and procedural learning: evidence from focal cerebellar lesions. Brain 1997;120:1753–1762.

Monger C, Carr JH, Fowler V. Evaluation of a home-based exercise and training programme to improve sit-to-stand in patients with chronic stroke. Clin Rehabil 2002;16:361–367.

Montgomery J. Assessment and treatment of locomotor deficits in stroke. In: Duncan PW, Badke MB. Stroke rehabilitation: the recovery of motor control. Chicago: Year Book, 1987:223–259.

Monzee J, Lamarre Y, Smith AM. The effects of digital anesthesia on force control using a precision grip. J Neurophysiol 2003;89:672–683.

Monzee J, Smith AM. Responses of cerebellar interpositus neurons to predictable perturbations applied to an object held in a precision grip. J Neurophysiol 2004;91:1230–1239.

Moore S, Brunt D, Nesbitt ML, Juarez T. Investigation of evidence for anticipatory postural adjustments in seated subjects who performed a reaching task. Phys Ther 1992;72:335–343.

Morasso P. Spatial control of arm movements. Exp Brain Res 1981;42:223–227.

Morgan M, Phillips JG, Bradshaw JL, et al. Age-related motor slowness: simply strategic? J Gerontol 1994;49:M133–M139.

Morgan P. The relationship between sitting balance and mobility outcomes in stroke. Aust J Physiother 1994;40:91–96.

Morris DM, Uswatte G, Crago JE, et al. The reliability of the Wolf motor function test for assessing upper extremity function after stroke. Arch Phys Med Rehabil 2001;82:750–755.

Morris JC, Rubin EH, Morris EJ. Senile dementia of the Alzheimer's type: an important risk factor for serious falls. J Gerontol 1987;42:412–417.

Morris ME, Iansek R, Matyas TA, Summers JJ. Stride length regulation in Parkinson's disease: normalization strategies and underlying mechanisms. Brain 1996;119:551–569.

Morris ME, Iansek R, Smithson F, Husham F. Postural instability in Parkinson's disease: a comparison with and without a concurrent task. Gait Posture 2000;12:205–216.

Morris ME, Martin CL, Schenkman ML. Striding out with Parkinson disease: Evidence based physical therapy for gait disorders. Phys Ther 2010;90:280–288.

Morris RGM, Anderson E, Lynch GS, Baudry M. Selective impairment of learning and blockage of long-term potentiation by an N-methyl-D-aspartate receptor antagonist, AP5. Nature 1986;319:774–776.

Morris SL, Dodd KJ, Morris ME. Outcomes of progressive resistance strength training following stroke: a systematic review. Clin Rehabil 2004;18(1):27–39.

Mortenson PA, Eng JJ. The use of casts in the management of joint mobility and hypertonia following brain injury in adults: a systematic review. Phys Ther 2003;83:648–658.

Morton SM, Bastian AJ. Cerebellar control of balance and locomotion. Neuroscientist 2004;10:247–259.

Morton SM, Bastian AJ. Mechanisms of cerebellar gait ataxia. Cerebellum 2007;6:79–86.

Morton SM, Bastian AJ. Relative contributions of balance and voluntary leg-coordination deficits to cerebellar gait ataxia. J Neurophysiol 2003;89:1844–1856.

Moseley AM, Lanzarone S, Bosman JM, et al. Ecological validity of walking speed assessment after traumatic brain injury: a pilot study. J Head Trauma Rehabil 2004;19:341–348.

Moseley AM, Stark A, Cameron ID, Pollock A. Treadmill training and body weight support for walking after stroke. Cochrane Database Syst Rev 2003;3:CD002840.

Mott FW, Sherrington CS. Experiments upon the influence of sensory nerves upon movement and nutrition of the limbs: preliminary communication. Proc R Soc Lond Biol 1895;57: 481–488.

Mouchnino L, Aurenty R, Massion J, Pedotti A. Coordination between equilibrium and head-trunk orientation during leg movement: a new strategy built up by training. J Neurophysiol 1992;67:1587–1599.

Mourey F, Grishin A, d'Athis P, et al. Standing up from a chair as a dynamic equilibrium task: a comparison between young and elderly subjects. J Gerontol 2000;55:B425–B431.

Msall ME, DiGaudio K, Rogers BT, et al. Functional Independence Measure for Children (WeeFIM): conceptual basis and pilot use in children with developmental disabilities. Clin Pediatr 1994;33:421–430.

Msall ME, Ottenbacher K, Duffy L, et al. Reliability and validity of the WeeFim in children with neurodevelopmental disabilities. Pediatr Res 1996;39(4):378.

Mudge S, Barber PA, Stott NS. Circuit-based rehabilitation improves gait endurance but not usual walking activity in chronic stroke: a randomized controlled trial. Arch Phys Med Rehabil 2009;90:1989–1994.

Mudge S, Stott NS, Walt SE. Criterion validity of the StepWatch Activity Monitor as a measure of walking activity in patients after stroke. Arch Phys Med Rehabil 2007;88:1710–1715.

Mudge S, Stott NS. Timed walking tests correlate with daily step activity in persons with stroke. Arch Phys Med Rehabil 2009;90:296–301.

Mudie MH, Matyas TA. Can simultaneous bilateral movement involve the undamaged hemisphere in reconstruction of neural networks damaged by stroke? Disabil Rehabil 2000; 22(1–2):23–37.

Mudie MH, Matyas TA. Reposnses of the densely hemiplegic upper extremity to bilateral training. Neurorehabil Neural Repair 2001;15: 129–140.

Muir RB, Lemon RN. Corticospinal neurons with a special role in precision grip. Brain Res 1983;261:312–316.

Muir SW, Berg K, Chesworth B, Speechley M. Use of the Berg Balance Scale for predicting multiple falls in community dwelling elderly people: A prospective study. Phys Ther 2008; 88:449–459.

Mulcahey MJ, Betz RR, Kozin SH, et al.. Implantation of the Freehand System during initial rehabilitation using minimally invasive techniques. Spinal Cord 2004a;42(3):46–55.

Mulcahey MJ, Smith BT, Betz RR. Psychometric rigor of the Grasp and Release Test for measuring functional limitation of persons with tetraplegia: a preliminary analysis. J Spinal Cord Med 2004b;27(1):41–46.

Mulder T, Berndt H, Pauwels J, Nienhuis B. Sensorimotor adaptability in the elderly and disabled. In: Stelmach G, Homberg V, eds. Sensori-motor impairment in the elderly. Dordrecht, the Netherlands: Kluwer, 1993.

Mulroy S, Gronley J, Weiss W, et al. Use of cluster analysis for gait pattern classification of patients in early and late recovery phases following stroke. Gait Posture 2003;18:114–125.

Mulroy SJ, Klassen T, Gronley JK, et al. Gait parameters associated with responsiveness to treadmill training with body weight support after stroke: an exploratory study. Phys Ther 2010;90:209–223.

Muratori LM, Dapul G, Bartels MN, Gordon AM. Effect of object transport on grasp coordination in multiple system atrophy. Mov Disord 2006;21:555–563.

Murray M, Kory R, Sepic S. Walking patterns of normal women. Arch Phys Med Rehabil 1970;51:637–650.

Murray MP, Kory RC, Clarkson BH, Sepic SB. Comparison of free and fast speed walking patterns of normal men. Am J Phys Med 1966; 45:8–24.

Murray MP, Kory RC, Clarkson BH. Walking patterns in healthy older men. J Gerontol 1969;24:169–178.

Murray MP, Mollinger LA, Gardner GM, Sepic SB. Kinematic and EMG patterns during slow, free, and fast walking. J Orthop Res 1984;2: 272–280.

Murray MP. Gait as a total pattern of movement. Am J Phys Med 1967;46:290–333.

Mushiake H, Inase M, Tanji J. Neuronal activity in the primate premotor, supplementary and precentral motor cortex during visually guided and internally determined sequential movements. J Neurophysiol 1991;66:705–718.

Mushiake H, Strick P. Preferential activity of dentate neurons during limb movements guided by vision. J Neurophysiol 1993;70:2660–2664.

Mutlu A, Livanelioglu A, Gunel K. Reliability of Ashworth and Modified Ashworth Scales in children with spastic cerebral palsy. BMC Musculoskel Disord 2008;9:44–51.

Mutsaarts M, Steenbergen B, Bekkering H. Anticipatory planning deficits and task context effects in hemiparetic cerebral palsy. Exp Brain Res 2006;172:151–162.

N

Nadeau S, Gravel D, Arsenault AB, et al. Dynamometric assessment of the plantarflexors in hemiparetic subjects: relations between muscular, gait and clinical parameters. Scand J Rehabil Med 1997;29:137–146.

Nagi S. Disability concepts revised: Implications for prevention. In IOM. Disability in America: Washington DC: National Academy Press, 1991. Toward a National Agenda for Prevention.

Nagi SZ. Some conceptual issues in disability and rehabilitation. In: Sussman MD, ed. Sociology and rehabilitation. Washington, DC: American Sociological Association, 1965:100–113.

Nambu A, Tokuno H, Takada M. Functional significance of the cortico-subthalamopallidal 'hyperdirect' pathway. Neurosci Res 2002;43:111–117.

Napier JR. The prehensile movement of the human hand. J Bone Joint Surg Br 1956;38:902–913.

Narici MV, Maffulli N, Maganaris CN. Ageing of human muscles and tendons. Disabil Rehabil 2008;30:1548–1554.

Nashner L. Adapting reflexes controlling the human posture. Exp Brain Res 1976;26:59–72.

Nashner L, Woollacott M. The organization of rapid postural adjustments of standing humans: an experimental-conceptual model. In: Talbott RE, Humphrey DR, eds. Posture and movement. New York: Raven, 1979:243–257.

Nashner L, Woollacott M, Tuma G. Organization of rapid responses to postural and locomotor-like perturbations of standing man. Exp Brain Res 1979;36:463–476.

Nashner LM. Fixed patterns of rapid postural responses among leg muscles during stance. Exp Brain Res 1977;30:13–24.

Nashner LM. Balance adjustment of humans perturbed while walking. J Neurophysiol 1980;44:650–664.

Nashner LM. Adaptation of human movement to altered environments. Trends Neurosci 1982;5:358–361.

Nashner LM. Sensory, neuromuscular, and biomechanical contributions to human balance. In: Duncan P, ed. Balance: Proceedings of the APTA Forum. Alexandria, VA: American Physical Therapy Association, 1989:5–12.

Nashner LM, Shumway-Cook A, Marin O. Stance posture control in select groups of children with cerebral palsy: deficits in sensory organization and muscular coordination. Exp Brain Res 1983;49:393–409.

Negrotti A, Secchi C, Gentilucci M. Effects of disease progression and L-dopa therapy on the control of reaching-grasping in Parkinson's disease. Neuropsychologia 2005;43:450–459.

Neistadt ME. A critical analysis of occupational therapy approaches for perceptual deficits in adults with brain injury. Am J Occup Ther 1990;44:299–304.

Nelson SR, DiFabio RP, Anderson JH. Vestibular and sensory interaction deficits assessed by dynamic platform posturography in patients with multiple sclerosis. Ann Otol Rhinol 1995;104:62–68.

Neptune RR, Kautz SA, Zajac FE. Contributions of the individual ankle plantar flexors to support, forward progression and swing initiation during walking. J Biomech 2001;34:1387–1398.

Neuhaus BE, Ascher B, Coullon M, et al. A survey of rationales for and against hand splinting in hemiplegia. Am J Occup Ther 1981;35:83–95.

Neumann O. Automatic processing: a review of recent findings and a plea for an old theory. In: Prinz W, Sanders AF, eds. Cognition and motor processes. Berlin: Springer Verlag, 1984:255–293.

Nevitt MC, Cummings SR, Kidd S, Black D. Risk factors for reMW recurrent nonsyncopal falls. JAMA 1989;261:2663–2668.

Newell A, Rosenbloom PS. Mechanisms of skill acquisition and the law of practice. In: Anderson JR, ed. Cognitive skills and their acquisition. Hillsdale, NJ: Erlbaum, 1981:1–55.

Newell K, van Emmerik REA. The acquisition of coordination: preliminary analysis of learning to write. Hum Mov Sci 1989;8:17–32.

Newell K. Degrees of freedom and the development of center of pressure profiles. In: Newell KM, Molenaar PMC, eds. Applications of nonlinear dynamics to developmental process modeling. Hillsdale, NJ: Erlbaum, 1997:63–84.

Newell KM. Motor skill acquisition. Annu Rev Psychol 1991;42:213–237.

Newell KM, Carlton LG, Hancock PA. Kinetic analysis of response variability. Psychol Bull 1984;96:133–151.

Newell KM, Kennedy JA. Knowledge of results and children's motor learning. Dev Psychol 1978;14:531–536.

Newell KM, Vaillancourt DE. Dimensional change in motor learning. Hum Move Sci 2001;20: 695–715.

Newton R. Validity of the Multi-Directional Reach Test: a practical measure for limits of stability in older adults. J Gerontol Med Sci 2001; 56A:M248–M252.

Ng SS, Hui-Chan CW. The Timed Up & Go test: its reliability and association with lower-limb impairments and locomotor capacities in people with chronic stroke. Arch Phys Med Rehabil 2005;86:1641–1647.

Nichols D, Case-Smith J. Reliability and validity of the Pediatric Evaluation of Disability Inventory. Ped Phys Ther 1996;8(1):15–24.

Nilsagård Y, Denison E, Gunnarsson LG, Boström K. Factors perceived as being related to accidental falls by persons with multiple sclerosis. Disabil Rehabil 2009a;31(16):1301–1310.

Nilsagård Y, Lundholm C, Denison E, Gunnarsson LG. Predicting accidental falls in people with multiple sclerosis – a longitudinal study. Clin Rehabil 2009b;23(3):259–269.

Nitsche MA, Fricke K, Henschke U, et al. Pharmacological modulation of cortical excitability shifts induced by transcranial direct current stimulation in humans. J Physiol 2003;553:293–301.

Nolan KJ, Savalia KK, Lequerica AH, Elovic EP. Objective assessment of functional ambulation in adults with hemiplegia using ankle foot orthotics after stroke. Arch Phys Med Rehabil 2009;1:524–529.

Norton BJ, Bromze HE, Saurmann SA, Eliasson SG. Correlation between gait speed and spasticity at the knee. Phys Ther 1975;55:355–359.

Noth J. Trends in the pathophysiology and pharmacotherapy of spasticity. J Neurol 1991;238:131–139.

Novacheck TF, Stout JS, Tervo R. Reliability and validity of the Gillette Functional Assessment Questionnaire as an outcome measure in children with walking disabilities. J Pediatr Orthop 2000;20(1):75–86.

Nowak DA, Glasauer S, Hermsdorfer J. Grip force efficiency in long-term deprivation of somatosensory feedback. Neuroreport 2003;14:1803–1807.

Nowak DA, Grefkes C, Dafotakis M, et al. Dexterity is impaired at both hands following unilateral subcortical middle cerebral artery stroke. Eur J Neurosci 2007;25:3173–3184.

Nowak DA, Topka H, Risch S, et al. The beneficial effects of subthalamic nucleus stimulation on manipulative finger force control in Parkinson's disease. Exp Neurol 2005;193:427–436.

Nudo RJ, Milliken GW, Jenkins WM, Merzenich MM. Use-dependent alterations of movement representations in primary motor cortex of adult squirrel monkeys. J Neurosci 1996;16:785–807.

Nudo RJ. Mechanisms for recovery of motor function following cortical damage. Curr Opin Neurobiol 2006;16:638–644.

Nudo RJ. Postinfarct cortical plasticity and behavioral recovery. Stroke 2007;38:840–845.

Nutt JG, Carter JH, Lea ES, Woodward WR. Motor fluctuations during continuous levodopa infusions in patients with Parkinson's disease. Mov Disord 1997;12:285–292.

Nutt JG, Carter JH, Woodward W, et al. Does tolerance develop to levodopa? Comparison of 2- and 21-H levodopa infusions. Mov Disord 1993;8:139–143.

Nutt JG, Woodward WR, Hammerstad JP, et al. The "on-off" phenomenon in Parkinson's disease. Relation to levodopa absorption and transport. N Engl J Med 1984;310:483–488.

Nwaobi OM, Brubaker CE, Cusick B, Sussman MD. Electromyographic investigation of extensor activity in cerebral-palsied children in different seating positions. Dev Med child Neurol 1983;25:175–183.

Nyberg L, Gustafson Y. Fall prediction index for patients in stroke rehabilitation. Stroke 1997;28:716–721.

O

O'Byrne JM, Jenkinson A, O'Brien TM. Quantitative analysis and classification of gait patterns in cerebral palsy using a three dimensional motion analyzer. J Child Neurol 1998;13:101–108.

O'Keefe J, Dostsrovsky J. The hippocampus as a spatial map: preliminary evidence from unit activity in the freely-moving rat. Brain Res 1971;34:171–175.

O'Shea S, Morris ME, Iansek R. Dual task interference during gait in people with Parkinson's disease: effects of motor versus cognitive secondary tasks. Phys Ther 2002;82:888–897.

O'Sullivan SB, Schmitz TJ. Physical rehabilitation assessment and treatment, 4th ed. Philadelphia: Davis, 2001.

Ochi M, Makino K, Wada F, et al. A walker with a device of partial suspension for patients with gait disturbance: body weight supported walker. J UOEH 2009;31:259–263.

Ochs AL, Newberry J, Lenhardt ML, Harkins SW. Neural and vestibular aging associated with falls. In: Birren JE, Schaie KW, eds. Handbook of psychology of aging. New York: Van Nostrand & Reinholdt, 1985:378–399.

Ogden R, Franz SI. On cerebral motor control: the recovery from experimentally produced hemiplegia. Psychobiology 1917;1:33–49.

Ohata K, Tsuboyama T, Haruta T, et al. Relation between muscle thickness, spasticity, and activity limitations in children and adolescents with cerebral palsy. Dev Med Child Neurol 2008;50:152–156.

Oie KS, Kiemel T, Jeka JJ. Human multisensory fusion of vision and touch: detecting nonlinearity with small changes in the sensory environment. Neurosci Lett 2001;315:113–116.

Oie KS, Kiemel T, Jeka JJ. Multisensory fusion: simultaneous re-weighting of vision and touch for the control of human posture. Cogn Brain Res 2002;14:164–176.

Okamoto T, Kumamoto M. Electromyographic study of the learning process of walking in infants. Electromyography 1972;12:149–158.

Okamoto T, Okamoto K, Andrew PD. Electromyographic study of newborn stepping in neonates and young infants. Electromyogr Clin Neurophysiol 2001;41:289–296.

Okamoto T, Okamoto K. Electromyographic characteristics at the onset of independent walking in infancy. Electromyogr Clin Neurophysiol 2001;41:33–41.

Oliver D, Britton M, Seed P, et al. Development and evaluation of evidence based risk assessment tool (STRATIFY) to predict which elderly inpatients will fall: case-control and cohort studies. BMJ 1997;315:1049–1053.

Oliver D, Daly F, Martin FC, McMurdo ME. Risk factors and risk assessment tools for falls in hospital in-patients: a systematic review. Age Ageing 2004;33(2):122–130.

Olivier I, Cuisinier R, Vaugoyeau M, et al. Dual-task study of cognitive and postural interference in 7-year-olds and adults. Neuroreport 2007;18:817–821.

Olivier I, Palluel E, Nougier V. Effects of attentional focus on postural sway in children and adults. Exp Brain Res 2008;185:341–345.

Olney SJ, Griffin MP, McBride ID. Multivariate examination of data from gait analysis of persons with stroke. Phys Ther 1998;78:814–828.

Olney SJ, Griffin MP, McBride ID. Temporal, kinematic and kinetic variables related to gait speed in subjects with hemiplegia: a regression approach. Phys Ther 1994;74:872–885.

Olney SJ, Griffin MP, Monga TN, McBride ID. Work and power in gait of stroke patients. Arch Phys Med Rehabil 1991;72:309–314.

Olney SJ, Monga TN, Costigan PA. Mechanical energy of walking of stroke patients. Arch Phys Med Rehabil 1986;67:92–98.

Olsen JZ. Handwriting without tears, 7th ed. Potomac MD: Olsen Publishing, 1998.

Onla-or S, Winstein CJ. Determining the optimal challenge point for motor skill learning in adults with moderately severe Parkinsons disease. Neurorehabil Neural Repair 2008;22:385–395.

Orendurff MS, Schoen JA, Bernatz GC, et al. How humans walk: bout duration, steps per bout, and rest duration. J Rehabil Res Dev 2008;45:1077–1089.

Orendurff MS, Segal AD, Klute GK, Berge JS. The effect of walking speed on center of mass displacement. J Rehabil Res Dev 2004;41:829–834.

Ornitz E. Normal and pathological maturation of vestibular function in the human child. In: Romand R, ed. Development of auditory and vestibular systems. New York: Academic Press, 1983:479–536.

Örnkloo H, von Hofsten, C. Fitting objects into holes: on the development of spatial cognition skills. Dev Psychol 2007;43:404–416.

Orr R, Raymond J, Fiatarone Singh M. Efficacy of progressive resistance training on balance performance in older adults: a systematic review of randomized controlled trials. Sports Med 2008;38:317–343.

Ostir GV, Volpato S, Fried LP, et al. Reliability and sensitivity to change assessed for a summary measure of lower body function: results from the Women's Health and Aging Study. J Clin Epidemiol 2002;55:916–921.

Ottenbacher KJ, Msall ME, Lyon NR, et al. Interrater agreement and stability of the functional independence measure for children (WeeFim™): use in children with developmental disabilities. Arch Phys Med Rehabil 1997;78:1309–1315.

Ouellette M, LeBrasseur NK, Beam JF, et al. High intensity resistance training improves muscle strength, self-reported function and disability in long term stroke survivors. Stroke 2004;35:1404–1409.

Overstall PW, Exton-Smith AN, Imms FJ, Johnson AL. Falls in the elderly related to postural imbalance. BMJ 1977;1:261–264.

Oxford GK, Vogel LV, Mitchell A, et al. Adult norms for a commercially available nine hold peg test for finger dexterity. Am J Occup Ther 2003;57:570–573.

P

Page S, Levine P. Forced use after TBI: promoting plasticity and function through practice. Brain Injury 2003;17:675–684.

Pai Y-C, Maki BE, Iqbal K, et al. Thresholds for step initiation induced by support-surface translation: a dynamic center-of-mass model provides much better prediction than a static model. J Biomech 2000;33:387–392.

Pai Y-C, Naughton BJ, Chang RW, Rogers MW. Control of body center of mass momentum during sit-to-stand among young and elderly adults. Gait Posture 1994;2:109–116.

Pai Y-C, Wening JD, Runtz EF, et al. Role of feedforward control of movement stability in reducing slip-related balance loss and falls among older adults. J Neurophysiol 2003;90: 755–762.

Paillard J. Cognitive versus sensorimotor encoding of spatial information. In: Ellen P, Thinus-Blanc C, eds. Cognitive processes and spatial orientation in animal and man: neurophysiology and developmental aspects, NARO ASI Series 37. The Hague: Martinus Nijhoff, 1987:43–77.

Paillard J. The contribution of peripheral and central vision to visually guided reaching. In: Ingle DJ, Goodale MA, Mansfield RJW, eds. Analysis of visual behavior. Cambridge, MA: MIT Press, 1982:367–385.

Pak S, Patten C. Strengthening to promote functional recovery poststroke: an evidence-based review. Top Stroke Rehabil 2008;15:177–199.

Palisano R, Rosenbaum P, Walter S, et al. Development and validation of a gross motor function classification system for children with cerebral palsy. Dev Med Child Neurol 1997;39: 214–223.

Palisano RJ. Neuromotor and developmental assessment. In: Wilhelm IJ, ed. Physical therapy assessment in early infancy. New York: Churchill Livingstone, 1993:173–224.

Palliyath S, Hallett M, Thomas SL, Lebiedowska MK. Gait in patients with cerebellar ataxia. Mov Disord 1998;13:958–964.

Palombaro KM, Craik RL, Mangione KK, Tomlinson JD. Determining meaningful changes in gait speed after hip fracture. Phys Ther 2006;86:809–816.

Pandyan AD, Price CIM, Rodgers H, et al. Biomechanical examination of a commonly used measure of spasticity. Clin Biomech 2001;16:859–865.

Pang MY, Lam T, Yang JF. Infants adapt their stepping to repeated trip-inducing stimuli. J Neurophysiol 2003;90:2731–2740.

Pang MY, Yang JF. The initiation of the swing phase in human infant stepping: importance of hip position and leg loading. J Physiol (Lond) 2000;528(Pt 2):389–404.

Pang MY, Yang JF. Interlimb co-ordination in human infant stepping. J Physiol 2001;533 (Pt 2):617–625.

Pang MY, Yang JF. Sensory gating for the initiation of the swing phase in different directions of human infant stepping. J Neurosci 2002;22:5734–5740.

Papa E, Cappozzo A. Sit-to-stand motor strategies investigated in able-bodied young and elderly subjects. J Biomech 2000;33:1113–1122.

Pare M, Dugas C. Developmental changes in prehension during childhood. Exp Brain Res 1999;125:239–247.

Pare N, Rabin L, Fogel J, Pepin M. Mild traumatic brain injury and its sequelae: characterisation of divided attention deficits. Neuropsychol Rehabil 2009;19:110–137.

Park ES, Park CI, Lee HJ, et al. The characteristics of sit-to-stand transfer in young children with spastic cerebral palsy based on kinematic and kinetic data. Gait Posture 2003;17:43–49.

Park S, Horak FB, Kuo AD. Postural feedback responses scale with biomechanical constraints in human standing. Exp Brain Res 2004;154:417–427.

Parker TM, Osternig LR, Lee HJ, et al. The effect of divided attention on gait stability following concussion. Clin Biomech 2005;20:389–395.

Parker VM, Wade DT, Langton Hewer R. Loss of arm function after stroke: measurement, frequency, and recovery. Int Rehabil Med 1986;8:69–73.

Partridge CJ, Edwards SM, Mee R, van Langenberghe HVK. Hemiplegic shoulder pain: a study of two methods of physiotherapy treatment. Clin Rehabil 1990;4:43–49.

Pascual-Leone A, Amedi A, Fregni F, Merabet LB. The plastic human brain cortex. Annu Rev Neurosci 2005;28:377–401.

Pascual-Leone A, Cammarota A, Wassermann EM, et al. Modulation of motor cortical outputs to the reading hand of Braille readers. Ann Neurol 1993;34:33–37.

Pascual-Leone A, Grafman J, Hallett M. Modulation of cortical motor output maps during development of implicit and explicit knowledge. Science 1994;263:1287–1289.

Passingham RE. Premotor cortex: sensory cues and movement. Behav Brain Res 1985;18:175–185.

Passinham RE, Chen YC, Thaler D. Supplementary motor cortex and self-initiated movement. In: Ito M, ed. Neural programming. Tokyo: Japan Scientific Society, 1989:13–24.

Pastalan LA, Mantz RK, Merrill J. The simulation of age-related sensory losses: a new approach to the study of environmental barriers. In: Preiser WFE, ed. Environment design research, vol. 1. Stroudsberg, PA: Dowden, Hutchinson & Ross, 1973:383–390.

Patla AE. Understanding the control of human locomotion: a prologue. In: Patla AE, ed. Adaptability of human gait. Amsterdam: North-Holland, 1991:3–17.

Patla AE. Age-related changes in visually guided locomotion over different terrains: major issues. In: Stelmach G, Homberg V, eds. Sensorimotor impairment in the elderly. Dordrecht: Kluwer, 1993:231–252.

Patla AE. Understanding the roles of vision in the control of human locomotion. Gait Posture 1997;5:54–69.

Patla AE. Strategies for dynamic stability during adaptive human locomotion. IEEE Eng Med Biol Mag 2003;22:48–52.

Patla AE, Adkin A, Martin C, et al. Characteristics of voluntary visual sampling of the environment for safe locomotion over different terrains. Exp Brain Res 1996;112:513–522.

Patla AE, Frank JS, Winter DA. Balance control in the elderly: implications for clinical assessment and rehabilitation. Can J Public Health 1992a;83 [Suppl 2]:S29–S33.

Patla PE, Ishac MG, Winter DA. Anticipatory control of center of mass and joint stability during voluntary arm movement from a standing posture: interplay between active and passive control. Exp Brain Res 2002;143:318–327.

Patla AE, Practor J, Morson B. Observations on aspects of visual gait assessment: a questionnaire study. Physiother Can 1987;39:311–316.

Patla AE, Prentice SD, Martin C, Rietdyk S. The bases of selection of alternate foot placement during locomotion in humans. In: Posture and gait: control mechanisms. Woollacott MH, Horak F, eds. Eugene: University of Oregon, 1992b:226–229.

Patla AE, Shumway-Cook A. Dimensions of mobility: defining the complexity and difficulty associated with community mobility. J Aging Phys Activity 1999;7:7–19.

Patla AE, Winter DA, Frank JS, et al. Identification of age-related changes in the balance-control system. In: Duncan P, ed. Balance: Proceedings of the APTA Forum, Alexandria, VA: American Physical Therapy Association, 1990:43–55.

Patrick E, Ada L. The Tardieu scale differentiates contracture from spasticity whereas the Ashworth Scale is confounded by it. Clin Rehabil 2006;20:173–182.

Patterson SL, Forrester LW, Rodgers MM, et al. Determinants of walking function after stroke: differences by deficit severity. Arch Phys Med Rehabil 2007;88:115–119.

Patton HD, Fuchs A, Hille B, et al. Textbook of physiology, vol 1, 21st ed. Philadelphia: Saunders, 1989.

Patton JL, Stoykov ME, Kovic M, Mussa-Ivaldi FA. Evaluation of robotic training forces that either enhance or reduce error in chronic hemiplegic stroke survivors. Exp Brain Res 2005;26:1–16.

Patton JL, Stoykov ME, Kovic M, Mussa-Ivaldi FA. Evaluation of robotic training forces that either enhance or reduce error in chronic hemiparetic stroke survivors. Exp Brain Res 2006;168:368–383.

Paulignan Y, McKenzie C, Marteniuk R, Jeannerod M. The coupling of arm and finger movements during prehension. Exp Brain Res 1990;79:431–436.

Paulus W, Straube A, Brandt T. Visual stabilisation of posture. Brain 1984;107:1143–1163.

Pause M, Kunesch E, Binkofski F, Freund HG. Sensorimotor disturbances in patients with lesions of the parietal cortex. Brain 1989; 112:1599–1625.

Pavol MJ, Owings TM, Foley KT, Grabiner MD. The sex and age of older adults influence the outcome of induced trips. J Gerontol 1999;54A:M103–M108.

Payton O, Melson C, Ozer M. Patient participation in program planning: a manual for therapists. Philadelphia: FA Davis, 1990.

Pearson K, Gordon J. Locomotion. In: Kandel E, Schwartz JH, Jessell TM, eds. Principles of neural science, 4th ed. New York: McGraw-Hill, 2000:737–755.

Pearson KG, Ramirez JM, Jiang W. Entrainment of the locomotor rhythm by group Ib afferents from ankle extensor muscles in spinal cats. Exp Brain Res 1992;90:557–566.

Pearson KG. Proprioceptive regulation of locomotion. Curr Opin Neurobiol 1995;5:786–791.

Peel C, Sawyer Baker P, Roth DL, et al. Assessing mobility in older adults: the UAB Study of Aging Life-Space Assessment. Phys Ther 2005;85:1008–1019.

Pehoski C. Object manipulation in infants and children. In: Henderson A, Pehoski C., eds. Hand function in the child: foundations for remediation. St.Louis: Mosby, 1995:136–153.

Peiper A. Cerebral functions in infancy and childhood. New York: Consultants Bureau, 1963.

Penfield W, Rassmussen T. The cerebral cortex of man: a clinical study of localization of function. New York: Macmillan, 1950.

Penfield W. Functional localization in temporal and deep Sylvian areas. Res Publ Assoc Res Nerv Ment Dis 1958;36:210–226.

Perell KL, Nelson A, Goldman RL, et al. Fall risk assessment measures: an analytic review. J Gerontol A Biol Sci Med Sci 2001;56:M761–M766.

Perenin MT, Jeannerod M. Residual vision in cortically blind hemifields. Neuropsychologia 1975;13:1–7.

Pérennou D. Weight bearing asymmetry in standing hemiparetic patients. J Neurol Neurosurg Psychiatry 2005;76:62.

Perera S, Mody SH, Woodman RC, Studenski SA. Meaningful change and responsiveness in common physical performance measures in older adults. J Am Geriatr Soc 2006;54:743–752.

Perkins-Ceccato N, Passmore SR, Lee TD. Effects of focus of attention depend on golfers' skill. J Sports Sci 2003;21:593–600.

Perry J, Burnfield JM. Gait analysis: normal and pathological function. Thorofare, NJ: Slack, 2010.

Perry J, Garrett M, Gronley JK, Mulroy, SJ. Classification of walking handicap in the stroke population. Stroke 1995;26:982–989.

Perry J. Gait analysis: normal and pathological function. Thorofare, NJ: Slack, 1992.

Perry SB. Clinical implications of a dynamical systems theory. Neurol Rep 1998;22:4–10.

Perry RJ, Hodges JR. Attention and executive deficits in Alzheimer's disease: a critical review. Brain 1999;122:383–406.

Peterka RJ, Black FO. Age-related changes in human posture control: sensory organization tests. J Vestib Res 1990–1991;1:73–85.

Peterka RJ, Loughlin PJ. Dynamic regulation of sensorimotor integration in human postural control. J Neurophysiol 2004;91:410–423.

Peterka RJ. Sensorimotor integration in human postural control. J Neurophysiol 2002;88:1097–1118.

Peterson EW, Cho CC, Finlayson ML. Fear of falling and associated activity curtailment among middle aged and older adults with multiple sclerosis. Mult Scler 2007;13:1168–1175.

Peterson EW, Cho CC, von Koch L, Finlayson ML. Injurious falls among middle aged and older adults with multiple sclerosis. Arch Phys Med Rehabil 2008;89:1031–1037.

Petit J, Giroux-Metges MA, Gioux M. Power developed by motor units of the peroneus tertius muscle of the cat. J Neurophysiol 2003;90:3095–3104.

Petrarca M, Zanelli G, Patanè F, et al. Reach-to-grasp interjoint coordination for moving object in children with hemiplegia. J Rehabil Med 2009;41:995–100.

Pettersson AF, Olsson E, Wahlund LO. Motor function in subjects with mild cognitive impairment and early Alzheimer's disease. Dement Geriatr Cogn Disord 2005;19(5–6):299–304.

Pfeiffer E. Short portable mental status questionnaire. J Am Geriatric Soc 1975;23:433–441.

Pham TM, Winblad B, Granholm AC, Mohammed AH. Environmental influences on brain neurotrophins in rats. Pharmacol Biochem Behav 2002;73:167–175.

Piaget J. The origins of intelligence in children. New York: Norton, 1954.

Pierce SR, Daly K, Gallagher KG, et al. Constraint-induced therapy for a child with hemiplegic cerebral palsy: a case report. Arch Phys Med Rehabil 2002; 83(10):1462–1463.

Pierce SR, Gallagher KG, Schaumburg SW, et al. Home forced use in an outpatient rehabilitation program for adults with hemiplegia: a pilot study. Neurorehabil Neural Repair 2003;17(4):214–219.

Pijnappels M, Bobbert MF, van Dieen JH. Control of support limb muscles in recovery after tripping in young and older subjects. Exp Brain Res 2005;160:326–333.

Pitts DG. The effects of aging on selected visual functions: dark adaptation, visual acuity, stereopsis, and brightness contrast. In: Sekular R, Kline D, Dismukes K, eds. Modern aging research: aging and human visual function. New York: Liss, 1982:131–160.

Platt JR. Strong inference. Science 1964;146:347–352.

Platz T, Eickhof C, Nuyens G, Vuadens P. Clinical scales for the assessment of spasticity, associated phenomena, and function: a systematic review of the literature. Disabil Rehabil 2005;27:7–18.

Plotnik M, Giladi N, Hausdorff JM. Bilateral coordination of gait and Parkinson's disease: the effects of dual tasking. J Neurol Neurosurg Psychiatry 2009;80:347–350.

Plummer-D'Amato P, Altmann LJP, Saracino D, et al. Interactions between cognitive tasks and gait after stroke: A dual task study. Gait Posture 2008;27:683–688.

Podsiadlo D, Richardson S. The timed "Up and Go" test: a test of basic functional mobility for frail elderly persons. J Am Geriatr Soc 1991;39:142–148.

Poewe WH. Clinical aspects of motor fluctuations in Parkinson's disease. Neurology 1994;44 (7 Suppl 6):S6–S9.

Pohl M, Werner C, Holzgraefe M, et al. Repetitive locomotor training and physiotherapy improve walking and basic activities of daily living after stroke: a single-blind, randomized multicentre trial (DEutsche GAngtrainerStudie, DEGAS). Clin Rehabil 2007;21:17–27.

Pohl PS, McDowd JM, Filion DL, et al. Implicit learning of a perceptual motor skill after stroke. Phys Ther 2001;81:1780–1789.

Pohl PS, Winstein CJ, Fisher BE. The locus of age-related movement slowing: sensory processing in continuous goal-directed aiming. J Gerontol 1996;51:P94–P102.

Pohl PS, Winstein CJ. Practice effects on the less-affected upper extremity after stroke. Arch Phys Med Rehabil 1999;80:668–675.

Poizner H, Mack L, Verfaellie M, et al. Three-dimensional computergraphic analysis of apraxia. Brain 1990;113:85–101.

Poldrack RA, Sabb FW, Foerde K, et al. Neural correlates of motor skill automaticity. J Neurosci 2005;25:5356–5364.

Polit A, Bizzi E. Characteristics of motor programs underlying arm movements in monkeys. J Neurophysiol 1979;42:183–194.

Pons TP, Garraghty PE, Mishkin M. Lesion induced plasticity in the second somatosensory cortex of adult macaques. Proc Natl Acad Sci USA 1988;85:5279–5281.

Pont K, Wallen M., Bundy A, Case-Smith J. Reliability and validity of the test of in-hand manipulation in children ages 5 to 6 years. Am J Occup Ther 2008;62:384–392.

Poole JL, Burtner PA, Torres TA, et al. Measuring dexterity in children using the nine-hole peg test. J Hand Ther 2005;18:348–351.

Poole JL, Whitney SL. Motor assessment scale for stroke patients: concurrent validity and interrater reliability. Arch Phys Med Rehabil. 1988;69(3 Pt 1):195–197.

Poole KE, Vedi S, Debiram I, Rose C, Power J, Loveridge N, Warburton EA, Reeve J, Compston J. Bone structure and remodelling in stroke patients: early effects of zoledronate. Bone 2009;44:629–633.

Porro G, van der Linden D, van Nieuwenhuizen O, Wittebol-Post D. Role of visual dysfunction in postural control in children with cerebral palsy. Neural Plast 2005;12:205–210.

Pound P, Gompertz P, Ebrahim S. A patient-centered study of the consequences of stroke. Clin Rehabil 1998;12:338–347.

Powell J, Pandyan AD, Granat M, et al. Electrical stimulation of wrist extensors in poststroke hemiplegia. Stroke 1999;30:1384–1389.

Powell LE, Myers AM. The Activities-specific Balance Confidence (ABC) Scale. J Gerontol Med Sci 1995;50A(1):M28–M34.

Powers RK, Campbell DL, Rymer WZ. Stretch reflex dynamics in spastic elbow flexor muscles. Ann Neurol 1989;25:32–42.

Powers RK, Rymer WZ. Effects of acute dorsal spinal demisection on motor neuron discharge in the medial gastrocnemius of the decerebrate cat. J Neurophysiol 1988;59:1540–1556.

Pozzo T, Berthoz A, Lefort L. Head stabilization during various locomotor tasks in humans. 1. Normal subjects. Exp Brain Res 1990;82:97–106.

Pozzo T, Berthoz A, Lefort L, Vitte E. Head stabilization during various locomotor tasks in humans. II. Patients with bilateral peripheral vestibular deficits. Exp Brain Res 1991;85:208–217.

Pozzo T, Levik Y, Berthoz A. Head stabilization in the frontal plane during complex equilibrium tasks in humans. In: Woollacott M, Horak F, eds. Posture and gait: control mechanisms. Eugene: University of Oregon, 1992:97–100.

Prayson RA, Hannahoe BM. Clinicopathological findings in patients wtih infantile hemiparesis and epilepsy. Hum Pathol 2004;35:734–738.

Prechtl HF, Cioni G, Einspieler C, et al. Role of vision on early motor development: lessons from the blind. Dev Med Child Neurol 2001;43:198–201.

Prechtl HFR. Continuity and change in early neural development. In: Prechtl HFR, ed. Continuity of neural functions from prenatal to postnatal life. Clinics in Developmental Medicine 94. Oxford: Blackwell Scientific, 1984:1–15.

Prechtl HFR. Prenatal motor development. In: Wade MC, Whiting HTA, eds. Motor development in children: aspects of coordination and control. Dordrecht, the Netherlands: Martinus Nijhoff, 1986:53–64.

Price DD, McGrath PA, Rafii A, Buckingham B. The validation of visual analogue scales as ratio scale measure for chronic and experimental pain. Pain 1983;17:45–56.

Prigatano GP, Fordyce DJ. Cognitive dysfunction and psychological adjustment after brain injury, In: GP Prignatano, ed. Neuropychological rehabilitation after brain injury. Baltimore: Johns Hopkins University Press, 1986.

Priplata A, Niemi J, Salen M, et al. Noise enhanced human balance control. Phys Rev Lett 2002; 89(23):238101.

Prokop T, Berger W. Influence of optic flow on locomotion in normal subjects and patients with Parkinson's disease. Electroencephalogr Clin Neurophysiol 1996;99:402.

Puthoff ML, Janz KF, Nielson D. The relationship between lower extremity strength and power to everyday walking behaviors in older adults with functional limitations. J Geriatr Phys Ther 2008;31:24–31.

Pyoria O, Talvitie U, Villberg J. The reliability, distribution and responsiveness of the postural control and Balance For Stroke Test. Arch Phys Med Rehabil 2005;86:296–302.

Q

Qiu Q, Ramirez DA, Saleh S, et al. The New Jersey Institute of Technology Robot-Assisted Virtual Rehabilitation (NJIT-RAVR) system for children with cerebral palsy: a feasibility study. J Neuroeng Rehabil 2009;6:40.

Quaney BM, Perera S, Maletsky R, et al. Impaired grip force modulation in the ipsilesional hand after unilateral middle cerebral artery stroke. Neurorehabil Neural Repair 2005;19:338–349.

Quinn L, Gordon J. Functional outcomes: documentation for rehabilitation. Philadelphia: Saunders, 2003.

Quintana LA. Evaluation of perception and cognition. In: Trombly CA, ed. Occupational therapy for physical dysfunction, 4th ed. Baltimore: Williams & Wilkins, 1995.

R

Rabadi MH, Rabadi FM. Comparison of the Action Research Arm Test and the Fugl-Meyer Assessment as measures of upper-extremity motor weakness after stroke. Arch Phys Med Rehabil 2006;87:962–966.

Rabbitt P, Birren JE. Age and responses to sequences of repetitive and interruptive signals. J Gerontol 1967;22:143–150.

Rabbitt PM, Rogers M. Age and choice between responses in a self-paced repetitive task. Ergonomics 1965;8:435–444.

Rademaker GGJ. De Beteekenis der Roode Kernen en van the overige Mesencephalon voor Spiertonus, Lichaam-shouding en Labyrinthaire Reflexen. Leiden: Eduarol Ijdo, 1924.

Raghavan P. The nature of hand motor impairment after stroke and its treatment. Curr Treat Options Cardiovasc Med 2007;9:221–228.

Raghavan P, Krakauer JW, Gordon AM. Impaired anticipatory control of fingertip forces in patients with a pure motor or sensorimotor lacunar syndrome. Brain 2006;129: 1415–1425.

Raghavan P, Petra E, Krakaer JW, Gordon AM. Patterns of impairment in digit independence after subcortical stroke. J Neurophysiol 2005; 95:369–378.

Raibert M. Symmetry in running. Science 1986;231:1292–1294.

Ralston HJ. Energetics of human walking. In: Herman RM, Grillner S, Stein PSG, Stuart DG, eds. Neural control of locomotion. New York: Plenum, 1976:77–98.

Ramachandran VS, Stewart M, Rogers-Ramachandran DC. Perceptual correlates of massive cortical reorganization. Neuroreport 1992;3:583–586.

Ramnemark A, Nyberg L, Lorentzon R, et al. Progressive hemiosteoporosis on the paretic side and increased bone mineral density in the nonparetic arm the first year after severe stroke. Osteoporos Int 1999;9:269–275.

Ramon Y, Cajal S. Degeneration and regeneration of the nervous system. May RM, trans. London: Oxford University, 1928.

Rand MK, Lemay M, Squire LM, et al. Control of aperture closure initiation during reach-to-grasp movements under manipulations of visual feedback and trunk involvement in Parkinson's disease. Exp Brain Res 2009;November 10. 2010;201:509–525.

Rand MK, Shimansky Y, Stelmach GE, et al. Effects of accuracy constraints on reach-to-grasp movements in cerebellar patients. Exp Brain Res 2000;135:179–188.

Rand MK, Smiley-Oyen AL, Shimansky YP, et al. Control of aperture closure during reach-to-grasp movements in Parkinson's disease. Exp Brain Res 2006;168:131–142.

Rankin JK, Woollacott MH, Shumway-Cook A, Brown LA. Cognitive influence on postural stability: a neuromuscular analysis in young and older adults. J Gerontol 2000;55A:M112–M119.

Rantanen T, Guralnik JM, Ferrucci L, et al. Coimpairments: strength and balance as predictors of severe walking disability. J Gerontol 1999;54A:M172–M176.

Rasmussen IA, Xu J, Antonsen IK, et al. Simple dual tasking recruits prefrontal cortices in chronic severe traumatic brain injury patients, but not in controls. J Neurotrauma 2008;25:1057–1070.

Reber RJ, Squire LR. Encapsulation of implicit and explicit memory in sequence learning. J Cogn Neurosci 1998;10:248–263.

Redfern MS, Jennings JR, Martin C, Furman JM. Attention influences sensory integration for postural control in older adults. Gait Posture 2001;14:211–216.

Redfern MS, Muller MLTM, Jennings JR, Furman JM. Attentional dynamics in postural control during perturbations in young and older adults. J Gerontol Biol Sci 2002;57A:298–303.

Reed ES. An outline of a theory of action systems. J Motor Behav 1982;14:98–134.

Regnaux JP, David D, Daniel O, et al. Evidence for cognitive processes involved in the control of steady state of walking in healthy subjects and after cerebral damage. Neurorehabil Neural Repair 2005;19(2):125–132.

Reid KF, Naumova EN, Carabello RJ, et al. Lower extremity muscle mass predicts functional performance in mobility-limited elders. J Nutr Health Aging 2008;12:493–498.

Reilly D, van Donkelaar P, Saavedra S, Woollacott MH. The effects of dual task conditions: the interaction between the development of postural control and executive attention. J Motor Behav 2008a;40:90–102.

Reilly DS, Woollacott MH, van Donkelaar P, Saavedra S. The interaction between executive attention and postural control in dual-task conditions: children with cerebral palsy. Arch Phys Med Rehabil 2008b;89:834–842.

Reimers J. Clinically based decision making for surgery. In: Sussman M, ed. The diplegic child. Rosemont, IL: American Academy of Orthopedic Surgeons, 1992:155, 156, 158.

Reinbolt JA, Fox MD, Arnold AS, et al. Importance of preswing rectus femoris activity in stiff-knee gait. J Biomech. 2008;41:2362–2369.

Reinkensmeyer DJ, Maier MA, Guigon E, et al. Do robotic and non-robotic arm movement training drive motor recovery after stroke by a common neural mechanism? Experimental evidence and a computational model. Conf Proc IEEE Eng Med Biol Soc 2009;2009:2439–2441.

Reisman DS, Scholz JP. Aspects of joint coordination are preserved during pointing in persons with post-stroke hemiparesis. Brain 2003;126(Pt 11):2510–2527.

Remple MS, Bruneau RM, Vandenberg PM, et al. Sensitivity of cortical movement representations to motor experience: evidence that skill learning but not strength training induces cortical reorganization. Behav Brain Res 2001;123:133–141.

Rey A. Le freinage volontaire du mouvement graphique chez l'enfant. In: Epreuves d'intelligence pratique et de psychomotricite. Neuchatel: Delachaux & Niestle, 1968.

Riach CL, Hayes KC. Maturation of postural sway in young children. Dev Med Child Neurol 1987;29:650–658.

Riach CL, Starkes JL. Velocity of center of pressure excursions as an indicator of postural control systems in children. Gait Posture 1994;2: 167–172.

Rice MS, Newell KM. Interlimb coupling and left hemiplegia because of right cerebral vascular accident. Occup Ther J Res 2001;21:12–28.

Rice MS, Newell KM. Upper extremity interlimb coupling in persons with left hemiplegia due to stroke. Arch Phys Med Rehabil 2004;85: 629–634.

Richards CL, Malouin F, Bravo G, et al. The role of technology in task-oriented training in persons with subacute stroke: a randomized controlled trial. Neurorehabil Neural Repair 2004;18(4): 199–211.

Richards CL, Malouin F, Dumas F, et al. Early and intensive treadmill locomotor training for young children with cerebral palsy: a feasibility study. Pediatr Phys Ther 1997;9:158–165.

Richards CL, Malouin F, Dumas F, et al. Gait velocity as an outcome measure of locomotor recovery after stroke. In: Craik RL, Oatis C, eds. Gait analysis: theory and applications. St. Louis: Mosby, 1995:355–364.

Richards CL, Malouin F, Wood-Dauphinee S, et al. Task-specific physical therapy for optimization of gait recovery in acute stroke patients. Arch Phys Med Rehabil 1993;74:612–620.

Richardson D. Physical therapy in spasticity. Eur J Neurol 2002;9:17–26.

Richardson PK, Atwater SW, Crowe TK, Dietz JC. Performance of preschoolers on the Pediatric Clinical Test of Sensory Interaction for Balance. Am J Occup Ther 1992;46:793–800.

Richter A, Loscher W. Pathophysiology of idiopathic dystonia: findings from genetic animal models. Progr Neurobiol 1998;54:633–677.

Richter RR, VanSant AF, Newton RA. Description of adult rolling movements and hypothesis of developmental sequences. Phys Ther 1989; 69:63–71.

Ricken AX, Bennett SJ, Savelsbergh GJ. Coordination of reaching in children with spastic hemiparetic cerebral palsy under different task demands. Motor Control 2005;9:357–371.

Rikli R, Jones CJ. Senior Fitness Test Manual. Champaign, IL: Human Kinetics, 2001.

Riley MA, Baker AA, Schmit JM, Weaver E. Effects of visual and auditory short-term memory tasks on the spatiotemporal dynamics and variability of postural sway. J Motor Behav 2005;37:311–324.

Riley MA, Wong S, Mitra S, Turvey MT. Common effects of touch and vision on postural parameters. Exp Brain Res 1997;117:165–170.

Rine RM, Braswell J, Disher D, et al. Improvement of motor development and postural control following intervention in children with sensorineural hearing loss and vestibular impairment. Int J Pediatr Otorhinolaryngol 2004;68:1133–1232.

Ring C, Nayak USL, Isaacs B. Balance function in elderly people who have and who have not fallen. Arch Phys Med Rehabil 1988;69:261–264.

Riolo L, Fisher K. Is there evidence that strength training could help improve muscle function and other outcomes without reinforcing abnormal movement patterns or increasing reflex activity in a man who has had a stroke? Phys Ther 2003;83:844–851.

Risedal A, Zeng J, Johansson BB. Early training may exacerbate brain damage after focal brain ischemia in the rat. J Cereb Blood Flow Metab 1999;19:997–1003.

Rizzolatti G, Camarda R, Fogassi L, et al. Functional organization of inferior area 6 in the macaque monkey. Exp Brain Res 1988;71:491–597.

Roberts TDM. Neurophysiology of postural mechanisms. London: Butterworths, 1979.

Robertson SL, Jones LA. Tactile sensory impairments and prehensile function in subjects with left-hemisphere cerebral lesions. Arch Phys Med Rehabil 1994;75:1108–1117.

Robinson CA, Matsuda PN, Ciol MA, et al. Understanding the factors impacting participation in community mobility following stroke: physical characteristics of the individual. Abstract presented at the World Congress of Physical Therapy, Vancouver, BC, Canada, 2007.

Robinson CA. Identifying personal factors associated with participation in community walking following stroke. Unpublished doctoral dissertation. Seattle, WA: University of Washington, 2010.

Robinson JL, Schmidt GL. Quantitative gait evaluation in the clinic. Phys Ther 1981;61:351–353.

Rocchi L, Chiari L, Cappello A, et al. Comparison between subthalamic nucleus and globus pallidus internus stimulation for postural performance in Parkinson's disease. Gait Posture 2004;19:172–183.

Rocchi L, Chiari L, Cappello A, Horak FB. Identification of distinct characteristics of postural sway in Parkinson's disease: a feature selection procedure based on principal component analysis. Neurosci Lett 2006;394: 140–145.

Rocchi L, Chiari L, Horak FB. Effects of deep brain stimulation and levodopa on postural sway in Parkinson's disease. J Neurol Neurosurg Psychiatry 2002;73:267–274.

Rochester L, Hetherington V, Jones B, et al. Attending to the task: interference effects of functional tasks on walking in Parkinson's disease and the roles of cognition, depression, fatigue and balance. Arch Phys Med Rehabil 2004;85:1578–1585.

Roerdink M, de Haart M, Daffertshofer A, et al. Dynamical structure of center-of-pressure trajectories in patients recovering from stroke. Exp Brain Res 2006;174:256–269.

Roerdink M, Geurts A, de Haart M, Beek P. On the Relative Contribution of the paretic leg to the control of posture after stroke. Neurorehabil Neural Repair 2009;23:267–274.

Rogers MW. Control of posture and balance during voluntary movements in Parkinson's disease. In: Duncan P, ed. Balance: proceedings of the APTA Forum. Alexandria, VA: American Physical Therapy Association, 1990:79–86.

Rogers MW. Motor control problems in Parkinson's disease. In: Contemporary management of motor control problems. Proceedings of the II Step Conference. Alexandria, VA: American Physical Therapy Association, 1991:195–208.

Roland PE, Larsen B, Lassen NA, Skinhof E. Supplementary motor area and other cortical areas in organization of voluntary movements in man. J Neurophysiol 1980;43:118–136.

Roll JP, Bard C, Paillard, J. Head orienting contributes to directional accuracy of aiming at distant targets. Hum Mov Sci 1986;5:359–371.

Roll, JP, Roll R. From eye to foot: a proprioceptive chain involved in postural control. In: Amblard B, Berthoz A, Clarac F, eds. Posture and gait: development, adaptation and modulation. Amsterdam: Elsevier, 1988:155–164.

Romberg MH. Manual of nervous diseases of man. London: Sydenham Society, 1853:395–401.

Roncesvalles MN, Woollacott MW, Burtner PA. Neural factors underlying reduced postural adaptability in children with cerebral palsy. Neuroreport 2002;13:2407–2410.

Roncesvalles MNC, Jensen J. The expression of weight-bearing ability in infants between four and seven months of age. Sport Exer Psychol 1993;15:568.

Roncesvalles MNC, Woollacott MH, Jensen JL. Development of lower extremity kinetics for balance control in infants and young children. J Motor Behav 2001;33:180–192.

Roncesvalles MNC, Woollacott MH, Jensen JL. The development of compensatory stepping skills in children. J Motor Behav 2000;32:100–111.

Roncesvalles N, Woollacott M, Brown N, Jensen J. An emerging postural response: is control of the hip possible in the newly walking child? J Motor Behav 2003;36:147–159.

Ronnqvist L, Rosblad B. Kinematic analysis of unimanual reaching and grasping movements in children with hemiplegic cerebral palsy. Clin Biomech 2007;22:165–175.

Rosander K, von Hofsten C. Development of gaze tracking of small and large objects. Exp Brain Res 2002;146:257–264.

Rosander K, von Hofsten C. Visual-vestibular interaction in early infancy. Exp Brain Res 2000;133:321–333.

Rose D. Fall proof: a comprehensive balance and mobility program. Champaign, IL: Human Kinetics, 2003.

Rose DJ. A multilevel approach to the study of motor control and learning. Boston: Allyn & Bacon, 1997.

Rose DK, Winstein CJ. Bimanual training after stroke: are two hands better than one? Top Stroke Rehabil 2004;11:20–31.

Rose J, Wolff DR, Jones VK, et al. Postural balance in children with cerebral palsy. Dev Med Child Neurol 2002;44:58–63.

Rose SJ. Physical therapy diagnosis: role and function. Phys Ther 1989;69:535–537.

Rosen B, Lundborg G. Early use of artificial sensibility to improve sensory recovery after repair of the median and ulnar nerve. Scand J Plast Reconstr Surg Hand Surg 2003;37(1):54–57.

Rosenbaum D. Human motor control. New York: Academic Press, 1991.

Rosenhall U, Rubin W. Degenerative changes in the human vestibular sensory epithelia. Acta Otolaryngol 1975;79:67–81.

Rosenkranz K, Nitsche MA, Tergau F, Paulus W. Diminution of training-induced transient motor cortex plasticity by weak transcranial direct current stimulation in the human. Neurosci Lett 2000;296(1):61–63.

Rosenrot P, Wall JC, Charteris J. The relationship between velocity, stride time, support time and swing time during normal walking. J Hum Mov Stud 1980;6:323–335.

Rosenthal RB, Deutsch SD, Miller W, et al. A fixed-ankle, below-the-knee orthosis for the management of genu recurvatum in spastic cerebral palsy. J Bone Joint Surg Am 1975;57: 545–547.

Rosin R, Topka H, Dichgans J. Gait initiation in Parkinson's disease. Mov Disord 1997;12:682–690.

Ross SA, Engsberg JR. Relation between spasticity and strength in individuals with spastic diplegic cerebral palsy. Dev Med Child Neurol 2002;44(3):148–157.

Rossetti Y, Revol P, McIntosh R, et al. Visually guided reaching: bilateral posterior parietal lesions cause a switch from fast visuomotor to slow cognitive control. Neuropsychologia 2005;43:162–177.

Rothstein J. Disability and our identity. Phys Ther 1994;74:375–377.

Rothstein JM, Echternach JL, Riddle DL. The Hypothesis-Oriented Algorithm for Clinicians II (HOAC II): a guide for patient management. Phys Ther 2003;83:455–470.

Rothstein JM, Echternach JL. Hypothesis-oriented algorithm for clinicians: a method for evaluation and treatment planning. Phys Ther 1986;66:1388–1394.

Rothwell JC, Traub MM, Day BL, et al. Manual motor performance in a deafferented man. Brain 1982;105:515–542.

Rothwell JC. Brainstem myoclonus. Clin Neurosci 1995–1996;3(4):214–218.

Rothwell JC. Cerebral cortex. In: Rothwell JC, ed. Control of human voluntary movement, 2nd ed. 1994:293–286.

Rovee-Collier CK, Sullivan MW. Organization of infant memory. J Exp Psychol [Hum Learn] 1980;6:798–807.

Roy CW. Shoulder pain in hemiplegia: a literature review. Clin Rehabil 1988;2:35–44.

Rozendal RH. Biomechanics of standing and walking. Amsterdam: Elsevier, 1986.

Rozumalski A, Schwartz MH. Crouch gait patterns defined using k-means cluster analysis are related to underlying clinical pathology. Gait Posture 2009;30:155–160.

Rubenstein LZ. Falls in older people: epidemiology, risk factors and strategies for prevention. Age Ageing 2006;35-S2:ii37-ii41.

Rubenstein LZ, Josephson KR. Guidelines for prevention of falls in older persons. J Am Geriatr Soc 2001;49:664–672.

Rubenstein LZ, Robbins AS, Schulman BL, et al. Falls and instability in the elderly. J Am Geriatr Soc 1988;36:266–278.

Ruff HA. Infants' manipulative exploration of objects: effects of age and object characteristics. Dev Psychol 1984;20:9–20.

Runge CF, Shupert CL, Horak FB, Zajac FE. Postural strategies defined by joint torques. Gait Posture 1999;10:161–170.

Russell DJ, Rosenbaum PL, Gowland C, et al. Manual for the gross motor function measure. Hamilton, ON: McMaster University, 1993.

Rymer W, Katz RT. Mechanisms of spastic hypertonia. In: Katz RT, ed. Spasticity: state of the art review, vol. 8. Philadelphia: Hanley & Belfus, 1994:441–154.

S

Saavedra S, Joshi A, Woollacott M, van Donkelaar P. Eye hand coordination in children with cerebral palsy. Exp Brain Res 2009;192:155–165.

Saavedra S, Woollacott MH. Contributions of spinal segments to trunk postural control during typical development. Dev Med Child Neurol 2009;51(Suppl.5):82.

Sackett DL, Rosenberg WMC, Muir Gray JA, et al. Evidence-based medicine: what it is and what it isn't. BMJ 1996;312:71–72.

Sadeghi H, Allard P, Duhaime M. Contributions of lower limb muscle power in gait of people without impairments. Phys Ther 2000;80: 1188–1196.

Saenz M, Lewis LB, Huth AG, et al. Visual motion area mt+/v5 responds to auditory motion in human sight-recovery subjects. J Neurosci 2008;28:5141–5148.

Sahrmann SA. Diagnosis by the physical therapist: a prerequisite for treatment. Phys Ther 1988;68:1703–1706.

Sahrmann SA, Norton BJ. The relationship of voluntary movement to spasticity in the upper motor neuron syndrome. Arch Neurol 1977;2:460–465.

Said CM, Galea M, Lythgo N. Obstacle crossing performance does not differ between the first and subsequent attempts in people with stroke. Gait Posture 2009;30:455–458.

Said CM, Goldie PA, Culham E, et al. Control of lead and trail limbs during obstacle crossing following stroke. Phys Ther 2005;85: 413–427.

Said CM, Goldie PA, Patla AE, et al. Balance during obstacle crossing following stroke. Gait Posture 2008;27:23–30.

Sainburg RL. Evidence for a dynamic-dominance hypothesis of handedness. Exp Brain Res 2002;142(2):241–258.

Sainburg RL. Handedness: differential specializations for control of trajectory and position. Exer Sport Sci Rev 2005;33(4):206–213.

Sainburg RL, Duff SV. Does motor lateralization have implications for stroke rehabilitation? J Rehabil Res Dev 2006; 4:311–322.

Sainburg RL, Ghilardi MF, Poizner H, Ghez C. Control of limb dynamics in normal subjects and patients without proprioception. J Neurophysiol 1995;73:820–835.

Sainburg RL, Poizner H, Ghez C. Loss of proprioception produces deficits in interjoint coordination. J Neurophysiol 1993;70:2136–2147.

Sainburg RL, Wang J. Interlimb transfer of visuomotor rotations: independence of direction and final position information. Exp Brain Res 2002;145:437–447.

Sakata H, Shibutani H, Kawano K, Harrington TL. Neural mechanisms of space vision in the parietal association cortex of the monkey. Vision Res 1985;25:453–463.

Salbach NM, Mayo NE, Higgins J, et al. Responsiveness and predictability of gait speed and other disability measures in acute stroke. Arch Phys Med Rehabil 2001;82:1204–1212.

Salbach NM, Mayo NE, Robichaud-Ekstrand S, et al. Balance self-efficacy and its relevance to physical function and perceived health status after stroke. Arch Phys Med Rehabil 2006;87: 364–370.

Salbach NM, Mayo NE, Wood-Dauphinee S, et al. A task oriented intervention enhances walking distance and speed in the first year post stroke: a randomized controlled trial. Clin Rehabil 2004;18:509–519.

Salimi I, Brochier T, Smith AM. Neuronal activity in somatosensory cortex of monkeys using a precision grip. II. Responses To object texture and weights. J Neurophysiol 1999a;81:835–844.

Salimi I, Brochier T, Smith AM. Neuronal activity in somatosensory cortex of monkeys using a precision grip. III. Responses to altered friction perturbations. J Neurophysiol 1999b;81: 845–857.

Salmoni AW, Schmidt RA, Walter CB. Knowledge of results and motor learning: a review and critical reappraisal. Psychol Bull 1984;95: 355–386.

Sandin KJ, Smith BS. The measure of balance in sitting in stroke rehabilitation prognosis. Stroke 1990;21:82–86.

Sanes JN, LeWitt PA, Mauritz KH. Visual and mechanical control of postural and kinetic tremor in cerebellar system disorders. J Neurol Neurosurg Psychiatry 1988;51:934–943.

Sanes JN, Mauritz KH, Dalakas MC, Evarts EV. Motor control in humans with large-fiber sensory neuropathy. Hum Neurobiol 1985;4: 101–114.

Sanford J, Moreland J, Swanson LR, et al. Reliability of the Fugl-Meyer assessment for testing motor performance in patients following stroke. Phys Ther 1993;73:447–454.

Sarnacki SJ. Rising from supine on a bed: a description of adult movement and hypothesis of developmental sequences. Richmond, VA: Virginia Commonwealth University; 1985. Master's thesis.

Satkunam LE. Rehabilitation medicine: 3. Management of adult spasticity CMAJ 2003;169:1173–1179.

Saunders D. Evaluation, treatment and prevention of musculoskeletal disorders. Minneapolis: Viking Press, 1991.

Sauvage LR, Myklebust BM, Crow-Pan J, et al. A clinical trial of strengthening and aerobic exercise to improve gait and balance in elderly male nursing home residents. Am J Phys Med Rehabil 1992;71:333–342.

Schaechter JD, Kraft E, Hilliard TS, et al. Motor recovery and cortical reorganization after constraint-induced movement therapy in stroke patients: a preliminary study. Neurorehabil Neural Repair 2002;16(4):1–13.

Schallert T, Fleming SM, Woodlee MT. Should the injured and intact hemispheres be treated differently during the early phases of physical restorative therapy in experimental stroke or parkinsonism? Phys Med Rehabil Clin 2003;14:1–20.

Schallert T, Leasure JL, Kolb B. Experience associated structural events, subependymal cellular proliferative activity and functional recovery after injury to the central nervous system. J Cereb Blood Flow Metab 2000;20:1513–1528.

Schaltenbrand G. The development of human motility and motor disturbances. Arch Neurol Psychiatry 1928;20:720.

Scheker LR, Chesher SP, Ramirez S. Neuromuscular electrical stimulation and dynamic bracing as a treatment for upper extremity spasticity in children with cerebral palsy. Br J Hand Surg 1999;2: 226–232.

Schenkman M. Interrelationships of neurological and mechanical factors in balance control. In: Duncan P, ed. Balance: proceedings of the APTA Forum. Alexandria, VA: American Physical Therapy Association, 1990:29–41.

Schenkman MA, Berger RA, Riley PO, et al. Whole-body movements during rising to standing from sitting. Phys Ther 1990;10:638–651.

Schenkman M, Butler RB. "Automatic Postural Tone" in posture, movement, and function. Forum on physical therapy issues related to cerebrovascular accident. Alexandria, VA: American Physical Therapy Association, 1992:16–21.

Schenkman M, Butler RB. A model for multisystem evaluation, interpretation, and treatment of individuals with neurologic dysfunction. Phys Ther 1989;69:538–547.

Schenkman M, Cutson TM, Zhu CW, Whetten-Goldstein K. A longitudinal evaluation of patients' perceptions of Parkinson's disease. Gerontologist 2002;42:790–798.

Schenkman M, Deutsch JE, Gill-Body KM. An integrated framework for decision making in neurologic physical therapist practice. Phys Ther 2006;86:1681–1702.

Schieber MH. Muscular production of individuated finger movements: the roles of extrinsic finger muscles. J Neurosci 1995;15(1 Pt 1): 284–297.

Schieppati M, Hugon M, Grasso M, et al. The limits of equilibrium in young and elderly normal subjects and in Parkinsonians. Electroencephalogr Clin Neurophysiol 1994;93:286–298.

Schillings AM, van Wezel BM, Mulder T, Duysens J. Muscular responses and movement strategies during stumbling over obstacles. J Neurophysiol 2000;83:2093–2102.

Schloon H, O'Brien MJ, Scholten CA, Prechtl HE. Muscle activity and postural behavior in newborn infants: a polymyographic study. Neuropadiatrie 1976;7:384–415.

Schmid A, Duncan PW, Studenski S, et al. Improvements in speed based gait classification are meaningful. Stroke 2007;6:2096–2100.

Schmidt R. Motor and action perspectives on motor behaviour. In: Meijer OG, Roth K, eds. Complex movement behavior: the motor-action controversy. Amsterdam: Elsevier, 1988a:3–44.

Schmidt RA. A schema theory of discrete motor skill learning. Psychol Rev 1975;82:225–260.

Schmidt RA. Motor control and learning, 2nd ed. Champaign, IL: Human Kinetics, 1988b.

Schmidt RA. Motor learning principles for physical therapy. Contemporary management of motor control problems. Proceedings of the II Step Conference. Alexandria, VA: American Physical Therapy Association, 1991.

Schmidt RA, Lee TD. Motor control and learning: a behavioral emphasis. Champaign, IL: Human Kinetics, 2005.

Schmidt RA, Young DE, Swinnen S, Shappiro DC. Summary knowledge of results for skill acquisition: support for the guidance hypothesis. J Exp Psychol Learn Mem Cogn 1989;15: 352–359.

Schmitz TJ. Coordination assessment. In: O'Sullivan S, Schmitz TM, eds. Physical rehabilitation: assessment and treatment, 4th ed. Philadelphia: FA Davis, 2001:212.

Schmitz, TJ. Gait training with assistive devices. In: O'Sullivan S, Schmitz TM, eds. Physical rehabilitation: assessment and treatment. 2nd ed. Philadelphia: FA Davis 1998.

Schneck CM, Henderson A. Descriptive analysis of the developmental progression of grip position for pencil and crayon control in nondysfunctional children. Am J Occup Ther 1990;44:893–900.

Schneiberg S, Sveistrup H, McFadyen B, et al. The development of coordination for reach-to-grasp movements in children. Exp Brain Res 2002;146(2):142–154.

Schneider K, Zernicke RF. Jerk-cost modulations during the practice of rapid arm movements. Biol Cybern 1989;60:221–230.

Schnitzler A, Kessler KR, Benecke R. Transcallosally mediated inhibition of interneurons within human primary motor cortex. Exp Brain Res 1996;112:381–391.

Scholtes VAB, Becher JG, Beelen A, Lankhorst GJ. Clinical assessment of spasticity in children with cerebral palsy: a critical review of available instruments. Dev Med Child Neurol 2006;48:64–73.

Scholz JP, Danion F, Latash ML, Schöner G. Understanding finger coordination through analysis of the structure of force variability. Biol Cybern 2002;86:29–39.

Scholz JP, Schöner G, Hsu WL, et al. Motor equivalent control of the center of mass in response to support surface perturbations. Exp Brain Res 2007;180:163–179.

Scholz, JP, Schöner G. The uncontrolled manifold concept: Identifying control variables for a functional task. Experimen Brain Res 1999;126:289–306.

Schöner G. 1995. Recent developments and problems in human movement science and their conceptual implications. Ecol Psychol 1995; 7:291–314.

Schultz A, Alexander NB, Gu MJ, Boismier T. Postural control in young and elderly adults when stance is challenged: clinical versus laboratory measurements. Ann Otol Rhinol Laryngol 1993;102:508–517.

Schultz AB. Muscle function and mobility biomechanics in the elderly: an overview of some recent research. J Gerontol 1995;50A(special issue):60–63.

Schwab RS. Progression and prognosis in Parkinson's disease. J Nerv Ment Dis 1960; 130:556–572.

Schwartz I, Sajin A, Fisher I, et al. The effectiveness of locomotor therapy using robotic-assisted gait training in subacute stroke patients: a randomized controlled trial. Phys Med Rehabil 2009;1:516–523.

Schwartz MF, Reed ES, Montgomery M, et al. The quantitative description of action disorganization after brain damage: a case study. Cogn Neuropsychol 1991;8:381–414.

Scianni A, Butler JM, Ada L, Teixeira-Salmela LF. Muscle strengthening is not effective in children and adolescents with cerebral palsy: a systematic review. Aust J Physiother. 2009;55(2):81–87.

Sea MJC, Henderson A, Cermak SA. Patterns of visual spatial inattention and their functional significance in stroke patients. Arch Phys Med Rehabil 1993;74:355–360.

Seeger BR, Caudrey DJ, O'Mara NA. Hand function in cerebral palsy: the effect of hip flexion angle. Dev Med Child Neurol 1984;26: 601–606.

Seidel B, Krebs DE. Base of support is not wider in chronic ataxic and unsteady patients. J Rehabil Med 2002;34(6):288–292.

Serrien DJ, Nirkko AC, Wiesendanger M. Role of the corpus callosum in bimanual coordination: a comparison of patients with congenital and acquired callosal damage. Eur J Neurosci 2001;14:1897–1905.

Serrien DJ, Wiesendanger M. Temporal control of a bimanual task in patients with cerebellar dysfunction. Neuropsychologia 2000;38:558–565.

Shaltenbrand G. The development of human motility and motor disturbances. Arch Neurol Pyschiatr 1928;20:720–730.

Shambes GM, Gibson JM, Welker W. Fractured somatotopy in granule cell tactile areas of rat cerebellar hemispheres revealed by micromapping. Brain Behav Evol 1978;15:94–140.

Shapiro DC, Schmidt RA. The schema theory: recent evidence and developmental implications. In: Kelso FAS, Clark JE, eds. The development of movement control and coordination. New York: Wiley, 1982:113–173.

Shaughnessy M, Michael KM, Sorkin JD, Macko RF. Steps after stroke: capturing ambulatory recovery. Stroke 2005;23:1305–1307.

Shea CH, Shebilske W, Worchel S. Motor learning and control. Englewood Cliffs, NJ: Prentice Hall, 1993.

Shea SL, Aslin RN. Oculomotor responses to step-ramp targets by young infants. Vision Res 1990;30:1077–1092.

Sheldon JH. On the natural history of falls in older age. BMJ 1960;4:1685–1690.

Sheldon JH. The effect of age on the control of sway. Gerontol Clin 1963;5:129–138.

Shellenkens JM, Scholten CA, Kalverboer AF. Visually guided hand movements in children with minor neurological dysfunction: Response time and movement organization. J Child Psych Psychiatry 1983;24:89–102.

Shepard K. Theory: criteria, importance and impact. In: Contemporary management of motor control problems: proceedings of the II Step Conference. Alexandria, VA: American Physical Therapy Association, 1991:5–10.

Shepherd RB, Crosbie J, Squires T. The contribution of the ipsilateral leg to postural adjustments during fast voluntary reaching in sitting. Abstract of International Society for Biomechanics, 14th Congress, Paris, 1993.

Sherrard RM, Bower AJ. BDNF and NT3 extend the critical period for developmental climbing fiber plasticity. Neuroreport 2001;12:2871–2874.

Sherrington C, Whitney J, Lord SR, et al. Effective exercise for the prevention of falls: a systematic review and meta-analysis. J Am Geriatr Soc 2008;56:2234–2243.

Sherrington CS. Decerebrate rigidity, and reflex coordination of movements. J Physiol Lond 1898;22:319–332.

Sherrington C. The integrative action of the nervous system, 2nd ed. New Haven: Yale University, 1947.

Sherrington C. The integrative action of the nervous system. New Haven: Yale University, 1906.

Shiavi R, Limbird T, Frazer M, et al. Helical motion analysis of the knee–I. Methodology for studying kinematics during locomotion. J Biomech 1987;20:459–469.

Shik ML, Severin FV, Orlovsky GN. Control of walking and running by means of electrical stimulation of the mid-brain. Biophysics 1966;11:756–765.

Shumway-Cook A. Equilibrium deficits in children. In: Woollacott M, Shumway-Cook A, eds. Development of posture and gait across the life span. Columbia: University of South Carolina, 1989:229–252.

Shumway-Cook A, Anson D, Haller S. Postural sway biofeedback for pretraining postural control following hemiplegia. Arch Phys Med Rehabil 1988;69:395–400.

Shumway-Cook A, Baldwin M, Pollisar N, Gruber W. Predicting the probability of falls in community dwelling older adults. Phys Ther 1997a;77:812–819.

Shumway-Cook A, Gruber W, Baldwin M, Liao S. The effect of multidimensional exercises on balance, mobility and fall risk in community dwelling older adults. Phys Ther 1997b;77: 46–57.

Shumway-Cook A, Brauer S, Woollacott M. Predicting the probability for falls in community-dwelling older adults using the Timed Up and Go Test. Phys Ther 2000;80:896–903.

Shumway-Cook A, Ciol M, Gruber W, Robinson C. Incidence and risk factors for falls following hip fracture in community dwelling older adults. Phys Ther 2005a;85:648–655.

Shumway-Cook A, Ciol MA, Hoffman J, et al. Falls in the Medicare population: incidence, associated factors, and impact on health care. Phys Ther 2009;89:324–332.

Shumway-Cook A, Guralnik JM, Phillips CL, et al. Age-associated declines in complex walking task performance: the Walking InChianti Toolkit. J Am Geriatr Soc 2007;55:58–65.

Shumway-Cook A, Horak F. Assessing the influence of sensory interaction on balance. Phys Ther 1986;66:1548–1550.

Shumway-Cook A, Horak FB. Vestibular rehabilitation: an exercise approach to managing symptoms of vestibular dysfunction. Semin Hearing 1989;10:196–205.

Shumway-Cook A, Horak FB. Rehabilitation strategies for patients with vestibular deficits. Neurol Clin 1990;8:441–457.

Shumway-Cook A, Horak F. Balance rehabilitation in the neurologic patient: course syllabus. Seattle: Neuroscience Education and Research Associates, 1992.

Shumway-Cook A, Hutchinson S, Kartin D, et al. Effect of balance training on recovery of stability in children with cerebral palsy. Dev Med Child Neurol 2003;45:591–602.

Shumway-Cook A, McCollum G. Assessment and treatment of balance disorders in the neurologic patient. In: Montgomery T, Connolly B, eds. Motor control and physical therapy: theoretical framework and practical applications. Chattanooga, TN: Chattanooga, 1990:123–138.

Shumway-Cook A, Olmscheid R. A systems analysis of postural dyscontrol in traumatically brain-injured patients. J Head Trauma Rehabil 1990;5:51–62.

Shumway-Cook A, Patla A, Stewart A, et al. Environmental components of mobility disability in community-living older persons. J Am Geriatr Soc 2003;51:393–398.

Shumway-Cook A, Patla A, Stewart A, et al. Environmental demands associated with community mobility in older adults with and without mobility disability. Phys Ther 2002;82: 670–681.

Shumway-Cook A, Patla A, Stewart A, et al. Assessing environmentally determined mobility disability: self-report versus observed community mobility. J Am Geriatr Soc 2005b;53:700–704.

Shumway-Cook A, Woollacott M. The growth of stability: postural control from a developmental perspective. J Motor Behav 1985a;17:131–147.

Shumway-Cook A, Woollacott M. Postural control in the Down's syndrome child. Phys Ther 1985b;9:211–235.

Shumway-Cook A, Woollacott M. Theoretical issues in assessing postural control. In: Wilhelm I, ed. Physical therapy assessment in early infancy. New York: Churchill Livingstone, 1993:161–171.

Shumway-Cook A, Woollacott M. Attentional demands and postural control: the effect of sensory context. J Gerontology 2000;55A:M10–M16.

Shumway-Cook A, Woollacott M, Baldwin M, Kerns K. The effects of cognitive demands on postural control in elderly fallers and nonfallers. J Gerontol 1997c;52:M232–M240.

Silsupadol P, Lugade V, Shumway-Cook A, et al. Training-related changes in dual-task walking performance of elderly persons with balance impairment: a double-blind, randomized controlled trial. Gait Posture 2009a;29:634–639.

Silsupadol P, Shumway-Cook A, Lugade V, et al. Effects of single-task versus dual-task training on balance performance in older adults: a double-blind, randomized controlled trial. Arch Phys Med Rehabil 2009b;90:381–387.

Silsupadol P, Shumway-Cook A, Woollacott M. Training of balance under single and dual task conditions in older adults with balance impairment: three case reports. Phys Ther 2006;86: 269–281.

Simoneau GG, Cavanagh PR, Ulbrecht JS, et al. The influence of visual factors on fall-related kinematic variables during stair descent by older women. J Gerontol 1991;46:188–195.

Simonsick EM, Kasper JD, Guralnik JM, et al. Severity of upper and lower extremity functional limitation: scale development and validation with self-report and performance-based measures of physical function. Women's Health and Aging Study Research Group. J Gerontol B Psychol Sci Soc Sci 2001;56:S10–S19.

Singer RN. Motor learning and human performance, 3rd ed. New York: Macmillan, 1980.

Sinkjaer T, Andersen JB, Larsen B. Soleus stretch reflex modulation during gait in humans. J Neurophysiol 1996;76:1112–1120.

Sinkjaer T, Magnussen I. Passive, intrinsic and reflex mediated stiffness in the ankle extensors of hemiparetic patients. Brain 1994;117: 355–363.

Sjostrom M, Fugl-Meyer AR, Nordin G, Wahlby L. Post stroke hemiplegia: muscle strength and structure. Scand J Rheumatol 1980;7:53–67.

Slavin MD, Held JM, Basso DM, et al. Fetal brain tissue transplants and recovery of locomotion following damage to sensorimotor cortex in rats. Prog Brain Res 1988;78:33–38.

Slijper H, Latash, ML, Rao N, Aruin AS. Task-specific modulation of anticipatory postural adjustments in individuals with hemiparesis. Clin Neurophysiol 2002;113:642–655.

Sloane P, Baloh RW, Honrubia V. The vestibular system in the elderly. Am J Otolaryngol 1989;1:422–429.

Slobounov SM, Moss SA, Slobounova ES, Newell KM. Aging and time to instability of posture. J Geronotol Biol Sci 1998;53:71–78.

Small SL, Hlustik P, Noll DC, et al. Cerebellar hemispheric activation ipsilateral to the paretic hand correlates with functional recovery after stroke. Brain 2002;125:1544–1557.

Smania N, Martini MC, Gambina G, et al. The spatial distribution of visual attention in hemineglect and extinction patients. Brain 1998;121:1759–1770.

Smania N, Picelli A, Gandolfi M, et al. Rehabilitation of sensorimotor integration deficits in balance impairment of patients with stroke hemiparesis: a before/after pilot study. Neurol Sci 2008;29:313–319.

Smidt GL, Rogers MW. Factors contributing to the regulation and clinical assessment of muscular strength. Phys Ther 1982;62:1283–1290.

Smith BT, Mulcahey MJ, Betz RR. An implantable upper extremity neuroprosthesis in a growing child with a C5 spinal cord injury. Spinal Cord 2001;39:118–123.

Smith GV, Silver KH, Goldberg AP, Macko RF. "Task-oriented" exercise improves hamstring strength and spastic reflexes in chronic stroke patients. Stroke 1999;30(10):2112–2118.

Smith JL, Smith LA, Dahms KL. Motor capacities of the chronic spinal cat: recruitment of slow and fast extensors of the ankle. Neurosci Abstr 1979;5:387.

Smith JL, Zernicke RF. Predictions for neural control based on limb dynamics. Trends Neurosci 1987;10:123–128.

Smith JL. Programming of stereotyped limb movements by spinal generators. In: Stelmach GE, Requin J, eds. Tutorials in motor behavior. Amsterdam: North-Holland, 1980:95–115.

Smith LH, Harris SR. Upper extremity inhibitive casting for a child with cerebral palsy. Phys Occup Ther Ped 1985;5:71–79.

Snijders AH, Weerdesteyn V, Hagen YJ, et al. Obstacle avoidance to elicit freezing of gait during treadmill walking. Mov Disord 2010;25:57–63.

Snow BJ, Tsui JK, Bhart MH, et al. Treatment of spasticity with botulinum toxin: a double blind study. Ann Neurol 1990;28:512–515.

Sofuwa O, Nieuwboer A, Desloovere K, et al. Quantitative gait analysis in Parkinson's disease: comparison with a healthy control group. Arch Phys Med Rehabil 2005;86:1007–1013.

Sohlberg MM, Mateer CA. Introduction to cognitive rehabilitation. New York: Guilford Press, 1989.

Sollerman C. Assessment of grip function: evaluation of a new method. Sweden: MITAB, 1984.

Son K, Miller JAA, Schultz AB. The mechanical role of the trunk and lower extremities in a seated weight moving task in sagittal plane. J Biomech Eng 1988;110:97–103.

Southard D, Higgins T. Changing movement patterns: effects of demonstration and practice. Res Q Exer Sport 1987;58:77–80.

Speechley M, Tinetti M. Assessment of risk and prevention of falls among elderly persons: role of the physiotherapist. Physiother Can 1990;2:75–79.

Speechley M, Tinetti M. Falls and injuries in frail and vigorous community elderly persons. J Am Geriatr Soc 1991;39:46–52.

Speers RA, Kuo AD, Horak FB. Contributions of altered sensation and feedback responses to changes in coordination of postural control in aging. Gait Posture 2002;16:20–30.

Sperle PA, Ottenbacher KJ, Braun SL, et al. Equivalence reliability of the functional independence measure for children (WeeFIM) administration methods. Am J Occup Ther 1997;51(1):35–41.

Spirduso W, Francis K, MacRae PG. Physical dimensions of aging. Champaign, IL: Human Kinetics, 2005.

Squire LR. Mechanisms of memory. Science 1986;232:1612–1619.

Stalvey B, Owsley C, Sloane ME, Ball K. The Life Space Questionnaire: a measure of the extent of mobility of older adults. J Appl Gerontol 1999;18:479–498.

Stapley PJ, Drew T. The pontomedullary reticular formation contributes to the compensatory postural responses observed following removal of the support surface in the standing cat. J Neurophysiol 2009;101:1334–1350.

Stapley PJ, Ting LH, Hulliger M, Macpherson JM. Automatic postural responses are delayed by pyridoxine-induced somatosensory loss. J Neurosci 2002;22:5803–5807.

Steenbergen B, Hulstijn W, Lemmens IHL, Meulenbroek RGJ. The timing of prehensile movements in subjects with cerebral palsy. Dev Med Child Neurol 1998;40:108–114.

Stehouwer DJ, Farel PB. Development of hindlimb locomotor behavior in the frog. Dev Psychobiol 1984;17:217–232.

Stein DG, Brailowsky S, Will B. Brain repair. New York: Oxford, 1995.

Stein J, Krebs HI, Frontera WR, et al. Comparison of two techniques of robot-aided upper limb exercise training after stroke. Am J Phys Med Rehabil 2004;83:720–728.

Stein RB. Reflex modulation during locomotion: functional significance. In: Patla A, ed. Adaptability of human gait. Amsterdam: North Holland, 1991:21–36.

Stephens MJ, Yang JF. Loading during the stance phase of walking in humans increases the extensor EMG amplitude but does not change the duration of the step cycle. Exp Brain Res 1999;124:363–370.

Stergiou N, Harbourne R, Cavanaugh J. Optimal movement variability: a new theoretical perspective for neurologic physical therapy. J Neurol Phys Ther 2006;30:120–129.

Stern EB. Stability of the Jebsen-Taylor hand function test across three test sessions. Am J Occup Ther 1992;7:647–649.

Stern GM, Lander CM, Lees AJ. Akinetic freezing and trick movements in Parkinson's disease. J Neural Transm Suppl 1980;16:137–141.

Stern Y, Mayeux R, Rosen J, Ilson J. Perceptual motor dysfunction in Parkinson's disease: a deficit in sequential and predictive voluntary movement. J Neurol Neurosurg Psychiatry 1983;46:145–51.

Steward O. Reorganization of neuronal connections following CNS trauma: principles and experimental paradigms. J Neurotrauma 1989;6:99–151.

Stillman B, McMeeken J. A video-based version of the pendulum test: technique and normal response. Arch Phys Med Rehabil 1995;76(2):166–176.

Stockmeyer S. An interpretation of the approach of Rood to the treatment of neuromuscular dysfunction. Am J Phys Med 1967;46:950–955.

Stoffregen TA, Adolph K, Thelen T, et al. Toddlers' postural adaptations to different support surfaces. Mot Control 1997;1:119–137.

Stoffregen TA, Pagulayan RJ, Bardy BG, Hettinger LJ. Modulating postural control to facilitate visual performance. Hum Mov Sci 2000;19:203–220.

Stoffregen TA, Riccio GE. An ecological theory of orientation and the vestibular system. Psychol Rev 1988;95(1):3–14.

Stone JH. Sensibility. In: Casanova J, ed. Clinical assessment recommendations, 2nd ed. Chicago: American Society of Hand Therapists, 1992:71–84.

Stoykov ME, Stojakovich M, Stevens JA. Beneficial effects of postural intervention on prehensile action for an individual with ataxia resulting from brainstem stroke. Neurorehabilitation 2005;20(2):85–89.

Strick PL. Anatomical organization of multiple areas of frontal lobe: implications for recovery of function. Adv Neurol 1988;47:293–312.

Strub RL, Black FW. The mental status examination in neurology. Philadelphia: FA Davis, 1977.

Strupp M, Arbusow V, Pereira DB, et al. Subjective straight ahead during neck muscle vibration: effect of aging. Neuroreport 1999;10: 3191–3194.

Studenski S, Duncan PW, Chandler J. Postural responses and effector factors in persons with unexplained falls: results and methodologic issues. J Am Geriatr Soc 1991;39:229–234.

Sturnieks DL, St George R, Lord SR. Balance disorders in the elderly. Clin Neurophysiol 2008;38:467–478.

Sudarsky L, Ronthal M. Gait disorders among elderly patients: a survey study of 50 patients. Arch Neurol 1983;40:740–743.

Sudarsky L, Ronthal M. Gait disorders in the elderly: assessing the risk for falls. In: Vellas B, Toupet M, Rubenstein L, et al., eds. Falls, balance and gait disorders in the elderly. Amsterdam: Elsevier, 1992:117–127.

Sudsawad P, Trombly CA, Henderson A, Tickle-Degnen L. The relationship between the Evaluation Tool of Children's Handwriting and teacher's perceptions of handwriting legibility. Am J Occup Ther 2001;55(5):518–523.

Sudsawad P, Trombly CA, Henderson A, Tickle-Degnen L. Testing the effect of kinesthetic training on handwriting performance in first-grade students. Am J Occup Ther 2002;56(1):26–33.

Sugden DA. Movement speed in children. J Motor Behav 1980;12:125–132.

Sullivan E, Rose E, Pfefferbaum A. Effect of vision, touch and stance on cerebellar vermian-related sway and tremor: a quantitative physiological and MRI study. Cerebral Cortex 2006;16: 1077–1086.

Sullivan JE, Hedman LD. A home program of sensory and neuromuscular electrical stimulation with upper-limb task practice in a patient 5 years after a stroke. Phys Ther 2004;84: 1045–1054.

Sullivan KJ, Knowlton BJ, Dobkin BH. Step training with body weight support: effect of treadmill speed and practice paradigms on poststroke locomotor recovery. Arch Phys Med Rehabil 2002;83:683–691.

Sunderland A. Recovery of ipsilateral dexterity after stroke. Stroke 2000;31(2):430–433.

Sundermeier L, Woollacott M, Jensen J, Moore S. Postural sensitivity to visual flow in aging adults with and without balance problems. J Gerontol A Biol Sci Med Sci 1996;51: M45–M52.

Sundermier L, Woollacott M, Roncesvalles N, Jensen J. The development of balance control in children: comparisons of EMG and kinetic variables and chronological and developmental groupings. Exp Brain Res 2001;136:340–350.

Sur M, Pallas SL, Roe AW. Cross-modal plasticity in cortical development: differentiation and specification of sensory neocortex. Trends Neurosci 1990;13:227–233.

Surberg PR. Aging and effect of physical-mental practice upon acquisition and retention of a motor skill. J Gerontol 1976;31:64–67.

Surrey LR, Hodson J, Robinson E, et al. Pinch strength norms for 5-to 12-year-olds. Phys Occup Ther Pediatr 2001;21(1):37–49.

Surrey LR, Nelson K, Delelio C, et al. A comparison of performance outcomes between the Minnesota Rate of Manipulation Test and the Minnesota Manual Dexterity Test. Work 2003;20(2):97–102.

Sutherland DH, Olshen R, Cooper L, Woo S. The development of mature gait. J Bone Joint Surg Am 1980;62:336–353.

Suzuki E, Chen W, Kondo T. Measuring unilateral spatial neglect during stepping. Arch Phys Med Rehabil 1997;78:173–178.

Suzuki M, Miyai I, Ono T, et al. Prefrontal and premotor cortices are involved in adapting walking and running speed on the treadmill: an optical imaging study. Neuroimage 2004;23: 1020–1026.

Svehlík M, Zwick EB, Steinwender G, et al. Gait analysis in patients with Parkinson's disease off dopaminergic therapy. Arch Phys Med Rehabil 2009;90:1880–1886.

Sveistrup H, Woollacott M. Practice modifies the developing automatic postural response. Exp Brain Res 1997;114:33–43.

Sveistrup H, Woollacott MH. Longitudinal development of the automatic postural response in infants. J Motor Behav 1996;28:58–70.

Sveistrup H, Woollacott MH. Systems contributing to the emergence and maturation of stability in postnatal development. In: Savelsbergh GJP, ed. The development of coordination in infancy. Amsterdam: Elsevier, 1993:324.

Swanson AB, Goran-Hagert C, Swanson, GD. Evaluation of impairment of hand function. In: Hunter JM, Schneider LH, Mackin EJ, Bell JA, eds. Rehabilitation of the hand. St. Louis: Mosby, 1978:31–69.

Sweatt JD, Kandel ER. Persistent and transcriptionally-dependent increase in protein phosphorylation in long-term facilitation of Aplysia sensory neurons. Nature 1989;339:51–54.

T

Taguchi K, Tada C. Change of body sway with growth of children. In: Amblard B, Berthoz A, Clarac F, eds. Posture and gait: development, adaptation and modulation. Amsterdam: Elsevier, 1988:59–65.

Taira M, Milne S, Georgopoulos AP, et al. Parietal cortex neurons of the monkey related to the visual guidance of hand movement. Exp Brain Res 1990;83:29–36.

Takahashi M, Tsujita N, Akiyama I. Evaluation of the vestibulo-ocular reflex by gaze function. Acta Otolaryngol 1988;105:7–12.

Takakusaki K, Saitaoh K, Harada H, Kashiwayanagi M. Role of the basal ganglia-brainstem pathways in the control of motor behaviors. Neurosci Res 2004;50:137–151.

Takakusaki K, Tomita N, Yano M. Substrates for normal gait and pathophysiology of gait disturbances with respect to the basal ganglia dysfunction. J Neurol 2008;255:19–29.

Takebe D, Kukulka C, Narayan G, et al. Peroneal nerve stimulator in rehabilitation of hemiplegic patients. Arch Phys Med Rehabil 1975;56: 237–239.

Tang A, Rymer WZ. Abnormal force—EMG relations in paretic limbs of hemiparetic human subjects. J Neurol Neurosurg Psychiatry 1981;44:690–698.

Tang PF, Woollacott MH, Chong RKY. Control of reactive balance adjustments in perturbed human walking: roles of proximal and distal postural muscle activity. Exp Brain Res 1998;119:141–152.

Tang PF, Woollacott MH. Inefficient postural responses to unexpected slips during walking in older adults. J Gerontol 1998;53:M471–M480.

Tang PF, Woollacott MH. Phase-dependent modulation of proximal and distal postural responses to slips in young and older adults. J Gerontol 1999;54:M89–M102.

Tardieu C, Lespargot A, Tabary C, Bret MD. For how long must the soleus muscle be stretched each day to prevent contracture? Dev Med Child Neurol 1988;30(1):3–10.

Tatton WG, Eastman MJ, Bedingham W, et al. Defective utilization of sensory input as the basis for bradykinesia, rigidity and decreased movement repertoire in Parkinson's disease: a hypothesis. Can J Neurol Sci 1984;11:136–143.

Taub E. Motor behavior following deafferentation in the developing and motorically mature monkey. In: Herman S, Grillner R, Ralston HJ, et al., eds. Neural control of locomotion. New York: Plenum, 1976:675–705.

Taub E. Some anatomical observations following chronic dorsal rhizotomy in monkeys. Neuroscience 1980;5:389–401.

Taub E. Technique to improve chronic motor deficit after stroke. Arch Phys Med Rehabil 1993;74:347–354.

Taub E, Berman AJ. Movement and learning in the absence of sensory feedback. In: Freedman SJ, ed. The neurophysiology of spatially oriented behavior. Homewood, NJ: Dorsey, 1968: 173–192.

Taub E, Miller NE, Novack TA, et al. Technique to improve chronic motor deficit after stroke. Arch Phys Med Rehabil 1993;74:347–354.

Taub E, Crago JE, Uswatte G. Constraint-induced movement therapy: a new approach to treatment in physical rehabilitation. Rehab Psychol 1998;43(2):152–170.

Taub E, Ramey SL, DeLuca S, Echols K. Efficacy of constraint-induced movement therapy for children with cerebral palsy with asymmetric motor impairment. Pediatrics 2004;113: 305–312.

Taylor N, Sand PL, Jebsen RH. Evaluation of hand function in children. Arch Phys Med Rehabil 1973;54(3):129–135.

Teasdale N, Bard C, LaRue J, Fleury M. On the cognitive penetrability of postural control. Exp Aging Res 1993;19:1–13.

Teasdale N, Simoneau M. Attentional demands for postural control: the effects of aging and sensory reintegration. Gait Posture 2001; 14:203–210.

Teasdale N, Stelmach GE, Breunig A. Postural sway characteristics of the elderly under normal and altered visual and support surface conditions. J Gerontol 1991;46:B238–B244.

Teasell R, McRae M, Foley N, Bhardwaj A. The incidence and consequences of falls in stroke patients during inpatient rehabilitation: factors associated with high risk. Arch Phys Med Rehabil 2002;83:329–333.

Teixeira-Salmela LF, Olney SJ, Nadeau S, Brouwer B. Muscle strengthening and physical conditioning to reduce impairment and disability in chronic stroke survivors. Arch Phys Med Rehabil 1999;80:1211–1218.

Tessier-Lavigne M. Visual processing by the retina. In: Kandel ER, Schwartz JH, Jessell TM, eds. Principles of neural science, 4th ed. New York: McGraw-Hill, 2000:507–522.

Teulings HL, Contreras-Vidal JL, Stelmach GE, Adler CH. Parkinsonism reduces coordination of fingers, wrist, and arm in fine motor control. Exp Neurol 1997;146:159–170.

Thelen DG, Schultz AB, Alexander NB, Ashton-Miller JA. Effects of age on rapid ankle torque development. J Gerontol Med Sci 1996;51: M226–M232.

Thelen E, Corbetta D, Kamm K, et al. The transition to reaching: mapping intention and intrinsic dynamics. Child Dev 1993;64:1058–1098.

Thelen E, Fisher DM, Ridley-Johnson R. The relationship between physical growth and a newborn reflex. Infant Behav Dev 1984;7:479–493.

Thelen E, Fisher DM. Newborn stepping: an explanation for a disappearing reflex. Dev Psychol 1982;18:760–775.

Thelen E, Kelso JAS, Fogel A. Self-organizing systems and infant motor development. Dev Rev 1987;7:39–65.

Thelen E, Spencer JP. Postural control during reaching in young infants: a dynamic systems approach. Neurosci Biobehav Rev 1998;22: 507–514.

Thelen E, Ulrich BD. Hidden skills: a dynamic systems analysis of treadmill stepping during the first year. Monogr Soc Res Child Dev 1991;56(1):1–104.

Thelen E, Ulrich, BD, Jensen JL. The developmental origins of locomotion. In: Woollacott MH, Shumway-Cook A, eds. Development of posture and gait across the life span. Columbia: University of South Carolina, 1989:25–47.

Thielman G, Kaminski T, Gentile AM. Rehabilitation of reaching after stroke: comparing 2 training protocols utilizing trunk restraint. Neurorehabil Neural Repair 2008;22:697–705.

Thielman GT, Dean CM, Gentile AM. Rehabilitation of reaching after stroke: task-related training versus progressive resistive exercise. Arch Phys Med Rehabil 2004;85:1613–1618.

Thilmann AF, Fellows SJ, Garms E. The mechanism of spastic muscle hypertonus. Brain 1991; 114:233–244.

Thomas RL, Williams AK, Lundy-Ekman L. Supine to stand in elderly persons: relationship to age, activity level, strength and range of motion. Issues Aging 1998;21:9–18.

Thorstensson A, Roberthson H. Adaptations to changing speed in human locomotion: speed of transition between walking and running. Acta Physiol Scand 1987;131:211–214.

Tiffin J. Purdue pegboard examiner manual. Chicago: Science Research Associates, 1968.

Tilson JK, Sullivan KJ, Cen SY, et al. Meaningful gait speed improvement during the first 60 days poststroke: minimal clinically important difference. Phys Ther 2010;90:196–208.

Timiras P. Aging of the skeleton, joints and muscles. In: Timiras PS, ed. Physiological basis of aging and geriatrics, 2nd ed. Ann Arbor, MI: CRC Press, 1994.

Tinetti ME. Performance-oriented assessment of mobility problems in elderly patients. J Am Geriatr Soc 1986;34:119–126.

Tinetti ME, Doucette JT, Claus EB.The contribution of predisposing and situational risk factors to serious fall injuries. J Am Geriatr Soc 1995;43:1207–1213.

Tinetti ME, Ginter SF. Identifying mobility dysfunctions in elderly patients: standard neuromuscular examination or direct assessment? JAMA 1988;259:1190–1193.

Tinetti ME, Richman D, Powell L. Falls efficacy as a measure of fear of falling. J Gerontol 1990;45:P239–P243.

Tinetti ME, Speechley M, Ginter SF. Risk factors for falls among elderly persons living in the community. N Engl J Med 1988;319:1701–1707.

Tinetti ME, Williams TF, Mayewski R. Fall risk index for elderly patients based on numbers of chronic disabilities. Am J Med 1986;80:429–434.

Ting LH, Macpherson JM. A limited set of muscle synergies for force control during a postural task. J Neurophysiol 2005;93:609–613.

Ting LH, Macpherson JM. Ratio of shear to load ground-reaction force may underlie the directional tuning of the automatic postural response to rotation and translation. J Neurophysiol 2004;92:808–823.

Titus MND, Gall NG, Yerxa EJ, et al. Correlation of perceptual performance and activities of daily living in stroke patients. Am J Occup Ther 1991;45:410–418.

Tobis JS, Lowenthal M. Evaluation and management of the brain damaged patient. Springfield IL: Charles C Thomas, 1960.

Toffola ED, Sparpaglione D, Pistorio A, Buonocore M. Myoelectric manifestations of muscle changes in stroke patients. Arch Phys Med Rehabil 2001;82:661–665.

Toro B, Nester CJ, Farren PC. The status of gait assessment among physiotherapists in the United Kingdom. Arch Phys Med Rehabil 2003;84:1878–1884.

Torres-Aleman I. Insulin like growth factors as mediators of functional plasticity in the adult brain. Horm Metab Res 1999;31:114–119.

Torres-Oviedo G, Macpherson JM, Ting LH. Muscle synergy organization is robust across a variety of postural perturbations. J Neurophysiol 2006;96:1530–1546.

Torres-Oviedo G, Ting LH. Muscle synergies characterizing human postural responses. J Neurophysiol 2007;98:2144–2156.

Toupet M, Gagey PM, Heuschen S. Vestibular patients and aging subjects lose use of visual input and expend more energy in static postural control. In: Vellas B, Toupet M, Rubenstein L, et al., eds. Falls, balance and gait disorders in the elderly. Paris: Elsevier, 1992:183–198.

Towen B. Neurological development in infancy. Clinics in Developmental Medicine 58. Philadelphia: JF Lippincott, 1976.

Travis AM, Woolsey CN. Motor performance of monkeys after bilateral partial and total cerebral decortication. Am J Phys Med 1956;35:273–310.

Treisman A. Solutions to the binding problem: progress through controversy and convergence. Neuron 1999;24:105–110, 111–125.

Tretriluxana J, Gordon J, Fisher BE, Winstein CJ. Hemisphere specific impairments in reach-to-grasp control after stroke: effects of object size. Neurorehabil Neural Repair 2009;23: 679–691.

Tretriluxana J, Gordon J, Winstein CJ. Manual asymmetries in grasp pre-shaping and transport-grasp coordination. Exp Brain Res 2008;188:305–315.

Trombly C. Anticipating the future: assessment of occupational function. Am J Occup Ther 1993;47:253–257.

Trombly CA, Ma HI. A synthesis of the effects of occupational therapy for persons with stroke. Part I: Restoration of roles, tasks, and activities. Am J Occup Ther 2002;56(3):250–259.

Trombly CA, Radomski MV, Trexel C, Burnet-Smith SE. Occupational therapy and achievement of self-identified goals by adults with acquired brain injury: phase II. Am J Occup Ther 2002;56(5):489–498.

Trombly CA. Theoretical foundations for practice. In: Trombly CA, ed. Occupational therapy for physical dysfunction, 4th ed. Baltimore: Williams & Wilkins, 1995:15–28.

Twitchell T. Reflex mechanisms and the development of prehension. In: Connolly K, ed. Mechanisms of motor skill development. New York: Academic, 1970.

Twitchell TE. The restoration of motor function following hemiplegia in man. Brain 1951; 74:443.

Tyson SF. The support taken through walking aids during hemiplegic gait. Clin Rehabil 1998;12:395–401.

U

Ugur C, Gucuyener D, Uzuner N, et al. Characteristics of falling in patients with stroke. J Neurol Neurosurg Psychiatry 2000;69:649–651.

Ullman MT. Contributions of memory circuits to language: the declarative/procedural model. Cognition 2004;92:231–270.

Ulrich DA, Ulrich BD, Angulo-Kinzler RM, Yun J. Treadmill training of infants with Down syndrome: evidence-based developmental outcomes. Pediatrics 2001;108(5):E84.

Ungerleider LG, Brody BA. Extrapersonal spatial orientation: the role of posterior parietal, anterior frontal, and inferotemporal cortex. Exp Neurol 1977;56:265–280.

Uswatte G, Taub E, Morris D, Light K, Thompson PA. The Motor Activity Log-28: assessing daily use of the hemiparetic arm after stroke. Neurology 2006;67:1189–1194.

Utley A, Sugden D. Interlimb coupling in children with hemiplegic cerebral palsy during reaching and grasping at speed. Dev Med Child Neurol 1998;40:396–404.

V

Valero-Cuevas FJ, Smaby N, Venkadesan M, et al. The strength-dexterity test as a measure of dynamic pinch performance. J Biomech 2002;36(2):265–270.

Vallée M, McFadyen BJ, Swaine B, et al. Effects of environmental demands on locomotion after traumatic brain injury. Arch Phys Med Rehabil 2006;87:806–813.

Vallis LA, McFadyen BJ. Children use different anticipatory control strategies than adults to circumvent an obstacle in the travel path. Exp Brain Res 2005;167:119–127.

Van de Port I, Kwakkel G, Lindeman E. Community ambulation in patients with chronic stroke:

how is it related to gait speed? J Rehabil Med 2008;40:23–27.

Van der Fits IB, Lip AW, van Eykern LA, Hadders-Algra M. Postural adjustments during spontaneous and goal-directed arm movements in the first half year of life. Behav Brain Res 1999;106:75–90.

van der Heide JC, Begeer C, Fock JM, et al. Postural control during reaching in preterm children with cerebral palsy. Dev Med Child Neurol 2004;46:253–266.

van der Heide JC, Otten B, Stremmelaar E, Hadders-Algra M. Kinematic characteristics of reaching movements in preterm children with cerebral palsy. Pediatr Res 2005;57:883–889.

Van der Krogt M, Doorenbosch, A, Becher JG, Harlaar J. Walking speed modifies spasticity effects in gastrocnemius and soleus in cerebral palsy gait. Clin Biomech 2009;24:422–428.

van der Lee JH, Beckerman H, Lankhorst GJ, Bouter LM. The responsiveness of the Action Research Arm Test and the Fugl-Meyer Assessment Scale in chronic stroke patients. J Rehabil Med 2001;33:110–113.

van der Meer AL, van der Weel FR, Lee DN. The functional significance of arm movements in neonates. Science 1995;267:693–695.

van der Putten JJMF, Hobart JC, Freeman JA. Measuring change in disability after inpatient rehabilitation: comparison of the responsiveness of the Barthel Index and the Functional Independence Measure. J Neurol Neurosurg Psychiatry 1999;66:480–484.

Van Donkelaar P, Lee RG. Interactions between the eye and hand motor systems: disruptions due to cerebellar dysfunction. J Neurophysiol 1994;72:1674–1684.

van Peppen RPS, Kortsmit M, Lindeman E, Kwakkel G. Effects of visual feedback therapy on postural control in bilateral standing after stroke: a systematic review. J Rehabil Med 2006;38:3–9.

van Praag H. Exercise and the brain: something to chew on. Trends Neurosci 2009;32:283–90.

van Roon D, Steenbergen B, Meulenbroek RGJ. Trunk use and co-contraction in cerebral palsy as a regulatory mechanism for accuracy control. Neuropsychologia 2005;43:497–508.

Van Thiel E, Meulenbroek RG, Hulstijn W, Steenbergen B. Kinematics of fast hemiparetic aiming movements toward stationary and moving targets. Exp Brain Res 2000;132: 230–242.

Van Thiel E, Steenbergen B. Shoulder and hand displacements during hitting, reaching, and grasping movements in hemiparetic cerebral palsy. Motor Control 2001;5:166–182.

van Vliet PM, Sheridan MR. Ability to adjust reach extent in the hemiplegic arm. Physiotherapy 2009;95:176–184.

van Vliet PM, Sheridan MR. Coordination between reaching and grasping in patients with hemiparesis and healthy subjects. Arch Phys Med Rehabil 2007;88:1325–1331.

van Wegen EE, van Emmerik RE, Wagenaar RC, Ellis T. Stability boundaries and lateral postural control in Parkinson's disease. Motor Control 2001;5,:254–269.

Van Woerkom TC, Minderhoud JM, Gottschal T, Micolai G. Neurotransmitters in the treatment of patients with severe head injuries. Eur Neurol 1982;21:227–234.

Vandervoort AA, Chesworth BM, Cunningham DA, et al. Age and sex effects on mobility of the human ankle. J Gerontol 1992;47:17–21.

VanSant AF. Age differences in movement patterns used by children to rise from a supine position to erect stance. Phys Ther 1988a;68:1130–1138.

VanSant AF. Concepts of neural organization and movement. In: Connolly BH, Montgomery PC, eds. Therapeutic exercise in developmental disabilities. Chattanooga, TN: Chattanooga, 1987:1–8.

VanSant AF. Life-span development in functional tasks. Phys Ther 1990;70:788–798.

VanSant AF. Rising from a supine position to erect stance: description of adult movement and a developmental hypothesis. Phys Ther 1988;68:185–192.

Vaughan CL, Sussman MD. Human gait: From clinical interpretation to computer simulation. In: Grabiner MD, ed. Current issues in biomechanics. Champaign, IL: Human Kinetics, 1993:53–68.

Vearrier LA, Langan J, Shumway-Cook A, Woollacott M. An intensive massed practice approach to retraining balance post-stroke. Gait Posture 2005;22:154–163.

Venglar M. Case report: Tai Chi and Parkinsonism. Physiother Res Int 2005;10(2):116–121.

Verbrugge L, Jette A. The disablement process. Soc Sci Med 1994;38:1–14.

Vercher JL, Gauthier GM, Guedon O, et al. Self-moved target eye tracking in control and deafferented subjects: roles of arm motor command and proprioception in arm-eye coordination. J Neurophysiol 1996;76:1133–1144.

Vereijken B, van Emmerik REA, Whiting HTA, Newell KM. Freezing degrees of freedom in skill acquisition. J Motor Behav 1992;24:133–142.

Verrel J, Bekkering H, Steenbergen B. Eye-hand coordination during manual object transport with the affected and less affected hand in adolescents with hemiparetic cerebral palsy. Exp Brain Res 2008;187:107–116.

Viitasalo MK, Kampman V, Sotaniemi KA, et al. Analysis of sway in Parkinson's disease using a new inclinometry-based method. Mov Disord 2002;17:663–669.

Vilenchik MM, Knudson AG. Inverse radiation dose-rate effects on somatic and germ-line mutations and DNA damage rates. Proc Natl Acad Sci 2000;97:5381–5386.

Vilis T, Hore J. Central neural mechanisms contributing to cerebellar tremor produced by limb perturbations. J Neurophysiol 1980;43: 279–291.

Vinter A. Manual imitations and reaching behaviors: an illustration of action control in infancy. In: Bard C, Fleury M, Hay L, eds. Development of eye-hand coordination across the lifespan. Columbia: University of South Carolina, 1990:157–187.

Viosca E, Martinez JL, Almagro PL, et al. Proposal and validation of a new functional ambulation classification scale for clinical use. Arch Phys Med Rehabil 2005;86:1234–1238.

Visser H. Gait and balance in senile dementia of Alzheimer's type. Age Ageing 1983;12: 296–301.

Vitório R, Pieruccini-Faria F, Stella F, et al. Effects of obstacle height on obstacle crossing in mild Parkinson's disease. Gait Posture 2010;31:143–146.

Voelcker-Rehage C, Alberts JL. Age-related changes in grasping force modulation. Exp Brain Res 2005;166:61–70.

Voelcker-Rehage C, Alberts JL. Effect of motor practice on dual-task performance in older adults. J Gerontol B Psychol Sci Soc Sci 2007;62: P141–P148.

Voepel-Lewis T, Merkel S, Tait AR, et al. The reliability and validity of the Face, Legs, Activity, Cry, Consolability observational tool as a measure of pain in children with cognitive impairment. Anesth Analg 2002;95:1224–1229.

Vollmer B, Holmström L, Forsman L, et al. Evidence of validity in a new method to measure dexterity in children and adolescents. Dev Med Child Neurol 2010; May 24 [Epub ahead of print].

von Hofsten C. Eye-hand coordination in the newborn. Dev Psychol 1982;18:450–461.

von Hofsten C. Developmental changes in the organization of pre-reaching movements. Dev Psychol 1984;3;378–388.

von Hofsten C. Studying the development of goal-directed behavior. In: Kalverboer AF, Hopkins B, Geuze R, eds. Motor development in early and later childhood: longitudinal approaches. Cambridge, UK: Cambridge University, 1993:109–124.

von Hofsten C. On the development of perception and action. In: Valsiner J, Connolly K, eds. Handbook of developmental psychology. Thousand Oaks, CA: Sage, 2003.

von Hofsten C. Action in development. Dev Sci 2007;10:54–60.

von Hofsten C, Fazel-Zandy S. Development of visually guided hand orientation in reaching. J Exp Child Psychol 1984;38:208–219.

von Hofsten C, Lindhagen K. Observations on the development of reaching for moving objects. J Exp Child Psychol 1979;28:158–173.

von Hofsten C, Ronnqvist L. Preparation for grasping an object: a developmental study. J Exp Psychol 1988;14:610–621.

von Hofsten C, Rosander K. Development of smooth pursuit tracking in young infants. Vision Res 1997;37:1799–1810.

von Hofsten C, Rosander K. The development of gaze control and predictive tracking in young infants. Vision Res 1996;36:81–96.

von Hofsten C, Woollacott M. Anticipatory postural adjustments during infant reaching. Neurosci Abstr 1989;15:1199.

Voss D, Ionata M, Myers B. Proprioceptive neuromuscular facilitation: patterns and techniques, 3rd ed. Philadelphia: Harper & Row, 1985.

Vrtunski PB, Patterson MB. Psychomotor decline can be described by discontinuities in response trajectories. Int J Neurosci 1985;27:265–275.

Vuillerme N, Nafati G. How attentional focus on body sway affects postural control during quiet standing. Psychol Res 2007;71:192–200.

Vygotsky LS. Mind in society: the development of higher psychological processes. Cambridge, MA: Harvard University Press, 1978.

W

Waagfjord J, Levangle PK, Certo CME. Effects of treadmill training on gait in a hemiparetic patient. Phys Ther 1990;70:549–558.

Wade MG, Lindquist R, Taylor JR, Treat-Jacobson D. Optical flow, spatial orientation, and the control of posture in the elderly. J Gerontol 1995;50B:P51–P58.

Wadsworth PT, Krishman R. Intrarater reliability of manual muscle testing and hand held dynamometric muscle testing. Physiol Rev 1987;67:1342–1347.

Wagenaar RC, Beek WJ. Hemiplegic gait: a kinematic analysis using walking speed as a basis. J Biomech 1992;25:1007–1015.

Wakeling J, Delaney R, Dudkiewicz I. A method for quantifying dynamic muscle dysfunction in children and young adults with cerebral palsy. Gait Posture 2007;25:580–589.

Waksvik K, Levy R. An approach to seating for the cerebral palsied. Can J Occup Ther 1979;46:147–152.

Walker N, Mellick D, Brooks CA, Whiteneck GG. Measuring participation across impairment groups using the Craig Handicap Assessment Reporting Technique. Am J Phys Med Rehabil 2003 Dec;82(12):936–941.

Walker-Batson D, Smith P, Unwin H, et al. Use of amphetamine in the treatment of aphasia. Restor Neurol Neurosci 1992;4:47–50.

Wallace PS, Whishaw IQ. Independent digit movements and precision grip patterns in 1–5-month-old human infants: hand-babbling,

including vacuous then self-directed hand and digit movements, precedes targeted reaching. Neuropsychologia 2003;41:1912–1918.
Wallace SA, Weeks DL, Kelso JAS. Temporal constraints in reaching and grasping behavior. Hum Mov Sci 1990;9:69–93.
Wallen P. Cellular bases of locomotor behaviour in lamprey: coordination and modulatory control of spinal circuitry. In: Ferrell WR, Proske U, eds. Neural control of movement. New York: Plenum, 1995:125–133.
Wang CH, Hsieh CL, Dai MH, et al. Interrater reliability and validity of the Stroke Rehabilitation Assessment of Movement (STREAM) instrument. J Rehabil Med 2002;34(1):20–24.
Wang J, Bohan M, Leis BC, Stelmach GE. Altered coordination patterns in parkinsonian patients during trunk-assisted prehension. Parkinsonism Relat Disord 2006;12:211–222.
Wang J, Sainburg RL. Interlimb transfer of novel inertial dynamics is asymmetrical. J Neurophysiol 2004a;92:349–360.
Wang J, Sainburg RL. Interlimb transfer of visuomotor rotations depends on handedness. Exp Brain Res 2006a;175(2):223–230.
Wang J, Sainburg RL. Limitations in interlimb transfer of visuomotor rotations. Exp Brain Res 2004b;155:1–8.
Wang J, Sainburg RL. The symmetry of interlimb transfer depends on workspace locations. Exp Brain Res 2006b;170:464–471.
Wanning T. Healing and the mind/body arts: massage, acupuncture, yoga, t'ai chi, and Feldenkrais. AAOHN J 1993;41(7):349–351.
Warburg CL. Assessment and treatment planning strategies for perceptual deficits. In: O'Sullivan S, Schmitz T, eds. Physical rehabilitation: assessment and treatment, 2nd ed. Philadelphia: FA Davis, 1994.
Ward AB. A summary of spasticity management—a treatment algorithm. Eur J Neurol 2002;9:48–55.
Ward NS, Brown MM, Thompson AJ, Frackowiak RS. Neural correlates of motor recovery after stroke: a longitudinal fMRI study. Brain 2003;126:2476–2496.
Ward NS, Cohen LG. Mechanisms underlying recovery of motor function after stroke. Arch Neurol 2004;61:1844–1848.
Warren WH. Action modes and laws of control for the visual guidance of action. In: Meijer OG, Roth K, eds. Complex movement behavior: the motor-action controversy. Amsterdam: North-Holland, 1988:339–380.
Wartenberg R. Pendulousness of the legs as a diagnostic test. Neurology 1951;1:8–24.
Washington K, Shumway-Cook A, Price R, et al. Muscle responses to seated perturbations for typically developing infants and those at risk for motor delays. Dev Med Child Neurol 2004;46:681–688.
Waters R, McNeal DR, Tasto J. Peroneal nerve conduction velocity after chronic electrical stimulation. Arch Phys Med Rehabil 1975;56:240–243.
Waters RL, Barnes G, Husserl T, et al. Comparable energy expenditure after arthrodesis of the hip and ankle. J Bone Joint Surg Am 1988;70:1032–1037.
Waters RL, Mulroy S. The energy expenditure of normal and pathologic gait. Gait Posture 1999;9:207–231.
Waters RL, Wilson DJ, Savinelli R. Rehabilitation of the upper extremity following stroke. In: Hunter J, Schneider LH, Mackin EJ, Bell JA, eds. Rehabilitation of the hand. St. Louis: Mosby, 1978:505–520.
Webber A, Virji-Babul N, Edwards R, Lesperance M. Stiffness and postural stability in adults with Down syndrome. Exp Brain Res 2004;155:450–458.
Weber PC, Cass SP. Clinical assessment of postural stability. Am J Otol 1993;14:566–569.
Weiller C, Chollet F, Friston KJ, et al. Functional reorganization of the brain in recovery from striato-capsular infarction in man. Ann Neurol 1992;31:463–472.
Weiller C, Ramsay SC, Wise RJS, et al. Individual patterns of functional reorganization in the human cerebral cortex after capsular infarction. Ann Neurol 1993;33:181–189.
Weiskrantz L, Warrington ER, Sanders MD, Marshall J. Visual capacity in the hemianopic field following a restricted occipital ablation. Brain 1974;97:709–728.
Weiss A, Herman T, Plotnik M, et al. Can an accelerometer enhance the utility of the Timed Up & Go Test when evaluating patients with Parkinson's disease? Med Eng Phys 2010;32:119–125.
Weisz S. Studies in equilibrium reaction. J Nerv Ment Dis 1938;88:150–162.
Welch TD, Ting LH. A feedback model reproduces muscle activity during human postural responses to support-surface translations. J Neurophysiol 2008;99:1032–1038.
Welford AT. Motor performance. In: Birren G, Schaie K, eds. Handbook of the psychology of aging. New York: Van Nostrand Reinhold, 1977:3–20.
Welford AT. Motor skills and aging. In: Mortimer J, Pirozzolo FJ, Maletta G, eds. The aging motor system. New York: Praeger, 1982:152–187.
Werner C, von Frankenberg S, Treig T, et al. Treadmill training with partial body weight support and an electromechanical gait trainer for restoration of gait in subacute stroke patients. Stroke 2002;33:2895–2901.
Westlake KP, Patten C. Pilot study of Lokomat versus manual-assisted treadmill training for locomotor recovery post-stroke. J Neuroeng Rehabil 2009;6:18–29.
Westling G, Johansson RS. Factors influencing the force control during precision grip. Exp Brain Res 1984;53:277–284.
Wetter S, Poole JL, Haaland KY. Functional implications of ipsilesional motor deficits after unilateral stroke. Arch Phys Med Rehabil 2005;86:776–781.
Whanger A, Wang HS. Clinical correlates of the vibratory sense in elderly psychiatric patients. J Gerontol 1974;29:39–45.
Whipple RH, Wolfson LI, Amerman PM. The relationship of knee and ankle weakness to falls in nursing home residents: an isokinetic study. J Am Geriatr Soc 1987;35:13–20.
Whitall J, McCombe Waller S, Silver KH, Macko RF. Repetitive bilateral arm training with rhythmic auditory cueing improves motor function in chronic hemiparetic stroke. Stroke 2000;31:2390–2395.
White BL, Castle P, Held R. Observations on the development of visually-directed reaching. Child Dev 1964;35:349–364.
Whiteneck GG, Charlifue SW, Gerhart KA, et al. Quantifying handicap: a new measure of long-term rehabilitation outcomes. Arch Phys Med Rehabil 1992;73:519–526.
Whitney S, Wrisley D, Furman J. Concurrent validity of the Berg Balance Scale and the Dynamic Gait Index in people with vestibular dysfunction. Physiotherapy Res Int 2003;8:178–186.
Whitney SL, Hudak MT, Marchetti GF. The dynamic gait index relates to self reported fall history in individuals with vestibular dysfunction. J Vestib Res 2000;10:99–105.
Whitney SL, Wrisley DM. The influence of footwear on timed balance scores of the modified clinical test of sensory interaction and balance. Arch Phys Med Rehabil 2004;85:439–443.
Wickens CD. Attention and skilled performance. In: Holding DH, ed. Human skills. New York: Wiley, 1989:71–105.
Wielinski CL, Erickson-Davis C, Wichmann R, et al. Falls and injuries resulting from falls among patients with Parkinson's disease and other Parkinsonian syndromes. Mov Disord 2005;20:410–415.
Wiener-Vacher SR, Toupet F, Narcy P. Canal and otolith vestibulo-ocular reflexes to vertical and off vertical axis rotations in children learning to walk. Acta Otolaryngol 1996;116:657–656.
Wiesendanger M, Serrien DJ. Neurological problems affecting hand dexterity. Brain Res Rev 2001;36:161–168.
Wiesendanger M, Serrien DJ. Neurological problems affecting hand dexterity. Brain Res Rev 2001;36:161–168.
Wiley ME, Damiano DL. Lower-extremity strength profiles in spastic cerebral palsy. Dev Med Child Neurol 1998;40:100–107.
Wilk K. Dynamic muscle strength testing. In: Amundsen LR, ed. Muscle strength testing: instrumented and non-instrumented systems. New York: Churchill Livingstone, 1990.
Wilkins AJ, Shallice T, McCarthy R. Frontal lesions and sustained attention. Neuropsychologia 1987;25:359–365.
Williams EN, Carrll SG, Reddihough DS, et al. Investigation of the timed "up and go" test in children. Dev Med Child Neurol 2005;47:518–524.
Williams G, Robertson V, Greenwood K, et al. The concurrent validity and responsiveness of the high-level mobility assessment tool for measuring the mobility limitations of people with traumatic brain injury. Arch Phys Med Rehabil 2006a;87:437–442.
Williams GP, Greenwood KM, Robertson VJ, et al. High-Level Mobility Assessment Tool (HiMAT): interrater reliability, retest reliability, and internal consistency. Phys Ther 2006b;86:395–400.
Williams GP, Morris ME. High-level mobility outcomes following acquired brain injury: a preliminary evaluation. Brain Inj 2009;23:307–312.
Williams H. Aging and eye-hand coordination. In: Bard C, Fleury M, Hay L, eds. Development of eye-hand coordination across the lifespan. Columbia: University of South Carolina, 1990:327–357.
Williamson GL, Leiper CI, Mayer NH. Beaver College Assessment of speed and accuracy of movement in older adults using Fitts' tapping test. Neurosci Abstr 1993;19:556.
Wilmut K, Wann JP, Brown JH. Problems in the coupling of eye and hand in the sequential movements of children with Developmental Coordination Disorder. Child Care Health Dev 2006;32:665–678.
Wilson DM. The central nervous control of flight in a locust. J Exp Biol 1961;38:471–490.
Wing AM, Frazer C. The contribution of the thumb to reaching movements. Q J Exp Psychol 1983;35A:297–309.
Winograd CH, Lemsky CM, Nevitt MC, et al. Development of a physical performance and mobility examination. J Am Geriatr Soc 1994;42:743–749.
Winstein CJ. Designing practice for motor learning: clinical implications: contemporary management of motor control problems. Proceedings of the II Step Conference. Alexandria, VA: American Physical Therapy Association, 1991.
Winstein C, Gardner ER, McNeal DR, et al. Standing balance training: effect on balance and locomotion in hemiparetic adults. Arch Phys Med Rehabil 1989;70:755–762.
Winstein C, Wolf SL. Task-oriented training to promote upper extremity recovery. In: Stein J, ed. Stroke recovery and rehabilitation. New York: Demos, 2009.
Winstein CJ, Merians AS, Sullivan KJ. Motor learning after unilateral brain damage. Neuropsychologia 1999;27:975–987.

Winstein CJ, Miller JP, Blanton S, et al. Methods for a multisite randomized trial to investigate the effect of constraint-induced movement therapy in improving upper extremity function among adults recovering from a cerebrovascular stroke. Neurorehabil Neural Repair 2003;17:137–172.

Winstein CJ, Pohl PS. Effects of unilateral brain damage on the control of goal directed hand movements. Exp Brain Res 1995;105:163–174.

Winstein CJ, Rose DK, Tan SM, et al. A randomized controlled comparison of upper-extremity rehabilitation strategies in acute stroke: a pilot study of immediate and long-term outcomes. Arch Phys Med Rehabil 2004;85:620–628.

Winstein CJ, Schmidt RA. Reduced frequency of knowledge of results enhances motor skill learning. J Exp Psychol Learn Memory Cogn 1990;16:677–691.

Winter DA. Overall principle of lower limb support during stance phase of gait. J Biomech 1980;13:923–927.

Winter D. Energy generation and absorption at the ankle and knee during fast, natural and slow cadences. Clin Orthop Relat Res 1983a;175:147–154.

Winter DA. Biomechanical motor patterns in normal walking. J Motor Behav 1983b;15:302–330.

Winter DA. Kinematic and kinetic patterns of human gait: variability and compensating effects. Hum Mov Sci 1984;3:51–76.

Winter DA. Biomechanics and motor control of human movement. New York: Wiley, 1990: 80–84.

Winter DA. Knowledge base for diagnostic gait assessments. Med Prog Technol 1993;19:61–81.

Winter DA. A.B.C. of balance during standing and walking. Waterloo (Ont): Waterloo Biomechanics; 1995.

Winter DA, McFadyen BJ, Dickey JP. Adaptability of the CNS in human walking. In: Patla AE, ed. Adaptability of human gait. Amsterdam: Elsevier, 1991:127–144.

Winter DA, Patla AE, Frank JS, Walt SE. Biomechanical walking pattern changes in the fit and healthy elderly. Phys Ther 1990;70: 340–347.

Winter DA, Prince F, Frank JS, et al. Unified theory regarding A/P and M/L balance in quiet stance. J Neurophysiol 1996;75: 2334–2343.

Winter DA, Prince F, Steriou P, Powell C. Medial-lateral and anterior-posterior motor responses associated with centre of pressure changes in quiet standing. Neurosci Res Commun 1993;12:141–148.

Winters TF, Gage JR, Hicks R. Gait patterns in spastic hemiplegia in children and young adults. J Bone Joint Surg Am 1987;69:437–441.

Wise RA, Brown CD. Minimal clinically important differences in the six-minute walk test and the incremental shuttle walking test. COPD 2005;2:125–129.

Wisleder D, Zernicke RF, Smith JL. Speed-related changes in hindlimb intersegmental dynamics during the swing phase of cat locomotion. Exp Brain Res 1990;79:651–660.

Witherington DC, von Hofsten C, Rosander K, et al. The development of anticipatory postural adjustments in infancy. Infancy 2002;3: 495–517.

Witney AG, Wing A, Thonnard JL, Smith AM. The cutaneous contribution to adaptive precision grip. Trends Neurosci 2004;27:638–643.

Wolf SL. A method for quantifying ambulatory activities. Phys Ther 1979;59:767–768.

Wolf SL, Catlin PA, Ellis M, et al. Assessing Wolf Motor Function Test as outcome measure for research in patients after stroke. Stroke 2001;32:1635.

Wolf SL, LeCraw DE, Barton LA. Comparison of motor copy and targeted biofeedback training techniques for restitution of upper extremity function among patients with neurologic disorders. Phys Ther 1989a;69:719–735.

Wolf SL, Lecraw DE, Barton LA, Jann BB. Forced use of hemiplegic upper extremities to reverse the effect of learned nonuse among chronic stroke and head injured patients. Exp Neurol 1989b;104(2):125–132.

Wolf SL, McJunkin JP, Swanson ML, Weiss PS. Pilot normative database for the Wolf Motor Function Test. Arch Phys Med Rehabil 2006;87(2):443–445.

Wolf SL, Thompson PA, Morris DM, et al. The EXCITE trial: attributes of the Wolf motor function test in patients with subacute stroke. Neurorehabil Neural Repair 2005;19(3):194–205.

Wolf SL, Winstein CJ, Miller JP, et al. Retention of upper limb function in stroke survivors who have received constraint-induced movement therapy: the EXCITE randomized trial. Lancet Neurol 2008;7(1):33–40.

Wolfson L, Whipple R, Amerman P, et al. Gait and balance in the elderly. Clin Geriatr Med 1985;1:649–659.

Wolfson L, Whipple R, Amerman P, Tobin JN. Gait assessment in the elderly: a gait abnormality rating scale and its relation to falls. J Gerontol 1990;45:M12–M19.

Wolfson L, Whipple R, Derby C, et al. Balance strength training in older adults: Intervention gains and Tai Chi maintenance. J Am Geriatr Soc 1996;44:498–506.

Wolfson L, Whipple R, Derby CA, et al. A dynamic posturography study of balance in healthy elderly. Neurology 1992;42:2069–2075.

Wong DL, Baker CM. Pain in children: comparison of assessment scales. Pediatr Nurs 1988;14:9–17.

Wood BH, Bilclough JA, Bowron A, Walker RW. Incidence and predition of falls in Parkinson's disease: a prospective multidisciplinary study. J Neurol Neurosurg Psychiatry 2002;72: 721–725.

Wood DE, Burridge JH, VanWijck FM, et al. Biomechanical approaches applied to the lower and upper limb for the measurement of spasticity: a systematic review of the literature. Disabil Rehabil 2005;27:19–32.

Woodbury ML, Velozo CA, Richards LG, et al. Dimensionality and construct validity of the Fugl-Meyer assessment of the upper extremity. Arch Phys Med Rehabil 2007;88:715–723.

Wood-Dauphinee SL, Williams JI, Shapiro SH. Examining outcome measures in a clinical study of stroke. Stroke 1990 May;21(5):731–739.

Woodford H, Walker R. Emergency hospital admissions in idiopathic Parkinson's disease. Mov Disord 2005;20:1104–1108.

Woollacott M. Gait and postural control in the aging adult. In: Bles W, Brandt T, eds. Disorders of posture and gait. Amsterdam:Elsevier, 1986:325–336.

Woollacott M. Aging, posture control and movement preparation. In: Woollacott MH, Shumway-Cook A, eds. Development of posture and gait across the life span. Columbia: University of South Carolina, 1989:155–175.

Woollacott M. Unbounded potentialities of resonance—the dynamic interface between mind and brain: perspectives from neuroscience and meditative traditions, and research at their common frontiers. Masters thesis, University of Oregon, 2005.

Woollacott M, Burtner P, Jensen J, et al. Development of postural responses during standing in healthy children and in children with spastic diplegia. Neurosci Biobehav Rev 1998;22:583–589.

Woollacott M, Debu B, Mowatt M. Neuromuscular control of posture in the infant and child: is vision dominant? J Motor Behav 1987;19:167–186.

Woollacott M, Roseblad B, von Hofsten C. Relation between muscle response onset and body segmental movements during postural perturbations in humans. Exp Brain Res 1988;72: 593–604.

Woollacott M, Shumway-Cook A, Hutchinson S, et al. The effect of balance training on the organization of muscle activity used in the recovery of stability in children with cerebral palsy: a pilot study. Dev Med Child Neurol 2005;47:455–461.

Woollacott M, Shumway-Cook A. Attention and the control of posture and gait: a review of an emerging area of research. Gait Posture 2002;16:1–14.

Woollacott M, Shumway-Cook A. Changes in posture control across the life span: a systems approach. Phys Ther 1990;70:799–807.

Woollacott M, Shumway-Cook A. Clinical research methodology for the study of posture and balance. In: Masdeu JC, Sudarsky L, Wolfson L, eds. Gait disorders of aging: falls and therapeutic strategies. Philadelphia: Lippincott-Raven, 1997:107–121.

Woollacott M, Shumway-Cook A. The development of the postural and voluntary motor control system in Down's syndrome children. In: Wade M, ed. Motor skill acquisition of the mentally handicapped: issues in research and training. Amsterdam: Elsevier, 1986:45–71.

Woollacott MH, Jensen J. Posture and locomotion. In: Heuer H, Keele S, eds. Handbook of perception and action, vol. 2. New York: Academic Press, 1996:333–403.

Woollacott MH, Shumway-Cook A, Nashner L. Aging and posture control: changes in sensory organization and muscular coordination. Int J Aging Hum Dev 1986;23:97–114.

Woollacott MH, Sveistrup H. Changes in the sequencing and timing of muscle response coordination associated with developmental transitions in balance abilities. Hum Mov Sci 1992;11:23–36.

World Health Organization. International classification of functioning, disability and health. Geneva: World Health Organization, 2001.

World Health Organization. International Classification of Impairment, Activity and Participation ICIDH-2. Geneva: World Health Organization, 1980.

Wright BD, Masters GN. Rating scale analysis. Chicago: MESA, 1982.

Wright DL, Kemp TL. The dual-task methodology and assessing the attentional demands of ambulation with walking devices. Phys Ther 1992;72:306–315.

Wright JM von. A note on the role of 'guidance' in learning Br J Psychol 1957;48:133–137.

Wright PA, Granat MH. Therapeutic effects of functional electrical stimulation of the upper limb of eight children with cerebral palsy. Dev Med Child Neurol 2000;42:724–727.

Wrisley DM, Kumar NA. Functional gait assessment: concurrent, discriminative, and predictive validity in community-dwelling older adults. Phys Ther 2010;Apr 1. 2010;90: 761–773.

Wrisley DM, Marchetti GF, Kuharsky DK, Whitney SL. Reliability, internal consistency and validity of data obtained with the functional gait assessment. Phys Ther 2004;84:906–918.

Wrisley DM, Walker ML, Echternach JL, Strasnick B. Reliability of the Dynamic Gait Index in people with vestibular disorders. Arch Phys Med Rehabil 2003;84:1528–1533.

Wrisley DM, Whitney SL, Furman JM. Vestibular rehabilitation outcomes in patients with a history of migraine. Otol Neurotol 2002;23: 483–487.

Wu C, Trombly CA, Lin K, Tickle-Degnen L. Effects of object affordances on reaching in persons with and without cerebrovascular accident. Am J Occup Ther 1998;52:447–456.

Wu CY, Chou SH, Kuo MY, et al. Effects of object size on intralimb and interlimb coordination during a bimanual prehension task in patients with left cerebral vascular accidents. Motor Control 2008;12:296–310.

Wu CY, Trombly CA, Lin KC. The relationship between occupational form and occupational performance: a kinematic perspective. Am J Occup Ther 1994;48:679–687.

Wu T, Hallett M. Neural correlates of dual task performance in patients with Parkinsons disease. J Neurol Neurosurg Psychiatry 2008;79:760–766.

Wu T, Hallett M. The influence of normal human aging on automatic movements. J Physiol 2005;562:605–615.

Wu T, Kansaku K, Hallett M. How self-initiated memorized movements become automatic: a functional MRI study. J Neurophysiol 2004a;91:1690–1698.

Wu YW, Day SM, Strauss DJ, Shavelle RM. Prognosis for ambulation in cerebral palsy: a population-based study. Pediatrics 2004b;114: 1264–1271.

Wulf G, Prinz W. Directing attention to movement effects enhances learning: a review. Psychon Bull Rev 2001;8:648–660.

Wulf G, Shea C, Park JH. Attention and motor performance: preferences for and advantages of an external focus. Res Q Exerc Sport 2001;72: 335–244.

Wulf G, Weigelt C. Instructions about physical principles in learning a complex motor skill: to tell or not to tell. Res Q Exerc Sport 1997;68:362–367.

Wurtz RH, Kandel ER. Central visual pathways. In: Kandel ER, Schwartz JH, Jessell TM, eds. Principles of neural science, 4th ed. New York: McGraw-Hill, 2000a:523–547.

Wurtz RH, Kandel ER. Perception of motion, depth and form. In: Kandel ER, Schwartz JH, Jessell TM, eds. Principles of neural science, 4th ed. New York: McGraw-Hill, 2000b:548–571.

X

Xue Q, Fried LP, Glass TA, et al. Life-space constriction, development of frailty, and the competing risk of mortality. Am J Epidemiol 2008;167:240–248.

Y

Yan K, Fang J, Shahani BT. An assessment of motor unit discharge patterns in stroke patients using surface electromyographic technique. Muscle Nerve 1998a;21:946–947.

Yan K, Fang J, Shahani BT. Motor unit discharge behaviors in stroke patients. Muscle Nerve 1998b;21:1502–1506.

Yang JF, Stephens MJ, Vishram R. Transient disturbances to one limb produce coordinated, bilateral responses during infant stepping. J Neurophysiol 1998;79:2329–2337.

Yang YR, Chen Y, Lee C, et al. Dual task related gait changed in individuals with stroke. Gait Posture 2007a;25:185–190.

Yang YR, Wang RY, Chen YC, Kao MJ. Dual-task exercise improves walking ability in chronic stroke: a randomized controlled trial. Arch Phys Med Rehabil 2007b;88:1236–1240.

Yasukawa A. Upper extremity casting: adjunct for a child with cerebral palsy hemiplegia. J Occup Ther 1990;4:840–846.

Yasukawa A. Upper-extremity casting: adjunct treatment for the child with cerebral palsy. In: Case-Smith J, Pehoski C, eds. Development of hand skills in children. Rockville, MD: American Occupational Therapy Association, 1992: 111–123.

Yim SY, Cho JR, Lee IY. Normative data and developmental characteristics of hand function for elementary school children in Suwon area of Korea: grip, pinch and dexterity study. J Korean Med Sci 2003;18:552–558.

Yogev G, Plotnik M, Peretz C. Gait asymmetry in patients with Parkinson's disease and elderly fallers: when does the bilateral coordination of gait require attention? Exp Brain Res 2007;177:336–346.

Yorkston KM, Kuehn CM, Johnson KL, et al. Measuring participation in multiple sclerosis: a comparison of the domains of frequency, importance, and self-efficacy. Disabil Rehabil 2008;30;88–97.

Young A. Exercise physiology in geriatric practice. Acta Scand 1986;711(Suppl): 227–232.

Young JL, Mayer RF. Physiological alternation of motor units in hemiplegia. J Neurol Sci 1982;54:401–412.

Z

Zackowski KM, Dromerick AW, Sahrmann SA, et al. How do strength, sensation, spasticity and joint individuation relate to the reaching deficits of people with chronic hemiparesis? Brain 2004;127:1035–1046.

Zaino CA, McCoy SW. Reliability and comparison of electromyographic and kinetic measurements during a standing reach task in children with and without cerebral palsy. Gait Posture 2008;27:128–137.

Zampieri C, Salarian A, Carlson-Kuhta P, et al. An Instrumented Timed Up and Go Test characterizes gait and postural transitions in untreated Parkinson's disease. J Neurol Neurosurg Psychiatry 2009;September 2. 2010;81:171–176.

Zarro VJ. Mechanisms of inflammation and repair. In: Michlovitz SL, ed. Thermal agents in rehabilitation. Philadelphia: Davis, 1986.

Zarrugh MY, Todd FN, Ralston HJ. Optimization of energy expenditure during level walking. Eur J Appl Physiol 1974;33:293–306.

Zee DS. Vertigo. In: Johnson RT ed, Current therapy in neurologic disease. St. Louis: CV Mosby 1985;8–13.

Zehr EP, Duysens J. Regulation of arm and leg movement during human locomotion. Neuroscientist 2004;10:347–361.

Zehr EP, Komiyama T, Stein RB. Cutaneous reflexes during human gait: electromyographic and kinematic responses to electrical stimulation. J Neurophysiol 1997;77:3311–3325.

Zeller W. Konstitution und Entwicklung. Gottingen: Verlag fur Psychologic, 1964.

Zettel JL, McIlroy WE, Maki BE. Gaze behavior of older adults during rapid balance-recovery reactions. J Gerontol 2008;63A:885–891.

Zeuner KE, Shill HA, Sohn YH, et al. Motor training as treatment in focal hand dystonia. Mov Disord 2005;20:335–341.

Zihl J, Werth R. Contributions to the study of "blindsight": 2. The role of specific practice forsaccadiclocalizationinpatientswithpostgeniculate visual field defects. Neuropsychologia 1984;22:13–22.

Zucker RS, Regehr WG. Short term synaptic plasticity. Annu Rev Physiol 2002;64:355–405.

INDEX

A

D

H

I

J

N

O

P

Q

R

V

W

Y

Z